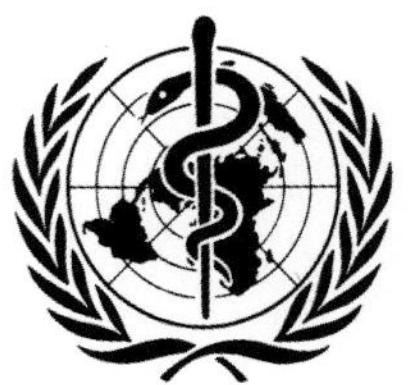

AF479090

World Health Organization Classification of Tumours

WHO 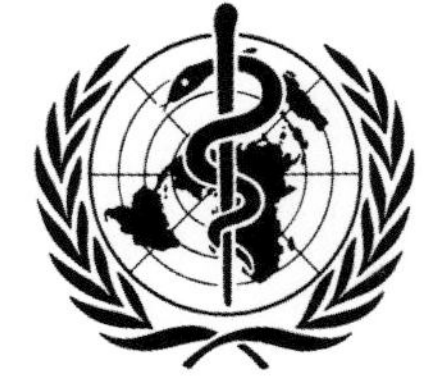 OMS

International Agency for Research on Cancer (IARC)

4th Edition

# WHO Classification of Skin Tumours

Edited by

David E. Elder
Daniela Massi
Richard A. Scolyer
Rein Willemze

International Agency for Research on Cancer
Lyon, 2018

## World Health Organization Classification of Tumours


Series Editors
Fred T. Bosman, MD, PhD
Elaine S. Jaffe, MD
Sunil R. Lakhani, MD, FRCPath
Hiroko Ohgaki, PhD


## WHO Classification of Skin Tumours


| | |
|---|---|
| Editors | David E. Elder, MB ChB, FRCPA<br>Daniela Massi, MD, PhD<br>Richard A. Scolyer, MD, FRCPA, FRCPath<br>Rein Willemze, MD |
| IARC Editor | Ian A. Cree, MB ChB, PhD, FRCPath |
| Project Coordinator | Asiedua Asante |
| Assistant | Anne-Sophie Hameau |
| Technical Editor | Jessica Cox |
| Database | Alberto Machado |
| Layout | Markus Fessler |
| Printed by | Naturaprint<br>74370 Argonay, France |
| Publisher | International Agency for<br>Research on Cancer (IARC)<br>69372 Lyon Cedex 08, France |

**The WHO Classification of Skin Tumours presented in this book reflects the views of a Working Group that convened for a Consensus and Editorial Meeting at the International Agency for Research on Cancer, Lyon, 24–26 September 2017.**

Members of the Working Group are indicated in the list of contributors on pages 398–408.

Published by the International Agency for Research on Cancer (IARC),
150 Cours Albert Thomas, 69372 Lyon Cedex 08, France



Distributed by
WHO Press, World Health Organization, 20 Avenue Appia, 1211 Geneva 27, Switzerland
Tel.: +41 22 791 3264; Fax: +41 22 791 4857; email: bookorders@who.int



First print run (15 000 copies)

**Format for bibliographic citations:**
Elder DE, Massi D, Scolyer RA, Willemze R, editors (2018).
WHO classification of skin tumours. 4th ed.
Lyon: IARC.

**IARC Library Cataloguing-in-Publication Data**

WHO classification of skin tumours / edited by David E. Elder, Daniela Massi, Richard A. Scolyer, Rein Willemze. – 4th edition.

(World Health Organization classification of tumours)

1. Skin neoplasms – pathology    2. Skin neoplasms – genetics

I. Elder, David E. II. Series

ISBN 978-92-832-2440-2    (NLM Classification: WR 500)

# Contents

# WHO classification of skin tumours

| Keratinocytic/epidermal tumours | |
|---|---|
| *Carcinomas* | |
| Basal cell carcinoma NOS | 8090/3 |
| Nodular basal cell carcinoma | 8097/3 |
| Superficial basal cell carcinoma | 8091/3 |
| Micronodular basal cell carcinoma | 8097/3 |
| Infiltrating basal cell carcinoma | 8092/3 |
| Sclerosing/morphoeic basal cell carcinoma | 8092/3 |
| Basosquamous carcinoma | 8094/3 |
| Pigmented basal cell carcinoma | 8090/3 |
| Basal cell carcinoma with sarcomatoid differentiation | 8092/3 |
| Basal cell carcinoma with adnexal differentiation | 8090/3 |
| Fibroepithelial basal cell carcinoma | 8093/3 |
| Squamous cell carcinoma NOS | 8070/3 |
| Keratoacanthoma | 8071/3* |
| Acantholytic squamous cell carcinoma | 8075/3 |
| Spindle cell squamous cell carcinoma | 8074/3 |
| Verrucous squamous cell carcinoma | 8051/3 |
| Adenosquamous carcinoma | 8560/3 |
| Clear cell squamous cell carcinoma | 8084/3 |
| Other (uncommon) variants | |
| Squamous cell carcinoma with sarcomatoid differentiation | 8074/3 |
| Lymphoepithelioma-like carcinoma | 8082/3 |
| Pseudovascular squamous cell carcinoma | 8074/3 |
| Squamous cell carcinoma with osteoclast-like giant cells | 8035/3 |
| Squamous cell carcinoma in situ (Bowen disease) | 8070/2 |
| Merkel cell carcinoma | 8247/3 |
| | |
| *Carcinoma precursors and benign simulants* | |
| Premalignant keratoses | |
| Actinic keratosis | 8070/0* |
| Arsenical keratosis | 8070/0* |
| PUVA keratosis | 8070/0* |
| Verrucae | |
| Verruca vulgaris | |
| Verruca plantaris | |
| Verruca plana | |
| Benign acanthomas/keratoses | |
| Seborrhoeic keratosis | 8052/0 |
| Solar lentigo | 8052/0 |
| Lichen planus–like keratosis | 8052/0 |
| Clear cell acanthoma | 8084/0* |
| Large cell acanthoma | 8072/0* |
| Warty dyskeratoma | 8054/0* |
| Other benign keratoses | 8052/0 |

| Melanocytic tumours | |
|---|---|
| *Melanocytic tumours in intermittently sun-exposed skin* | |
| Low-CSD melanoma (superficial spreading melanoma) | 8743/3 |
| Simple lentigo and lentiginous melanocytic naevus | 8742/0* |
| Junctional naevus | 8740/0 |
| Compound naevus | 8760/0 |
| Dermal naevus | 8750/0 |
| Dysplastic naevus | 8727/0 |
| Naevus spilus | 8720/0 |
| Special-site naevi (of the breast, axilla, scalp, and ear) | |
| Halo naevus | 8723/0 |
| Meyerson naevus | 8720/0 |
| Recurrent naevus | |
| Deep penetrating naevus | 8720/0 |
| Pigmented epithelioid melanocytoma | 8780/1* |
| Combined naevus, including combined *BAP1*-inactivated naevus/melanocytoma | 8720/0 |
| | |
| *Melanocytic tumours in chronically sun-exposed skin* | |
| Lentigo maligna melanoma | 8742/3 |
| Desmoplastic melanoma | 8745/3 |
| | |
| *Spitz tumours* | |
| Malignant Spitz tumour (Spitz melanoma) | 8770/3 |
| Spitz naevus | 8770/0 |
| Pigmented spindle cell naevus (Reed naevus) | 8770/0 |
| | |
| *Melanocytic tumours in acral skin* | |
| Acral melanoma | 8744/3 |
| Acral naevus | 8744/0* |
| | |
| *Genital and mucosal melanocytic tumours* | |
| Mucosal melanomas (genital, oral, sinonasal) | 8720/3 |
| Mucosal lentiginous melanoma | 8746/3 |
| Mucosal nodular melanoma | 8721/3 |
| Genital naevus | 8720/0 |
| | |
| *Melanocytic tumours arising in blue naevus* | |
| Melanoma arising in blue naevus | 8780/3 |
| Blue naevus NOS | 8780/0 |
| Cellular blue naevus | 8790/0 |
| Mongolian spot | |
| Naevus of Ito | |
| Naevus of Ota | |

*Melanocytic tumours arising in congenital naevi*

| | |
|---|---|
| Melanoma arising in giant congenital naevus | 8761/3 |
| Congenital melanocytic naevus | 8761/0* |
| Proliferative nodules in congenital melanocytic naevus | 8762/1 |

*Ocular melanocytic tumours*

| | |
|---|---|
| Uveal melanoma | |
| Epithelioid cell melanoma | 8771/3 |
| Spindle cell melanoma, type A | 8773/3 |
| Spindle cell melanoma, type B | 8774/3 |
| Conjunctival melanoma | |
| Melanoma NOS | 8720/3 |
| Conjunctival primary acquired melanosis with atypia/melanoma in situ | 8720/2 |
| Conjunctival naevus | 8720/0 |

*Nodular, naevoid, and metastatic melanomas*

| | |
|---|---|
| Nodular melanoma | 8721/3 |
| Naevoid melanoma | 8720/3 |
| Metastatic melanoma | 8720/6 |

**Appendageal tumours**

*Malignant tumours with apocrine and eccrine differentiation*

| | |
|---|---|
| Adnexal adenocarcinoma NOS | 8390/3 |
| Microcystic adnexal carcinoma | 8407/3 |
| Porocarcinoma | 8409/3* |
| Porocarcinoma in situ | 8409/2 |
| Malignant neoplasms arising from spiradenoma, cylindroma, or spiradenocylindroma | 8403/3 |
| Malignant mixed tumour | 8940/3 |
| Hidradenocarcinoma | 8402/3 |
| Mucinous carcinoma | 8480/3 |
| Endocrine mucin-producing sweat gland carcinoma | 8509/3 |
| Digital papillary adenocarcinoma | 8408/3 |
| Adenoid cystic carcinoma | 8200/3 |
| Apocrine carcinoma | 8401/3 |
| Squamoid eccrine ductal carcinoma | 8560/3 |
| Syringocystadenocarcinoma papilliferum | 8406/3* |
| Secretory carcinoma | 8502/3 |
| Cribriform carcinoma | 8201/3 |
| Signet-ring cell/histiocytoid carcinoma | 8490/3 |

*Benign tumours with apocrine and eccrine differentiation*

| | |
|---|---|
| Hidrocystoma/cystadenoma | 8404/0 |
| Syringoma | 8407/0 |
| Poroma | 8409/0 |
| Syringofibroadenoma | 8392/0 |
| Hidradenoma | 8402/0 |
| Spiradenoma | 8403/0 |
| Cylindroma | 8200/0 |
| Tubular adenoma | 8211/0 |
| Syringocystadenoma papilliferum | 8406/0 |
| Mixed tumour | 8940/0 |
| Myoepithelioma | 8982/0 |

*Malignant tumours with follicular differentiation*

| | |
|---|---|
| Pilomatrical carcinoma | 8110/3 |
| Proliferating trichilemmal tumour | 8103/1* |
| Trichoblastic carcinoma/carcinosarcoma | 8100/3* |
| Trichilemmal carcinoma | 8102/3 |

*Benign tumours with follicular differentiation*

| | |
|---|---|
| Trichoblastoma | 8100/0 |
| Pilomatricoma | 8110/0 |
| Trichilemmoma | 8102/0 |
| Trichofolliculoma | 8101/0 |
| Pilar sheath acanthoma | 8104/0* |
| Tumour of the follicular infundibulum | 8104/0* |
| Melanocytic matricoma | 8110/0 |
| Spindle cell–predominant trichodiscoma | 8391/0 |

*Tumours with sebaceous differentiation*

| | |
|---|---|
| Sebaceous carcinoma | 8410/3 |
| Sebaceous adenoma | 8410/0 |
| Sebaceoma | 8410/0 |

*Site-specific tumours*

| | |
|---|---|
| Mammary Paget disease | 8540/3 |
| Extramammary Paget disease | 8542/3 |
| Adenocarcinoma of anogenital mammary-like glands | 8500/3 |
| Hidradenoma papilliferum | 8405/0 |
| Fibroadenoma of anogenital mammary-like glands | 9010/0 |
| Phyllodes tumour of anogenital mammary-like glands | 9020/0 |

**Tumours of haematopoietic and lymphoid origin**

| | |
|---|---|
| *Mycosis fungoides* | 9700/3 |
| Folliculotropic mycosis fungoides | 9700/3 |
| Granulomatous slack skin | 9700/3 |
| Pagetoid reticulosis | 9700/3 |
| Sézary syndrome | 9701/3 |

*Primary cutaneous CD30+ T-cell lymphoproliferative disorders*

| | |
|---|---|
| Lymphomatoid papulosis | 9718/1 |
| Primary cutaneous anaplastic large cell lymphoma | 9718/3 |
| Cutaneous adult T-cell leukaemia/lymphoma | 9827/3 |
| Subcutaneous panniculitis-like T-cell lymphoma | 9708/3 |

*Cutaneous manifestations of chronic active EBV infection*

| | |
|---|---|
| Hydroa vacciniforme–like lymphoproliferative disorder | 9725/1 |

| | |
|---|---|
| Extranodal NK/T-cell lymphoma, nasal type | 9719/3 |

*Primary cutaneous peripheral T-cell lymphomas, rare subtypes*

| | |
|---|---|
| Primary cutaneous gamma-delta T-cell lymphoma | 9726/3 |

| | |
|---|---|
| Primary cutaneous CD8+ aggressive epidermotropic cytotoxic T-cell lymphoma | 9709/3 |
| Primary cutaneous acral CD8+ T-cell lymphoma | 9709/3 |
| Primary cutaneous CD4+ small/medium T-cell lymphoproliferative disorder | 9709/1 |
| *Secondary cutaneous involvement in T-cell lymphomas and leukaemias* | |
| Systemic anaplastic large cell lymphoma, ALK-positive | 9714/3 |
| Systemic anaplastic large cell lymphoma, ALK-negative | 9715/3 |
| Angioimmunoblastic T-cell lymphoma | 9705/3 |
| T-cell prolymphocytic leukaemia | 9834/3 |
| Primary cutaneous marginal zone (MALT) lymphoma | 9699/3 |
| Primary cutaneous follicle centre lymphoma | 9597/3 |
| Primary cutaneous diffuse large B-cell lymphoma, leg type | 9680/3 |
| Intravascular large B-cell lymphoma | 9712/3 |
| EBV-positive mucocutaneous ulcer | 9680/1 |
| Lymphomatoid granulomatosis | |
| Grade 1–2 | 9766/1 |
| Grade 3 | 9766/3 |
| *Cutaneous involvement in primarily extracutaneous B-cell lymphomas and leukaemias* | |
| Mantle cell lymphoma | 9673/3 |
| Burkitt lymphoma | 9687/3 |
| Chronic lymphocytic leukaemia/ small lymphocytic lymphoma | 9823/3 |
| *T-lymphoblastic and B-lymphoblastic leukaemia/lymphoma* | |
| T-lymphoblastic leukaemia/lymphoma | 9837/3 |
| B-lymphoblastic leukaemia/lymphoma | 9811/3 |
| Blastic plasmacytoid dendritic cell neoplasm | 9727/3 |
| Cutaneous involvement in myeloid leukaemia | 9930/3 |
| Cutaneous mastocytosis | 9740/1 |
| Mast cell sarcoma | 9740/3 |
| Indolent systemic mastocytosis | 9741/1 |
| Aggressive systemic mastocytosis | 9741/3 |
| Systemic mastocytosis with an associated haematological neoplasm | 9741/3 |
| Mast cell leukaemia | 9742/3 |
| *Histiocytic and dendritic cell neoplasms* | |
| Langerhans cell histiocytosis | 9751/1 |
| Indeterminate cell histiocytosis/ indeterminate dendritic cell tumour | 9757/3 |
| Rosai–Dorfman disease | |
| Juvenile xanthogranuloma | |
| Erdheim–Chester disease | 9749/3 |
| Reticulohistiocytosis | 8831/0 |

**Soft tissue and neural tumours**

| | |
|---|---|
| *Adipocytic tumours* | |
| Atypical lipomatous tumour | 8850/1 |
| Dedifferentiated liposarcoma | 8858/3 |
| Pleomorphic liposarcoma | 8854/3 |
| Lipoma | 8850/0 |
| Spindle cell/pleomorphic lipoma | 8857/0 |
| Angiolipoma | 8861/0 |
| Naevus lipomatosus superficialis | |
| *Fibroblastic, myofibroblastic, and fibrohistiocytic tumours* | |
| Myxoinflammatory fibroblastic sarcoma | 8811/1 |
| Dermatofibrosarcoma protuberans | 8832/1 |
| Giant cell fibroblastoma | 8834/1 |
| Bednar tumour | 8833/1 |
| Fibrosarcomatous dermatofibrosarcoma protuberans | 8832/3 |
| Plexiform fibrohistiocytic tumour | 8835/1 |
| Superficial fibromatosis | 8813/1 |
| Dermatofibroma (fibrous histiocytoma) | 8832/0 |
| Epithelioid fibrous histiocytoma | 8830/0 |
| Fibromas | |
| Fibroma of tendon sheath | 8813/0 |
| Calcifying aponeurotic fibroma | 8816/0 |
| Sclerotic fibroma | 8823/0* |
| Nuchal-type fibroma | 8810/0 |
| Gardner fibroma | 8810/0 |
| Pleomorphic fibroma | 8832/0 |
| Elastofibroma | 8820/0 |
| Collagenous fibroma | 8810/0 |
| Superficial acral fibromyxoma | 8811/0 |
| Cutaneous myxoma | 8840/0 |
| Dermatomyofibroma | 8824/0 |
| Myofibroma | 8824/0 |
| Myofibromatosis | 8824/1 |
| Plaque-like CD34+ dermal fibroma | 8810/0 |
| Nodular fasciitis | 8828/0 |
| *Smooth muscle tumours* | |
| Cutaneous leiomyoma | 8890/0 |
| Cutaneous leiomyosarcoma (atypical smooth muscle tumour) | 8897/1 |
| *(Myo)pericytic tumours* | |
| Glomus tumour | 8711/0 |
| Glomuvenous malformation (glomangiomyoma) | 8713/0 |
| Glomus tumour of uncertain malignant potential | 8711/1* |
| Malignant glomus tumour | 8711/3 |
| Myopericytoma | 8824/0 |
| Angioleiomyoma | 8894/0 |

| | |
|---|---|
| *Vascular tumours* | |
| Cutaneous angiosarcoma | 9120/3 |
| *Haemangioendotheliomas* | |
| Composite haemangioendothelioma | 9136/1 |
| Kaposiform haemangioendothelioma | 9130/1 |
| Pseudomyogenic haemangioendothelioma | 9138/1 |
| Retiform haemangioendothelioma | 9136/1 |
| Epithelioid haemangioendothelioma | 9133/3 |
| Kaposi sarcoma | 9140/3 |
| Atypical vascular lesion | 9126/0* |
| Cutaneous epithelioid angiomatous nodule | 9125/0 |
| *Haemangiomas* | |
| Cherry haemangioma | 9120/0 |
| Sinusoidal haemangioma | 9120/0 |
| Microvenular haemangioma | 9120/0 |
| Hobnail haemangioma | 9120/0 |
| Glomeruloid haemangioma | 9120/0 |
| Spindle cell haemangioma | 9120/0 |
| Epithelioid haemangioma | 9125/0 |
| Tufted haemangioma | 9161/0 |
| Angiokeratoma | 9141/0 |
| Infantile haemangioma | 9131/0 |
| Rapidly involuting congenital haemangioma | 9131/0 |
| Non-involuting congenital haemangioma | 9131/0 |
| Lobular capillary haemangioma | 9131/0 |
| Verrucous venous malformation | 9142/0 |
| Arteriovenous malformation | 9123/0 |
| Lymphangioma (superficial lymphatic malformation) | 9170/0 |
| | |
| *Neural tumours* | |
| Neurofibroma | 9540/0 |
| Solitary circumscribed neuroma | 9570/0 |
| Dermal nerve sheath myxoma | 9562/0 |
| Perineurioma | 9571/0 |
| Malignant perineurioma | 9571/3 |
| Granular cell tumour | 9580/0 |
| Malignant granular cell tumour | 9580/3 |
| Schwannoma | 9560/0 |
| Malignant peripheral nerve sheath tumour | 9540/3 |
| Epithelioid malignant peripheral nerve sheath tumour | 9542/3 |
| Malignant triton tumour | 9561/3 |
| | |
| *Tumours of uncertain differentiation* | |
| Atypical fibroxanthoma | 8830/1 |
| Pleomorphic dermal sarcoma | 8802/3 |
| Myxofibrosarcoma | 8811/3 |
| Epithelioid sarcoma | 8804/3 |
| Dermal clear cell sarcoma | 9044/3 |
| Ewing sarcoma | 9364/3 |
| Primitive non-neural granular cell tumour | 8990/1 |
| Cellular neurothekeoma | 9562/0 |

---

The morphology codes presented here are from the International Classification of Diseases for Oncology (ICD-O) {826A}.

Behaviour is coded /0 for benign tumours; /1 for tumours with unspecified, borderline, or uncertain behaviour; /2 for carcinoma in situ and grade 3 intraepithelial neoplasia; /3 for malignant tumours; and /6 for malignant tumours at a metastatic site.

This classification is modified from the previous WHO classification, taking into account changes in our understanding of these lesions.

* These new codes were approved by the IARC/WHO Committee for ICD-O.

CSD, cumulative sun damage; NOS, not otherwise specified; PUVA, psoralen and ultraviolet A.

# TNM classification of skin tumours

## Carcinoma of Skin (excluding eyelid, head and neck, perianal, vulva, and penis)

(ICD-O-3 C44.5-7, C63.2)

### TNM Clinical Classification

#### T – Primary Tumour

TX Primary tumour cannot be identified
T0 No evidence of primary tumour
Tis Carcinoma in situ
T1 Tumour 2 cm or less in greatest dimension
T2 Tumour > 2 cm and ≤ 4 cm in greatest dimension
T3 Tumour > 4 cm in greatest dimension or minor bone erosion or perineural invasion or deep invasion*
T4a Tumour with gross cortical bone/marrow invasion
T4b Tumour with axial skeleton invasion including foraminal involvement and/or vertebral foramen involvement to the epidural space

Note
*Deep invasion is defined as invasion beyond the subcutaneous fat or > 6 mm (as measured from the granular layer of adjacent normal epidermis to the base of the tumour); perineural invasion for T3 classification is defined as clinical or radiographic involvement of named nerves without foramen or skull base invasion or transgression.
In the case of multiple simultaneous tumours, the tumour with the highest T category is classified and the number of separate tumours is indicated in parentheses, e.g. T2(5).

#### N – Regional Lymph Nodes

NX Regional lymph nodes cannot be assessed
N0 No regional lymph node metastasis
N1 Metastasis in a single lymph node 3 cm or less in greatest dimension
N2 Metastasis in a single ipsilateral lymph node, more than 3 cm but not more than 6 cm in greatest dimension or in multiple ipsilateral lymph nodes none more than 6 cm in greatest dimension
N3 Metastasis in a lymph node more than 6 cm in greatest dimension

#### M – Distant Metastasis

M0 No distant metastasis
M1 Distant metastatic disease*

Note
*Contralateral nodes in non-melanoma non-head and neck cancer are distant metastases.

### pTNM Pathological Classification

The pT and pN categories correspond to the T and N categories.

pN0 Histological examination of a regional lymphadenectomy specimen will ordinarily include 6 or more lymph nodes. If the lymph nodes are negative, but the number ordinarily examined is not met, classify as pN0.

#### pM – Distant Metastasis*

pM1 Distant metastasis microscopically confirmed

Note
*pM0 and pMX are not valid categories.

### Stage

| | | | |
|---|---|---|---|
| Stage 0 | Tis | N0 | M0 |
| Stage I | T1 | N0 | M0 |
| Stage II | T2 | N0 | M0 |
| Stage III | T3 | N0 | M0 |
| | T1, T2, T3 | N1 | M0 |
| Stage IVA | T1, T2, T3 | N2, N3 | M0 |
| | T4 | Any N | M0 |
| Stage IVB | Any T | Any N | M1 |

## Skin Carcinoma of the Head and Neck

(ICD-O-3 C44.0, C44.2-4)

### TNM Clinical Classification

**T – Primary Tumour**

| | |
|---|---|
| TX | Primary tumour cannot be identified |
| T0 | No evidence of primary tumour |
| Tis | Carcinoma in situ |
| T1 | Tumour 2 cm or less in greatest dimension |
| T2 | Tumour > 2 cm and ≤ 4 cm in greatest dimension |
| T3 | Tumour > 4 cm in greatest dimension or minor bone erosion or perineural invasion or deep invasion* |
| T4a | Tumour with gross cortical bone/marrow invasion |
| T4b | Tumour with skull base or axial skeleton invasion including foraminal involvement and/or vertebral foramen involvement to the epidural space |

Note

*Deep invasion is defined as invasion beyond the subcutaneous fat or > 6 mm (as measured from the granular layer of adjacent normal epidermis to the base of the tumour), perineural invasion for T3 classification is defined as clinical or radiographic involvement of named nerves without foramen or skull base invasion or transgression.

**N – Regional Lymph Nodes**

- N0 No regional lymph node metastasis
- N1 Metastasis in a single ipsilateral lymph node, 3 cm or less in greatest dimension without extranodal extension
- N2 Metastasis described as:
  - N2a Metastasis in a single ipsilateral lymph node more than 3 cm but not more than 6 cm in greatest dimension without extranodal extension
  - N2b Metastasis in multiple ipsilateral lymph nodes, none more than 6 cm in greatest dimension, without extranodal extension
  - N2c Metastasis in bilateral or contralateral lymph nodes, none more than 6 cm in greatest dimension, without extranodal extension
- N3a Metastasis in a lymph node more than 6 cm in greatest dimension without extranodal extension
- N3b Metastasis in a single or multiple lymph nodes with clinical extranodal extension*

Note

*The presence of skin involvement or soft tissue invasion with deep fixation/tethering to underlying muscle or adjacent structures or clinical signs of nerve involvement is classified as clinical extranodal extension.

**M – Distant Metastasis**

| | |
|---|---|
| M0 | No distant metastasis |
| M1 | Distant metastasis |

### pTNM Pathological Classification

The pT categories correspond to the clinical T categories.

**pN – Regional Lymph Nodes**

Histological examination of a selective neck dissection specimen will ordinarily include 10 or more lymph nodes. Histological examination of a radical or modified radical neck dissection specimen will ordinarily include 15 or more lymph nodes.

- pNX Regional lymph nodes cannot be assessed
- pN0 No regional lymph node metastasis
- pN1 Metastasis in a single ipsilateral lymph node, 3 cm or less in greatest dimension without extranodal extension
- pN2 Metastasis described as:
  - pN2a Metastasis in a single ipsilateral lymph node, less than 3 cm in greatest dimension with extranodal extension, or more than 3 cm but not more than 6 cm in greatest dimension without extranodal extension
  - pN2b Metastasis in multiple ipsilateral lymph nodes, none more than 6 cm in greatest dimension, without extranodal extension
  - pN2c Metastasis in bilateral or contralateral lymph nodes, none more than 6 cm in greatest dimension, without extranodal extension
- pN3a Metastasis in a lymph node more than 6 cm in greatest dimension without extranodal extension
- pN3b Metastasis in a lymph node more than 3 cm in greatest dimension with extranodal extension or multiple ipsilateral, or any contralateral or bilateral node(s) with extranodal extension

**pM – Distant Metastasis***

| | |
|---|---|
| pM1 | Distant metastasis microscopically confirmed |

Note

*pM0 and pMX are not valid categories.

### Stage

| | | | |
|---|---|---|---|
| Stage 0 | Tis | N0 | M0 |
| Stage I | T1 | N0 | M0 |
| Stage II | T2 | N0 | M0 |
| Stage III | T3 | N0 | M0 |
| | T1, T2, T3 | N1 | M0 |
| Stage IVA | T1, T2, T3 | N2, N3 | M0 |
| | T4 | Any N | M0 |
| Stage IVB | Any T | Any N | M1 |

The information presented here has been excerpted from the 8th edition of the *TNM classification of malignant tumours* (2017) {311A}.
A help desk for specific questions about the TNM classification is available at http://www.uicc.org/resources/tnm/helpdesk.

## Carcinoma of Skin of the Eyelid

(ICD-O C44.1)

### TNM Clinical Classification

**T – Primary Tumour**

T0 No evidence of primary tumour

Tis Carcinoma in situ

T1 Tumour 10 mm or less in greatest dimension

- T1a Not invading the tarsal plate or eyelid margin
- T1b Invades tarsal plate or eyelid margin
- T1c Involves full thickness of eyelid

T2 Tumour > 10 mm, but 20 mm or less in greatest dimension

- T2a Not invading the tarsal plate or eyelid margin
- T2b Invades the tarsal plate or eyelid margin
- T2c Involves full thickness of eyelid

T3 Tumour > 20 mm in greatest dimension

- T3a Not invading the tarsal plate or eyelid margin
- T3b Invades tarsal plate or eyelid margin
- T3c Involves full thickness of eyelid

T4 Any eyelid tumour that invades adjacent ocular, or orbital, or facial structures

- T4a Tumour invades ocular or intraorbital structures
- T4b Tumour invades (or erodes through) the bony walls of orbit or extends to paranasal sinuses or invades the lacrimal sac/nasolacrimal duct or brain

**N – Regional Lymph Nodes**

NX Regional lymph nodes cannot be assessed

N0 No evidence of lymph node involvement

N1 Metastasis in a single ipsilateral regional lymph node, 3 cm or less in greatest dimension

N2 Metastasis in a single ipsilateral lymph node more than 3 cm in greatest dimension or in bilateral or contralateral lymph nodes

**M – Distant Metastasis**

M0 No distant metastasis

M1 Distant metastasis

### pTNM Pathological Classification

The pT and pN categories correspond to the T and N categories.

**pM – Distant Metastasis***

pM1 Distant metastasis microscopically confirmed

Note

*pM0 and pMX are not valid categories.

### Stage

| | | | |
|---|---|---|---|
| Stage 0 | Tis | N0 | M0 |
| Stage IA | T1 | N0 | M0 |
| Stage IB | T2a | N0 | M0 |
| Stage IIA | T2b, T2c, T3 | N0 | M0 |
| Stage IIB | T4 | N0 | M0 |
| Stage IIIA | Any T | N1 | M0 |
| Stage IIIB | Any T | N2 | M0 |
| Stage IV | Any T | Any N | M1 |

The information presented here has been excerpted from the 8th edition of the *TNM classification of malignant tumours* (2017) {311A}.
A help desk for specific questions about the TNM classification is available at http://www.uicc.org/resources/tnm/helpdesk.

## Malignant Melanoma of Skin

(C00.0-C00.2, C00.6, C44.0-C44.9, C51.0-C51.2, C51.8-C51.9, C60.0-C60.2, C60.8-C60.9, C63.2)

### TNM Clinical Classification

**T – Primary Tumour**
The extent of the tumour is classified after excision, see pT.

**N – Regional Lymph Nodes**

- NX Regional lymph nodes cannot be assessed
- N0 No regional lymph node metastasis
- N1 Metastasis in one regional lymph node or intralymphatic regional metastasis *without* nodal metastases
  - N1a Only microscopic metastasis (clinically occult)
  - N1b Macroscopic metastasis (clinically apparent)
  - N1c Satellite or in-transit metastasis *without* regional nodal metastasis
- N2 Metastasis in two or three regional lymph nodes, or intralymphatic regional metastasis *with* lymph node metastasis
  - N2a Only microscopic nodal metastasis
  - N2b Macroscopic nodal metastasis
  - N2c Satellite or in-transit metastasis *with* only one regional nodal metastasis
- N3 Metastasis in four or more regional lymph nodes, or matted metastatic regional lymph nodes, or satellite(s) or in-transit metastasis *with* metastasis in two or more regional lymph nodes
  - N3a Only microscopic nodal metastasis
  - N3b Macroscopic nodal metastasis
  - N3c Satellite(s) or in-transit metastasis with two or more regional nodal metastases

Note
Satellites are tumour nests or nodules (macro- or microscopic) within 2 cm of the primary tumour. In-transit metastasis involves skin or subcutaneous tissue more than 2 cm from the primary tumour but not beyond the regional lymph nodes.

**M – Distant Metastasis**

- M0 No distant metastasis
- M1 Distant metastasis*
  - M1a Skin, subcutaneous tissue or lymph node(s) beyond the regional lymph nodes
  - M1b Lung
  - M1c Other non-central nervous system sites
  - M1d Central nervous system

Notes
*Suffixes for M category:
(0) lactic dehydrogenase (LDH) – not elevated
(1) LDH – elevated
so that M1a(1) is metastasis in skin, subcutaneous tissue, or lymph node(s) beyond the regional lymph nodes with elevated LDH.
No suffix is used if LDH is not recorded or is unspecified.

### pTNM Pathological Classification

**pT – Primary Tumour**

- pTX Primary tumour cannot be assessed*
- pT0 No evidence of primary tumour
- pTis Melanoma in situ (Clark level I)

Note
*pTX includes shave biopsies and curettage that do not fully assess the thickness of the primary.

- pT1 Tumour 1 mm or less in thickness
  - pT1a less than 0.8 mm in thickness without ulceration
  - pT1b less than 0.8 mm in thickness with ulceration or 0.8 mm or more but no more than 1 mm in thickness, with or without ulceration
- pT2 Tumour more than 1 mm but not more than 2 mm in thickness
  - pT2a without ulceration
  - pT2b with ulceration
- pT3 Tumour more than 2 mm but not more than 4 mm in thickness
  - pT3a without ulceration
  - pT3b with ulceration
- pT4 Tumour more than 4 mm in thickness
  - pT4a without ulceration
  - pT4b with ulceration

**pN – Regional Lymph Nodes**
The pN categories correspond to the N categories.

- pN0 Histological examination of a regional lymphadenectomy specimen will ordinarily include 6 or more lymph nodes. If the lymph nodes are negative, but the number ordinarily examined is not met, classify as pN0. Classification based solely on sentinel node biopsy without subsequent axillary lymph node dissection is designated (sn) for sentinel node, e.g. (p)N1(sn).

**pM – Distant Metastasis***

- pM1 Distant metastasis microscopically confirmed

Note
*pM0 and pMX are not valid categories.

### Clinical Stage

(Continued on next page)

## Malignant Melanoma of Skin

(Continued)

### Clinical Stage

| | | | |
|---|---|---|---|
| Stage 0 | pTis | N0 | M0 |
| Stage IA | pT1a | N0 | M0 |
| Stage IB | pT1b | N0 | M0 |
| | pT2a | N0 | M0 |
| Stage IIA | pT2b | N0 | M0 |
| | pT3a | N0 | M0 |
| Stage IIB | pT3b | N0 | M0 |
| | pT4a | N0 | M0 |
| Stage IIC | pT4b | N0 | M0 |
| Stage III | Any pT | N1, N2, N3 | M0 |
| Stage IV | Any pT | Any N | M1 |

### Pathological Stage*

| | | | |
|---|---|---|---|
| Stage 0 | pTis | N0 | M0 |
| Stage IA | pT1a | N0 | M0 |
| | pT1b | N0 | M0 |
| Stage IB | pT2a | N0 | M0 |
| Stage IIA | pT2b | N0 | M0 |
| | pT3a | N0 | M0 |
| Stage IIB | pT3b | N0 | M0 |
| | pT4a | N0 | M0 |
| Stage IIC | pT4b | N0 | M0 |
| Stage IIIA | pT1a, T1b, T2a | N1a, N2a | M0 |
| Stage IIIB | pT1a, T1b, T2a | N1b, N1c, N2b | M0 |
| | pT2b, T3a | N1, N2a, N2b | M0 |
| Stage IIIC | pT1a, T1b, T2a, T2b, T3a | N2c, N3 | M0 |
| | pT3b, T4a | N1, N2, N3 | M0 |
| | pT4b | N1, N2 | M0 |
| Stage IIID | pT4b | N3 | M0 |
| Stage IV | Any pT | Any N | M1 |

Note

* If lymph node(s) are identified with no apparent primary the stage is as below

| | | | |
|---|---|---|---|
| Stage IIIB | pT0 | N1b, N1c | M0 |
| Stage IIIC | pT0 | N2b, N2c, N3b, N3c | M0 |

The information presented here has been excerpted from the 8th edition of the *TNM classification of malignant tumours* (2017) {311A}.
A help desk for specific questions about the TNM classification is available at http://www.uicc.org/resources/tnm/helpdesk.

## Merkel Cell Carcinoma of Skin

(ICD-O-3 C44.0-9, C63.2)

### TNM Clinical Classification

#### T – Primary Tumour

| | |
|---|---|
| TX | Primary tumour cannot be assessed |
| T0 | No evidence of primary tumour |
| Tis | Carcinoma in situ |
| T1 | Tumour 2 cm or less in greatest dimension |
| T2 | Tumour more than 2 cm but not more than 5 cm in greatest dimension |
| T3 | Tumour more than 5 cm in greatest dimension |
| T4 | Tumour invades deep extradermal structures, i.e. cartilage, skeletal muscle, fascia or bone |

#### N – Regional Lymph Nodes

| | |
|---|---|
| NX | Regional lymph nodes cannot be assessed |
| N0 | No regional lymph node metastasis |
| N1 | Regional lymph node metastasis |
| N2 | In-transit metastasis *without* lymph node metastasis |
| N3 | In-transit metastasis *with* lymph node metastasis |

Note
In-transit metastasis: a discontinuous tumour distinct from the primary lesion and located between the primary lesion and the draining regional lymph nodes or distal to the primary lesion.

#### M – Distant Metastasis

| | | |
|---|---|---|
| M0 | No distant metastasis | |
| M1 | Distant metastasis | |
| | M1a | Skin, subcutaneous tissues or non-regional lymph node(s) |
| | M1b | Lung |
| | M1c | Other site(s) |

### pTNM Pathological Classification

The pT category corresponds to the T category.

#### pN – Regional Lymph Nodes

| | | |
|---|---|---|
| pN0 | Histological examination of a regional lymphadenectomy specimen will ordinarily include 6 or more lymph nodes. If the lymph nodes are negative, but the number ordinarily examined is not met, classify as pN0. | |
| pNX | Regional lymph nodes cannot be assessed | |
| pN0 | No regional lymph node metastasis | |
| pN1 | Regional lymph node metastasis | |
| | pN1a(sn) | Microscopic metastasis detected on sentinel node biopsy |
| | pN1a | Microscopic metastasis detected on node dissection |
| | pN1b | Macroscopic metastasis (clinically apparent) |
| pN2 | In-transit metastasis *without* lymph node metastasis | |
| pN3 | In-transit metastasis *with* lymph node metastasis | |

Note
In-transit metastasis: a discontinuous tumour distinct from the primary lesion and located between the primary lesion and the draining regional lymph nodes or distal to the primary lesion.

#### pM – Distant Metastasis*

| | |
|---|---|
| pM1 | Distant metastasis microscopically confirmed |

Note
*pM0 and pMX are not valid categories.

#### Clinical Stage

| | | | |
|---|---|---|---|
| Stage 0 | Tis | N0 | M0 |
| Stage I | T1 | N0 | M0 |
| Stage IIA | T2, T3 | N0 | M0 |
| Stage IIB | T4 | N0 | M0 |
| Stage III | Any T | N1, N2, N3 | M0 |
| Stage IV | Any T | Any N | M1 |

#### Pathological Stage

| | | | |
|---|---|---|---|
| Stage 0 | Tis | N0 | M0 |
| Stage I | T1 | N0 | M0 |
| Stage IIA | T2, T3 | N0 | M0 |
| Stage IIB | T4 | N0 | M0 |
| Stage IIIA | T0 | N1b | M0 |
| | T1, T2, T3, T4 | N1a, N1a(sn) | M0 |
| Stage IIIB | T1, T2, T3, T4 | N1b, N2, N3 | M0 |
| Stage IV | Any T | Any N | M1 |

The information presented here has been excerpted from the 8th edition of the *TNM classification of malignant tumours* (2017) {311A}.
A help desk for specific questions about the TNM classification is available at http://www.uicc.org/resources/tnm/helpdesk.

## Soft Tissue Sarcoma of Skin

(ICD-O-3 C49)

In the 8th edition of the *TNM classification of malignant tumours* {311A}, the T categories for soft tissue tumours are defined somewhat differently depending on the site of origin:

- Extremity and superficial trunk
- Retroperitoneum
- Head and neck
- Thoracic and abdominal viscera

The excerpted TNM classification of tumours of soft tissues information shown below can be applied to skin soft tissue sarcomas originating at the anatomical sites indicated below.

## Tumours of Soft Tissues

(ICD-O-3 C38.1, 2, C47-49)

### TNM Clinical Classification

**T – Primary Tumour**

TX Primary tumour cannot be assessed
T0 No evidence of primary tumour

***Extremity and Superficial Trunk***

T1 Tumour 5 cm or less in greatest dimension
T2 Tumour more than 5 cm but no more than 10 cm in greatest dimension
T3 Tumour more than 10 cm but no more than 15 cm in greatest dimension
T4 Tumour more than 15 cm in greatest dimension

***Head and Neck***

T1 Tumour 2 cm or less in greatest dimension
T2 Tumour more than 2 cm but no more than 4 cm in greatest dimension
T3 Tumour more than 4 cm in greatest dimension
T4a Tumour invades the orbit, skull base or dura, central compartment viscera, facial skeleton, and/or pterygoid muscles
T4b Tumour invades the brain parenchyma, encases the carotid artery, invades prevertebral muscle or involves the central nervous system by perineural spread

**N – Regional Lymph Nodes**

NX Regional lymph nodes cannot be assessed
N0 No regional lymph node metastasis
N1 Regional lymph node metastasis

**M – Distant Metastasis**

M0 No distant metastasis
M1 Distant metastasis

### pTNM Pathological Classification

The pT and pN categories correspond to the T and N categories.

**pM – Distant Metastasis***

pM1 Distant metastasis microscopically confirmed

Note
*pM0 and pMX are not valid categories.

### Stage – Extremity and Superficial Trunk

| | | | | |
|---|---|---|---|---|
| Stage IA | T1 | N0 | M0 | G1, GX Low Grade |
| Stage IB | T2, T3, T4 | N0 | M0 | G1, GX Low Grade |
| Stage II | T1 | N0 | M0 | G2, G3 High Grade |
| Stage IIIA | T2 | N0 | M0 | G2, G3 High Grade |
| Stage IIIB | T3, T4 | N0 | M0 | G2, G3 High Grade |
| | Any T | N1* | M0 | Any G |
| Stage IV | Any T | Any N | M1 | Any G |

### Stage – Head and Neck

There is no stage for soft tissue sarcoma of the head and neck.

The information presented here has been excerpted from the 8th edition of the *TNM classification of malignant tumours* (2017) {311A}.
A help desk for specific questions about the TNM classification is available at http://www.uicc.org/resources/tnm/helpdesk.

## Primary Cutaneous Lymphomas

(Mycosis fungoides and Sézary syndrome)

The Union for International Cancer Control (UICC) does not provide a TNM classification of primary cutaneous lymphomas, but the International Society for Cutaneous Lymphomas (ISCL) and the European Organisation of Research and Treatment of Cancer (EORTC) have proposed the following classification system for mycosis fungoides and Sézary syndrome {1946}.

### ISCL/EORTC revision to the classification of mycosis fungoides and Sézary syndrome

Reproduced, with permission, from Olsen E et al. {1946}.

| TNMB stages | |
|---|---|
| **Skin** | |
| $T_1$ | Limited patches,* papules, and/or plaques† covering < 10% of the skin surface. May further stratify into $T_{1a}$ (patch only) vs $T_{1b}$ (plaque ± patch). |
| $T_2$ | Patches, papules or plaques covering ≥ 10% of the skin surface. May further stratify into $T_{2a}$ (patch only) vs $T_{2b}$ (plaque ± patch). |
| $T_3$ | One or more tumors‡ (≥ 1-cm diameter) |
| $T_4$ | Confluence of erythema covering ≥ 80% body surface area |
| **Node** | |
| $N_0$ | No clinically abnormal peripheral lymph nodes§; biopsy not required |
| $N_1$ | Clinically abnormal peripheral lymph nodes; histopathology Dutch grade 1 or NCI $LN_{0-2}$ |
| $N_{1a}$ | Clone negative# |
| $N_{1b}$ | Clone positive# |
| $N_2$ | Clinically abnormal peripheral lymph nodes; histopathology Dutch grade 2 or NCI $LN_3$ |
| $N_{2a}$ | Clone negative# |
| $N_{2b}$ | Clone positive# |
| $N_3$ | Clinically abnormal peripheral lymph nodes; histopathology Dutch grades 3-4 or NCI $LN_4$; clone positive or negative |
| $N_X$ | Clinically abnormal peripheral lymph nodes; no histologic confirmation |
| **Visceral** | |
| $M_0$ | No visceral organ involvement |
| $M_1$ | Visceral involvement (must have pathology confirmation¶ and organ involved should be specified) |
| **Blood** | |
| B0 | Absence of significant blood involvement: ≤ 5% of peripheral blood lymphocytes are atypical (Sézary) cells‖ |
| $B_{0a}$ | Clone negative# |
| $B_{0b}$ | Clone positive# |
| B1 | Low blood tumor burden: > 5% of peripheral blood lymphocytes are atypical (Sézary) cells but does not meet the criteria of $B_2$ |
| $B_{1a}$ | Clone negative# |
| $B_{1b}$ | Clone positive# |
| B2 | High blood tumor burden: ≥ 1000/μL Sézary cells‖ with positive clone# |

* For skin, patch indicates any size skin lesion without significant elevation or induration. Presence/absence of hypo- or hyperpigmentation, scale, crusting, and/or poikiloderma should be noted.

† For skin, plaque indicates any size skin lesion that is elevated or indurated. Presence or absence of scale, crusting, and/or poikiloderma should be noted. Histologic features such as folliculotropism or large-cell transformation (> 25% large cells), CD30+ or CD30−, and clinical features such as ulceration are important to document.

‡ For skin, tumor indicates at least one 1-cm diameter solid or nodular lesion with evidence of depth and/or vertical growth. Note total number of lesions, total volume of lesions, largest size lesion, and region of body involved. Also note if histologic evidence of large-cell transformation has occurred. Phenotyping for CD30 is encouraged.

§ For node, abnormal peripheral lymph node(s) indicates any palpable peripheral node that on physical examination is firm, irregular, clustered, fixed or 1.5 cm or larger in diameter. Node groups examined on physical examination include cervical, supraclavicular, epitrochlear, axillary, and inguinal. Central nodes, which are not generally amenable to pathologic assessment, are not currently considered in the nodal classification unless used to establish N3 histopathologically.

¶ For viscera, spleen and liver may be diagnosed by imaging criteria.

‖ For blood, Sézary cells are defined as lymphocytes with hyperconvoluted cerebriform nuclei. If Sézary cells are not able to be used to determine tumor burden for B2, then one of the following modified ISCL criteria along with a positive clonal rearrangement of the TCR may be used instead: (1) expanded CD4+ or CD3+ cells with CD4/CD8 ratio of 10 or more, (2) expanded CD4+ cells with abnormal immunophenotype including loss of CD7 or CD26.

\# A T-cell clone is defined by PCR or Southern blot analysis of the T-cell receptor gene.

NCI, US National Cancer Institute; TCR, T-cell receptor; TNMB, tumour, node, metastasis, blood.

### Histopathological staging of lymph nodes in mycosis fungoides (MF) and Sézary syndrome

Reproduced, with permission, from Olsen et al. {1946}.

| Updated ISCL/ EORTC classification | Dutch system {2339A} | NCI-VA classification {496A,512A,2325A} |
|---|---|---|
| $N_1$ | Grade 1: dermatopathic lymphadenopathy (DL) | $LN_0$: no atypical lymphocytes<br>$LN_1$: occasional and isolated atypical lymphocytes (not arranged in clusters)<br>$LN_2$: many atypical lymphocytes or in 3-6 cell clusters |
| $N_2$ | Grade 2: DL; early involvement by MF (presence of cerebriform nuclei > 7.5 μm) | $LN_3$: aggregates of atypical lymphocytes; nodal architecture preserved |
| $N_3$ | Grade 3: partial effacement of LN architecture; many atypical cerebriform mononuclear cells (CMCs)<br>Grade 4: complete effacement | $LN_4$: partial/complete effacement of nodal architecture by atypical lymphocytes or frankly neoplastic cells |

LM, lymph node; NCI-VA, US National Cancer Institute–Veterans Administration.

## Primary Cutaneous Lymphomas

(Other than mycosis fungoides and Sézary syndrome)

The Union for International Cancer Control (UICC) does not provide a TNM classification of primary cutaneous lymphomas, but the International Society for Cutaneous Lymphomas (ISCL) and the European Organisation of Research and Treatment of Cancer (EORTC) have proposed the following classification system for primary cutaneous lymphomas other than mycosis fungoides and Sézary syndrome {1368A}.

### ISCL/EORTC proposal on TNM classification of cutaneous lymphoma other than mycosis fungoides and Sézary syndrome

Reproduced, with permission, from Kim YH et al. {1368A}.

| | Classification |
|---|---|
| **T** | |
| T1: | Solitary skin involvement |
| T1a: | a solitary lesion <5 cm diameter |
| T1b: | a solitary >5 cm diameter |
| T2: | Regional skin involvement: multiple lesions limited to 1 body region or 2 contiguous body regions* |
| T2a: | all-disease-encompassing in a <15-cm-diameter circular area |
| T2b: | all-disease-encompassing in a >15- and <30-cm-diameter circular area |
| T2c: | all-disease-encompassing in a >30-cm-diameter circular area |
| T3: | Generalized skin involvement |
| T3a: | multiple lesions involving 2 noncontiguous body regions |
| T3b: | multiple lesions involving ≥3 body regions |
| **N** | |
| N0 | No clinical or pathologic lymph node involvement |
| N1 | Involvement of 1 peripheral lymph node region† that drains an area of current or prior skin involvement |
| N2 | Involvement of 2 or more peripheral lymph node regions† or involvement of any lymph node region that does not drain an area of current or prior skin involvement |
| N3 | Involvement of central lymph nodes |
| **M** | |
| M0 | No evidence of extracutaneous non–lymph node disease |
| M1 | Extracutaneous non–lymph node disease present |

* Definition of body regions (see Figure 1 of Kim YH et al. {1368A}): Head and neck: inferior border—superior border of clavicles, T1 spinous process. Chest: superior border—superior border of clavicles; inferior border—inferior margin of rib cage; lateral borders—mid-axillary lines, glenohumeral joints (inclusive of axillae). Abdomen/genital: superior border—inferior margin of rib cage; inferior border—inguinal folds, anterior perineum; lateral borders—mid-axillary lines. Upper back: superior border—T1 spinous process; inferior border—inferior margin of rib cage; lateral borders—mid-axillary lines. Lower back/buttocks: superior border—inferior margin of rib cage; inferior border—inferior gluteal fold, anterior perineum (inclusive of perineum); lateral borders—mid-axillary lines. Each upper arm: superior borders—glenohumeral joints (exclusive of axillae); inferior borders—ulnar/radial-humeral (elbow) joint. Each lower arm/hand: superior borders—ulnar/radial-humeral (elbow) joint. Each upper leg (thigh): superior borders—inguinal folds, inferior gluteal folds; inferior borders—mid-patellae, mid-popliteal fossae. Each lower leg/foot: superior borders—mid-patellae, mid-popliteal fossae.

† Definition of lymph node regions is consistent with the Ann Arbor system: Peripheral sites: antecubital, cervical, supraclavicular, axillary, inguinal-femoral, and popliteal. Central sites: mediastinal, pulmonary hilar, paraortic, iliac.

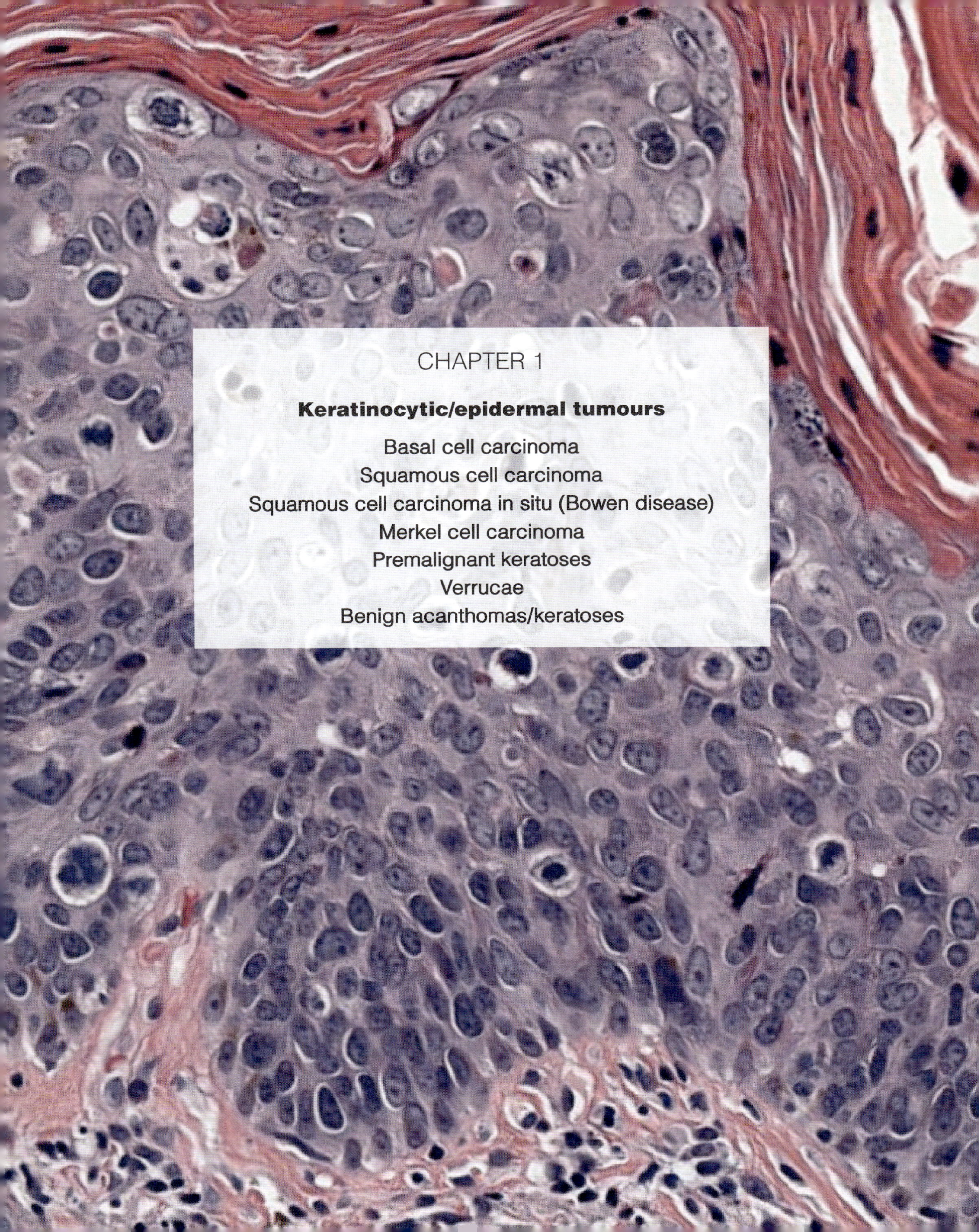

CHAPTER 1

# Keratinocytic/epidermal tumours

Basal cell carcinoma
Squamous cell carcinoma
Squamous cell carcinoma in situ (Bowen disease)
Merkel cell carcinoma
Premalignant keratoses
Verrucae
Benign acanthomas/keratoses

# Keratinocytic/epidermal tumours: Introduction

Scolyer R.A.
Armstrong B.
Berti E.
Damian D.
Elder D.E.
Massi D.
Messina J.

Keratinocytic tumours comprise a broad range of benign, premalignant, and malignant lesions arising from keratinocytes of the epidermis and adnexae. Benign lesions include verrucae, acanthomas, and seborrhoeic keratoses. Actinic, arsenical, and PUVA keratoses are premalignant lesions with the potential for transformation to squamous cell carcinoma. Keratinocytic malignancies (basal cell carcinomas and squamous cell carcinomas) are collectively more common than all other cancers combined, and are therefore the most frequently encountered malignancies in routine clinical and pathology practice. Merkel cell carcinoma is far less common, but because it is considered to be a malignancy of skin-derived neuroendocrine cells, it is now included here in the *Keratinocytic/epidermal tumours* chapter of the 4th edition. Another important change since the 3rd edition is the categorization of keratoacanthoma as a variant of squamous cell carcinoma. The pathological criteria for the diagnosis of micronodular, infiltrating, sclerosing/morphoeic (high-risk), and some other variants of basal cell carcinoma have also been refined and clarified since the 3rd edition.

## *Carcinomas*

### Etiology

Ultraviolet (UV) radiation – specifically, UVB radiation (with a wavelength of 290–320 nm) and UVA radiation (with a wavelength of 320–400 nm) – is estimated to cause 95% of keratinocytic cancers {94}. Exposure to artificial sources of UV radiation is a risk factor for keratinocytic cancers. One study found that the incidence rate of cutaneous squamous cell carcinoma (SCC) among psoriasis patients who had received 351–450 PUVA treatments was 6 times the rate among patients who had received < 50 treatments; there was also a (more modest) increase in the risk of basal cell carcinoma (BCC) {2508}. Indoor tanning, especially among individuals aged < 25 years, is also associated with an increased risk of SCC and BCC {2794}. Immunosuppression is another potent promoter of skin carcinogenesis. Among individuals who are chronically and profoundly immunosuppressed, such as solid-organ transplant recipients, the rate of SCC is 50–80 times as high as among immunocompetent individuals, and the rate of BCC is about 5–10 times as high {1815,2134}. Other etiological factors associated with elevated risk of keratinocytic cancers include exposure to ionizing radiation, environmental exposure to arsenic, HPV infection, and smoking {1559,1585,2124}. Increased risk of keratinocytic cancer is also associated with a variety of uncommon genetic syndromes. Patients with xeroderma pigmentosum, a disorder of nucleotide excision repair, have extreme sensitivity to sunlight and a risk of skin cancer about 10 000 times that in the general population, with keratinocytic cancers developing from an average age of < 10 years {627}.

### Basal cell carcinoma

Carcinoma derived from keratinocytes is the most common malignancy in fair-skinned populations worldwide {1588}. In populations with high levels of UV radiation exposure, such as in Australia, keratinocytic cancer is more than 4 times as common as all other cancers combined {2499}. The majority of keratinocytic cancers that occur in immunocompetent individuals are BCCs, which grow over months to years and only rarely metastasize {2758}. Dysregulation of the hedgehog pathway, as a result of deletion of the *PTCH1* gene or overactivation of the smoothened (SMO) protein, is central in the pathogenesis of BCCs {1962}. This pathway is affected by UV radiation–induced mutations in the majority of cases. Individuals with naevoid BCC syndrome (typically caused by *PTCH1* mutation) develop multiple BCCs, beginning in childhood or adolescence {2081}.

BCC is histopathologically diverse, and the recognition of more than 20 patterns in the literature makes the creation of a classification system challenging {2285}. It is well recognized that the various histological subtypes of BCC, including nodular, superficial, micronodular, infiltrating, and sclerosing/morphoeic tumours, have different clinical presentations and responses to treatment {2513}. In this volume, we emphasize a classification that recognizes BCC subtypes with lower and higher risks of recurrence. Low-risk subtypes include nodular, superficial, pigmented, and fibroepithelial BCC, as well as other variants. The diverse patterns of nodular BCC, although of no distinct clinical consequence, have strikingly varied morphologies, including adenoid, cystic, and keratotic variants. Because patient management is largely stratified by risk of recurrence, emphasis is placed on more-stringent histological criteria for diagnosis of the high-risk subtypes, specifically micronodular, infiltrating, and sclerosing/morphoeic BCC. Accordingly, basosquamous carcinoma, an oft-controversial entity with a higher risk of recurrence than other BCC variants, is more strictly defined as a malignancy with features of both BCC and SCC. Rare subtypes of BCC such as BCC with adnexal differentiation and BCC with sarcomatoid differentiation may be difficult to distinguish from adnexal neoplasms; illustrative examples and differential diagnostic considerations are therefore emphasized in this volume.

### Squamous cell carcinoma

SCC, which is more common than BCC in immunosuppressed populations {2084}, has metastatic potential and tends to grow more rapidly (within weeks to months) than does BCC. The various SCC histological subtypes and differentiation grades have important implications for management and prognosis. SCC in situ (Bowen disease), characterized by full-thickness epidermal atypia, presents as erythematous, scaling plaques, which can remain unchanged for many years. An estimated 4% of SCC in situ lesions progress to invasive SCC {541}. Molecular and cytogenetic studies provide

supporting evidence that actinic keratoses and SCC in situ are precursors of invasive SCC {463}. The role of UV radiation in the pathogenesis of SCC is well established {94}.
Some variants of invasive SCC have distinctive clinical settings as well as prognosis. Low-grade variants include keratoacanthoma (which is now considered to be a well-differentiated variant of SCC with distinctive clinical behaviour) and verrucous SCC. These variants can be locally destructive but have little if any potential to metastasize.
More-aggressive forms include adenosquamous carcinoma, spindle cell SCC, and some other rare variants. Acantholytic SCC and adenosquamous carcinoma can be difficult to distinguish from primary and metastatic adenocarcinoma, whereas spindle cell SCC must be distinguished from other spindle cell malignancies, including atypical fibroxanthoma, pleomorphic dermal sarcoma, and melanoma. Some variants of SCC, in particular clear cell SCC, can be difficult to distinguish from adnexal carcinomas, and are therefore highlighted in this volume.
Several grading and staging systems for SCC have been promulgated; the most commonly used staging criteria are those set forth by the American Joint Committee on Cancer (AJCC). In addition to tumour size, nodal status, and metastasis, the AJCC criteria recognize the high-risk histological features of tumour thickness > 2 mm, Clark level IV or V invasion, perineural invasion, primary site on the ear or lip, and poor differentiation. The National Comprehensive Cancer Network (NCCN) has a high-risk stratification system that includes additional clinical factors (poorly defined tumours, recurrent tumours, immunosuppression, site of prior radiation or chronic inflammation, rapid growth, and neurological symptoms) as well as the aforementioned high-risk histological subtypes, perineural invasion, and lymphovascular invasion {477}.

### Merkel cell carcinoma

Merkel cell carcinoma (MCC) is much less common than BCC and SCC, with an estimated 1600 new cases per year in the USA, but its incidence seems to be increasing {1677}. There is ongoing debate as to the cell of origin, but this tumour is likely derived from a cutaneous epithelial cell or cutaneous-residing stem cell. Therefore, MCC is included here in the *Keratinocytic/epidermal tumours* chapter of the 4th edition. MCC is more common in immunosuppressed patients and tends to be more aggressive in the setting of immunosuppression {1949}. MCC typically involves the head and neck region of elderly patients, and it is strongly associated with chronic UV radiation exposure. Clonal integration of the Merkel cell polyomavirus (MCPyV) is present in approximately 80% of cases in regions of the world with lower sun exposure. Molecular studies have revealed marked differences in the types and frequencies of mutations in MCPyV-positive and MCPyV-negative MCCs, suggesting that distinct transformation pathways are associated with these mechanisms. Compared with virus-positive tumours, MCPyV-negative tumours have more mutations in the *TP53* and *RB1* genes, a UV radiation signature mutation profile with many C>T substitutions, and a higher total mutation burden {900,2107}. Accurate diagnosis of MCC usually requires immunohistochemical evaluation and exclusion of metastatic neuroendocrine carcinoma from other primary sites. Adequate staging is paramount for appropriate decision-making regarding management.

## Carcinoma precursors and benign simulants

### Premalignant keratoses

Actinic keratoses (AKs) affect > 60% of fair-skinned individuals aged > 40 years who live in regions with high ambient ultraviolet (UV) irradiance {1664}. The absolute risk of malignant transformation in AKs is unknown, but seems to be very low; malignant transformation is estimated to occur in only 1 in 1000 to 1 in 10 000 lesions {213}. Many AKs regress, either spontaneously or in response to reduced UV radiation exposure. A prospective study of almost 8000 AKs found a clinical regression rate of > 50% at 1 year without treatment, increasing to 70% at 5 years {546}. Daily sunscreen use can reduce the rate of new facial AKs and enhance the regression of existing lesions, and AK counts are reported to decrease by about 25% in winter compared with summer {827,2608}. Other environmental exposures include exposure to arsenic (usually in well-water or through occupational exposure), which can also cause arsenical keratosis, and UV radiation therapy administered in conjunction with psoralens, which can also cause PUVA keratosis {2508}.

### Benign lesions

Benign keratinocytic neoplasms, including seborrhoeic keratosis, solar lentigo, and large cell acanthoma, are the most common tumours affecting the skin. Mostly related to sun exposure, they can become inflamed, and thus may be clinically and histopathologically difficult to distinguish from malignancy. Lichen planus–like keratosis is the most distinctive form of inflamed benign keratinocytic neoplasm, and can occasionally be difficult to distinguish from a melanocytic neoplasm. Other (less common) lesions, grouped under the rubric "acanthoma", are similarly benign but display a variety of distinguishing histological features: acantholysis, epidermolytic hyperkeratosis, hypergranulosis, glycogen deposition, and melanocyte hyperplasia. Verrucae (caused by HPV infection), as squamoproliferative lesions occasionally resembling benign and malignant keratinocytic neoplasms, are also included in this chapter.

# Basal cell carcinoma

Messina J.
Epstein E.H. Jr
Kossard S.
McKenzie C.
Patel R.M.
Patterson J.W.
Scolyer R.A.

## Definition
Basal cell carcinoma (BCC) is a carcinoma derived from basal cells of the interfollicular epidermis and/or hair follicle. BCCs exhibit morphological variability, but they invariably contain islands or nests of peripherally palisaded basaloid cells with hyperchromatic nuclei and scant cytoplasm.

## ICD-O code
Basal cell carcinoma NOS 8090/3

## Synonyms
Basal cell epithelioma; basalioma

## Epidemiology
BCC is the most common malignancy in humans {1588,2252}. Incidence rates are inversely related to geographical latitude and are higher in lighter-skinned populations {2735}. Rates are highest in Australia (where one in two residents develops BCC before the age of 70 years) and lowest in parts of Africa {1588}. Worldwide, the incidence of BCC is increasing everywhere except for Australia, where it seems to have reached a plateau {1588}. In the USA, the incidence rate is approximately 576 cases per 100 000 person-years {108}. The male-to-female ratio is approximately 1.5:1 {1461}. Patients with two or more BCCs are at high risk of developing subsequent tumours, which are more likely to be of the superficial subtype. Multiple BCCs disproportionately occur in men {1461}. The risk of BCC steadily increases with age {422}. However, incidence rates are increasing faster in younger age groups, particularly among women. Exposure to indoor tanning is a risk factor for early-onset BCC {1284}.

## Etiology
The finding that ultraviolet (UV) radiation exposure is the most important risk factor for BCC carcinogenesis is supported by abundant evidence {2735}, including higher incidence rates of BCC in regions closer to the equator and among individuals with relatively high sun exposure, and the tumours' predilection for anatomical sites exposed to more sunlight. These tumours harbour many UV radiation signature mutations. Intermittent acute UV radiation exposure, particularly during childhood, is implicated in the development of BCC. However, unlike in squamous cell carcinoma (SCC), the increase in BCC incidence peaks at approximately 30 000 hours of cumulative sun exposure and then flattens; in contrast, SCC risk increases indefinitely with increasing cumulative sun exposure {2242}. Ionizing radiation and systemic arsenic exposure are also known environmental insults associated with BCC carcinogenesis, and organ transplant recipients may develop a risk of BCC as much as 10 times that in the general population {2735}.

**Table 1.01** Histological subtypes of basal cell carcinoma (BCC) stratified by risk of recurrence

| Lower risk | Higher risk |
|---|---|
| Nodular BCC | Basosquamous carcinoma |
| Superficial BCC | Sclerosing/morphoeic BCC |
| Pigmented BCC | Infiltrating BCC |
| Infundibulocystic BCC (a variant of BCC with adnexal differentiation) | BCC with sarcomatoid differentiation |
| Fibroepithelial BCC | Micronodular BCC |

## Localization
BCC is predominantly found in sun-exposed skin; in one review, 64% of cases were found on the head, and 24% on the trunk {2092}. However, BCC has also been reported in the perianal and genital region, nail unit, palm, and sole. Different histological subtypes have predilections for different anatomical locations: superficial BCC occurs mainly on the trunk (overall), whereas nodular BCC is the predominant subtype of the head and neck. Superficial BCC is most common in females, in whom it is more often found on the legs than at other sites {167}.

## Clinical features
The variety of clinical presentations seen in BCC reflects the variety of the histopathological variants of these tumours. The classic feature is a pearly, telangiectatic papule, which may be eroded or ulcerated. Superficial BCC may present as an annular, mildly scaly plaque resembling tinea corporis. Sclerosing/morphoeic BCC and infiltrating BCC can have a scar-like appearance; pigmented BCC can resemble melanoma.

## Histopathology
The various BCC variants all contain aggregates of basaloid cells with scant cytoplasm, as well as hyperchromatic nuclei surrounded by fibromyxoid stromal change that produces retraction of tumour from the stroma. Apoptotic tumour cells are often present; melanocytes may be found in tumour nests, and keratinization may be seen. The surrounding stroma may show amyloid deposition.

## Differential diagnosis
The differential diagnosis includes other follicular-derived basaloid tumours (chiefly trichoepithelioma) and basaloid SCC. Immunohistochemically, BCC is distinguished from trichoepithelioma by more frequent diffuse BCL2 expression and more frequent CD10 expression in tumour cells, which shows an inverse relationship with stromal staining. Trichoepithelioma shows a higher frequency of peripheral staining of tumour nests for CK15, CK20, and podoplanin (recognized by D2-40) {1057,2589}. Sclerosing/morphoeic BCC shows more frequent expression of androgen receptor and fewer CK20-positive cells than does desmoplastic trichoepithelioma {1291}. BCC expresses BerEP4 and is negative for EMA (epithelial membrane antigen), whereas the converse is true for SCC.

## Histogenesis

Sporadic trichoepitheliomas have been genetically linked to BCCs by their shared characteristic of frequent deletions of *PTCH1* {1700}. However, this characteristic is not found in trichoblastoma {981}; therefore, considerable debate remains as to the relationship of these tumours.

## Genetic profile

BCC has one of the highest prevalence rates of somatic mutations of all cancers, and most of these mutations show the UV radiation signature of cytosine to thymine substitutions (C>T or CC>TT) {1219}. Loss of heterozygosity of the *PTCH1* gene on chromosome 9q22.3 is found in 58–69% of sporadic BCCs, as well as in all BCCs in patients with naevoid BCC syndrome (NBCCS) {2735}. About 40% of the *PTCH1* mutations found in sporadic BCCs show the UV radiation signature {2149}. Mutations in the *TP53* gene on chromosome 17p13.1 are found in 44–65% of BCCs. Loss of function of this gene is implicated in dysregulation of cell-cycle arrest, senescence, apoptosis, and DNA repair {2735}. *MC1R* variants are also implicated in BCC pathogenesis, and the risk is independent of skin and hair colour {998}.

## Genetic susceptibility

NBCCS (see p. 388) is an autosomal dominant disorder characterized by multiple BCCs, odontogenic keratocysts of the jaws, palmar and/or plantar pits, and skeletal abnormalities. Patients with NBCCS develop one to more than a thousand BCCs, starting in puberty. The risk is increased following UV radiation exposure. Patients with NBCCS typically have germline mutations in the *PTCH1* gene, which encodes a receptor for the sonic hedgehog (SHH) protein. *PTCH1* mutation leads to increased release of the transmembrane protein smoothened (SMO), which leads to downstream activation of the GLI1 transcriptional pathway {1484}. Other genetic abnormalities that predispose individuals to BCC include xeroderma pigmentosum, Bazex–Dupré–Christol syndrome, and Rombo syndrome {801}.

## Prognosis and predictive factors

There is no formal staging system for risk stratification specific to patients with BCC. In the *American Joint Committee on Cancer (AJCC) Cancer Staging Manual*, BCC is typically grouped with other cutaneous malignancies, including SCC {68}; however, TNM staging is rarely reported for this tumour, which usually remains localized. The National Comprehensive Cancer Network (NCCN) guidelines stratify the BCC variants by low versus high risk of recurrence, on the basis of clinical and pathological parameters, chiefly histological type (Table 1.01) {1882}.

# *Nodular basal cell carcinoma*

## Definition

Nodular basal cell carcinoma (BCC), the most common BCC variant, is characterized by large tumour nodules in the dermis.

## ICD-O code 8097/3

## Localization

Nodular BCC is most common in the head and neck region.

## Clinical features

Nodular BCC presents as a pearly plaque or nodule, often with telangiectasia. On dermoscopy, a pattern of arborizing vessels is seen {2907}. The cystic variant may appear as a translucent cystic nodule, and mucin-filled cystic cavities may resemble hidrocystoma. Ulceration is frequent in larger lesions, historically termed "rodent ulcers".

## Histopathology

Islands of basaloid cells with peripheral palisading extend into the dermis; centrally, a haphazard nuclear arrangement with frequent apoptosis is seen. Retraction spaces form between tumour islands and stroma, and amyloid deposition may be seen. Some tumours show prominent, keloidal-type collagenous stroma.

Variants of nodular BCC include keratotic BCC, with tumour nests showing central mature keratinization; nodulocystic or cystic BCC, with cystic degeneration within tumour islands; and adenoid BCC, with cribriform nests. Nodular BCC tumour tissue may exhibit a rippled, labyrinthine, or trabecular pattern. Clear, signet-ring, granular, and giant (monster) cell types have been described. The aforementioned cellular variants can also occur with other subtypes of BCC.

## Differential diagnosis

Nodular BCC can be difficult to distinguish from benign and malignant trichoblastic tumours, especially trichoblastic tumours

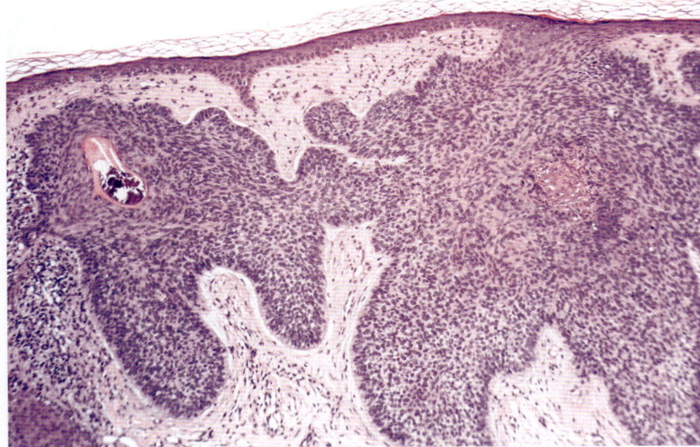

**Fig. 1.01** Nodular basal cell carcinoma. Peripheral palisading, central keratinization, and dystrophic calcification of tumour nests.

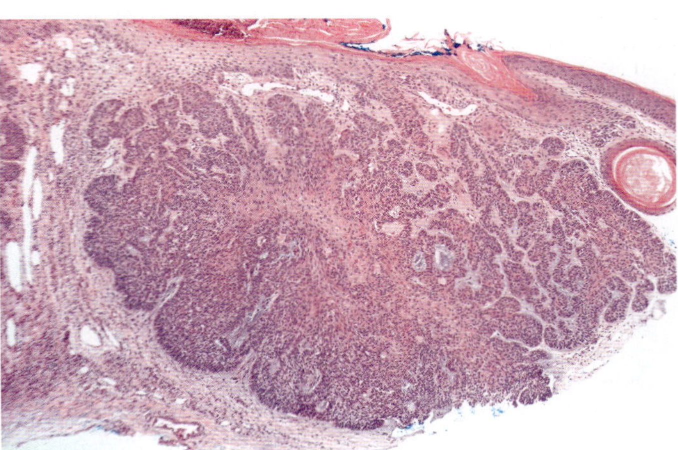

**Fig. 1.02** Nodular basal cell carcinoma (BCC), keratotic variant (keratotic BCC). Central keratinization within tumour nodules.

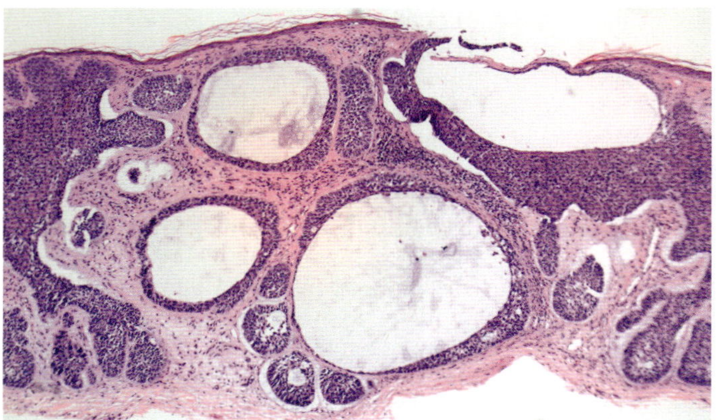

**Fig. 1.03** Nodular basal cell carcinoma (BCC), nodulocystic variant (nodulocystic BCC). Cystic degeneration within some of the tumour islands.

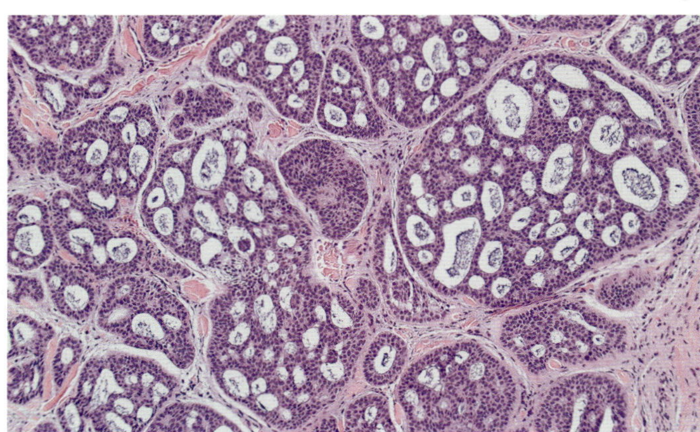

**Fig. 1.04** Nodular basal cell carcinoma (BCC), adenoid variant (adenoid BCC). Cribriform tumour islands.

in sun-damaged skin (see *Trichoblastic carcinoma/carcinosarcoma*, p. 197, and *Trichoblastoma*, p. 201). Lesions with cystic change may be difficult to distinguish from adnexal tumours, particularly adenoid cystic carcinoma. Merkel cell carcinoma may also be considered; immunohistochemically, BCC can be positive for markers of neuroendocrine differentiation (usually chromogranin or synaptophysin) but is negative for CK20, which is positive in Merkel cell carcinoma.

### Prognosis and predictive factors

Nodular BCC is considered to be a low-risk variant of BCC. After adequate surgical excision (with the appropriate method determined by location and tumour size), recurrence and metastasis are exceedingly rare.

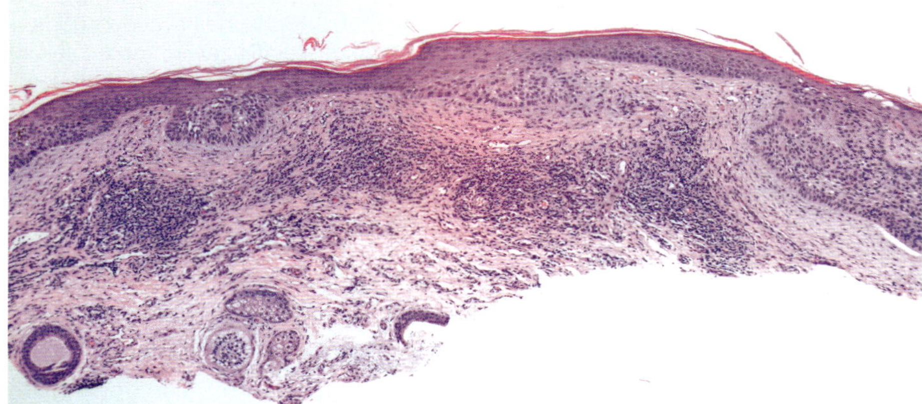

**Fig. 1.05** Superficial basal cell carcinoma. Nests of basaloid cells project from the epidermis. Note the separation artefact.

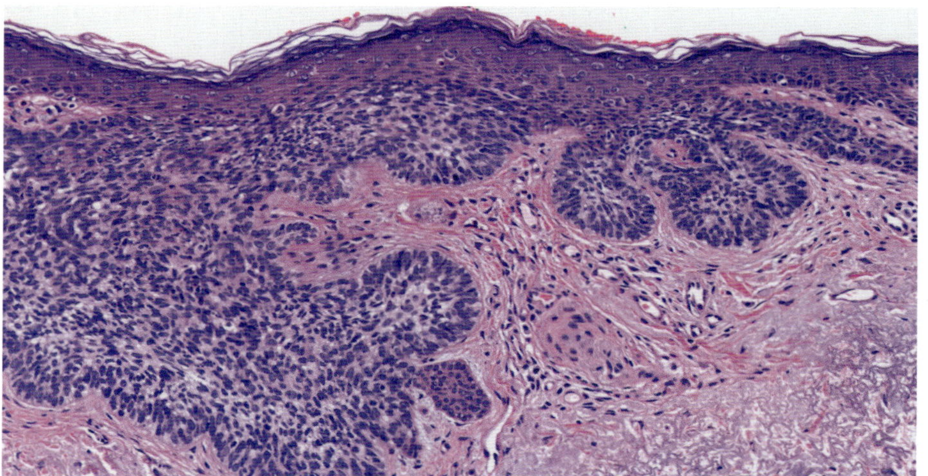

**Fig. 1.06** Superficial basal cell carcinoma. Nests of basaloid cells are attached to the undersurface of the epidermis.

## *Superficial basal cell carcinoma*

### Definition

Superficial basal cell carcinoma (BCC) is a BCC variant with epidermal connection, confined to the papillary dermis.

### ICD-O code 8091/3

### Synonym

Superficial multifocal basal cell carcinoma

### Clinical features

Superficial BCC is characterized by erythematous patches ranging from a few millimetres to > 10 cm in diameter. It accounts for 10–30% of BCCs and occurs most frequently on the trunk. Areas of regression appear as pale patches or fibrosis {1676}. Clinically, this is a low-risk histological subtype {1779}.

### Histopathology

This variant consists of superficial lobules of basaloid cells that project from the epidermis or from the sides of follicles or eccrine ducts into the dermis, typically surrounded by loose myxoid stroma. Usually, the lobules are confined to the papillary dermis and are < 1 mm thick {1716}. Some examples of superficial BCC appear multifocal on vertical sections but can be shown to be connected by stroma using 3D digital imaging techniques {1488}. Mixed patterns with a nodular, micronodular, or infiltrating component are seen in some tumours.

### Differential diagnosis
BerEP4 positivity can help distinguish superficial BCC from actinic keratosis.

## *Micronodular basal cell carcinoma*

### Definition
Micronodular basal cell carcinoma (BCC) is a high-risk variant of BCC; it is characterized by small nests, which often extend deeply into the dermis.

### ICD-O code 8097/3

### Clinical features
Micronodular BCC presents as an elevated or flat, poorly defined lesion, and is most common on the head and neck. It is classified as a high-risk tumour, with the potential to recur after surgery {288}.

### Histopathology
Micronodular BCC shows tumour micronodules often scattered throughout the dermis and subcutis; these may appear as separate satellites outlined by a thin rim of stroma, separated by a normal dermis. The tumours have an irregular, tentacular, and infiltrative deep or peripheral edge, composed predominantly (i.e. >50%) of small discrete nodules (<0.15 mm in diameter) {1719}. The tumours can reach a large size and may demonstrate perineural involvement. This pattern is frequently mixed with others, such as nodular BCC. Punch biopsies have a significant false-negative rate for detecting micronodular BCC in mixed tumours {1275}. Section misorientation and the lack of strict definitions in terms of the size and number of micronodules may contribute to poor interobserver reproducibility in the diagnosis of this variant reported in some studies {1719}.

### Differential diagnosis
The differential diagnosis includes nodular BCC with focal micronodular architecture, but such tumours are encased by a common stroma and lack the satellite pattern seen in micronodular BCC.

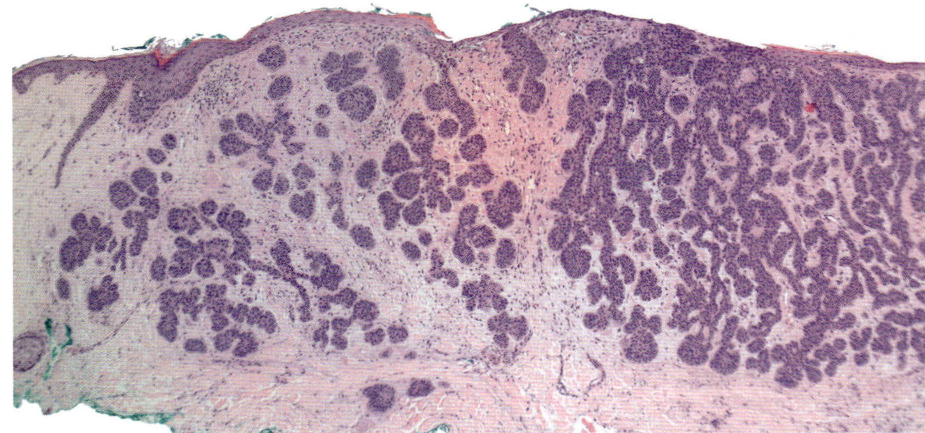

**Fig. 1.07** Micronodular basal cell carcinoma. A small example showing separate small tumour islands at the base of the lesion.

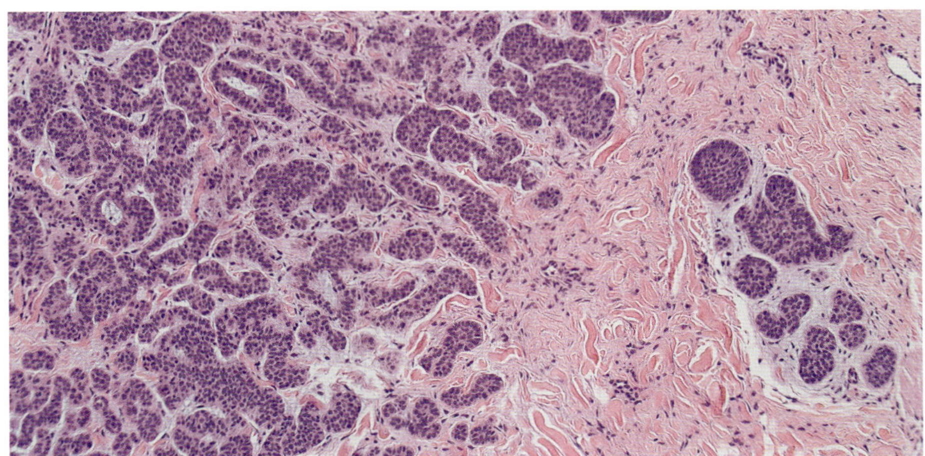

**Fig. 1.08** Mixed micronodular and adenoid basal cell carcinoma. This lesion shows a micronodular pattern (right) and an adenoid pattern (left).

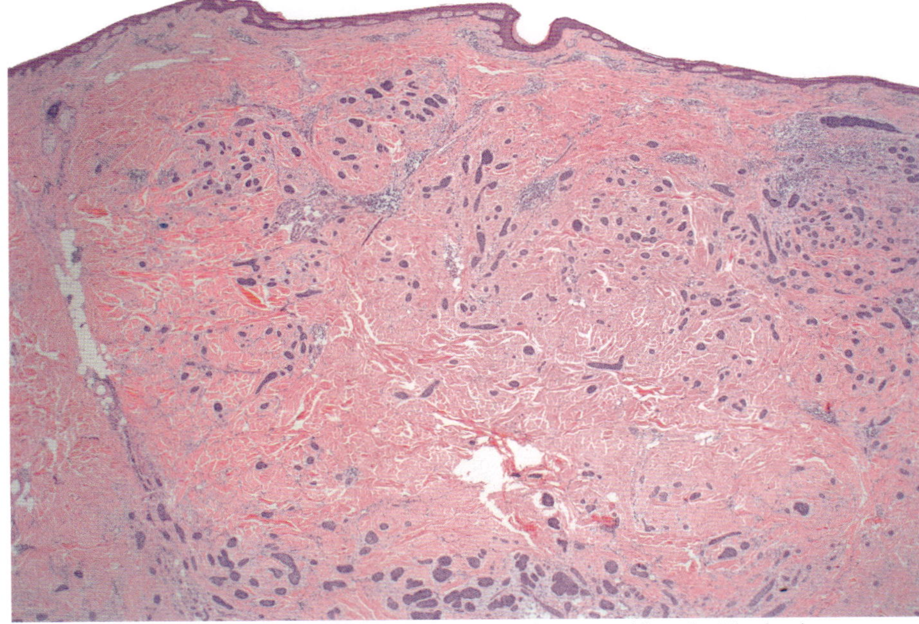

**Fig. 1.09** Micronodular basal cell carcinoma. Small, discrete nodules scattered throughout the dermis.

## Infiltrating basal cell carcinoma

### Definition
Infiltrating basal cell carcinoma (BCC) is a BCC variant characterized by narrow tumour cords and nests with an irregular, infiltrative growth pattern.

### ICD-O code 8092/3

### Synonym
Basal cell carcinoma with aggressive growth pattern

### Clinical features
These tumours have a scar-like presentation, and are most frequent on the upper trunk, head, and neck. They are more common in patients aged <35 years than older patients {1541}. Biopsy should include deep reticular dermis for most accurate diagnosis {506}.

### Histopathology
Variably sized, sometimes jagged nests of basaloid tumour cells infiltrate the normal dermal collagen. The tumour has an irregular/tentacular infiltrative/permeating pattern of invasion at the deep tumour edge {1719}. Tumour nests are typically >5–8 cells thick, and approximately one third of infiltrating BCCs are admixed with a nodular BCC component {550}. Perineural invasion is more frequent in this subtype {1544}. There is often overlap with sclerosing/morphoeic BCC.

### Prognosis and predictive factors
This subtype has a high risk of recurrence, necessitating surgery with strict margin control. Infiltrating BCC is often admixed with low-risk subtypes (e.g. nodular BCC and superficial BCC), but the presence of infiltrative morphology defines the risk of the tumour.

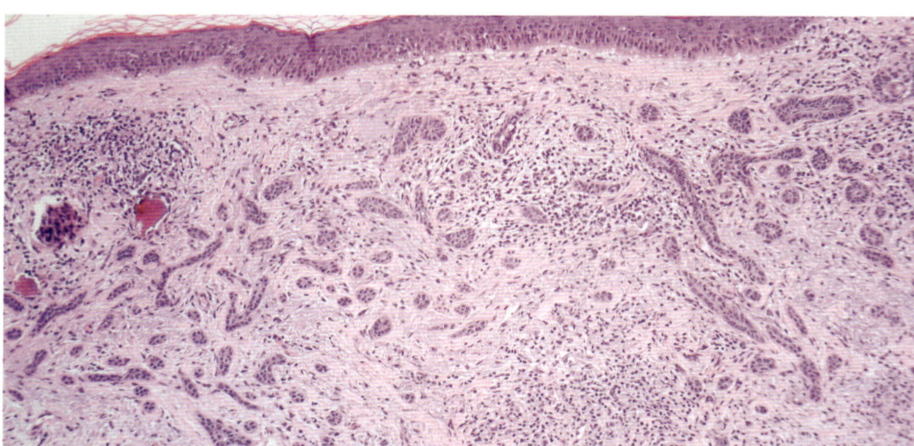

**Fig. 1.10** Infiltrating basal cell carcinoma. Variably sized narrow strands of basaloid cells surrounded by abundant tumour stroma.

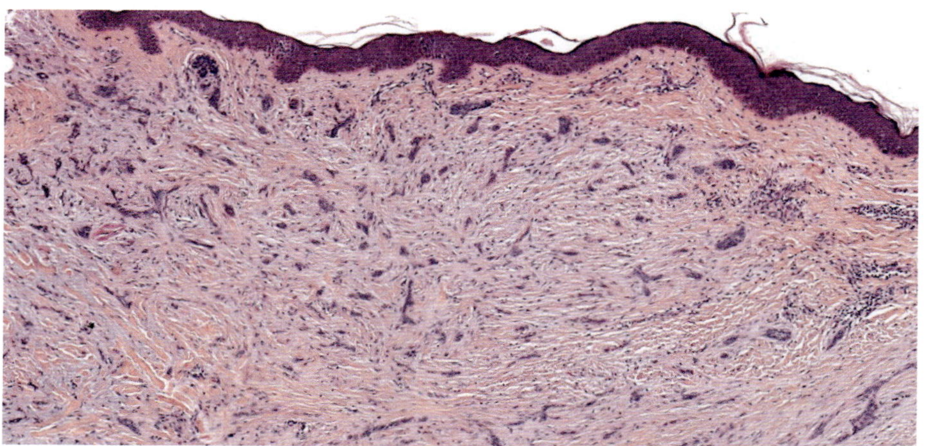

**Fig. 1.11** Infiltrating basal cell carcinoma. Infiltrative cords and nests of epithelial cells are present within fibrotic stroma.

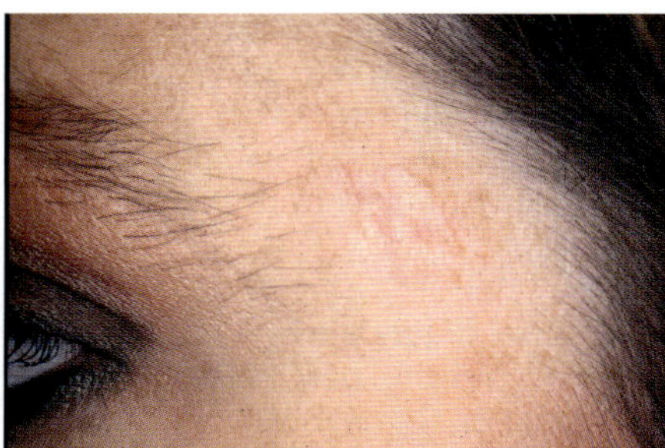

**Fig. 1.12** Sclerosing/morphoeic basal cell carcinoma. A scar-like plaque on sun-damaged skin.

## Sclerosing/morphoeic basal cell carcinoma

### Definition
Sclerosing/morphoeic basal cell carcinoma (BCC) is a BCC variant characterized by very thin cords of basaloid cells surrounded by abundant collagenous stroma.

### ICD-O code 8092/3

### Synonym
Morpheaform basal cell carcinoma

### Clinical features
This subtype presents as a poorly defined, scar-like plaque that rarely ulcerates or bleeds {550}.

### Histopathology
Narrow cords of tumour (1–5 cells thick) are compressed by induced sclerotic collagenous stroma, disrupting the normal dermal architecture. Retraction artefact is uncommon. These tumours penetrate deeply and show an irregular/tentacular, deeply infiltrative border with the surrounding stroma. There is often overlap with infiltrating BCC, which lacks the prominent induced collagenous stroma.

### Differential diagnosis
Sclerosing/morphoeic BCC can be difficult to distinguish from desmoplastic trichoepithelioma and microcystic adnexal carcinoma; immunostaining may facilitate this distinction. Fibroblast activation protein is positive in stromal fibroblasts of BCC but not desmoplastic trichoepithelioma {5}. BerEP4 is expressed in BCC but not microcystic adnexal carcinoma {2377}.

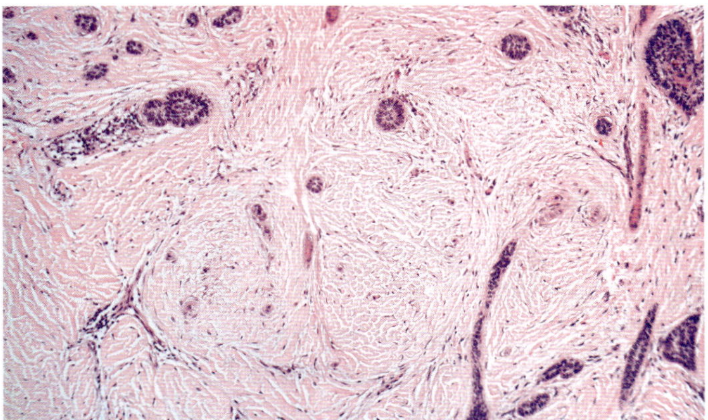

**Fig. 1.13** Sclerosing/morphoeic basal cell carcinoma. Narrow nests of tumour cells are surrounded by abundant collagen.

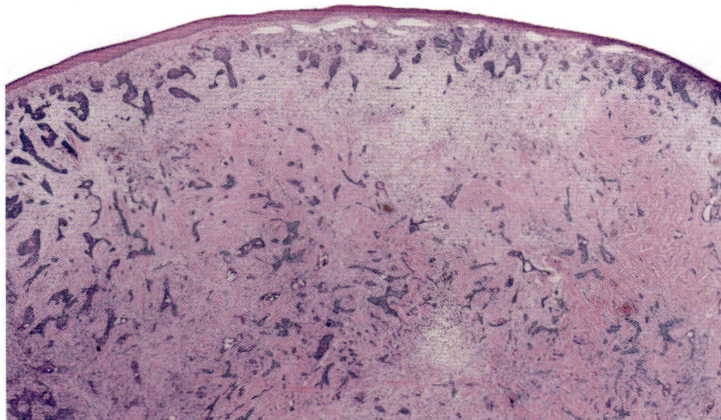

**Fig. 1.14** Sclerosing/morphoeic basal cell carcinoma. A deeply infiltrating tumour is present within sclerotic stroma.

### Prognosis and predictive factors

Like infiltrating BCC, micronodular BCC and basosquamous carcinoma, this variant of BCC is a high-risk subtype, prone to increased frequency of perineural invasion and local recurrence, and necessitating surgical excision with strict margin control.

## *Basosquamous carcinoma*

### Definition

Basosquamous carcinoma is considered to be an aggressive variant of basal cell carcinoma (BCC); it has features of both BCC and squamous cell carcinoma (SCC), as well as transition zones between the two.

### ICD-O code

8094/3

### Synonym

Metatypical basal cell carcinoma

### Epidemiology

Basosquamous carcinoma arises most commonly in the sun-exposed skin of older, fair-skinned White men.

### Clinical features

The lesion presents as a slowly evolving papule or nodule, which may ulcerate. Dermoscopic features include a keratin mass, surface scaling, ulceration, and white structureless areas. The lesion combines the polymorphous vascular pattern of BCC with white circles, which are also a diagnostic clue to keratoacanthoma and other SCCs {36}. Basosquamous carcinoma has a metastatic rate of 5–8.4%, which is comparable to that of SCC and higher than that of conventional BCC (< 0.1%) {47}. Metastases are most frequent in regional lymph nodes, followed by lung {2568}.

### Histopathology

Islands of basaloid cells are comingled with atypical squamous cells with abundant eosinophilic cytoplasm; the atypical squamous cells can be focal or scattered throughout the lesion. Transition zones contain cells with features intermediate between the two. Perineural invasion is found in about 10% of cases. There is often a cellular fibrotic stroma. The basaloid component stains positively for BerEP4, whereas squamous areas express EMA (epithelial membrane antigen). BerEP4 shows a gradation of staining in transition zones, with gradual loss of reactivity towards squamous cell areas {1247}. Higher cyclin D1 expression and lower BCL2 expression are noted in basosquamous carcinoma and other aggressive subtypes of BCC than in conventional, non-aggressive subtypes {2457}.

### Differential diagnosis

Basosquamous carcinoma can be distinguished from keratotic BCC (a subtype of nodular BCC) by the presence of cytologically malignant squamous epithelium and the absence of central mature squamous pearls in tumour nodules. It must

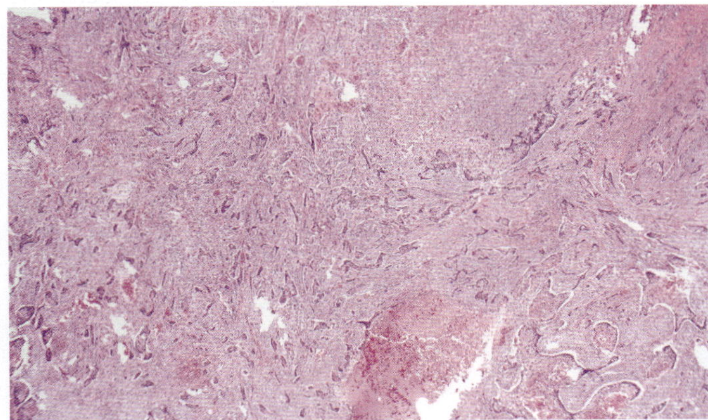

**Fig. 1.15** Basosquamous carcinoma. Basaloid areas (upper portion of the field) intermingled with areas of malignant squamous epithelium (lower portion of the field).

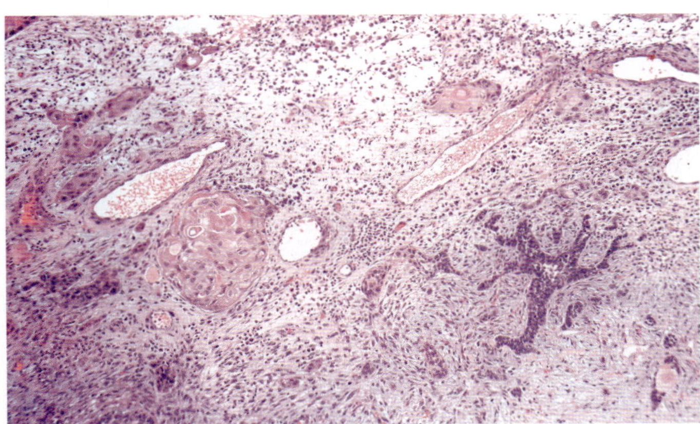

**Fig. 1.16** Basosquamous carcinoma. Infiltrative basaloid strands intermixed with islands of polygonal atypical squamous cells.

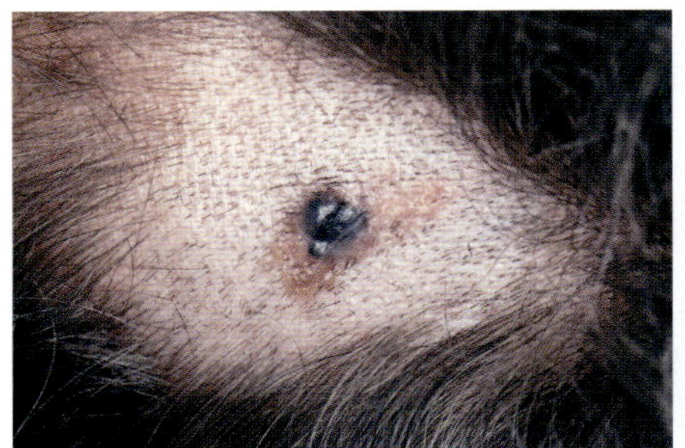

**Fig. 1.17** Pigmented basal cell carcinoma. A pigmented papulonodule surrounded by erythematous plaque.

also be distinguished from a collision of SCC and BCC, where the two tumours are more clearly delineated from one another.

### Prognosis and predictive factors

This is an aggressive BCC subtype; the local recurrence rate may be as high as 4.5%, and lymph node metastasis occurs in 5% of cases {2808}. Patients with metastatic disease have a median survival of 6.5 years and an overall 5-year survival rate of 54% {2936}.

## Pigmented basal cell carcinoma

### Definition

Pigmented basal cell carcinoma (BCC) is a BCC variant that contains melanin pigment.

### ICD-O code 8090/3

### Epidemiology

Pigmented BCC has a predilection for individuals of African, Hispanic, and Asian descent {2452}.

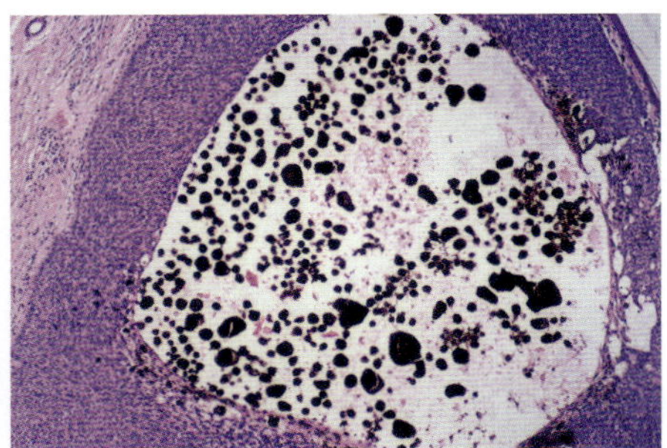

**Fig. 1.18** Pigmented basal cell carcinoma. A cystic basaloid nodule filled with melanophages; dendritic melanocytes can be seen within a basaloid nest.

### Clinical features

Pigmented BCC shows pigmentation, usually superimposed on other classic clinical BCC features (tumours without classic BCC features can be difficult to distinguish from melanoma). The pigmentation can be focal and dot-like or can involve the entire tumour. Dermoscopy can improve diagnostic accuracy. Dermoscopic features include large blue-grey ovoid nests, blue-grey globules, and leaf-like areas {1161}.

### Histopathology

Both nodular and superficial BCC variants can contain pigment, and are considered to fall into the category of pigmented BCC. Pigmented BCC contains increased numbers of benign dendritic melanocytes within tumour islands. There is phagocytosed melanin within tumour cells of the BCC, as well as within peritumoural macrophages {292}.

### Differential diagnosis

The clinical differential diagnosis includes melanoma, pigmented squamous cell carcinoma in situ, and pigmented seborrhoeic keratosis. Nodular variants may be difficult to distinguish from adnexal tumours such as pigmented trichoblastoma, porocarcinoma, and melanocytic matricoma {890}. BCC can occur in collision with melanoma, whereas the term "basomelanocytic tumour" has been proffered to describe a tumour arising from a progenitor cell with both basal and melanocytic differentiation {70}. However, the existence of basomelanocytic tumour as a bona fide entity remains controversial.

## Basal cell carcinoma with sarcomatoid differentiation

### Definition

Basal cell carcinoma (BCC) with sarcomatoid differentiation is a BCC variant that has a basaloid epithelial component and sarcomatous stroma, which can exhibit a variety of histologies.

### ICD-O code 8092/3

### Synonyms

Metaplastic carcinoma; carcinosarcomatous basal cell carcinoma;
sarcomatoid basal cell carcinoma

### Clinical features

These carcinomas occur predominantly in elderly men, in sun-exposed areas of the head, neck, chest, and forearms {2662}. The tumours tend to be large (averaging 2.8 cm) at presentation {2912}.

### Histopathology

A BCC component is admixed with a malignant mesenchymal component, which may consist of pleomorphic undifferentiated sarcoma, osteosarcoma, chondrosarcoma, leiomyosarcoma, and/or rhabdomyosarcoma {2662}. The stromal component is thought to be the result of divergent mesenchymal differentiation of the epithelial component, but is typically negative for epithelial markers.

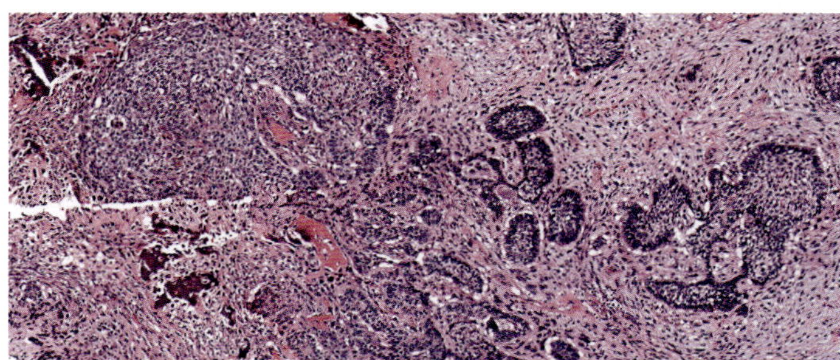

**Fig. 1.19** Basal cell carcinoma (BCC) with sarcomatoid differentiation. Nests of BCC are surrounded by a hypercellular, predominantly spindle cell sarcomatoid stromal component; a focal area shows osteosarcomatous differentiation.

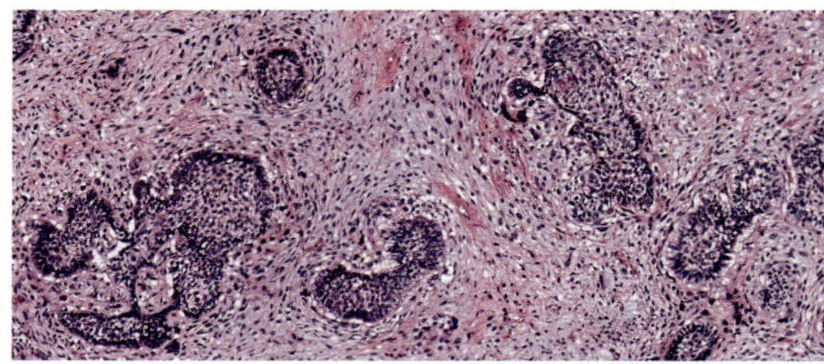

**Fig. 1.20** Basal cell carcinoma (BCC) with sarcomatoid differentiation. Higher magnification detailing nests of BCC surrounded by hypercellular sarcomatoid stroma, which includes atypical plump and spindle cells in a fibromyxoid background.

### Histogenesis
A small series showed similar chromosomal changes in epithelial and mesenchymal components, supporting divergent differentiation of the epithelial component {1013}.

### Prognosis and predictive factors
The rarity of this tumour makes determination of prognosis difficult {2912}.

## *Basal cell carcinoma with adnexal differentiation*

### Definition
Basal cell carcinoma (BCC) with adnexal differentiation is a BCC variant with differentiation towards follicular, sebaceous, apocrine, or eccrine glands {478}.

### ICD-O code 8090/3

### Clinical features
Infundibulocystic BCC and BCC with ductal differentiation have a predilection for periocular skin {199,1795}.

### Histopathology
BCC with matrical differentiation contains shadow cells indicative of hair matrix differentiation {66,1039}. Infundibulocystic BCC shows differentiation towards the follicular infundibulum, with anastomosing cords and nests of basaloid cells, punctuated by small infundibular cyst-like structures {1290,2637,2763}. BCC with sebaceous differentiation shows mature sebocytes, which stain for EMA (epithelial membrane antigen) {1796}. BCC with ductal differentiation contains ducts resembling those found in apocrine or eccrine sweat glands. BCC with apocrine differentiation often shows decapitation secretion. BCC with eccrine differentiation has ducts with a distinct cuticle, which stain positively for polyclonal CEA and EMA {550,1055,1795,2283}.

### Differential diagnosis
BCC with matrical differentiation must be distinguished from pilomatrical carcinoma. The differential diagnosis of infundibulocystic BCC includes basaloid follicular hamartoma and trichoepithelioma. BCC with sebaceous differentiation should be differentiated from sebaceous carcinoma, sebaceous adenoma, and sebaceoma {550}. BCC with ductal differentiation must be distinguished from

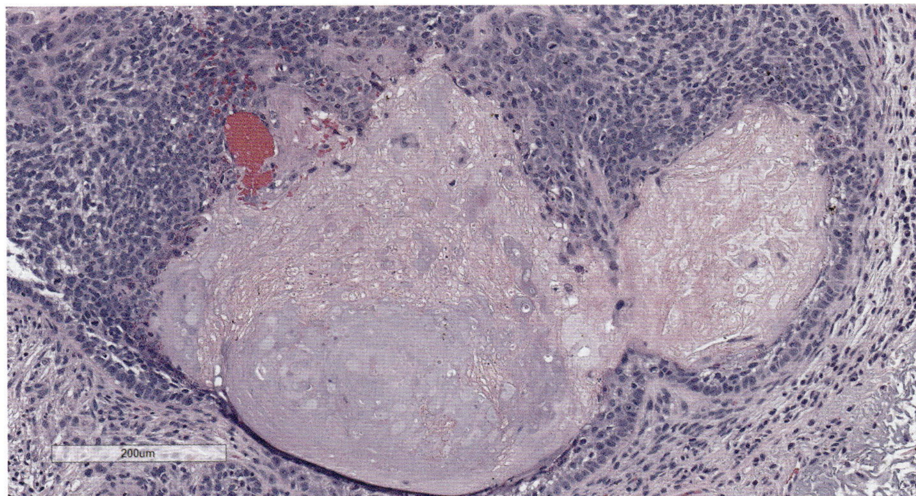


**Fig. 1.21** Basal cell carcinoma with matrical differentiation. Infiltrative basaloid tumour containing islands of shadow cells indicative of hair matrix differentiation.

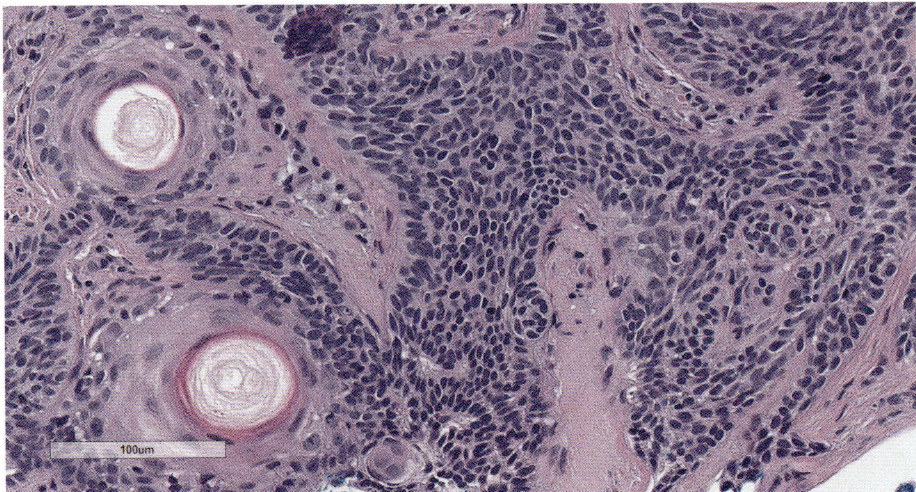


**Fig. 1.22** Infundibulocystic basal cell carcinoma. Anastomosing cords of basaloid tumour cells punctuated by small keratin-filled cysts.

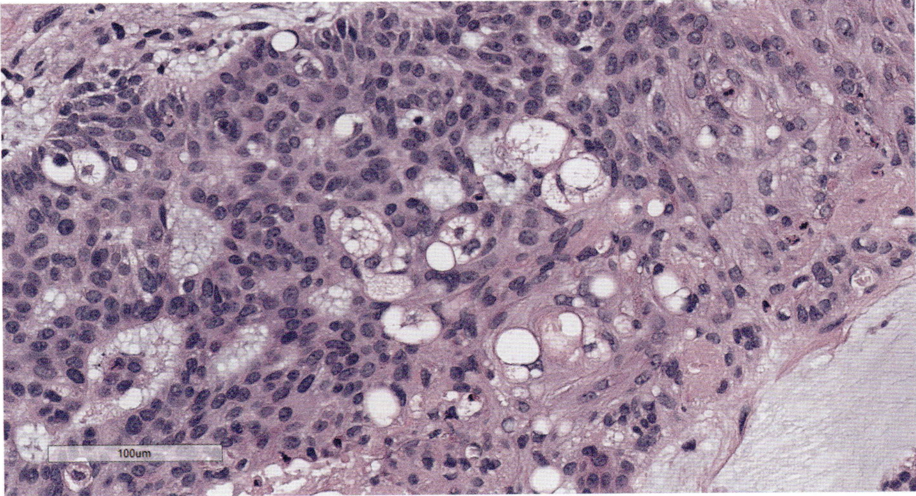


**Fig. 1.23** Basal cell carcinoma with sebaceous differentiation. Basaloid tumour containing multivacuolated mature sebocytes, consistent with sebaceous differentiation.

sweat gland carcinomas. Entrapped native eccrine ducts may mimic eccrine ductal differentiation. Carcinomas in the differential diagnosis of BCC with adnexal differentiation have a higher risk for aggressive biological behaviour than do typical BCCs. In some instances, distinguishing BCC with adnexal differentiation from true adnexal tumours can be exceedingly difficult.

### Genetic profile

A small series of BCCs with matrical differentiation showed molecular abnormalities in *CTNNB1*, *KIT*, *CDKN2A*, *TP53*, *SMAD4*, *ERBB4*, and *PTCH1*, providing supporting evidence that these tumours may be variants of BCC {1476}.

### Genetic susceptibility

Multiple infundibulocystic BCCs can occur in the familial setting, and can also occur in naevoid BCC syndrome {545,2354}. BCC with sebaceous differentiation may be seen in Muir–Torre syndrome, and often has significant histological overlap with other sebaceous neoplasms {550}.

### Prognosis and predictive factors

Adnexal BCC variants do not have prognostic significance.

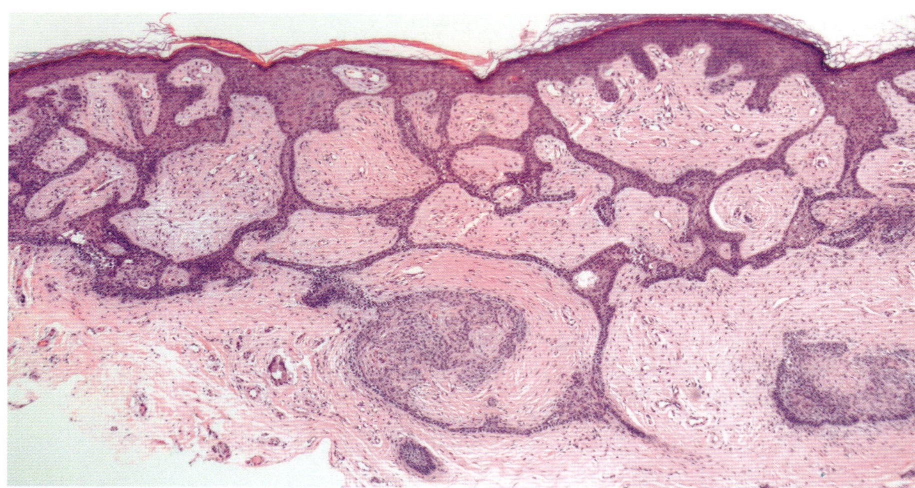

**Fig. 1.24** Fibroepithelial basal cell carcinoma. Basaloid strands emanate from the epidermis and are surrounded by fibroblastic stroma.

## *Fibroepithelial basal cell carcinoma*

### Definition

Fibroepithelial basal cell carcinoma (BCC) is a BCC variant composed of delicate, interanastomosing strands of basaloid cells surrounded by abundant fibroblastic stroma.

### ICD-O code 8093/3

### Synonyms

Fibroepithelioma of Pinkus;
Pinkus tumour

### Localization

These lesions most commonly involve the trunk, in particular the back. They are rarely multiple.

### Clinical features

Fibroepithelial BCC presents as a flesh-coloured nodule.

### Histopathology

Fibroepithelial BCC shows anastomosing basaloid strands emanating downwards from the epidermis. There are strands of basaloid cells that surround fibrotic stroma. In some lesions, basaloid islands are present {2507}.

### Differential diagnosis

Fibroepithelial BCC is distinguished from eccrine syringofibroadenoma by the absence of eccrine ductal epithelium and cuticle in the basaloid strands, and by its predominantly truncal versus acral location {1049}. There is controversy as to whether fibroepithelial BCC constitutes a variant of BCC or a skin adnexal tumour {283,978,2376}.

# Squamous cell carcinoma

Murphy G.F.
Beer T.W.
Cerio R.
Kao G.F.
Nagore E.
Pulitzer M.P.

## *Squamous cell carcinoma*

### Definition

Cutaneous squamous cell carcinoma (SCC) is a malignancy of epidermal keratinocytes that exhibits various degrees of differentiation that partially recapitulate the cytology of squamous cells of the epidermal stratum spinosum. The lesions can be in situ or invasive with the potential for metastasis.

### ICD-O code

Squamous cell carcinoma NOS 8070/3

### Epidemiology

The incidence of SCC is difficult to establish, but data on non-melanoma skin cancer suggest that there were an estimated 701 000 SCC tumours affecting 430 500 people in the USA in 2006 (assuming that 20% of tumours are SCC) {2216}. SCC is the second most common form of skin cancer (after basal cell carcinoma) and is more common in men than in women. Most cases occur in sun-exposed skin of elderly individuals, most commonly individuals with lighter skin pigmentation.

### Etiology

In addition to ultraviolet (UV) radiation, other factors that have been implicated in the etiology of SCC include chronic immunosuppression, other forms of radiation, topical carcinogens, burn scars, chronic inflammation, sinus tracts, HPV infection, arsenic, and coal tar. Cutaneous SCC was the first occupational cancer to be identified, described in the scrotal skin of British chimney sweeps in 1775 by Percivall Pott.

### Localization

The sites most often affected are chronically sun-exposed areas, including the face and lips, ears, balding scalp, arms, trunk, and (particularly in women) legs. More widespread sites may be affected in those who have used indoor tanning {2794}. In rare lesions associated with HPV infection or immunosuppression, the genitalia and distal digits (particularly the subungual region) are commonly involved.

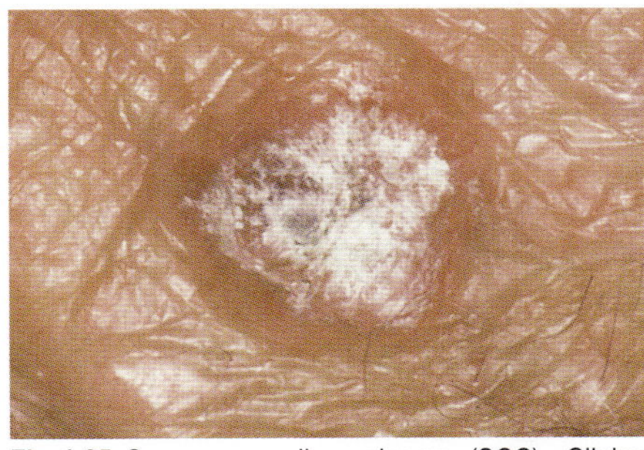

**Fig. 1.25** Squamous cell carcinoma (SCC). Clinical appearance of typical invasive SCC forming a nodule surmounted by hyperkeratotic scale, arising in chronically sun-damaged skin.

### Clinical features

SCC in situ may appear as roughened hyperkeratotic lesions mimicking benign keratoses, dermatoses (e.g. psoriasis), or lichen simplex chronicus. With invasion and progressive growth, hyperkeratotic nodules may develop ulceration. The well-differentiated keratoacanthoma variant of SCC (see p. 36) forms crateriform lesions with central keratin plugs. Less well differentiated tumours produce irregular, erythematous scaling nodules and plaques. Lesions with perineural spread may produce pain or paraesthesias. Lymph node spread is the primary route of metastasis. When visceral lesions develop, they most commonly affect the lung, followed by the bone, CNS, and liver.

### Histopathology

Many SCCs progress from in situ lesions to progressively more deeply invasive tumours. Classic SCC in situ (see p. 46) shows full-thickness keratinocytic atypia. Some SCCs have no identifiable in situ precursor. Lesions vary from well to poorly differentiated, with most classified as well to moderately differentiated. Some well-differentiated forms are classified as keratoacanthomas (see p. 36), which are now considered to be a specific variant of SCC. The staging of SCC is based on lesion diameter, invasion depth, differentiation, and perineural invasion.

Immunohistochemistry is generally not required, except for some poorly differentiated SCCs. Cutaneous SCC is typically positive for p63, p40, EMA (epithelial membrane antigen), CK5/6, MNF116, and high-molecular-weight 34βE12. Unlike in basal cell carcinoma, BerEp4 is negative. Some SCCs show morphological evidence of neuroendocrine differentiation, which can be confirmed by immunohistochemistry.

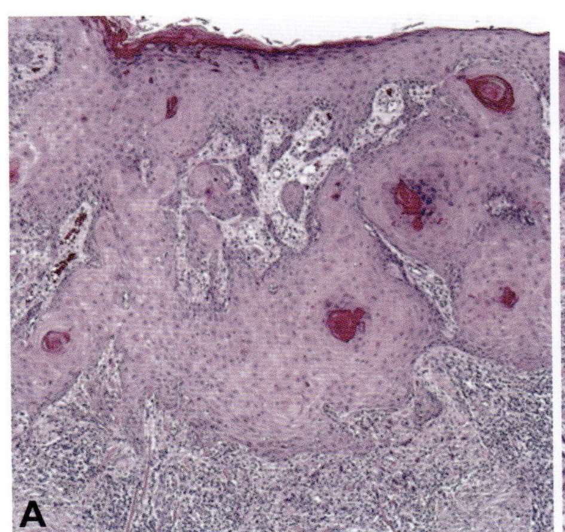

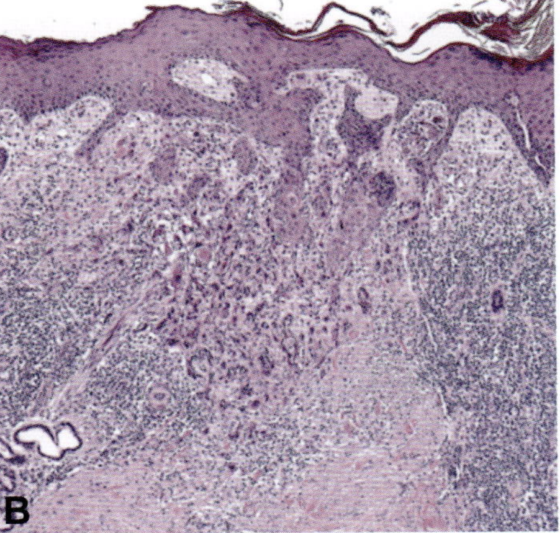

**Fig. 1.26** Squamous cell carcinoma (SCC). Histological appearance of two well-differentiated SCCs. **A** Blunt-type intradermal invasion. **B** A more infiltrative pattern of invasion.

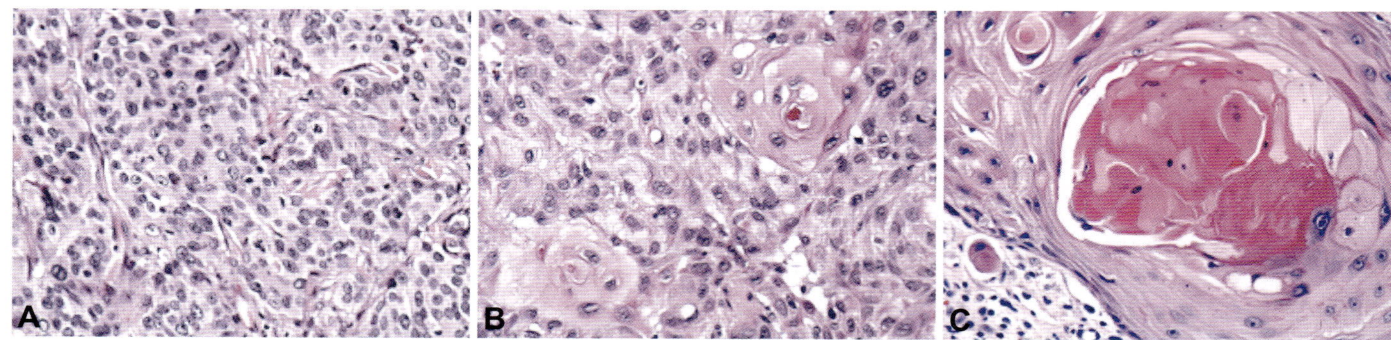

**Fig. 1.27** Squamous cell carcinoma (SCC). Degrees of cytological differentiation in invasive SCC, ranging from poorly differentiated SCC (**A**) with crowded sheets formed by rounded cells with high N:C ratios; to moderately differentiated SCC (**B**) showing foci with distinct squamous morules and occasional minute foci of keratin formation; to well-differentiated SCC (**C**) with regions formed by relatively large polyhedral cells with abundant, glassy eosinophilic cytoplasm with abundant keratin formation.

### Differential diagnosis

Well-differentiated SCC must be distinguished from pseudoepitheliomatous hyperplasia, syringometaplasia, cells traumatically introduced into scars, perineural hyperplasia, endophytic keratoses, warts, and squamoid adnexal tumours. Poorly differentiated SCC must be differentiated from conditions such as melanoma, atypical fibroxanthoma, sarcoma, and lymphoma, which often requires immunohistochemistry.

### Histogenesis

Most UV radiation–related cutaneous SCCs appear to develop through a multistep process in actinic keratoses or in fields of squamous dysplasia. Common mutations involve tumour suppressor genes such as *TP53*, *NOTCH1*, and *NOTCH2* {1800}. Activating mutations in genes such as *HRAS* and *KRAS* are also frequently involved. UV radiation–induced *TP53* mutations likely occur early on in the process. Advanced age, immunosuppression, and environmentally determined defects in the epigenome appear to contribute to impaired elimination of precursors of malignant transformation. Cutaneous SCC probably arises from an epidermal or follicular stem cell {1136}.

### Genetic profile

Recent genetic expression profile studies suggest that the differentially expressed genes *CXCL8* (IL-8), *MMP1*, *HIF1A*, *ITGA6*, and *ITGA2* are promising diagnostic and therapeutic targets {2403}.

### Genetic susceptibility

Patients with xeroderma pigmentosum, vitiligo, and albinism are at increased risk of SCC. A recent two-stage genome-wide association study of a large number of SCCs revealed 11 susceptibility loci. Of these, 7 are related to pigmentation: *MC1R*, *ASIP*, *TYR*, *SLC45A2*, *OCA2*, *IRF4*, and *BNC2*. The other 4 are involved in tumour immune evasion, apoptosis inhibition, or other oncogenic pathways: 11q23.3 (*CADM1*), 2p22.3, 7p21.1 (*AHR*), and 9q34.3 (*SEC16A*) {421}.

### Prognosis and predictive factors

Confirmed high-risk prognostic features are tumour thickness > 2 mm, Clark level IV or V invasion, perineural invasion, primary site on the ear or lip, and poor differentiation. Perineural invasion of nerves ≥ 0.1 mm in diameter correlates with higher disease-specific death rates {2235}.

## Keratoacanthoma

### Definition

Keratoacanthoma is a common, rapidly growing squamoproliferative tumour that may spontaneously regress. It is histologically indistinguishable from (and likely a variant of) well-differentiated cutaneous invasive squamous cell carcinoma, with distinct clinical behaviour {1474}.

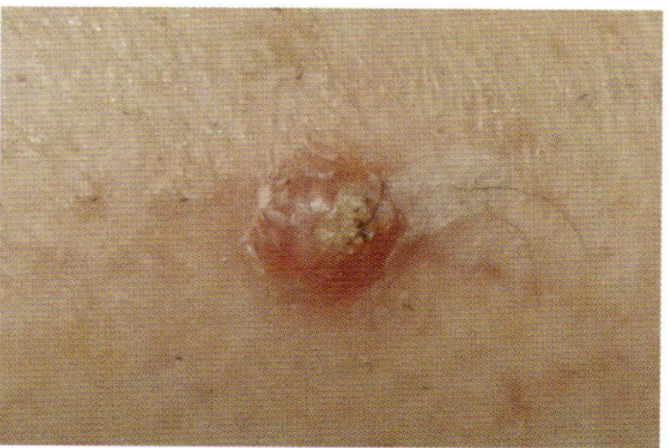
**Fig. 1.28** Proliferative-stage solitary keratoacanthoma. An evolving, 2.0 cm keratoacanthoma of 4 weeks' duration on the lower leg of a 56-year-old woman, presenting as a well-defined erythematous nodule with a central tan-yellow keratin plug.

### ICD-O code 8071/3

### Synonyms

Well-differentiated squamous cell carcinoma, keratoacanthoma type; keratoacanthoma-like squamous cell carcinoma

### Epidemiology

Keratoacanthomas typically arise in the sun-exposed skin of older, fair-skinned individuals between the sixth and seventh decades of life {2641} and have a slight predilection for men. Rare cases occur in childhood and adolescence in association with organoid naevus or xeroderma pigmentosum {749}.

### Etiology

Ultraviolet (UV) radiation, photon radiation, trauma (e.g. at sites of a skin graft or vaccination), infections, and chemical carcinogens have been linked to the development of keratoacanthoma lesions, with solar damage being the predominant risk factor. Other factors include immunosuppression/immunodeficiency, tattoos, and BRAF inhibitors. Human polyomavirus 6 (HPyV6) DNA was recently detected in keratoacanthomas {188}, and other serotypes (HPyV19 and HPyV48) have been isolated in giant keratoacanthomas and keratoacanthomas in HIV-infected patients.

### Localization

Keratoacanthomas most commonly occur in facial skin (in as many as 70% of cases in temperate climates); they also commonly occur on the dorsum of the hands and forearms among men and on the legs among women.

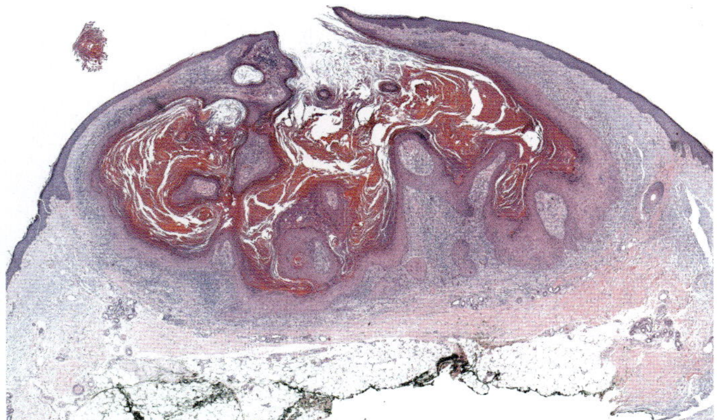

**Fig. 1.29** Mature-stage solitary keratoacanthoma. A scanning view showing a characteristic crateriform architecture with a central keratin core and the hallmarks of keratoacanthoma. A well-defined border and peripheral epidermal lipping are visible.

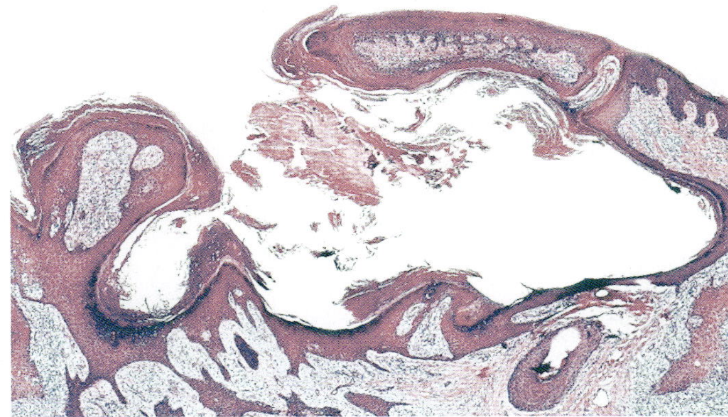

**Fig. 1.30** Regressing-stage solitary keratoacanthoma. The flattened crateriform architecture with central keratin debris remains. There also remain a few lobules of residual proliferative squamous cells with horn cysts surrounded by an inflammatory infiltrate (right). Underlying dermal fibrosis (scarring) and irregular strands of squamous cells at the base are evident.

## Clinical features

*Solitary keratoacanthoma*

This is the most common variant. It presents as a symmetrical, dome-shaped tumour, capped with keratin. It evolves rapidly and may involute over the course of several months. The size ranges from a few millimetres to 20 cm. Giant keratoacanthomas (> 5 cm) have a predilection for the nose and the dorsum of the hands; they can reach up to 15 cm, with destruction of underlying tissues. Three clinical stages have been observed: a proliferative stage (a rapidly enlarging erythematous papule or nodule with a smooth surface), a mature stage (a central whitish-yellow nodule with a crateriform keratotic core), and a regressing stage (a keratotic nodule that progressively flattens in association with elimination of the central keratotic plug, sometimes followed by the formation of a hypopigmented scar).

*Multiple keratoacanthomas*

These rare tumours can be sporadic or familial. Sporadic multiple keratoacanthomas may be associated with prurigo nodularis, usually on the sun-damaged lower legs of elderly women.

*Multiple familial keratoacanthomas of Ferguson-Smith type*

These keratoacanthomas, also known as multiple self-healing squamous epithelioma, were first described in Scottish families with an autosomal dominant inheritance pattern with variable penetrance {1278}. Patients may have hundreds of keratoacanthomas, each with characteristics similar to those seen in solitary keratoacanthoma.

*Multiple keratoacanthoma centrifugum marginatum*

Theses rare skin tumours show persistent growth with an annular, coral reef–like appearance. The lesions involve the back of the hands and can become very large, approaching 20 cm.

*Generalized eruptive keratoacanthomas of Grzybowski*

Affected patients have a generalized eruption of hundreds to thousands of small, well-demarcated papules (some with keratotic centres), predominantly in unexposed skin. The condition is exceedingly rare, and familial clustering has been described {1474}

*Subungual keratoacanthoma*

This rapidly growing and locally destructive tumour originates in the distal nail bed, separating it from the nail plate. The thumb, middle finger, and big toe are most commonly involved.

## Histopathology

The microscopic features of keratoacanthoma vary by clinical stage {2559}. In the early proliferative stage, the tumour is symmetrical and composed of invaginations of interconnecting follicular infundibular/isthmus-type squamous epithelium. The squamous cells contain pale, glassy, eosinophilic cytoplasm and show abrupt (trichilemmal) keratinization devoid of an intervening granular cell layer. At the base, there are irregular strands of mildly atypical keratinocytes; rare mitoses; a dense mixed neutrophilic, lymphocytic, and eosinophilic infiltrate; and intraepithelial microabscesses. Perineural and lymphovascular invasion have been reported to occur in keratoacanthomas.

Mature-stage keratoacanthoma has a typical crateriform architecture. Well-differentiated squamous lobules showing follicular differentiation with trichilemmal keratinization surround a central keratin core. Epidermal lipping is present on both sides of the keratin core.

Regressing-stage keratoacanthomas retain a central invagination and crateriform appearance, although the tumour becomes thinner and flattened, with fewer squamous lobules and horn cysts around the crater. A dense mixed inflammatory infiltrate and dermal scar-like fibrosis are present at the base.

Immunohistochemically, keratoacanthoma is positive for cellular markers seen in the infundibulum and isthmus of follicular structures {1791}. Biomarkers have been reported to be of no predictive value in terms of whether a lesion is destined for progression or regression {1474}.

## Differential diagnosis

Unlike non-keratoacanthoma well-differentiated squamous cell carcinomas, keratoacanthomas show a cup-shaped architecture, trichilemmal keratinization, transepithelial elimination of elastic and collagen fibres in resolving lesions, and intraepithelial microabscesses. Depending on the evolutionary stage and the nature of the biopsy, differential diagnoses may include verrucae, irritated

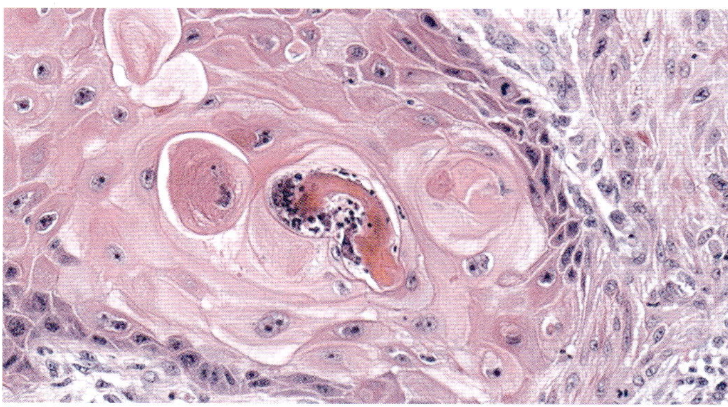

**Fig. 1.31** Keratoacanthoma. A small microabscess is present within a nest of large keratinocytes with pale and glassy eosinophilic cytoplasm; there is minimal nuclear atypia.

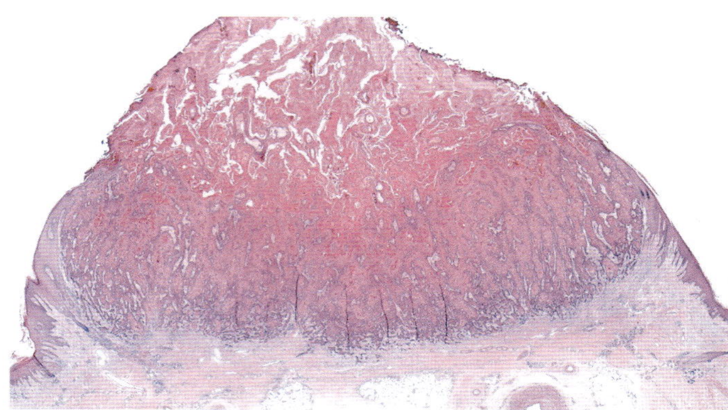

**Fig. 1.32** Keratoacanthoma. A well-differentiated squamoproliferative lesion is present, with a central keratin crater.

seborrhoeic keratoses, inverted follicular keratoses, prurigo nodularis, molluscum contagiosum, and deep fungal infections with pseudoepitheliomatous hyperplasia.

### Histogenesis

Most examples of keratoacanthoma affect hair-bearing skin, and are most likely to be derived from follicular infundibular/isthmus keratinocytes. Rare tumours located on glabrous skin and mucous membranes are probably derived from epithelial keratinocytes.

### Genetic profile

The *MAP3K8* (*TPL2*) oncogene may be a driver common to the development of both keratoacanthoma and squamous cell carcinoma {1526}. Patients with multiple familial keratoacanthomas of Ferguson-Smith type have DNA repair failures associated with Muir–Torre syndrome and xeroderma pigmentosum. Disease-specific mutations in *TGFBR1* have also been identified in patients with multiple familial keratoacanthomas of Ferguson-Smith type {1278}. There is a possible role of *TP53* in the development of some keratoacanthomas; mutant p53 oncoproteins are found in about 10% of tested lesions.

### Genetic susceptibility

Rarely, there is a genetic predisposition to developing keratoacanthomas, in particular multiple familial keratoacanthomas of Ferguson-Smith type. Muir–Torre syndrome is commonly associated with keratoacanthoma lesions, suggesting that the genetic defect (or defects) that causes the syndrome also plays an etiological role in keratoacanthoma {749}.

### Prognosis and predictive factors

Many (if not most) keratoacanthomas eventually undergo resolution, but central facial giant keratoacanthoma and subungual keratoacanthoma may be locally aggressive. It is impossible to predict with certainty the behaviour of a well-differentiated squamoproliferative lesion on the basis of a partial biopsy, or when margins are involved.

## *Acantholytic squamous cell carcinoma*

### Definition

Acantholytic squamous cell carcinoma (SCC) is a histological variant of invasive SCC characterized by impaired intercellular adhesion that may result in the formation of pseudoglandular spaces.

### ICD-O code

8075/3

### Synonyms

Adenoid squamous cell carcinoma; pseudoglandular squamous cell carcinoma

### Epidemiology

The acantholytic variant accounts for <5% of all SCCs, although the criteria for this designation (focal versus widespread acantholysis) are not well established. Older male patients are most frequently affected {940}, and an increased incidence has been reported in organ transplant recipients {2466}.

### Etiology

Given that most acantholytic SCCs occur in chronically sun-exposed sites, ultraviolet (UV) radiation–induced damage is likely a causative factor. The known association with chronic immunosuppression {2466} implies a role for defective immunosurveillance.

### Localization

The lesions often involve skin of the head, neck, face, and ears. Other sun-exposed sites can also be involved. In one review, about 60% of lesions involved the head and neck, and 40% involved the trunk and extremities {2111}.

### Clinical features

The clinical appearance of acantholytic invasive SCC is the same as that of its non-acantholytic counterpart (SCC-NOS).

### Histopathology

At scanning magnification, the overall architecture of invasive acantholytic SCC does not differ substantially from that of ordinary non-acantholytic variants. The overlying epidermis is often thickened and hyperkeratotic or ulcerated, and full-thickness carcinoma in situ may be absent (a factor to consider when evaluating superficial shave biopsies). The hallmark of this variant is acantholysis resulting in variably sized spaces within the invasive tumour lobules. At higher magnification, it is apparent that these spaces result from cell separation due to acantholysis of tumour cells, which often appear to float within the resultant defects. Acantholytic cells are rounded in contour and may exhibit premature keratinization (dyskeratosis) or necrosis. When the spaces formed within invasive tumour islands are round to ovoid and bordered by an intact layer of tumour cells at the perimeter, a pseudoglandular pattern may develop. Such patterns of acantholysis may produce apparent lumina, reminiscent of glandular or vascular spaces (pseudovascularization). Immunohistochemically, acantholytic SCC shows reactivity typical of ordinary invasive SCC: pseudoglandular spaces are negative for mucin, CK7, and CEA {2000}, and pseudovascular regions are negative for CD31 and ERG.

### Differential diagnosis

Lesions with extensive acantholysis can mimic either primary cutaneous (adnexal) or metastatic adenocarcinoma, and pseudoglandular spaces must be differentiated from the expression of true glands, as seen in the adenosquamous carcinoma variant (see p. 42). Pseudovascular regions may superficially resemble angiosarcoma. Generally, acantholytic SCC variants are not sufficiently well differentiated to elicit consideration of acantholytic benign keratosis (e.g. warty dyskeratoma).

### Histogenesis

The histogenetic factors are most often the same genomic, molecular, and causative factors that are applicable to ordinary invasive SCC. Compared with non-acantholytic SCCs, the acantholytic variant has been shown to have decreased expression of desmoglein 3 and E-cadherin {940}. Defective desmosomal protein expression has been confirmed {1933} and is probably largely responsible for the acantholytic pattern observed histologically. The genetic profile of and potential susceptibility loci for acantholytic SCC are not yet understood.

### Prognosis and predictive factors

It has been suggested that acantholytic SCC is a more aggressive variant of SCC {940}, with a mortality rate at follow-up of 19% {1874}, although more-recent data conflict with this interpretation {2111}. Histological attributes that may confer aggressive behaviour have recently been comparatively evaluated for acantholytic versus non-acantholytic SCC {2111}; these included microscopic tumour diameter, depth of invasion, degree of differentiation, and presence of perineural invasion. No significant differences between acantholytic and non-acantholytic ordinary SCCs were identified; overall, the notion that acantholytic SCC is a biologically and clinically more aggressive variant of SCC has not been substantiated {848}.

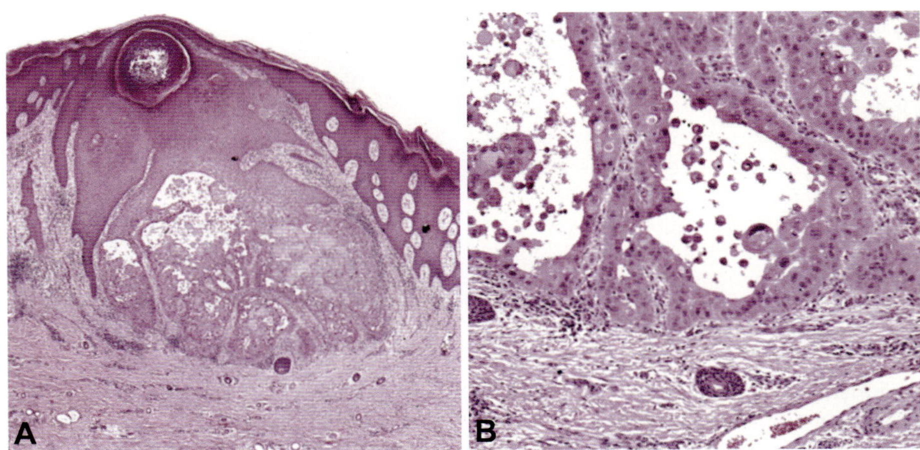


**Fig. 1.33** Invasive squamous cell carcinoma with acantholysis. **A** Scanning magnification shows clear spaces within infiltrative tumour lobules. **B** Higher magnification reveals pseudoglandular spaces bordered by several layers of squamous epithelium enclosing regions where acantholytic cells appear to float within central defects.

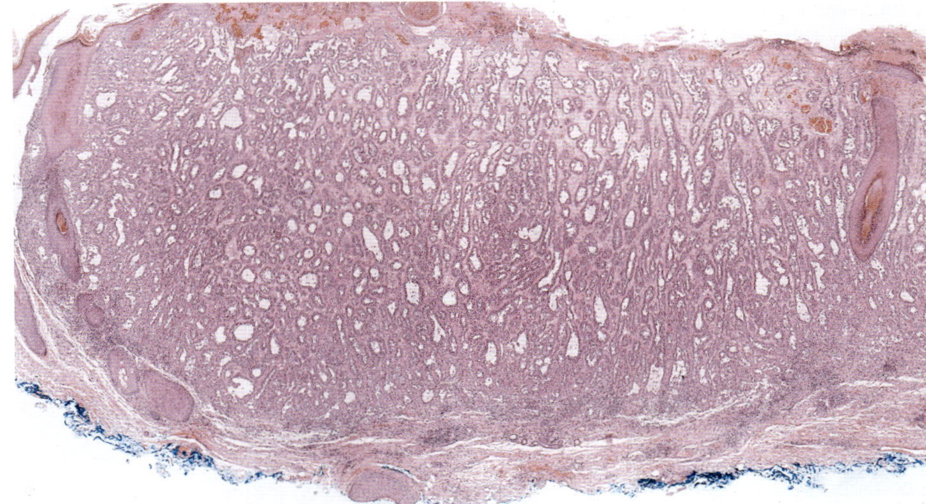

**Fig. 1.34** Acantholytic squamous cell carcinoma. At low magnification, acantholytic spaces are visible within much of the tumour.

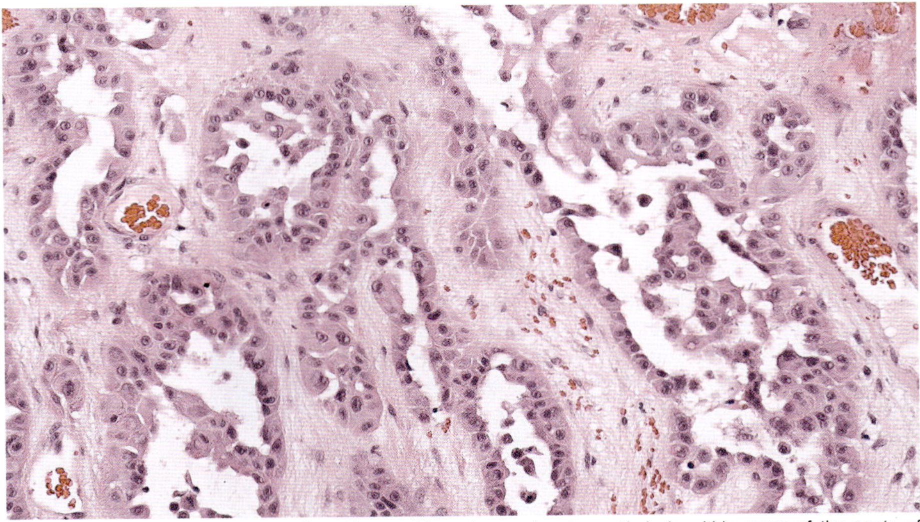

**Fig. 1.35** Acantholytic squamous cell carcinoma. There is prominent acantholysis within many of the nests of invasive squamous cells.

## *Spindle cell squamous cell carcinoma*

### Definition

Spindle cell squamous cell carcinoma (SCC) is a rare, poorly differentiated variant of SCC; it is composed predominantly of spindled tumour cells with partial or complete loss of morphological squamous differentiation.

### ICD-O code 8074/3

### Synonyms

Pseudosarcomatous squamous cell carcinoma; sarcomatoid squamous cell carcinoma

### Epidemiology

These skin tumours arise most commonly in elderly White men, and rarely in Asian populations. The incidence is highest among individuals aged >70 years. The reported age range for penile tumours is broad (28–81 years).

### Etiology

Ultraviolet (UV) radiation exposure, iatrogenic ionizing irradiation, scarring burns, solid-organ transplantation, and immunosuppression predispose individuals to this variant. Penile tumours are frequently associated with high- or low-grade squamous intraepithelial dysplasia or lichen sclerosus.

### Localization

Spindle cell SCC typically arises in the sun-exposed skin of the face and head, neck, chest, and upper extremities. Similar tumours are found in mucocutaneous regions of the head and neck (e.g. the larynx, hypopharynx, oropharynx, and nasal cavity) {241}, as well as within the urogenital tract, and are well described on the distal penis (e.g. the glans/prepuce and foreskin).

### Clinical features

Spindle cell SCC is typically a raised or exophytic plaque, nodule, or tumour, and is indistinguishable from classic SCC. It is often about 2 cm in largest dimension, and can reach up to 10 cm. Patients often present with bleeding or ulceration, and may report a history of rapid tumour growth.

### Histopathology

Spindle cell SCC typically occurs in a background of severe solar elastosis, and is composed of closely packed fascicles of pleomorphic spindle cells, with frequent mitotic activity. There may be a background of actinic keratosis or SCC in situ. Keratinization is usually absent. The tumour involves the dermis and may extend into the subcutis and along interlobular fat septa.

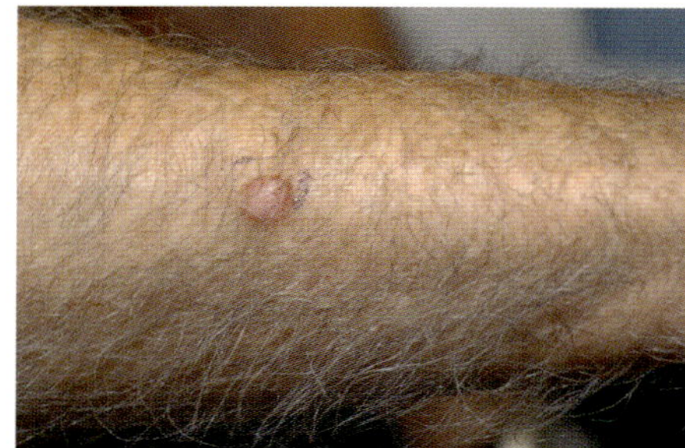

**Fig. 1.36** Spindle cell squamous cell carcinoma occurring as a nodule on the arm.

### Differential diagnosis

The most common differential diagnoses are atypical fibroxanthoma, superficial undifferentiated pleomorphic sarcoma, desmoplastic and spindle cell melanomas, leiomyosarcoma, and less-common tumours such as spindle cell and sarcomatoid lymphomas. The finding of an overlying in situ or intermingled keratinizing component can be helpful, but immunohistochemistry is required to establish the diagnosis in most cases. Specifically, positive staining for p63, p40, 34βE12, CK5/6, and/or MNF116 is usually required for diagnosis, particularly if no epithelioid squamous component is present {241}. EMA (epithelial membrane antigen), AE1/AE3, and CAM5.2 are less sensitive. S100-positive intratumoural dendritic cells must not be confused with the cells of spindle cell melanoma; other melanoma-specific stains can facilitate this distinction.

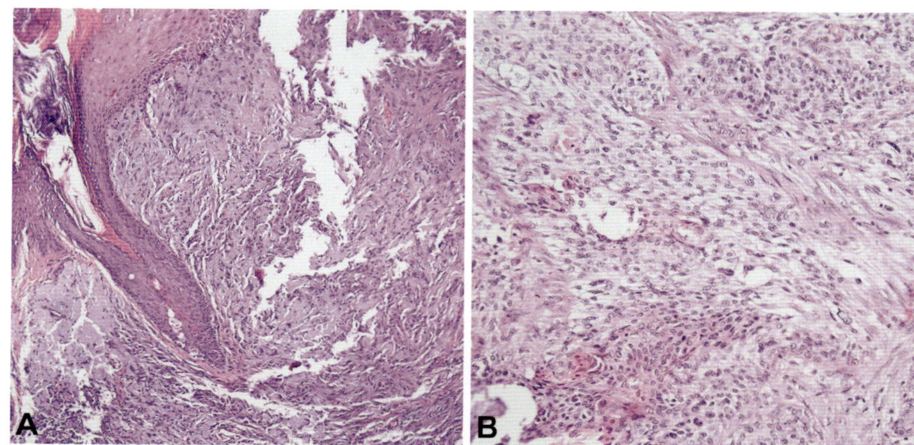

**Fig. 1.37** Spindle cell squamous cell carcinoma. **A** Note the edge of a tumour nodule with marked solar elastosis. **B** Epithelioid, vaguely nested cells in transition to a fusiform elongated spindled morphology.

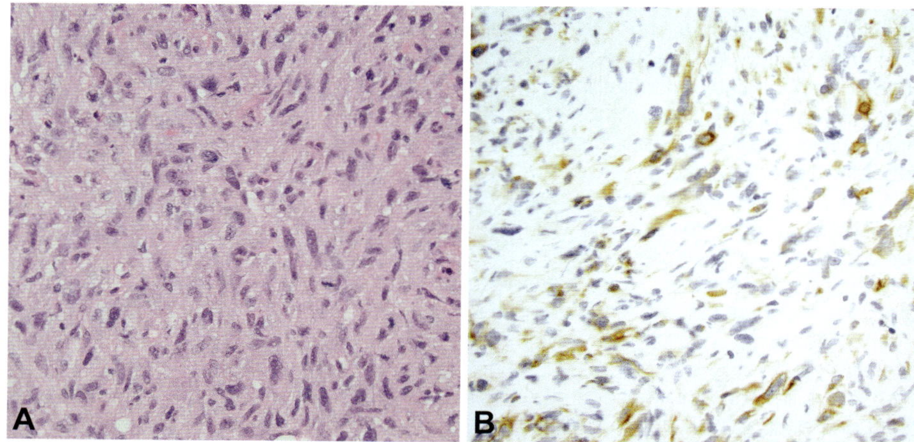

**Fig. 1.38** Spindle cell squamous cell carcinoma. **A** Closely packed pleomorphic spindle cells. **B** Pancytokeratin immunostaining is positive in scattered lesional cells.

## Histogenesis

A monoclonal origin for these tumours is the currently accepted theory {470}. The morphological changes have been postulated to be caused by epithelial–mesenchymal transition, in which the precursor squamous cells lose polarity and cohesiveness and transform into spindle-shaped cells {241}, acquiring increased motility and invasiveness {2419}.

## Prognosis and predictive factors

Spindle cell morphology itself may be a predictor of poor prognosis. Depth of invasion (particularly invasion into bone or muscle), as well as origination at the site of a burn or radiation damage (including sun damage) may be associated with worse outcome or death. Positive margins are associated with significantly higher rates of recurrence and metastasis, and with significantly poorer survival. Penile variants have a high rate of metastasis and are associated with a high rate of death due to metastatic disease {2297}.

# *Verrucous squamous cell carcinoma*

## Definition

Verrucous squamous cell carcinoma (SCC) is a rare, well-differentiated variant of cutaneous SCC; it has a characteristically undulant architecture and often exhibits locally aggressive behaviour, yet has low potential for metastasis. Similar lesions also affect mucosal surfaces.

## ICD-O code 8051/3

## Synonyms

Oral florid papillomatosis;
Ackerman tumour {338,488};
epithelioma cuniculatum {34,2349,2357};
Buschke–Löwenstein tumour {1178};
giant condyloma acuminatum;
papillomatosis cutis carcinoides

## Epidemiology

Verrucous SCC is predominantly a tumour of older men, with 75% of patients aged ≥ 60 years {1401}.

## Etiology

Chronic irritation, inflammation, HPV infection, and impaired immunity have been proposed as possible etiological factors {533,1169}. As with other forms of cutaneous SCC, chemical carcinogens and environmental exposures have also been implicated. However, the precise inciting factors responsible for this uncommon variant remain unknown.

## Localization

Verrucous SCC can affect both oral mucosa and skin. The mucosal site of predilection is the oral cavity (Ackerman tumour); cutaneous lesions most often involve the palms, soles (epithelioma cuniculatum), distal digits, and anogenital region (Buschke–Löwenstein tumour) {533}, but isolated reports indicate that verrucous SCC can arise at virtually any cutaneous site, including the skin of the scalp, face, back, and extremities, sometimes in association with chronic ulcers and scars, such as in the pretibial variant (papillomatosis cutis carcinoides).

## Clinical features

The clinical appearance of cutaneous verrucous SCC varies according to its site of occurrence. Palmoplantar lesions tend to grow and evolve slowly, forming hyperkeratotic plaques that may be confused with verrucae or callosities. Anogenital lesions form exophytic, condylomatoid excrescences that may be deeply invasive and difficult to eradicate, particularly in the setting of immunocompromise. Occasionally, tumours can have a more nodular clinical appearance {533}.

## Histopathology

The histopathology of verrucous SCC is similar at all sites of occurrence. The lesions show a complex exophytic and endophytic architecture, with hyperkeratosis (often prominent) and characteristic deep tongues of intradermal growth that are club-like in contour. Cytological atypia is minimal, apart from several layers at the interface of the bulbous tips of the endophytic extensions. Characteristically, the inter-rete spaces are greatly diminished, with apparently reduced vascularity. The associated stroma may be inflamed, and fields of verrucous epidermal acanthosis and lichen simplex chronicus may flank lesions. Viral cytopathic alterations are generally not present in verrucous SCC, although they may be seen in the adjacent hyperplastic epidermis.

## Differential diagnosis

The most frequent diagnostic challenge is differentiation from exuberant reactive processes. Penile lesions of verruciform xanthoma have been described as simulants of verrucous SCC {591}. Verrucoid and endophytic squamous proliferations associated with fungal, leishmanial, and non-tuberculous mycobacterial infections may bear some resemblance to verrucous SCC {2257,2289}. Confusion with fields of plantar verrucae may occasionally result in patients receiving less-aggressive therapy than is required for verrucous SCC {918}. Overall, the finding of deeply endophytic, club-shaped tongues with pushing borders of well-differentiated squamous epithelium with only one or two cell layers (at most) at the advancing border showing atypia should raise suspicion for verrucous SCC.

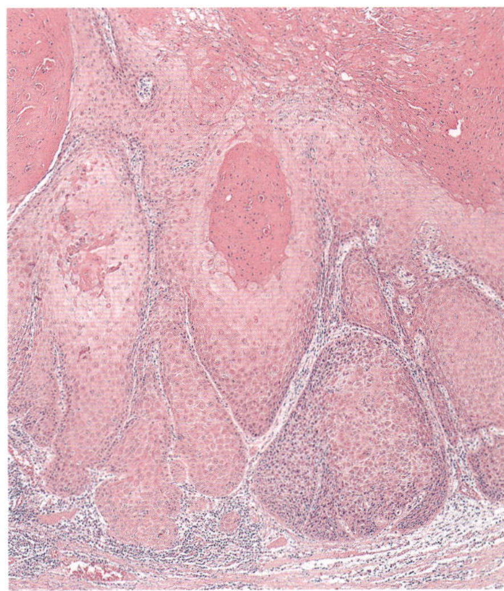

**Fig. 1.39** Verrucous squamous cell carcinoma. Scanning magnification shows a well-differentiated, keratinizing field giving rise to exuberant hyperkeratosis; the endophytic component forms invasive tongues with a characteristic club-shaped architecture.

## Histogenesis

Verrucous SCC has been described in association with a variety of reactive and inflammatory conditions, including vulvar lichen planus {2619}, although the precise histogenesis remains unclear. The role of HPV is controversial, in part because of diagnostic confusion between condylomatous and hyperplastic lesions and true verrucous SCC. An analysis of 13 rigorously defined verrucous SCCs from head and neck, anogenital, and extragenital skin using PCR-based HPV detection failed to implicate a causal role for HPV {605}. However, there is a clear association between certain oncogenic HPV types and cutaneous SCC,

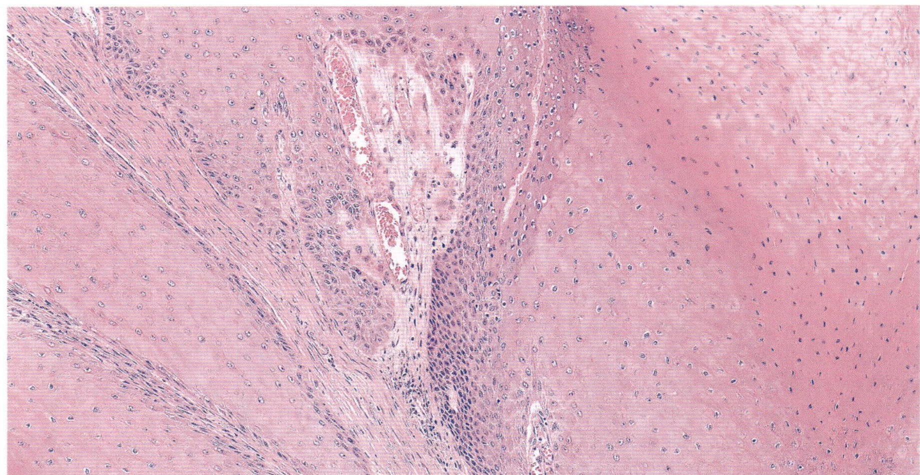

**Fig. 1.40** Verrucous squamous cell carcinoma. The epithelial–stromal interface is mostly smooth, but focally irregularly contoured.

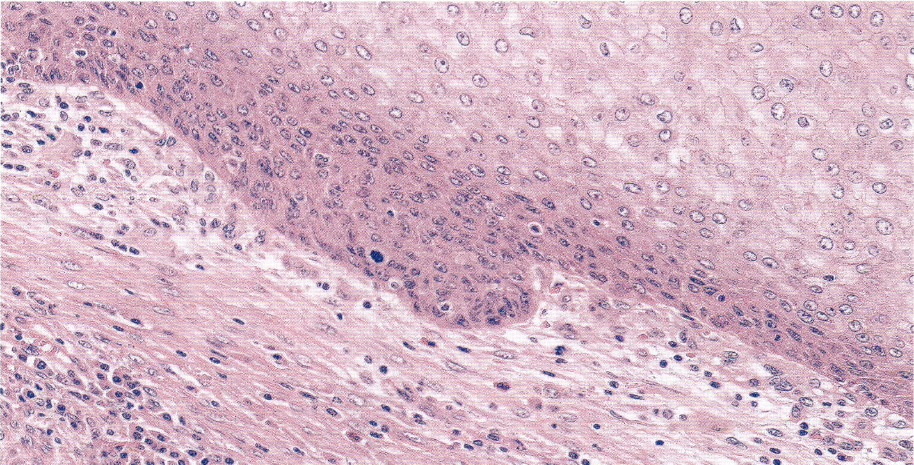

**Fig. 1.41** Verrucous squamous cell carcinoma. The advancing front of the tumour is formed by several cell layers of smaller atypical cells with mitotic figures in this otherwise cytologically bland and well-differentiated lesion.

particularly in the setting of immunosuppression {654}, and the potential role of HPV in verrucous SCC warrants further investigation.

### Genetic profile

Overexpression of MDM2, a negative regulator of p53, has been implicated {1963}.

### Prognosis and predictive factors

Incompletely excised lesions have a high recurrence rate, and recurrences can be more aggressive than the initial tumour. Metastasis generally does not occur, although transformation to more-aggressive forms of SCC has been described in patients who had received irradiation or chemotherapy.

## *Adenosquamous carcinoma*

### Definition

Adenosquamous carcinoma is a rare squamous cell carcinoma (SCC) variant that exhibits mixed squamous and glandular differentiation and aggressive clinical behaviour.

### ICD-O code 8560/3

### Etiology

Although this is considered to be a variant of SCC with divergent glandular differentiation, the pathogenesis is unknown. Malignant transformation from epithelial stem cells differentiating into both squamous and glandular-like cells is a plausible explanation.

### Clinical features

These tumours occur mostly in the head and neck of elderly patients, most frequently in men {140,398,831}. Clinically, they can be indistinguishable from typical SCC, presenting as an indurated keratotic plaque. The incidence is likely higher among immunosuppressed patients.

### Histopathology

The tumour is composed of small to large interconnecting nests of anaplastic squamoid cells displaying cytoplasmic cornification and (in some cases) keratinizing cysts and desmoplastic stroma. The tumour mass is connected with the epidermis, indicating its epidermal origin. Glandular differentiation is variable, constituting 5–80% of the total tumour area, and can include both ductular and glandular elements {831}. The glandular elements can be highlighted with CEA and CK7 immunostaining. These tumours frequently show severe nuclear atypia, a high mitotic rate, and an infiltrative pattern, with involvement of nerve, subcutis, muscle, and bone.

### Differential diagnosis

Other aggressive primary SCCs (particularly those with infiltrative and desmoplastic features) and metastatic carcinomas should be excluded. The differential diagnosis may also include mucoepidermoid carcinoma, a low-grade neoplasm that rarely arises as a primary cutaneous tumour and that is characterized by various proportions of well-differentiated mucinous, squamous, and intermediate cells; however, this concept is controversial. Notably, mucoepidermoid carcinoma shows less cellular atypia and mitotic activity than is seen in adenosquamous carcinoma. The low number of reported cases raises the possibility that primary cutaneous mucoepidermoid carcinoma may constitute a less aggressive form of adenosquamous carcinoma. There is also controversy regarding the relationship of this tumour to squamoid eccrine ductal carcinoma (p. 176), and in particular as to whether the two are in fact the same entity.

### Prognosis and predictive factors

This variant has been associated with an aggressive clinical course, with a high rate of recurrence and metastasis. Because of the relative frequency of

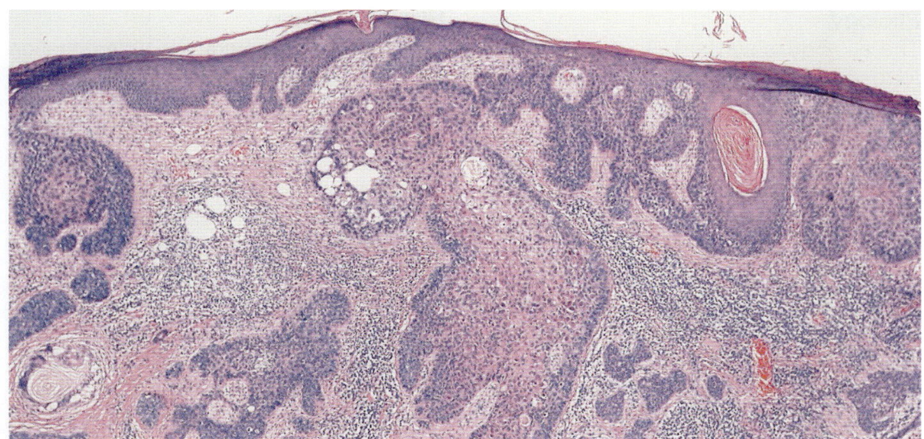

**Fig. 1.42** Adenosquamous carcinoma. Overt squamous differentiation is present in parts of the tumour.

**Fig. 1.43** Adenosquamous carcinoma. Well-formed glandular structures containing mucinous secretion in the glandular areas of the tumour.

nerve involvement and subclinical extension, meticulous examination of all resection margins to assess the adequacy of excision is required.

## Clear cell squamous cell carcinoma

### Definition
Clear cell squamous cell carcinoma (SCC) is a histological variant of SCC that microscopically shows abundant clear cytoplasm. There is no consensus on the required proportion of clear cells for the definition of clear cell SCC, but >25% has been suggested {528}. The tumours may be invasive or in situ {39}.

### ICD-O code
8084/3

### Epidemiology
This rare SCC variant often occurs on sun-damaged skin of older men.

### Etiology
The risk factors appear to be similar to those for conventional SCC.

### Localization
The head and neck are affected most frequently. Similar tumours on the glans penis may behave aggressively {2296}.

### Clinical features
These tumours, which often present in elderly men, have no clinical features to distinguish them from conventional SCC.

### Histopathology
The tumours contain malignant squamoid epithelial cells with cytoplasmic vacuolation and focal keratinization. Intracytoplasmic vacuoles are typically unilocular, unlike in sebaceous neoplasms (which show a characteristic microvesicular pattern). The clear material is largely glycogen, with a diastase-sensitive positive periodic acid–Schiff (PAS) reaction {567}. Some clear cell SCCs without glycogen have been identified {1462}, with vesiculation possibly representing a degenerative phenomenon or artefact. Rarely, a single cytoplasmic vacuole compresses the nucleus; such lesions may be designated as signet-ring cell SCC {544,671,1720,1868}. Gland formation is not seen.

The immunohistochemistry is similar to that of conventional SCC; BerEP4 is negative.

### Differential diagnosis
There is some morphological similarity between the histological appearances of clear cell SCC, signet-ring cell SCC, and trichilemmal carcinoma. Trichilemmal carcinoma is usually deeply seated with no connection to the epidermis, and may show peripheral palisading, basement membrane prominence, and pilar keratinization {2850}. Sebaceous gland carcinoma shows multivacuolated cytoplasm with frequent positivity for perilipin, adipophilin, androgen receptor, and BerEP4 {1961}. Clear cell basal cell carcinoma is BerEP4-positive.

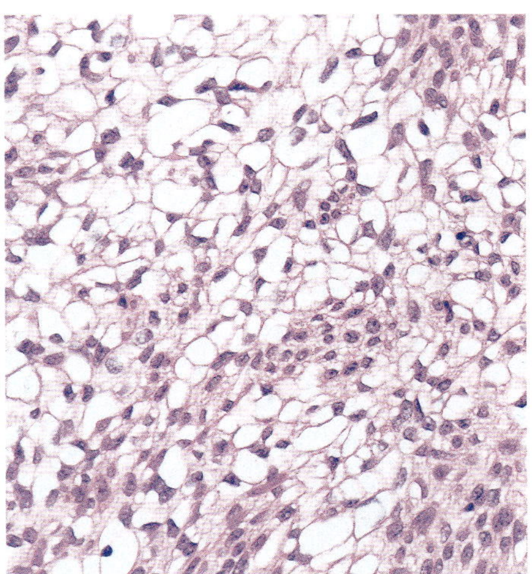

**Fig. 1.44** Clear cell squamous cell carcinoma. Cytoplasmic vacuolation is prominent in areas with some signet-ring cells.

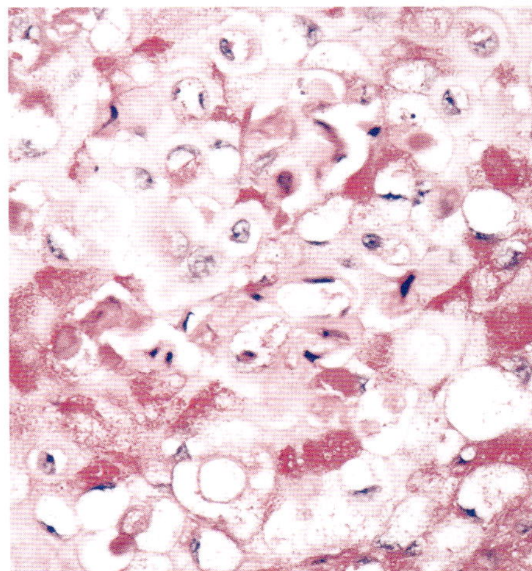

**Fig. 1.45** Clear cell squamous cell carcinoma. The cells have glycogen-rich cytoplasm and give a positive periodic acid–Schiff (PAS) reaction.

The presence of ducts, highlighted by staining for CEA and EMA (epithelial membrane antigen), helps to identify porocarcinoma, hidradenocarcinoma, and dermal duct tumours. In clear cell atypical fibroxanthoma, cytokeratin staining is negative and keratinization is absent {1899}. Clear cell and balloon cell melanomas stain for melanocyte markers.

If there is no evidence of epidermal origin, metastatic carcinomas should be considered, especially from the kidney (PAX8-positive) {1502}.

### Genetic susceptibility

The genetic susceptibilities are unknown beyond those associated with conventional SCC.

### Prognosis and predictive factors

The prognosis of clear cell SCC is comparable to that of other SCC types {398}.

## Other (uncommon) variants

### Definition

The other variants of cutaneous squamous cell carcinoma (SCC) are a poorly defined group of uncommon tumours that exhibit differentiation characteristics or stromal responses that result in diagnostic ambiguity.

### ICD-O codes

| | |
|---|---|
| Squamous cell carcinoma with sarcomatoid differentiation | 8074/3 |
| Lymphoepithelioma-like carcinoma | 8082/3 |
| Pseudovascular squamous cell carcinoma | 8074/3 |
| Squamous cell carcinoma with osteoclast-like giant cells | 8035/3 |

### Synonyms

For SCC with sarcomatoid differentiation: carcinosarcoma; metaplastic carcinoma; pseudosarcomatous squamous cell carcinoma;
sarcomatoid squamous cell carcinoma;
For pseudovascular SCC: pseudoangiosarcomatous squamous cell carcinoma; pseudovascular adenoid squamous cell carcinoma; pseudoangiomatous squamous cell carcinoma {1410}

### Epidemiology

These SCC variants are exceedingly rare.

### Etiology

The etiology is similar to that of common forms of SCC.

### Localization

SCC with sarcomatoid differentiation typically involves sun-exposed skin of the face and head, neck, chest, and upper extremities. Lymphoepithelioma-like carcinoma (LELC) of the skin typically involves sun-exposed skin, most often of the head and neck. Pseudovascular SCC affects ultraviolet (UV) radiation–damaged skin of the head and scalp, and typically occurs in elderly individuals {1866}. SCC with osteoclast-like giant cells (SCC-OGC) generally involves the head and neck of elderly individuals {482}.

### Clinical features

These rare variants of SCC typically show rapid growth but have no individually characteristic features.

### Histopathology

SCCs with sarcomatoid differentiation typically have a component of SCC with classic morphology demonstrating keratinization along with a sarcomatous component. The sarcomatous component accounts for a variable proportion of the tumour, and thorough sampling may be necessary to establish the diagnosis. In non-genital sites, a background of severe solar elastosis is typical. Heterologous elements may include chondroblastic, osteoblastic, rhabdomyosarcomatous, and myoid differentiation. Elements with myoid differentiation are rarely positive for markers of epithelial differentiation.

LELC of the skin is characterized by poorly differentiated tumour cells islands surrounded and infiltrated by lymphocytes and variable numbers of plasma cells. Accordingly, the lesions resemble undifferentiated nasopharyngeal carcinoma (lymphoepithelioma). Immunohistochemistry (pancytokeratin, CK5/6, or

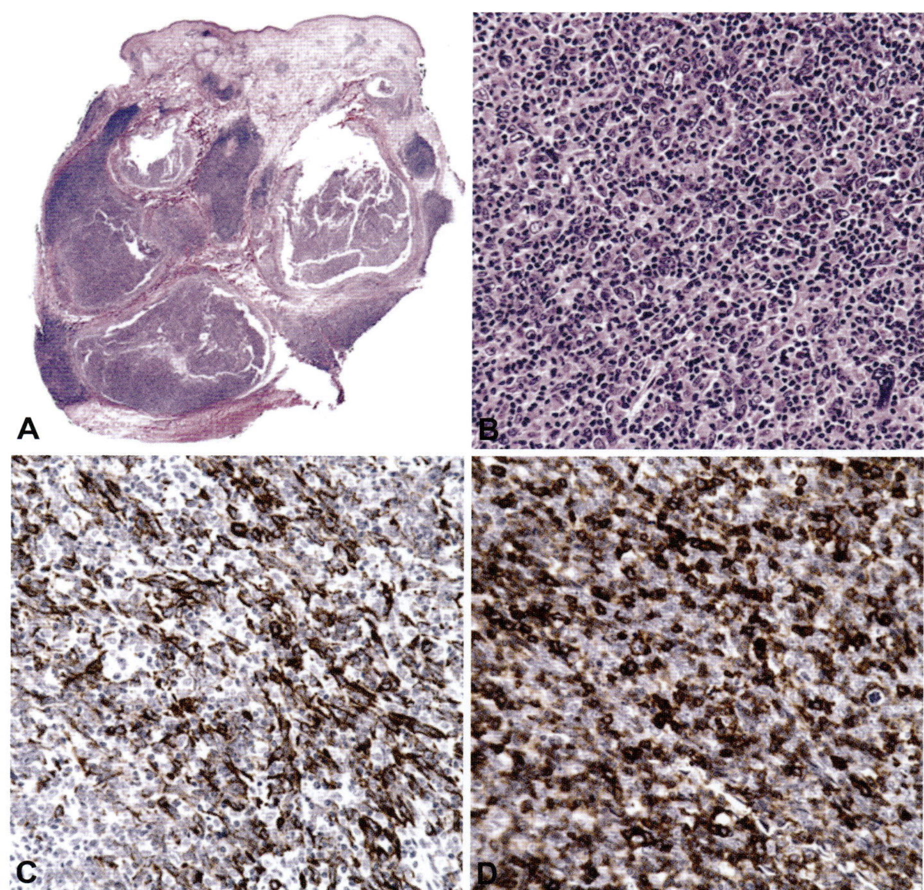


**Fig. 1.46** Lymphoepithelioma-like carcinoma of the skin. The tumour shows a dermal architecture, composed of multiple nodules (**A**) consisting of lymphocytes and plasma cells in which malignant infiltrative squamous epithelial elements are embedded (**B**). Immunostaining for pancytokeratin (**C**) and the T-cell co-receptor CD3 (**D**) aids in distinguishing the two components of this rare neoplasm.

p63) confirms the presence of epithelial elements that may be masked by the lymphoid component.

Pseudovascular SCC is a higher-grade SCC with an infiltrative architecture formed by cords of cytokeratin and p63-immunoreactive cells with intercellular lumen-like spaces (possibly a result of acantholysis), resulting in potential diagnostic confusion with angiosarcoma; but in angiosarcoma, the neoplastic cells are positive for vascular markers such as CD31, CD34, and ERG. The stroma of pseudovascular SCC may show myxoid change.

The epithelial component of SCC-OGC tends to be of higher grade, with moderate to poor differentiation {482}. The inflammatory stroma contains multinucleated non-tumoural giant cells that resemble osteoclasts and show immunoexpression of osteoclast/histiocytic markers {482}.

## Differential diagnosis

LELC of the skin must be distinguished from reactive and neoplastic lymphoid infiltrates of the skin. Lymphadenoma has a banal epithelial component {1176}. Pseudovascular SCC must be distinguished from vascular lesions (including angiosarcoma and SCC-OGC), histiocytic reactions, and infections with inductive squamous proliferation.

## Histogenesis

The rarity of these uncommon variants precludes definitive data regarding histogenetic pathways. Although LELC of the skin histologically resembles undifferentiated nasopharyngeal carcinoma (lymphoepithelioma), a strong association with EBV has not been demonstrated, which facilitates this variant's distinction from lymphoepithelioma.

## Prognosis and predictive factors

Some pseudovascular SCCs and SCC-OGCs demonstrate more-aggressive biological behaviour than do other SCC variants {1866}.

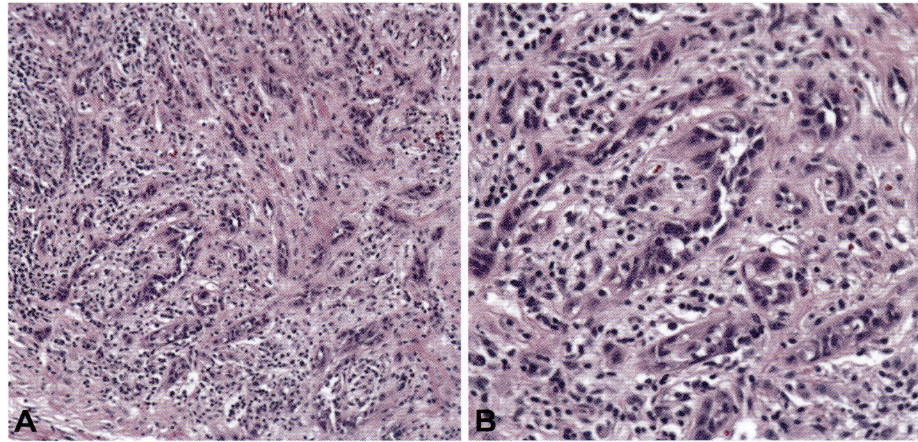


**Fig.1.47** Pseudovascular squamous cell carcinoma. Intermediate magnification (**A**) and high magnification (**B**) show infiltrative cords of malignant squamous cells that are centrally dyshesive, producing lumen-like spaces.

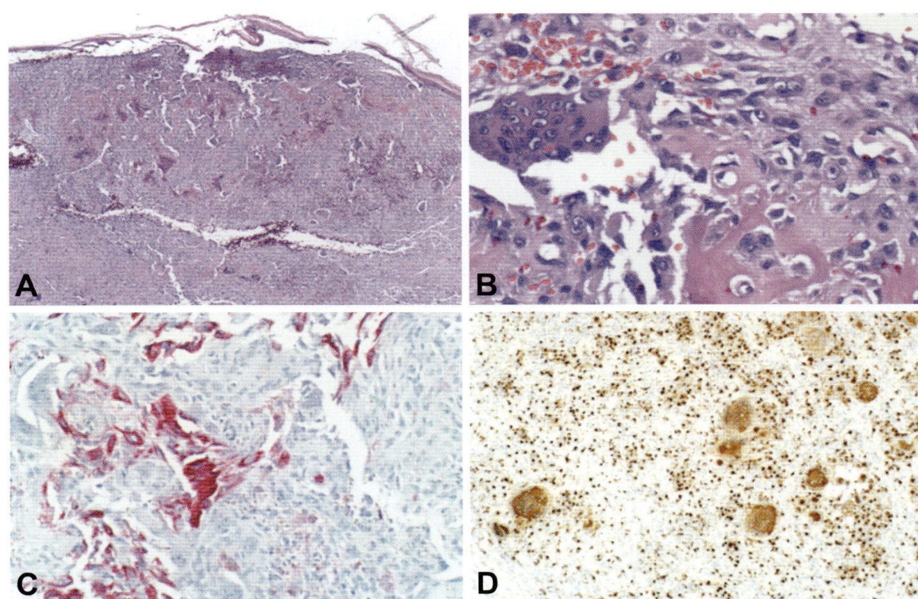


**Fig. 1.48** Squamous cell carcinoma with osteoclast-like giant cells. The tumour forms a nodule composed of a pandermal infiltrate (**A**) of malignant squamous elements admixed with giant cells resembling osteoclasts (**B**); the two components are further distinguished by immunostaining for pancytokeratin (**C**) and CD68 (**D**).

# Squamous cell carcinoma in situ (Bowen disease)

Pulitzer M.P.
Beer T.W.
Cerio R.
Kao G.F.
Murphy G.F.
Nagore E.
Scolyer R.A.

## Definition

Squamous cell carcinoma (SCC) in situ, also known as Bowen disease, is SCC confined to the epidermis and superficial adnexal epithelium, further characterized by full-thickness involvement of the epidermis by dysplastic squamous cells. The term "Bowen disease" was originally used specifically to describe SCC in situ in sun-protected skin as a harbinger of internal malignancy, but the terms "Bowen disease" and "SCC in situ" are now used interchangeably to describe epidermal SCC in situ of both sun-damaged and sun-protected skin.

## ICD-O code 8070/2

## Synonyms

Intraepidermal carcinoma;
Bowenoid papulosis; keratinocytic intraepidermal neoplasia (KIN III)

Vulvar intraepithelial neoplasia (VIN III), penile intraepithelial neoplasia (PeIN III), erythroplasia of Queyrat, and anal intraepithelial neoplasia (AIN III) are discussed in the relevant WHO classifications of tumours of the corresponding organ systems.

## Epidemiology

Most cases present in the sun-exposed skin of elderly White patients with higher cumulative sun exposure, with a median age of presentation >60 years. Specific populations at higher risk of SCC in situ include organ transplant recipients on immunosuppressive regimens and populations with long-term exposure to high levels of arsenic in drinking-water. Ultraviolet (UV) radiation exposure from tanning beds has resulted in an increased number of young people presenting with SCC in situ, but the finding of SCC in situ in a young person with minimal sun damage should prompt consideration of arsenic exposure.

## Etiology

Most cases of SCC in situ (Bowen disease) are caused by UV radiation exposure, including UVB and UVA radiation exposure from sunlight or tanning beds. Radiotherapy and photochemotherapy are also etiological. High-risk (alpha genus) HPV infection is the major cause of SCC in situ involving the periungual region and genital skin. The terms "VIN III" and "PeIN III" are used for genital lesions. Beta genus papillomaviruses may have synergistic effects with UV radiation in the setting of immunosuppression due to organ transplant or HIV infection in causing some cutaneous SCCs in situ. Arsenic ingestion can play a role in SCC in situ in non–sun-exposed skin.

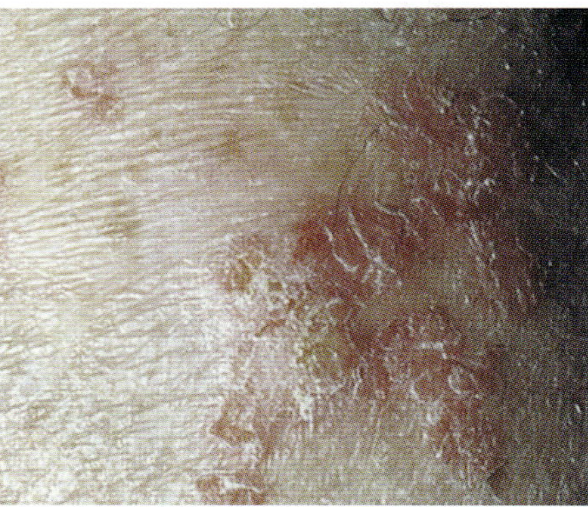

**Fig. 1.49** Bowen disease. Erythematous, scaly, fissuring plaques on lower leg of a middle-aged woman.

## Localization

SCC in situ predominantly involves sun-exposed skin, but also occurs in non–sun-exposed skin. Typical sites of involvement include the lower limbs, head, neck, and hands. Less commonly affected regions include subungual, periungual, genital (VIN III, PeIN III, and erythroplasia of Queyrat), and perianal (AIN III) sites.

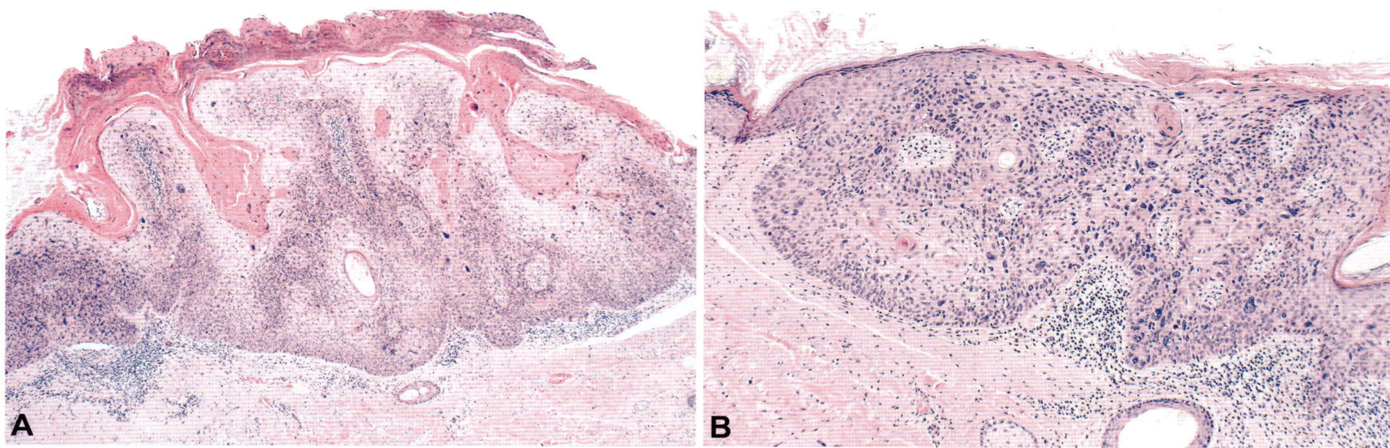


**Fig. 1.50** Squamous cell carcinoma in situ (Bowen disease). **A** There is full-thickness epidermal dysplasia associated with acanthosis and parakeratotic hyperkeratosis. **B** Full-thickness epidermal dysplasia is present; the superficial dermis shows severe solar elastosis and a patchy lymphocytic inflammatory cell infiltrate, but there is no dermal invasion.

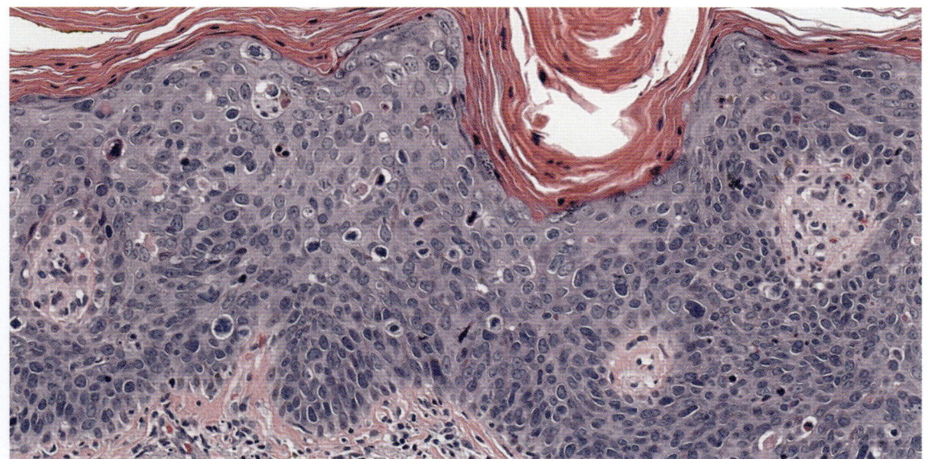

**Fig. 1.51** Squamous cell carcinoma in situ (Bowen disease). Full-thickness epidermal dysplasia is present.

## Clinical features

SCC in situ usually presents as a solitary, slow-growing, scaly, erythematous patch or plaque, which can remain unchanged for many years. Clinical features include crusting, pigmentation, and a verrucous appearance. Dermoscopic features include scale, glomerular vessels, yellow crust, haemorrhage, hypopigmentation, and linear irregular vessels {2879}.

## Histopathology

SCC in situ is characterized pathologically by full-thickness epidermal dysplasia, involvement of superficial skin adnexal epithelium, and no invasion of the underlying dermis. The stratum corneum is usually hyperparakeratotic, but may demonstrate orthokeratosis. Epidermal thickness is variable, but acanthosis is common. Atypical squamous cells (which are enlarged and pleomorphic and demonstrate hyperchromatic nuclei) replace the full thickness of the epidermis, often showing a loss of polarity. Mitotic figures are increased in number and typically extend to the epidermal surface. The granular layer is frequently absent. The basal layer may be retained (the so-called eyeliner sign). Occasional cases demonstrate single or nested atypical squamous cells dispersed throughout the full thickness of the epidermis, imparting a pagetoid appearance.

In some cases, cytological atypia is more subtle, and demonstration of full-thickness epidermal staining with Ki-67 is helpful for confirming the diagnosis of SCC in situ. p16 may be similarly helpful in assessing the degree of dysplasia in genital lesions {2186}.

## Differential diagnosis

SCC in situ with a pagetoid growth pattern must be distinguished (often requiring immunohistochemistry) from mammary and extramammary Paget disease, melanoma in situ, and less-common benign simulants such as clonal seborrhoeic keratosis and hidroacanthoma simplex.

Actinic keratosis is distinguished from SCC in situ by the lack of full-thickness epidermal dysplasia. Whereas SCC in situ shows parakeratosis (which is often confluent), actinic keratoses spare the epithelium of adnexal structures, correlating with a so-called flag sign of alternating orthokeratosis and parakeratosis. Microinvasive SCC may be difficult to distinguish from SCC in situ, especially when lichenoid inflammation is present, but careful examination of the dermoepidermal junction in SCC reveals jagged, often keratinizing dermal invasive foci.

## Histogenesis

UV radiation–induced mutations of *TP53* play a role in the development of many SCCs. SCC in situ in the context of arsenic exposure arises from oxidative stress, depletion of natural antioxidants, immune dysfunction, genotoxicity, impaired DNA repair, and disrupted signal transduction {1155}.

## Genetic profile

UV radiation–induced mutations of the gene encoding p53, which is centrally involved in cellular apoptosis, proliferation, and DNA repair, are present in 40% of SCC in situ cases {2141}. Amplification and activating mutations of *HRAS*, *NRAS*, and *KRAS*, likely due to UVB radiation exposure, are common {2525}. Molecular and cytogenetic studies provide supporting evidence that SCC in situ and actinic keratoses are precursors of invasive SCCs.

## Prognosis and predictive factors

Approximately 3–5% of all SCC in situ lesions progress to invasive SCC; among erythroplasia of Queyrat lesions specifically, the proportion is 10% {2879}.

# Merkel cell carcinoma

Busam K.J.
Walsh N.
Wood B.A.

## Definition

Merkel cell carcinoma (MCC) is the eponymous name for primary cutaneous neuroendocrine carcinoma.

## ICD-O code 8247/3

## Synonyms

Trabecular carcinoma {2620};
Toker tumour; primary neuroendocrine carcinoma of the skin

## Epidemiology

MCC predominantly affects elderly White individuals. In the USA, according to the SEER Program database, 95% of MCC cases are in White patients {273}. The median age at diagnosis is 75 years {273}, and <5% of patients are diagnosed before the age of 50 years. The reported incidence of MCC is 0.13 cases per 100 000 person-years in Europe {2692}, 0.79 cases per 100 000 person-years in the USA {783}, and 1.6 cases per 100 000 person-years in Australia {2897}. The incidence has been increasing worldwide. MCC is associated with immunosuppression. Compared with the rate in the general population, the incidence is 10 times as high among HIV-infected individuals {690}, 5–10 times as high among solid-organ transplant recipients {328}, and approximately 40 times as high among patients with chronic lymphocytic leukaemia {1053}. However, fewer than 10% of patients with MCC are severely immunocompromised {1053}.

## Etiology

Both ultraviolet (UV) radiation exposure and clonal integration of the Merkel cell polyomavirus (MCPyV) are strongly associated with MCC, with increasing evidence that somewhat distinct pathways to transformation are associated with these mechanisms.

## Localization

Most MCCs occur in sun-damaged skin. The most commonly affected sites, in order of frequency of involvement, are the head and neck, extremities, and trunk.

## Clinical features

The tumour typically presents as a rapidly growing flesh-coloured or violaceous nodule or plaque {1053}. The clinical differential diagnosis includes basal cell carcinoma, squamous cell carcinoma, amelanotic melanoma, atypical fibroxanthoma, lymphoma, and cyst. Metastatic disease may develop in the absence of detectable or prior history of primary MCC; in such cases, the primary tumour may have spontaneously regressed {2766}.

## Histopathology

The tumour typically presents as a so-called blue nodule in the dermis and/or subcutis. A spectrum of cytological features from small to intermediate and large cells has been described; the intermediate cell type is most common {2106,2765}. The nuclei of the tumour cells characteristically display a fine granular salt-and-pepper chromatin pattern. Nuclear moulding is common. Rosette-like structures may be seen.

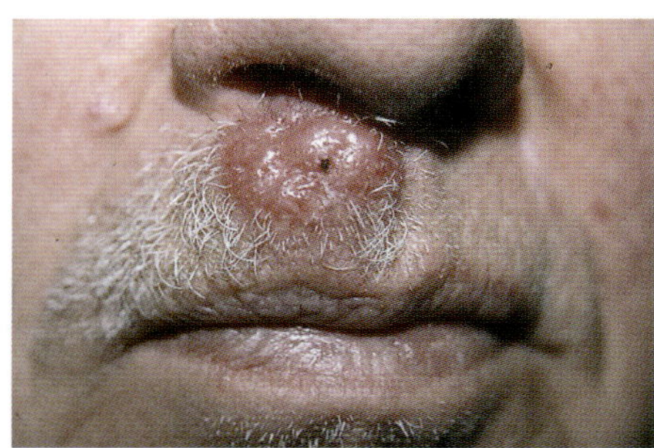

**Fig. 1.52** Merkel cell carcinoma. Nodule on the upper lip.

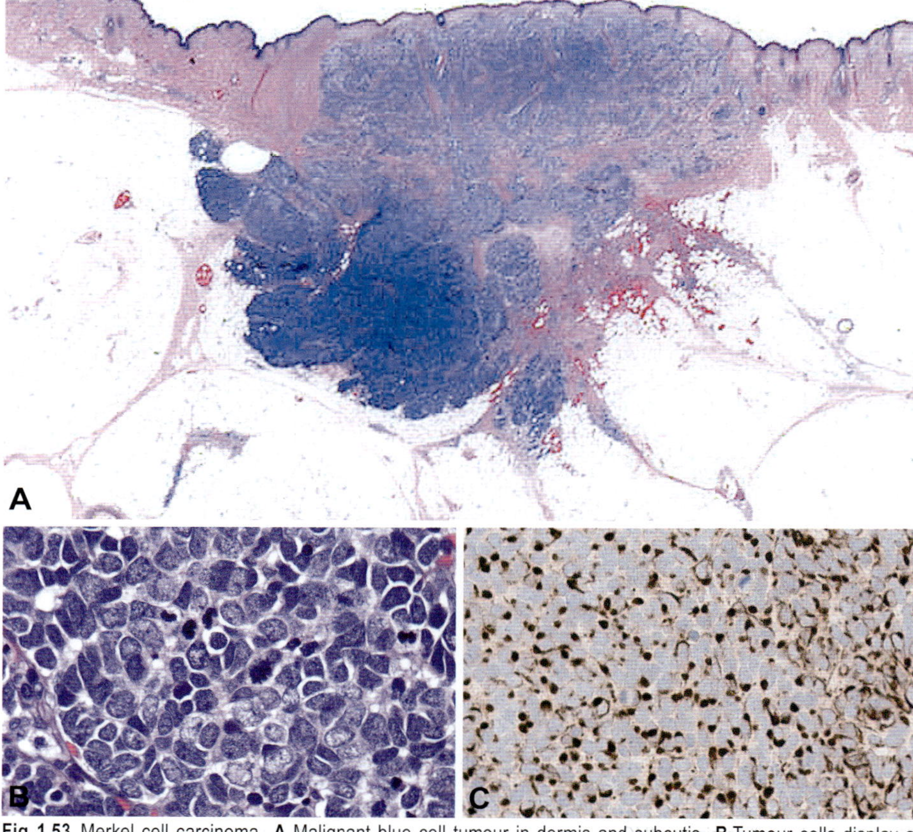

**Fig. 1.53** Merkel cell carcinoma. **A** Malignant blue-cell tumour in dermis and subcutis. **B** Tumour cells display a salt-and-pepper chromatin pattern, nuclear moulding, and mitoses. **C** Tumour cells are immunoreactive for CK20 in a perinuclear dot-like pattern.

Mitotic figures and apoptotic bodies tend to be numerous. Lymphatic invasion is frequently seen. Some MCCs show a tumour cell component within the epidermis (epidermotropic MCC). In very rare cases, the tumour is confined to the epidermis or follicles, which may constitute MCC in situ.

Most tumours develop de novo. However, a small number of primary cutaneous neuroendocrine carcinomas are associated with squamous cell carcinoma or (more rarely) basal cell carcinoma or an adnexal tumour. Although collision tumours may occur, there is also evidence that biphenotypic and multiphenotypic tumours exist. For example, a primary cutaneous neuroendocrine carcinoma may sometimes represent a differentiation pathway of another tumour, particularly squamous cell carcinoma. MCPyV is usually absent in combined tumours {343}.

Immunohistochemically, the tumour cells are positive for epithelial markers such as CAM5.2, AE1/AE3, CK20, 34βE12, BerEP4, EMA (epithelial membrane antigen), and sometimes CK7, as well as for neuroendocrine markers (chromogranin, synaptophysin, and CD56) {576}. They also express NFP. Perinuclear dot-like staining for CK20 and/or NFP reliably confirm the diagnosis of MCC {1707}. TTF1 staining is almost always negative. The monoclonal antibody CM2B4 can confirm the presence of the MCPyV large T antigen {343}. The reported rates of MCPyV positivity are variable, which may reflect variation in the sensitivity of detection as well as geographical etiological heterogeneity {559}.

## Differential diagnosis

MCC must be distinguished from metastatic neuroendocrine neoplasms of extracutaneous origin. On small biopsies, MCC may be confused with basal cell carcinoma, lymphoma, or round cell sarcomas such as cutaneous Ewing sarcoma. Epidermotropic MCC may also be confused with melanoma or sebaceous carcinoma. Carcinoid tumours (primary or metastatic) must also be distinguished from MCC.

## Histogenesis

The cell of origin of MCC is unknown. Initially, the discovery of cytoplasmic neuroendocrine granules in trabecular carcinomas (as MCCs were called at the time), led to the conclusion that the tumours arose from normal Merkel cells. But this assumption is now in doubt, and alternative histogenetic contenders include cutaneous stem cells, pro-/pre-B cells, and either cancer stem cells or lineage-specific cancer cells capable of neometaplasia. The histogenesis of pure MCCs likely differs from that of combined or biphenotypic tumours. Hair follicle stem cells have recently been linked with biphenotypic tumours, but conclusive data are lacking.

## Genetic profile

Divergent genetic profiles have been reported in MCPyV-positive and MCPyV-negative MCCs, supporting the postulated ontological dichotomy in this group of tumours. In particular, compared with virus-positive tumours, MCPyV-negative tumours have more mutations in the

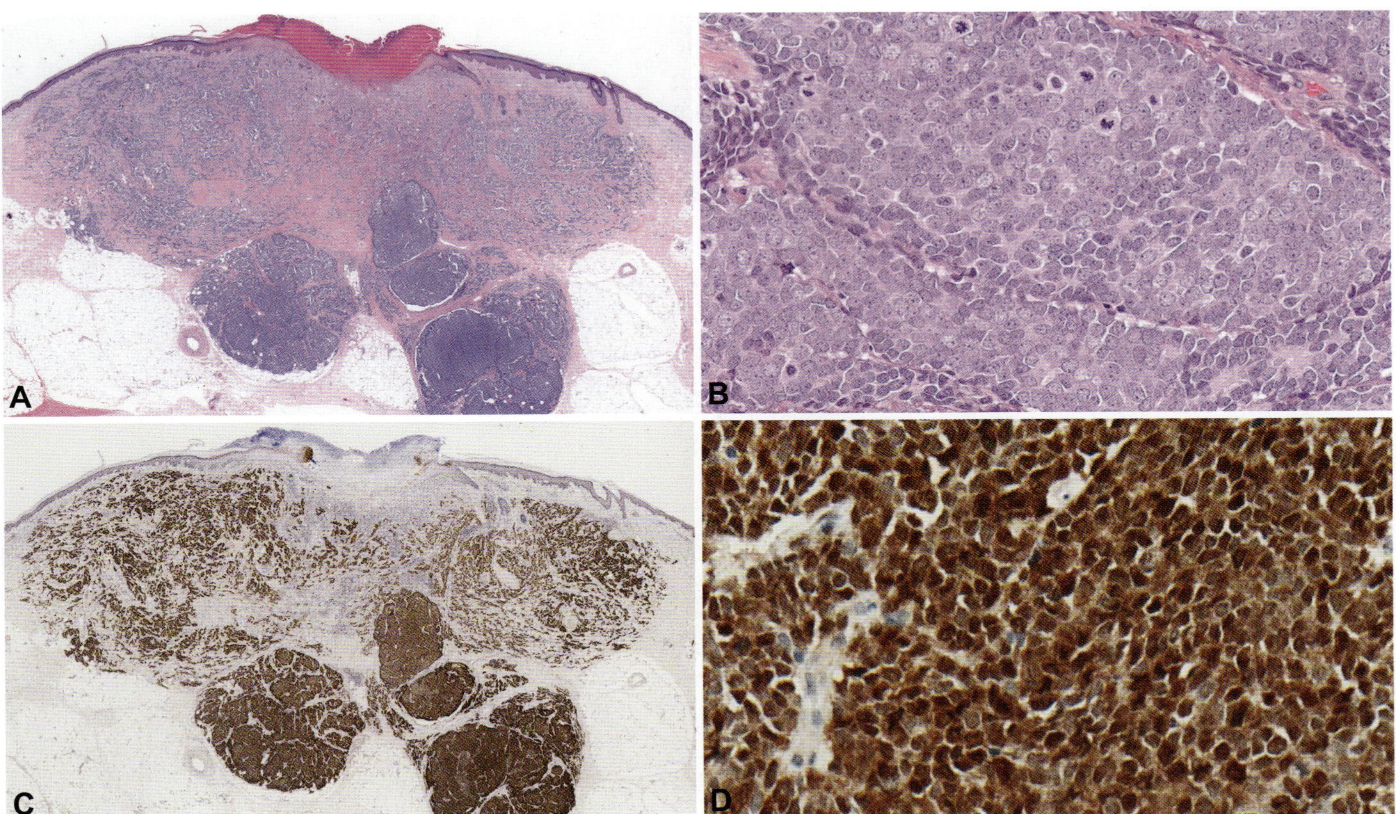


**Fig. 1.54** Merkel cell carcinoma (MCC). **A** MCC in dermis and subcutis. **B** The tumour cells display a finely stippled chromatin pattern; there is focal rosette-like arrangement of the nuclei; and several mitotic figures are present. **C** The tumour cells are uniformly immunoreactive with CM2B4 (an antibody to the Merkel cell polyomavirus large T antigen). **D** Higher magnification shows nuclear labelling with CM2B4.

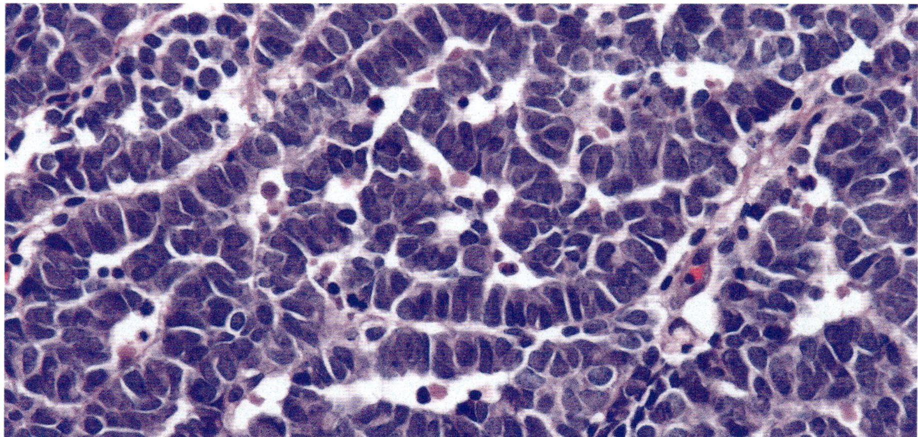

**Fig. 1.55** Merkel cell carcinoma. The tumour cells display a trabecular growth pattern.

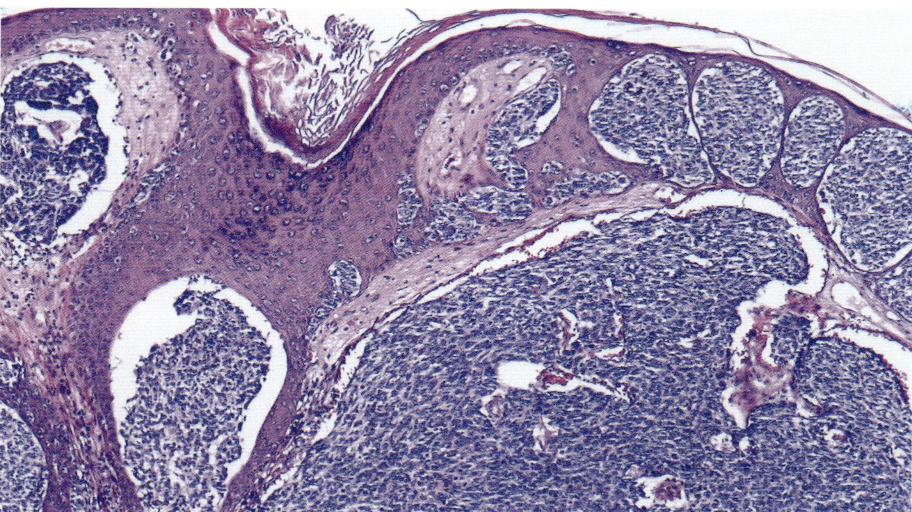

**Fig. 1.56** Epidermotropic Merkel cell carcinoma. The tumour cells are present in the epidermis and dermis; the nesting pattern may result in confusion with other tumours such as melanoma.

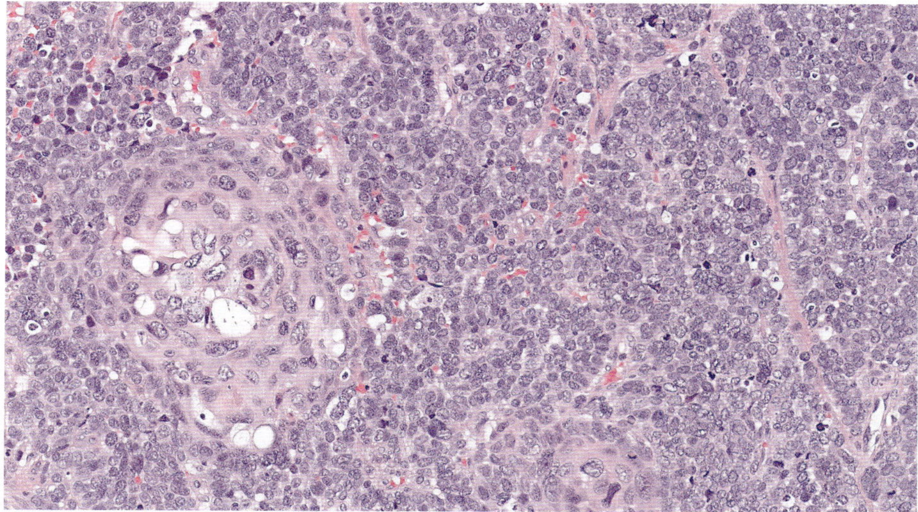

**Fig. 1.57** Combined neuroendocrine and squamous cell carcinoma (SCC). This tumour shows mixed features of neuroendocrine carcinoma and SCC.

*TP53* and *RB1* genes, a UV radiation signature mutation profile with many C>T substitutions, and a higher total mutation burden. These findings suggest that separate UV radiation–related and MCPyV-related tumorigenic molecular pathways exist in MCC {900,2107}.

## Prognosis and predictive factors

The 5-year overall survival rates for patients with MCC are estimated to be 51% for patients with localized disease, 35% for patients with regional metastasis, and 14% for patients with distant metastasis {1012}. However, because so many patients affected by MCC are elderly, overall survival data have limited value. In a large single-institution dataset, the disease-specific death rate at 5 years was 30% {778}. In patients with localized disease, tumour size and extent of invasion correlate with prognosis. The American Joint Committee on Cancer (AJCC) developed a staging system with four stages based on tumour size and involvement of nearby tissues – T1 (≤ 2 cm), T2 (> 2 cm, ≤ 5 cm), T3 (> 5 cm), and T4 (involvement of deep soft tissue layers) – as well as spread to regional lymph nodes (N categories) and distant sites (M categories) {1012}. Reports of the prognostic value of lymphatic invasion and sentinel lymph node status have been inconsistent. Patients presenting with nodal disease alone (with no identifiable cutaneous primary) seem to have a better prognosis than do patients with an identifiable primary lesion and nodal metastasis. Tumour-infiltrating lymphocytes have been suggested to be a stage-independent predictor of survival {2014}.

# Premalignant keratoses

Mihm M.C. Jr
James C.
Martinka M.
Soyer H.P.

## Actinic keratosis

### Definition
Actinic keratosis (AK) is an intraepithelial neoplastic lesion that may progress into invasive squamous cell carcinoma (SCC) or may spontaneously regress {500,2359,2908}.

### ICD-O code
8070/0

### Synonyms
Solar keratosis; keratinocytic intraepithelial neoplasia; senile keratosis

### Epidemiology
AKs occur more commonly in more sun-exposed regions, in people with fair skin, and in males; their incidence increases with advancing age {827,833,2237,2490}.

### Etiology
Risk factors include cumulative intermittent sun exposure, chronic immunosuppression, arsenic exposure, PUVA therapy, and chronic cutaneous inflammation {833,2640,2908}. Exposure to ultraviolet (UV) radiation (UVB and to a lesser extent UVA radiation) plays the major role in carcinogenesis {833}.

### Localization
The lesions occur on sun-exposed areas such as the face, lower lip (actinic cheilitis), bald scalp, lateral neck, forearms, and dorsal hands, as well as on the lower legs and trunk {833,2237,2359,2490}.

### Clinical features
AK commonly presents as an asymptomatic scaly erythematous patch or plaque, usually 2–10 mm in diameter, surmounted with a rough adherent scale often resembling sandpaper. There are often multiple lesions, flesh-coloured and confluent, with a background of chronic sun damage {833,2237,2514}.

### Histopathology
There is focal parakeratosis, atypia of the basal cell layer, irregularity in size of the nucleus, hyperchromasia, and pleomorphism. Parakeratosis is present over the atypical epidermis but often spares the acrosyringium and the hair follicle {1576}.

**Table 1.02** Actinic keratosis variants and their histologies

| Variant | Histology |
|---|---|
| Hypertrophic/acanthotic | Epidermal hyperplasia, increased hyperkeratosis and parakeratosis {245} |
| Bowenoid | Almost full-thickness atypia of squamous cells {2005} |
| Atrophic | One or two layers of atypical squamous cells and parakeratosis |
| Acantholytic | Suprabasal cell acantholysis and dyskeratosis {1549,2237} |
| Epidermolytic | Characteristic granular changes {2237} |
| Lichenoid | Band-like infiltrate of lymphocytes with basal epidermal damage {2237,2567} |
| Pigmented | Increased melanin in basal cells, with dermal melanophages {1211,2237}; the possibility of associated lentigo maligna should be considered and excluded |

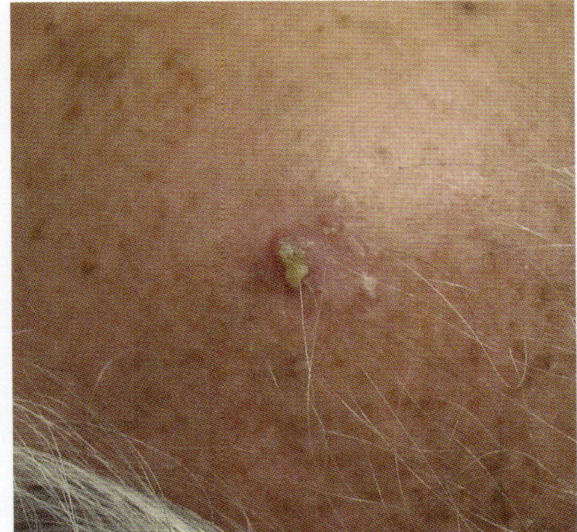

**Fig. 1.58** Actinic keratosis (AK). Scaling AK in a background of severe sun damage, with scattered solar lentigines.

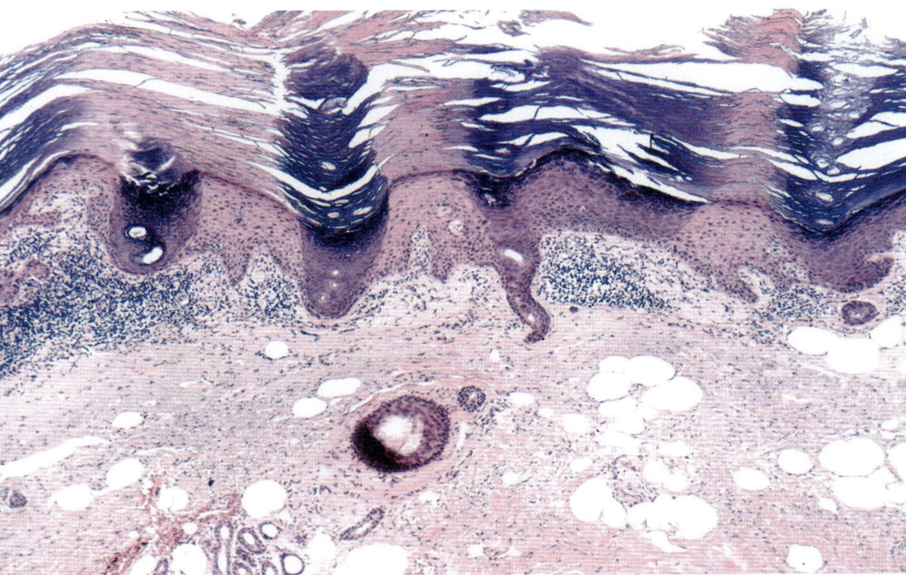

**Fig. 1.59** Actinic keratosis (AK). Striking alternation of parakeratosis and orthokeratosis due to sparing of appendageal keratin. This feature is a diagnostic sign of AK. Note the hyperplasia of the epidermis, with disordered maturation.

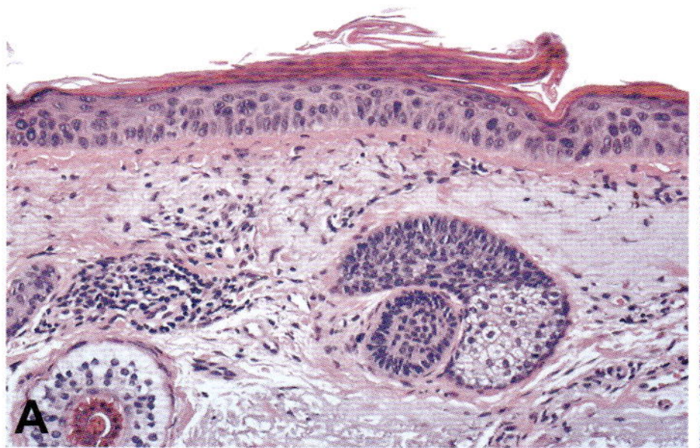

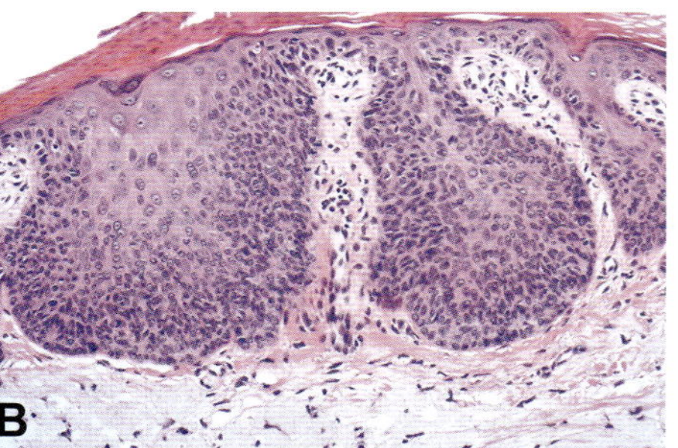


**Fig. 1.60** Actinic keratosis. **A** Atrophic type. Striking effacement of the rete ridges. The basal cells of the flattened epidermis show characteristic atypia, with only a few layers of atypical keratinocytes beneath the parakeratotic scale. **B** Bowenoid type. Prominent proliferative epidermis, with thickening of the squamous cell layer and bulging of the rete ridges. There is a residual granular cell layer, a feature that distinguishes the lesion from squamous cell carcinoma in situ (Bowen disease).

Dysplasia of the spinous-layer keratinocytes gives rise to a loss of polarity, mitotic activity, and disordered granular cell layer. The keratinocytic dysplasia is variable and may extend from the basal epidermis to involve the upper layers of the epidermis, with variable loss of the granular layer. AK in which the keratinocytic atypia extends beyond the basal layer but is not full-thickness involvement has been termed Bowenoid AK; if the epidermal dysplasia is full-thickness, the lesion is categorized as SCC in situ (Bowen disease). Solar elastosis is present {500,2237}. There are multiple variants of AK (see Table 1.02, p. 51). AKs can occur in association with other lesions, including seborrhoeic keratosis, solar lentigo, and melanocytic tumours. Most AKs express cyclin D, BCL2, and p53 {1576}.

### Differential diagnosis

The differential diagnosis includes solar lentigo, seborrhoeic keratosis, discoid lupus erythematosus, verrucous naevi, warty dyskeratoma, SCC in situ (Bowen disease), SCC (including keratoacanthoma), basal cell carcinoma, and porokeratosis {2237,2441}. AKs may occur in association with other lesions.

### Genetic profile

*TP53* mutations are the most common genetic alteration in AK {833,1892,2359, 2493}. Other mutations include mutations of *CDKN2A* on chromosome 9p21 – the gene encoding p16 (p16INK4a) and p14ARF – and mutations of *CDKN2B* – the gene encoding p15 (p15INK4b) {635,1833,2148}. Loss of heterozygosity has been documented in as many as four loci and several chromosomes {1576}.

### Genetic susceptibility

The genetic factors associated with an increased risk for the development of AK are those that result in constitutional sensitivity to sunlight, such as childhood freckling, blue eyes, and blond or red hair. Oculocutaneous albinism; Rothmund–Thomson, Cockayne, and Bloom syndromes; and xeroderma pigmentosum are associated with the development of AKs in earlier life {833,2359,2514,2908}.

### Prognosis and predictive factors

AK may regress spontaneously, remain stable, or progress to invasive SCC {2441}; cases in which there are > 5 AKs have an increased risk of progression. The annual rate of malignant transformation is usually cited as < 1 per 1000 cases, but transformation rates are higher among the higher-risk cases {2490,2512}.

## *Arsenical keratosis*

### Definition

Arsenical keratosis (ASK) is a hyperkeratotic lesion that occurs in patients with previous exposure to arsenic {351,404,2358,2935}.

### ICD-O code 8070/0

### Epidemiology

Lesions develop after a latency period of 20–30 years {46,404,2358}. Some drinking-water (from wells) and naturopathic medicines contain high arsenic levels {46,2277,2887}.

### Clinical features

Melanosis, followed by yellowish, pinpoint, verrucous papules 2–10 mm in diameter, typically occurs on the thenar and lateral borders of the palms; the base and lateral surfaces of the fingers; and the soles, heels, and toes {46,1522,2358}.

### Histopathology

Variable histological changes include compact hyperkeratosis, acanthosis, and papillomatosis {351,404,1522,2055}. Bowenoid ASK may display vacuolated, dyskeratotic cells with abnormal mitoses and multinucleated giant cells, but the dysplastic keratinocytes do not involve the full thickness of the epidermis {1522,2887}.

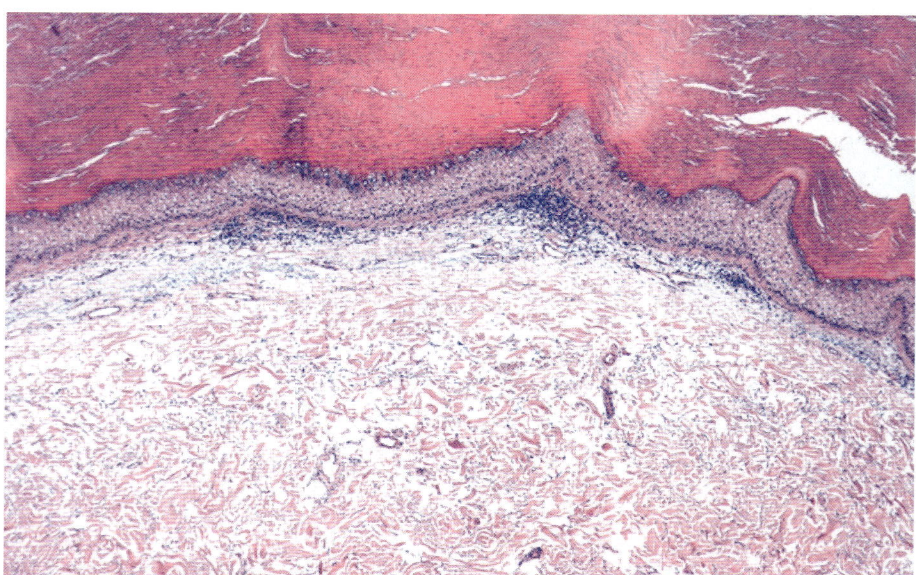

**Fig. 1.61** Arsenical keratosis. Almost full-thickness atypia of the epidermis, with dysregulated granular cell layer. Note the marked vacuolization of the cells, which is a helpful (although not diagnostic) feature.

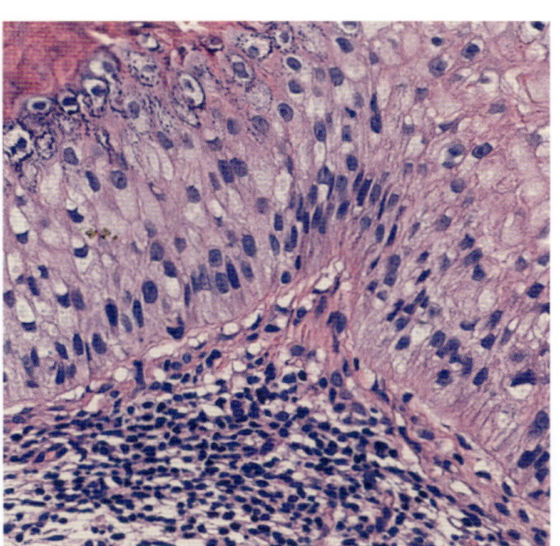

**Fig. 1.62** Arsenical keratosis. Marked hyperkeratosis with a hyperplastic, highly dysregulated epidermis; there is slight papillomatosis.

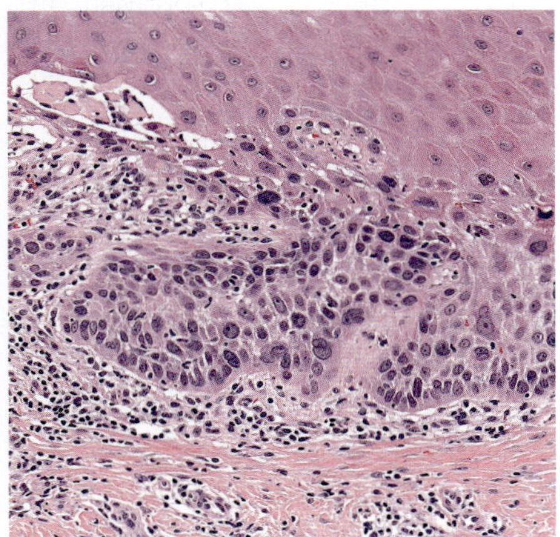

**Fig. 1.63** Arsenical keratosis. Biopsy of the sole reveals basaloid hyperplasia with marked atypia, budding downward into the inflamed dermis. The lichenoid infiltrate is associated with apoptosis and clustered dyskeratosis of cells. Note that the overlying squamous cells are hyperplastic but without marked atypia.

### Differential diagnosis

The differential diagnosis includes actinic keratosis, seborrhoeic keratosis, and squamous cell carcinoma in situ (Bowen disease) {1577}.

### Histogenesis

Exposure to arsenic and its compounds results in chromosomal abnormalities and gene amplification {404,2055}, with impairment of cellular DNA repair mechanisms {138,1155,1522,2011}; β1 integrin expression appears to be decreased {1521}. HPV may be a cofactor in the pathogenesis of ASK {876}.

### Genetic profile

Many arsenical skin cancers express p53 {271}.

### Prognosis and predictive factors

ASK may grow over years, and can also lead to invasive (often metastatic) squamous cell carcinoma. Pain, bleeding, fissuring, and ulceration predict progression {46,404,2358,2887}.

## *PUVA keratosis*

### Definition

PUVA keratosis is a hyperkeratotic lesion that occurs after prolonged exposure to psoralen and ultraviolet A (PUVA) therapy.

### ICD-O code 8070/0

### Synonym

Psoralen and ultraviolet A keratosis

### Epidemiology

PUVA therapy is associated with a dose-dependent risk of acquiring PUVA keratoses (with a prevalence of 2–5%), and with their transformation to squamous cell carcinoma and basal cell carcinoma; the incidence of such transformation is 15–30% after 5–8 years of exposure {1115,2508,2698}.

### Etiology

PUVA therapy, which is used for the treatment of psoriasis and other disorders {1114}, may be associated with DNA damage and PUVA-induced immunosuppression.

### Clinical features

PUVA keratosis presents as a characteristic raised papule with a broad base and a scaly, often warty appearance, on PUVA-treated skin {2698}.

### Histopathology

There is variable acanthosis, orthokeratosis, parakeratosis, and keratinocytic atypia, with possible papillomatosis {2698}. The presence of solar elastosis depends on the cutaneous site and degree of ultraviolet (UV) radiation–induced damage {2698}. The histopathological features are not specific, and diagnosis of PUVA keratosis requires clinical correlation.

### Differential diagnosis

The differential diagnosis includes actinic keratosis {2698}.

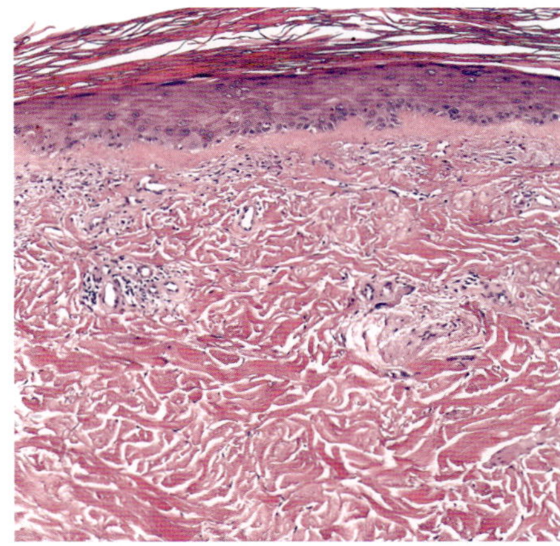

**Fig. 1.64** PUVA keratosis. Hyperkeratosis with scattered parakeratosis. Note the effacement of the epidermal rete ridges, with atypia of the basal layer cells.

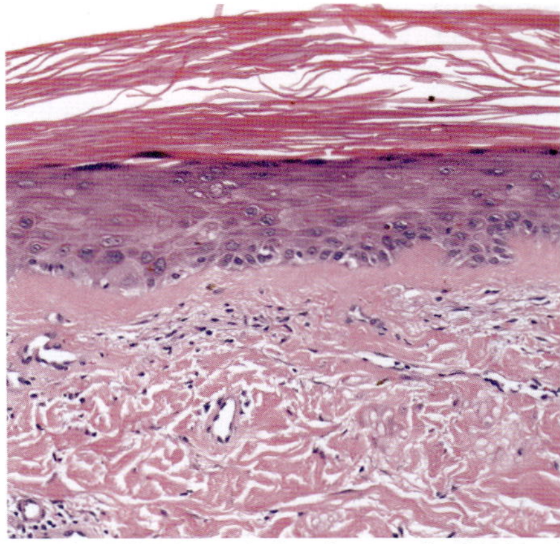

**Fig. 1.65** PUVA keratosis. Prominent atypia of the basal layer, with variably sized nuclei and focal squamatization. The squamous cells show dysmaturation with a variable increase in size and pallor; the granular cell layer is retained.

### Genetic profile

PUVA therapy may induce p53 expression and phosphorylation, as well as apoptosis {611}.

### Prognosis and predictive factors

Exposure to > 350 PUVA treatments has been found to increase the risk of squamous cell carcinoma {2508,2698}.

# Verrucae

Grayson W.
Tan K.B.
Tommasino M.

## Verruca vulgaris

### Definition
Verruca vulgaris is a common HPV-induced benign cutaneous squamoproliferative lesion.

### Synonym
Common viral wart

### Epidemiology
The reported prevalence is as high as 16% in children and 3.5% in adults {236,1359}. Immunosuppression is a risk factor {375}. Verrucae have been reported to account for 10% of skin lesions in renal transplant recipients {813}.

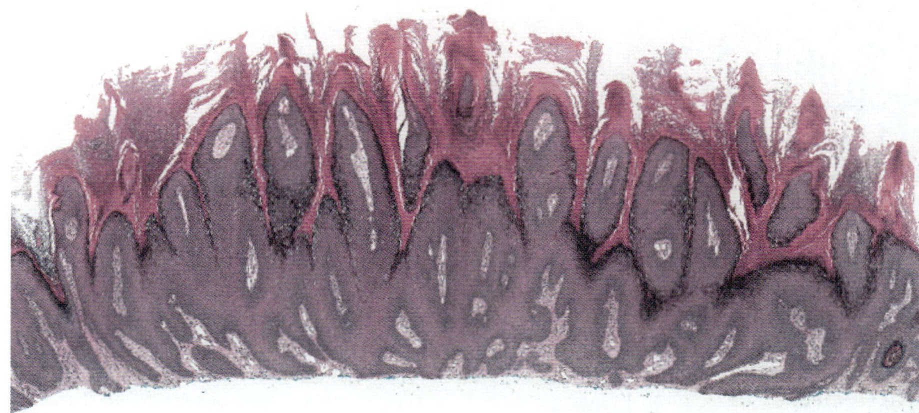

**Fig. 1.66** Verruca vulgaris. A characteristic inward proliferation of the rete ridges is evident in this low-power view of a shave excision biopsy.

### Etiology
Verruca vulgaris is caused by various subtypes of HPV. The main HPV types implicated in common warts are HPV1, HPV2, and HPV4 {375}. Others include HPV7, and HPV26–29 {499}. HPV75–77 have been detected in immunosuppressed patients {1643}. Genital HPV types HPV6 and HPV11 have rarely been detected in common warts among children {2021}. HPV16 (a genital type with oncogenic potential) was detected in 6.6% of non-genital warts in 45 immunocompetent patients {2020}. Verrucae sometimes occur on the vulva in children and adults {957}.

### Localization
There is a predilection for the hands and fingers {375}. Other sites include the elbows, knees, flexures, face, and genitalia {375,1359}.

### Clinical features
The lesions present as single or multiple verrucous, keratotic papules or nodules, 1–20 mm in diameter {375,1359}. Facial lesions may appear filiform {1736}. Occasional verrucae present as a cutaneous horn.

### Histopathology
There is hyperkeratosis, acanthosis, and papillomatosis, with prominent, inwardly proliferating rete ridges. Columns of parakeratosis overlie foci of papillomatosis. There is hypergranulosis, with coarse keratohyaline granules. Koilocytes are often present in the superficial epidermis {375,1359}. Dilated, tortuous capillaries occupy the papillary dermis. A lichenoid inflammatory infiltrate is sometimes present, and may correlate with regression/involution {1436}. Routine HPV subtyping is not indicated.

### Differential diagnosis
The utility of immunostaining for the diagnosis of verrucae is currently limited. Verrucae should be distinguished from seborrhoeic keratoses and verrucous psoriasis; this is particularly challenging when koilocytes are absent, which is more common in older warts {752,1352}. Occasionally, the distinction of inflamed seborrhoeic keratosis from verruca is not possible; a variety of terms have been used in such cases, such as "verruciform keratosis", "benign squamous papilloma", and "benign squamous keratosis". Keratoacanthoma may share architectural features with a crateriform verruca {1934}.

### Histogenesis
HPV infects the suprabasal keratinocytes, as well as the interappendageal epidermis and the stem cells of the follicular bulge {666}. HPV DNA synthesis takes place in the superficial prickle cell layer. Full virus assembly with capsid production occurs within the accentuated granular cell layer. Viral particles are released via desquamated cornified cells {499}.

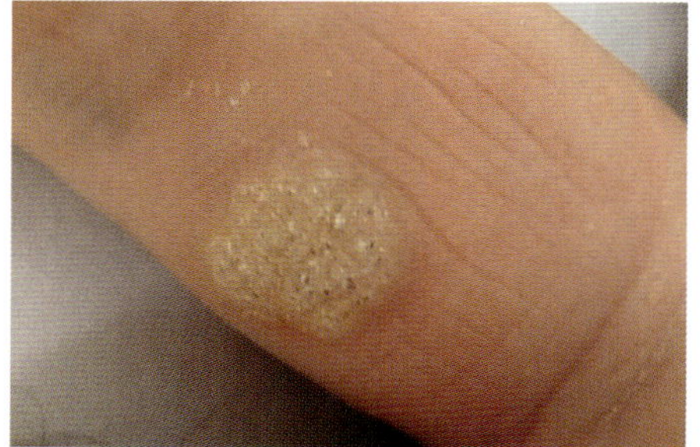

**Fig. 1.67** Verruca vulgaris. A hyperkeratotic digital lesion with dark punctate speckles on its surface.

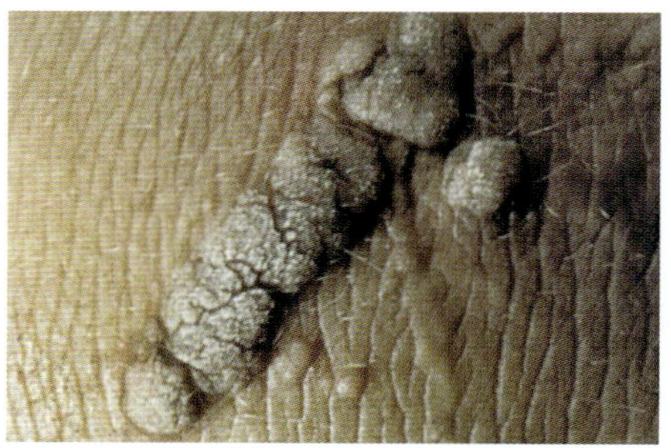

**Fig. 1.68** Verruca vulgaris showing the Koebner phenomenon. Linear arrangement of the lesions as consequence of scratching.

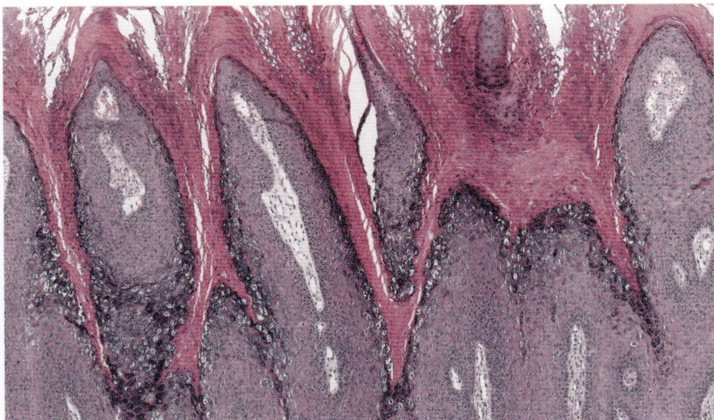

**Fig. 1.69** Verruca vulgaris. There is striking papillomatosis, hyperkeratosis, parakeratosis, and hypergranulosis.

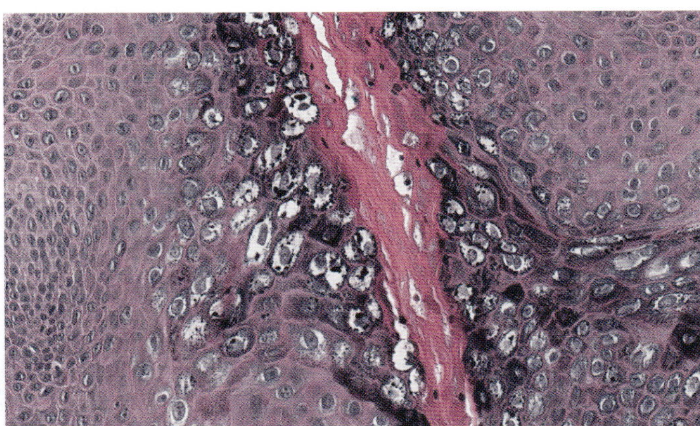

**Fig. 1.70** Verruca vulgaris. High-power photomicrograph demonstrating hypergranulosis and koilocytosis.

### Prognosis and predictive factors

Spontaneous involution may occur {1359}, although less often in immunocompromised patients {375}. In HIV-infected patients, antiretroviral therapy often expedites regression {2670}. Squamous dysplasia occasionally supervenes {258,1183}. Rare verrucae may progress to squamous cell carcinoma, especially in the setting of immunosuppression {1913}.

## *Verruca plantaris*

### Definition

Verruca plantaris is a common HPV-induced benign epidermal proliferative lesion affecting the soles or palms.

### Synonyms

Plantar wart; palmoplantar wart; plantar verruca

### Epidemiology

Children are affected more frequently than adults, with a reported prevalence of 1.8–20% {2694,2864}.

### Etiology

HPV1, HPV2, and HPV4 usually predominate {375,1501}. HPV27 and HPV57 have been recorded in cases from Spain and California {590,1374}. HPV60 has been linked to verruca plantaris and epidermal cysts {1112,1287}. Primary hyperhidrosis and communal showers are risk factors {1237,2762}. HIV-infected patients may have larger and more numerous lesions {1728}.

### Localization

Verruca plantaris occurs on the soles and palms.

### Clinical features

The lesions can be single or multiple, and are often painful. The myrmecial form (associated with HPV1) presents as a hard, slightly elevated keratotic papule or nodule on the plantar or palmar surface. The more superficial mosaic form (associated with HPV4 and HPV2) exhibits its confluent growth and is resistant to therapy {375,1501}. Black surface dots reflect intralesional vascular thrombosis.

### Histopathology

There is marked hyperkeratosis, acanthosis, hypergranulosis, and koilocytosis {375}. Papillomatosis is usually mild.

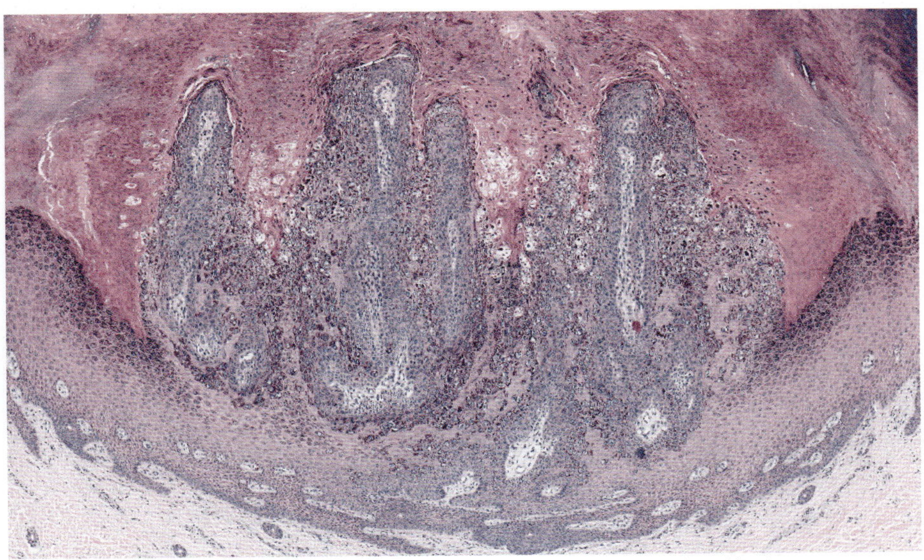

**Fig. 1.71** Verruca plantaris. Low-power photomicrograph depicting a typical endophytic architecture.

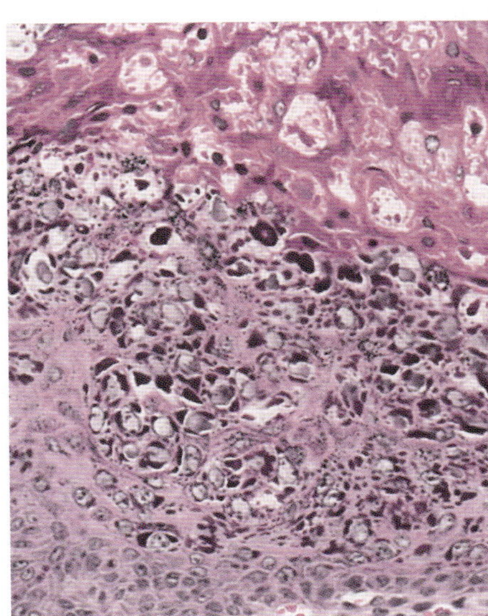

**Fig. 1.72** Verruca plantaris. The characteristic coarse eosinophilic intracytoplasmic inclusions are clearly demonstrated in this high-power photomicrograph.

The myrmecial (so-called ant-hill) variant shows endophytic growth and vacuolated keratinocytes containing coarse eosinophilic keratohyaline granules. Regressing lesions exhibit haemorrhage, necrosis, thrombosis, and a mixed inflammatory infiltrate {215}.

### Differential diagnosis

Callosities occur on pressure points and are also endophytic and hyperkeratotic, but lack koilocytes and coarse keratohyaline granules {2904}. Molluscum contagiosum also displays endophytic growth and intracytoplasmic inclusions, but the inclusions are basophilic and less heterogeneous {2162}.

### Histogenesis

See the *Histogenesis* subsection (p. 54) of *Verruca vulgaris*.

### Prognosis and predictive factors

Verruca plantaris often regresses spontaneously. Lesions in children tend to resolve more rapidly {375}. Verrucous carcinoma is a very rare complication {1718}.

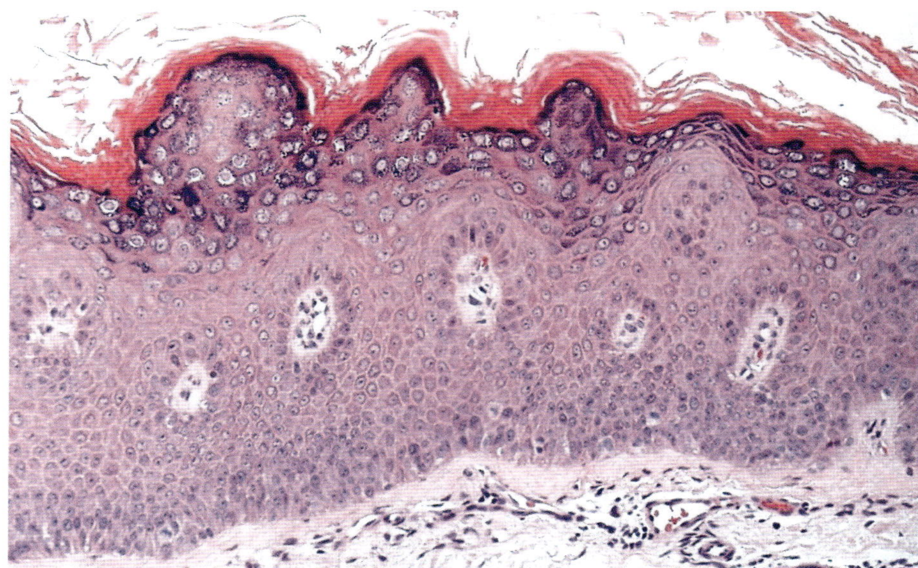

**Fig. 1.74** Verruca plana. Only minimal papillomatosis is evident, and there is associated acanthosis, mild hyperkeratosis, hypergranulosis, and perinuclear clearing of some superficial keratinocytes.

## *Verruca plana*

### Definition

Verruca plana is an HPV-induced benign epidermal proliferation characterized by flat-topped cutaneous papules.

### Synonyms

Plane wart; flat wart

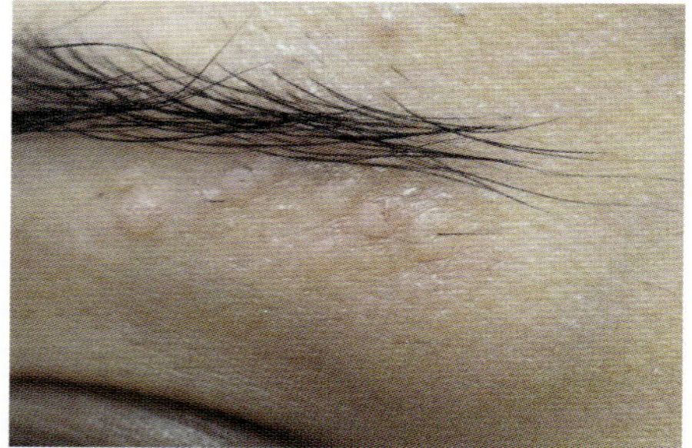

**Fig. 1.73** Verruca plana. Multiple skin-coloured, flat-topped cutaneous papules are present.

### Epidemiology

Verruca plana most commonly affects children. In adults, there is a predilection for women {375}.

### Etiology

The most frequently implicated HPV types are HPV3 and HPV10 {375}. Immunosuppression is a risk factor {375}. Multiple plane warts occupying > 5% of the body surface area are a potential harbinger of underlying HIV infection {1594}. In HIV-infected patients, a sudden eruption of lesions may herald the immune reconstitution inflammatory syndrome {1163}.

### Localization

The lesions occur most frequently on the face, hands, and shins {375}.

### Clinical features

The lesions present as several smooth-surfaced, skin-coloured to light-brown papules. Associated Koebnerization can occur {375}. Redness or depigmentation is often indicative of regression {214}.

### Histopathology

There is orthokeratosis, mild acanthosis, and variable hypergranulosis, but only minimal papillomatosis. Scattered koilocytes (some with grey-blue cytoplasm) are present in the upper third of the epidermis {375}. Owl's-eye intranuclear inclusions may be found. Regression is associated with a superficial perivascular lymphocytic infiltrate, lymphocytic exocytosis, and keratinocytic apoptosis {2217,2556}.

### Differential diagnosis

Epidermodysplasia verruciformis shows enlarged keratinocytes with abundant bluish-grey, often vacuolated cytoplasm {1927}. Seborrhoeic keratoses tend to be more scattered, and are dermoscopically and histologically distinctive {1572,2556}.

### Histogenesis

See the *Histogenesis* subsection (p. 54) of *Verruca vulgaris*.

### Prognosis and predictive factors

The lesions may be persistent or recurrent despite treatment {402}. In a 1977 study of plane warts that had regressed, 64% were found to have done so spontaneously; the other 36% underwent regression following various forms of treatment {2556}.

# Benign acanthomas/keratoses

Brenn T.
Elgart G.W.
Howard V.
Piris A.
Tallon B.

## *Seborrhoeic keratosis*

### Definition

Seborrhoeic keratosis is a benign intraepidermal neoplasm that most commonly occurs in ageing skin.

### ICD-O code 8052/0

### Synonyms

Senile wart; seborrhoeic wart

### Epidemiology

These lesions are very common. In an Australian population, seborrhoeic keratoses were present in 12% of people aged 15–25 years, 79% of people aged 26–50 years, and 100% of people aged >50 years {2881}. The lesions increase in number with age and are found less commonly in more-pigmented skin. There is no apparent sex predilection.

### Etiology

Ultraviolet (UV) radiation exposure is related to the etiology of some seborrhoeic keratoses. Other possible causes under investigation include genetic and metabolic factors.

### Localization

Seborrhoeic keratoses have a predilection for the trunk, head, and neck, but can occur on any skin surface other than the palms, soles, and mucosal surfaces {983}. They tend to group together in skin creases, such as under the breast or in the groin.

### Clinical features

Seborrhoeic keratoses typically present as solitary or multiple flat-based papules or plaques with a filiform surface. A brown or black appearance is typical, but some lesions are pale or grey. Macular seborrhoeic keratoses remain thin, with subtle scale. Stucco keratoses, which are considered a variant of seborrhoeic keratosis, form distinctive small keratoses that are largely restricted to the lower limbs. Dermoscopy reveals multiple brown or white clods, representing plugs of keratin, and thick ridges impart a cerebriform pattern {363}. The acute appearance of multiple seborrhoeic keratoses associated with an internal malignancy is called the Leser–Trélat sign.

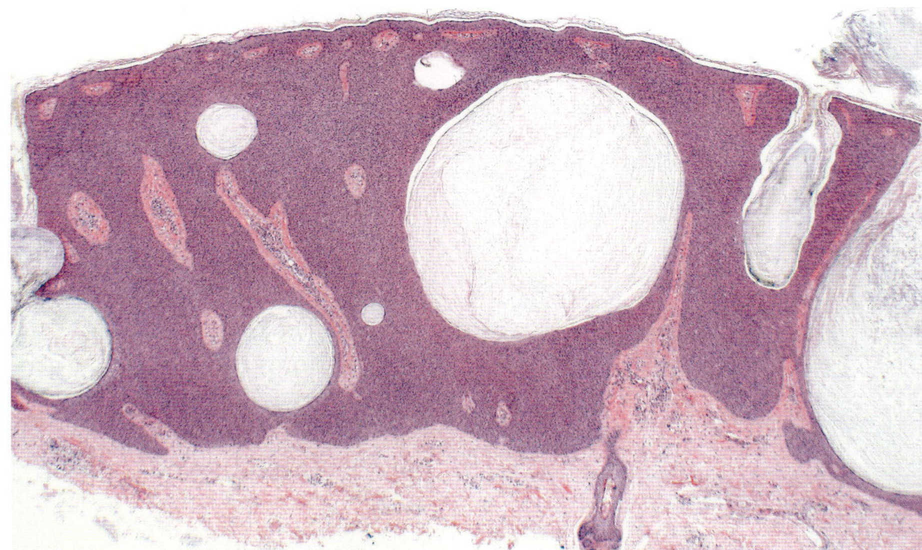

**Fig. 1.75** Acanthotic (regular) seborrhoeic keratosis. This variant is characterized by a regular architecture composed of broad columns of acanthotic epidermis; note the flat base and the presence of multiple so-called horn cysts.

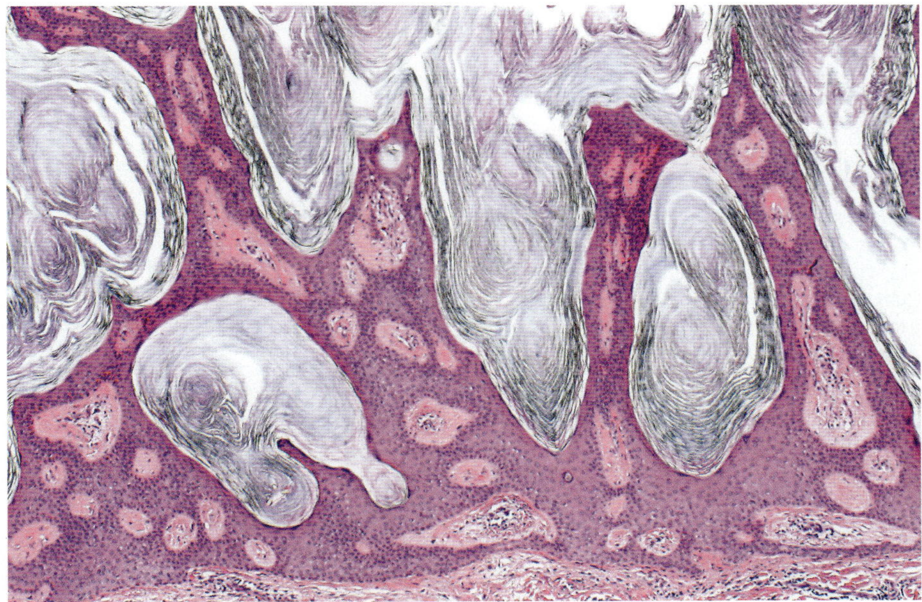

**Fig. 1.76** Keratotic (papillomatous) seborrhoeic keratosis. This variant shows a papillomatous architecture and marked hyperkeratosis.

### Histopathology

Seborrhoeic keratoses are well-demarcated intraepidermal neoplasms composed of a proliferation of basaloid keratinocytes. They are characterized by a papillomatous architecture with a flat base. There is overlying hyperkeratosis, and so-called horn cyst formation is seen on cross-sectioning. Increased basal cell layer pigmentation is common. The profile may be variably exophytic, flat, or endophytic, and several histological variants are recognized:

*Acanthotic (regular) type:*
This variant, the most common form of seborrhoeic keratosis, shows broad adjoining columns of hyperplastic epidermis.

*Keratotic (papillomatous) type*
In this variant, there is prominent hyperkeratosis with variable papillomatosis and acanthosis. When there is a prominent inflammatory infiltrate, there may be significant overlap with the irritated variant.

*Reticulated (adenoid) type*
This variant has an architecture with more-subtle, thin, elongated rete ridges and small horn cysts.

*Clonal type*
Intraepidermal nests of benign pale keratinocytes (the Borst–Jadassohn phenomenon) are characteristic of this variant.

*Irritated type:*
In this variant, the hyperkeratotic stratum corneum contains superficial scale crust. The keratinocytes may show foci of squamatization and squamous eddies. There is evidence of increased apoptosis, consistent with increased cell turnover {2034}. Lichenoid degeneration of the basal layer is seen, with scattered necrotic keratinocytes and a superficial lichenoid lymphocytic infiltrate.

*Pigmented type:*
In this variant, the presence of increased keratinocyte pigmentation and scattered melanophages is the basis of the clinical pigmented appearance.

*Macular type*
Clinically and histologically, macular seborrhoeic keratoses can be difficult to distinguish from some solar lentigines. The acanthosis is mild with subtle clonal nests, a helpful clue in difficult cases. Increased basal layer pigmentation creates a dirty-socks appearance. Horn cysts are not seen.

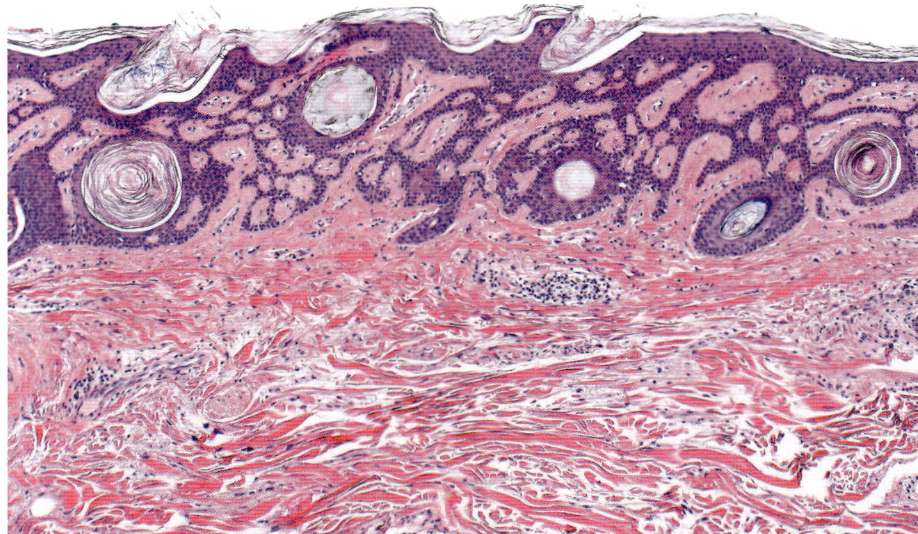

**Fig. 1.77** Reticulated (adenoid) seborrhoeic keratosis. This variant shows a complex and anastomosing proliferation of narrow elongated rete ridges, also showing horn cyst formation.

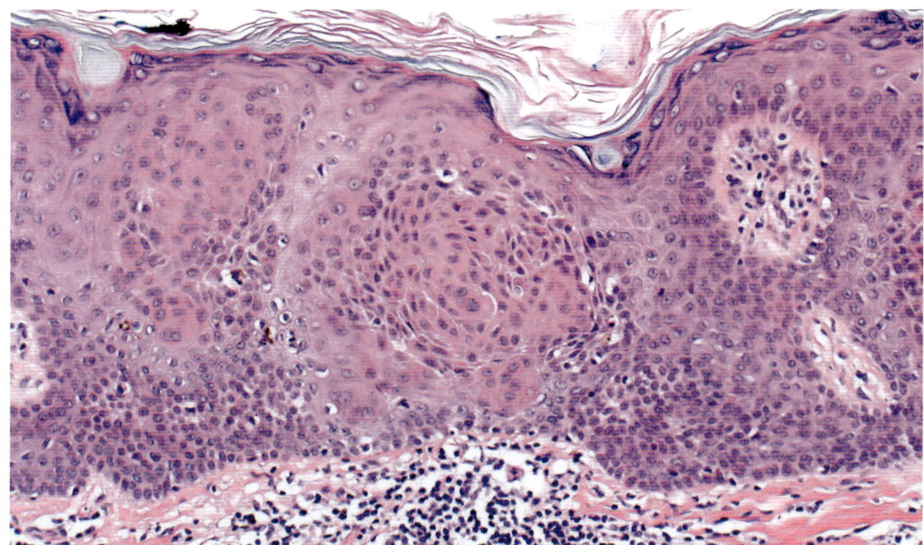

**Fig. 1.78** Clonal seborrhoeic keratosis. Intraepidermal keratinocyte nests are characteristic of this variant.

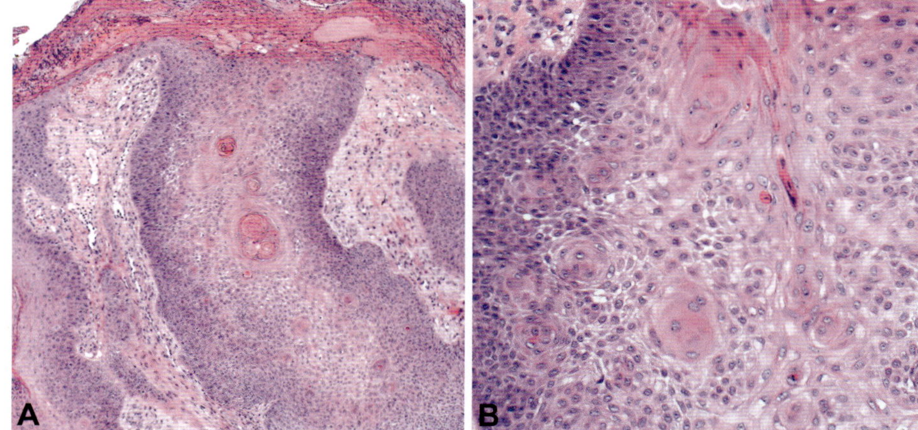


**Fig. 1.79** Irritated seborrhoeic keratosis. **A** This variant shows irregular growth with hyperparakeratosis. **B** Higher magnification reveals spongiosis and numerous squamous eddies.

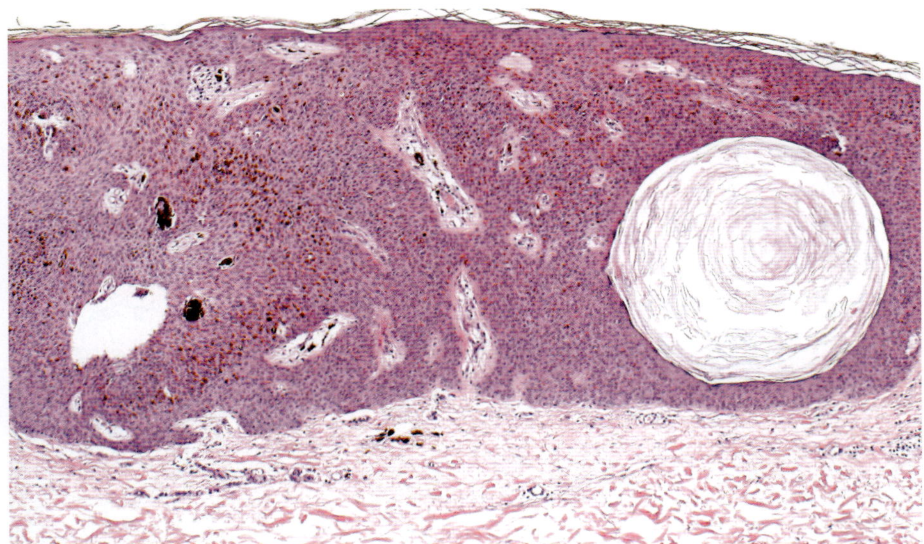

**Fig. 1.80** Pigmented seborrhoeic keratosis. Abundant melanin pigment is seen in this variant.

### Differential diagnosis

The keratotic variant shows significant histological overlap with verruca vulgaris, but seborrhoeic keratoses lack the inward-bending rete, koilocytosis, prominent superficial vascularity, and cap-like haemorrhage. Dowling–Degos disease and some epidermal naevi may appear very similar, and can be overlooked when clinical details are not available. Actinic keratosis and squamous cell carcinoma in situ are characterized by varying degrees of squamous dysplasia not seen in seborrhoeic keratosis. Reactive keratinocytic atypia in irritated seborrhoeic keratosis can often mimic squamous dysplasia, and reliable distinction is challenging, especially on small and fragmented biopsies. However, true squamous dysplasia or squamous cell carcinoma in situ can occur in association with seborrhoeic keratoses.

### Histogenesis

Seborrhoeic keratoses arise from epidermal keratinocytes. They have an increased proliferation rate and decreased apoptosis compared with normal keratinocytes {2446}.

### Genetic profile

Somatic mutations are seen in *FGFR3*, *PIK3CA*, the *TERT* promoter, the *DPH3* promoter, *HRAS*, *KRAS*, *EGFR*, and *AKT1*.

### Prognosis and predictive factors

Seborrhoeic keratoses are benign, but a search for internal malignancy should be performed in response to the sudden appearance of multiple lesions.

## *Solar lentigo*

### Definition

Solar lentigo is a benign keratinocytic proliferation associated with ultraviolet (UV) radiation exposure. It is closely related to seborrhoeic keratosis.

### ICD-O code 8052/0

### Synonyms

Senile lentigo; actinic lentigo

### Epidemiology

Solar lentigines are markers of chronic sun damage, and increase with age. Middle-aged to elderly adults are affected, with a predilection for White populations.

### Etiology

Solar lentigo is caused by chronic UV radiation exposure {166}.

### Localization

Solar lentigo occurs at sites of chronic sun exposure, with a predilection for the face, dorsum of the hands, and forearms.

### Clinical features

Solar lentigines present as tan to brown, uniformly pigmented but not always sharply demarcated macules, measuring a few millimetres in diameter. So-called ink-spot lentigines are characterized by their dark pigmentation.

### Histopathology

Solar lentigines are well-circumscribed, with elongated rete ridges showing budding and basal cell layer hyperpigmentation. Fusion of rete ridges may also be seen. Overlying hyperkeratosis is common, and a background of solar elastosis is characteristic. Mildly increased numbers of junctional melanocytes may also be found {73}. Ink-spot lentigines are small and sharply demarcated, with prominent basal cell layer hyperpigmentation accentuated at the tips of the rete ridges.

### Differential diagnosis

The histopathological features of solar lentigo and seborrhoeic keratosis may overlap. Pigmented actinic keratoses show keratinocytic dysplasia. Lentigo maligna is characterized by confluent growth of junctional melanocytes, with melanocyte atypia. Evaluation of melanocyte density using melan-A, MITF, or SOX10 staining is helpful in difficult cases {1364}.

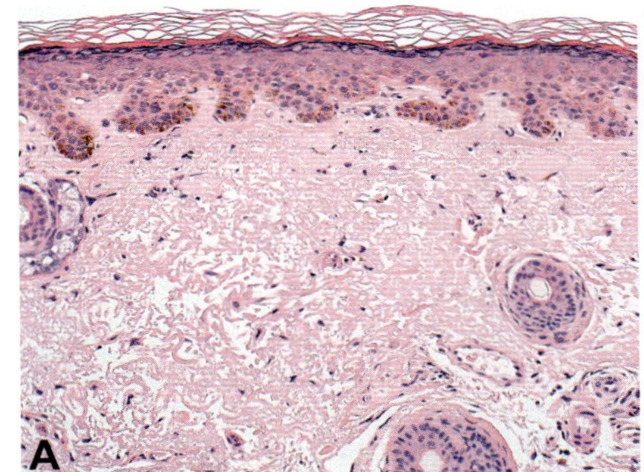


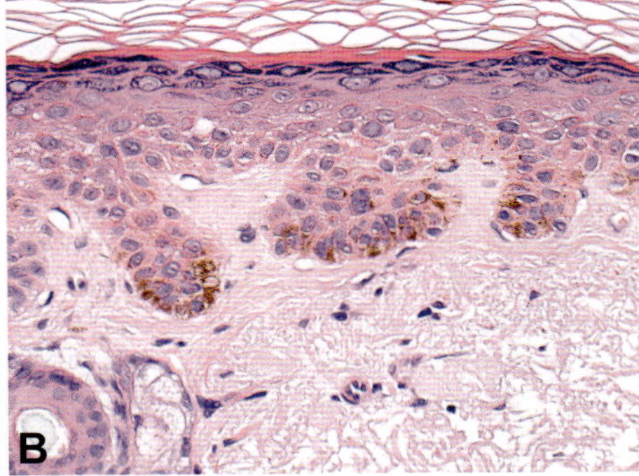


**Fig. 1.81** Solar lentigo. **A** Elongated rete ridges with basal cell layer hyperpigmentation are characteristic; overlying orthohyperkeratosis is an additional finding. **B** Higher magnification demonstrates the absence of keratinocytic atypia.

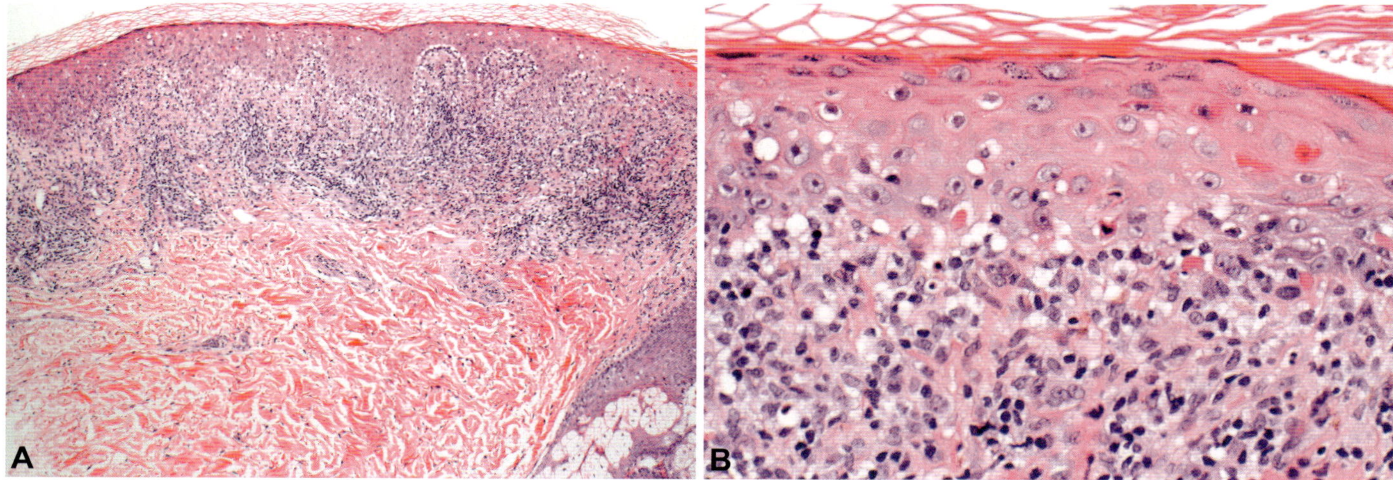


**Fig. 1.82** Lichen planus–like keratosis. **A** There is epidermal hyperplasia and a band-like superficial dermal chronic inflammatory cell infiltrate. **B** Higher magnification highlights the interface change with numerous apoptotic keratinocytes, some of which are also found in the upper layers of the epidermis. There is an associated lymphohistiocytic infiltrate within the superficial dermis showing pigmentary incontinence.

### Histogenesis

Solar lentigo is an intraepidermal proliferation of keratinocytes.

### Genetic profile

Little is known about the genetic profile. *FGFR3* and *PIK3CA* mutations are seen in a subset of cases, but solar lentigo consistently lacks *BRAF* mutation {982}.

### Prognosis and predictive factors

Solar lentigines are benign. Their number increases with age, and they may be an indicator of sun damage to the skin.

## *Lichen planus–like keratosis*

### Definition

Lichen planus–like keratosis is a benign squamoproliferative lesion showing chronic inflammation and interface changes (likely representing active regression).

### ICD-O code 8052/0

### Synonym

Lichenoid keratosis

### Epidemiology

This common lesion presents in adulthood (mean age: 59 years), with a female-to-male ratio of 2:1 {1831}. Lichen planus–like keratosis most frequently occurs in White populations.

### Localization

Lichen planus–like keratoses present as solitary lesions, most commonly on the trunk (in 76% of cases), followed by the limbs (in 33%), and uncommonly on the head and neck (in 3%) {1831}.

### Clinical features

Lichen planus–like keratoses are erythematous plaques with variable scale, measuring 5–20 mm. Dermoscopy shows irregular telangiectatic vessels and uniform clusters of grey dots {330,2788}.

### Histopathology

The lesions are well demarcated and show variable irregular acanthosis, with overlying hyperkeratosis and parakeratosis. There is an associated prominent band-like chronic inflammatory cell infiltrate within the superficial dermis, resulting in interface change with scattered necrotic keratinocytes and basal layer vacuolar degeneration of the overlying epidermis. The inflammatory cell infiltrate is composed of lymphocytes, histiocytes, and often melanophages. Eosinophils and plasma cells may be admixed. Prominent keratinocytic degeneration may result in a subepidermal cleft and blister formation. Late atrophic lesions exhibit a thinned epidermis and superficial dermal fibrosis.

### Differential diagnosis

A regressed melanocytic lesion (in particular a regressed melanoma) may be difficult to exclude. Complete loss of melanocytes in the involved epidermis and prominent dermal melanophages suggest a pre-existing melanocytic lesion {425}. Examining deeper levels and immunostaining for melanocytic markers is often helpful to investigate for a residual melanocytic lesion. The clinical context, as well as the presence of parakeratosis and a deeper perivascular infiltrate, distinguishes lichen planus–like keratosis from lichen planus. Lichenoid actinic keratoses demonstrate basal layer keratinocytic atypia.

### Histogenesis

Lichen planus–like keratosis is a benign intraepidermal keratotic neoplasm.

### Prognosis and predictive factors

Lichen planus–like keratosis is entirely benign.

## *Clear cell acanthoma*

### Definition

Clear cell acanthoma is a benign squamous lesion composed of keratinocytes with pale to clear cytoplasm.

### ICD-O code 8084/0

### Synonyms

Pale cell acanthoma; Degos acanthoma

### Epidemiology

This uncommon lesion is typically found in middle-aged or elderly individuals, with a median age of 63 years. It rarely presents in younger patients. There is no sex or race preference {2089}.

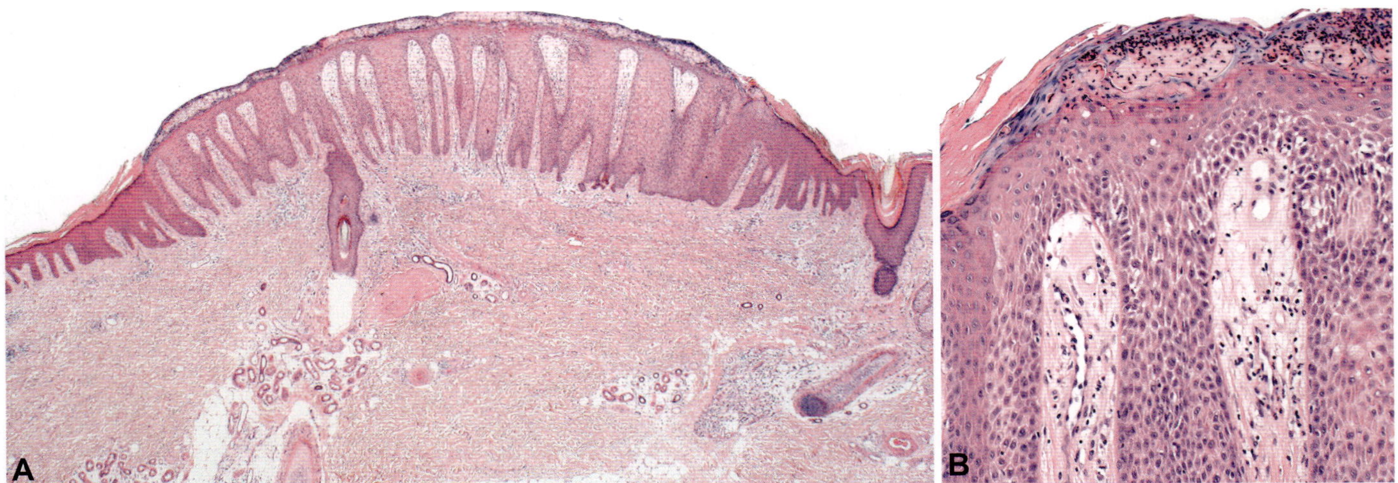


**Fig. 1.83** Clear cell acanthoma. **A** The lesion is sharply demarcated and shows regular, psoriasiform epidermal hyperplasia. **B** The lesional keratinocytes contain palely eosinophilic cytoplasm. There is overlying parakeratosis containing neutrophils; also note the sharp demarcation with the adjacent epidermis.

### Localization
The lower extremities are mainly affected.

### Clinical features
Clear cell acanthoma presents as a sharply delineated pink, red, or brown papule or nodule, 0.5–4 cm in size. Polypoid lesions as large as 6 cm have been reported. Clear cell acanthoma is usually solitary, but multiple eruptive lesions have been described. Additional findings include an inflamed scale crust with vascular puncta that bleed when traumatized {519}.

### Histopathology
A well-circumscribed psoriasiform intraepidermal squamous proliferation composed of glycogen-rich cells with bland cytological features is characteristic. The lateral edges are well defined, with sharp demarcation from the background epidermis. There are scattered intralesional neutrophils, which can aggregate in a superficial scale crust. The rete ridges are fused, with thinning of papillary plates. The dermis shows prominent vessels and a mixed inflammatory infiltrate. Adnexal structures are spared.

### Differential diagnosis
The differential diagnosis includes seborrhoeic keratosis and psoriasis. The finding of pseudohorn cysts, a papillary architecture, and an absence of pale cells favours a diagnosis of seborrhoeic keratosis. The sharp demarcation and lack of adnexal involvement helps to rule out psoriasis.

### Prognosis and predictive factors
The clinical course is benign.

## *Large cell acanthoma*

### Definition
Large cell acanthoma is a benign squamous lesion on the same morphological spectrum as solar lentigo and seborrhoeic keratosis {819,1734}.

### ICD-O code 8072/0

### Epidemiology
Large cell acanthoma presents on sun-damaged skin of middle-aged to elderly adults and mainly occurs in fair-skinned individuals {819,1734}.

### Etiology
This lesion is caused by chronic ultraviolet (UV) radiation exposure.

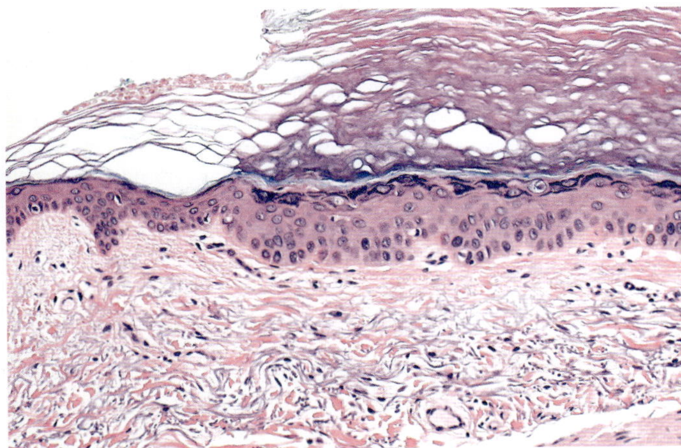

**Fig. 1.84** Large cell acanthoma. This epidermal tumour is sharply demarcated and shows acanthosis and overlying orthohyperkeratosis.

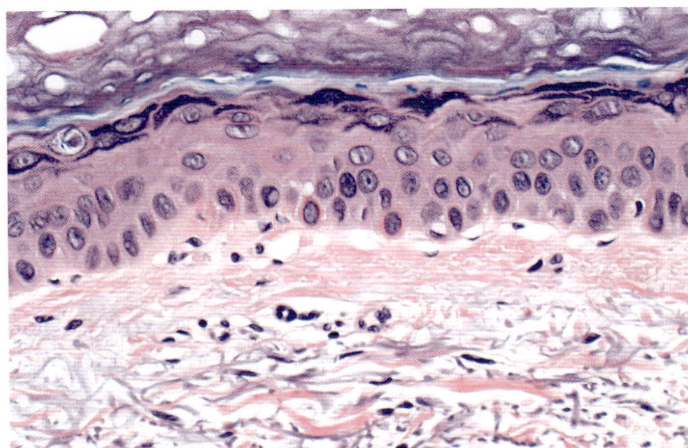

**Fig. 1.85** Large cell acanthoma. The hallmark feature is the presence of large keratinocytes with smooth nuclear contours and no signs of keratinocytic dysplasia.

## Localization
The face and arms are most commonly affected; presentation on the trunk and lower limbs is less common.

## Clinical features
Large cell acanthoma presents as tan to brown, well-demarcated macules and plaques with a discrete scale, typically < 1 cm in diameter. Rarely, larger lesions have been described.

## Histopathology
Large cell acanthoma is well circumscribed and characterized by a mildly acanthotic epidermis, which may be flattened or show bulbous rete ridges. The hallmark feature is the presence of enlarged keratinocytes with nuclei twice the normal size. The lesional cells contain abundant cytoplasm, and the nuclear contours are smooth. Cytological atypia is not a feature, and mitotic activity is rare. In addition, there is basal cell layer hyperpigmentation, and orthohyperkeratosis is frequently present. A background of solar elastosis is commonly observed. A papillomatous variant has also been reported.

## Differential diagnosis
Actinic keratoses are characterized by intraepidermal keratinocytic dysplasia with cytological atypia and nuclear pleomorphism; the presence of parakeratosis is a further clue. Lentigo maligna is composed of a confluent growth of atypical melanocytes at the dermoepidermal junction; differentiation from large cell acanthoma may be challenging on histology alone, and immunohistochemistry for melan-A or SOX10 may be helpful.

## Histogenesis
Large cell acanthoma is an intraepidermal proliferation of distinctive enlarged keratinocytes.

## Prognosis and predictive factors
Large cell acanthoma is benign.

# *Warty dyskeratoma*

## Definition
Warty dyskeratoma is a benign endophytic squamoproliferative lesion arising in association with pilosebaceous units and showing prominent acantholytic dyskeratosis.

## ICD-O code 8054/0

## Synonyms
Isolated dyskeratosis follicularis; follicular dyskeratoma

## Epidemiology
Warty dyskeratoma occurs across a wide age range, with a predilection for elderly individuals (median age: 61 years, range: 3–88 years) and a female predominance {1259}.

## Localization
The head and neck area is typically involved, but warty dyskeratoma can also occur on the trunk, extremities, and oral and genital mucosa {61,1259}.

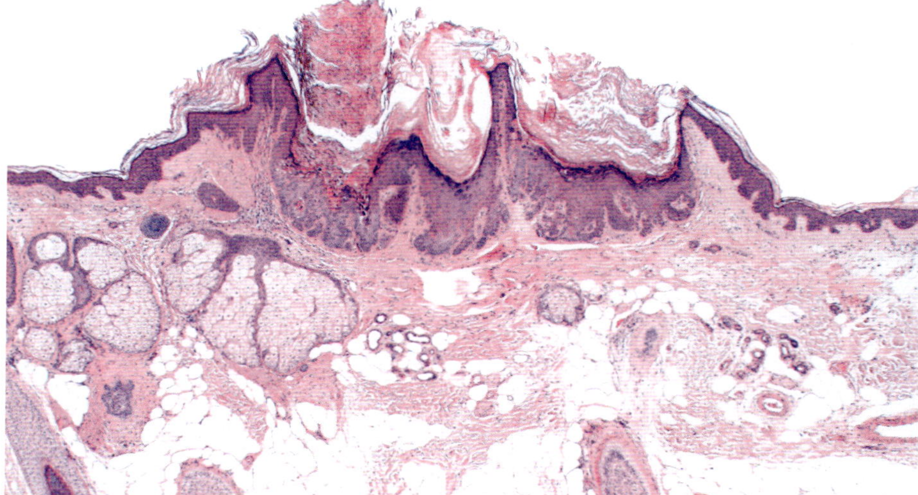
**Fig. 1.86** Warty dyskeratoma. This epidermal tumour shows an endophytic growth with a cup-shaped architecture; there is marked overlying hyperkeratosis and parakeratosis.

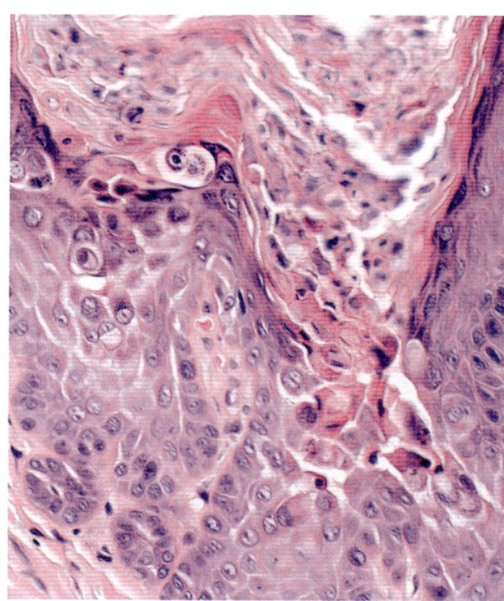
**Fig. 1.87** Warty dyskeratoma. The keratinocytes show acantholysis and dyskeratosis, with an overlying parakeratotic column.

## Clinical features
Warty dyskeratomas present as solitary tan to light-brown papules or small nodules, and may appear umbilicated. They are rarely multiple. Mucosal lesions are white.

## Histopathology
Warty dyskeratoma is a well-circumscribed cup-shaped epidermal invagination. It is composed of a proliferation of keratinocytes, with budding into surrounding papillary dermis. There is prominent acantholysis, with suprabasal clefting, dyskeratosis, corps ronds, corps grains, and an overlying parakeratotic plug. Mitoses are common. The surrounding epidermis may be hyperplastic or papillomatous, and an epidermal collarette may also be seen. A connection with a pilosebaceous unit is common. The surrounding stroma is often hyalinized and contains stromal clefts and a chronic inflammatory cell infiltrate, as well as melanophages. Rarely, cystic and nodular variants are encountered, and a combination of the various patterns may be present in an individual neoplasm.

## Differential diagnosis
Darier disease and Grover disease can be excluded on clinical grounds. Acantholytic squamous cell carcinoma shows keratinocytic atypia; it lacks the circumscription and well-demarcated outlines, and commonly shows an infiltrative growth.

### Histogenesis

This neoplasm is believed to show hair follicle differentiation.

### Prognosis and predictive factors

Warty dyskeratoma is benign and nonrecurring.

## Other benign keratoses

### Definition

Benign keratoses with distinctive morphological patterns that do not meet the criteria for any of the entities described in the previous sections include acantholytic acanthoma, acantholytic dyskeratotic acanthoma, epidermolytic acanthoma, granular parakeratotic acanthoma, psoriasiform keratosis, and melanoacanthoma.

### ICD-O code 8052/0

### Epidemiology, localization, and clinical features

Acantholytic acanthomas present as solitary papules or nodules (0.5–1.2 cm), with a predilection for the trunk of adults (median age: 60 years) {322}. Males are more commonly affected. Multiple lesions have been reported in the setting of immunosuppression {2133}.

Acantholytic dyskeratotic acanthomas are solitary lesions (< 1 cm) that affect the trunk of adults, with a slight female predominance. The nail may also be affected {1394,2243,2321}.

Epidermolytic acanthomas are verrucous papules or plaques (0.2–1.2 cm) that may be solitary or multiple. The anatomical distribution is wide and includes genital and mucosal sites. A wide age range is affected {507,669,1807,2400}.

Granular parakeratotic acanthomas are rare solitary lesions affecting mainly the trunk and extremities and occurring in adults {2175}.

Psoriasiform keratoses are solitary scaly erythematous papules or plaques (≤ 3 cm). The anatomical distribution is wide, with a predilection for the extremities of adults {1856,2767}.

Melanoacanthomas are dark-brown, well-circumscribed plaques or nodules measuring as much as several centimetres. They have a wide anatomical distribution and affect adults {1799,2101}.

### Histopathology

Acantholytic acanthoma is a well-circumscribed keratosis characterized by epidermal acanthosis, a papillomatous growth pattern, and overlying hyperkeratosis. There is prominent acantholysis affecting various levels of the epidermis and resembling pemphigus vulgaris, pemphigus foliaceus, or benign chronic pemphigus (Hailey–Hailey disease). Focal dyskeratosis may also be present, and there is an associated superficial dermal chronic inflammatory cell infiltrate.

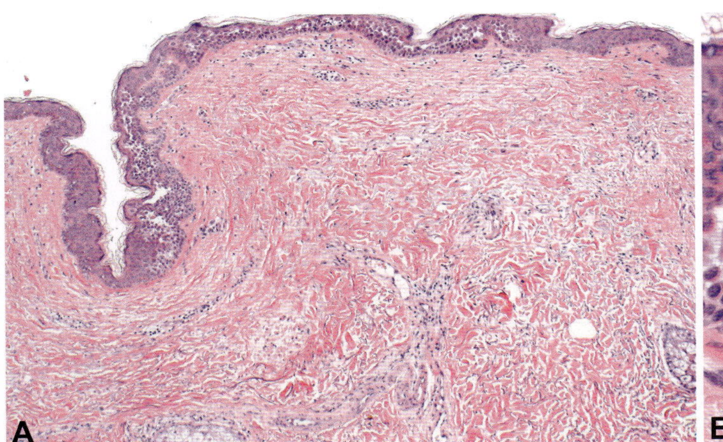

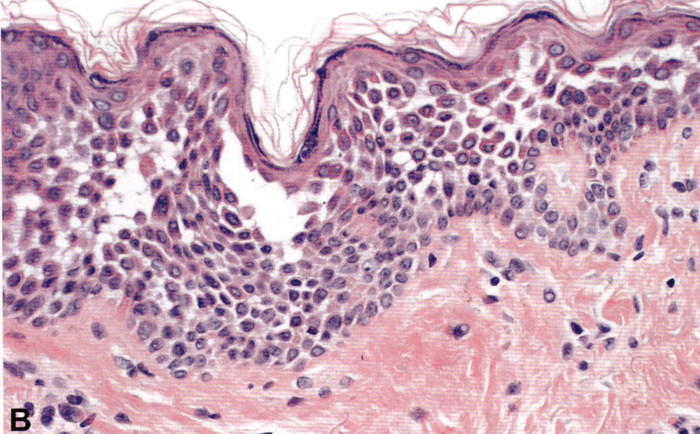

**Fig. 1.88** Acantholytic acanthoma. **A** Well-circumscribed keratosis characterized by epidermal thickening and acantholysis. **B** Higher magnification reveals prominent acantholysis with lack of dyskeratosis, reminiscent of benign chronic pemphigus (Hailey–Hailey disease).

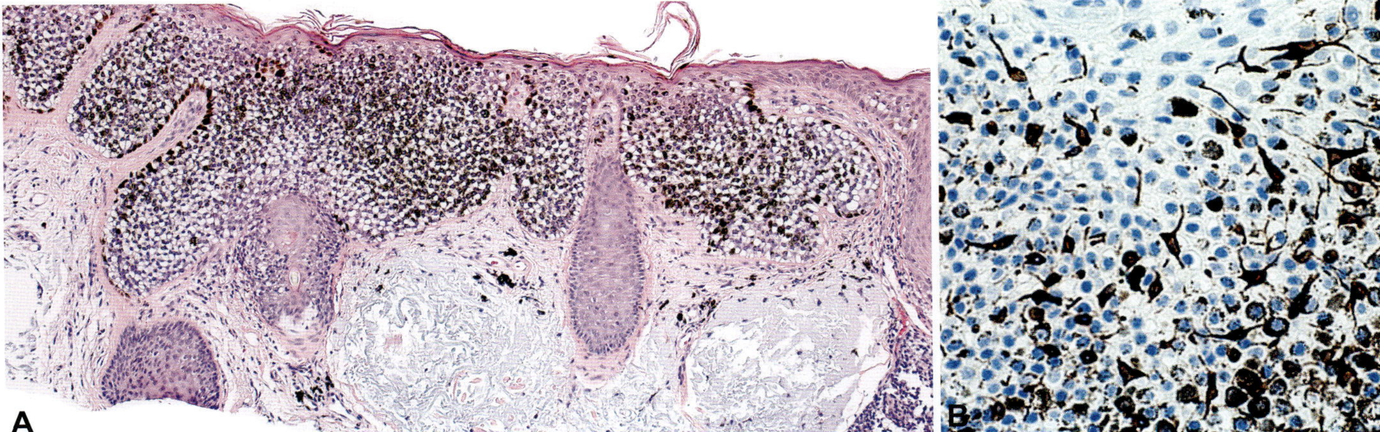

**Fig. 1.89** Melanoacanthoma. **A** The prominent intralesional melanin pigment may lead to an erroneous diagnosis of a melanocytic lesion. **B** Immunohistochemistry for melan-A highlights colonization by dendritic melanocytes.

Acantholytic dyskeratotic acanthoma is sharply demarcated and shows acanthosis with prominent acantholytic dyskeratosis with corps grains and corps ronds.

Epidermolytic acanthoma is a well-delineated keratosis with verrucous epidermal hyperplasia showing striking epidermolytic hyperkeratosis.

Granular parakeratotic acanthoma is a well-circumscribed epidermal proliferation with a growth pattern reminiscent of adenoid seborrhoeic keratosis but showing marked granular parakeratosis.

Psoriasiform keratosis is characterized by verrucous irregular epidermal hyperplasia with hyperkeratosis, parakeratosis, and intracorneal neutrophils. Dilated vessels and a chronic inflammatory cell infiltrate are apparent in the superficial dermis.

Melanoacanthoma is microscopically similar to seborrhoeic keratosis or other benign squamoproliferative lesions, but shows colonization by numerous dendritic melanocytes with bland cytological features. In addition, there is marked melanin deposition within keratinocytes. Immunohistochemistry for melan-A or HMB45 antigen highlights the dendritic melanocytes.

### Differential diagnosis

The above-mentioned keratoses closely resemble the various dermatoses reflected in their names. Because they may be indistinguishable histologically, their clinical presentation as solitary papules, nodules, and plaques is the key to correct diagnosis. Melanoacanthoma may be mistaken for melanoma; immunohistochemistry for melanocytic markers demonstrates the colonization of a keratosis by dendritic melanocytes.

### Prognosis and predictive factors

These are benign keratoses.

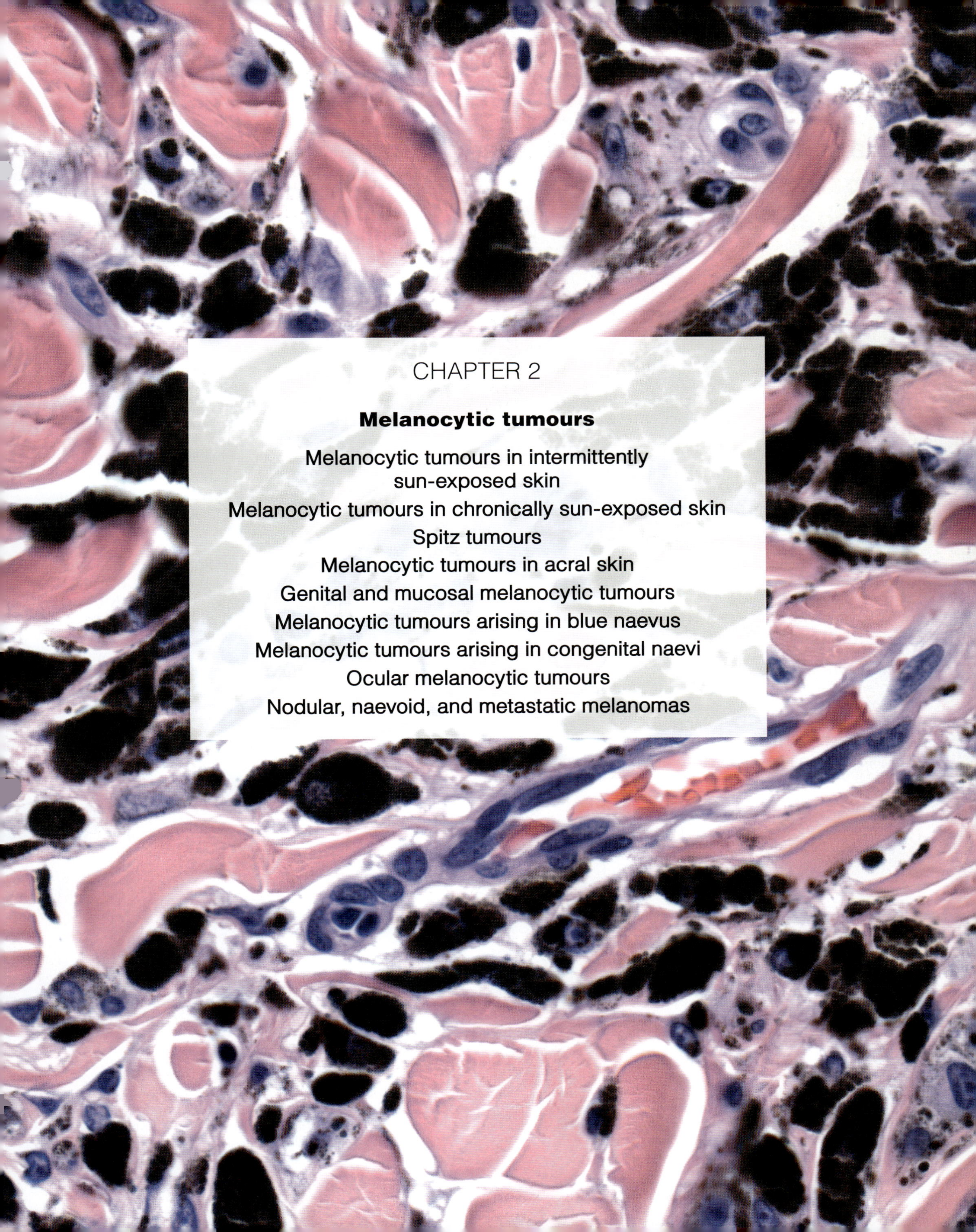

CHAPTER 2

# Melanocytic tumours

Melanocytic tumours in intermittently sun-exposed skin

Melanocytic tumours in chronically sun-exposed skin

Spitz tumours

Melanocytic tumours in acral skin

Genital and mucosal melanocytic tumours

Melanocytic tumours arising in blue naevus

Melanocytic tumours arising in congenital naevi

Ocular melanocytic tumours

Nodular, naevoid, and metastatic melanomas

# Melanocytic tumours: Introduction

## Melanocytic tumour classification and the pathway concept of melanoma pathogenesis

Elder D.E.
Barnhill R.L.
Bastian B.C.
Cook M.G.
de la Fouchardière A.
Gerami P.
Lazar A.J.
Massi D.
Mihm M.C. Jr
Nagore E.
Scolyer R.A.
Yun S.J.

### Clinical features

Despite the advent of large-scale and high-resolution genomics, the gold standard for melanoma diagnosis continues to be histopathology, which also remains the primary tool for classification, in conjunction with clinical characteristics. The clinicopathological classification was contemporaneously proposed by McGovern {1714} and Clark et al. {493}, and led to the recognition that melanomas evolve through stages of tumour progression, beginning as spreading patch- and plaque-like lesions in the epidermis and superficial dermis. Such lesions are considered to be in the radial growth phase (RGP), because they expand along the radii of an imperfect circle in the skin; the term "horizontal growth phase" has sometimes been used to describe the appearance in tissue sections. RGP melanomas (Fig. 2.01) have a good prognosis until deeper/thicker invasion of the dermis occurs with formation of a tumour mass, termed the vertical growth phase (VGP) (Fig. 2.02). Over time, it has been recognized that these melanomas may be associated with specific precursor lesions, some of which are intermediate (both morphologically and genomically) between wholly benign lesions and established melanomas {489,2394}.

Three major categories of melanoma were initially recognized, based on the presence or absence of the RGP and its variants: nodular melanoma is defined as a VGP melanoma without an identifiable RGP {493}; the initially recognized RGP variants were superficial spreading melanoma (also called pagetoid melanoma) and lentigo maligna melanoma. The distinctions between these categories were later supplemented by epidemiological and genomic observations, leading to the concept of alternative pathways in the development of melanoma {555,1524,1645,2813}. Of the two major pathways, which account for the majority of melanomas in populations with skin that is susceptible to solar damage, one (leading to superficial spreading melanoma and a subset of nodular melanoma) is associated with a low degree of cumulative sun damage (CSD) as assessed by the degree of solar elastosis on biopsy (see Fig. 2.03); the other pathway (leading to lentigo maligna melanoma and another subset of nodular melanoma) is associated with a high degree of CSD. Other melanomas (e.g. melanoma in acral skin or mucosa) arise via pathways in which solar damage does not appear to play any role.

Crucial observations related to genomic pathogenesis followed the seminal discovery of *BRAF* as a commonly mutated oncogene in melanoma {580}. BRAF p.V600 mutations (in particular p.V600E mutations) are the most frequently found oncogenic alterations in melanomas in skin with a low degree of CSD (low-CSD melanomas), whereas *NF1*, *NRAS*, other *BRAF* (non-p.V600E), and perhaps *KIT* mutations (all mutually exclusive) predominate in melanomas in skin with a high degree of CSD (high-CSD melanomas) {168,1445,2746}. The *TERT* promoter is commonly mutated at an early stage in melanoma evolution {2392}. Other oncogenes are more rarely involved, particularly in the melanomas occurring

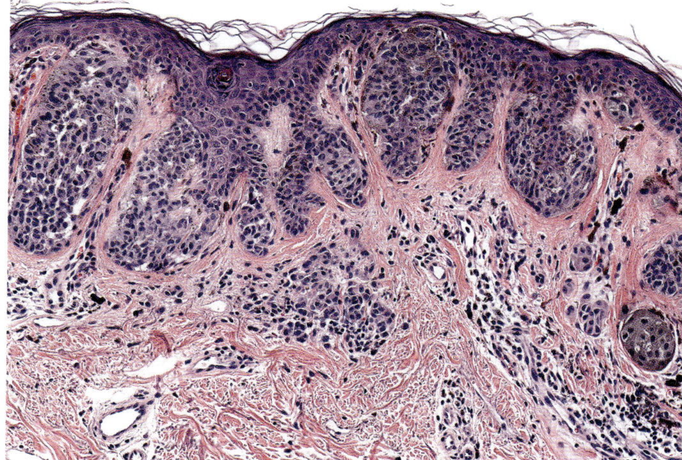

**Fig. 2.01** Superficial spreading melanoma, radial growth phase. There are atypical melanocytes with pagetoid scatter in the epidermis, as well as clusters of cells in the dermis resembling those in the epidermis and lacking evidence of tumorigenic proliferation or mitotic activity (see Table 2.02, p. 69).

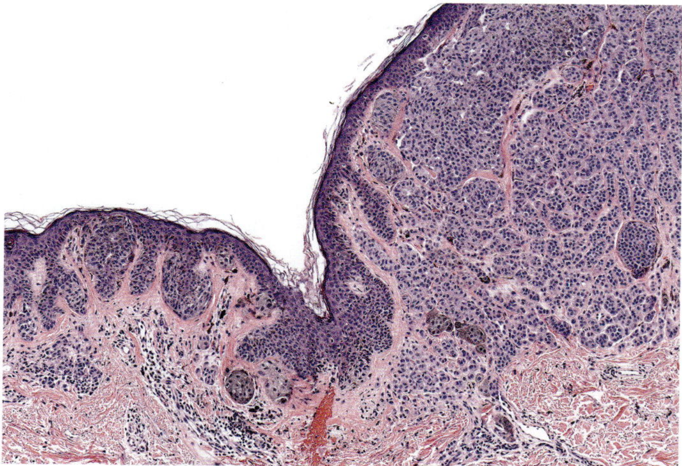

**Fig. 2.02** Superficial spreading melanoma, radial (also called horizontal) growth phase (RGP, left) and vertical growth phase (VGP, right). The VGP is composed of uniformly atypical cells that fill and expand the papillary dermis and infiltrate the reticular dermis, constituting a mass or so-called tumorigenic lesion. Unlike the cells of a naevus, these cells do not mature and do not disperse into the reticular dermis.

in sun-shielded sites. Tumour suppressor genes such as *CDKN2A* (encoding p16) are also implicated in melanoma pathogenesis {2392}. One group recently linked the concepts of tumour progression and evolutionary pathways by demonstrating that progression from benign lesions to advanced melanomas depends on sequential acquisition of abnormalities involving oncogenes and tumour suppressors, as well as other classes of genes {2394}; the study also provided a genomic definition of so-called intermediate lesions (such as dysplastic naevus), which had more than one genomic abnormality. Dysplastic naevus is characterized by cytological and architectural atypia, and is a potential precursor of melanoma, albeit with a very low individual lesion risk {680}. Other lesions in this category include deep penetrating naevus, pigmented epithelioid melanocytoma, and the *BAP1*-inactivated tumours, all of which can present as components of combined naevi and for which the consensus meeting Working Group proposes the general term "melanocytomas". See the relevant sections for detailed discussion.

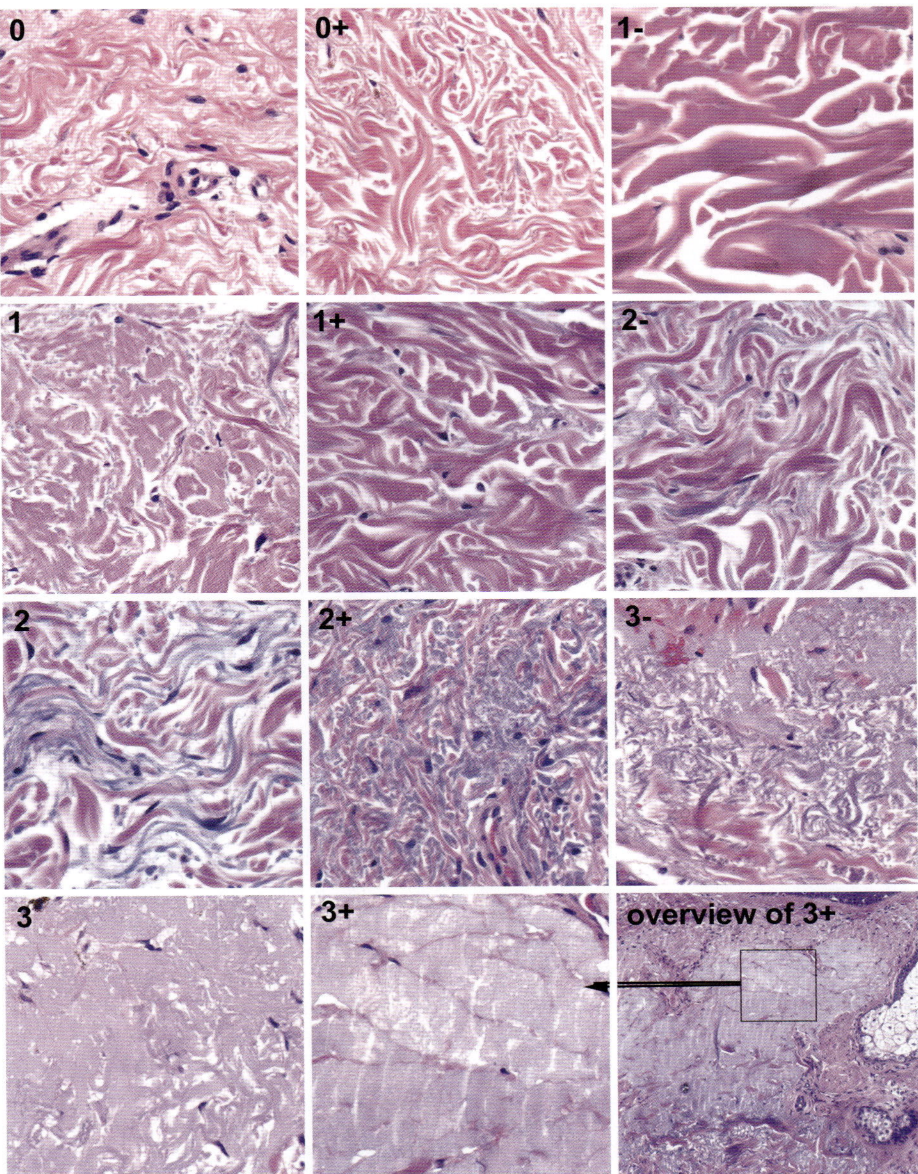


**Fig. 2.03** Grades of solar elastosis. Grade 1 is distinguished by the presence of single elastic fibres, grade 2 by bunches of fibres, and grade 3 by basophilic material that has lost its fibrillary texture.

### Multidimensional pathway classification

Bastian {168} has proposed a multidimensional classification for melanocytic lesions based on the role of ultraviolet (UV) radiation, the cell (or tissue) of origin, and characteristic recurrent genomic alterations. In biopsies, UV radiation exposure is assessed in terms of solar elastosis, as a measure of CSD (Fig. 2.03) {1486A}. Most melanomas in Northern Hemisphere populations occur in skin with either a low or high degree of CSD. But some types of melanoma occur in skin or mucous membranes either with no CSD or with variable CSD that is not considered to be etiologically relevant (e.g. because of the absence of UV radiation signature mutations), and these tumours account for the majority of melanomas in non-White populations, at a much lower absolute incidence rate. Non-malignant melanocytic tumours include both naevi/tumours that are wholly benign and lesions that are intermediate between benign tumours and melanomas. The benign lesions included in this category are neoplasms because they are clonal proliferations of cells with mutated oncogenes; they are potential precursors in many cases, and are also simulants of the corresponding melanomas, necessitating accurate diagnostic distinction. The pathways (or classes) of melanoma are listed in Table 2.01 (p. 68).

### Melanomas arising in sun-exposed skin

Epidemiologically, these melanomas are associated with sun exposure in susceptible individuals. Clinically and histologically, they are associated with varying degrees of CSD.

*Low-CSD melanoma (including superficial spreading melanoma and low-CSD nodular melanoma)*

Also known as pagetoid melanoma {1714}, this class of RGP lesions is associated epidemiologically with intermittent sun exposure in a relatively young age group, with a low to moderate degree of CSD in the affected skin. Naevi and dysplastic naevi are precursors and risk factors, as well as simulants. The use of tanning beds is also a significant risk factor, and has been associated with the occurrence of multiple superficial spreading melanomas at a young age {556}.

**Table 2.01** Classification of melanoma

| | | |
|---|---|---|
| Melanomas arising in sun-exposed skin | **Pathway I**: | Low-CSD melanoma/superficial spreading melanoma |
| | **Pathway II**: | High-CSD melanoma/lentigo maligna melanoma |
| | **Pathway III**: | Desmoplastic melanoma |
| Melanomas arising at sun-shielded sites or without known etiological associations with UV radiation exposure | **Pathway IV**: | Malignant Spitz tumour (Spitz melanoma) |
| | **Pathway V**: | Acral melanoma |
| | **Pathway VI**: | Mucosal melanoma |
| | **Pathway VII**: | Melanoma arising in congenital naevus |
| | **Pathway VIII**: | Melanoma arising in blue naevus |
| | **Pathway IX**: | Uveal melanoma |

Low/high-CSD melanoma, melanoma in skin with a low/high degree of cumulative sun damage.
Various: Nodular, naevoid, and metastatic melanomas.

These lesions are defined by the patterns of RGP; a VGP may or may not be present. Histopathologically, there is nested proliferation and pagetoid scatter of large neoplastic cells with prominent pigmentation; genomically, BRAF p.V600 mutations predominate {1524,1645,2746,2813}. A subset of nodular melanomas also belong in this category, probably arising as a pure VGP in a telescoped RGP (i.e. short-lived and overwhelmed by the rapidly growing nodule), and the same applies to all the RGP categories. Nodular melanoma (defined by a VGP without an RGP) is discussed along with its simulants (naevoid melanoma and cutaneous metastatic melanoma) in the *Nodular, naevoid, and metastatic melanomas* section (p. 145).

*High-CSD melanoma (including lentigo maligna melanoma and high-CSD nodular melanoma)*

Associations include chronic sun exposure in an older age group, freckles/lentigines, and Fitzpatrick skin type I/II as risk factors; lentiginous proliferation of the neoplastic cells in the RGP; neoplastic cells that may appear smaller with minimal cytoplasm and less pigment; and predominant mutations of *NF1*, *NRAS*, and perhaps *KIT* {1524,1645,2746,2813}. Rather than originating from naevi, these melanomas originate from melanoma in situ, which may overlap with indeterminate, often diagnostically uncertain, proliferations that may be precursors and are risk markers and simulants. High-CSD nodular melanoma may share attributes with the VGP of lentigo maligna melanoma.

*Desmoplastic melanoma*

This rare tumour is a VGP variant that may arise in an RGP of lentigo maligna type (associated with CSD) or less commonly of another lentiginous type, i.e. acral or mucosal melanoma (not associated with CSD). It can also arise de novo. In the CSD-associated lesions, there is a high mutation burden, with a very strong UV radiation signature {2392}; inactivating *NF1* mutations are common {2825}, and exome sequencing has identified recurrent *NFKBIE* promoter mutations and remarkably diverse activating mutations in the MAPK (ERK) pathway {2392}. The less common non-CSD desmoplastic melanomas are not expected to share these characteristics.

### Melanomas arising at sun-shielded sites or without known etiological associations with UV radiation exposure

These melanomas can occur in skin with or without CSD; they have no consistent relationship with sun exposure, which appears to have relatively little (or no) relevance to their pathogenesis.

*Malignant Spitz tumour (Spitz melanoma)*

The relationship of malignant Spitz tumours with benign Spitz naevi is uncertain, and diagnostic distinction from these simulants is often difficult. Histologically, the lesions are composed of large spindle and/or epithelioid melanocytes {1974}. These tumours occur in a younger age group than do most other melanomas, and they are usually less aggressive in terms of lethal behaviour than are similarly staged conventional melanomas. CSD is usually absent or minimal. Genetic alterations are also distinctive, including mutations in *HRAS* and kinase fusions in *ROS1*, *NTRK1*, *NTRK3*, *ALK*, *BRAF*, *MET*, and *RET*, as well as *TERT* promoter mutations in rare highly aggressive or lethal variants of Spitz melanoma {1532}. Certain variants are less stable than others. For example, *HRAS* mutation and copy-number gains are fairly common in benign Spitz naevi but very unusual in Spitz melanomas; in contrast, *BRAF* fusion is seen both in Spitz naevi and (less frequently, but on occasion) in Spitz melanomas {170,1383,2824,2882}. Homozygous 9p21 deletion in atypical Spitz tumours may be associated with clinically aggressive behaviour and death due to disease {872}.

*Acral melanoma (including nodular melanoma in acral skin)*

Risk factors may include trauma; there is no apparent etiological relationship with sun exposure {1251,1784}. CSD is typically absent. Acral melanomas typically begin as melanoma in situ (which can be subtle in its early phases), as a field of genomically unstable, clonally related melanocytes {169}. The relationship with other precursors is unclear; benign acral naevi are typically simulants rather than precursors. Acral melanomas are characterized histologically in the RGP, usually by lentiginous proliferation, whereas the VGP may be composed of spindle cells and may be desmoplastic. Genomically, these lesions have a comparatively low point-mutation burden and a high degree of copy-number variation, often with multiple amplifications of genes such as *CCND1*, *KIT*, and *TERT*, and mutations of *BRAF*, *NRAS*, and *KIT* among other oncogenes {554,555,839}. Some acral melanomas have kinase fusions of *ALK* {1912} or *RET* {2671}. Nodular melanoma in acral skin may share attributes with the VGP of acral melanoma.

*Mucosal melanoma*

These tumours have no etiological relationship with sun exposure. CSD is typically absent. Poorly defined lentiginous proliferations may be precursors and simulants. The VGP may be spindled and may be desmoplastic. The somatic-mutation burden is considerably lower than in melanoma arising in sun-exposed skin, with more numerous copy-number and structural variations. *KIT* and *NRAS* mutations have been described in a substantial proportion of tumours (varying by site), and *BRAF* mutations are relatively uncommon {554,555,838,2861}.

*Melanoma arising in congenital naevus*
The risk factors for congenital naevi are largely unknown, but there is no apparent etiological relationship with sun exposure. CSD is typically absent. Proliferations that occur in congenital naevi are simulants, and may be precursors. *NRAS* mutation is the predominant somatic event in giant congenital naevi {440}, as well as in the melanomas that arise therein, at least in childhood {180,1595}. Activating *TERT* promoter hypermethylation and promoter mutations are also common {731}. The genetic profile of small and medium congenital naevi is different, with a higher proportion of cases bearing *BRAF* mutations {180,440}; there is also an older age profile and a significant role for sun exposure in the melanomas that develop in small and medium congenital naevi.

*Melanoma arising in blue naevus*
The risk factors for blue naevi and the melanomas that arise in them are largely unknown, but there is no apparent etiological relationship with sun exposure. CSD is typically absent; if present, it can be regarded as an incidental finding. Blue naevi and cellular blue naevi are simulants and potential precursors. Their genetic alterations overlap extensively with those seen in uveal melanoma {2700}. Initiating mutations in the Gαq signalling pathway, mainly affecting the genes *GNAQ* and *GNA11*, are common to both blue naevi and their associated melanomas. Copy-number aberrations in aggressive variants include monosomy 3 (which is associated with loss of *BAP1*) and gains of chromosome 8q {1642,2394}. Additional secondary copy-number aberrations include mutations in *SF3B1* and *EIF1AX* {428,532}.

*Uveal melanoma*
There is no identified relationship with sun exposure, as evidenced by a low mutation burden with no clear UV radiation signature. Benign naevi are simulants and may be precursors. Mutations in the Gαq pathway affecting *GNAQ*, *GNA11*, *PLCB4*, and *CYSLTR2* predominate and are mutually exclusive {1232,1823,1823,2700}. *BAP1*, *SF3B1*, and *EIF1AX* mutations occur during tumour progression in an almost mutually exclusive manner and are associated with different levels of metastatic risk {1009,1670}. Similar biology is shared by leptomeningeal primary melanocytic tumours and by melanomas associated with blue naevi {588}.

**Table 2.02** Definitions of terms related to melanoma progression

| Term | Definition |
| --- | --- |
| **Radial growth phase (RGP)** | An atypical melanocytic proliferation confined to the epidermis and superficial dermis, meeting the criteria for melanoma (in situ or invasive), but lacking a VGP. |
| **Vertical growth phase (VGP)** | A melanocytic proliferation in the dermis characterized by expansile growth (tumorigenic proliferation) and/or mitotic activity, meeting the criteria for melanoma. In the limiting case, there is a nest in the dermis larger than the largest intraepidermal nest. In a lentiginous melanoma with no nests, this criterion is necessarily more subjective. |
| **Superficial atypical melanocytic proliferation of uncertain significance (SAMPUS)**[a] | An atypical melanocytic proliferation confined to the epidermis and superficial dermis, with features insufficient for definitive diagnosis but not ruling out RGP malignancy, lacking a tumorigenic VGP. |
| **Melanocytic tumour of uncertain malignant potential (MELTUMP)**[a] | An atypical melanocytic proliferation in the dermis that is tumorigenic but lacks the specific criteria needed to distinguish between benign and malignant proliferations. |
| **Intermediate lesion** | A junctional and sometimes also superficial dermal lesion considered to be benign or equivocal that is characterized by cytological and architectural atypia, intermediate between wholly benign and fully malignant lesions, and characterized genomically by mutations of two or more genes (but fewer than in fully evolved malignancy). |
| **Melanocytic neoplasm of low malignant potential (provisional)** | A proliferation that may fulfil traditional criteria for invasive melanoma but is not likely to be associated with melanoma-specific death. Provisionally, these lesions are thinner than 1 mm; lack a VGP, mitotic activity, ulceration, and regression; and occur in individuals aged < 55 years. |
| **Melanocytoma** | A tumorigenic neoplasm of melanocytes that generally has increased cellularity and/or atypia (compared with a common naevus) and an increased (although generally still low) probability of neoplastic progression. |

[a] The differential diagnosis and potentially applicable microstaging attributes should be described, and the terms should be written out in full.

## Paediatric melanoma

Knowledge concerning paediatric melanomas is important, in particular because of the propensity for both underdiagnosis and overdiagnosis of melanoma in this age group {155,2492}. Underdiagnosis can occur because of the rarity of paediatric melanomas, particularly in prepubertal children. Overdiagnosis can occur because of confusion with simulants of melanoma in this age group; for example, congenital naevi with pagetoid melanocytosis and proliferative nodules {2888}, spitzoid neoplasms, and special-site naevi (e.g. of the acral, scalp, and genital regions) {155,2492}. The histopathological criteria for the diagnosis of paediatric melanomas are essentially the same as those for the diagnosis of adult melanomas {155,2098}.

Patient age can be used to classify paediatric melanomas into two subtypes (which differ substantially with respect to prevalence, etiology, and histomorphology): prepubertal (congenital and childhood) paediatric melanomas occur in patients aged ≤ 10–12 years; postpubertal (adolescent) paediatric melanomas occur in patients aged between 10–12 years and 19 years. Prepubertal paediatric melanomas differ from adult melanomas in a number of important respects, including the increased frequency of melanomas originating from congenital naevi and spitzoid neoplasms, the increased frequency of *NRAS* mutations, and the limited role of UV radiation and *BRAF* mutations in these melanomas {130,1595}. There are four major histopathological subtypes:

*De novo melanomas*
These arise at birth or in prepubertal (and sometimes older) individuals; they commonly develop in the dermis,

**Table 2.03** The Melanocytic Pathology Assessment Tool and Hierarchy for Diagnosis (MPATH-Dx)/therapeutic classification of melanocytic tumours {2057}

| | |
|---|---|
| **Class 1** | Melanocytic tumours with very low risk of progression<br>(e.g. common and mildly dysplastic naevi)<br>No further treatment generally recommended[a] |
| **Class 2** | Melanocytic tumours with low (but currently unquantifiable) risk of progression<br>(e.g. Spitz naevus without atypia and moderately dysplastic naevi)<br>May warrant complete excision with narrow (e.g. < 5 mm) margins[a] |
| **Class 3** | Melanocytic tumours with higher risk of progression<br>(e.g. severely dysplastic naevi and melanoma in situ)<br>Usually warrants complete excision with wider (e.g. 5 mm) margins[a] |
| **Class 4** | AJCC stage pT1a and pT1b invasive melanomas<br>Usually warrants wide excision (e.g. 1 cm margins), with consideration of sentinel lymph node biopsy according to national guidelines[a] |
| **Class 5** | AJCC stage pT2 (or higher) invasive melanomas, posing higher risk of metastasis<br>Usually warrants wide excision (e.g. > 1 cm margins), additional prognostic/staging work-up (e.g. sentinel lymph node biopsy), and/or adjuvant therapy, according to national guidelines[a] |

AJCC, American Joint Committee on Cancer.

[a] The guidelines assume that the biopsy is representative and the margin is positive.

with an undifferentiated or so-called blast-like cytomorphology, and show small, medium, or large cell phenotypes {155,2098,2524}. These melanomas often develop rapidly and require immunohistochemical and molecular evaluation for distinction from other poorly differentiated or undifferentiated malignant neoplasms. Comparable melanomas are rare in adults. Some small cell melanomas in children may be indistinguishable from naevoid melanomas in adults {155}.

*Melanomas arising in congenital naevi*
These usually arise in large or giant congenital naevi, at birth, in childhood, or (sometimes) in older individuals {155,2098,2524}. These melanomas often develop in the dermis or subcutis. Comparable melanomas are seen in adults.

*Spitz melanomas*
These can arise in patients of any age.

*Conventional adult-type melanomas*
These usually have an epithelioid cell phenotype corresponding to the superficial spreading and nodular subtypes in adults {155,2098}.

## Prognostic classification

The prognosis of melanoma can be assessed in terms of prognostic attributes. The most commonly used attributes are those defined in the American Joint Committee on Cancer (AJCC)/Union for International Cancer Control (UICC) staging model {135}, which includes tumour thickness, ulceration, microscopic satellites, and mitotic rate (still recommended for inclusion in reports in the 2017 *AJCC Staging Manual*, 8th edition {68}). Other attributes that may be used in decision-making in specific circumstances include tumour-infiltrating lymphocytes, lymphovascular invasion (especially lymphatic invasion {1350}), perineural invasion, regression, and (to a lesser extent) Clark level of invasion and lesional location. Localized primary melanomas constitute TNM stages I and II; regional metastasis defines stage III, and non-regional metastasis defines stage IV. Stage 0 constitutes melanomas in situ, which generally have no capability to metastasize. For stage I (thickness < 1 mm) tumours, which are the most prevalent, the overall survival is excellent, with a 10-year survival rate of about 95%. However, within stage I, a subset of patients can be identified as being at greater risk, on the basis of unfavourable microstaging attributes. There is also a subset of stage I cases (accounting for ~40% of all cases) with an associated survival rate of essentially 100% {884}. These lesions are typically characterized by a low tumour thickness (< 0.8 mm) and an absence of mitoses, ulceration, and regression; they are confined to the RGP and Clark level II invasion; therefore, they often lack strong diagnostic features to distinguish them from precursor or simulant lesions (including dysplastic naevi), and the diagnostic reproducibility for such distinctions is poor {1592}. These lesions likely contribute to the overdiagnosis of melanoma, which has resulted in dramatic increases in incidence rates over the past several decades with little or no corresponding increase in mortality {2807}. Therefore, pending the results of future research and consensus, it may be appropriate to consider using alternative terminology for these lesions, which could be regarded as severe dysplasias; by analogy with other tumour systems, they could also be termed "melanocytic proliferations of low malignant potential".

## Diagnostic reproducibility

Despite best efforts to provide clear criteria for diagnosis, there is evidence that pathologists use diagnostic terms differently depending on individual, local, and regional practices and the influence of different schools of thought {682}. In addition, the reproducibility of diagnoses between pathologists is poor, especially for intermediate lesions and melanocytic neoplasms of low malignant potential {684}. This can result in uncertainty as to the most appropriate management for different lesions, especially when patients are referred between centres with different practice patterns. The consensus meeting Working Group supports the use of descriptive and provisional terminology for lesions that are characterized by conflicting criteria; such terms may include "superficial atypical melanocytic proliferation of uncertain significance (SAMPUS)" and "intraepidermal atypical melanocytic proliferation of uncertain significance (IAMPUS)" for lesions whose differential diagnosis is limited to thin non-mitogenic and non-tumorigenic RGP and to melanoma in situ, respectively. These terms are applicable for diagnostically problematic lesions whose differential diagnosis could include a melanoma with essentially no potential for metastasis, but perhaps with potential for local persistence, recurrence, and progression if not completely excised. These lesions have a very good prognosis following excision. In this context, "of uncertain significance" means with risk of local regrowth and further progression. The term "melanocytic tumour of uncertain malignant potential (MELTUMP)" can be used for tumorigenic lesions whose differential diagnosis includes VGP melanoma as a leading consideration (see the definitions listed in Table 2.02). "Malignant potential" in this context means risk of metastasis and potential death from disease even after complete excision. These lesions can occur via any of the pathways described above. It is therefore recommended that the above provisional terms for intermediate or indeterminate lesions be used with reference to the respective pathway; for example, "MELTUMP intermediate between blue naevus and melanoma arising in blue naevus" (or one or the other may be favoured). For clarity, the acronyms specified above should always be spelled out in formal reports. In general, the treatment of these cases should be planned with the differential diagnosis of melanoma taken into consideration, and staging attributes should be supplied {682}. The terms discussed here should not be used to completely replace the descriptive terminology, which may in due course achieve higher levels of observer agreement and therefore be more valuable. In terms of the behaviour codes of the ICD-O classification, benign neoplasms are coded /0; intermediate neoplasms (including SAMPUS, IAMPUS, and MELTUMP) are coded /1; the provisional category of melanocytic neoplasms of low malignant potential and melanomas in situ are coded /2; and invasive melanomas are coded /3.

### Management-based classification

One of the most important uses of a diagnosis is to guide management. The specific diagnosis is particularly important for melanomas, but also guides the management of intermediate lesions that have been incompletely excised; in general, these lesions should be completely removed in order to enable full histological evaluation and to minimize the potential for local persistence, recurrence, and progression. In terms of accuracy and reproducibility, the diagnosis of intermediate lesions is challenging using current criteria, and there is considerable variation in the use of terminology across institutions {684,1592,2057}. The Melanocytic Pathology Assessment Tool and Hierarchy for Diagnosis (MPATH-Dx) schema has been proposed in an effort to reduce uncertainty and promote consistent management practices, and its efficacy has been evaluated {684,1592,2057}. In addition to a traditional text-based diagnosis, this schema proposes the additional categorization of each case into one of five classes based on treatment options (see Table 2.03). This classification is designed to offer guidelines for consideration, but not mandatory standards of care, given that pathologists are not likely to be aware of all the factors that may influence management in individual cases. These are general guidelines that should be interpreted in accordance with local and national standards where such standards exist, and clinical factors should also be considered. In most countries, there are formal evidence-based national guidelines for classes 3–5 (the melanomas) {511}, but not for classes 1 and 2. Therefore, these guidelines do not impact the current recommendations for management of melanomas, but are intended to guide the management of benign tumours (including intermediate lesions), which are associated with the most diagnostic difficulty and inconsistency.

# Genomic landscape of melanoma

Bastian B.C.
de la Fouchardière A.
Elder D.E.
Gerami P.
Lazar A.J.
Massi D.
Nagore E.
Scolyer R.A.
Yun S.J.

Like other cancers, melanomas arise through the accumulation of mutations that constitutively activate growth-promoting signalling pathways and ablate tumour-suppressive mechanisms. The mutational mechanisms causing these genetic alterations vary considerably, depending on the type of melanoma. Melanomas arising in skin with some degree of cumulative sun damage (CSD) harbour an extraordinarily high number of point mutations, mostly cytosine to thymidine (C>T) transitions at dipyrimidine sites, a hallmark of ultraviolet (UV) radiation–induced mutations {867}. Melanomas in skin with a high degree of CSD (high-CSD melanomas) carry the highest mutation burdens, and rank among the most highly mutated cancers overall, with approximately 100 000 somatic mutations per genome (equivalent to 30 mutations/Mb of DNA) {1445}. This rate is exceeded only in desmoplastic melanomas, which have a median of 62 mutations/Mb {2392}. Melanomas in skin with a low degree of CSD (low-CSD melanomas) have about 15 mutations/Mb. In contrast, melanomas arising in the glabrous skin, nail apparatus, or mucous membranes have low mutation burdens, typically without a UV radiation signature. Instead, these melanomas are characterized by abundant copy-number changes, including multiple high-level amplifications {555}. Unlike in other solid tumours, these amplifications arise early on in the melanomas' progression and appear to be the dominant force shaping their genomes. Uveal melanomas, as well as the likely closely biologically related melanomas arising in blue naevus and primary melanomas of the CNS, also have a very low mutation burden, but lack the highly rearranged genomes of acral and mucosal melanomas (see Table 2.04) {168}.

In cutaneous melanomas, genetic alterations disrupt a common set of key signalling pathways. These include the MAPK pathway, which is activated by mutations of the upstream receptor at the level of KIT, RAS family members acting immediately downstream of receptors, negative regulators of RAS (e.g. NF1, RASA2, and SPRED1), and RAS effectors acting further downstream (e.g. BRAF, MEK, and cyclin D1). Alterations in the genes encoding these proteins tend to be mutually exclusive of each other in untreated melanomas, but they can co-occur in melanomas after targeted therapy and contribute to resistance to therapy. The G1/S checkpoint is also a common target of mutations, which override its ability to restrain cell-cycle entry. Inactivation of *CDKN2A* (encoding p16) by deletion or mutation is very common in cutaneous melanomas; alternative events in melanoma progression include amplification or mutation of *CDK4* (which encodes p16's target kinase) and loss of RB1. These alterations are infrequent in uveal melanoma. *CDKN2A* and *CDK4* mutations are also seen in the form of germline alterations, which predispose individuals to melanoma with high penetrance {2090}.

Other signalling pathways recurrently mutated in melanomas include pathways implicated in chromatin modifications, such as those related to the SWI/SNF chromatin remodelling complex {867,1098,2393} (affecting genes such as *ARID2*, *ARID1A*, and *EZH2*), and inactivation of the histone modifier *BAP1*, which is a frequent event in uveal melanoma {1009}.

The most common mutations in cutaneous melanomas are found in the *TERT* promoter {1141}; these cause increased expression of telomerase, resulting in cell immortalization by extension of the replicative lifespan of cells, allowing them to avoid replicative senescence in response to critical telomere shortening. Germline mutations of the *TERT* promoter and other genes encoding proteins involved in telomere maintenance (e.g. *POT1*, *ACD*, and *TERF2IP*) result in longer telomeres and are another cause of melanoma susceptibility {2090}.

Although the melanoma subtypes share alterations in these pathways, the manner in which the pathways are deregulated shows considerable variation among the

**Table 2.04** Characteristic attributes of various types of melanomas

| Attribute | Type of melanoma | | | | |
|---|---|---|---|---|---|
| | High-CSD | Low-CSD | Acral/mucosal | Uveal | Spitz |
| Mutation burden | Very high | High | Low | Very low | Probably low |
| UV radiation signature | Strong | Strong | Absent | Absent | Variable |
| DNA copy-number changes | Multiple | Multiple | Numerous | Few | Multiple |
| Type of aberrations | Typically chromosomal arms or entire chromosomes | Typically chromosomal arms or entire chromosomes | Multiple focused amplifications and deletions | Typically chromosomal arms or entire chromosomes | Typically chromosomal arms or entire chromosomes |

High/low-CSD melanoma, melanoma in skin with a high/low degree of cumulative sun damage.

**Table 2.05** Genetic alterations within common signalling pathways in various types of melanomas; the affected genes are listed in order of frequency

| Pathway(s) | Type of melanoma | | | | |
|---|---|---|---|---|---|
| | High-CSD | Low-CSD | Acral/mucosal | Uveal | Spitz |
| MAPK pathway activation | *NF1* (loss), *NRAS*, *BRAF* (non-p.V600E), *KIT* | *BRAF* (p.V600E), *NRAS* | *NRAS*, *KIT*, *NF1* (loss), *SPRED1* (loss), *BRAF* (p.V600E), *CCND1* (amplification); kinase fusions of *ALK*, *ROS1*, *RET*, *NTRK1* | *GNAQ*, *GNA11*, *CYSLTR2*, *PLCB4* | *HRAS*; fusions of *ROS1*, *NTRK1*, *NTRK3*, *ALK*, *RET*, *MET*, *BRAF* |
| G1/S checkpoint | *CDKN2A* (loss) | *CDKN2A* (loss) | *CDKN2A* (loss), *CDK4* (amplification) | | *CDKN2A* (loss) |
| p53 pathway | *CDKN2A* (loss), *TP53* | *CDKN2A* (loss), *TP53* | *CDKN2A* (loss), *TP53* | | *CDKN2A* (loss) |
| Chromatin modifiers | SWI/SNF | SWI/SNF | SWI/SNF | *BAP1* | |
| Other alterations | *TERT* (promoter mutations) | *TERT* (promoter mutations) | *TERT* (amplification) | *SF3B1*, *EIF1AX* | *TERT* (promoter mutations) |

High/low-CSD melanoma, melanoma in skin with a high/low degree of cumulative sun damage.

subtypes (see Table 2.05). In low-CSD melanomas, BRAF p.V600E mutations account for the majority of MAPK pathway–activating mutations. In contrast, high-CSD melanomas rarely harbour BRAF p.V600E mutations, but instead have other *BRAF* mutations or (more frequently) loss-of-function mutations in *NF1* or activating mutations of *NRAS* or occasionally *KIT*. These differences in genetic alterations, along with the different age distributions (low-CSD melanomas tend to arise in younger individuals) and the associations with different precursors (low-CSD melanomas often arise in naevi; high-CSD melanomas do not), gave rise to the dual pathway hypothesis and the proposal to classify these melanoma types into two separate categories, broadly corresponding to the traditional subtypes of superficial spreading melanoma and lentigo maligna melanoma {1645,2813}.

Uveal melanoma stands out in that it has Gαq signalling pathway mutations, most (~90%) of which affect two closely related genes, *GNAQ* and *GNA11*, which encode α-subunits of heterotrimeric G proteins. Less commonly, mutations affect the G protein–coupled receptor CYSLTR2 (which signals through Gαq) or *PLCB4* (which encodes the Gαq effector phospholipase Cβ4). Additional mutations that coincide with malignant progression to melanoma are inactivating mutations in the histone deubiquitinase *BAP1* and mutations that change the function of the splicing factor SF3B1 or the translation elongation factor EIF1AX. *GNAQ* or *GNA11* mutations, followed by progression mutations in *BAP1*, *EIF1AX*, or *SF3B1*, are also found in melanomas arising in blue naevus, as well as in primary leptomeningeal melanomas and melanocytomas {1468,1849,2699,2700}. The similarities between the genetic alterations found in uveal melanoma, melanoma arising in blue naevus, and leptomeningeal melanomas gave rise to the proposal that these melanomas represent a clade of closely biologically related tumours that originate from a developmentally distinct type of melanocyte that does not reside within an epithelial structure {168}.

The multiple pathogenic mutations found in fully evolved melanomas arise in a typical sequence. Benign naevi typically harbour a single MAPK pathway mutation, such as a BRAF p.V600E mutation (in acquired naevi) {2077}; an *NRAS* mutation (in congenital and some acquired naevi) {386}; an *HRAS* mutation {170} or a kinase fusion of *ALK*, *BRAF*, *ROS1*, *NTRK1*, *NTRK3*, *MET*, or *RET* {279,2824,2882,2886} (in Spitz naevi); or a *GNAQ* or *GNA11* mutation (in blue naevi), but no additional mutations. Therefore, these mutations, as a single event, appear to be sufficient for naevus initiation, at least in some individuals {2394}, but the proliferation of their constituent cells is limited by several mechanisms subsumed under the term "senescence". The clonal expansion of these partially transformed melanocytes increases the likelihood that one of them acquires an additional pathogenic mutation that overrides one or more mechanisms that constrain unlimited proliferation in naevi. Such a mutation then leads to a further clonal expansion of the cell that acquired the new mutation, with increasing risk of additional mutations. This process has been exemplified in atypical spitzoid proliferations arising in common acquired naevi (typically harbouring BRAF p.V600E mutations) in which biallelic loss of *BAP1* in one of the *BRAF*-mutant cells of the acquired naevus results in the formation of a second clone of larger epithelioid cells that are *BRAF*-mutant and *BAP1* null {2827}.

Naevi can thus be melanoma precursors because they are composed of partially transformed melanocytes that already harbour one of the multiple mutations required for melanoma formation. The numerical expansion of the original melanocyte that first acquired the oncogenic mutation into hundreds of thousands of daughter cells carrying the same mutation then increases the probability of one of those cells acquiring an additional pathogenic mutation on top of the first one. UV irradiation of naevus cells is the major driver generating these secondary and subsequent mutations that ultimately lead to melanoma {2394}.

Categories of neoplasms are now emerging that have more pathogenic mutations than found in benign naevi and fewer mutations than found in melanomas; the atypical spitzoid proliferations with

**Table 2.06** Classification of melanomas and precursor lesions on the basis of epidemiological, clinical, pathological, and genomic attributes

| | Low UV radiation exposure/CSD | | | | High UV radiation exposure/CSD | |
|---|---|---|---|---|---|---|
| **Pathway** | I | | | | II | III |
| **Endpoint of pathway** | Low-CSD melanoma/SSM | | | | High-CSD melanoma/LMM | Desmoplastic melanoma |
| **Benign neoplasms (naevi)** | Naevus | | | | ?<br>IMP | ?<br>IMP |
| **Intermediate/low-grade dysplasias and melanocytomas** | Low-grade dysplasia | BIN | DPN | | ?<br>IAMP/dysplasia | ?<br>IAMP/dysplasia |
| **Intermediate/high-grade dysplasias and melanocytomas** | High-grade dysplasia/MIS | *BAP1*-inactivated melanocytoma/ MELTUMP | Deep penetrating melanocytoma/ MELTUMP | PEM/MELTUMP | Lentigo maligna (MIS) | MIS |
| **Malignant neoplasms** | Low-CSD melanoma/SSM (VGP) | Melanoma in BIN (rare) | Melanoma in DPN (rare) | Melanoma in PEM (rare) | LMM (VGP) | Desmoplastic melanoma |
| **Common mutations**[a,b] | **BRAF p.V600E** or ***NRAS***<br><br>*TERT*; *CDKN2A*; *TP53*; *PTEN* | ***BRAF*** or ***NRAS*** + ***BAP1*** | ***BRAF***, ***MAP2K1***, or ***NRAS*** + ***CTNNB1*** or ***APC*** | ***BRAF*** + ***PRKAR1A*** or ***PRKCA*** | ***NRAS***; **BRAF (non-p.V600E)**; ***KIT***; or *NF1*<br><br>*TERT*; *CDKN2A*; *TP53*; *PTEN*; *RAC1* | ***NF1***; *ERBB2*; *MAP2K1*; *MAP3K1*; *BRAF*; *EGFR*; *MET*<br><br>*TERT*; *NFKBIE*; *NRAS*; *PIK3CA*; *PTPN11* |

**BIN**, *BAP1*-inactivated naevus; **BN**, blue naevus; **CBN**, cellular blue naevus; **CN**, congenital naevus; **CSD**, cumulative sun damage; **DPN**, deep penetrating naevus; **IAMP**, intraepidermal atypical melanocytic proliferation; **IAMPUS**, intraepidermal atypical melanocytic proliferation of uncertain significance; **IMP**, intraepidermal melanocytic proliferation without atypia; **LMM**, lentigo maligna melanoma; low/high-CSD melanoma, melanoma in skin with a low/high degree of cumulative sun damage; **MELTUMP**, melanocytic tumour of uncertain malignant potential; **MIS**, melanoma in situ; **PEM**, pigmented epithelioid melanocytoma; **SSM**, superficial spreading melanoma; **STUMP**, spitzoid tumour of uncertain malignant potential; **UV**, ultraviolet; **VGP**, vertical growth phase (tumorigenic and/or mitogenic melanoma).

*BAP1* mutations mentioned above are one example. A recent study identified a genetically intermediate state in a subset of preneoplastic lesions adjacent to primary melanomas {2394}. These areas were classified as ambiguous by multiple pathologists, and interobserver agreement was significantly lower than for lesions with only one oncogenic alteration. These observations challenge the notion that melanocytic neoplasms can be only either benign or malignant, and indicate that a biologically intermediate progression stage exists, encompassing junctional and superficial dermal lesions that are benign but atypical/ dysplastic, as well as melanoma in situ. Also included in this category are lesions such as *BAP1*-inactivated naevus, deep penetrating naevus, and pigmented epithelioid melanocytoma, which form papulonodular tumorigenic dermal proliferations; for these lesions, the consensus meeting Working Group proposes the general term "melanocytomas". Additional studies are needed to determine the histopathological correlates and the risk of recurrence and progression of lesions within this category, such as superficial atypical melanocytic proliferation of uncertain significance (SAMPUS) and melanocytic tumour of uncertain malignant potential (MELTUMP), introduced in the previous section.

The landscape of genomic abnormalities in the context of UV radiation exposure, CSD, and precursor lesions is presented in Table 2.06.

| Low to no (or variable/incidental) UV radiation exposure / CSD | | | | | |
|---|---|---|---|---|---|
| **IV** | **V** | **VI** | **VII** | **VIII** | **IX** |
| Malignant Spitz tumour / Spitz melanoma | Acral melanoma | Mucosal melanoma | Melanoma in CN | Melanoma in BN | Uveal melanoma |
| Spitz naevus | ? Acral naevus | ? Melanosis | CN | Blue naevus | ? Naevus |
| Atypical Spitz tumour (melanocytoma) | IAMP / dysplasia | Atypical melanosis / dysplasia / IAMPUS | Nodule in CN (melanocytoma) | (Atypical) CBN (melanocytoma) | ? |
| STUMP / MELTUMP | Acral MIS | Mucosal MIS | MIS in CN | Atypical CBN | ? |
| Malignant Spitz tumour/ Spitz melanoma (tumorigenic) | Acral melanoma (VGP) | Mucosal lentiginous melanoma (VGP) | Melanoma in CN (tumorigenic) | Melanoma in blue naevus (tumorigenic) | Uveal melanoma |
| ***HRAS***; ***ALK***; ***ROS1***; ***RET***; ***NTRK1***; ***NTRK3***; ***BRAF***; or ***MET*** | ***KIT***; ***NRAS***; ***BRAF***; ***HRAS***; ***KRAS***; ***NTRK3***; ***ALK***; or ***NF1*** | ***KIT***, ***NRAS***, ***KRAS***, or ***BRAF*** | ***NRAS***; **BRAF p.V600E** (small lesions); or ***BRAF*** | ***GNAQ***; ***GNA11***; or ***CYSLTR2*** | ***GNAQ***, ***GNA11***, ***CYSLTR2***, or ***PLCB4*** |
| *CDKN2A* | *CDKN2A*; *TERT*; *CCND1*; *GAB2* | ***NF1***; *CDKN2A*; *SF3B1*; *CCND1*; *CDK4*; *MDM2* | | *BAP1*; *EIF1AX*; *SF3B1* | *BAP1*; *SF3B1*; *EIF1AX* |

Definitions: *Melanocytoma* is a tumorigenic neoplasm of melanocytes that generally has increased cellularity and/or atypia (compared with a common naevus) and an increased (although generally still low) probability of neoplastic progression; *tumorigenic* means forming a mass of neoplastic cells.

[a] Common mutations in each pathway are listed; mutations already identified in benign or borderline low lesions are shown in bold.
[b] Blue, loss-of-function mutation; red, gain-of-function mutation; green, change-of-function mutation; orange, amplification; purple, rearrangement; grey, promoter mutation.

# Melanocytic tumours in intermittently sun-exposed skin

## Low-CSD melanoma (superficial spreading melanoma)

Duncan L.M.
Bastian B.C.
Elder D.E.
Mihm M.C. Jr

### Definition

Low-CSD melanoma – melanoma in skin with a low degree of cumulative sun damage (CSD) as assessed by the degree of solar elastosis – is characterized by pagetoid and/or lentiginous intraepidermal components {492,493}; both of these major patterns are encompassed by the term "superficial spreading melanoma (SSM)". Melanomas arising via other pathways (e.g. melanoma arising in blue naevus) can occasionally also occur in low-CSD skin and should be interpreted accordingly.

### ICD-O code

8743/3

### Synonyms

Superficial spreading melanoma; non-CSD melanoma

### Epidemiology

Low-CSD melanomas/SSMs account for nearly two thirds of cases occurring in lighter-skinned people (Fitzpatrick skin type I–III), and they are significantly less common in darker-skinned people. Males and females are affected similarly.

### Etiology

Low-CSD melanoma/SSM is epidemiologically linked to sun exposure, and genomic analyses have revealed a high mutation burden with an ultraviolet (UV) radiation mutation signature {1094}. Repeated sunburns in childhood and intermittent sun exposure throughout life are associated with an increased risk of developing SSM. Tanning bed use has been linked to an increased rate of melanoma in young women {1508}.

### Localization

Low-CSD melanoma/SSM can occur at any cutaneous site, but is most common in locations with intermittent sun exposure, including women's legs and men's backs and shoulders.

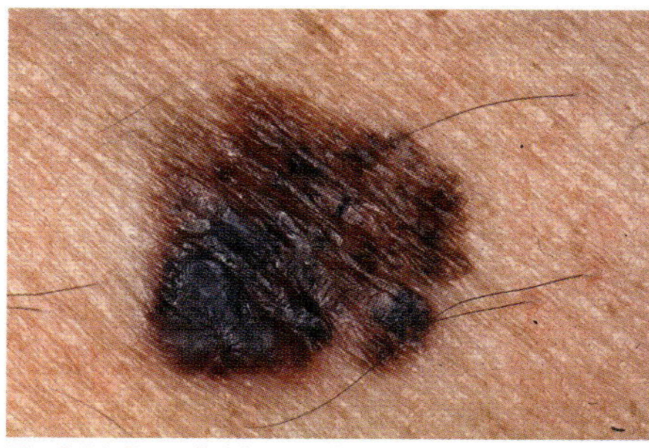

**Fig. 2.04** Superficial spreading melanoma. This tumour has a radial-growth-phase component (plaque-like, predominantly tan, at the upper-right of the lesion) and a tumorigenic vertical growth phase (raised, predominantly black in this example).

### Clinical features

In situ, low-CSD melanoma/SSM occurs as a pigmented macule with an irregular outline; with the onset of invasion, a papule or plaque develops. The borders of SSM are usually sharply delimited from the surrounding skin, but may be poorly defined. The pigmentation is quite variable; multiple shades of brown are often seen, ranging from tan to nearly black. There may be white areas corresponding to regression, and red foci correlate with increased vascularity and inflammation. Occasionally, the melanoma may be amelanotic and mimic a keratinocytic neoplasm, but more commonly, pigment is present (often to a marked degree). The radial growth phase (RGP) may reach > 1 cm in diameter before developing an invasive component. Dermal invasion often presents as a papule, which rarely may ulcerate and bleed. In rare cases, satellite metastases occur in close proximity to the primary tumour. Most cases are asymptomatic, but some patients experience itching, ulceration with oozing, crusting, and bleeding.

### Histopathology

In the pagetoid pattern of melanoma in situ, there is an intraepidermal proliferation of individual cells at many levels of the epidermis and variably sized nests along the dermoepidermal junction. The atypical melanocytes have large nuclei, irregularly clumped or dense chromatin, prominent nucleoli, and eosinophilic or lightly pigmented cytoplasm. A confluence of intraepidermal nests and

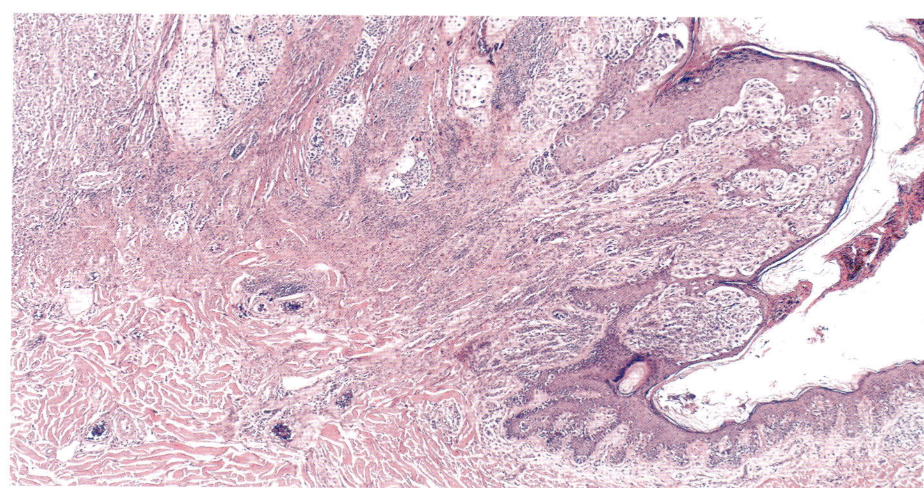

**Fig. 2.05** Superficial spreading melanoma. Individual cells and nests are present at all levels of the epidermis and extend as a shoulder beyond the invasive dermal tumour. A benign naevus is present in the epidermis and dermis (lower right).

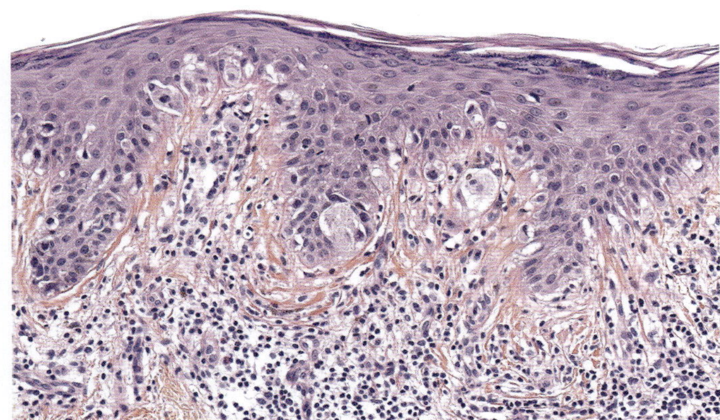

**Fig. 2.06** Low-CSD melanoma. Lentiginous junctional proliferation of large atypical melanocytes with a pigmented cytoplasm without pagetoid scatter (in this instance).

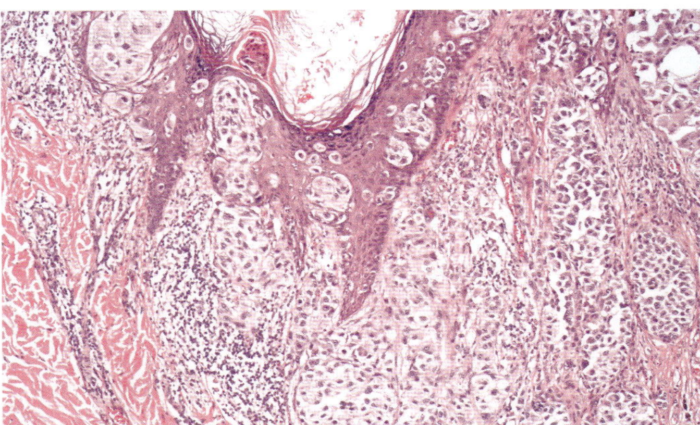

**Fig. 2.07** Superficial spreading melanoma. The dermal invasive melanoma has cytological features similar to those of the intraepidermal tumour cells. Individual cells in the epidermis display a pagetoid growth pattern.

prominent so-called buck-shot pagetoid spread is seen. Slight epidermal hyperplasia is associated with the intraepidermal tumour. Occasionally, the tumour cells may extend down hair follicle epithelium or eccrine ducts. In the lentiginous pattern of low-CSD melanomas, there is a predominance of smaller cells, with less or no pagetoid scatter, and fewer nests; these cases are distinguishable from lentigo maligna and are included within the general category of low-CSD melanoma (SSM).

Invasive low-CSD melanoma/SSM presents as a dermal proliferation of cytologically atypical melanocytes with features resembling those seen in the overlying in situ tumour. The melanoma may invade as only a few scattered cells in the superficial papillary dermis without mitotic activity (invasive RGP), or may form expansile nests larger than those seen in the epidermis, often with mitoses (vertical growth phase; VGP). A lymphocytic infiltrate may be present along the advancing margin of the VGP or throughout the VGP (brisk tumour-infiltrating lymphocytes), or there may be patchy infiltration of the VGP (non-brisk tumour-infiltrating lymphocytes) or no lymphocytic infiltration of the VGP (absent tumour-infiltrating lymphocytes). The lesions may be ulcerated. Microscopic satellite metastases may be seen in the dermis. Lymphovascular invasion, when present, can be confirmed using combined D2-40 and S100 staining. Regression may occur in the RGP, with a focal absence of tumour in the epidermis and dermis flanked by tumour in the epidermis and dermis; the dermis in the intervening area devoid of tumour has rich vascularity, stromal oedema, and pigment-laden macrophages.

## Differential diagnosis

The differential diagnosis of the pagetoid form of low-CSD melanoma/SSM in situ includes Paget disease, carcinoma in situ, spitzoid neoplasms, and other tumours that may display a pagetoid intraepidermal growth pattern. On immunohistochemical evaluation, the tumour cells in melanoma in situ stain positively for the melanocytic markers SOX10 and MITF. Staining for other melanocytic markers also highlights the intraepidermal tumour in melanoma, but may highlight other intraepidermal structures as well, including pigment in keratinocytes (e.g. HMB45 antigen and melan-A) and Langerhans cells (e.g. S100 protein). The dermal component in low-CSD melanoma is composed of cytologically atypical melanocytes that are usually mitotically active and display minimal reduction in nuclear size or amount of cytoplasm, with increased dermal depth; this is distinct from the maturation seen in the dermal component of naevi. Mitoses are rarely observed in benign naevi. The few rare types of benign naevi that display mitoses are not associated with an overlying/adjacent RGP.

## Histogenesis

A benign naevus is found in association with SSM in approximately 30% of cases {1564}.

## Genetic profile

BRAF p.V600E mutations are the most common mutations known to activate the MAPK pathway in melanoma, and they are the earliest pathogenic mutations identified in > 50% of low-CSD melanomas/SSMs and associated naevi {1645}. *TERT* promoter mutations are found in the majority of SSMs. Mutation of *CDKN2A*, which encodes p16 (p16INK4a) is common in SSM, and biallelic inactivation of *CDKN2A* is limited to invasive melanomas {934}. *PTEN* and *TP53* mutations occur in advanced primary melanomas. The point-mutation burden increases with tumour progression from naevus to melanoma; a UV radiation signature is detectable at all stages {2394}. Chromosomal abnormalities are common, most often involving loss at chromosomes 9, 10, 6q, and 20, and gains of chromosomes 1q, 6p, 7, 8q, 17q, and 20q {171}.

## Genetic susceptibility

Melanoma susceptibility genes include *CDKN2A*, *CDK4*, and several genes of the shelterin complex, which plays a role in telomere maintenance.

## Prognosis and predictive factors

The prognosis of low-CSD melanoma/SSM does not differ significantly from that of other forms of cutaneous melanoma. Predictive factors include tumour thickness, ulceration, mitogenicity, tumour-infiltrating lymphocytes, lymphovascular invasion, and microscopic satellites.

# Simple lentigo and lentiginous melanocytic naevus

Wick M.R.
Elenitsas R.
Kim J.
Kossard S.

## Definition

Simple lentigo and lentiginous melanocytic naevus are typically pigmented macules, and may represent early stages in the development of so-called ordinary melanocytic naevi. In simple lentigo (also called lentigo simplex), an increased number of melanocytes is seen at the basal layer, but no junctional nests of such cells are evident {1545}. In contrast, lentiginous junctional melanocytic naevus does contain small melanocytic nests at the epidermal base, as well as lentiginous single-cell melanocytic proliferation. Lentiginous compound naevi additionally contain small groups of lesional melanocytes in the papillary dermis {2460}.

## ICD-O code

Simple lentigo and lentiginous melanocytic naevus 8742/0

## Synonyms

Jentigo; naevus incipiens

## Epidemiology

Simple lentigines and acquired melanocytic naevi (of which lentiginous melanocytic naevus is an example) are predominantly seen in White populations; people of colour develop them much less commonly. Typically, the lesions first appear around the age of 2 years, and accrue steadily thereafter. Risk factors include fair skin (commonly with red hair, blue eyes, and an inability to tan), a tendency to burn with sun exposure, and concurrent ephelides {1545,2460}.

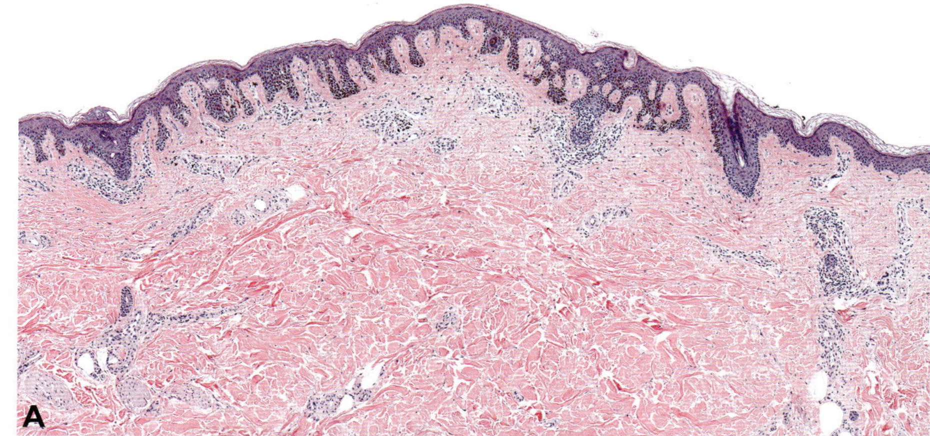

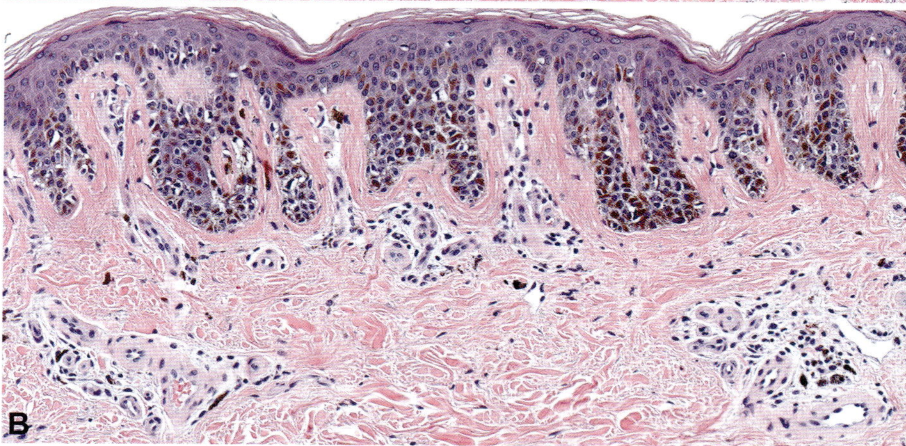

**Fig. 2.09** Lentiginous junctional naevus. **A** This lesion measures <4 mm in diameter and has a regular pattern of elongated rete ridges with nests of naevoid melanocytes, mainly near the tips and sides of the rete, with a few bridging nests. In the dermis, there is a patchy perivascular lymphocytic infiltrate with a few scattered melanophages. **B** Cytologically, the lesional cells are naevoid (larger than melanocytes but smaller than epithelioid cells) and have nuclei that are generally not larger than the nucleus of a resting keratinocyte. The architectural features in this lesion may overlap with those of a dysplastic naevus, except for small size and lack of marked cytological atypia.

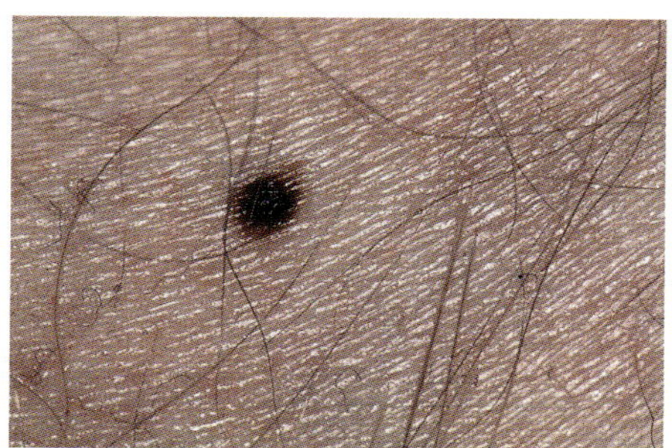

**Fig. 2.08** Lentiginous junctional naevus. A small, symmetrical macular or slightly raised uniformly pigmented lesion.

## Localization

Simple lentigo can occur anywhere on the skin or mucous membranes, and the lesions become more numerous with increasing age.

## Clinical features

The lesions are round or oval macules 3–15 mm in diameter, with irregular or smooth margins and homogeneous colour. They are not painful or pruritic and do not darken with sun exposure {1545,2460}. Very rarely, multiple simple lentigines can cover the majority of one half of the body, a condition known as partial unilateral lentiginosis {2066}; another uncommon disorder is familial eruptive lentiginosis, in which first-degree relatives abruptly develop numerous lentigines over the entire body {1860}. Neither of these two conditions is associated with systemic syndromes. In contrast, Noonan syndrome with multiple lentigines is part of a group called RAS/MAPK pathway syndromes. It is an autosomal dominant, multisystem disease caused by a *PTPN11* mutation. In addition to multiple simple lentigines, individuals with Noonan syndrome with multiple lentigines have aberrations in the skeletal and cardiovascular systems {2320}.

Sporadic, single lentiginous naevi may be either macular or papular; they are usually <6 mm in diameter and symmetrical. Lesional coloration is uniformly light brown to dark brown. Individuals with darker skin types often have more-heavily pigmented naevi. The trunk and extremities are favoured locations.

## Histopathology

Simple lentigo shows an increased number of single melanocytes at the basal aspect of the epidermis, with variably elongated and hyperpigmented rete ridges. Constituent melanocytes have small, round to oval, monomorphous nuclei. The cells are spaced equally from one another but are more pronounced at the tips of the rete ridges. Associated melanin pigment is potentially found throughout the epidermis, including the stratum corneum. Melanophages may be present in the papillary dermis, and giant melanosomes can be seen in the lesional cells in some cases.

When one or more small nests of melanocytes are observed in a lesion that otherwise has the appearance of simple lentigo, the lesion is called a lentiginous melanocytic naevus.

## Differential diagnosis

The two most important differential diagnoses for this group of melanocytic lesions are lentiginous melanoma and dysplastic naevus. Both feature the presence of cytologically atypical melanocytic proliferations in the epidermal base. Cell growth to confluence is present in lentiginous melanoma but not in dysplastic naevus.

## Histogenesis

According to Cramer {542}, common forms of acquired melanocytic naevus derive from pluripotent cells in the nerve-sheath precursor stage of the embryological melanocytic differentiation pathway. Such precursors mature to varying degrees, producing the various clinicopathological forms of recognized melanocytic naevi.

## Genetic profile

Acquired melanocytic naevi, including lentiginous melanocytic naevi, frequently harbour activating *BRAF* mutations (most commonly p.V600E mutations), as is seen in some melanomas; these mutations are present in about 80% of naevi {618}. However, the initial growth of melanocytic naevi is followed by cell-cycle arrest, with the induction of *CDKN2A* (encoding p16) and acidic β-galactosidase activity, and eventual oncogene-induced senescence {1769}. *BRAF* mutations are not sufficient by themselves to produce malignant change in melanocytic populations.

## Genetic susceptibility

No genetic susceptibility factors are recognized for either sporadic simple lentigo or lentiginous melanocytic naevus. The genetic features of Noonan syndrome with multiple lentigines are mentioned above.

## Prognosis and predictive factors

Simple lentigo and lentiginous melanocytic naevus are benign proliferations, regardless of their anatomical locations. They tend to show minimal change over a long period of time, and they have minimal potential for malignant transformation.

# Junctional, compound, and dermal naevi

Elder D.E.
Barnhill R.L.
Duncan L.M.
Massi D.
Mihm M.C. Jr
Piepkorn M.
Rabkin M.
Scolyer R.A.
Wick M.R.

## Definition
Junctional, compound, and dermal naevi are benign localized neoplastic proliferations of naevus cells (a type of melanocyte) {2390}. Like all melanocytic naevi, these lesions are defined by the presence of nests of melanocytes.

## ICD-O codes

| | |
|---|---|
| Junctional naevus | 8740/0 |
| Compound naevus | 8760/0 |
| Dermal naevus | 8750/0 |

## Synonyms
Common acquired naevi; banal naevi

## Epidemiology
Acquired naevi appear during childhood and reach maximum number in adolescence, declining in number thereafter in cross-sectional studies {2336}. This finding may be due to a cohort effect, a process of senescence and disappearance over time, or both.

## Etiology
The prevalence of naevi in various populations depends on phenotypic factors (in particular sun susceptibility), sun exposure patterns, and genetic susceptibility {1896}, resulting in mutations of a single oncogene in a single cell, which expands to form a clone {2390}.

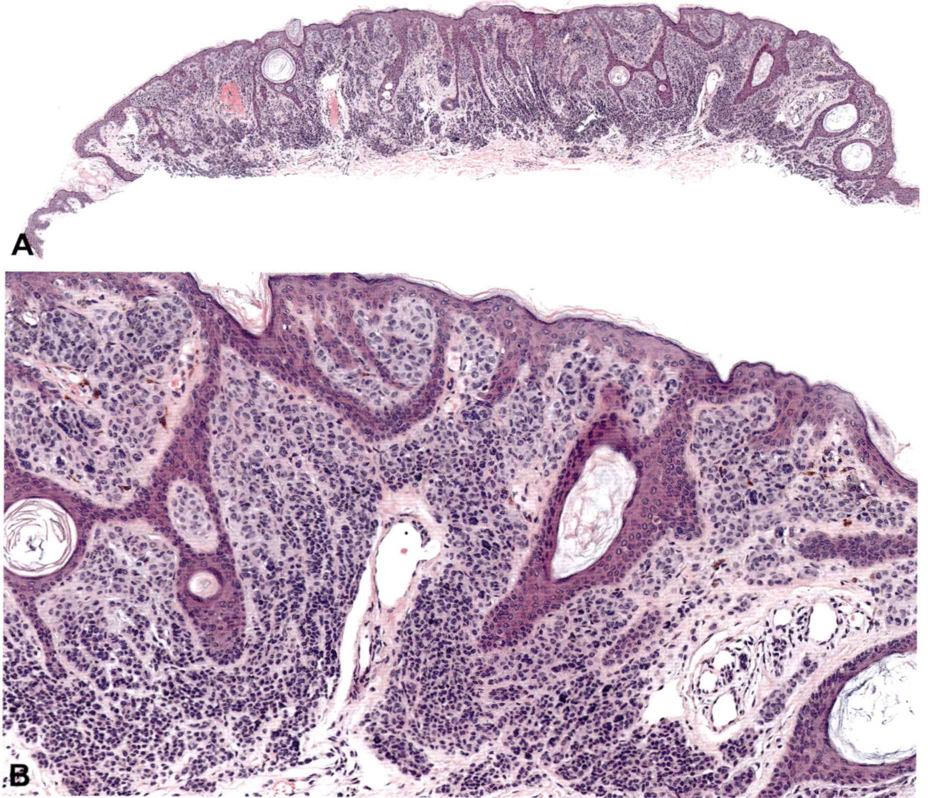

**Fig. 2.10** Compound naevus. **A** Well-circumscribed, symmetrical, moderately cellular proliferation of naevoid and naevoid-to-epithelioid melanocytes, with expansion of the papillary dermis and infiltration of the reticular dermis. There is no adjacent junctional component (shoulder). As seen here, complex elongation of rete ridges is seen in some naevi. **B** Higher magnification shows that there are a few nested naevoid-to-epithelioid type A naevus cells in the epidermis and superficial dermis. These blend with small lymphocyte-like type B naevus cells, which disperse into the reticular dermis at the base of the lesion. The lesional cell nuclei are small, without atypia, and there are no mitoses.

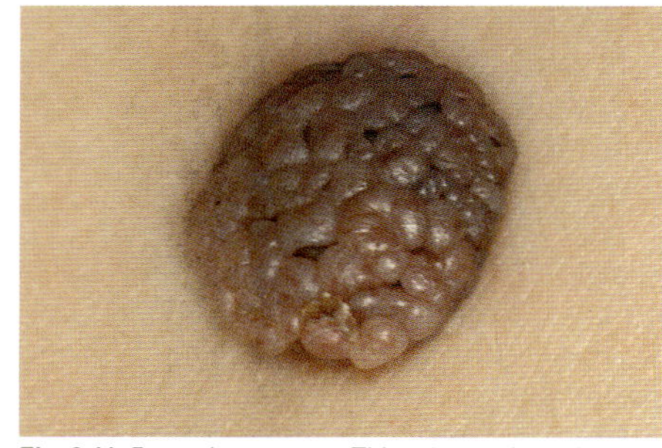

**Fig. 2.11** Dermal naevus. This dome-shaped, non-ulcerated, clinically stable lesion is generally skin-coloured and has likely lost its junctional component. The mammillated surface pattern is common in these lesions.

## Localization
Naevi are widely distributed over the body, with the most frequent site being the trunk {2180}.

## Clinical features
These are localized, generally symmetrical and uniformly pigmented lesions, typically <5 mm in diameter. They have been assumed to evolve from initial junctional proliferations to compound and then dermal naevi with accompanying development of a papular component, loss of the junctional component, and loss of pigment; however, a more complex model of separate evolution has been proposed {2028}.

## Histopathology
The naevoid melanocyte is larger than the native melanocyte population from which it has evolved, generally has less-prominent dendrites, and often contains pigment (in particular when junctional or in the superficial dermis) {2390}. In a junctional naevus, nests are present by definition and often admixed with single cells. In a compound naevus, nests are also present in the dermis. In a dermal naevus, there is no junctional component and there is often loss of pigment. Cells in the dermis may evolve from large epithelioid type A naevus cells (often arranged in nests in the upper dermis) to small lymphocyte-like type B cells to spindled type C cells, which often have

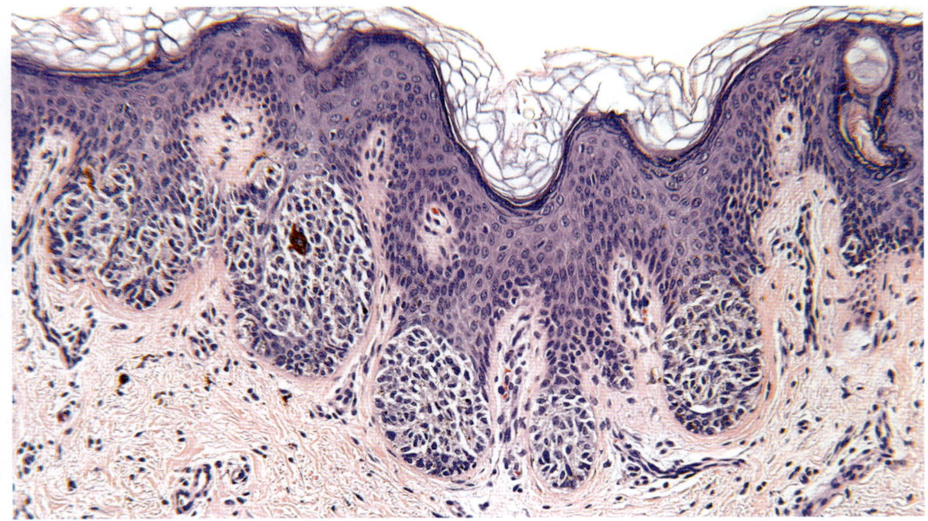

**Fig. 2.12** Junctional naevus with evenly distributed nests of uniform size (predominantly nested pattern).

signs of Schwannian differentiation, such as wavy fibre bundles, serpentine nuclei, structures mimicking sensory nerve end organs, and a lesser tendency to nesting. Although usually called maturation, the underlying mechanism of this phenotypic change is unclear. Maturation may reflect cytological changes that are induced by factors secreted by epithelial structures, such as the epidermis and appendages. WNT pathway activation has been implicated in this mechanism and can induce increased pigmentation and cell size, which diminish with increasing distance from the epithelia, from the superficial into the deeper components {2018,2884}.

## Differential diagnosis

The most important differential diagnosis is with melanoma, discussed in the specific sections. The major criteria that distinguish melanoma from common acquired naevi include size, symmetry, circumscription, ulceration, cellularity, pagetoid scatter, continuous basal (lentiginous) proliferation, cytological atypia, mitotic activity, failure of dermal cell maturation, and lymphovascular and perineural invasion. The differential diagnosis with other naevi, which is clinically less important, is discussed in the respective sections.

## Histogenesis

These lesions are thought to evolve as junctional proliferations of melanocytes, related to the mutation of a single oncogene as a driver mutation in actinically altered skin {2390}, and to evolve through the stages of compound and dermal naevi as described above.

## Genetic profile

Most acquired naevi have activating mutations of the oncogene *BRAF* (typically BRAF p.V600E) and less often mutations of *NRAS*. Different mutations are associated with distinct forms of naevi of other types, discussed in the respective sections {2390,2394}. *BAP1*-inactivated melanocytic lesions must be distinguished from Spitz naevi and atypical Spitz tumours, and are more akin to naevi with partial transformation by a second genomic event (i.e. *BAP1* loss). They usually lack epidermal hyperplasia, are usually epithelioid rather than spindled, often include a second naevus cell component, lack BAP1 expression, and are usually *BRAF*-mutant {2827,2828}.

## Genetic susceptibility

Several so-called naevus susceptibility genes have been described {1952}, but this information has not yet been translated into clinical practice.

## Prognosis and predictive factors

Naevi have medical significance in relation to melanoma, as simulants, potential precursors, and risk markers (discussed in the sections on dysplastic naevi and melanomas). Briefly, individuals with an increased total number of naevi or an increased number of large naevi are at increased risk of melanoma as determined in case–control and prospective cohort studies {845}. It has been shown that about one third of melanomas arise in compound naevi {379,1679}. Although many melanomas are associated with precursor naevi {237,2390}, the risk of progression for individual lesions is very low {2394,2660}.

# Dysplastic naevus

Elder D.E.
Barnhill R.L.
Bastian B.C.
Duncan L.M.
Massi D.
Mihm M.C. Jr
Piepkorn M.
Rabkin M.
Scolyer R.A.

## Definition

Dysplastic naevi are a subset of melanocytic naevi that are clinically atypical and characterized histologically by architectural disorder and cytological atypia, always involving their junctional component. In terms of their clinical and microscopic morphology, as well as genomic aspects, dysplastic naevi are intermediate between common acquired naevi and radial-growth-phase melanoma {678}.

## ICD-O code 8727/0

## Synonyms

Atypical naevus; large atypical naevus; B-K mole; atypical mole; melanocytic dysplasia; naevus with architectural disorder and melanocytic atypia

The term "Clark naevus" is not a synonym, because its definition does not include cytological atypia or a size criterion {1758}. The term "atypical naevus" is the most commonly used synonym; however, this term encompasses a broad range of unusual lesions, unless strictly defined.

## Epidemiology

Dysplastic naevi were first described in members of hereditary melanoma kindreds {495} and later in patients with non-familial melanoma {681} and in people unaffected by melanoma {2122}. The lesions typically develop in adolescence. The prevalence declines in older age groups, perhaps in part as a cohort effect and also because of involution {995}. In a case–control study, one or more clinically dysplastic naevi were found in 43% of 658 patients with melanoma and in 10% of 1009 control subjects; the most common number of naevi found was two among the patients and one among the controls {2667}. In a study of histological dysplasia, the prevalence of moderate or severe dysplasia was 24% in patients with melanoma and 12% in spouse controls {2434}.

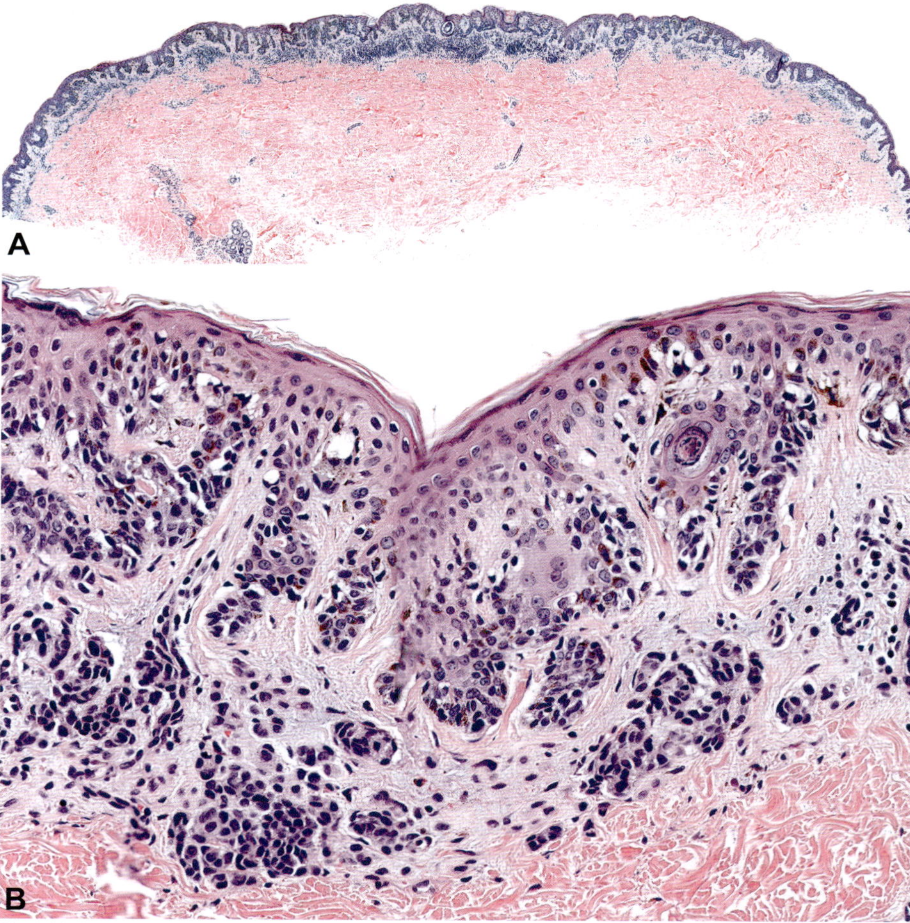

**Fig. 2.14** Compound dysplastic naevus, low grade. **A** Broad lesion characterized by relative symmetry and reasonably uniformly elongated rete ridges. In the centre, a dermal component partly fills the expanded papillary dermis; at the periphery, there are junctional shoulders. There is a patchy perivascular lymphocytic infiltrate. **B** High-power view of the edge of the dermal component and the beginning of the adjacent shoulder. The junctional component is moderately cellular and is composed of naevoid to epithelioid melanocytes; the nuclear size of these cells is < 1.5× that of resting (i.e. with the smallest nuclei) basal keratinocytes, constituting moderate random cytological atypia.

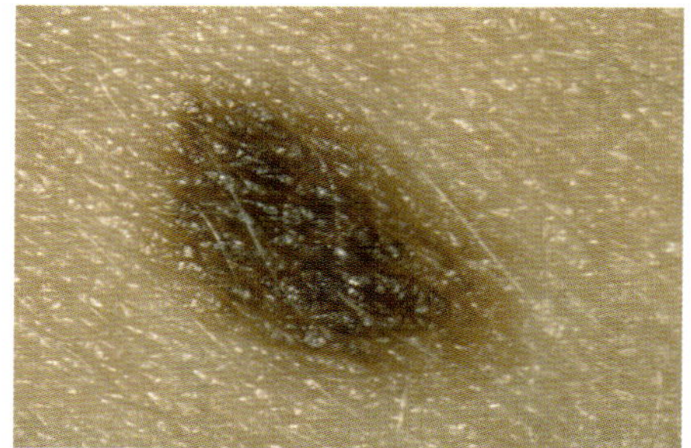

**Fig. 2.13** Dysplastic naevus. This lesion is broad, somewhat irregular, raised in the centre, and flat at the periphery. It has variegated shades of tan and dark brown, and an indefinite border.

## Etiology

Like other melanocytic tumours {160} (including melanomas), dysplastic naevi arise because of genetic, environmental, and phenotypic factors, in particular factors related to sun susceptibility and exposure. There is evidence of a genetic component to naevogenesis; genome-wide association studies of naevus counts have implicated several loci, but germline susceptibility loci unique to dysplastic naevi have not been reported

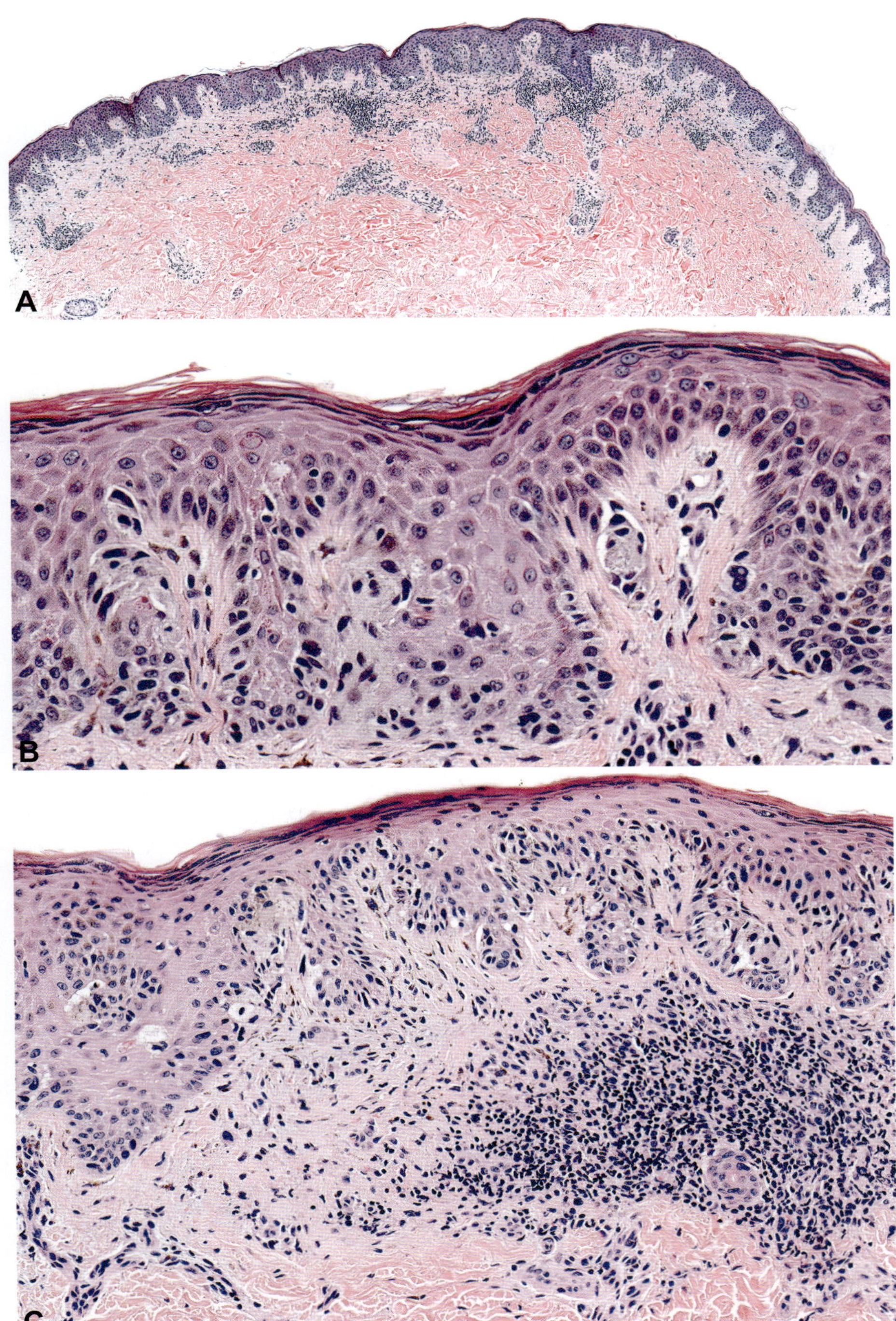

**Fig. 2.15** Compound dysplastic naevus, high grade. **A** Broad lesion, slightly >4 mm in diameter on the slide, with changes present at the left specimen edge. The rete ridges are somewhat irregularly thickened, although relatively uniformly elongated. There is a patchy to focally more dense lymphocytic infiltrate in the dermis, mostly perivascular and partly interstitial. Nests of melanocytes can be seen near the tips and sides of rete ridges, with some bridging nests. **B** Higher magnification shows that some of the lesional cells have a nuclear size >1.5× that of resting basal keratinocytes, and have irregular hyperchromatic nuclei, constituting severe random cytological atypia. There is a focal tendency to confluence of lesional cell nests in the epidermis with only minimal evidence of upward scatter in this field. In the dermis, there are perivascular lymphocytes and melanophages, with subtle concentric fibroplasia at the tip of some rete. **C** In this focal area of the same lesion, there are changes that raise concern for evolving melanoma (at least in situ); there are large cells with similar cytology as seen in panel B, and there is a focal tendency to upward pagetoid scatter near the middle of the lesion, not beyond the mid-spinous layer. A few cells in the dermis (left of centre) resemble those in the epidermis, with an associated focus of diffuse fibroplasia. The lymphocytic infiltrate is focally band-like; there is well-developed eosinophilic fibroplasia around rete ridges on the right.

{908}. It is possible that stimuli from chronic ultraviolet (UV) radiation exposure and the resulting cumulative sun damage (CSD) acting on a naevus can promote the attributes of clinical and histological atypia.

## Localization

The anatomical distribution of dysplastic naevi, like that of other naevi, only partially overlaps with that of melanoma, paralleling the distribution of melanoma in skin with a low degree of CSD (low-CSD melanoma) rather than that of high-CSD melanoma. Dysplastic naevi tend to arise in skin that is intermittently (rather than chronically) sun-exposed; the most common site is the back {456}.

## Clinical features

A widely adopted definition published by the International Agency for Research on Cancer (IARC) in 1990 (and subsequently modified) recommends the following criteria to identify atypical (dysplastic) naevi: there must be a macular component in at least one area; in addition, at least three of the following features must be present: a non–well-defined border, size ≥ 5 mm, colour variegation, uneven peripheral contour, and erythema {845}. The lesions almost always have a flat component (representing junctional proliferation), and there is often a central raised portion constituting a dermal component, resulting in a resemblance to a fried egg or a target. These criteria partially overlap with those for melanoma. Lesions with markedly atypical attributes, as well as new or changing lesions, should be submitted for histological evaluation to rule out melanoma. Dermoscopy and photographic follow-up and image analysis may be used to improve the specificity of clinical diagnosis {2840}.

## Histopathology

Melanocytic dysplasia comprises alterations of architectural disorder and cytological atypia {678}. The term "architectural disorder" refers to deviation from a stereotypical junctional naevus pattern (in which uniform nests of naevoid melanocytes are present at the tips of rete ridges uniformly across the lesion) and also indicates increased size of the lesions relative to common acquired naevi. There may be single cells between the nests, suggesting the evolution of a junctional naevus from a pre-existing simple lentigo and forming a lentiginous naevus. Attributes of architectural disorder include the presence of junctional shoulders (lateral extension) adjacent to a dermal component (or the lesion may be entirely junctional), bridging of nests between adjacent elongated rete ridges, subtle suprabasal scatter of melanocytes confined to the lower epidermal levels (typically less pronounced than in melanoma), concentric and lamellar fibroplasia around elongated rete ridges, and a patchy lymphocytic infiltrate. Cytological atypia is characterized by enlargement of nuclei (with varying degrees of irregularity), chromatin clumping and hyperchromatism, and variably prominent nucleoli. Mitoses of intraepidermal lesional melanocytes are uncommon; if present, they constitute a severe cytological feature, raising the differential diagnosis of melanoma in situ.

Like other naevi, dysplastic naevi are immunolabelled for the melanocytic markers S100 protein, melan-A, MITF, tyrosinase, and SOX10 {1162,1810,2555}. HMB45 staining is useful because it can reveal stratification considered to be an attribute of maturation/senescence {1803}, with staining typically confined to superficial cells. The Ki-67 proliferation index is typically <5% in the dermal hotspot. Ki-67 staining can also be used to evaluate the junctional component; in dysplastic naevi, most cells are unlabelled, whereas the Ki-67 proliferation index can be >30% in melanoma in situ {989}. Staining for the tumour suppressor p16 can be useful for ruling out homozygous loss of *CDKN2A*. Although p16 inactivation is almost ubiquitous in invasive melanomas, it can occur by mechanisms other than deletion, so positive p16 staining does not rule out melanoma {2455}. A recent comprehensive molecular analysis showed that dysplastic naevi differ from common naevi in many respects and can be distinguished from common naevi at the molecular level {1803}. Other studies have found overlapping results between dysplastic and common naevi {1162}.

Diagnostic criteria for dysplastic naevi have been developed and validated by the International Melanoma Pathology Study Group (IMPSG) {2434,2868} (see Tables 2.07–2.12).

Other naevus variants, melanoma in situ, and invasive melanoma must be excluded. Lentiginous naevi that are junctional or compound (formerly known as mildly dysplastic naevi) are not associated with increased melanoma risk, are very common in the general population, have a very low probability of progression to melanoma, and have poor diagnostic reproducibility {1592}. Therefore, the consensus meeting Working Group recommends against the continued use of the term "mildly dysplastic naevus", and instead recommends using only two grades of dysplasia: low-grade and high-grade dysplasia, as defined in Table 2.13 (p. 86).

**Table 2.07** International Melanoma Pathology Study Group (IMPSG) diagnostic criteria for dysplastic naevus. Reproduced from: Shors AR et al. {2434} and Xiong MY et al. {2868}

**Dysplastic naevus**
- Width >4 mm in fixed sections (>5 mm clinically)
- Presence of architectural disorder, which requires both of the following:
  - Irregular (i.e. horizontally oriented, bridging adjacent rete, and/or varying in shape and size) and/or dyscohesive nests of intraepidermal melanocytes
  - Increased density of non-nested junctional melanocytes (e.g. more melanocytes than keratinocytes in an area ≥ 1 mm$^2$)
- Presence of cytological atypia, which is graded on the basis of the highest degree of cytological atypia present in more than a few melanocytes (see Table 2.13)

**Table 2.08** Diagnostic criteria for simple lentigo

**Simple lentigo**
- Width usually <4 mm in fixed sections
- Increased density of junctional melanocytes, mainly around the tips and sides of (often elongated) rete
- No nests (by definition)
- No to mild cytological atypia

Exclusions: Moderate or severe atypia of more than a few melanocytes suggests atypical lentigo or lentigo maligna, but not dysplastic naevus (use descriptive diagnosis, e.g. atypical lentiginous melanocytic proliferation).

**Table 2.09** Diagnostic criteria for lentiginous junctional naevus/lentigo

**Lentiginous junctional naevus/lentigo**
- Width usually <4 mm in fixed sections
- Increased density of non-nested junctional melanocytes around the tips and sides of (usually elongated) rete
- Nested junctional melanocytes range from collections of a few melanocytes to well-formed nests
- Usually symmetrical, but with poorly defined borders
- No to mild cytological atypia
- Minor/variable features (also seen in dysplastic and shoulder naevi): elongated rete, epidermal hyperpigmentation, pigment incontinence, papillary dermal fibrosis, patchy lymphocytic inflammation, adnexal involvement, lichenification, and upward spread of bland melanocytes to the mid-spinous layer

Exclusions: Moderate or severe atypia of more than a few melanocytes plus high solar elastosis – indicating cumulative sun damage (CSD) – suggests atypical lentiginous naevus or lentigo maligna, but not dysplastic naevus (use descriptive diagnosis); moderate or severe atypia of more than a few melanocytes plus irregularity and high cellularity with pagetoid scatter in the setting of a low degree of CSD suggests early melanoma.

**Table 2.10** Diagnostic criteria for lentiginous compound naevus

**Lentiginous compound naevus**
- Any width
- Increased density of non-nested melanocytes between junctional nests, often extending out along the shoulders of the nested junctional and/or intradermal components
- Junctional nests are prominent, well formed, and usually round
- Nested melanocytes are often larger than non-nested melanocytes, with larger nuclei and more-abundant cytoplasm
- Nuclei of nested melanocytes are uniform and not greatly enlarged or hyperchromatic

Exclusions: Moderate or severe atypia of more than a few melanocytes plus irregular and dyscohesive nesting without cumulative sun damage (CSD) suggests dysplastic naevus or early melanoma, especially if there is also pagetoid scatter; moderate or severe atypia of more than a few melanocytes plus CSD suggests atypical lentiginous naevus or lentigo maligna, but not dysplastic naevus (use descriptive diagnosis).

**Table 2.11** Diagnostic criteria for naevus with architectural disorder and minimal or mild cytological atypia

**Naevus with architectural disorder and minimal or mild cytological atypia**
- Width often < 4 mm in fixed sections
- Architectural features of dysplastic naevus
- Grade of cytological atypia and/or density of atypical melanocytes below the threshold for dysplastic naevus (see Table 2.13)

**Table 2.12** Modified International Melanoma Pathology Study Group (IMPSG) diagnostic criteria for melanoma. Reproduced from: Shors AR et al. {2434} and Xiong MY et al. {2868}

**Superficial spreading melanoma in situ**
- Contiguous proliferation of uniformly (e.g. > 50%) moderately to severely atypical melanocytes in an area ≥ 0.5 $mm^2$
  *and/or*
- Upward intraepidermal spread of moderately to severely atypical melanocytes involving the superficial spinous and granular layers in an area ≥ 0.5 $mm^2$
  *and/or*
- Large irregular junctional nests of different sizes, with focal confluence and variable nuclear atypia together with lesion asymmetry (so-called nested melanoma) {1472}

Note: Minimal/equivocal involvement may be reported as, for example, "severely dysplastic naevus with focal superficial atypical melanocytic proliferation of uncertain significance (SAMPUS) – cannot rule out evolving or early established melanoma in situ, superficial spreading melanoma type".

Exclusions: Recurrent naevus, traumatized naevus, recent ultraviolet (UV) radiation exposure and other reactive processes

**Lentigo maligna**
- Prominent solar elastosis
- Epidermal atrophy and flattened rete, at least focally
- Increased number of basal naevoid to epithelioid melanocytes, usually with contiguous proliferation in an area ≥ 0.5 $mm^2$
- Usually some pagetoid scatter
- Irregularly distributed junctional nests
- Uniform cytological atypia of nested and non-nested junctional melanocytes
- Often involves adnexa, especially hair follicles
- Sometimes atypical multinucleated melanocytes (starburst cells)

Note: Minimal/equivocal involvement may be reported as "lentiginous naevus with focal superficial proliferation of uncertain significance – cannot rule out evolving or early established melanoma in situ, lentigo maligna type".

## Differential diagnosis

The differential diagnosis includes simple lentigo (not strictly a naevus but considered to be in the developmental pathway of a naevus), lentiginous junctional naevus/lentigo, lentiginous compound naevus, and naevus with architectural disorder and minimal or mild cytological atypia. See Tables 2.08 to 2.11 for a summary of the diagnostic criteria for these entities. Solar lentigo, which is considered to be a primarily keratinocytic neoplasm, is characterized by some combination of elongated rete ridges, hyperpigmentation of basal keratinocytes, and a slight increase in the number of melanocytes {73}.

In addition to benign junctional and compound naevi, the differential diagnosis of dysplastic naevus also includes melanoma in situ and superficially invasive melanoma, most commonly superficial spreading and lentigo maligna melanomas. Acral naevi and melanomas can also simulate dysplasia; a melanocytic proliferation in acral skin is much more likely to be an acral naevus (or even a melanoma) than a dysplastic naevus. A modified version of the IMPSG diagnostic criteria for melanoma {2434,2868} is summarized in Table 2.12.

## Histogenesis

Dysplastic naevi are benign neoplasms of melanocytes. Melanocytic dysplasia may occur de novo or in association with congenital-pattern dermal naevi (defined as naevi that have a dermal component within the reticular dermis) or with common dermal naevi that are confined to the papillary dermis. It is likely that the dysplasia develops as a secondary change in relation to the pre-existing dermal naevus as a result of sequential acquisition of genetic abnormalities {2391}.

## Genetic profile

Like common acquired naevi, dysplastic naevi are associated with activating mutations of an oncogene, most commonly *BRAF* or *NRAS*. A category of intermediate lesions has recently been identified that is characterized by cytological and architectural atypia and the presence of more than one genomic abnormality (in contrast to common acquired naevi, which have only a single mutated oncogene). Mutation of the *TERT* promoter is a frequent early event in the progression towards melanoma in situ, and there is occasionally hemizygous loss of *CDKN2A* {2394}. The correlation of these genetic alterations with the degree of morphological dysplasia is still unknown.

## Genetic susceptibility

Dysplastic naevi are commonly found in members of hereditary melanoma kindreds. However, the transmission of dysplastic naevus does not conform to expectations of dominant Mendelian inheritance. Associations between naevi and various susceptibility genes have been identified, but these findings have little or no clinical utility at this time {908}.

## Prognosis and predictive factors

Dysplastic naevi have significance mainly in relation to melanoma, in three ways: as simulants of melanoma, as potential precursors of melanoma, and as biomarkers of increased risk for melanoma {678}. Their role as morphological simulants relates to the differential diagnosis of melanoma, discussed above.

In various studies, remnants of a dysplastic naevus have been described in 20–30% of melanomas {491,2274}, and a recent prospective study found that naevus remnants (of any type) were associated with 54.2% of melanomas {980}. Dysplastic naevi adjacent to melanomas have an increased frequency of *TERT* promoter mutations {2394}, indicating that they have genetically evolved beyond conventional naevi (in which such mutations are typically absent). This indicates that some dysplastic naevi represent biologically intermediate states between benign naevus and melanomas. There are currently insufficient data to

**Table 2.13** Nuclear features in the varying grades of dysplasia

| WHO classification (2018) | Former grade | Nuclear size vs resting basal cells | Chromatism | Variation in nuclear size and shape | Nucleoli |
|---|---|---|---|---|---|
| Not a dysplastic naevus | 0 (mild dysplasia) | 1× | May be hyperchromatic | Minimal | Small or absent |
| Low-grade dysplasia | 1 (moderate dysplasia[a]) | 1–1.5× | Hyperchromatic, or dispersed chromatin | Prominent in a small minority of cells (random atypia) | Small or absent |
| High-grade dysplasia | 2 (severe dysplasia[a]) | ≥1.5× | Hyperchromatic, coarse granular chromatin, or peripheral condensation | Prominent in a larger minority of cells | Prominent, often lavender |

[a] Architectural features are required for the diagnosis of dysplasia (see Table 2.07) and also contribute to grade; attributes that indicate a diagnosis of high-grade (severe) dysplasia even when cytological atypia is low-grade include pagetoid scatter above the basal layer (but to a lesser degree than in melanoma, usually not above the middle third, and focal, i.e. contained within an area < 0.5 $mm^2$), focal continuous basal proliferation, and intraepidermal mitoses (any dermal mitosis or anything more than a rare mitosis should raise concern for melanoma).

determine what proportion of non–melanoma-adjacent dysplastic naevi harbour similar alterations. Dysplastic naevi are much more common than melanomas, and the risk of progression of any given lesion is very low {2660}. However, naevi that show high-grade dysplasia and/or have additional genetic alterations such as *TERT* promoter mutation should be considered for complete excision.

Dysplastic naevi have been associated with increased melanoma risk in numerous clinically based case–control studies; in a meta-analysis of 46 studies, the relative risk associated with the presence of 5 dysplastic/atypical naevi (vs 0) was found to be 6.4 {845}. In a histological study of melanoma cases and spouse controls, moderate to severe dysplasia was associated with an increased risk of melanoma (odds ratio: 3.99, 95% CI: 1.02–15.71), whereas mild dysplasia was not associated with an increased risk {2434}. In a subsequent study using the same database, much of the increased relative risk associated with histological dysplasia was found to be conferred by lesional size alone (> 4.4 mm), which could therefore serve as a reasonable surrogate indicator of cytological and architectural atypia {2868}. In a retrospective review of pathology reports on 20 275 naevi, a personal history of melanoma was present in 5.7% of patients with mild atypia, 8.1% with moderate atypia, and 19.7% with severe atypia. The odds ratios as a measure of association between a dysplastic naevus and a personal history of melanoma were 4.1 for severe versus mild dysplasia, 2.8 for severe versus moderate dysplasia, and 1.5 for moderate versus mild dysplasia {2260}, again suggesting that the risk associated with mild dysplasia (i.e. mild versus no dysplasia, not studied presumably because of the large numbers involved) is not significantly different from baseline.

# Naevus spilus

Elenitsas R.
Lazova R.

## Definition

Naevus spilus is a melanocytic naevus composed of benign naevoid melanocytes in the epidermis and superficial dermis, presenting as a patch of hyperpigmented skin containing a variable number of darkly pigmented macules and papules {2337,2338}.

## ICD-O code 8720/0

## Synonym

Speckled lentiginous naevus

## Epidemiology

The prevalence rate of naevus spilus (0.2–2.8% depending on age) is similar to that of congenital melanocytic naevi {1428,1739,2443}. There is no race or sex predilection.

## Localization

Naevus spilus can occur at any anatomical site.

## Clinical features

Naevus spilus presents as a patch of light- to medium-brown hyperpigmentation with a variable number of black, brown, or reddish-brown macules and papules within it. The background pigmented patch is usually 3–6 cm in diameter (but can range from 1 cm to > 60 cm). The speckles are most commonly 2–3 mm (but can range from 1 mm to 9 mm). Approximately 80% of these lesions appear at birth or during early infancy. They may present as lightly coloured café-au-lait macules at birth, which later become hyperpigmented with darkly pigmented macules and papules over months, years, or sometimes decades.

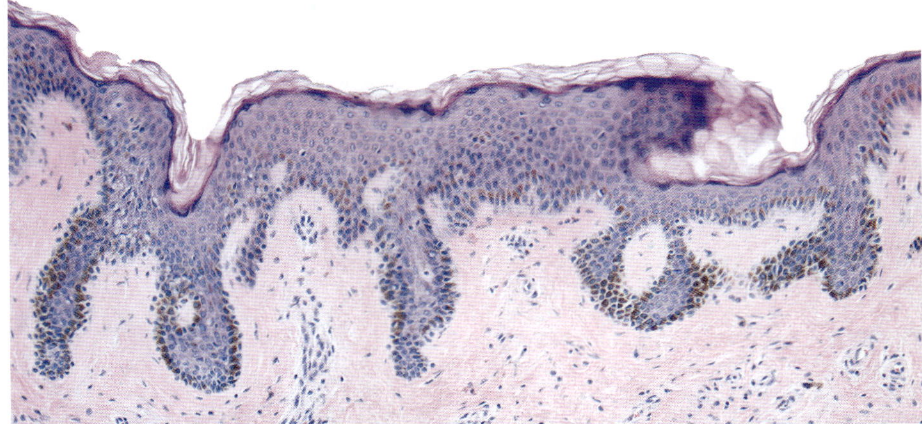

**Fig. 2.16** Naevus spilus. A background hyperpigmented patch, with elongated pigmented rete ridges and slightly increased numbers of single melanocytes at the dermoepidermal junction.

## Histopathology

The background hyperpigmented patch has elongated hyperpigmented rete ridges with slightly increased numbers of melanocytes. The speckles show variable findings, including lentiginous junctional naevi, compound and intradermal naevi, compound or intradermal naevi with congenital features, Spitz naevi, blue naevi, and naevi with cytological atypia (dysplastic naevi).

## Differential diagnosis

The differential diagnosis includes café-au-lait macules, agminated melanocytic naevi, and partial unilateral lentiginosis.

## Histogenesis

Naevus spilus may represent a defect in the melanoblasts that populate a localized area of the skin. Genetic and environmental factors may also play a role in its occurrence.

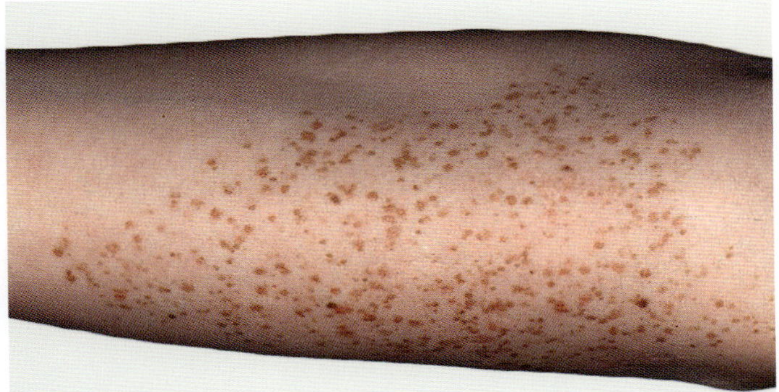

**Fig. 2.17** Naevus spilus. In a localized area, there is a lesion characterized by a speckled pattern of tan pigmented macules and papules in a pale-tan background.

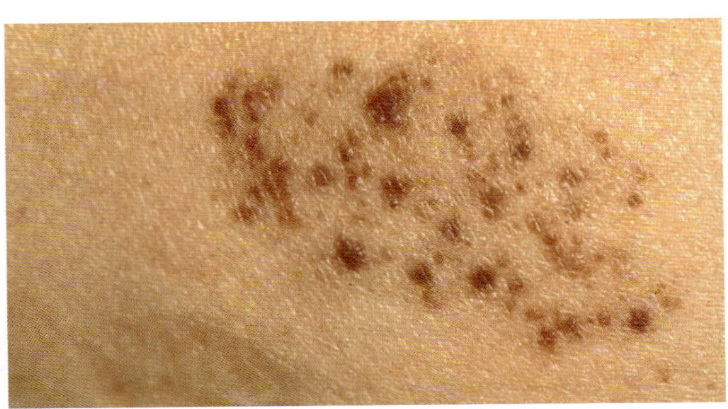

**Fig. 2.18** Naevus spilus. Speckled macules and papules in a pale-tan background.

### Genetic profile

The melanocytes within naevus spilus harbour oncogenic *HRAS* mutations, mostly c.37G>C (p.G13R). The melanocytes in the background patch carry a single mutant allele, which is amplified in the more cellular areas, constituting the speckles {1376,2318}.

### Genetic susceptibility

Speckled lentiginous naevus syndrome has been characterized as a distinct neurocutaneous phenotype in which ipsilateral neurological abnormalities are present in association with naevus spilus {1007,2131,2731}.

### Prognosis and predictive factors

Naevus spilus is a benign neoplasm. Predictors of the risk of malignant transformation for a naevus spilus have yet to be determined. Melanoma may develop within naevus spilus, with at least 20 cases reported in the literature to date {878,1609,2725,2931}.

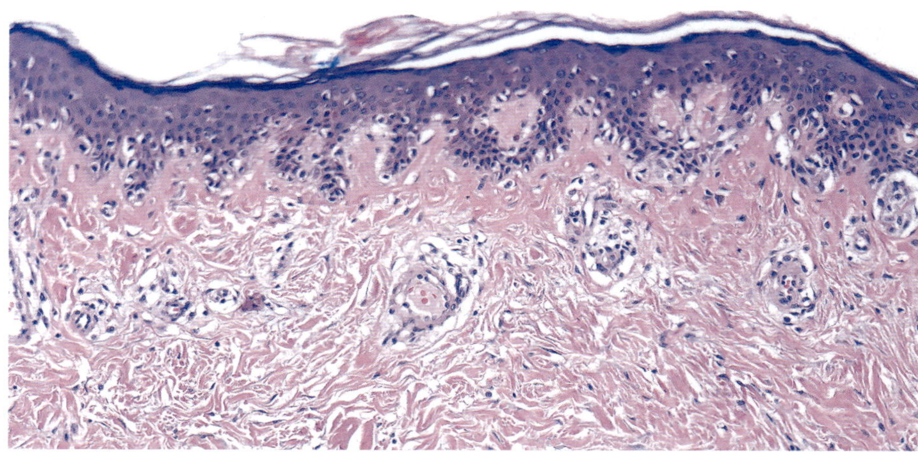

**Fig. 2.19** Junctional melanocytic naevus within a naevus spilus. Small nests of melanocytes and lentiginous melanocytic proliferation at the dermoepidermal junction.

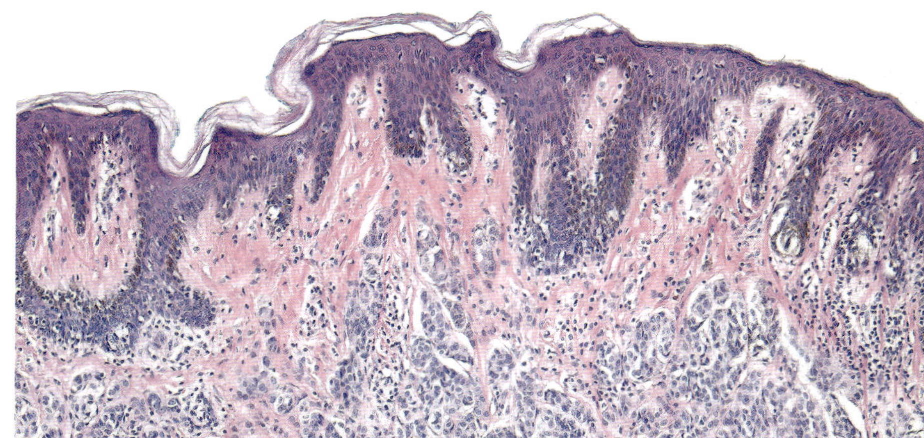

**Fig. 2.20** Compound melanocytic naevus within a naevus spilus. There are nests of uniform melanocytes in the epidermis and dermis. The rete ridges are elongated, with prominent melanin pigment in the basal layer of the epidermis.

# Special-site naevi (of the breast, axilla, scalp, and ear)

Brenn T.
Lazova R.
Massi D.
Rongioletti F.
Zalaudek I.

## Definition

Special-site naevi are melanocytic naevi located at specific anatomical sites (e.g. the breast, axilla and other flexural sites, scalp, ear, umbilicus, genital skin, and acral skin) that, although benign, show atypical or unusual histopathological features that can make them difficult to distinguish from melanoma, leading to misdiagnosis and/or unnecessarily high rates of re-excision {677}.

## Synonyms

Melanocytic naevi of special sites;
naevi with site-related atypia

## Epidemiology

The epidemiology of special-site naevi is unclear. Atypical naevi of the breast occur in both males and females {2226}. Atypical naevi of the scalp occur more frequently in younger patients {725}.

## Etiology

The etiology is unknown. The impact of embryological, hormonal, and physical influences – for example, ultraviolet (UV) radiation exposure and trauma – on the genesis of the atypical microscopic findings of special-site naevi in relationship with the specific anatomical sites remains to be elucidated.

Estrogenic factors, which exert an important influence on breast tissue and milk line areas, can also play a role in melanocytic proliferation; repetitive friction and rubbing can result in reactive morphological changes {683,1885}.

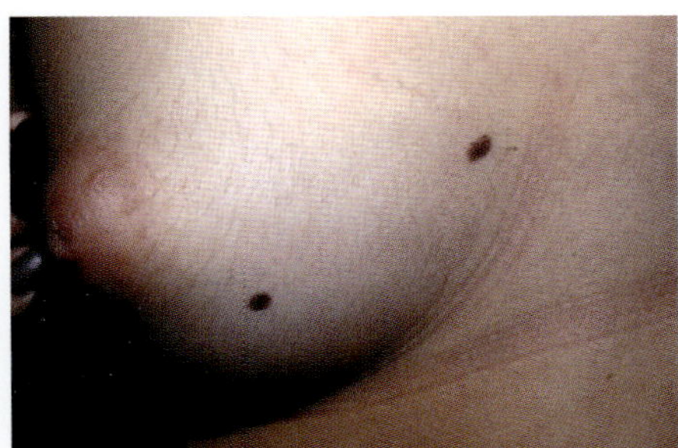

**Fig. 2.21** Special-site naevi of the breast.

It is unclear whether special-site naevi are distinct clinicopathological entities or represent microscopic variation along a biological spectrum.

## Localization

The best-known special-site naevi are those of acral sites and genitalia, which are addressed in separate sections (see *Acral naevus*, p. 119, and *Genital naevus*, p. 123). Other special-site naevi include naevi located on the breast, axilla and other flexural sites, scalp, ears, or umbilicus.

## Clinical features

Special-site naevi that present with atypical histopathological features are clinically innocuous, except for the large size of the lesions, which are usually >6 mm and have irregular borders {1103}. Most patients are not aware of any morphological changes.

## Histopathology

Special-site naevi have architectural features that deviate from those of ordinary acquired naevi and overlap with those of dysplastic naevi and melanomas, including asymmetry, irregular nesting arrangement, cytological atypia, pagetoid spread, dermal fibroplasia, and lymphocytic infiltrate {31}. In particular, breast naevi have been found to exhibit significantly more atypical features than naevi from other sites, and tend to show nesting irregularities, prominent intraepidermal melanocytes, melanocytic atypia, and dermal fibroplasia {2226}. Naevi of flexural sites may show a papillomatous so-called mushroom pattern, with variably sized nests located along the tips and sides of rete ridges and mild cytological junctional atypia. A second pattern is more similar to atypical naevi from the breast {31}. A primarily nested and discohesive pattern has also been described, characterized by irregular junctional nests in which there is lack of cellular cohesion, with floating melanocytes similar to those seen in atypical genital naevi {2223}. Naevi of the scalp may also exhibit architectural disorders that overlap with those of the special-site naevi, including lentiginous growth, large pleomorphic dyscohesive nests, random melanocytes with large nuclei and abundant pale cytoplasm, placement of nests along the lateral side of the rete ridges, follicular involvement, rare suprabasal melanocytes, and superficial fibroplasia. Features overlapping with those of dysplastic naevi and superficial congenital naevi are also observed {782}. Naevi on the ear share many features with those from the scalp, breast, umbilicus, genitalia, flexural sites, and acral skin {1505}.

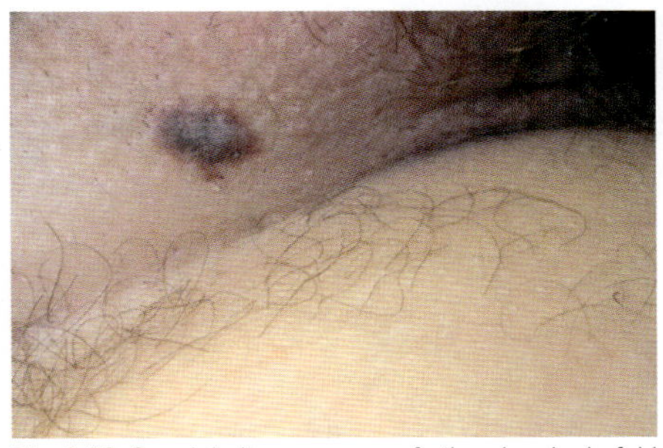

**Fig. 2.22** Special-site naevus of the inguinal fold (flexural naevus).

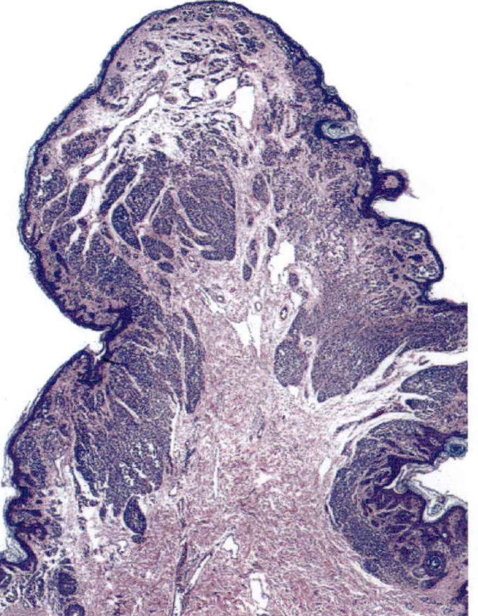

**Fig. 2.23** Special-site naevus of the groin showing a papillomatous mushroom pattern.

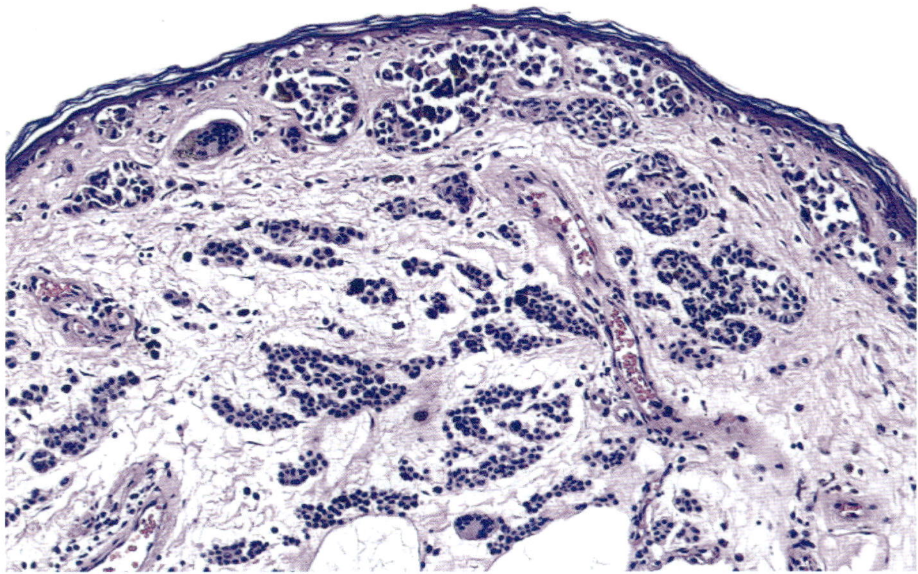

**Fig. 2.24** Special-site naevus of the groin. Nested and discohesive pattern with irregular junctional nests. Note the lack of cellular cohesion, with floating melanocytes similar to those seen in atypical genital naevi.

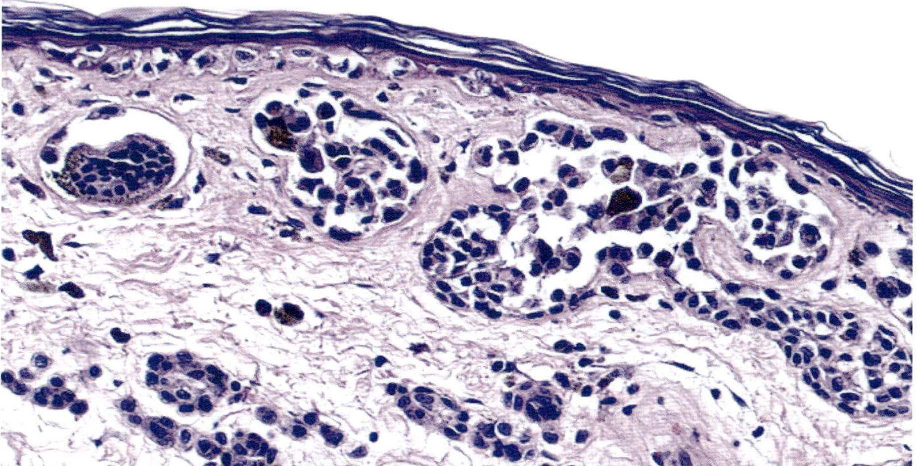

**Fig. 2.25** Special-site naevus of the groin. Cytological atypia restricted to the junctional and papillary dermis.

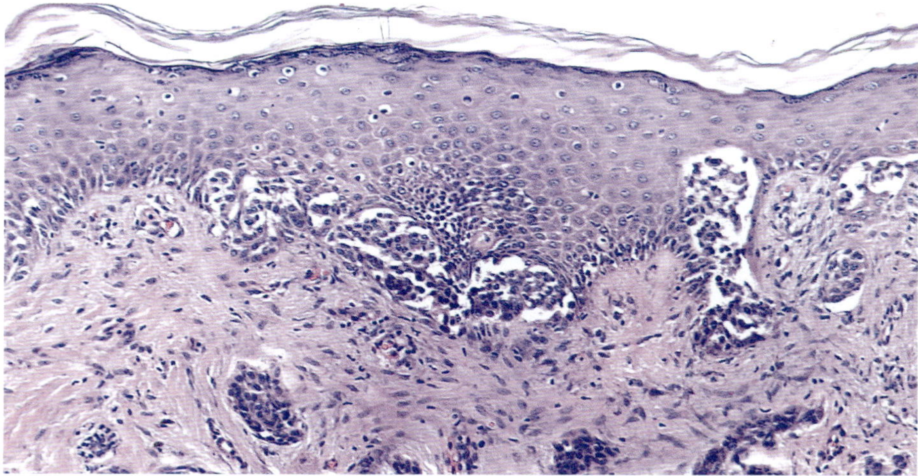

**Fig. 2.26** Special-site naevus of the umbilicus. Irregular nesting arrangement with a dyscohesive pattern, cytological junctional atypia, slight pagetoid spreading, and dermal fibroplasia.

## Differential diagnosis

Special-site naevi have architectural features mimicking those of melanomas; however, the naevi do not show increased mitotic activity or individual necrotic melanocytes, and the cells demonstrate maturation with descent into the deeper dermis. Melanomas show prominent pagetoid spread, greater cytological atypia, and a more developed host response. Lesions not considered to be melanomas may be classified as dysplastic naevi. In fact, all of the atypical or unusual histopathological features that may be found in special-site naevi are also seen in dysplastic naevi (also called atypical naevi or naevi with architectural disorder). In such cases, the specific anatomical site and sometimes the clinically unremarkable characteristics of special-site naevi that are often removed for cosmetic reasons may help. Dermoscopy is useful in distinguishing acral naevi from acral melanoma {1492}. However, the dermoscopic features may be misleading, because acral naevi can show a prominent pigment network with bizarre lines, as well as large globules, mimicking features of melanoma {1754}.

## Prognosis and predictive factors

Special-site naevi are considered to be benign lesions, and their atypical histopathological features do not correspond to any unusual or malignant biological behaviour. In particular, no evidence of increased melanoma risk has ever been confirmed. The importance of these naevi is related to the recognition of their existence and their distinction from melanoma. It is important for dermatologists and dermatopathologists to distinguish special-site melanocytic naevi from melanoma in order to prevent misdiagnosis and avoid unnecessary wide excisions.

# Halo naevus

Xu X.
Chu E.

## Definition

Halo naevus is a naevus with circumferential depigmentation, often associated with a brisk lymphocytic infiltrate histopathologically.

## ICD-O code 8723/0

## Synonyms

Sutton naevus; leukoderma acquisitum centrifugum; perinaevoid vitiligo; perinaevoid leukoderma

## Epidemiology

In the general population, the incidence of halo naevi is estimated to be 1% {1066}. Halo naevi are most commonly found in children and young adults; the average age at presentation is about 15 years. There is no sex or race predilection.

## Etiology

Antigen-presenting cells and CD8+ T cells have been identified in the inflammatory infiltrates of halo naevi, implicating cytotoxic mechanisms in the destruction of naevus cells {2913}. Affected individuals also show activated lymphocytes in their peripheral blood {143}, as well as T-cell clonal expansion {1855} and naevus-reactive IgM antibodies {2623}. These findings are consistent with the idea that halo naevi represent the immunologically mediated rejection of a naevus. Treatment with the IL-6 inhibitors tocilizumab and imatinib has been associated with the development of halo naevi {741,1452}.

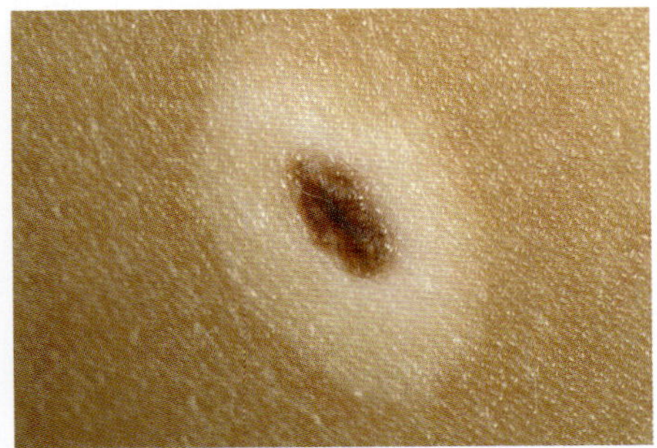

**Fig. 2.27** Halo naevus. Papular pigmented lesion surrounded by a symmetrical depigmented halo, in a background of tan skin.

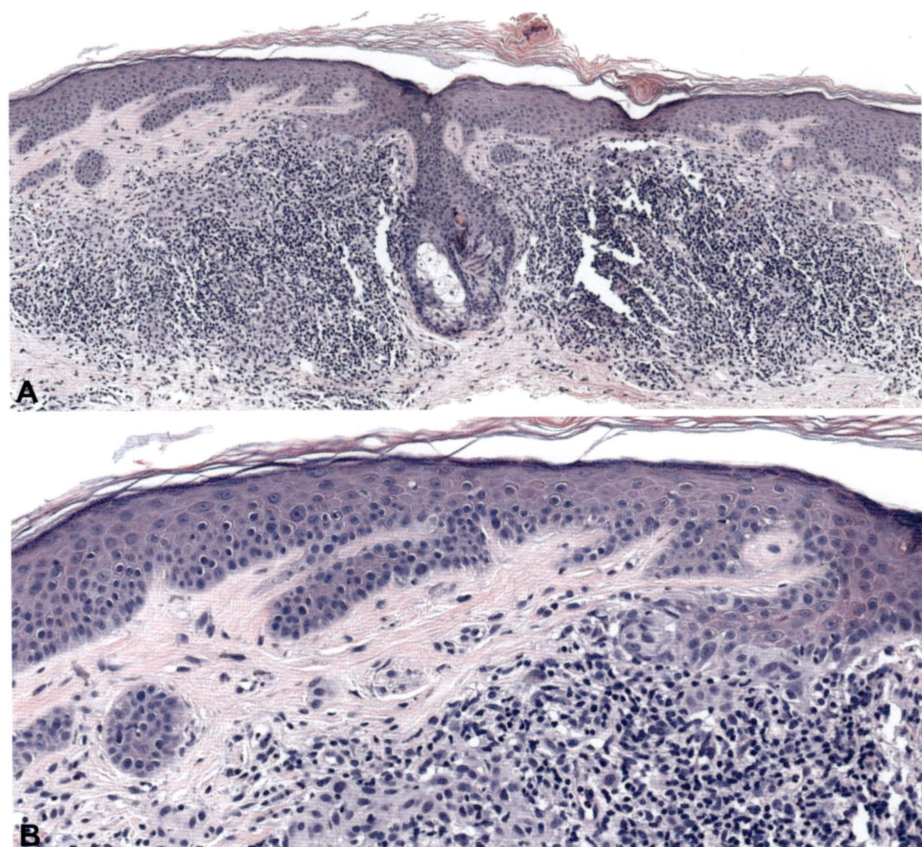

**Fig. 2.28** Halo naevus. **A** Well-circumscribed lesion that at first glance could be mistaken for a lymphocytic infiltrate. Infiltrating lymphocytes are intimately admixed with naevus cells; this leads to apoptosis and ultimately the disappearance of the naevus cells. In later examples, the naevus cells are less conspicuous than in this field. **B** At higher magnification, the epithelioid melanocytes can be distinguished more clearly from the surrounding smaller lymphocytes.

## Localization

Halo naevi are most common on the trunk but can occur anywhere on the body.

## Clinical features

Halo naevi often present during the summer, perhaps because the halo contrasts better with tanned skin. They are most common in teenagers and young adults; in these cases, they are sometimes associated with dysplastic naevi, and are sometimes multiple. Less often, a solitary halo lesion develops in an older adult; in this setting, the possibility of melanoma should be ruled out histologically, in particular if the central pigmented lesion is clinically atypical or if the halo is eccentric or asymmetrical in contour. Serial follow-up of halo naevi reveals a characteristic time sequence, beginning with the appearance of the halo around a compound naevus, followed by fading and disappearance of the naevus. The most common overall dermoscopic patterns are the uniform globular pattern and the structureless pattern {1274}.

## Histopathology

Early halo naevi present as a small circumscribed lesion composed of naevus cells located in the papillary dermis and usually also the epidermis. The lesion is symmetrical and is composed of cells that are uniform from one side of

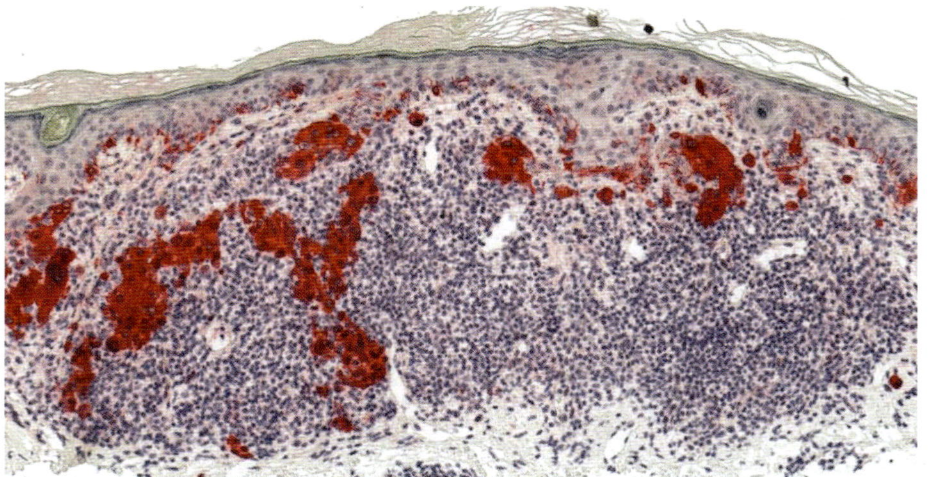

**Fig. 2.29** Halo naevus. Melan-A (MART1) immunostaining highlights the naevus cells, but not the lymphocytic inflammatory infiltrate.

the lesion to the other and that tend to become smaller (i.e. more mature) from the top to the bottom. The epidermis may be hyperkeratotic, with follicular plugging {2791}. The lymphocytic infiltrate partially or completely obscures the naevus cells. Melanin-laden histiocytes and mast cells may be present. Occasional halo naevi contain a few giant cells, or there may be a frankly granulomatous response. Over the subsequent weeks or months, the dermal naevus cells disappear; then the histological differential diagnosis may include lichenoid inflammatory dermatoses. Over a period of 1–2 years, the inflammatory cells disappear; histological examination of the site of a completely resolved halo naevus may reveal essentially normal skin, with little or no evidence of scarring or residual pigment {2791}. In most halo naevi, there is little or no readily observable melanocytic abnormality in the epidermis at the shoulder of the lesion beyond the lateral border of the dermal component, even though it is in this region where the striking halo is apparent clinically. The clinically depigmented areas may show complete absence of junctional melanocytes histologically, and there may be a few scattered lymphocytes at the dermoepidermal interface.

In most halo naevi, the lesional cells are unremarkable dermal naevus cells with large pigmented (type A) or small nonpigmented (type B) cytology. Pigment is located in naevus cells and in melanophages superficially, and is usually coarse in texture. In some lesions, the dermal cells have nuclei that are larger than is usual in common naevi; there is sometimes hyperchromatism and a degree of pleomorphism (with or without nucleoli) constituting cytological atypia, which is present in about 50% of halo naevi and is usually mild or at worst moderate in degree {1822}. This cytological atypia may represent a form of inflammatory or reactive atypia. Mitotic figures are not usually seen; their presence should prompt more careful examination to rule out melanoma, with deeper sections and embedding of any residual gross tissue {2146}. Findings suggestive of melanoma in a lesion simulating a halo naevus include the presence of a separate population of cells with an expansile pattern of growth; severe uniform cytological atypia; and the presence of frequent mitoses, ulceration, or tumour necrosis. The halo phenomenon may occasionally involve other types of naevi, including dysplastic naevi {2635}, Spitz naevi {1033}, and congenital naevi {2623}, as well as melanomas {2346}.

In most lesions, there is no intraepidermal melanocytic proliferation adjacent to the dermal component, but in a few lesions an adjacent component of melanocytic dysplasia may be observed. If an in situ or microinvasive (radial-growth-phase) component diagnostic of melanoma is present adjacent to a dermal lesion simulating halo naevus, the entire lesion is most likely to constitute melanoma with brisk inflammation.

### Differential diagnosis

The most important differential diagnosis is melanoma. Compared with nodular melanoma or the tumorigenic (vertical-growth-phase) component of superficial spreading melanoma, a halo naevus is usually smaller. However, some small melanomas may have naevoid characteristics, but with diffuse cellular atypia combined with mitotic activity and a prominent pattern of diffuse lymphocytic infiltration. If there is a junctional component, its character is that of a naevus rather than a melanoma. Epidermotropic metastatic melanoma has been reported to resemble a halo naevus in the setting of anti-PD1 therapy {1034}.

Some halo naevi may be difficult to distinguish from dysplastic naevi that have an unusually brisk lymphocytic infiltrate. If the characteristic patterns of dysplasia are seen at the shoulder of the compound portion of a lesion whose other features are consistent with a halo naevus, the diagnosis of dysplastic naevus with halo reaction can be made. When naevus cells are inconspicuous among a dense infiltrate of lymphocytes, inflammatory dermatoses such as lichenoid keratoses may be simulated {896}; in such cases, S100, melan-A, or HMB45 staining may reveal the hidden naevus cells. Finally, there are lesions that have an infiltrative lymphocytic response similar to that of a halo naevus but there is no clinical halo. These lesions may be signed out descriptively as "compound (or dermal) naevi with halo reaction" {2146}. Conversely, some naevi with a clinical halo may lack a lymphocytic infiltrate of the type seen in halo naevi {863}. These can be termed non-inflammatory halo naevi.

### Histogenesis

The histogenesis of halo naevus is related to the immunological mechanisms by which an immune response develops to existing aggregates of naevus cells.

### Genetic susceptibility

Patients with Turner syndrome have been reported to have an increased incidence of halo naevi {296}.

### Prognosis and predictive factors

Halo naevi are benign lesions. Morbidity is minimal (limited to cosmetic appearance).

# Meyerson naevus

Messina J.
Lowe L.

## Definition

Meyerson naevus is a benign naevus with superimposed eczematous dermatitis, characterized histologically by spongiosis.

## ICD-O code 8720/0

## Synonyms

Halo eczema; halo dermatitis

## Epidemiology

Meyerson naevus typically occurs in young adults, with an equal sex distribution {753}.

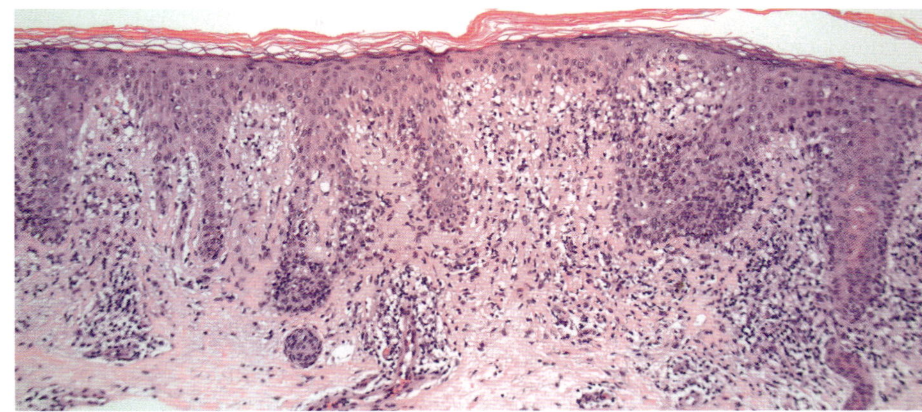

**Fig. 2.31** Meyerson naevus. Acanthosis and exocytosis of lymphocytes masking a subtle melanocytic proliferation.

## Etiology

The eczematous reaction is likely triggered by factors within the naevus, because excision of the naevus has been reported to lead to regression of the accompanying inflammation {540}. Other postulated etiological factors include ultraviolet (UV) radiation exposure, chemotherapy, and interferon alfa-2b, but none has been proven {753}.

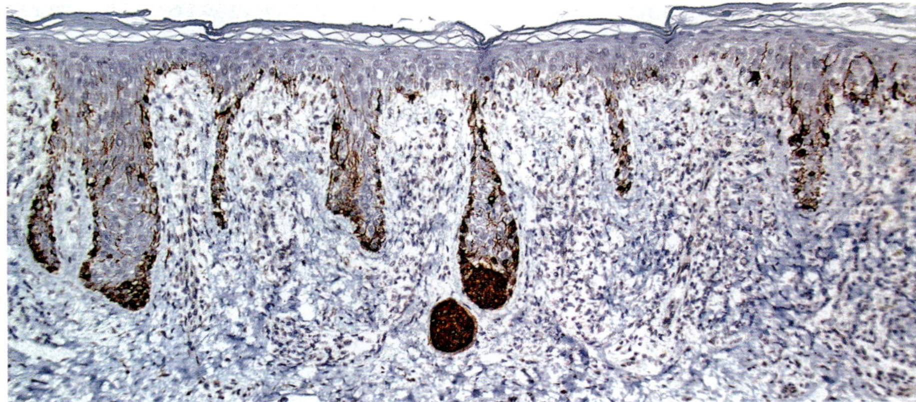

**Fig. 2.32** Meyerson naevus. Melan-A immunohistochemical stain reveals rare nests of benign melanocytes in epidermis and dermis.

## Localization

Meyerson naevus occurs predominantly on the trunk and proximal extremities {753}.

## Clinical features

First described by Meyerson in 1971, the Meyerson phenomenon produces an inflammatory reaction around a pre-existing naevus or other lesion, such as sebaceous naevus and even melanoma {759,1761}. Erythema and scaling symmetrically surround and extend beyond the borders of the central naevus, with the scaling producing a halo. In two thirds of cases, multiple naevi are involved {1586}. The lesions may be pruritic. In some cases, the inflammation may subside with topical corticosteroid treatment; in other cases, excision is necessary to cause the inflammation to subside.

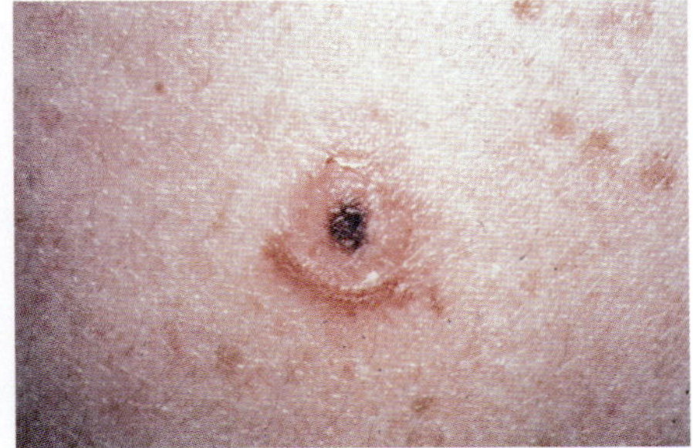

**Fig. 2.30** Meyerson naevus with an eczematous halo around a pigmented naevus.

## Histopathology

Parakeratosis with serum overlies epidermal acanthosis with spongiosis. There is a superficial perivascular lymphocytic infiltrate, which is predominantly CD4-positive {1586}. Eosinophils may be present. The infiltrate may obscure the underlying naevus, which may be acquired or congenital.

## Differential diagnosis

Halo naevi lack the changes of spongiotic dermatitis that are characteristic of Meyerson naevi. They are also characterized by a predominant infiltrate of CD8+ lymphocytes, whereas Meyerson naevi show a predominance of CD4+ T cells {757}.

## Genetic susceptibility

Although typically an isolated lesion, Meyerson naevus may be associated with atopic dermatitis {2220}.

# Recurrent naevus

Zalaudek I.
Brenn T.
Elenitsas R.
Helm K.F.
Shea C.

## Definition

Recurrent naevus is a naevus that recurs after incomplete surgical removal, biopsy, or trauma.

## Synonyms

Persistent naevus; traumatized naevus; pseudomelanoma

## Epidemiology

Recurrent naevi commonly occur after partial surgical removal by shave excision. They are most frequently found in females, on the back, but can occur at any location. More than 50% of recurrent naevi arise within the first 6 months after biopsy, but recurrences may not be biopsied until many years later {1093,1375,1991,2385,2479}. Compound or intradermal naevi are the most common types of naevi to recur, possibly because their deeper component can persist after superficial removal {1991}. Recurrent naevi most commonly involve common acquired naevi, but in principle any type of naevus can recur.

## Etiology

The term "recurrent naevus" can be considered a misnomer; most experts believe that the naevus cells were always present (because of incomplete removal) but were not clinically evident until the naevus recurred on examination. Therefore, some clinicians prefer the term "persistent naevus". Naevi are more likely to recur if the original naevus was > 1 cm in size, had positive margins, was located on the back, and was removed by shave excision {2479}. Proliferation of residual melanocytes located in the deep dermis around adnexal structures, or occasionally in the epidermis at the periphery of incompletely excised naevi, is the possible etiology.

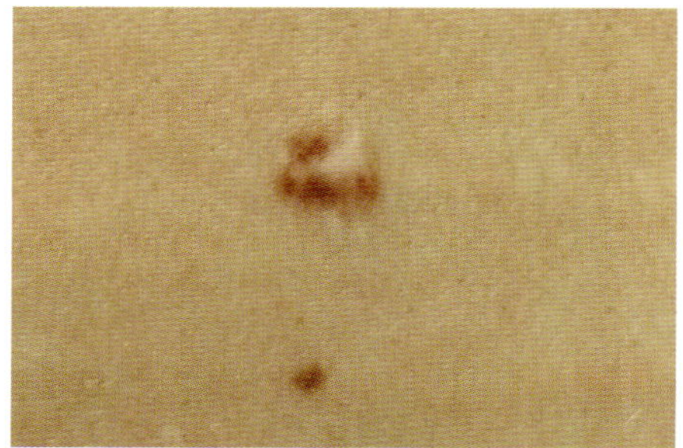

**Fig. 2.33** Recurrent naevus characterized by asymmetrical mottled hyper- and hypopigmented macules within a scar.

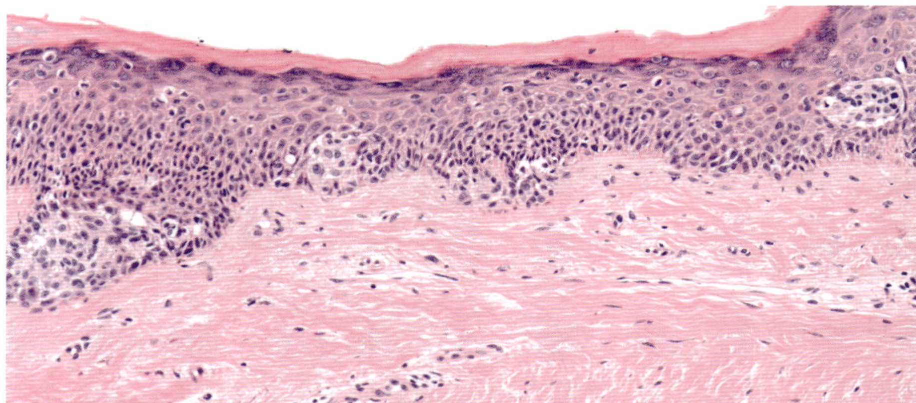

**Fig. 2.34** Recurrent naevus with asymmetrical distribution of pleomorphic single melanocytes and nests of melanocytes within an epidermis overlying a scar.

## Clinical features

Recurrent naevi can be recognized by the finding of pigmentation within a scar on clinical inspection. The morphological appearance can vary, from uniform symmetrical tan macules to asymmetrical hyper- and hypopigmented macules raising concern for melanoma. The potential clinical similarity to melanoma is an important diagnostic pitfall. Recurrent naevi can resemble melanoma both clinically and histologically. Dermoscopy reveals symmetry, radial lines, and a centrifugal growth pattern {259}. Unsuspecting pathologists have mistaken recurrent naevi for melanoma, hence the synonym "pseudomelanoma" {817,1432}.

## Histopathology

The key histopathological feature is a dermal scar characterized by parallel fibroblasts embedded in sclerotic collagen bundles, with vertically oriented blood vessels and an overlying epidermis with attenuation of the rete ridge pattern. Like all naevi, recurrent naevi can be compound, junctional, or intradermal. The classic description is of a trizonal lesion with a junctional epidermal component, a scar component, and an underlying benign dermal component {817}. The junctional component can vary from single melanocytes located along the dermoepidermal junction, to a predominance of nests, to occasional pagetoid spread of pleomorphic cells resembling melanoma (so-called pseudomelanoma) {1991,2479}. There may also be a few atypical cells in the superficial portion of the scar. Cytological atypia is usually mild, but occasionally moderate to severe. Mitotic figures can occasionally be seen. The atypia in the recurrence seems to be independent of the type of naevus that was originally biopsied {2479}. A helpful feature in distinguishing a recurrent naevus from melanoma is that the atypical melanocytic proliferation is usually localized to the area of the scar {1375}. There may be persistent benign junctional naevus extending beyond the scar. In diagnostically challenging cases, reviewing the prior pathology can be helpful.

## Differential diagnosis

The histological differential diagnosis includes other pigmented lesions, such as melanoma, dysplastic naevus, traumatized naevus, sclerosing naevus {726}, and dysplastic naevus with florid fibroplasia {1395}.

### Histogenesis

Immunohistochemistry indicates a low proliferation rate in recurrent naevi; maturation of the melanocytes within the dermis is evidenced either morphologically or by immunohistochemistry for tyrosinase or HMB45 antigen {1093}, showing decreased immunoreactivity in the deepest cells. S100-positive fibroblast-like cells can be found in and surrounding the scar, around blood vessels, and around eccrine glands {102}.

### Genetic profile

The genetic profile is identical to that of a non-recurrent naevus.

### Prognosis and predictive factors

Definitive diagnosis of a recurrent naevus requires a biopsy that demonstrates the transition from the skin affected by the scar to the adjacent normal skin. If this cannot be confirmed, or if the precise nature of the lesion previously removed from the site cannot be determined, complete excision of the recurrence should be considered.

# Deep penetrating naevus and melanocytoma

Barnhill R.L.
Bastian B.C.
Gerami P.
Magro C.
Scolyer R.A.

### Definition

Deep penetrating naevus (DPN) is an acquired melanocytic neoplasm composed of pigmented spindled and/or epithelioid melanocytes with distinctive deep architecture. The biological significance of these naevi lies in their frequent simulation of melanoma, the frequent uncertainty about their malignant potential, and their rare metastatic progression.

### ICD-O code

| | |
|---|---|
| Deep penetrating naevus | 8720/0 |

### Epidemiology

DPNs are uncommon. They occur in patients of all ages but have a predilection for women aged <40 years (mean age: 26 years, range: 3–63 years) {2205,2369}.

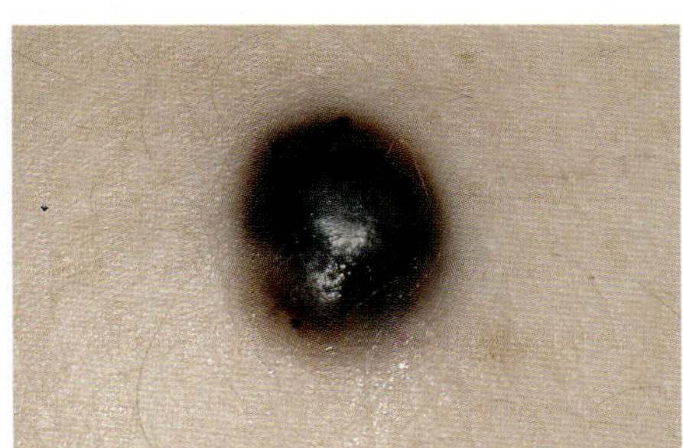

**Fig. 2.35** Deep penetrating naevus. A pigmented nodule that is generally symmetrical and not ulcerated. Biopsy and histopathological examination are needed to distinguish this lesion from a nodular melanoma.

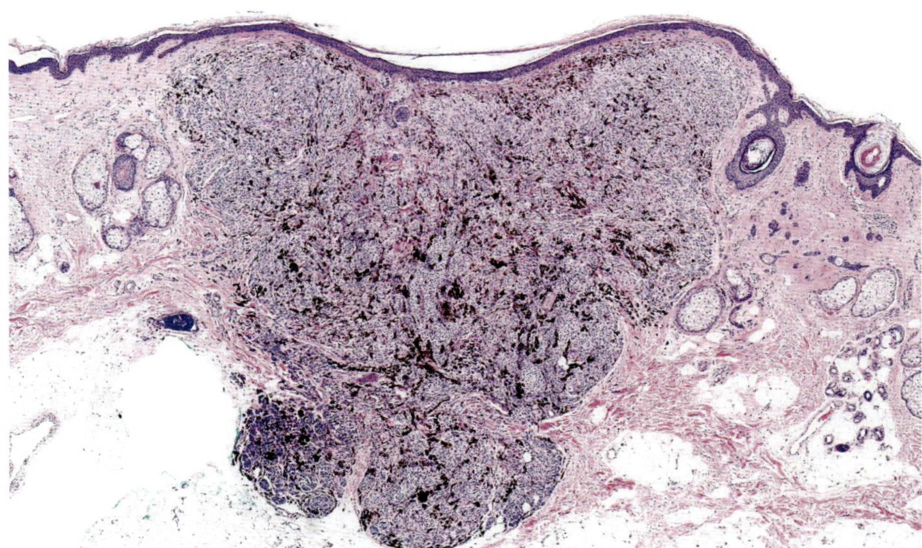

**Fig. 2.36** Deep penetrating naevus. The proliferation exhibits a small diameter, sharp circumscription, and symmetry. Note the wedge-shaped architecture and deep extension into subcutaneous fat.

### Localization

DPNs most commonly involve the head and neck, upper trunk, and proximal extremities {2369}.

### Clinical features

The lesions often present as symmetrical, well-circumscribed, dark-brown, bluish-brown, or bluish-black papules, sometimes with colour variegation. They are typically <5 mm in diameter (range: 2–10 mm) {524,2205,2369}. Atypical DPNs, which are rare, are usually larger and show atypical features.

### Histopathology

DPNs are almost always well-circumscribed, symmetrical, dermal-based melanocytic tumours defined by a population of enlarged pigmented spindle and epithelioid cells often in a distinctive deep wedge-shaped (or V-shaped) configuration {524,1733,1733,2205,2369}. A diffusely cellular superficial dermal

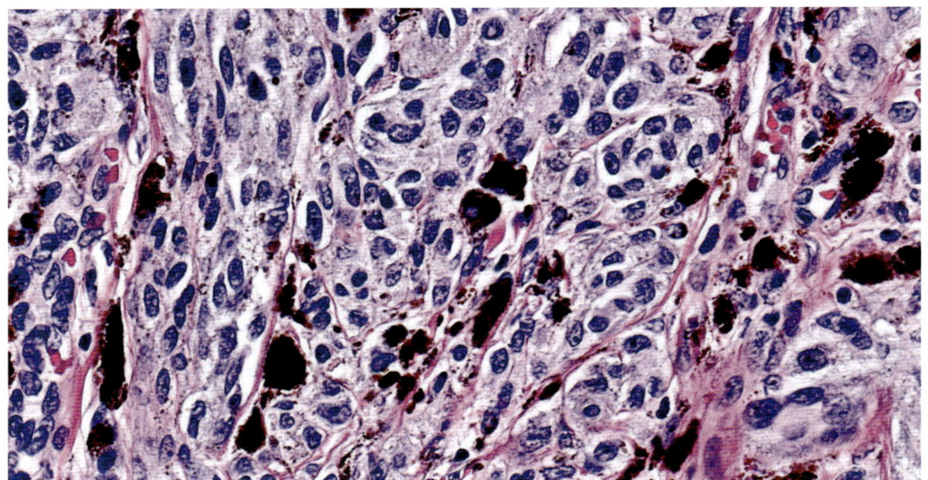

**Fig. 2.37** Deep penetrating naevus. Slightly enlarged fusiform melanocytes are arranged in bundles. These melanocytes contain scant, finely granular cytoplasmic melanin and enlarged nuclei with slight pleomorphism; the mitotic rate is 0–1 mitosis/mm$^2$.

component often gives way to distinct fascicles of enlarged, pigmented melanocytes present near the surface of the lesion and extending in most cases into the mid- to deep reticular dermis and in some cases into the subcutis. These fascicles are usually associated with neurovascular and adnexal structures and may have bulbous contours. There is usually an admixture of epithelioid cells, elongated cells, and melanophages. Cytologically, the melanocytes are slightly pigmented and often exhibit mild to moderate nuclear enlargement, pleomorphism, and some hyperchromatism. Pseudonuclear inclusions are common. Mitoses are absent or rare (e.g. 1–2 mitoses/mm$^2$). Additional features include frequent junctional nests and conventional naevus components (i.e. as part of a combined naevus).

Atypical DPNs (melanocytomas) have atypical features such as large size, asymmetry, aberrant architecture (e.g. sheet-like arrangements of melanocytes), increased mitotic rates, and severe cytological atypia {1629}.

DPNs express S100 protein and SOX10, as well as the melanocyte differentiation antigens HMB45 antigen, melan-A (MART1), tyrosinase, and MITF {147}. Diffuse HMB45 staining is particularly useful for the recognition of DPN.

## Differential diagnosis

Although DPN and its atypical variants are frequently confused with melanoma, standard histopathological criteria usually enable their distinction. Immunohistochemistry and genomic analysis may also facilitate interpretation. The term "atypical DPNs with uncertain malignant potential" connotes rare neoplasms defying definitive diagnosis as benign or malignant. The differential diagnosis also includes plexiform spindle cell naevus, Spitz naevus, cellular blue naevus, and pigmented epithelioid melanocytoma (also called epithelioid blue naevus). DPN and plexiform spindle cell naevus – *Pigmented spindle cell naevus (Reed naevus)*, p. 114 – show some overlap and form a histological continuum, analogous to that formed by pigmented spindle cell naevus and Spitz naevus. The essential differences are related to architecture (i.e. plexiform vs wedge-shaped configuration) and depth (i.e. DPNs exhibit greater depth than do plexiform spindle cell naevi). β-catenin staining is useful in identifying DPNs and distinguishing them from common acquired naevi, blue naevi, and Spitz naevi.

## Histogenesis and genetic profile

DPNs show activation of the WNT pathway through gain-of-function mutations of the gene encoding β-catenin (*CTNNB1*) or loss of *APC*. These alterations are typically present in combination with MAPK-activating mutations of genes such as *BRAF* (p.V600E), *MAP2K1* (*MEK1*), or *HRAS*. Most DPNs arise from common acquired naevi (which only carry the MAPK-activating mutation) through the acquisition of WNT pathway activation {2884}. However, a residual common naevus is not always found in sections, which may indicate that the precursor is not present in the planes of the sections examined, that the precursor has regressed, or that this stage has been skipped. WNT signalling increases the cell size and pigmentation of melanocytes, explaining the lack of apparent maturation in DPNs with pigmented and enlarged melanocytes that can extend deep into the dermis. Lesions with the typical morphology of DPN do not usually have *GNAQ* and *GNA11* mutations {205}, but those with overlapping features of blue naevus do {2884}.

## Genetic susceptibility

Several so-called naevus susceptibility genes have been described {1952}, but this information has not yet been translated into clinical practice.

## Prognosis and predictive factors

DPN and atypical DPN/melanocytomas are important simulants of melanoma. There is evidence that increasing age and atypical histological features may correlate with metastatic/neoplastic progression and increased risk for aggressive behaviour associated with these neoplasms, but this finding requires more-detailed study {1151,1629}. Melanomas that share histological features with DPN may also share the genetic hallmark of DPN (i.e. activation of the WNT pathway), indicating that some DPNs can progress to melanoma {2884}. Lesions with intermediate features (e.g. increased cellularity, relatively subtle atypia, and a few mitoses) that fall short of fulfilling the definitive criteria for melanoma may be termed "melanocytomas" (with varying degrees of atypia), to distinguish them from the wholly benign naevi and the fully malignant melanomas. However, DPNs appear for the most part to be very stable lesions, and their progression to melanoma is rare.

# Pigmented epithelioid melanocytoma

Zembowicz A.
Calonje E.
Mihm M.C. Jr

## Definition

Pigmented epithelioid melanocytoma (PEM) is a melanocytic neoplasm composed of heavily pigmented epithelioid and dendritic cells, with metastatic potential limited to regional lymph nodes. It can occur as a sporadic lesion {941,1655,1829,1931,2926} or in patients with Carney complex {384}.

## ICD-O code 8780/1

## Synonyms

Epithelioid blue naevus; animal-type melanoma (not recommended)

## Epidemiology

PEM is a rare tumour with a predilection for young people, including children; however, it can occur at any age. All racial groups are affected.

## Etiology

Other than an association with Carney complex, the etiology of PEM is unknown.

## Localization

PEM has a generalized distribution, including localization to the extremities, head and neck, and trunk.

## Clinical features

These lesions occur as a slow-growing pigmented nodule or papule.

## Histopathology

PEM can be a pure lesion or a component of a combined naevus with an adjacent common acquired naevus {2926}. PEM is usually a heavily pigmented, predominantly dermal tumour, with an inverted wedge or bulbous configuration. Small junctional nests can be seen in 30% of cases. Many PEMs induce epidermal hyperplasia. Some lesions are separated from the epidermis by a zone of uninvolved papillary dermis. Tumours tend to be more cellular in the centre and have infiltrative borders. Substantial stromal fibroplasia is usually absent. PEM is composed of varying proportions of pigmented dendritic and epithelioid melanocytes admixed with melanophages. The dendritic cells have long cytoplasmic projections. Unlike in blue naevus, the dendritic cells' nuclei are vesicular, with prominent nucleoli. The diagnostic epithelioid cells are round, polygonal, or elongated, and they range in size from medium to large, sometimes resembling Reed–Sternberg cells. The epithelioid cells can show substantial nuclear polymorphism and multinucleation. Mitotic

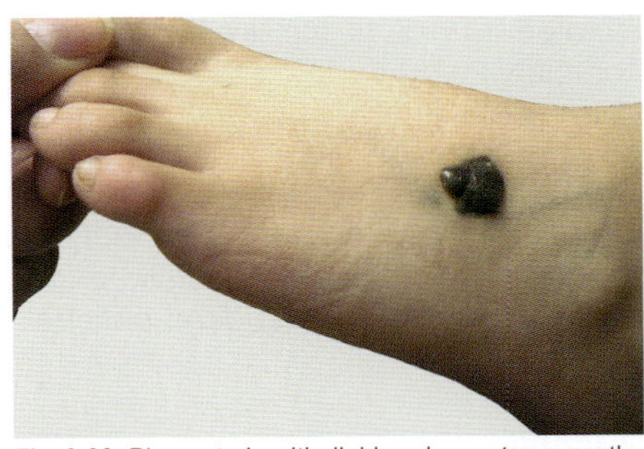

**Fig. 2.39** Pigmented epithelioid melanocytoma on the foot of a 7-year-old boy.

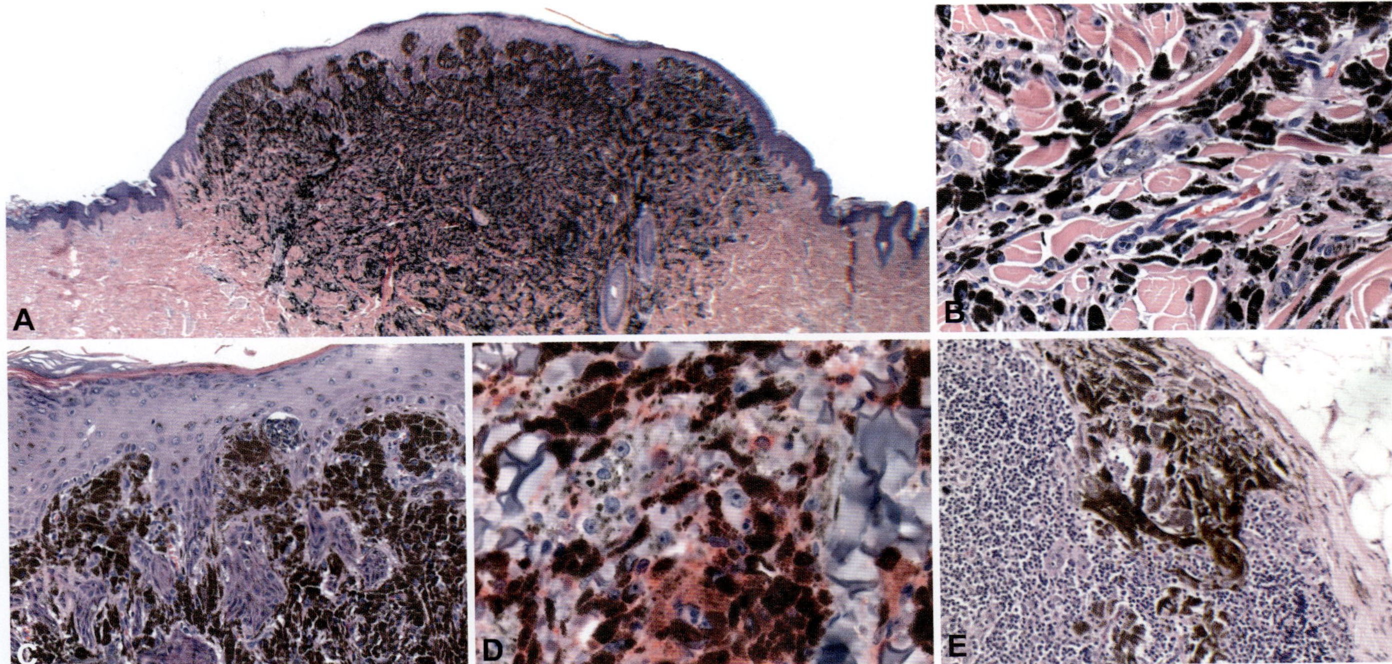

**Fig. 2.38** Pigmented epithelioid melanocytoma, pure. **A** Low-magnification showing epidermal hyperplasia, a wedge-shape configuration, and an infiltrative border. **B** Cellular composition including pigmented dendritic cells, epithelioid cells, and melanophages. **C** Junctional component. **D** Loss of PRKAR1A expression in large epithelioid cells. **E** Lymph node metastasis.

activity is low but can be observed. Large PEMs can be associated with ulceration or tumour necrosis. Immunostaining shows expression of melanocytic markers, including melan-A, S100 protein, HMB45 antigen, and SOX10. A subset of PEMs show loss of expression of the protein product of *PRKAR1A*, which is mutated in 62% of families with Carney complex {2928}.

## Differential diagnosis

The differential diagnosis includes blue naevus with epithelioid cells {2880}, pigmented melanoma (metastatic or primary), Spitz naevus, and deep penetrating naevus.

## Histogenesis

PEM may be a neoplasm of dorsal neural crest–derived melanocytes rather than of the melanocytic precursors originating from ventral neural crest believed to give rise to blue naevus.

## Genetic profile

Combined PEMs harbour both BRAF p.V600 mutations and loss-of-function alterations affecting *PRKAR1A*, including missense (p.P210L) and splice-site (c.178-1G>A) mutations and hemizygous deletion {504}, and therefore likely arise from common acquired naevi. A subset of pure PEMs harbour fusions of *PRKCA*, a gene located in the vicinity of *PRKAR1A* on chromosome 17, with one of two partners (resulting in *ATP2B4-PRKCA* or *RNF13-PRKCA* fusion) {132,504}. These pure PEMs may thus be more akin to Spitz naevi. Some pure PEMs show loss of expression of the PRKAR1A protein but no detectable mutations of the *PRKAR1A* gene {504,2928}. The genetic mechanisms involved in these lesions are unknown, but two lesions have shown mutations in *MAP2K1*, which encodes a kinase involved in MAPK signalling downstream of BRAF {132,504}. PEM does not show *TERT* promoter mutations or significant chromosomal copy-number changes {504}. PEM-like lesions harbouring *GNAQ* or *GNA11* mutation should be classified as blue naevi.

## Genetic susceptibility

PEM can occur in patients with Carney complex, but most cases are sporadic.

## Prognosis and predictive factors

PEM is an indolent melanocytic tumour with metastatic potential limited to regional lymph nodes and otherwise rare distant metastasis {2926}. Death from disease has not been reported. In most reported cases, lymph node deposits were discovered in sentinel lymph nodes, but patients have occasionally been reported with clinically detected lymph node metastases. Ulceration has been associated with lymphatic metastases {1655}.

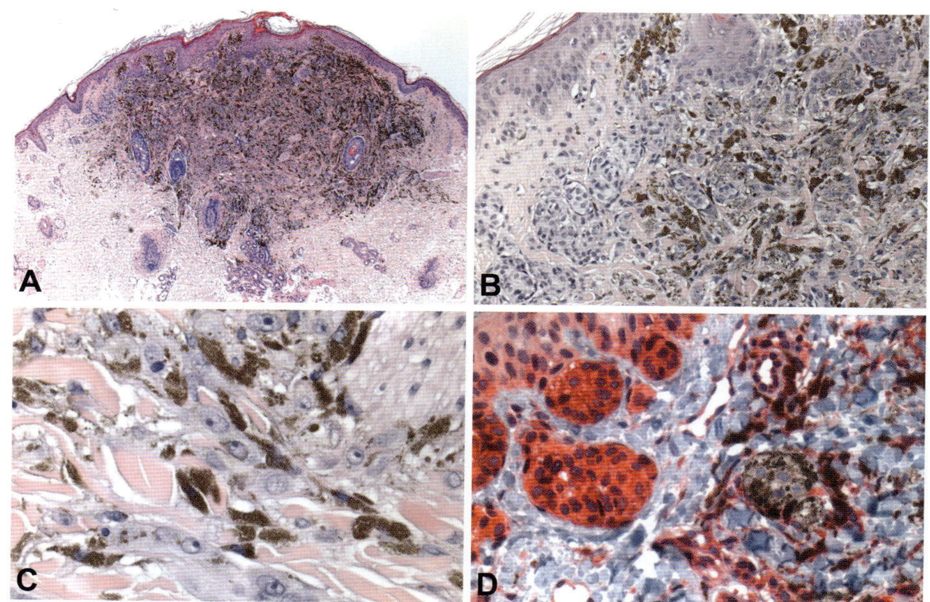


**Fig. 2.40** Pigmented epithelioid melanocytoma (PEM), combined. **A** Low-magnification view showing precursor naevus on the left. **B** Transition between common naevus (left) and PEM. **C** Large epithelioid cells, dendritic cells, and melanophages in the PEM component. **D** PRKAR1A expression in compound naevus but not PEM.

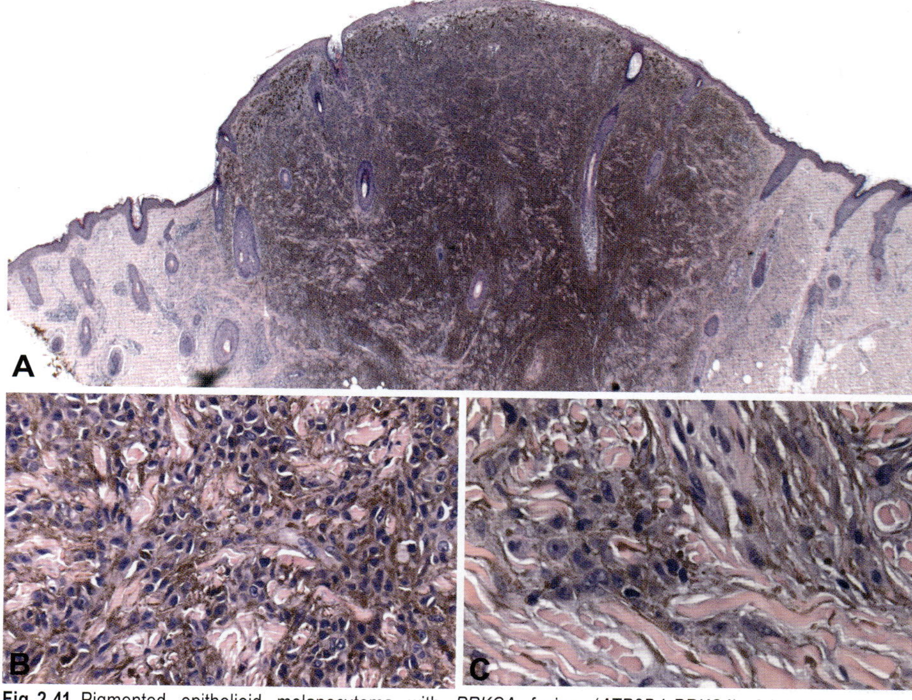


**Fig. 2.41** Pigmented epithelioid melanocytoma with *PRKCA* fusion (*ATP2B4-PRKCA*). **A** Low-magnification view. **B** Cellular area with epithelioid and dendritic cells in the centre of the lesion. **C** Large epithelioid cells at the periphery of the lesion.

# Combined naevus, including combined *BAP1*-inactivated naevus/melanocytoma

Wiesner T.
Mihm M.C. Jr
Scolyer R.A.

## Definition

A combined naevus contains two (or more) melanocytic naevus components in the same lesion. The cellular components can be any combination of any naevus variants, but most frequently, a common naevus component is combined with a blue naevus, deep penetrating naevus (DPN), or Spitz naevus component.

## ICD-O code 8720/0

## Synonyms

Clonal naevus; melanocytic naevus with phenotypic heterogeneity; naevus with dermal epithelioid component; inverted type A naevus; naevus with atypical dermal nodules {2366}

Combined *BAP1*-inactivated naevus {2743}: Wiesner naevus {1578}; *BAP1*-deficient tumour {875}; melanocytic *BAP1*-mutated atypical intradermal tumours {374}

## Epidemiology

The exact prevalence is unknown, but combined naevi are relatively uncommon; they have been found to account for < 1% of melanocytic naevi sampled for histopathological examination. Combined naevi can develop at any age, but typically present in young people, with a mean age of about 30 years {2366}.

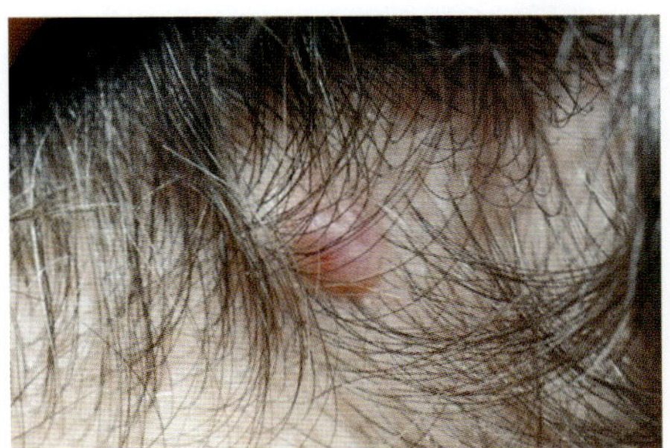

**Fig. 2.42** Combined *BAP1*-inactivated naevus. A symmetrical, pink, smooth-surfaced papule.

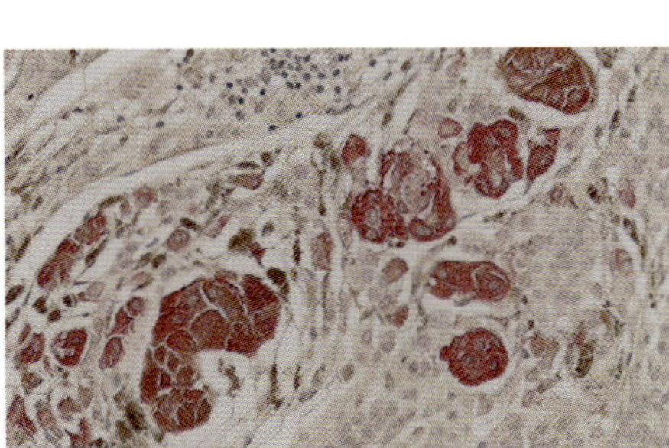

**Fig. 2.43** Combined naevus. HMB45-positive staining in the deep penetrating naevus component; the common naevus component (bottom of field) is negative.

## Etiology

The etiology is likely heterogeneous, but is unknown in most cases {2366}. Some combined naevi may develop by divergent cell differentiation, which might be triggered by the tumour microenvironment or by alterations in genes involved in chromatin modification or cell differentiation. Other combined naevi may represent collision tumours, with two naevus cell populations that have developed independently by distinct genomic aberrations. Some combined naevi evolve by the sequential acquisition of genomic aberrations; for example, in combined *BAP1*-inactivated naevi all melanocytes usually harbour BRAF p.V600E mutations, but only the epithelioid melanocytes

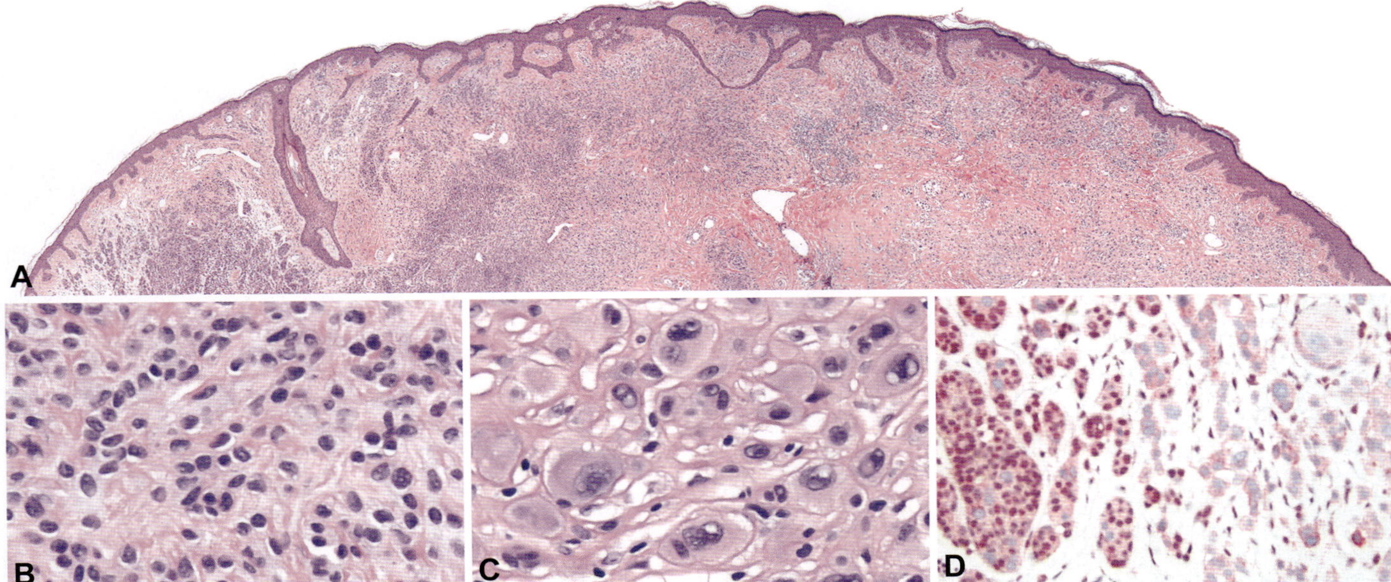

**Fig. 2.44** Combined *BAP1*-inactivated naevus. **A** Combined lesion with an area of (**B**) small, oval melanocytes (common acquired naevus) on the left and (**C**) large epithelioid melanocytes with large polymorphic nuclei, vesicular chromatin, abundant cytoplasm, distinct cell borders, and tumour-infiltrating lymphocytes on the right. **D** BAP1 immunohistochemistry shows nuclear staining in the common naevus component (left) and loss of nuclear staining in the epithelioid component (right).
Reprinted with permission from: Wiesner T et al. (2011) Nat Genet. 43:1018-21, Macmillan Publishers Ltd.

show a loss of BAP1 expression, indicating that the epithelioid component represents a progression from the common naevus component {2828}.

## Localization

Combined naevi are commonly observed on the head and neck region (accounting for ~25% of cases), but they can occur on any anatomical skin site; they occur on the trunk in about 35% of cases and on the extremities in about 35% of cases {2366}.

## Clinical features

The clinical picture of combined naevi is heterogeneous, determined by the combination and distribution of the cellular components. In general, combined naevi are usually well-circumscribed, asymmetrical papules with a diameter < 6 mm. They usually show two or more colours, ranging from skin-coloured, reddish, or brown to black and blue. Combined naevi with a blue naevus or DPN component often exhibit small blue or bluish-black dots within otherwise brown, reddish, or skin-coloured lesions. Combined *BAP1*-inactivated naevi are typically skin-coloured to reddish, dome-shaped papules, sometimes with small areas of brown colour at their periphery. Patients sometimes report a sudden change in a longstanding naevus, such as colour changes or increased growth, which may raise concern for melanoma {1682,2366}.

## Histopathology

Combined naevi are defined by two or more distinct naevus components, which may encompass any mixture and proportion of the entire phenotypic spectrum of melanocytic naevi. Most combined naevi have two cellular components, which may be either intimately admixed or next to each other. The most frequent combinations are common naevus with blue naevus, common naevus with DPN, and common naevus with Spitz naevus. In all of these lesions, the common naevus component is usually composed of small, plump, round to oval melanocytes. In common naevus with blue naevus, the blue naevus component of pigmented dendritic, spindled-shaped melanocytes is usually intermingled with the common naevus component, along with densely pigmented melanophages. Common naevus with DPN is characterized by large, oval or polygonal, lightly pigmented cells with pale vacuolated cytoplasm and often large, irregular nuclei. These cells are usually located within the common naevus component and interspersed melanophages. In common naevus with Spitz naevus, large spindle or epithelioid melanocytes with large, atypical nuclei are present. The spitzoid component is typically located within a circumscribed area rather than scattered among the common naevus cells. Tumour-infiltrating lymphocytes are often observed. In combined *BAP1*-inactivated naevi, the epithelioid cells present with well-defined cytoplasmic borders, amphophilic cytoplasm, vesicular nuclei, and prominent nucleoli. Other histological features of Spitz naevi, such as epidermal hyperplasia, hypergranulosis, clefting around junctional nests, and Kamino bodies, are usually absent. The spitzoid component in combined *BAP1*-inactivated naevi frequently shows loss of BAP1 on immunohistochemistry, along with *BRAF* mutations {346,1682,2366}.

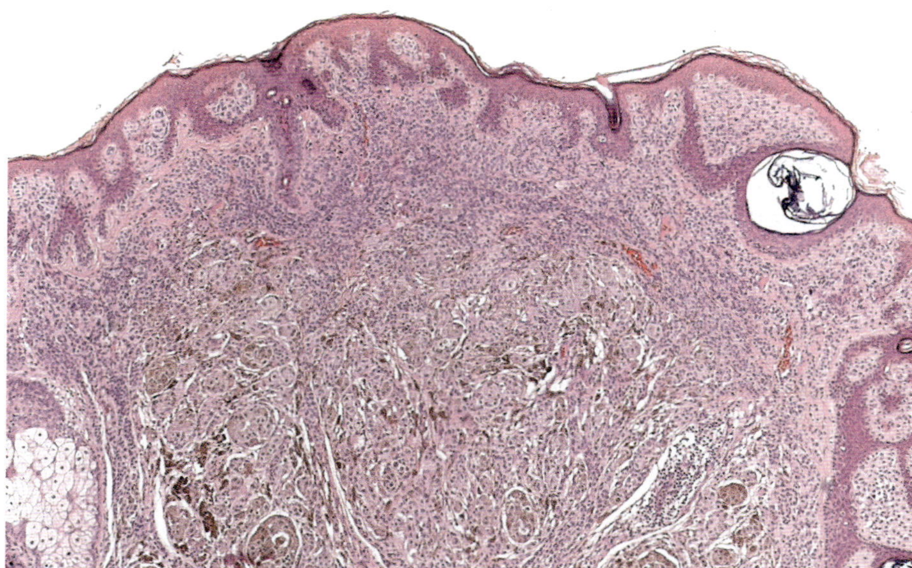

**Fig. 2.45** Combined naevus. A large nodular lesion comprising two populations of cells. A component of larger pigmented melanocytes is present in a background of small banal naevus cells.

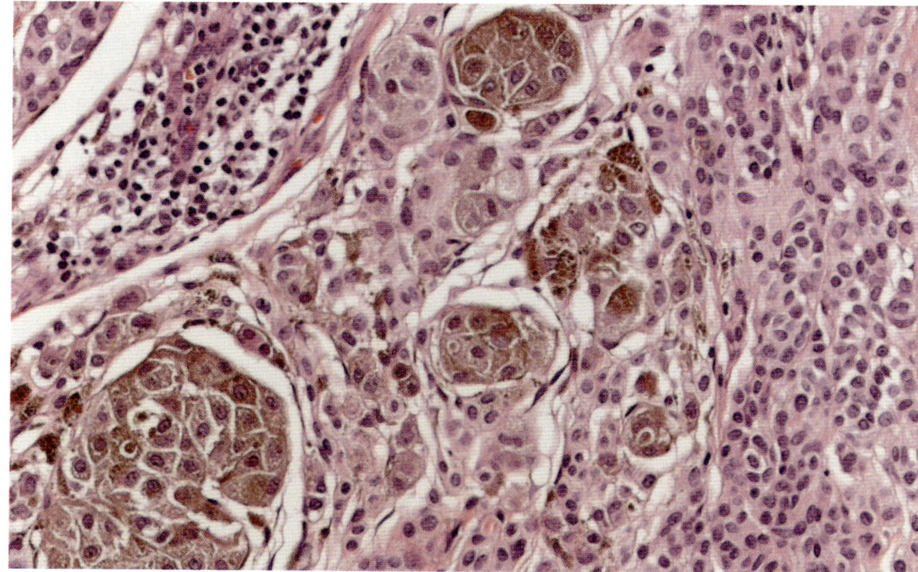

**Fig. 2.46** Combined naevus. One of the cell types, at the periphery on the right, is a small naevoid cell, extending into the reticular dermis and around skin appendages as is seen in a congenital-pattern naevus. The other cell type (left) is more voluminous and has pigmented cytoplasm.

## Differential diagnosis

Combined naevi, especially those with spitzoid or DPN components, can easily be confused with melanoma arising in a naevus. Helpful clues in the differential diagnosis are that, unlike melanomas, combined naevi usually display the following characteristics: occurrence in young patients (mean age: ~30 years); a diameter of ≤ 6 mm, ≤ 1 mitosis/mm², and ≤ 3 mitoses in the entire lesion; low cellularity; monomorphous cytological atypia; no (non-traumatic) ulceration; no necrosis; no solar elastosis; no thinning of the epidermis; and no pagetoid spread or any other pattern resembling melanoma in situ at the junction.

Unlike in melanoma, where at least one cellular component appears asymmetrical or poorly circumscribed, both of the cellular components of combined naevi (when evaluated independently from each other) are usually relatively symmetrical and well circumscribed (although the overall appearance is often asymmetrical). Also unlike in melanoma, where expansible-looking nodules appear to compress the naevoid component, the large cell component of combined naevi has no growth advantage and does not compress the naevoid component {141,1682,2366}.

## Genetic profile

For most combined naevi, the genetic profile is unknown. A substantial proportion of combined naevi with a spitzoid component show inactivation of *BAP1* (combined *BAP1*-inactivated naevus) {1578,2827}. Most lesions with BAP1 loss also have BRAF p.V600E mutations, but some with *NRAS* mutations have also been reported; combined naevi with BAP1 loss and *NRAS* mutations seem to arise from naevi similar to DPNs and are appropriately grouped in the low-CSD (i.e. arising in skin with a low degree of cumulative sun damage) category. Sporadic lesions have two additional alterations: the inactivation of both healthy *BAP1* alleles. Syndromic lesions have only one additional genomic abnormality, because one inactivating mutation of *BAP1* is already present in all cells.

## Genetic susceptibility

Patients with germline *BAP1* mutations (i.e. *BAP1* tumour predisposition syndrome) typically develop multiple combined *BAP1*-inactivated naevi and melanocytomas {347,2823}.

## Prognosis and predictive factors

Combined naevi are by definition benign; apart from cosmetic concerns, they cause no clinical problems. As is the case with some cellular blue naevi, DPNs, and Spitz naevi, and consistent with the tumour progression model {2826}, some atypical combined naevi/tumours have overlapping features with melanoma, but lack sufficient evidence for a histopathological diagnosis of melanoma. Atypical combined tumours may be potential precursor lesions of melanoma, rarely metastasize, and may be best designated as biologically indeterminate. For such lesions, the consensus meeting Working Group proposes the use of the term "melanocytoma", to distinguish them from the more banal lesions called naevi. Clinical information and molecular data (along with pathological criteria) may help to predict the biological behaviour of these atypical variants more accurately.

# Melanocytic tumours in chronically sun-exposed skin

## Lentigo maligna melanoma

Elder D.E.
Bastian B.C.
Kim J.
Massi D.
Mihm M.C. Jr
Scolyer R.A.
Wood B.A.

### Definition

High-CSD melanomas – melanomas in skin with a high degree of cumulative sun damage (CSD) as evidenced by severe solar elastosis – have distinctive clinical and genetic features. Lentigo maligna melanoma (LMM) is a type of high-CSD melanoma characterized by a lentiginous in situ component called lentigo maligna (also sometimes called LMM in situ) with a proliferation of mostly single cytologically atypical melanocytes in the basilar epidermis {493,1714}.

### ICD-O code

8742/3

### Synonym

Melanoma in Hutchinson melanotic freckle

### Epidemiology

Compared with superficial spreading melanoma, this form of melanoma occurs in a somewhat older population, and it occurs in skin sites that are chronically exposed to the sun, often because of outdoor work or daily exposure in the course of normal activity. Patients with LMM tend to have a high count of solar lentigines and a lower count of naevi {1524,1645,2103,2813}.

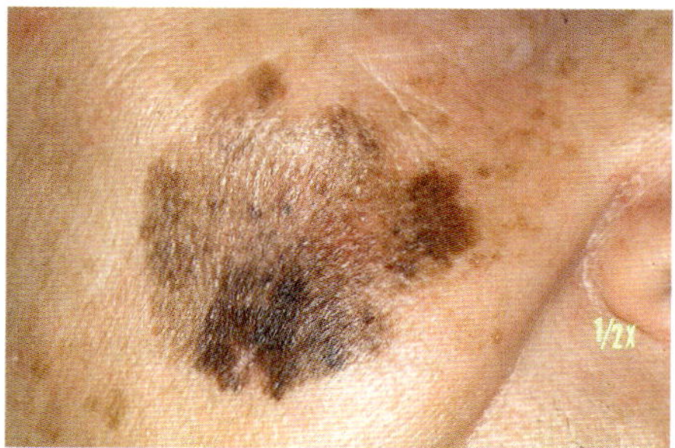


**Fig. 2.47** Lentigo maligna melanoma. Radial-growth-phase lesions usually present as a variegated patch/plaque in the skin; unlike in superficial spreading melanoma, the border is poorly defined in some areas and non-palpable.

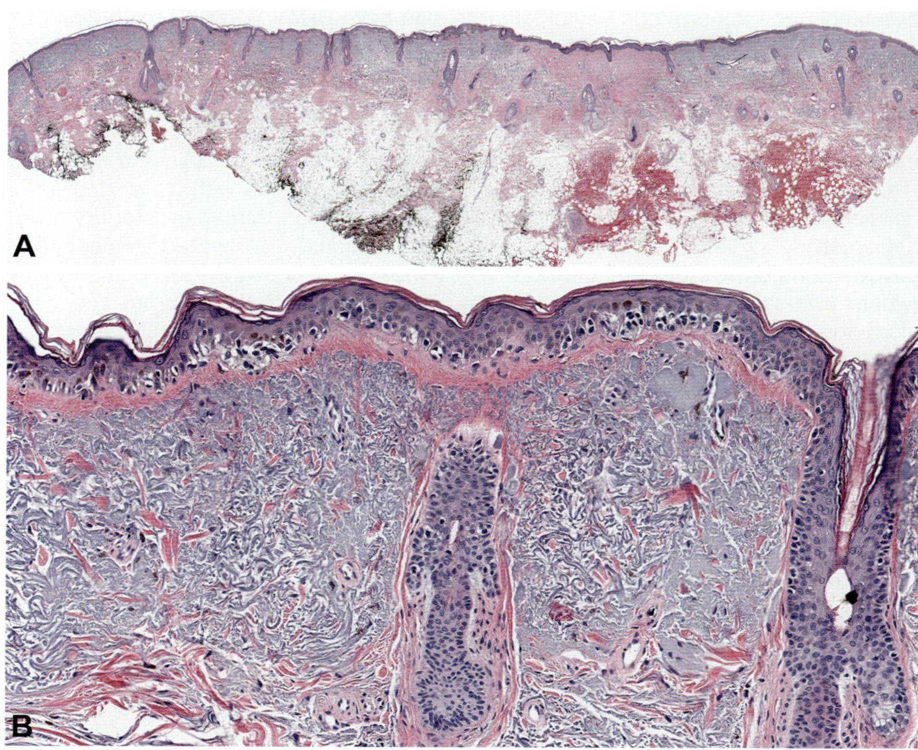


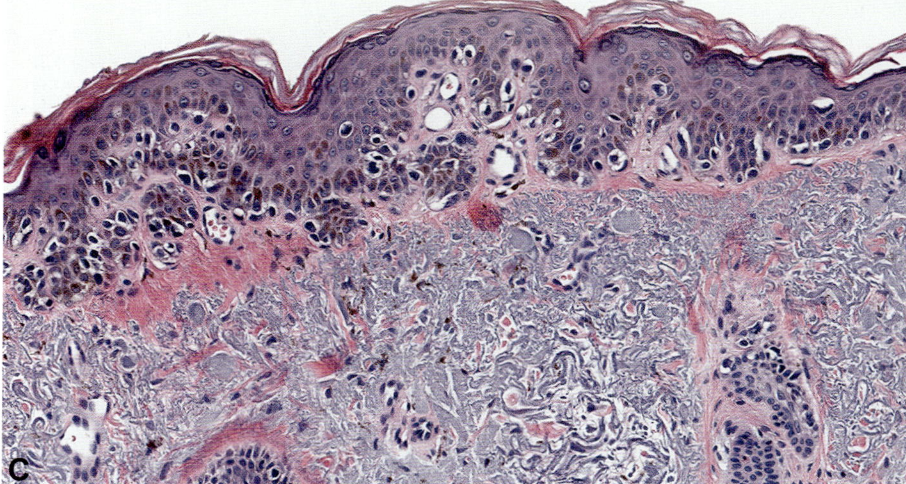


**Fig. 2.48** Lentigo maligna. **A** Broad resection specimen with a pink biopsy site scar, extensive solar elastosis, and irregularities of the epidermal contour including patchy rete ridge effacement. **B** This field shows the so-called classic pattern, with continuous basal (lentiginous) proliferation of uniformly atypical naevoid to epithelioid melanocytes. **C** Another field shows the dysplastic naevus-like (or naevoid lentigo maligna) pattern. Although this single field is not diagnostic of lentigo maligna, it is part of the larger lesion illustrated in panels A and B.

## Etiology

These lesions are related to cumulative sun exposure, which results in a very high mutation burden (see *Genetic profile*).

## Localization

Lentigo maligna and LMM occur in chronically sun-exposed skin, most frequently that of the head and neck region; in men, the ears and bald scalp are commonly affected, likely related to the loss of protection by a covering of hair {676}.

## Clinical features

Like other melanomas that arise through a radial growth phase (RGP), lentigo maligna usually presents as a patch or plaque that meets the ABCDE criteria for the clinical diagnosis of melanoma: asymmetry, border irregularity, colour variegation, diameter enlargement, and evolution (history of change). On occasion, the lesions are essentially completely amelanotic, and therefore lack colour variegation and present as an erythematous patch, simulating an inflammatory condition. As opposed to solar lentigines, the lesions are poorly circumscribed, histologically often extending beyond the clinical margin {700}. Lentigo maligna lesions are often indolent or slow-changing, and patients may regard them as stable, although photographic documentation (if available) typically demonstrates evolution. There may be patchy areas of regression, appearing as grey or flesh-coloured regions within the lesion. The vertical growth phase (VGP; the tumorigenic component) presents as a region of thickening, often occurring as a palpable and visible nodule or as a plaque-like area of skin thickening within the lesion. In advanced lesions, there may be ulceration and a history of bleeding.

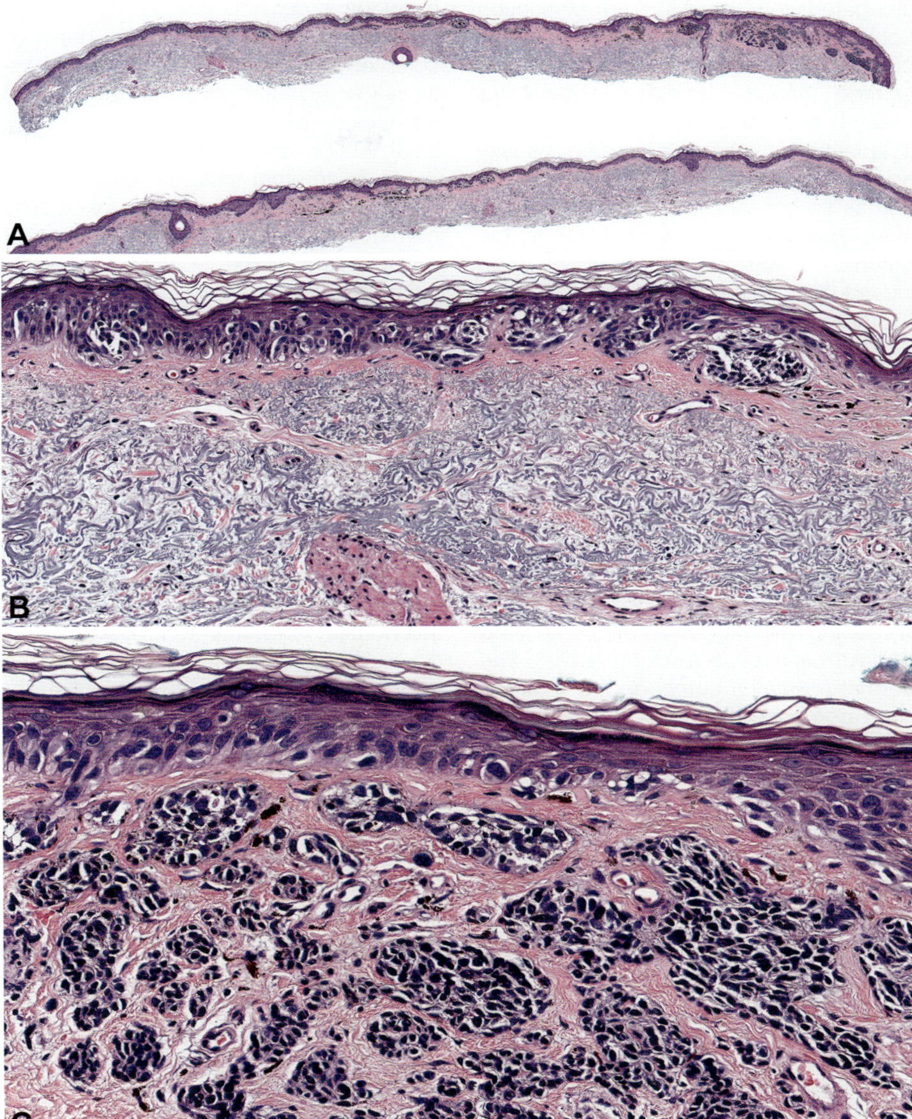


**Fig. 2.49** Lentigo maligna melanoma (LMM), invasive. **A** Broad excision specimen in sun-damaged skin; there is a papule in the upper dermis to the right, and there is irregular thickening and thinning of the epidermis, with a few nests near the dermoepidermal junction visible at this power. **B** Predominantly basal proliferation of moderately and uniformly atypical naevoid to epithelioid and spindle melanocytes; there is focal low-level suprabasal scatter and there are a few nests that appear to hang down from the epidermis in a droplet-like pattern; the process is in situ in this field. **C** There is a collection of cells in the papillary dermis, filling and expanding it. The cells have a somewhat naevoid morphology (relatively small, scant cytoplasm), and there is evidence suggesting maturation to a smaller cell type at the base, but the nuclei are hyperchromatic and irregular. There are no mitoses; the invasive component in LMM is often somewhat naevoid, as in this case; the tumour thickness is 0.3 mm, indicative of a lesion at minimal risk of metastasis.

## Histopathology

Compared with superficial spreading melanoma, LMM is often characterized by a more indefinite border, with epidermal thinning and loss of rete ridges, and by basal (lentiginous) rather than pagetoid proliferation of atypical melanocytes in the epidermis, with a lesser degree of nesting and with less pigment {2746}. Two major patterns of the RGP can be distinguished, and both are associated with severe solar elastosis in the dermis. The first pattern is so-called classic lentigo maligna, which is characteristically a broad lesion with a continuous proliferation of uniformly atypical naevoid to epithelioid melanocytes along the dermoepidermal junction. There may be a few irregularly distributed nests, which typically appear to hang down from the junction in a droplet-like pattern. These cells have enlarged, irregular, and hyperchromatic nuclei, constituting moderate to severe cytological atypia. There may be scattered mitoses within the junctional component. The second pattern has been variously described as naevoid lentigo maligna {1435} and dysplastic naevus-like lentigo maligna {740}. This pattern is characterized by a stronger tendency towards nest formation, and some nests may bridge adjacent elongated rete ridges. The distinction from dysplastic naevus can be difficult, particularly in partial biopsy specimens. Lentigo maligna lesions have greater breadth and more asymmetry, with the dysplastic naevus-like areas usually accounting for a minority of the lesion across its breadth. Dysplastic naevi are seen less commonly than LMM in the chronically sun-damaged skin of older individuals. Immunohistochemistry, for example using melan-A (MART1) and SOX10, can be useful in assessing the cellularity and degree of confluence of the junctional melanocytic proliferations {712,2603}, and can be used to detect occult invasion {181}; however, the results should be interpreted with caution, because dermal cells that are positive for melan-A but lack atypia likely do not represent invasive melanoma {572}. LMM is considerably less likely than superficial spreading melanoma to be associated with a true naevus remnant {2427}. The dermal (invasive) component of LMM is often composed of small to moderately enlarged, atypical ovoid, somewhat naevoid melanocytes, sometimes with a more spindled shape. On occasion, the dermal invasive component is partly or wholly desmoplastic (i.e. desmoplastic melanoma). Conversely, lentigo maligna is found overlying approximately 50% of desmoplastic melanomas.

## Differential diagnosis

LMM must be differentiated clinically and histologically from common pigmented lesions that occur at the same sites, including lentigines, naevi, and keratoses. The clinical differential diagnosis may be difficult, and biopsy is often needed to exclude malignancy. Dermoscopy (or confocal microscopy) may be helpful in the selection of lesions (or foci within larger lesions) for biopsy. Biopsies of small lesions should include the full breadth of the lesion, which can be accomplished with a wide and deep shave (saucerization) biopsy. The histological distinction is also often difficult, with overlapping histology between solar lentigines with atypia and dysplastic naevi. A heterogeneous appearance (or variety of appearances), including solar lentigo and dysplastic naevus-like areas, is common in larger lesions. Normal skin at chronically sun-exposed sites can show increased numbers of basilar melanocytes, some of which can have enlarged nuclei, which can make diagnosis difficult. These changes should be interpreted with caution when evaluating excision margins. Correlation with the size and other morphological features of the lesion and clinical context are important for avoiding misdiagnosis. Keratinocytic atypia, such as that occurring in a pigmented actinic keratosis, must be distinguished from melanocytic atypia. Dysplastic naevi do not commonly occur in chronically sun-damaged skin of older individuals, and this diagnosis should be made with caution, and with serious consideration of the possibility of a so-called naevoid lentigo maligna {1435} or dysplastic naevus-like lentigo maligna {740}. Occasionally, lymphocytic involvement of the basal epidermis in lichenoid inflammatory processes occurring in sun-damaged skin can be confused with lentigo maligna.

## Histogenesis

Lentigo maligna/LMM evolves through an RGP/in situ component of lentigo maligna type and may progress to a VGP and metastatic disease {493,1714}. It is not uncommon to see a lentigo maligna in contiguity with a solar lentigo, but is unclear whether this juxtaposition represents a precursor relationship or the collision of a melanoma with a pre-existing lentigo – a lesion very commonly present in chronically sun-damaged skin. Lesions can reach several centimetres in diameter without developing a deeply invasive component (VGP). The latency period of the evolution from lentigo maligna to LMM can vary from months to decades.

## Genetic profile

High-CSD melanoma has one of the highest mutation burdens of any cancer. The mutations carry an ultraviolet (UV) radiation signature of pyrimidine dimer formation {1445}. Genomically, the lesions are characterized by loss of the tumour suppressor *NF1* (which is more common in lentigo maligna than in other melanoma subtypes) or mutually exclusive activating mutations of the oncogenes *NRAS*, *BRAF* (generally non-p.V600E), or occasionally *KIT* {168,1445,2746}. In the VGP, there is typically loss of the tumour suppressor *CDKN2A* {2392}. *TERT* promoter mutations are also commonly present, and can be detected even in the in situ portion {2394}.

## Genetic susceptibility

Melanomas in sun-exposed skin, including LMM, occur in light-skinned individuals who are susceptible to sunburn and lack the ability to tan {1524}.

## Prognosis and predictive factors

When risk factors and microstaging attributes are taken into account, the prognosis of LMM is the same as that of other melanomas. However, there is a belief that the progression of lentigo maligna occurs more slowly than that of other melanoma subtypes, although this has not been clearly supported by rigorous observation. The major factors determining prognosis are tumour thickness and the presence or absence of ulceration. Other factors related to prognosis include the dermal mitotic rate, tumour-infiltrating lymphocytes in the VGP, and the presence or absence of lymphovascular and perineural invasion, although these attributes are not included in the current American Joint Committee on Cancer (AJCC) staging system {68}.

# Desmoplastic melanoma

Scolyer R.A.
Barnhill R.L.
Bastian B.C.
Busam K.J.
McCarthy S.W.

## Definition

Desmoplastic melanoma is a variant of spindle cell melanoma in which the malignant cells are separated by collagen fibres or fibrous stroma.

## ICD-O code 8745/3

## Epidemiology

Desmoplastic melanomas account for 1–4% of melanomas in populations with a predominance of pale-skinned individuals. As is the case with other melanoma subtypes, males are more often affected, with a male-to-female ratio of 1.75:1. The median age at diagnosis (~65 years) is slightly older for desmoplastic melanoma than for the most common melanoma subtypes.

## Etiology

Clinical, epidemiological, and genomic findings, including the common localization of desmoplastic melanoma in severely sun-damaged skin, very high mutation load, and ultraviolet (UV) radiation mutation signatures, implicate UV irradiation as the predominant etiological agent in the majority of cases.

## Localization

Desmoplastic melanoma most commonly involves chronically sun-exposed skin, most frequently that of the head and neck region (including the nose and lip). In men, the ears and bald scalp are commonly affected. However, these tumours can also occur at sites with minimal or no evidence of UV radiation–induced damage.

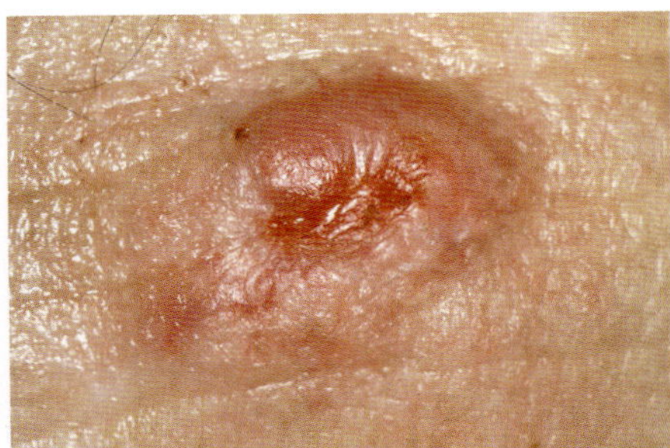

**Fig. 2.50** Desmoplastic melanoma. The range of appearances is broad; some examples arise in a pigmented patch; others, like this example, are amelanotic, level with the surface or elevated (as shown here), and (often) indurated.

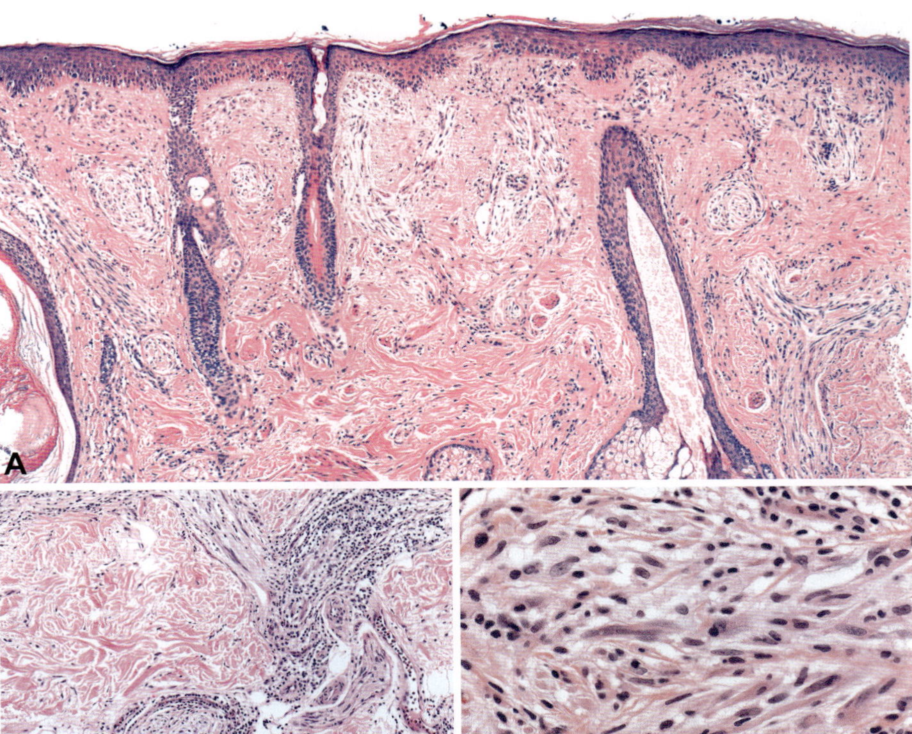


**Fig. 2.51** Desmoplastic neurotropic melanoma with so-called neural transforming areas in the lip of a 24-year-old woman. **A** Thick neuroid bundles are present in the upper dermis; there are also occasional atypical junctional melanocytes, a few subepidermal spindle cells, and scattered lymphocytes. **B** A neuroid bundle (top) contains atypical elongated spindle nuclei; intraneural and perineural involvement of a small nerve is also present. There is a prominent infiltrate of lymphocytes. **C** Abnormal spindle cells, some with elongated nuclei, are admixed with lymphocytes.

## Clinical features

Most cases present as a painless indurated plaque or poorly demarcated area of scar-like skin thickening; therefore, their clinical detection is often delayed. Some begin as a small papule or nodule. Almost half lack pigmentation. Clinically unpigmented tumours are particularly often mistaken for a scar, basal cell carcinoma, dermatofibroma, or other lesions. Pigmentation is usually due to an associated lentigo maligna. Unusual presenting features include a young age, an erythematous nodule, and alopecia.

## Histopathology

The dermal-based paucicellular tumours contain spindle-shaped melanocytes (which often resemble fibroblasts and are usually non-pigmented) in and between abundant fine, sclerotic or mature collagen bundles. The stroma often has a fibromyxoid appearance {1708}. The distribution of spindle cells is usually haphazard, but the cells occasionally form parallel bundles or storiform areas. The spindle cells often extend into the subcutis diffusely or in fibrous bands, and may involve deep fascia and interlobular

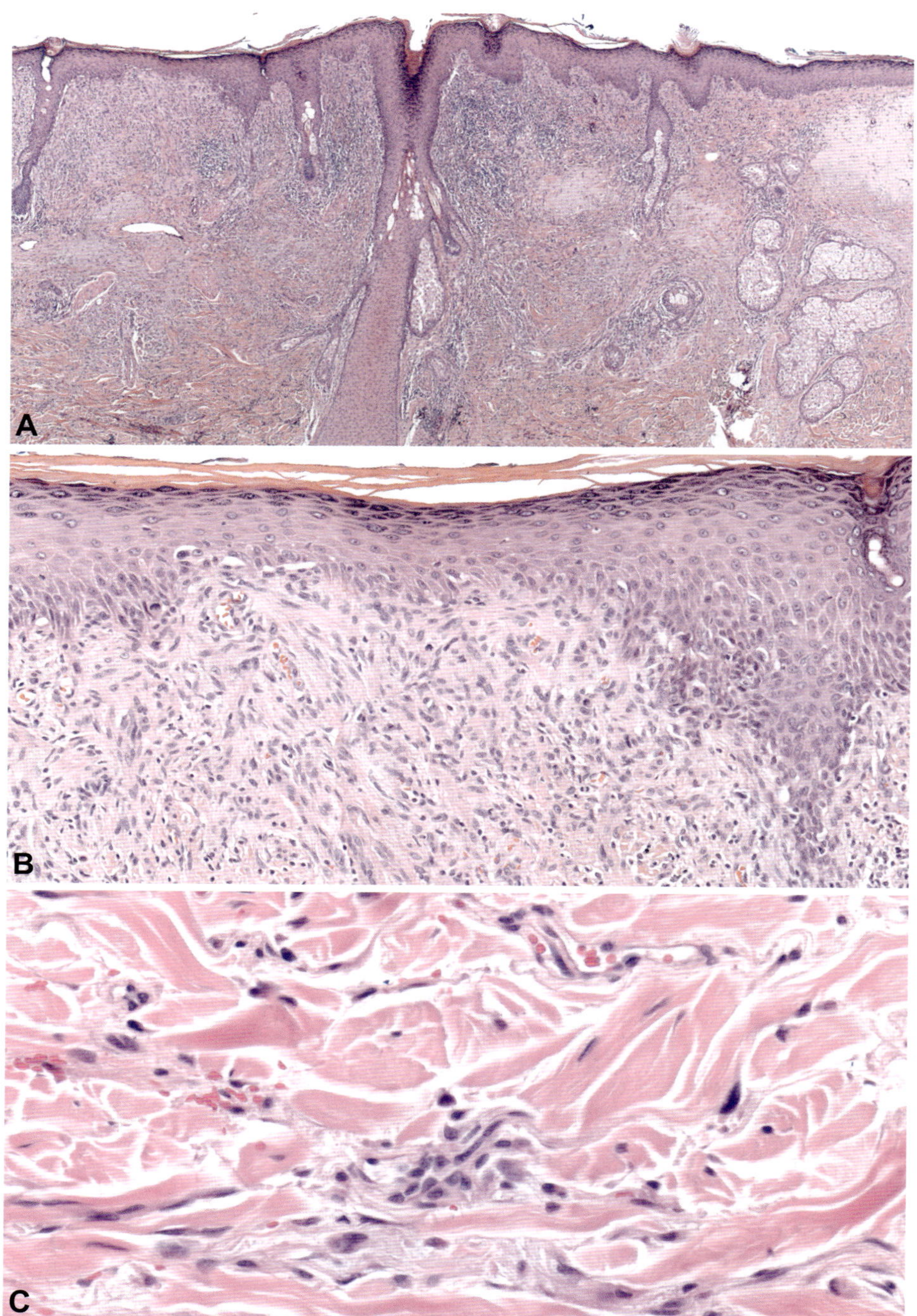

**Fig. 2.52** Desmoplastic neurotropic melanoma in the cheek of a 73-year-old man. **A** The increased cellularity in the dermis is due mainly to spindled melanocytes and lymphocytes; there is also patchy solar elastosis, deep acute haemorrhage, and epidermal thickening. **B** A few atypical enlarged melanocytes are present in the junctional zone. The fibrohistiocytic pattern is accompanied by scattered lymphocytes, some in clusters; mitoses are rare. **C** Malignant spindle cells with elongated nuclei appear to be within and between collagen bundles.

fibrous septa of the subcutis {341}. The overlying epidermis is usually thin and atrophic, and the adjacent superficial dermis usually shows severe solar elastosis. Characteristically, there are accompanying small aggregates of lymphocytes and occasional plasma cells within and/or at the edge of the tumour. The cytological atypia of the spindle cells usually varies from minimal to moderate, but can be severe. However, even in cases with mild atypia, there are usually a few larger or more-elongated hyperchromatic nuclei. The cytoplasm of the spindle cells is often poorly defined. In examples where the spindle cells are small, well scattered, and associated with solar elastosis, the lymphoid islands may be the main clue to the diagnosis. Paucicellular variants are easily missed on punch and shave biopsies, and more-cellular variants may be mistaken for a scar or a benign neural lesion. Lentigo maligna or an atypical epidermal melanocytic proliferation may be seen in the epidermis overlying desmoplastic melanoma, but junctional change is minimal or absent in about half of the cases. Neurotropism is a common accompanying feature (present in ~30% of cases) {2715}; it is characterized by tumour cells surrounding nerves in a circumferential fashion (termed perineural invasion) or (less commonly) by direct invasion of the endoneurium of nerves (termed intraneural invasion). Occasionally, desmoplastic melanoma may form nerve-like structures (termed neural transformation), which is regarded by some as a form of neurotropism. Neurotropism may also be present in melanomas without desmoplasia, but this is less common. There is sometimes an associated common acquired naevus. Vascular invasion is rare. In 2004, Busam and colleagues {344} proposed that desmoplastic melanoma could be classified as either pure desmoplastic melanoma or combined desmoplastic melanoma, and demonstrated that this classification correlated with clinical outcomes. Pure desmoplastic melanomas were defined as desmoplastic melanomas in which the overwhelming majority (> 90%) of invasive tumour was desmoplastic, whereas combined desmoplastic melanomas were defined as tumours in which typical areas of desmoplastic melanoma were mixed with non-desmoplastic melanoma foci, with the desmoplastic melanoma areas amounting to < 90% of the invasive melanoma {2364}. The spindle cells in desmoplastic melanoma are positive for S100 protein, SOX10, and NGFR, although only a few nuclei may be positive in some otherwise typical cases. HMB45 and melan-A (MART1) staining is usually negative, except in the non-desmoplastic areas of combined desmoplastic melanomas. SMA and CD10 may be positive. Desmoplastic melanomas may also present as a recurrence or occasionally as a metastasis from another type of melanoma {1851}.

## Differential diagnosis

The differential diagnosis includes desmoplastic naevus, which (like desmoplastic melanoma) may have perineural extension, but lacks asymmetry, mitotic activity, marked nuclear atypia, and lymphoid infiltrates, and is usually positive for melan-A. Well-established desmoplastic Spitz naevi may have many HMB45-negative spindle cells, but these naevi are usually symmetrical (with epidermal thickening), include at least a few plump cells, and have rare or absent mitoses. Sclerosing cellular blue naevi, which are most frequent on the scalp, also lack mitoses and are more or less diffusely HMB45-positive. Immature scars, especially in re-excision specimens, may focally resemble desmoplastic melanoma in that they may have some spindle cells that are positive for S100 protein and SOX10, as well as foci of lymphocytes and mitoses. Other differential diagnoses include dermatofibroma (fibrous histiocytoma), atypical fibroxanthoma/pleomorphic dermal sarcoma, sarcomatoid carcinoma, and leiomyosarcoma {1384}; these can usually be distinguished by morphology and appropriate immunohistochemistry.

## Histogenesis

Most desmoplastic melanomas have an exceedingly high mutation burden (median: > 60 mutations/Mb) with a strong signature of UV radiation as the primary mutagen. They appear to arise from melanocytes situated in a superficial location, likely the epidermis {2392}.

## Genetic profile

Desmoplastic melanomas typically lack strongly activating mutations in the MAPK pathway, such as BRAF p.V600E, *NRAS* c.181C>A (p.Q61K), and *NRAS* c.182A>G

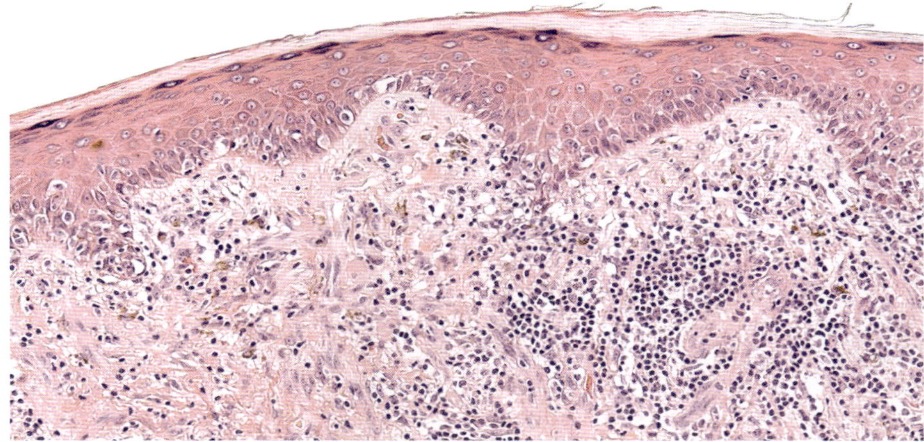

**Fig. 2.54** Desmoplastic melanoma in the forearm of a 76-year-old woman. Abnormal junctional melanocytes and dermal spindle cells with patchy lymphocytes.

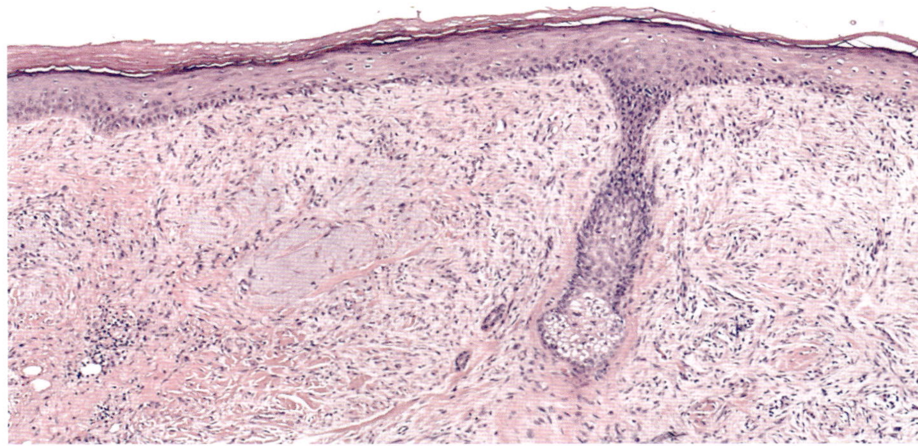

**Fig. 2.55** Desmoplastic melanoma in the scalp of a 68-year-old man. This punch biopsy specimen was originally diagnosed as a scar; only an occasional spindle cell was S100-positive, and no abnormal junctional melanocytes were found. A larger desmoplastic melanoma was removed from the same site 6 months later; clues to the diagnosis are the small foci of lymphocytes and the haphazard permeation of the dermal zone of elastosis by spindle cells.

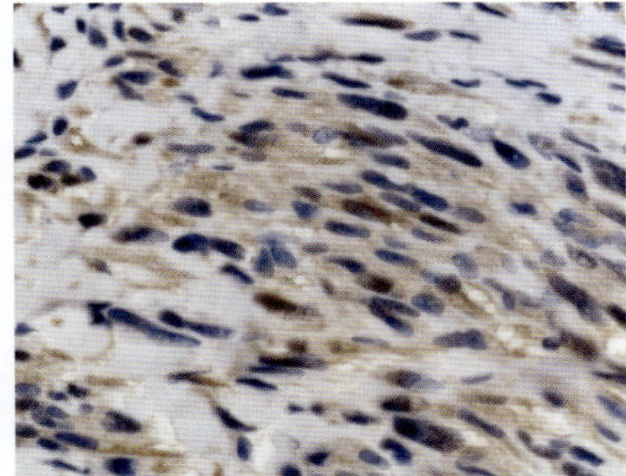

**Fig. 2.53** Desmoplastic melanoma in the upper lip of a 57-year-old man. Variable nuclear and cytoplasmic S100 positivity.

(p.Q61R) mutations. Instead, they frequently harbour *NF1* mutations (found in 55% of cases) {2392,2825,2825}, and they also show a diverse array of other MAPK-activating mutations that occur at low frequency and often in combination with *NF1* mutation, including amplification of receptor tyrosine kinase genes (e.g. *EGFR*, *MET*, and *ERBB2*) and inactivation of *CBL*. Several of these alterations are potential therapeutic targets. Mutations in the RB1 pathway are also common, primarily (i.e. in 47% of cases) affecting *CDKN2A*, and 48% of cases have *TP53* mutations. The exceedingly high mutation burden in desmoplastic melanomas makes them good candidates for immune checkpoint blockade therapy.

## Prognosis and predictive factors

Desmoplastic melanoma tends to be diagnosed at a more advanced local stage than other melanoma subtypes, with a median tumour thickness > 2.0 mm in most series. As is the case for other melanoma subtypes, prognosis is worse with increased tumour thickness, increased mitotic rate, male sex, and older age {1848}. However, desmoplastic melanomas tend to have a better prognosis than do other melanoma subtypes of similar tumour thickness. Local recurrences are common, in particular after incomplete excision or marginal excision < 10 mm, or when neurotropism is present {448}. Regional node field metastasis is less frequent in desmoplastic melanoma (in particular pure desmoplastic melanoma) than in other melanoma subtypes, and lung metastasis is more common as the initial site of metastasis. Wide local excision is the treatment of choice. Radiation therapy can help in achieving local control, in particular when neurotropism is present.

# Malignant Spitz tumour (Spitz melanoma)

Barnhill R.L.
Bahrami A.
Bastian B.C.
Busam K.J.
Cerroni L.
de la Fouchardière A.
Elder D.E.
Gerami P.
Lazova R.
Schmidt B.
Urso C.
Wiesner T.

## Definition

Malignant Spitz tumour (MST), the malignant form of Spitz naevus, is a rare variant of melanoma defined by characteristic clinical, histopathological, and genetic alterations {150,1532,2824,2826}. The term "spitzoid melanoma" is used for melanomas with some morphological resemblance to Spitz naevus; many such melanomas have characteristics of nodular melanomas in skin with a low degree of cumulative sun damage (low-CSD nodular melanomas) {1506}. In many cases, distinction from atypical Spitz tumour with uncertain malignant potential is impossible without knowledge of clinical evolution (i.e. the development of clinical – palpable – regional or distant metastases), death, or a distinctive molecular profile.

## ICD-O code

8770/3

## Synonyms

Spitz melanoma; spitzoid melanoma (a subset of cases); Spitz-like melanoma

## Epidemiology

Although the population-based prevalence of true MST has not been documented, MSTs are less common than Spitz naevi {1593}. They can occur at any age, but are more common among individuals aged > 40 years (mean age: 55 years) {1593,2764}. MST appears to be more common in men than in women.

## Localization

MST can occur at any anatomical site. The most common locations are the extremities and trunk {1593}.

## Clinical features

MST often presents as a changing or enlarging amelanotic or pigmented plaque, papule, or nodule {1593}. Other features suggesting melanoma are large size (often > 6 mm and particularly > 1 cm in diameter), asymmetry, irregular borders, colour variegation, ulceration, and bleeding {2465,2491,2764} (see Table 2.14).

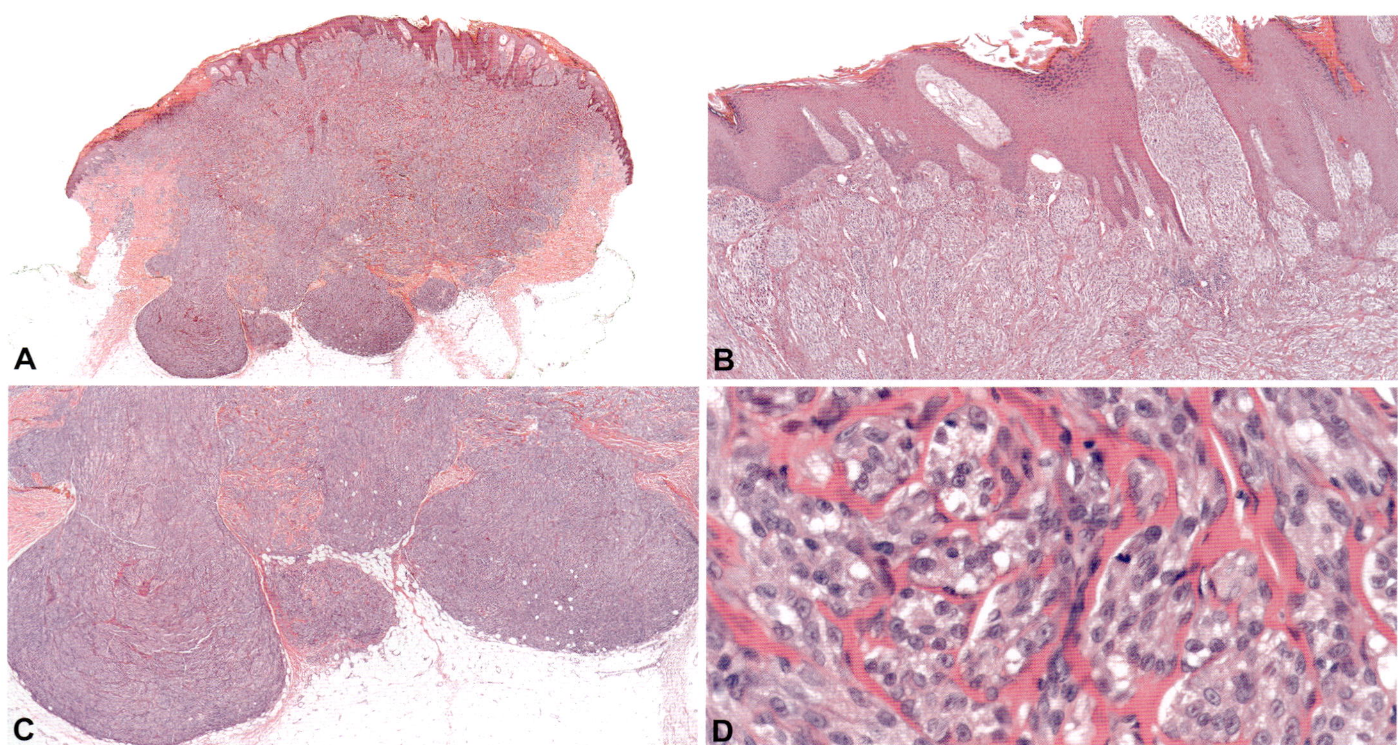


**Fig. 2.56** Malignant Spitz tumour. **A** Scanning magnification of a tumour that developed on the thigh of an 11-year-old girl shows an asymmetrical and ulcerated bulky neoplasm extending into subcutaneous fat. The tumour is 12 mm in diameter and 7 mm in thickness; no maturation is observed. **B** In this field, epidermal hyperplasia and vertically oriented nests of melanocytes are present, suggesting a spitzoid neoplasm. **C** The tumour extends into the subcutaneous fat without maturation; note the dense cellularity. **D** High magnification shows fascicles of spindle cells; the mitotic rate is 7 mitoses/mm$^2$; a *TERT* promoter mutation was confirmed. Following the initial diagnosis, the patient developed a regional clinical lymph node metastasis at 6 months and died from widespread metastases at 24 months.

**Table 2.14** Comparison of Spitz naevus, atypical Spitz tumour, and malignant Spitz tumour (Spitz melanoma)

| | Spitz naevus | Atypical Spitz tumour | Malignant Spitz tumour |
|---|---|---|---|
| **Clinical features** | Mean and median age: 21 years (range: 2–69 years)<br>Most commonly affects extremities<br>Pink or reddish plaque, papule, or nodule | Can occur at any age; more common in younger patients (<40 years)<br>Occurs on extremities, trunk<br>Plaque or nodule<br>Colour variegation | Can occur at any age (often >40 years)<br>Occurs on extremities, trunk<br>Asymmetrical<br>Enlarged plaque or nodule<br>Colour variegation<br>Changing lesion |
| **Histopathology** | <5 to 6 mm<br>Symmetrical<br>Well circumscribed<br>Epidermal hyperplasia<br>Vertically oriented nests with clefting<br>Central focal pagetoid spread (if any)<br>Often wedge-shaped<br>Maturation of dermal component<br>Few or no dermal mitoses (0–2/mm$^2$) | Often >5 to 10 mm<br>Symmetrical or asymmetrical<br>Well or poorly circumscribed<br>Ulceration possible<br>Irregular nesting<br>Increased cellularity<br>Greater pagetoid spread than in Spitz naevus<br>Deeper dermal extension than in Spitz naevus<br>Maturation may be partial or absent<br>2–6 dermal mitoses/mm$^2$<br>Deep mitoses<br>Possible necrosis | >5 mm; often >10 mm<br>Often asymmetrical<br>Often poorly circumscribed<br>Ulceration<br>Irregular and confluent nesting<br>Pagetoid spread may be extensive<br>Ulceration<br>Effacement of epidermis<br>Lack of maturation<br>Often >6 dermal mitoses/mm$^2$<br>Deep/marginal or atypical mitoses<br>Necrosis |
| **Cytology** | Enlarged epithelioid/spindle cells<br>Little or no nuclear pleomorphism<br>No high-grade cytological atypia | Enlarged epithelioid/spindle cells<br>Nuclear enlargement, pleomorphism, and hyperchromasia | Enlarged epithelioid/spindle cells<br>High-grade cytological atypia |
| **IHC** | HMB45 and Ki-67 staining diminished with depth in dermal component<br>Low Ki-67 proliferation index (<5%) | HMB45 and Ki-67 staining diminished or variable with depth<br>Low to intermediate Ki-67 proliferation index (5–15%) | HMB45 and Ki-67 deep staining common<br>Elevated Ki-67 proliferation index (>20%)<br>p16 expression may be diminished or absent |
| **Molecular pathology** | Array CGH: isolated gains of 7p and 11q, tetraploidy<br>Activating *HRAS* mutations<br>Kinase fusions | Array CGH: often ≥ 1 chromosomal abnormality<br>Kinase fusions<br>*PTEN* mutations<br>Heterozygous or homozygous loss of 9p21 may occur | Array CGH: >1 chromosomal abnormality<br>Kinase fusions<br>*BRAF* and *NRAS* mutations rare<br>*HRAS* mutations rare<br>*PTEN* mutations<br>Homozygous loss of 9p21<br>*TERT* promoter mutations |
| **Prognosis** | Very low (almost no) risk of progression | Low risk of progression<br>Almost always indolent<br>Clinical recurrences occur | Regional clinical lymph node metastases occur<br>Rare distant metastases and death |

CGH, comparative genomic hybridization; IHC, immunohistochemistry.

## Histopathology

The diagnosis of MST should be made in the context of the clinical features, including the patient's age. Lesions in adults should be viewed with higher suspicion of malignancy {2491}.

MSTs usually exhibit the morphological features of a Spitz naevus, and may be indistinguishable from atypical Spitz tumours (see *Spitz naevus*, p. 111). MSTs can be of any size but are often >1 cm. Additional features in the epidermal component suggesting melanoma include asymmetry; poor circumscription; effacement/consumption of the epidermis; ulceration; enlarged, irregular, and confluent nests; and pagetoid scatter {1532,2153,2764}. Aberrant morphological features in the dermal component commonly include asymmetry, nodular or sheet-like aggregates of melanocytes, diminished or absent maturation, deep localization of melanin, prominent lymphoid infiltrates, and necrosis {2153,2764}.

MSTs show some cytological similarities to Spitz naevi. In addition, there is conspicuous nuclear enlargement, with pleomorphism, thickening and irregularity of nuclear membranes, increased N:C ratios, hyperchromatism and clumping of chromatin, and enlarged eosinophilic nucleoli.

An increased mitotic rate (> 6 mitoses/mm$^2$ in a child aged > 1 year or > 2 mitoses/mm$^2$ in an adult {1532,2491}), deep mitoses, atypical forms, and mitoses localized in so-called hotspots suggest melanoma {409,2153}.

MST may demonstrate an abnormal pattern of HMB45 antigen and melan-A expression, with deep (rather than stratified) HMB45 staining and patchy (rather than diffuse) melan-A staining. p16 expression is often absent and the Ki-67 proliferation index is often > 20% {2676}.

## Differential diagnosis

The differential diagnosis includes Spitz naevus, atypical Spitz tumour, and conventional melanoma. Various immunomarkers and genomic findings (e.g. multiple chromosomal aberrations identified by array comparative genomic hybridization or FISH, *PTEN* mutations, and *TERT* promoter mutations {1532}), as well as gene expression profiling, may provide support for a diagnosis of MST {870,2826}. These findings must be interpreted within the clinical and histopathological context of each case.

## Histogenesis

The sequential acquisition of genetic alterations such as mutations of a single oncogene, kinase fusions, and additional aberrations (in particular loss of *CDKN2A*/p16 and *PTEN*, and *TERT* promoter mutations) is the likely mechanism of the pathogenesis of MST {2826}.

## Genetic profile

Mutually exclusive kinase fusions of *ROS1*, *ALK*, *BRAF*, *NTRK1*, *NTRK3*, *MET*, or *RET* have been reported in 39% of MSTs {2824}. In contrast, *BRAF*, *NRAS*, and *HRAS* mutations are usually absent or rare in MST {867,2826}. *TERT* promoter mutations, *PTEN* mutations, and DNA copy-number alterations may be observed in MSTs {1532,2824}.

## Prognosis and predictive factors

The prognosis of MST versus that of conventional melanoma is difficult to gauge, because of the substantial level of discordance in the diagnosis of MST. Factors reported to negatively influence the outcome of MST include older age, tumour diameter > 1 cm, ulceration, mitotic rate > 6 mitoses/mm$^2$ {1532,2491}, biallelic deletion of 9p21 {872}, and *TERT* promoter mutation {872,1532}.

# Spitz naevus

Barnhill R.L.
Bahrami A.
Bastian B.C.
Busam K.J.
Cerroni L.
de la Fouchardière A.
Elder D.E.
Gerami P.
Lazova R.
Schmidt B.
Urso C.
Wiesner T.

## Definition

Spitzoid melanocytic neoplasms are composed of large epithelioid and/or spindled cells with distinctive architecture {153}; they range from Spitz naevus to malignant Spitz tumour (MST; see *Malignant Spitz tumour*, p. 108), with an intermediate category termed "atypical Spitz tumour (AST)" (see Table 2.14, p. 109).

The term "Spitz naevus" is reserved for lesions lacking atypical features and with very low risk of neoplastic progression. AST is distinguished from prototypical Spitz naevus by the presence of one or more atypical features, and often by an uncertain malignant potential. The importance of AST lies in the need to distinguish them from melanoma – a distinction that is frequently uncertain. Histopathology remains the gold standard for assessing spitzoid neoplasms. Genetically, a Spitz naevus may be defined by a single alteration (e.g. a kinase fusion) and an AST by at least two genetic alterations. Studies designed to assess the features of spitzoid neoplasms associated with adverse events suggest that the frequency of such events is quite rare.

## ICD-O code 8770/0

## Synonyms

Spitz naevus: benign juvenile melanoma; epithelioid cell naevus; spindle cell naevus; spindle and epithelioid cell naevus; naevus of large spindle and/or epithelioid cells

Atypical Spitz tumour: atypical Spitz naevus; metastasizing Spitz naevus

## Epidemiology

The prevalence of Spitz naevus in the general population has not been reliably documented. In 1977, the incidence of Spitz naevus in Queensland, Australia, was estimated to be 1.4 cases per 100 000 person-years, compared with 25.4 cases of melanoma per 100 000 person-years {2792}. Spitz naevi constitute about 1% of all naevi excised from children {1726}, and 1–2% of all melanocytic lesions removed from patients of any age {156}. The lesions can occur at any age, but have a predilection for younger individuals. In one study of 342 patients, the mean and median age was 21 years, with 40% of the patients aged < 15 years and 77% < 30 years {2154}. Congenital Spitz naevi are exceedingly rare {2902}. Spitz naevi occur in all racial groups. Males and females are probably affected equally, although there is some evidence of a female predominance {1593} among young adults (i.e. with an approximate age range of 16–45 years) {2154}.

## Etiology

The etiology and pathogenesis of Spitz naevus are unknown. Eruptive Spitz naevi have been documented during pregnancy and puberty, suggesting a potential role for hormonal activation {584}.

## Localization

Spitz naevi can occur at any anatomical site. In a study of 484 patients, the most common site was the lower extremities {1593}. Other common locations are the face (in children) and the trunk (in adults) {2154,2792}.

## Clinical features

Conventional Spitz naevi are usually < 6 mm in diameter {2792}. They typically present as tan, pink, or reddish macular, plaque-like, or dome-shaped lesions that are symmetrical and well circumscribed and often have a smooth surface (see Table 2.14, p. 109). Some may be polypoid or verrucous. Brown or black papules or plaques are more common in adults, although heavily pigmented Spitz naevi can also occur in children. Ulceration is infrequent, but traumatic excoriation is common in children. Many variants of Spitz naevus have been described (see Table 2.15); the most common include pigmented, desmoplastic, and halo Spitz naevi {2154}.

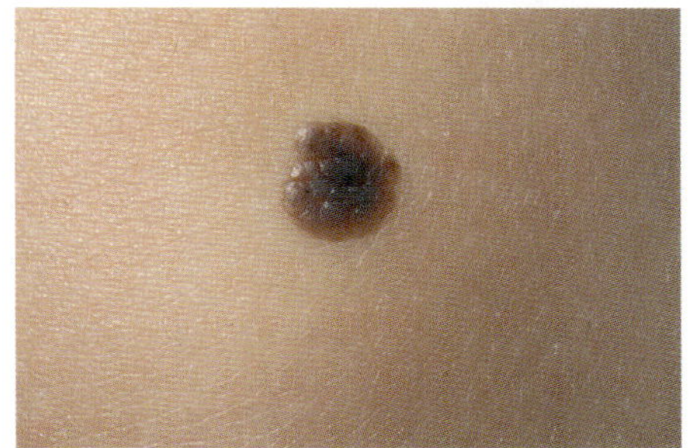

**Fig. 2.57** Spitz naevus. A more-or-less symmetrical nodule; this example has more pigment than most.

**Table 2.15** Variants of Spitz naevus

|  |
|---|
| Polypoid Spitz naevus |
| Agminated Spitz naevus |
| Pagetoid Spitz naevus |
| Dysplastic Spitz tumour |
| Desmoplastic Spitz naevus |
| Angiomatous Spitz naevus |
| Hyalinized Spitz naevus |
| Plexiform Spitz naevus |
| Halo Spitz naevus |
| Pseudogranulomatous Spitz naevus |
| Tubular Spitz naevus |
| Myxoid Spitz naevus |
| Pigmented epithelioid cell Spitz naevus |
| Combined Spitz naevus |
| Recurrent/persistent Spitz naevus |
| Pigmented spindle cell naevus |

Although Spitz naevi are typically solitary, multiple or agminated (grouped) Spitz naevi can occur in single or multiple areas {2911}. Multiple Spitz naevi, whether arising within a naevus spilus or outside that setting, are rare {2911}. Spitz naevi usually undergo a period of rapid growth lasting 3–6 months and then stabilize. Rarely, multiple Spitz naevi can develop in an eruptive fashion over the course of weeks or months {584}.

ASTs occur in patients of all ages, but are probably most common in adolescents and young adults. AST can be indistinguishable from melanoma on clinical grounds, because of large size (often > 6 mm and particularly > 1 cm in diameter), asymmetry, irregular borders, or colour variegation (see Table 2.14, p. 109) {150,2465,2491}.

## Histopathology

Prototypical (conventional) Spitz naevi are usually < 5 mm in diameter, symmetrical, and sharply circumscribed.

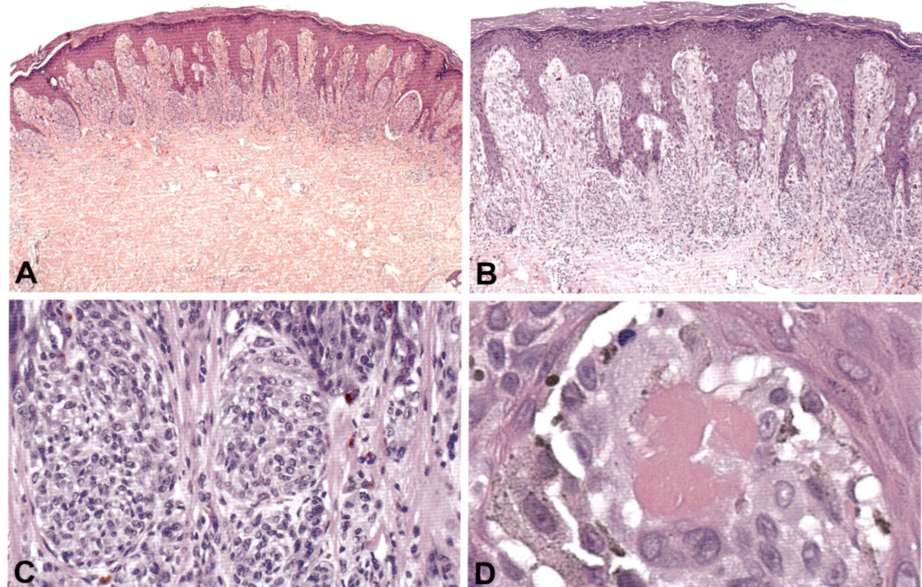

**Fig. 2.58** Spitz naevus. **A** The lesion measures 4.2 mm in diameter and 0.9 mm in thickness. Note the dome-shaped architecture with symmetry, sharp circumscription, uniform epidermal hyperplasia, and vertically oriented junctional nests of melanocytes. **B** Vertically oriented fascicles of spindled melanocytes at the dermoepidermal junction. The epidermis is hyperplastic, and clefting around some the junctional nests of melanocytes is present; melanocytes extend into the dermis with maturation; no mitoses are present. **C** Enlarged spindled and epithelioid cells with eosinophilic cytoplasm; the nuclei show uniformly dispersed chromatin and small nucleoli; no cytological atypia is seen. This neoplasm qualifies as a Spitz naevus on the basis of the characteristics described and the absence of atypical features; there has been no evidence of recurrence in > 15 years of follow-up. **D** Coalescent aggregates of eosinophilic homogeneous material (Kamino bodies) are surrounded by enlarged epithelioid and fusiform melanocytes. These cells exhibit abundant, slightly eosinophilic cytoplasm; the nuclei are enlarged, with dispersed chromatin patterns and distinct nucleoli.

They usually contain nests of large epithelioid cells, spindle cells, or both, usually extending from the epidermis into the reticular dermis in a wedge-shaped configuration {1974,2154,2792}. The junctional nests of closely opposed melanocytes often show clefting and separation from the surrounding epidermis. A hyperplastic epidermis and vertical orientation of junctional nests of spindled melanocytes contribute to the so-called raining-down appearance. Pagetoid scatter in the epidermis, if present, is usually focal, sparsely cellular, and limited to the centre of the lesion and the lower half of the epidermis {342,2047}. Additional intraepidermal findings may include discohesive junctional melanocytic nests, transepidermal elimination of entire nests of melanocytes, and Kamino bodies (eosinophilic hyaline globules) {2154}. Perivascular lymphoid infiltrates may be present.

In contrast, ASTs are usually larger (often > 5–10 mm in diameter) and may extend deeply into the dermis and the subcutaneous fat. They are often asymmetrical and not well circumscribed, may show effacement/consumption of the epidermis, and may be ulcerated {155,2465,2491}. AST may exhibit peripheral pagetoid scatter in single-cell or small nested patterns involving the upper layers of the epidermis. Although ASTs are usually plaque-like, they can uncommonly show features of dysplastic naevi (i.e. architectural disorder and cytological atypia); such cases have been termed dysplastic Spitz tumours {147}. ASTs often display high cellular density, with confluence of melanocytes in cellular aggregates or nodules that replace the dermis without maturation. A lack of uniformity from side to side and the persistence of melanocytic nests and fascicles of similar sizes within the deep dermis are abnormal features. Kamino bodies are less frequent, smaller, or absent.

In conventional Spitz naevi, melanocytes organized in junctional and/or superficial dermal nests progressively give way to smaller nests and eventually to single melanocytes deeper in the dermis. There is usually also a corresponding transition from larger to smaller cells and nuclei {1974,2154,2792}. There is usually single-cell dispersion at the base of the lesion.

Conventional Spitz naevus is composed of enlarged, relatively uniform spindle and/or epithelioid melanocytes with polyangular contours, abundant opaque or ground-glass cytoplasm, nuclei with delicately dispersed chromatin, occasional nuclear pleomorphism, and uniform nucleoli {1974,2792}. ASTs usually display a greater degree of nuclear enlargement, as well as nuclear pleomorphism, high N:C ratios, hyperchromatic nuclei, and large eosinophilic nucleoli {155,2465}.

Overall, the mitotic rate in conventional Spitz naevi is low (usually ≤ 2 mitoses/mm$^2$), or mitoses are absent {549,1974,2154,2792}. Mitoses are rare or absent in the deep dermis. In ASTs, the mitotic rate may be increased; a rate of > 6 mitoses/mm$^2$ is particularly concerning {2491}. Atypical mitoses may be present. Mitoses located at the deep margin (advancing front) also raise concern for malignancy {409,2491}.

Like other melanocytic naevi, Spitz naevus and AST express S100 protein and SOX10, as well as the melanocyte differentiation antigens melan-A (MART1), tyrosinase, and MITF {147}. A diminished gradient of HMB45 and Ki-67 staining with depth, along with a low Ki-67 proliferation index (< 5–10%), suggests a conventional Spitz naevus. In contrast, a Ki-67 proliferation index value > 20% suggests the possibility of melanoma {2676}, although exceptions to this rule of thumb are relatively common. p16 and other senescence markers alone do not allow distinction of naevi from melanoma {1678,2826}. Homozygous loss of the *CDKN2A* locus was associated with a lethal outcome in 3 of 11 ASTs in one study {869}, but this loss was not associated with distant metastasis in a second study {1532}. Loss of p16 in MSTs can occur with or without genomic *CDKN2A* loss, and immunohistochemical p16 aberrations favour a diagnosis of borderline Spitz tumour or MST (rather than Spitz naevus) {1014}.

### Differential diagnosis

Extensive clinical, histopathological, and genetic information is needed for the classification and risk stratification of spitzoid neoplasms as Spitz naevus, AST (often with uncertain malignant potential), or MST (see Table 2.14, p. 109). The most important differential diagnosis is melanoma. Suspicion for melanoma should be especially high in the presence of multiple major criteria, including age > 10 years (postpubertal), and particularly > 40 years; increased lesional diameter, particularly > 1 cm; ulceration; mitotic rates > 2 mitoses/mm$^2$, and particularly > 6 mitoses/mm$^2$ {2491}; and involvement of subcutaneous fat. Other important criteria are asymmetry; poor circumscription; increased cellularity of the lesion; diffuse, full-epidermal thickness and peripheral pagetoid spread; diminished or absent maturation of the dermal component; angiotropism {157}; lymphovascular invasion; and marked cytological atypia {151,1532,2491,2792}. Some non-Spitz melanomas may simulate MST with respect to some of these features. Certain immunomarkers and genomic alterations detected by FISH or array comparative genomic hybridization, or specific mutations such as *TERT* promoter mutations {1532}, may help to distinguish some ambiguous spitzoid neoplasms from melanoma {870,2826}.

*BAP1*-inactivated melanocytic lesions must also be distinguished from Spitz naevus and AST. They usually lack epidermal hyperplasia, are usually epithelioid rather than spindled, often include a second naevus cell component, lack BAP1 expression, and are usually *BRAF*-mutant {2827,2828}.

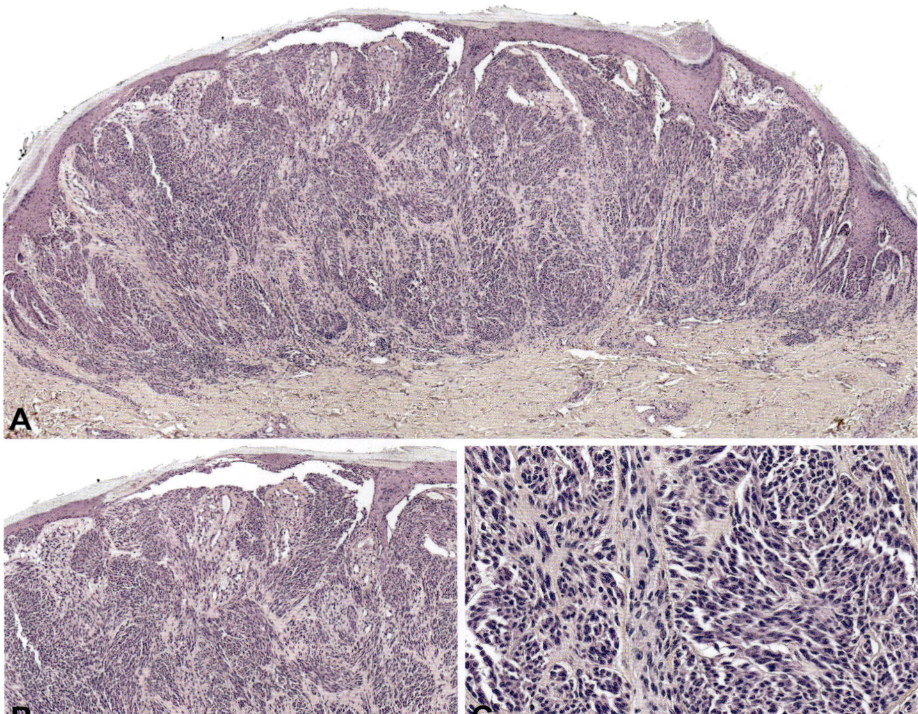

**Fig. 2.59** Atypical Spitz tumour of uncertain malignant potential. **A** Scanning magnification shows a small, reasonably symmetrical, and well-circumscribed tumour; however, the lesion exhibits effacement of the epidermis, absence of maturation, and dense cellularity. **B** Higher magnification discloses the effacement (or so-called consumption) of the epidermis; note the densely cellular fascicles of spindled melanocytes. **C** The neoplasm fails to show maturation with depth; compact nests of atypical melanocytes are present at the base of the tumour. Mitotic figures are noted in this deep nest and are present at the advancing front; the mitotic rate is 9 mitoses/mm$^2$. Focal necrosis is also present; sentinel lymph node biopsy was negative; the patient has shown no disease progression in 3 years of follow-up.

## Histogenesis

Spitz naevus lesions may evolve from junctional proliferations of melanocytes, which then extend into the dermis. Some Spitz naevi lack an epidermal component.

## Genetic profile

As many as 20% of Spitz naevi harbour activating *HRAS* mutations {170,2693}. In about 55% of Spitz naevi and ASTs, chromosomal rearrangement-induced fusions resulting in chimeric proteins have been identified in a mutually exclusive pattern {2824,2863,2882,2886}. These kinase fusions activate oncogenic signalling pathways and involve the kinase genes *ROS1*, *ALK*, *BRAF*, *NTRK1*, *NTRK3*, *MET*, and *RET*. *HRAS* mutations and kinase fusions are rare in melanoma {867}, and according to the tumour progression model, they can also be detected in MST {2826}. Unlike in melanoma, *BRAF* and *NRAS* mutations are usually absent in spitzoid neoplasms {2827}. In one study, homozygous somatic loss of 9p21 was observed in a small subset of AST cases resulting in locoregional or distant metastases or death {872}, but another study failed to confirm the significance of this finding {1532}.

## Prognosis and predictive factors

Spitz naevi, and ASTs even more so, are clinical and histological mimics of MST, and rarely potential precursors of melanoma.

# Pigmented spindle cell naevus (Reed naevus)

Barnhill R.L.
Bahrami A.
de la Fouchardière A.
Elder D.E.
Elenitsas R.
Gerami P.

## Definition

Pigmented spindle cell naevus (PSCN), also called Reed naevus, is a distinct variant of Spitz naevus {2146,2470}. Atypical pigmented spindle cell tumour (APSCT) is a PSCN with one or more atypical features {152}. Plexiform spindle cell naevus (PLEXSCN) is defined by fascicular–plexiform architecture in the reticular dermis {152,159,1151}. These three entities are of great importance because of their extremely frequent confusion with melanoma.

## ICD-O code 8770/0

## Synonyms

Pigmented spindle cell variant of Spitz naevus; Reed naevus; pigmented spindle cell tumour

## Epidemiology

PSCN, APSCT, and PLEXSCN are less common than Spitz naevus. PSCNs can occur at any age, but preferentially affect young people (mean age: 25 years, range: 3–66 years) {2275,2323}. Women are affected more often than men {2275,2323}. The mean patient age for PLEXSCN is about 33 years (range: 1–92 years).

## Etiology

As is the case with Spitz naevus, the etiology and pathogenesis of PSCN are unknown.

## Localization

PSCN and APSCT most commonly involve the extremities (affected in 75% of cases, most commonly the thigh), the trunk (20% of cases), and the head and neck (5% of cases) {152,2275,2323}. PLEXSCNs also have a predilection for the extremities (affected in 37% of cases), the head and neck (30% of cases), and the trunk (26% of cases) {152}.

## Clinical features

PSCNs are usually well-circumscribed, symmetrical, flat-topped papules or nodules averaging about 3 mm in diameter (range: 1.5–10 mm) {2275,2323}. They are usually a uniform dark brown, bluish-black, or black. There is often a history of recent onset or change. APSCTs are usually larger and asymmetrical, and they may show irregular borders and coloration {152}. PLEXSCNs are small, well-defined papules with dark-blue or bluish-black colour {152,159,1151}.

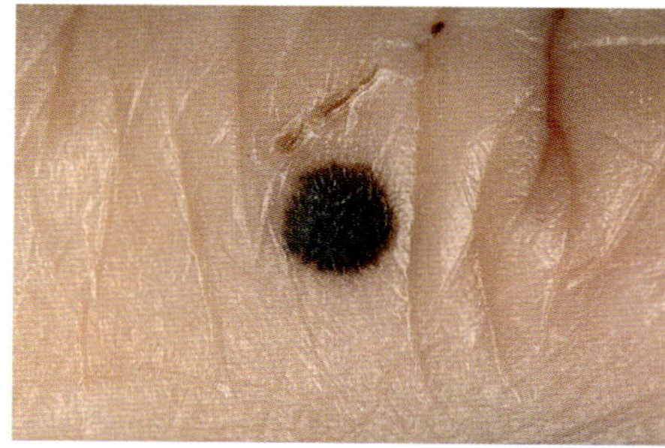

**Fig. 2.60** Pigmented spindle cell naevus presenting as symmetrical, uniformly darkly pigmented plaque. These lesions typically develop suddenly but are usually stable by the time they are excised.

## Histopathology

Prototypical PSCNs are small (mean diameter: 2.8 mm), well circumscribed, and symmetrical, with a slightly raised plate-like epidermal hyperplasia {2275,2323,2470}. Compact vertically oriented, whorled, or concentric fascicles of uniform, slender pigmented spindle cells constitute the junctional component. Clefting around junctional nests occurs. Pagetoid melanocytosis is relatively frequent but usually limited to the lower half of the epidermis. PSCNs may involve the papillary dermis and skin appendages. Hypercellular aggregates of smaller elongate to ovoid melanocytes may expand the papillary dermis. The spindle cells usually contain fine, granular melanin. The nuclei exhibit delicate chromatin and small inconspicuous nucleoli. PSCN and Spitz naevus form a histological continuum, with intermediate lesions (PSCN, spitzoid variant) manifesting larger pigmented spindle cells along with epithelioid cells more typical of Spitz naevus. Pigmented Kamino bodies may also be seen.

APSCTs are characterized by any of the following features: diameter > 6 mm (often); poor circumscription; asymmetry; effacement of the epidermis; ulceration; prominent single-cell melanocytic hyperplasia extending peripherally along the epidermal basal layer; and increasing degrees of pagetoid melanocytosis, mitotic activity, and cytological atypia {152}. Features of dysplastic naevus may be seen. The lesions may contain cellular aggregates or nodules of melanocytes that replace the dermis without maturation. Atypical variants may be

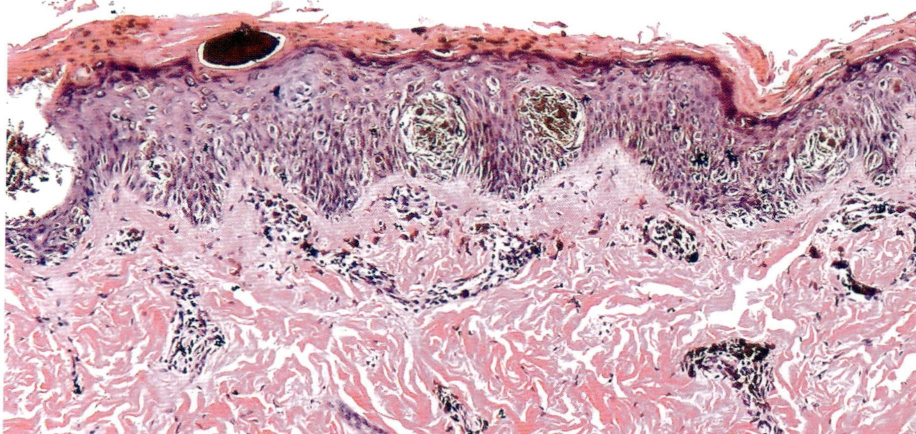

**Fig. 2.61** Pigmented spindle cell naevus. Discrete junctional nests containing heavily pigmented slender spindled melanocytes are present. In addition, scattered pagetoid melanocytes are noted in the lower half of epidermis, which is slightly hyperplastic, with a uniform plate-like configuration.

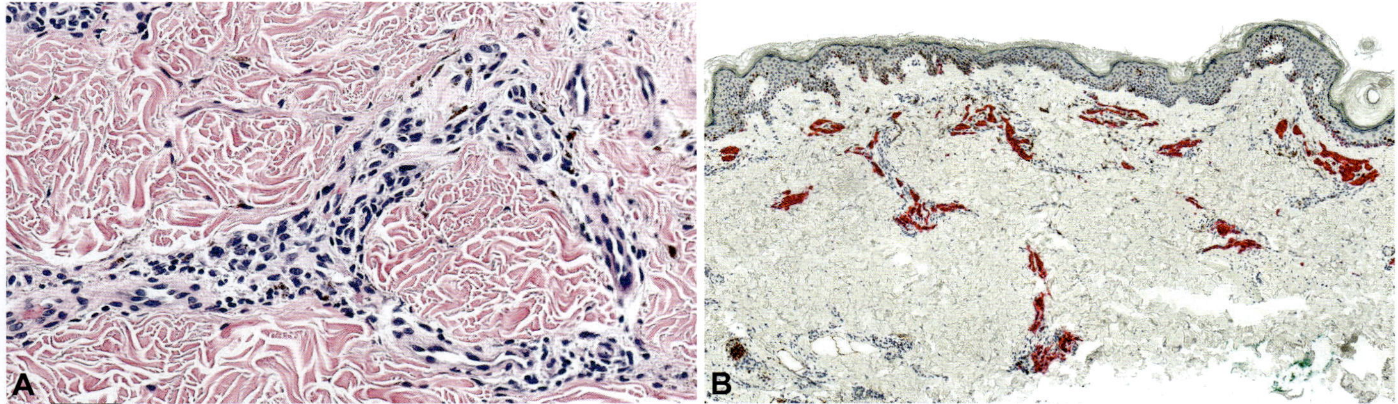


**Fig. 2.62** Plexiform spindle cell naevus. **A** Fascicles of spindled melanocytes are aligned along the abluminal surfaces of the vascular plexus (vascular channels) in the dermis. **B** HMB45 immunostain highlights plexiform architecture of naevus. The expression of HMB45 antigen is useful for the recognition of this entity.

distinctly biphasic, with nodules of large amelanotic spitzoid epithelioid cells present in a background PSCN.

PLEXSCNs are pigmented spindle cell proliferations characterized by small diameter (mean: 3 mm), sharp circumscription, symmetry, and a fascicular–plexiform (candelabra-like) architecture in the reticular dermis (corresponding to the neurovascular plexus); they are not necessarily deep or wedge-shaped {152,159,1151}. Junctional nests, epithelioid cells, other naevus components (combined naevus), low-grade cytological atypia, and mitotic activity (0–2 mitoses/mm$^2$) may be present. Atypical PLEXSCNs may show larger size, increased cellularity and cytological atypia, and mitotic rates of >3 mitoses/mm$^2$ {1151}. PSCN and APSCT express S100 protein and SOX10, as well as the melanocyte differentiation antigens melan-A (MART1), tyrosinase, and MITF {147}. A diminished gradient of HMB45 and Ki-67 staining is seen with depth. PLEXSCNs typically label with HMB45.

## Differential diagnosis

PSCN, APSCT, and PLEXSCN must be distinguished from melanoma; the distinction is based on the naevi's clinical features, typically small size, symmetry, sharp circumscription, predominantly nested pattern, and uniformity of cell type. PLEXSCN and deep penetrating naevus show some overlap and form a histological continuum analogous to that formed by PSCN and Spitz naevus. The essential differences are related to architecture and depth. In PLEXSCN, distinct fascicles of spindle cells are located along the neurovascular plexus, with intervening normal dermis. In deep penetrating naevus, the fascicles are often more cellular and more closely aggregated (with less intervening dermal collagen) in a wedge-shaped (or V-shaped) architecture. Deep penetrating naevi usually have greater depth than PLEXSCNs.

## Histogenesis

See *Spitz naevus* (p. 111).

## Genetic profile

The genetic profile has not yet been characterized. See *Spitz naevus* (p. 111).

## Prognosis and predictive factors

PSCN and its variants are important clinical and histological simulants of melanoma, and can (rarely) give rise to melanoma.

# Melanocytic tumours in acral skin

## Acral melanoma

Yun S.J.
Bastian B.C.
Duncan L.M.
Haneke E.
Uhara H.

### Definition
Acral melanoma is a melanoma occurring in glabrous acral skin, such as on the palms, soles, and nail apparatus. Many acral melanomas are of the acral lentiginous melanoma (ALM) form, which was first proposed by Reed in 1976 {2144}; histopathologically, this subtype is characterized by a lentiginous intraepidermal proliferation of atypical melanocytes. A predominantly lentiginous radial growth phase (RGP) evolves over months to years to an invasive and tumorigenic vertical growth phase (VGP). Acral melanoma also includes subungual melanoma, which was first described as melanotic whitlow, by Hutchinson in 1886 {498}.

### ICD-O code 8744/3

### Synonyms
Acral melanoma: acral lentiginous melanoma; plantar lentiginous melanoma {103}; palmar-plantar-subungual-mucosal melanoma {1777}
Subungual melanoma: nail apparatus melanoma

### Epidemiology
The relative incidence of acral melanoma versus other melanoma subtypes varies considerably with race, but the absolute incidence is similar. Acral melanoma is the most common melanoma subtype in Asian, Hispanic, and African populations {289,1663,2782}. In eastern Asia, acral melanoma accounts for > 50% of all cutaneous melanoma cases {431}. Subungual melanoma accounts for 10–20% of acral melanomas occurring in Asians {2054}. Acral melanoma increases in incidence with age, but can also occur in young people. Patients with acral melanoma are typically older than patients with other melanoma subtypes {2756}, with a mean age of 63 years {289,1451,2054}. The incidence rates among males and females are similar.

### Etiology
The etiology of acral melanoma has yet to be determined. Whereas ultraviolet (UV) radiation exposure is the major cause of non-acral melanoma, acral sites are not UV radiation–exposed. In a White population in Australia, acral melanoma was found to be strongly associated with high whole-body naevus counts, naevi on the soles, and sun exposure {932}. However, in Japan, a high whole-body count of acquired melanocytic naevi was found to be a risk factor for the development of non-acral melanoma, but not acral melanoma {2218}. The average number of melanocytic naevi on the soles of patients with acral melanoma did not differ from that of a control group {1409,2218}. The results of anatomical mapping of acral melanoma on the plantar surface suggest a possible association with mechanical or physical stress; the melanomas tend to occur on the weight-bearing portion of the sole {744,1251,1784}. Trauma may also be associated with subungual melanomas, given that they most commonly affect the nails of the thumb and great toe. Physical stress, pressure, friction, maceration, irritation, and trauma may play a role in the pathogenesis of acral melanoma, but further study is needed.

### Localization
Acral melanoma is melanoma occurring on the non–hair-bearing volar surface of hands and feet or the nail apparatus {744}. A few studies have also included the dorsal aspects of the hands and feet as acral sites. ALMs occur predominantly on volar surfaces, and superficial spreading melanoma occurs more commonly on dorsal surfaces {1451,2054}. Acral melanoma predominantly involves the soles (rather than the palms). Subungual melanoma accounts for about 20% of acral melanomas {744,1251,1451}. Acral melanoma on the sole primarily occurs on the weight-bearing portions of the sole, including the heel and forefoot areas {744,1251,1784}. Subungual melanomas affect the fingernails more frequently than the toenails, and right-side

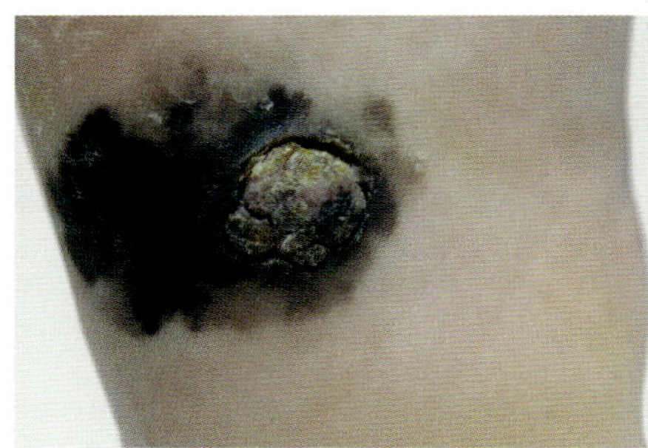

**Fig. 2.63** Acral melanoma. A large, irregular, black to brownish patch with elevated tumour on the sole.

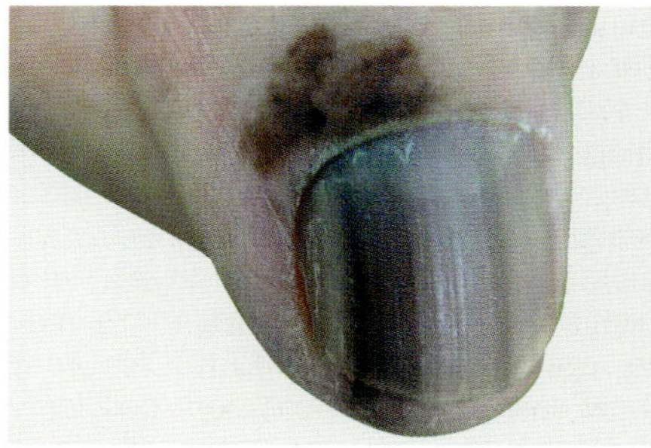

**Fig. 2.64** Subungual melanoma. Hutchinson's sign (i.e. dark pigmented macules beyond the proximal nail-fold and hyponychium) is remarkable.

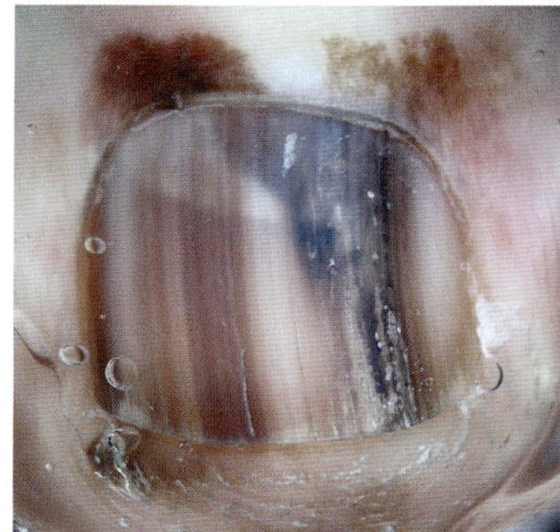

**Fig. 2.65** Subungual melanoma. A dermoscopic view shows multiple irregular longitudinal brown-to-black lines and Hutchinson's sign.

fingernails are more susceptible, as is the nail apparatus of the thumb and great toe.

## Clinical features

Acral melanoma presents as a large, asymmetrical, black, pigmented, irregular patch on acral sites. There is a long RGP; many patients have black patches for several months to years before developing elevated nodules correlating with the VGP. Surface ulceration over time is common. These features are characteristics of ALM {513}. However, acral melanoma sometimes manifests similarly to nodular melanoma: as a large nodule without a surrounding pigmented patch. Subungual melanoma often starts as longitudinal melanonychia, and then a pigmented patch spreads over the entire nail plate and into the skin beyond the nailfolds and hyponychium (a phenomenon called Hutchinson's sign) {2901}. Rare amelanotic acral melanomas, which show little or no black to brown pigmentation, are a diagnostic challenge; they are easily misdiagnosed as benign conditions {472}. Subungual melanomas may begin as longitudinal melanonychia or non-melanonychia lesions {1535}. Dermoscopy is an excellent tool to diagnose and differentiate acral melanoma. The parallel ridge pattern, which consists of a brown-to-black band-like pigmentation located on the ridges of the skin markings, is highly characteristic of early melanoma of the palms and soles {1935,2279,2280}. The dermoscopic features most indicative of early subungual melanoma are multiple irregular longitudinal brown-to-black lines on a brown background, micro-Hutchinson's sign, a wide pigmented band, and triangular pigmentation on the nail plate {294,1407,2222}.

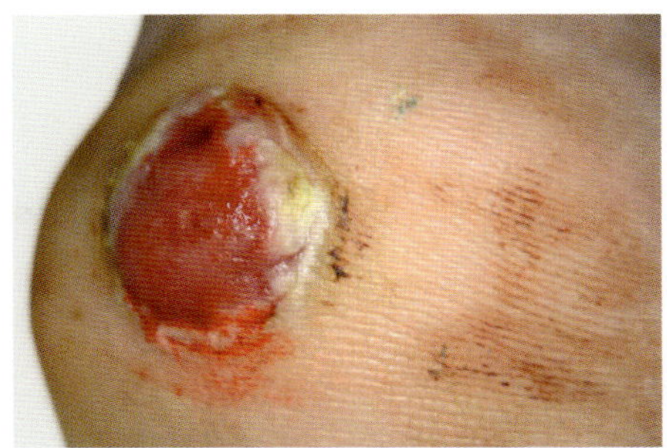

**Fig. 2.66** Amelanotic acral melanoma. An ulcerative erythematous nodule on the heel, without black pigment.

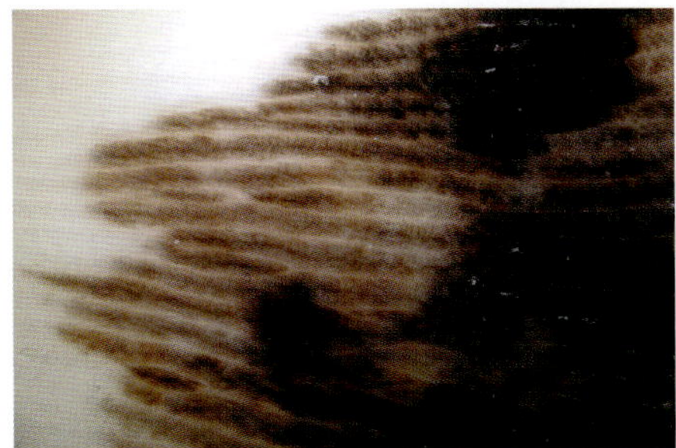

**Fig. 2.67** Acral melanoma. A dermoscopic view shows a parallel ridge pattern, with brown-to-black band-like pigmentation on the ridges of the skin markings: characteristics of acral melanoma on the sole.

## Histopathology

The most common histopathological subtype of acral melanoma is ALM, followed by nodular melanoma and superficial spreading melanoma {1251,1451,1608}. The RGP of ALM is characterized by a lentiginous proliferation (along the base of the epidermis) of atypical melanocytes with enlarged hyperchromatic nuclei and prominent dendrites {1366,2374}. In the very early stages of the RGP, there are only scattered (not confluent) lentiginous, atypical melanocytes in the epidermal basal layer {295,755}. The most common cell types are pigmented spindle cells. However, mixed cellular morphology, such as spindle cells and epithelioid cells, is frequently observed in VGP lesions. ALM is sometimes desmoplastic, neurotropic, and syringotropic {513,2374}. The histopathological features of nodular melanoma are similar to those of the VGP of acral melanoma, and those of superficial spreading melanoma at acral sites are similar to those of examples at other body sites. HMB45 and melan-A (MART1) staining highlights prominent dendritic processes of melanocytes. HMB45 is sometimes only focally positive or negative in amelanotic acral melanoma; HMB45 and melan-A are both negative in desmoplastic melanoma {472,1367}. SOX10 is a useful marker for revealing the nuclear variability of acral melanoma, and is also seen in desmoplastic variants. Subungual melanoma also begins with a scattered proliferation of atypical melanocytes in the nail matrix in its early stages {1199,1993,2569}. Over time, lymphocytic infiltrates, pagetoid scatter, cytological atypia with mitoses, and dermal invasion become evident. Interestingly, dermal invasive nodules are more conspicuous in the hyponychium, and dermal invasion in the nail matrix is a late event {1199,2422}. Immunostaining is helpful in differentiating histological mimics, such as poorly differentiated neoplasms of other lineages.

## Differential diagnosis

The most important differential diagnosis is acral naevus. Acral junctional naevus may be especially difficult to distinguish from acral melanoma in situ {295}.

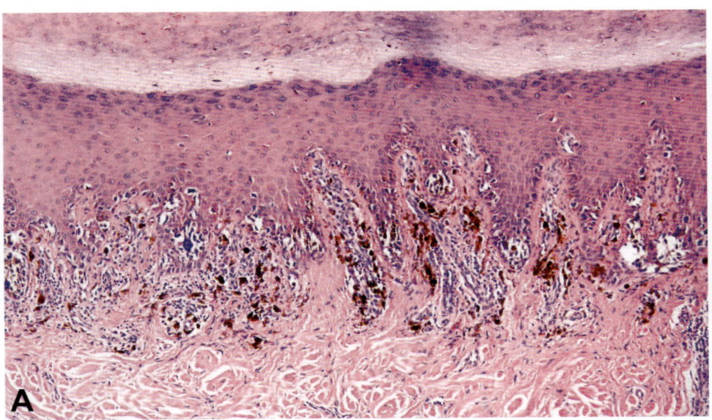



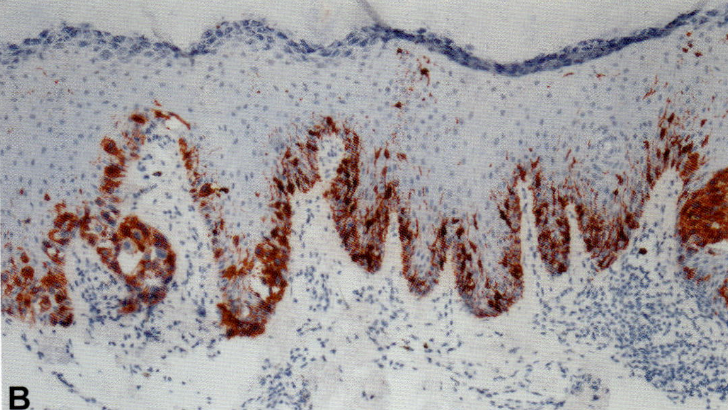



**Fig. 2.68** Acral melanoma. **A** There is a lentiginous proliferation of atypical hyperchromatic melanocytes in the epidermal basal layer, with mild lymphocytic infiltrates and many melanophages. **B** Immunostaining for melan-A highlights a lentiginous proliferation of atypical melanocytes with prominent dendritic processes.

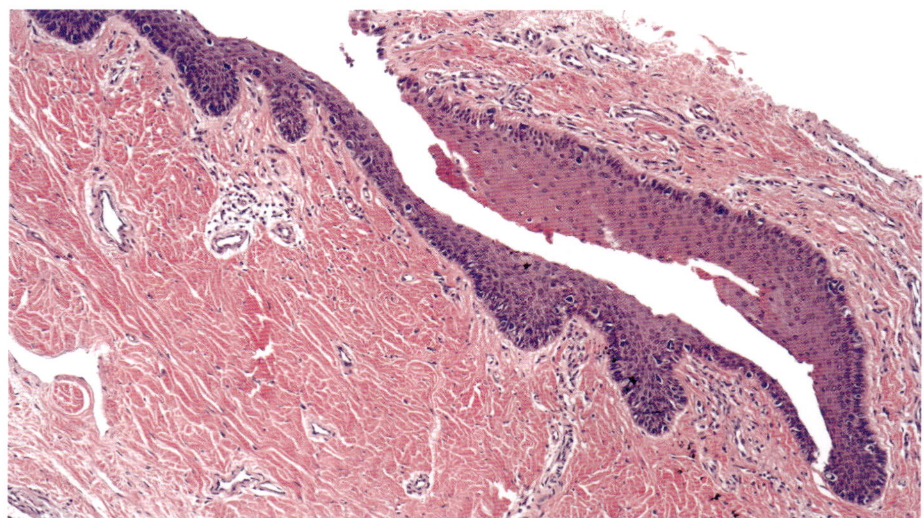

**Fig. 2.69** Subungual melanoma. This very early stage example shows only scattered proliferation of atypical hyperchromatic melanocytes in the nail matrix.

Pagetoid scatter may be seen in both lesions, but acral naevus does not typically exhibit marked cytological atypia or mitotic activity. Dermoscopic findings are usually helpful {2279,2280}. Patient age and the lesion size (and therefore, clinicopathological correlation) are also important. Amelanotic acral melanomas can clinically mimic benign conditions such as calluses, warts, onychomycosis, non-healing ulcers, and ingrown nails.

## Histogenesis

The secretory portion of eccrine sweat glands on the volar surface has been suggested to provide an anatomical niche for the melanocyte–melanoma precursor cells {1869,1941}.

## Genetic profile

Acral melanomas have a low mutation burden, typically without a UV radiation signature, and are characterized by many copy-number changes (including multiple high-level amplifications {555}) and structural rearrangements {1050}. *BRAF* mutations (found in 15% of cases), *NRAS* mutations (in 15% of cases), and *KIT* mutations or amplifications (in 15–40%) {168} occur in a mutually exclusive pattern, and focused gene amplifications of *CCND1* (found in 24% of cases) also tend to show this pattern. Other recurrently amplified genes include *TERT*, *CDK4*, *GAB2*, *PAK1*, and *RICTOR*. Loss-of-function mutations in *NF1*, *TP53*, and *CDKN2A* are common in acral melanoma {2090}.

## Genetic susceptibility

Only a relatively low proportion of patients with acral melanoma have any personal or family history of melanoma {2054}. One study found that patients with acral melanoma were more likely to have other cancers than were patients with other types of melanomas {127}.

## Prognosis and predictive factors

The prognosis is generally poor because of diagnostic delay associated with increased tumour thickness and frequent ulceration. In some populations, acral melanoma has been shown to have a worse outcome than other (stage-matched) melanomas {200,431}. However, a recent Japanese study found no difference in melanoma-specific and disease-free survival between acral melanoma and non-acral melanomas {2756}.

# Acral naevus

Yun S.J.
Bastian B.C.
Duncan L.M.
Haneke E.
Uhara H.

## Definition

Acral naevus is a melanocytic naevus occurring on the palms, soles, and nails. Nail matrix naevus (NMN) is an acral naevus occurring on the nail matrix.

## ICD-O code

8744/0

## Synonyms

Atypical or acral lentiginous naevus {1661}; naevus of special sites {31}; nail matrix naevus

## Epidemiology

In the USA, 36% of people have at least one acral naevus {1622}. Acral naevus is more common in individuals with higher constitutional pigmentation and many melanocytic naevi on the skin {1622,1968}. In Japan, the prevalence of plantar naevi is 10.9% and increases with age, peaking in the third and fourth decades of life {1409}. On average, females have more acral naevi than males do {1622}.

## Localization

Acral naevus occurs on the palms and soles {1808}. NMN affects the fingernails more commonly than the toenails, with the thumb being the most common site {2632}.

## Clinical features

Acral naevus presents as a brownish to black pigmented small macule or papule. NMN manifests as longitudinal melanonychia {2632}. In children, NMN is darker and multicoloured, and pseudo-Hutchinson's sign is frequently seen {1938}. Most acquired acral naevi have one of three major dermoscopic patterns: the parallel furrow pattern, the lattice-like pattern, and the fibrillar pattern {1935,2279,2280}. Dermoscopy of NMN shows regularly thick parallel lines without colour variation {204}. Dermoscopic patterns vary with age {738,1783,2539}. Acral naevi have a different distribution on volar sites than do acral melanomas, naevi primarily involving non–weight-bearing areas {1365}.

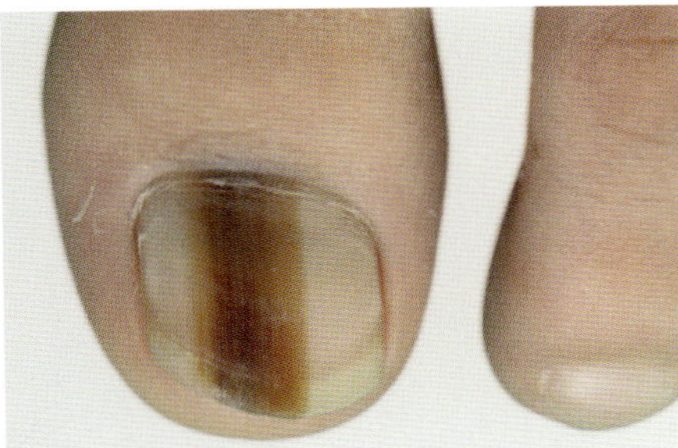

**Fig. 2.70** Nail matrix naevus. Longitudinal melanonychia on the left great toenail.

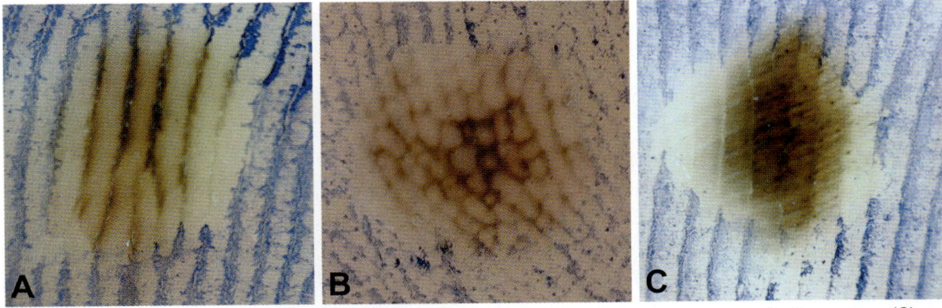


**Fig. 2.71** Acral naevus. The parallel furrow pattern (**A**), the lattice-like pattern (**B**), and the fibrillar pattern (**C**) are characteristic dermoscopic features of acral naevus on the sole. The application of blue ink highlights the furrows.

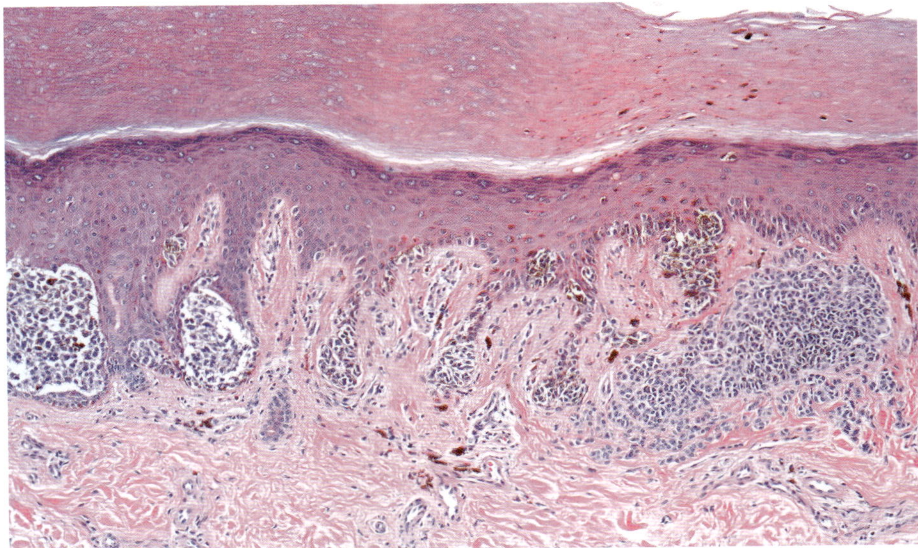

**Fig. 2.72** Acral compound naevus. There is single-cell proliferation, with variably sized nests in the epidermis. In the dermis, the naevus cells are small and show maturation.

## Histopathology

Compared with acral melanoma, acral naevus is relatively small and circumscribed. Pagetoid scatter, bridging between rete, and fibroplasia are not uncommon in acral naevus, but these features tend to be sparse and confined to the centre of the lesion. Naevus cells are disposed as single cells and in variably sized nests, often with confluence {31,286,722}. There may be random cytological atypia {677}. Acral naevus is often junctional; when it is compound, the dermal naevus cells display maturation to smaller cells with increasing dermal depth. NMN can be junctional or compound, and proper biopsy of the nail matrix is important {2184,2251}.

## Differential diagnosis

A confluent lentiginous intraepidermal proliferation of atypical melanocytes and a prominent inflammatory infiltrate are more common in acral melanoma than in acral naevus. NMN should be distinguished from other diseases causing melanonychia.

## Histogenesis

The histogenesis of acral naevus is similar to that of other cutaneous naevi.

## Prognosis and predictive factors

The lesions are benign, and progression to melanoma is rare. NMN in children initially shows a rapid increase in width and colour variegation, but it may undergo spontaneous regression (partial or complete) by adolescence {1357,1408,2631,2632}.

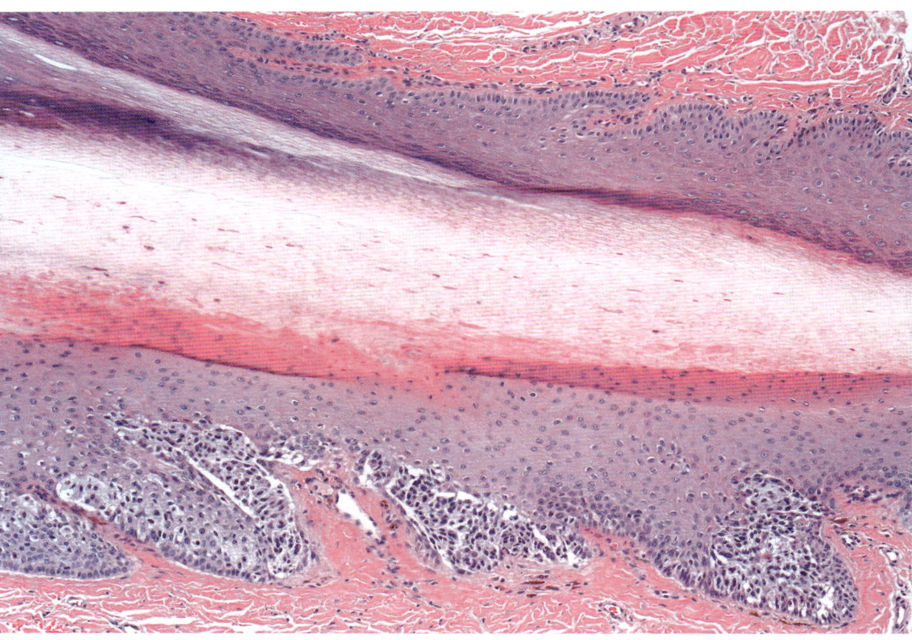

**Fig. 2.73** Nail matrix naevus. A biopsy of the case shown in Fig. 2.70 reveals variably sized nests in the nail matrix, consistent with junctional naevus. Clinicopathological correlation is necessary to completely rule out melanoma.

# Genital and mucosal melanocytic tumours

## Mucosal melanomas (genital, oral, sinonasal)

Prieto V.G.
Dehner L.P.
Pfeifer J.D.
Wick M.R.

### Definition

Mucosal melanomas are melanomas arising in a surface epithelium other than skin.

This section discusses the most common such lesions (excluding ocular lesions): melanomas that arise in non-cutaneous sites in the external female and male genital tracts, the distal urinary tract, the anorectal region, and the head and neck (oral cavity and nasal and paranasal sinuses).

### ICD-O codes

| | |
|---|---|
| Mucosal melanomas (genital, oral, sinonasal) | 8720/3 |
| Mucosal lentiginous melanoma | 8746/3 |
| Mucosal nodular melanoma | 8721/3 |

### Synonyms

Genital melanoma; oral melanoma; sinonasal melanoma

### Epidemiology

Only 0.03% of all cancer diagnoses are mucosal melanomas {2494}. In aggregate, mucosal melanomas account for 1.3% of all melanomas {430} among all racial groups {2582}. The mean age at diagnosis is 67 years, versus 55 years for cutaneous lesions {430}. About 65% of mucosal melanomas occur in women, versus 45% of cutaneous lesions.

### Etiology

Unlike cutaneous melanomas, mucosal melanomas have no apparent association with ultraviolet (UV) radiation exposure. Trauma has been suggested as a possible cause.

### Localization

Mucosal melanomas are localized in the head and neck region in 45–55% of all cases (of those, 50–80% occur in the nasal cavity and paranasal sinus), in the anorectal region in 25%, and in the vulvovaginal region in 15–20% (of those, 80–85% occur in the vulva) {430,951,2004,2582}. In both males and females, 5% of cases present in the distal urethra {673,1978}. The cervix is a very rare site of mucosal melanoma {1914}.

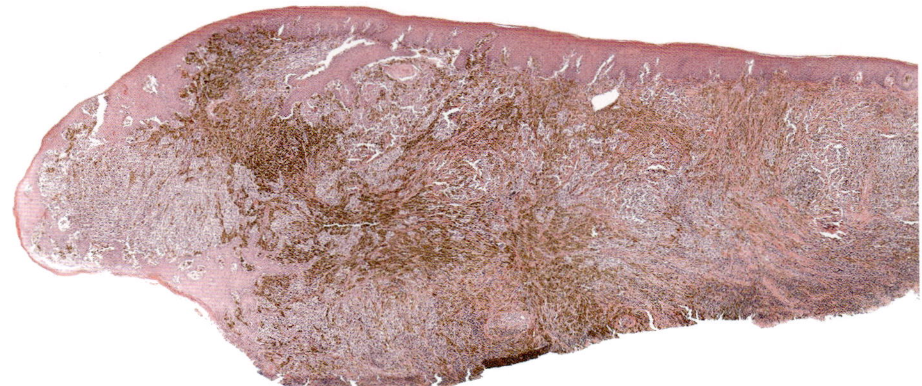

**Fig. 2.74** Mucosal melanoma presenting as bulky tumour in a mucous membrane. Melanomas of the oral cavity or the vulvovaginal or urethral mucosa could have this appearance.

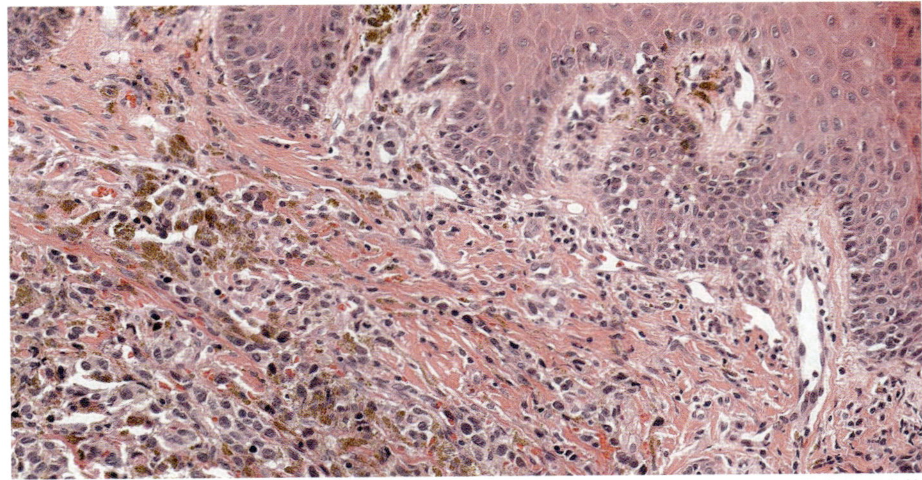

**Fig. 2.75** Mucosal melanoma. The invasive tumour is composed of uniformly atypical epithelioid cells (bottom left), admixed in this case with numerous melanophages. There is involvement of the overlying epithelium by atypical melanocytes, mostly basal in this field.

### Clinical features

Pigmentation is present in the great majority (85–90%) of mucosal melanomas overall, with one third of oral mucosal melanomas being pigmented {2371}. Other clinical features include blood streaking of nasal secretions, epistaxis, nasal stuffiness, proptosis, diplopia, and pain.

### Histopathology

The most common patterns are mucosal lentiginous and nodular. The lesions are composed of epithelioid and/or spindled melanocytes with amphophilic or eosinophilic cytoplasm with variable pigmentation, ovoid nuclei, and prominent nucleoli (rarely small cell or naevoid). The

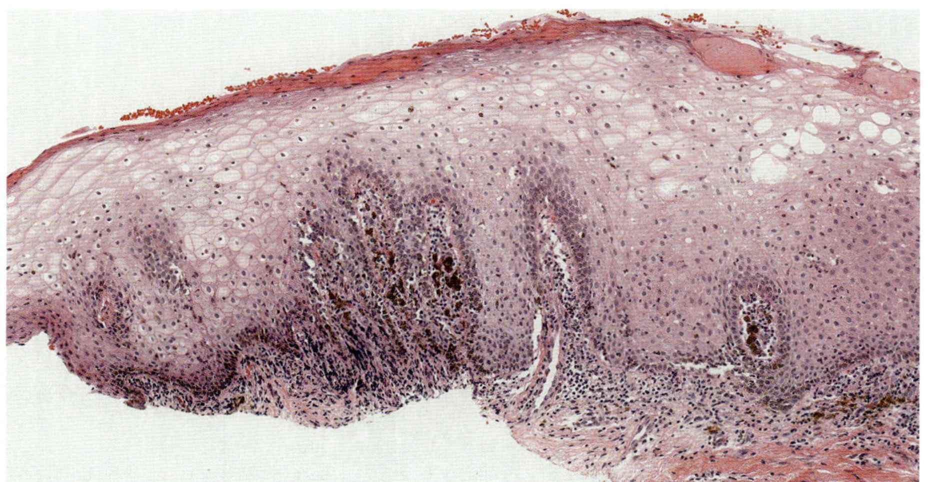

**Fig. 2.76** Mucosal melanoma. In the adjacent squamous epithelium, there is a basal (lentiginous) proliferation of atypical melanocytes (relatively subtle, as is often the case), with melanophages and lymphocytes in the subepithelial stroma.

overlying epidermis usually contains a lentiginous growth with single cells and small nests. Ulceration and vascular invasion are common in advanced lesions. Because of the often fragmented nature of the specimens, tangential sectioning may preclude the accurate measurement of thickness.

The tumour cells usually express melan-A (MART1), HMB45 antigen, SOX10, and MITF, supporting a melanocytic nature and possibly highlighting epidermotropism.

## Differential diagnosis

Mucosal lentigines have hyperpigmentation of basal keratinocytes without (or with only slightly increased numbers of) melanocytes. A possible mimic of mucosal lentigo is the presence, mostly in the oral mucosa, of focal areas of only slightly increased numbers of atypical melanocytes within obvious melanoma. Therefore, complete excision of any lesions resembling mucosal lentigo that extend to the tissue edges of the biopsy is needed for accurate diagnosis. Extramammary Paget disease also shows pagetoid migration, but the tumour cells express keratin (and usually CEA, CK7, and GCDFP15) in primary extramammary Paget disease and CK20 in secondary extramammary Paget disease (from the gastrointestinal tract). Amalgam tattoo shows pigmented macrophages in the lamina propria. Occasionally, melanoma may metastasize to the rectum, mimicking a primary lesion.

## Histogenesis

The histogenesis involves malignant transformation of the melanocytes normally occurring in these locations.

## Genetic profile

Mutations involving *KIT* and *NRAS* predominate {2248}.

## Genetic susceptibility

Anorectal melanomas are more frequent in patients with red hair {401}.

## Prognosis and predictive factors

There are no American Joint Committee on Cancer (AJCC) staging criteria for mucosal melanomas of the urethra, vagina, rectum, or anus. Head and neck lesions start in the T3 category. Melanoma of the vulva is AJCC-staged identically to cutaneous melanoma {1838,2588}.

The prognosis is poor, likely because of delayed detection. For vulvar melanoma, the median disease-specific survival is 74.2 months, with 5-year and 10-year disease-specific survival rates of 58.2% and 35.8%, respectively. Tumour thickness and dermal mitotic rate have been found to be most predictive of outcome {1863}. Early lesions (i.e. in situ or superficially invasive lesions) are typically expected to have a good prognosis after complete excision. Local recurrence and progression may occur after incomplete excision.

# Genital naevus

Prieto V.G.
Pfeifer J.D.
Wick M.R.

## Definition

Genital naevus is a benign melanocytic naevus located in the genital region.

## ICD-O code 8720/0

## Synonyms

Genital naevocytic naevus; naevus of the genital tract

## Epidemiology

About 20% of all women have pigmented lesions in the genital region, but <5% of such lesions are melanocytic naevi {403}.

## Localization

In women, the most commonly affected site is the labium minus, followed by the labium majus, clitoris, and vulvar vestibule. In men, the most common sites are the glans, shaft, and prepuce {403,494}.

## Clinical features

Genital naevi are flat or papular lesions, circumscribed and uniformly pigmented. They are usually solitary, typically occur in young adults, and can reach 1 cm in size.

## Histopathology

Although all melanocytic lesions occurring in this anatomical location are by definition genital, the term "genital naevus" is usually reserved for lesions with a junctional component of single cells and round or fusiform nests, with focal retraction artefact and dyscohesion. At scanning magnification, these lesions may have a mushroom-like silhouette. There may be focal pagetoid spread, limited to the centre of the lesion. The nests are usually distributed haphazardly along the epidermal rete ridges, often oriented parallel to the epidermal surface. The dermal component may show cytological atypia superficially, but shows maturation with increasing depth (i.e. the cells in the deep dermis are smaller than those at the dermoepidermal junction); mitotic figures are very rare and only superficial {888}. In pregnant women, genital naevi may show mitotic figures more commonly, but they are also only superficial. Some lesions have a dense lymphocytic infiltrate (the halo phenomenon), and some are associated with lichen sclerosus {381}.

## Differential diagnosis

The main differential diagnosis is melanoma. Genital melanomas are much more common in elder individuals (postmenopausal women). Melanomas have a higher degree of cytological atypia, lack maturation, and have more dermal mitotic figures. In melanomas, HMB45 staining is usually patchy, and Ki-67 staining indicates an increased proliferation rate throughout the lesion.

Dysplastic naevi share many features with genital naevi, in particular the architectural disorder (bridging and lamellar fibrosis) {2179}.

## Histogenesis

As is the case with other melanocytic lesions, there is still debate as to whether melanocytes in naevi (naevomelanocytes), come from the epithelium, migrate from the neural crest, or differentiate from cells in the dermal/mucosal nerves.

## Genetic profile

Unlike mucosal melanomas, most genital naevi contain BRAF p.V600E mutations {509,2664}.

## Prognosis and predictive factors

These are benign lesions. Very rarely, melanomas are seen associated with genital naevi.

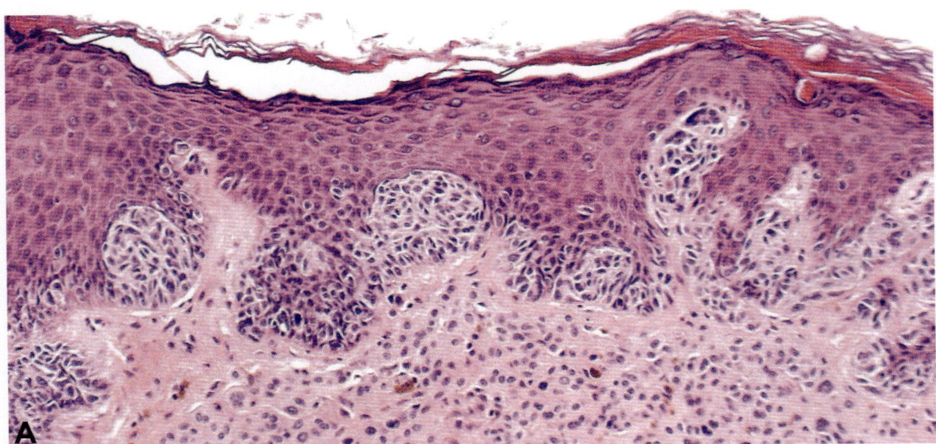


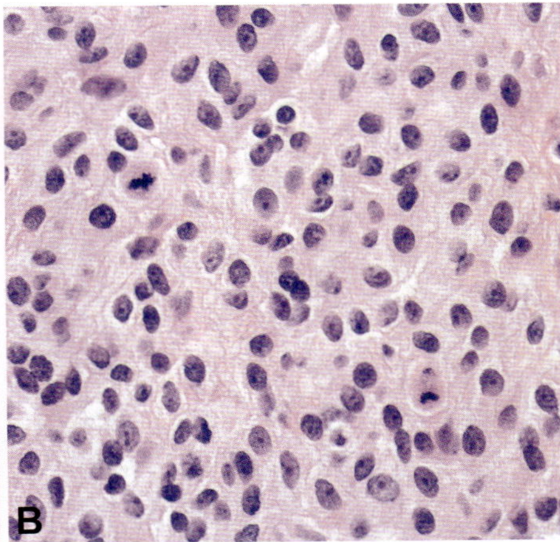


**Fig. 2.77** Genital naevus in a pregnant woman. **A** There is a junctional component of single cells and small nests. **B** The superficial dermal melanocytes display rare mitotic figures, limited to the upper half of the lesion.

# Melanocytic tumours arising in blue naevus

## Melanoma arising in blue naevus

de la Fouchardière A.
Scolyer R.A.
Calonje E.
Fullen D.R.
Gerami P.
Requena L.
Barnhill R.L.

### Definition

"Melanoma arising in blue naevus (MBN)" refers to melanoma arising in a pre-existing blue naevus, usually a cellular blue naevus. The term may also be used for melanoma arising at the site of a previously excised blue naevus, as well as for melanoma with cytoarchitectural features resembling (usually cellular) blue naevus but apparently arising de novo (and usually harbouring the specific mutations of these tumours).

### ICD-O code 8780/3

### Synonyms

Blue naevus–like melanoma; melanoma ex-blue naevus; melanoma mimicking cellular blue naevus; malignant blue naevus (not recommended)

### Epidemiology

MBN is rare.

### Localization

The scalp is the most common site of involvement, followed by the face, buttocks, back, and chest. Rarely, MBNs can occur in other locations {2883}.

### Clinical features

MBN usually occurs in individuals aged 20–60 years (often > 45 years), as a fast-growing, large (3–13 cm) nodule, which may show clinical evidence of a residual cellular blue naevus. When occurring in plaque-type blue naevi, these melanomas usually present as a new deep-growing firm nodule {2883}. There is no sex predilection.

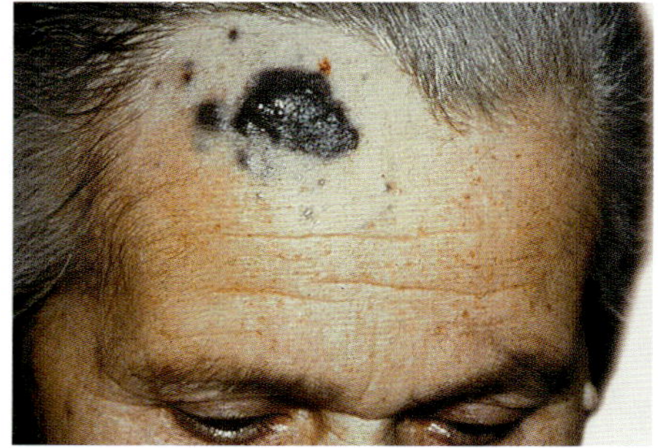

**Fig. 2.78** Melanoma arising in blue naevus. Note the presence of satellitosis.

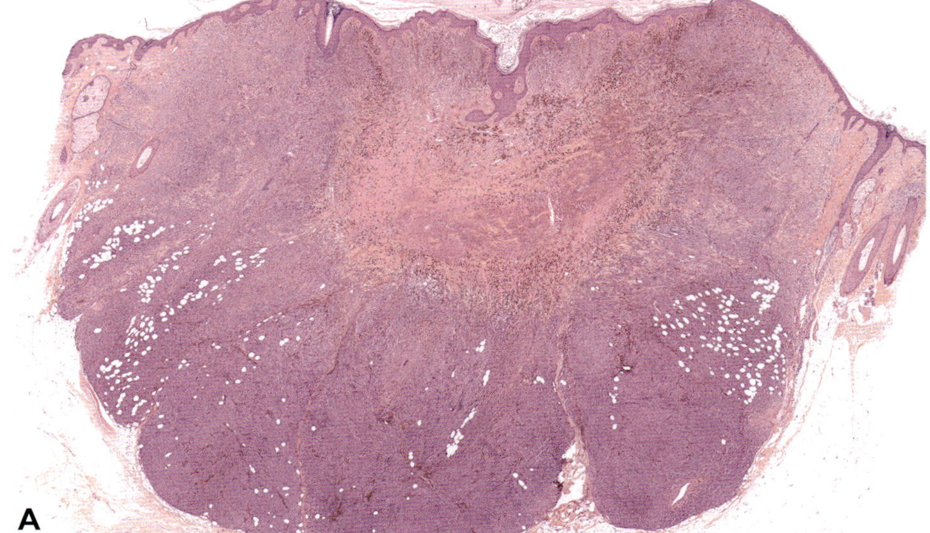

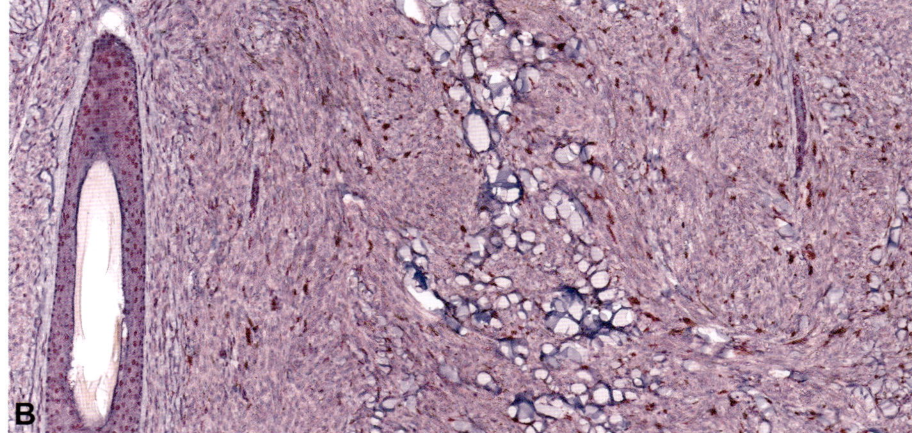

**Fig. 2.79** Melanoma arising in blue naevus. **A** Dense, destructive, sheet-like, pigmented dermal infiltration, with a central area of tumoural necrosis. **B** BAP1 immunostaining reveals loss of nuclear expression throughout the melanocytic lesion, with retention of expression in the follicular keratinocytes.

### Histopathology

The epidermis is usually uninvolved by melanoma but is sometimes ulcerated. The invasive tumour nodule often destroys surrounding adnexal structures and is usually arranged in dense dermal sheets of large spindled and epithelioid melanocytes with severe atypia and high mitotic activity. Occasional cases of MBN may be associated with a low mitotic rate, making the diagnosis of malignancy questionable. Loss of nuclear BAP1 immunoreactivity strongly supports the diagnosis of a

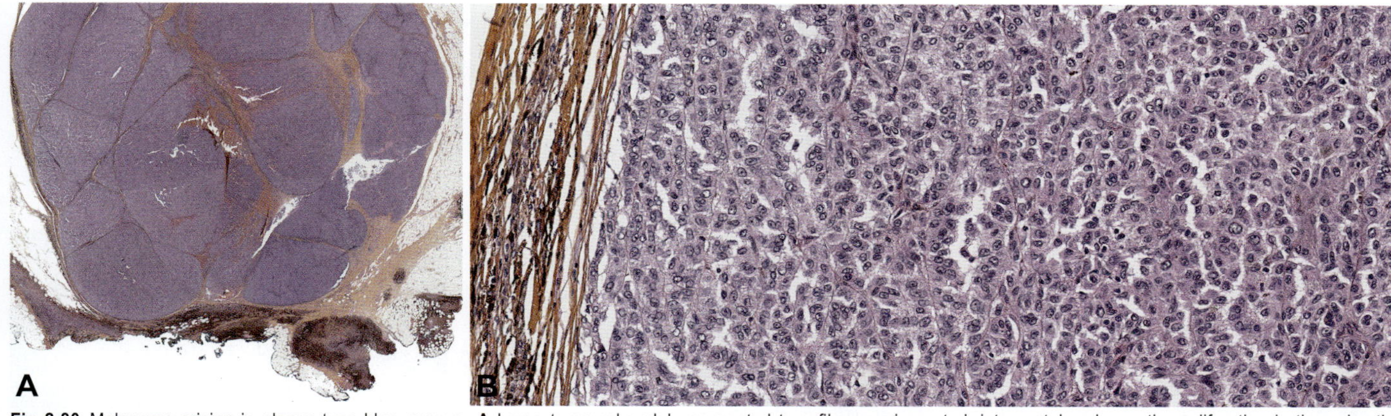


**Fig. 2.80** Melanoma arising in plaque-type blue naevus. **A** Large tumoural nodule connected to a fibrous, pigmented, intraseptal melanocytic proliferation in the subcutis. **B** Higher-magnification view shows sheets of large epithelioid melanocytes with multiple mitoses in the malignant area (right side), adjacent to small spindled melanocytes.

malignant neoplasm, even in the absence of marked cellular atypia and numerous mitoses {532}. Pigmentation is variable, sometimes only found within a subclone. Central areas of tumoural necrosis are frequent in large tumours. The pre-existing blue naevus, when not totally destroyed, can usually be found at the periphery of the tumour {1671}.

The Ki-67 (MIB1) proliferation index is often > 20% in the melanoma and < 5% in the naevus. When nuclear BAP1 staining is lost in the melanoma, the loss typically affects large contiguous populations of neoplastic cells. BAP1 staining is retained in the naevus portion when a naevus remnant is present {532}.

### Differential diagnosis

Diagnosis as a malignant neoplasm is usually straightforward; however, specific classification can be difficult when a benign blue naevus component is not identified. Bulky melanomas of various histological subtypes (nodular, superficial spreading melanoma) with extensive superficial regression can mimic MBN but usually contain a junctional melanocytic component. The diagnosis of metastatic melanoma and dermal relapses of melanoma relies on clinical history or adjacent scar tissue visualization. As a rule, MBNs do not have BRAF p.V600E mutations, and immunohistochemistry for BRAF oncoprotein can be useful to detect melanomas or cutaneous metastases mimicking MBN. Other hyperpigmented dermal mimics (e.g. atypical deep penetrating naevus, plexiform melanoma, and pigmented epithelioid melanocytoma) should be excluded, as should clear cell sarcoma in unpigmented cases. β-catenin immunohistochemistry is useful for identifying deep penetrating naevi and related melanomas {2884}.

### Histogenesis

MBNs evolve from blue naevi and related intradermal melanocytic proliferations, which are caused by somatic mutations of the Gαq signalling pathway. They are closely related biologically and genetically to uveal melanoma and other neoplasms arising from melanocytes not associated with epithelial structures (e.g. melanocytomas of the CNS and primary leptomeningeal melanomas).

### Genetic profile

MBNs harbour *GNAQ*, *GNA11*, *PLCB4*, or *CYSLTR2* mutations (usually already present in the associated blue naevus) in a mutually exclusive pattern {2700,2891}. Additional mutations can occur in *SF3B1* or *BAP1*. Array comparative genomic hybridization profiles show redundant patterns similar to those seen in uveal melanoma, with gains in 6p and/or 8q, monosomy 3, and loss in 1p {428,936}.

### Prognosis and predictive factors

MBNs are often aggressive, with frequent metastasis to the regional lymph nodes and liver; other common metastatic sites can also be affected. Monosomy 3 and loss of BAP1 immunoexpression have been proposed as indicators of a less favourable outcome {532}.

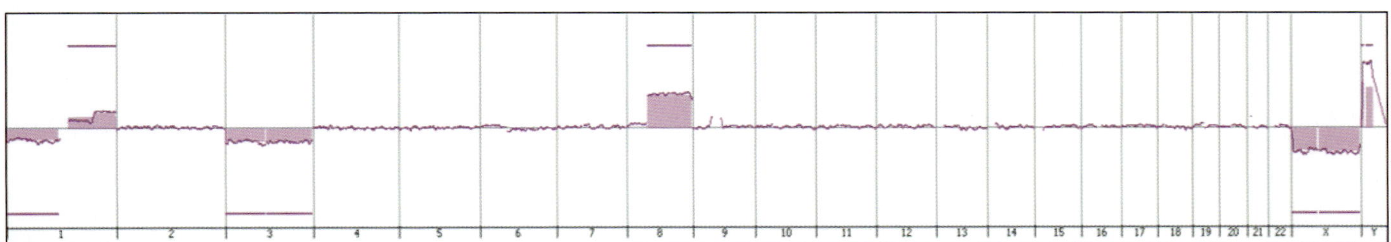


**Fig. 2.81** Melanoma arising in blue naevus. On a comparative genomic hybridization array, the high-level gain of 8q combined with monosomy 3 and loss of 1p suggests a melanoma arising in blue naevus with an adverse prognosis, comparable to that of a high-risk uveal melanoma.

# Blue naevus and cellular blue naevus

Scolyer R.A.
Calonje E.
de la Fouchardière A.
Fullen D.R.
Gerami P.
Requena L.

## Definition

Blue naevus is a dermal melanocytic tumour composed of dendritic, spindle, and/or ovoid cells associated with melanin pigment and stromal sclerosis; it has a blue tinctorial appearance clinically. There are two major subtypes: dendritic blue naevus (DBN) and cellular blue naevus (CBN).

## ICD-O codes

| | |
|---|---|
| Blue naevus NOS | 8780/0 |
| Cellular blue naevus | 8790/0 |

## Synonyms

Dendritic blue naevus: common blue naevus; dermal dendritic melanocytic naevus; naevus of Jadassohn; Tièche naevus; Jadassohn–Tièche blue naevus

## Epidemiology

Blue naevi occur less frequently than common acquired naevi but are not uncommon.

## Localization

Blue naevi can occur at any cutaneous site. DBNs most commonly involve the dorsal distal extremities and face, whereas CBNs typically involve the scalp, back, and buttocks. Blue naevi can also occur at many extracutaneous sites (including mucosal and subungual locations) and involve lymph nodes {1363}. The rare plaque-type blue naevus variant usually affects the scalp but can also occur elsewhere.

## Clinical features

Blue naevi can arise at any age but most commonly present in adults aged < 40 years. They characteristically exhibit a bluish-grey to bluish-black colour, attributed to the deep (dermal) location of abundant melanin pigment. DBNs usually present as well-demarcated, slightly raised papules, usually < 1 cm in diameter {2528}. CBNs more frequently affect females, with a female-to-male ratio of 2:1. CBNs usually present as pigmented nodules ranging from a few millimetres to several centimetres in size. Occasionally, cases are non-pigmented (called amelanotic or hypomelanotic blue naevi). The duration of the lesion prior to diagnosis ranges from months to years; in some cases, the lesion is present at birth. Plaque-type blue naevi usually present at birth or arise in early childhood, and may enlarge during puberty. Plaque-type blue naevus is often several centimetres in diameter and is composed of a single plaque or a confluence of several small macules and/or papules. Rarely, blue naevi may be grouped in a circumscribed anatomical area (so-called agminated

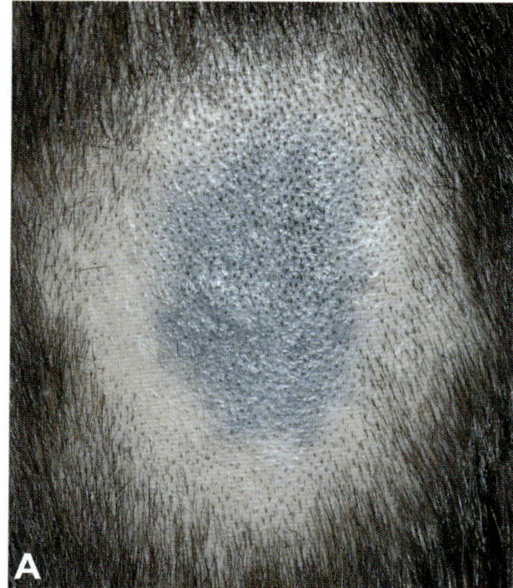

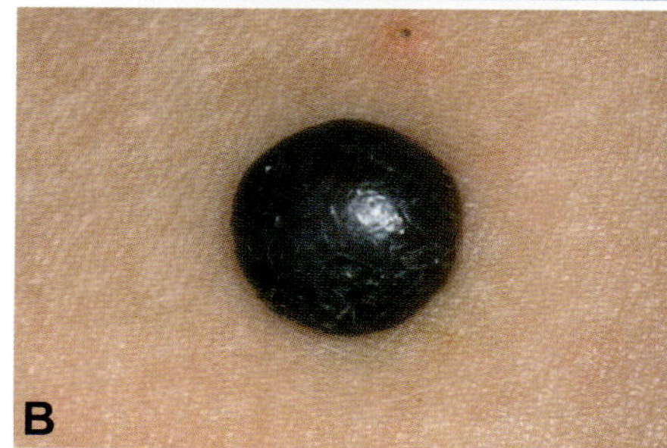

**Fig. 2.83 A** Blue naevus. This relatively large lesion exemplifies the characteristic colour due to the Tyndall effect of preferential blue colour transmission. **B** Cellular blue naevus. Symmetrical heavily pigmented nodule elevating the skin without ulceration.

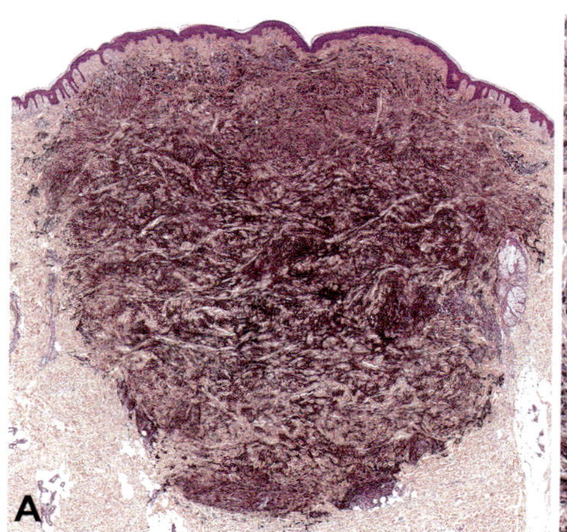

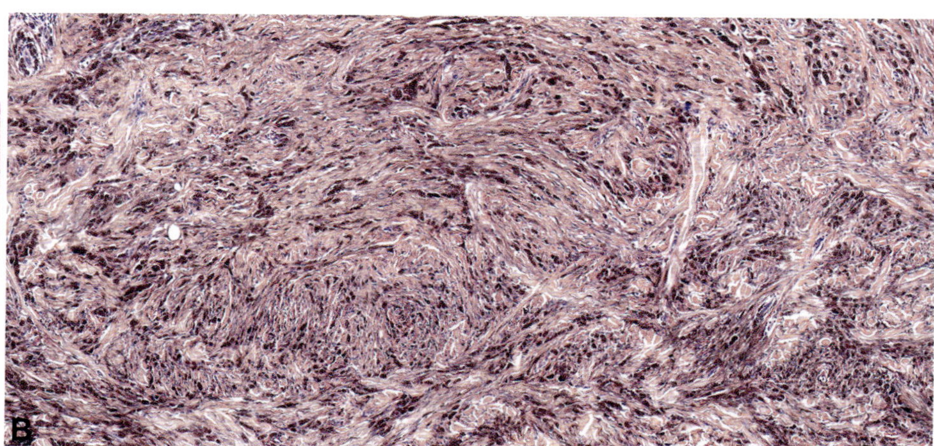

**Fig. 2.82** Dendritic blue naevus. **A** Poorly defined dermal hyperpigmented fibrosing proliferation. **B** There are small spindled and dendritic melanocytes in a fasciculated fibrotic background.

blue naevi); this is postulated to be due to perivascular spread of naevus cells, but without evidence of malignant behaviour. Other reported rare clinical variants include eruptive, linear, and targetoid blue naevi.

Pigmented epithelioid melanocytomas (also called epithelioid blue naevi) can occur in the context of Carney complex or as sporadic lesions.

## Histopathology

Blue naevi often include areas of both DBN and CBN, and are classified on the basis of the predominant component. DBNs are usually non-circumscribed dermal lesions composed predominantly of dendritic melanocytes associated with (and in areas separated by a variable amount of) sclerotic stromal collagen {1847}. When sclerotic stromal collagen is particularly prominent, the term "sclerosing blue naevus" may be used. The cells are bipolar and spindle-shaped, with elongated dendritic processes, sometimes grouped in short fascicles, often with an intervening grenz zone. The melanocytes contain variable amounts of melanin pigment in the cytoplasm, including within the dendritic processes. There are usually also scattered melanophages {2925}. Cellular atypia is absent, and mitotic figures are almost never seen.

CBNs are well-circumscribed nodular dermal tumours that are variably pigmented, with intact overlying epidermis. The majority of the pigment is in macrophages (melanophages); the melanocytes are usually only lightly pigmented. CBNs can show a variety of patterns, but a common feature is bulbous, vertically oriented extension of the lesion into the subcutaneous adipose tissue. In the most common pattern, well-defined nests of fusiform to ovoid cells are surrounded by collagen and numerous melanophages {1150}. The cells are usually oriented parallel to the long axis of the nests (often with central longitudinal nuclear grooves) and lack cell crowding, pleomorphism, nuclear atypia, and hyperchromasia. Sheets or fascicles of spindled to ovoid cells are also commonly present in CBNs. Occasionally, oedematous areas, myxoid stroma, or cystic change may occur (typically in the centre), but necrosis is generally absent. Mitotic activity is usually absent or low (< 1 mitosis/$mm^2$). Perineural extension and intralymphatic tumour may be seen in blue naevus and does

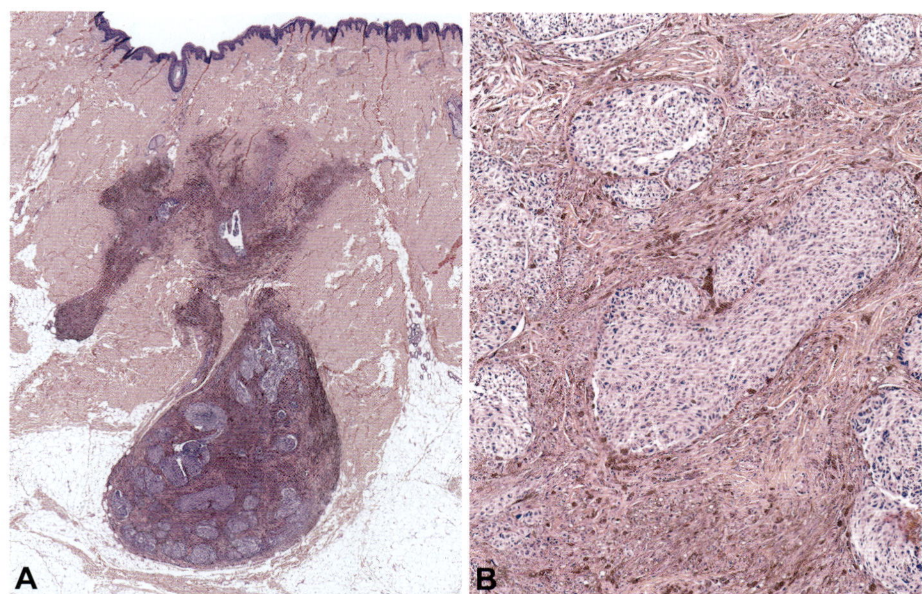

**Fig. 2.84** Cellular blue naevus. **A** Biphasic architecture with an upper intradermal, poorly delineated area of dendritic blue naevus and deep expansion pushing away the subcutis, with cellular nests of unpigmented melanocytes. **B** Higher magnification shows cellular nests of medium-sized fusiform to ovoid cells surrounded by heavily pigmented spindle cells.

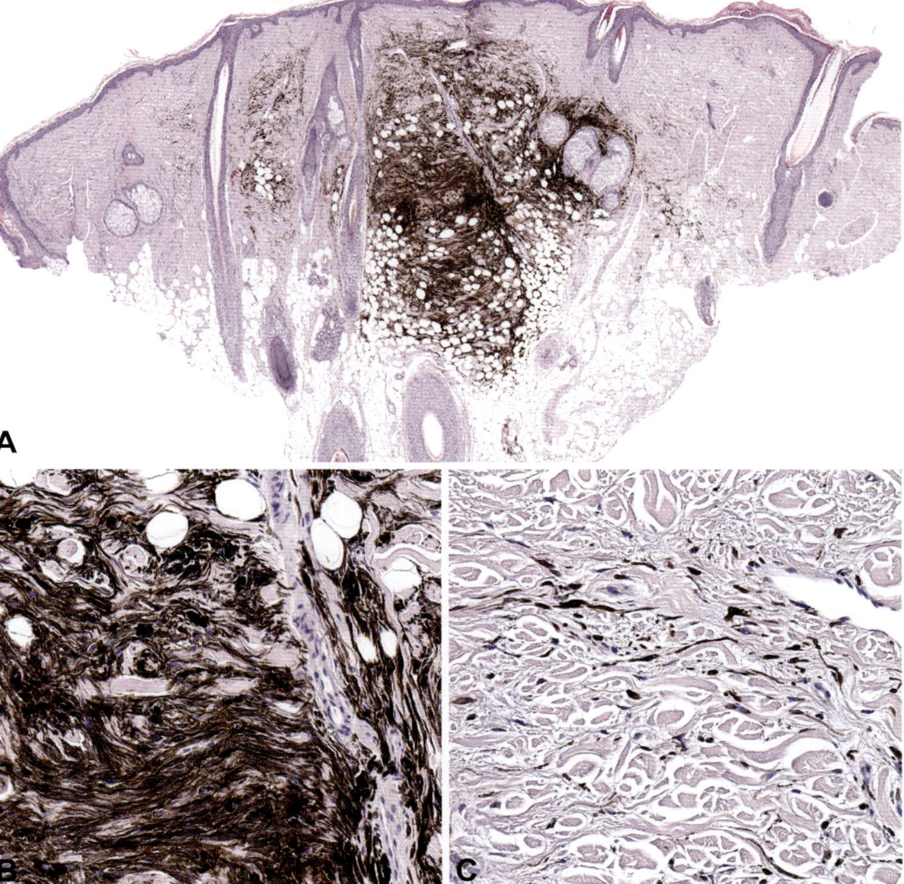

**Fig. 2.85** Dendritic blue naevus. **A** Poorly defined, hyperpigmented, fibrosing dermal proliferation. **B** Higher magnification shows small spindled and dendritic melanocytes in a fasciculated fibrotic background. **C** Small, poorly defined, spindled and dendritic dermal melanocytes.

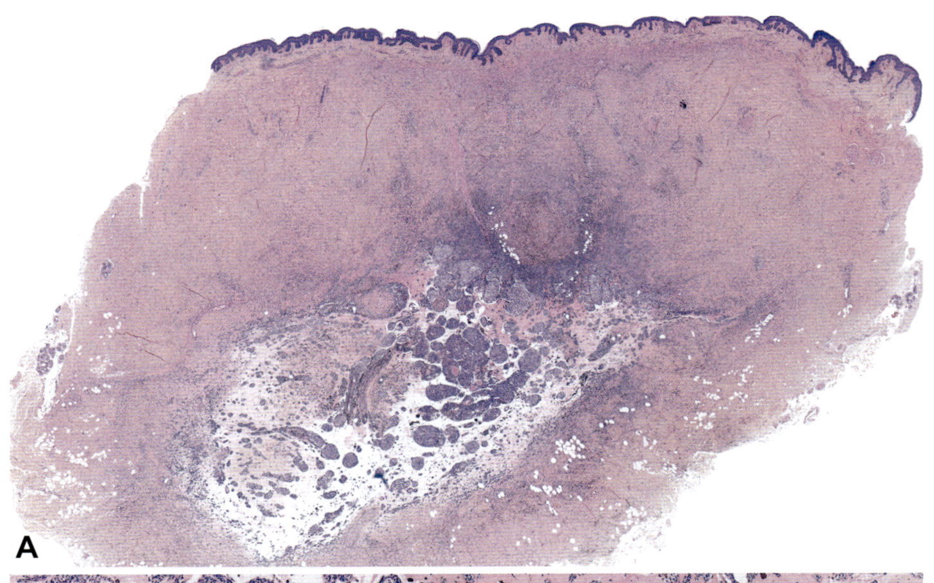

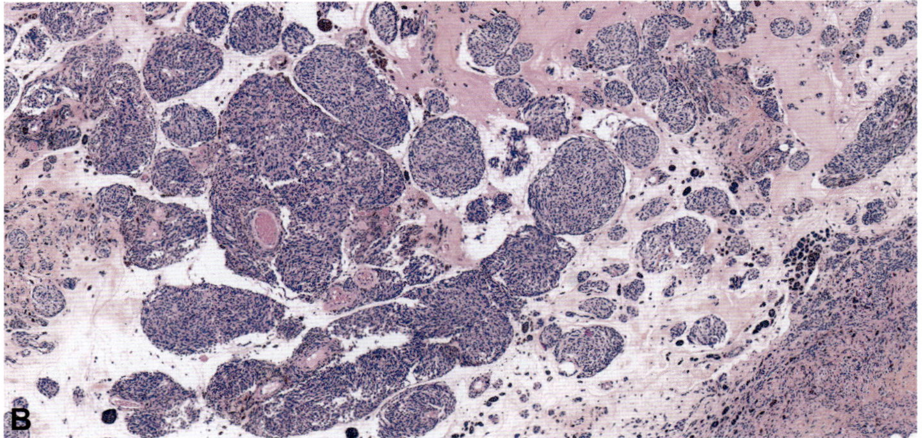

**Fig. 2.86** Cellular blue naevus. **A** Poorly delineated, spindled and fibrotic intradermal proliferation expanding deeply into the subcutis, with central myxoid/cystic changes surrounding cellular nests. **B** High-magnification view of the central area with myxoid/cystic changes surrounding cellular nests of bland, spindled, unpigmented melanocytes.

not indicate malignancy. Hypomelanotic and amelanotic blue naevi are uncommon variants of CBN, characterized by absent or minimal melanin pigment within the melanocytes and a paucity of melanophages. Plaque-type blue naevus is a clinicopathological variant of blue naevus characterized by large size, often with deep extension into the subcutis and along fascial planes; it shows a combination of the features seen in DBN and CBN {976}. Rarely, blue naevi may involve lymph nodes; such cases are usually located in the capsule and intranodal fibrous trabeculae, and they have cytological characteristics identical to those of their cutaneous counterparts. Unlike in many other naevi, the melanocytes in all blue naevus variants are usually positive for HMB45 antigen, SOX10, and melan-A, but may be negative for S100 protein.

Some blue naevi have large numbers of epithelioid melanocytes (epithelioid and fusiform blue naevi), and such lesions must be distinguished from pigmented epithelioid melanocytoma {2880}.

### Differential diagnosis

Typical examples of DBN and CBN are usually straightforward to diagnose. Hypopigmented DBNs may raise other bland spindle cell proliferations in the differential diagnosis, such as dermatofibroma or fibroblastic scar tissue. Immunohistochemistry for melanocytic markers will clarify the diagnosis in morphologically equivocal lesions. Sclerosing DBN may resemble desmoplastic melanoma or other dermal spindle cell proliferations, but it can be distinguished by its negligible cytological atypia and its characteristic dendritic cell positivity for HMB45 antigen, melan-A, SOX10, and often S100 protein; in contrast, desmoplastic melanoma is typically only positive for S100 protein and (frequently) SOX10. Amelanotic blue naevus may be misdiagnosed as dermatofibroma, scar, dermatofibrosarcoma protuberans, dermal Spitz naevus, desmoplastic naevus, or amelanotic melanoma, but each of these entities can be readily distinguished from blue naevus with a combination of clinical correlation, careful examination of the morphological features, and immunohistochemistry. CBNs show a range of histological features, which may lead to their misdiagnosis as melanoma {153}. Like melanoma, CBN is usually composed of large epithelioid and/or spindle cells, lacks maturation with depth, may extend deeply, may be pigmented, and may contain an occasional mitotic figure. Features favouring melanoma include tumoural necrosis, large pleomorphic epithelioid cells, cell crowding (usually associated with increased cell N:C ratios), cytological atypia and pleomorphism, frequent mitoses (> 2 mitoses/mm$^2$), and a infiltrative growth pattern (i.e. where the margins of the tumour are irregular, as opposed to the generally rounded or pushing margins of CBN). However, these criteria are not infallible, and there have been reported melanoma cases with some atypical features, such as one (or occasionally more) of the following: asymmetry, hypercellular foci, focal cytological atypia, and occasional mitoses (< 2 mitoses/mm$^2$) {1671}. In the absence of overtly malignant features, confident prediction of likely biological behaviour may not always be possible; such tumours may be called atypical CBNs of uncertain malignant potential (or atypical cellular blue melanocytomas). Ancillary investigations such as immunostaining for BAP1 (which is often lost in melanoma arising in blue naevus), as well as FISH and comparative genomic hybridization analysis to detect copy-number changes of chromosomes 3, 6, and 8, may be informative. Clear cell sarcoma can involve the skin and may be difficult to distinguish from CBN (including atypical CBN); both tumours are positive for S100 protein, HMB45 antigen, and melan-A. In most cases, clear cell sarcomas are larger than CBNs, have more nuclear atypia, and are composed of cells with pale or clear cytoplasm (often with scattered wreath-like giant cells); clear cell sarcoma may also show necrosis.

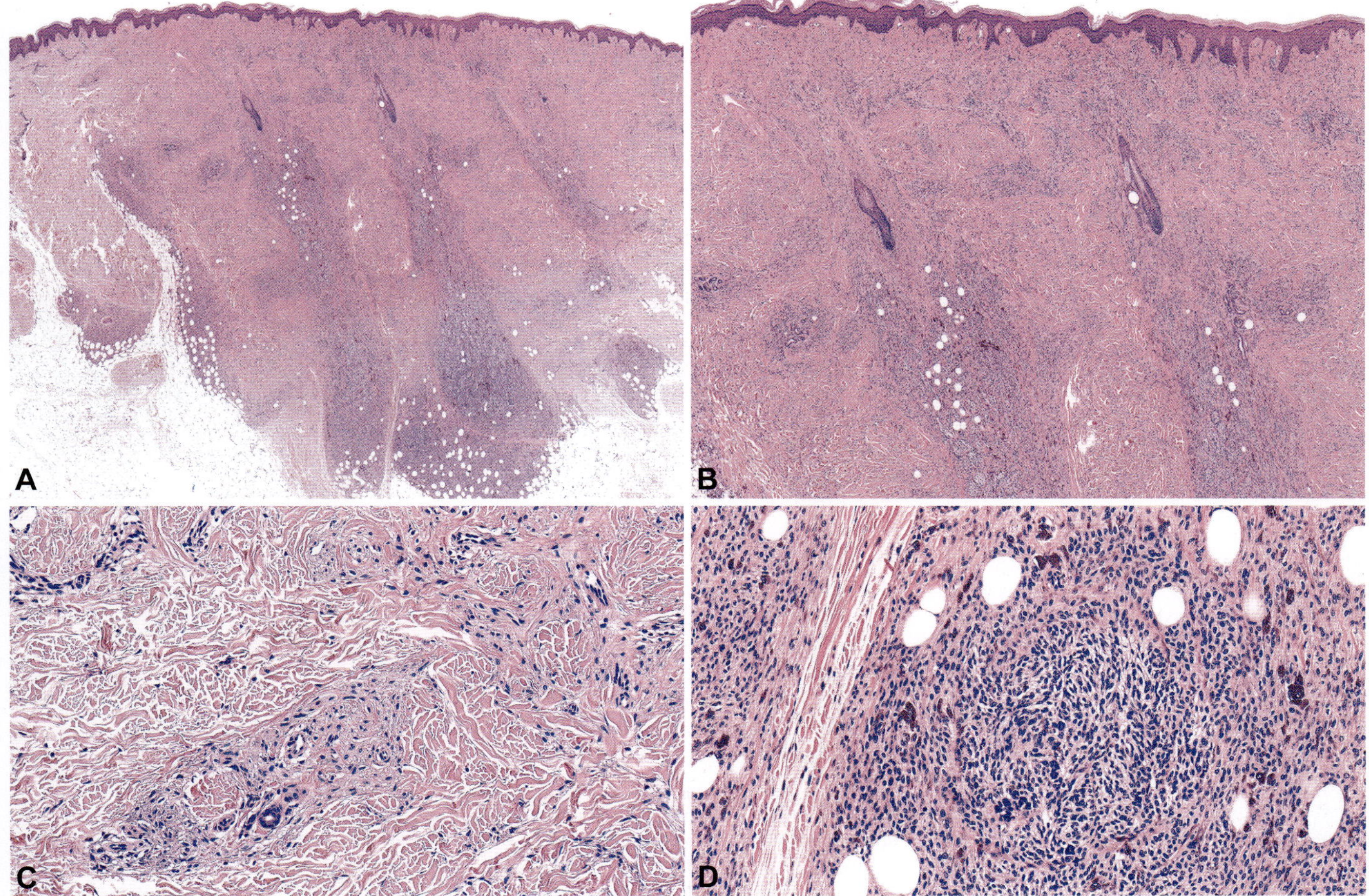

**Fig. 2.87** Cellular blue naevus. **A,B** Biphasic architecture, with a poorly delineated upper intradermal area of dendritic blue naevus and deep expansion extending into the subcutis with cellular nests of non-pigmented melanocytes. **C** Cellular blue naevus component, with nests of bland, spindled, unpigmented melanocytes associated with dispersed melanophages. **D** Plaque-type/cellular blue naevus component, with sheets and fascicles of pigmented spindled melanocytes with cellular nests surrounded by a fibro-oedematous stroma extending into the subcutis.

The finding of an *EWSR1* rearrangement or t(12;22) translocation favours clear cell sarcoma, whereas *GNAQ*, *GNA11*, or *CYSLTR2* mutation favours CBN. Other considerations include tumoural melanosis, haemosiderin deposition, tattoos, and blue naevus–like metastasis.

## Histogenesis

Blue naevi and intradermal melanocytic proliferations (melanocytic neoplasms of the uvea and leptomeninges) likely arise from a distinct type of melanocytes that originate from the neural crest through the ventromedial developmental pathway {168}.

## Genetic profile

Blue naevi frequently contain activating mutations in *GNAQ*, *GNA11*, or *PLCB4* (or less frequently, in *CYSLTR2*) in a mutually exclusive pattern (similar to that seen in uveal melanomas). They lack *BRAF*, *NRAS*, and *NF1* mutations {2699,2700}.

## Prognosis and predictive factors

Blue naevi are benign tumours that do not usually recur after complete excision. Recurrences occasionally occur after incomplete excision and usually resemble the original tumour. Incompletely excised blue naevi with atypical features warrant complete excision.

# Mongolian spot

Yun S.J.
Landman G.
Uhara H.

## Definition

Mongolian spot is dermal melanocytosis occurring on the lower back and buttocks.

## Epidemiology

Mongolian spots are most common in Asians and Africans {668,969,970,1942}. Most studies have found no sex predilection {1356,2177}.

## Localization

The most common site is the sacral area (affected in 78.9% of cases), followed by both sacral and extrasacral sites (18.3% of cases) and extrasacral sites alone (2.7% of cases) {969}.

## Clinical features

Mongolian spots present as bluish patches over the gluteal area, with somewhat variable colours according to the individual's race {969}. The blue colour is due to the Tyndall effect, a phenomenon in which light is scattered by dermal pigmentation and reflected to the skin surface {970}. Mongolian spot can be associated with cleft lip, supernumerary digits, lysosomal storage disease, inborn errors of metabolism, and Sjögren–Larsson syndrome {970,1004,1166,1177}. Phacomatosis pigmentovascularis is the association of extensive, aberrant, persistent Mongolian spots with vascular anomalies, such as naevus flammeus {758,988}.

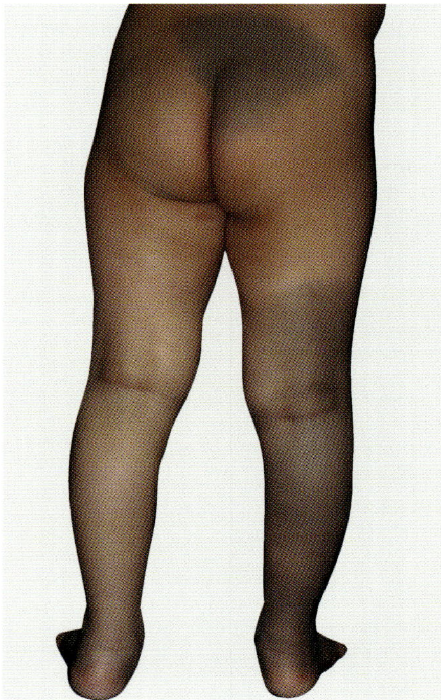

**Fig. 2.88** Mongolian spot. Bluish patches on the sacral area and right leg.

## Histopathology

Mongolian spots are composed of single pigmented dendritic melanocytes haphazardly dispersed in the dermis, tending to be parallel to the epidermis {644}.

## Differential diagnosis

The differential diagnosis includes blue naevi in which the cells occur in bundles of dendritic cells; in Mongolian spot, cells are scattered without disturbing the normal architecture {543}.

## Histogenesis

Mongolian spots arise because of an arrest of melanocyte migration in neural crest development to neurocutaneous units {543}.

## Genetic susceptibility

*GNA11* or *GNAQ* mutations are identified in patients with phacomatosis pigmentovascularis or extensive dermal melanocytosis {2606}.

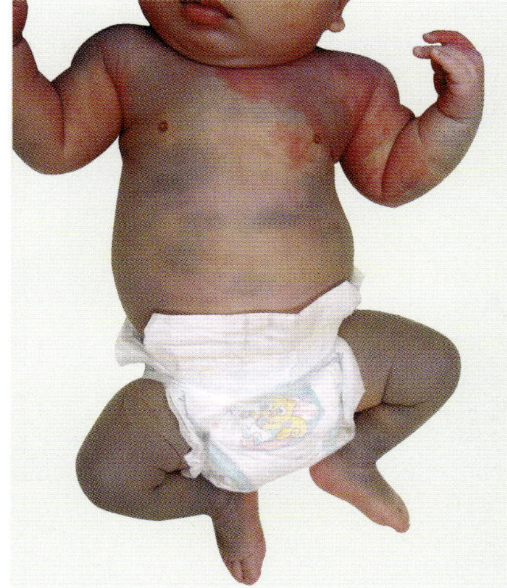

**Fig. 2.90** Phacomatosis pigmentovascularis. Aberrant Mongolian spots coexist with naevus flammeus on the trunk and extremities.

## Prognosis and predictive factors

Mongolian spots typically disappear by the age of 5–6 years. Extrasacral sites, multiple patches, size > 10 cm, and dark colour are markers of persistent Mongolian spots {969}.

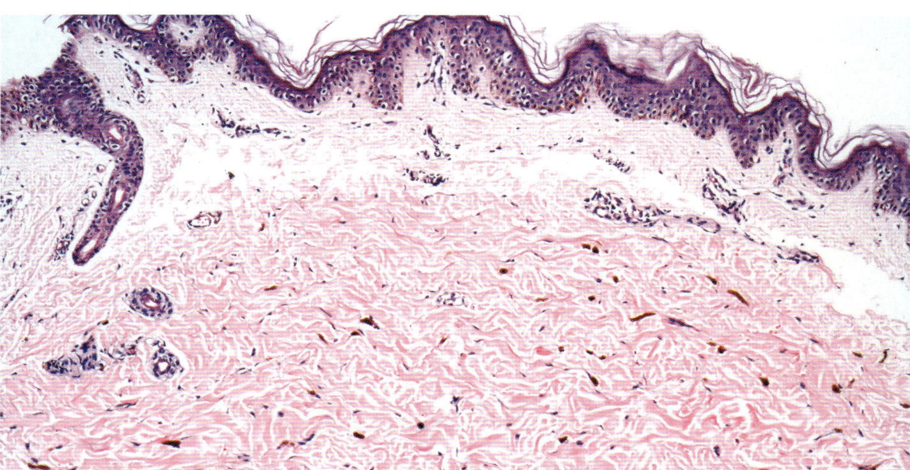

**Fig. 2.89** Mongolian spot. Pigmented dendritic melanocytes are scattered in the dermis.

# Naevus of Ito and naevus of Ota

Yun S.J.
Landman G.
Uhara H.

## Definition

Naevus of Ito, first described by Minor Ito in 1954, and naevus of Ota, described by Masao Ota in 1939, are dermal melanocytoses on the shoulders and arms (naevus of Ito) and on the face (naevus of Ota).

## Synonyms

Naevus of Ota: oculodermal melanocytosis; naevus fuscoceruleus ophthalmomaxillaris

## Epidemiology

Naevus of Ito is much less common than naevus of Ota {2842}. Both occur most commonly in Asians {1078}. Naevus of Ota is more frequent in females {1429,2070}.

## Localization

Naevus of Ito occurs on the side of the neck, supraclavicular and scapular areas, and shoulder region {820}. Naevus of Ota occurs on the face, in the distribution of the first two branches of the trigeminal nerve; it is unilateral in 90% of cases and bilateral in 10% {820,2669}. Naevus of Ito and naevus of Ota are present at birth in about 50% of cases. Most acquired lesions appear before adolescence; adult onset is rare {435,1692,2174}.

## Clinical features

The naevi appear as bluish patches at the locations specified above. Ocular manifestations occur in two thirds of naevus of Ota cases {2070,2114}. Ipsilateral deafness and meningeal and orbital melanocytoma may be associated with naevus of Ota {1972,2292,2421,2645,2716}. Phacomatosis pigmentovascularis can be associated {1872}. Malignant transformation is rare, with only 14 reported cases: 10 from naevus of Ota and 4 from naevus of Ito. More than 40 cases of primary melanoma in the orbital tissue and CNS have been reported in association with naevus of Ota {2663}.

## Histopathology

Single pigmented dendritic melanocytes are haphazardly dispersed in the upper dermis {644,1798,1842,1843}.

## Differential diagnosis

Acquired bilateral naevus of Ota–like macules, which were first described in 1984, are acquired dermal melanocytosis and differentiated clinically from naevus of Ota {1116,1992}.

## Histogenesis

These naevi arise because of an arrest of melanocyte migration in neural crest development to neurocutaneous units {543}.

## Genetic profile

*GNAQ* mutation has been detected in 6% of naevi of Ota {2699}. Gains in 6p25 and losses in 6q23 demonstrated by FISH; *GNAQ*, *BAP1*, and *TP53* mutations; and *BAP1* deletions have been reported in malignant transformed naevus of Ito and naevus of Ota {871,2663,2748}.

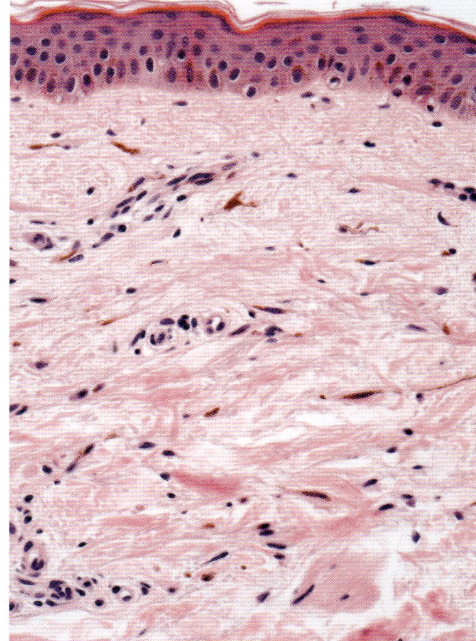

**Fig. 2.93** Naevus of Ota. Single dendritic melanocytes are dispersed in the dermis.

## Prognosis and predictive factors

Spontaneous regression does not occur; the naevi's colour darkens with puberty.

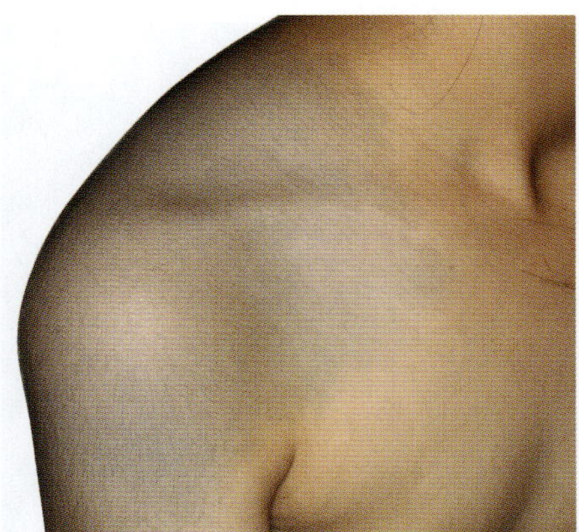

**Fig. 2.91** Naevus of Ito. A bluish patch on the right supraclavicular area and shoulder.

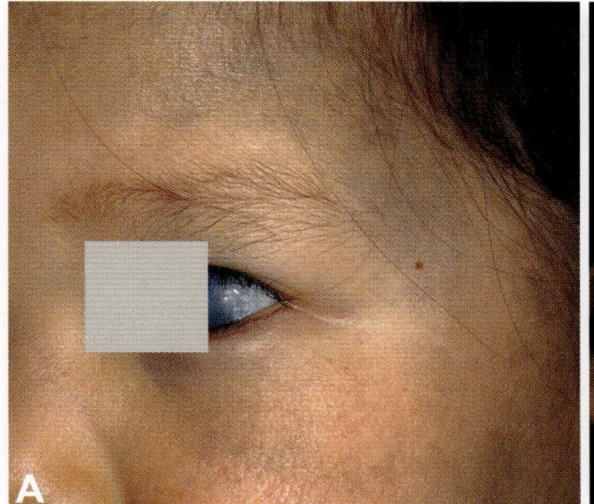



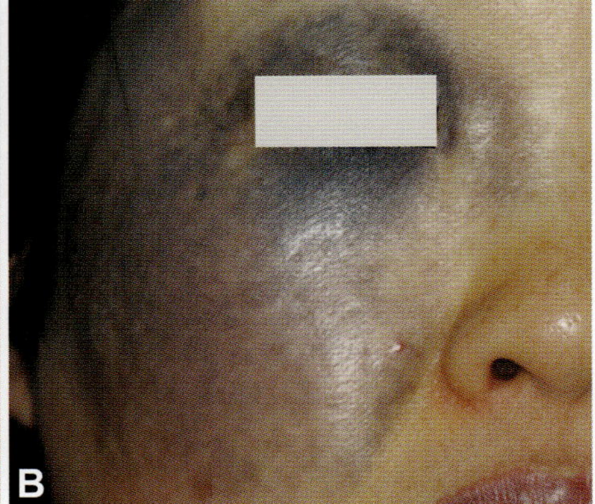



**Fig. 2.92** Naevus of Ota. **A** Bluish patch on the face with scleral involvement. **B** Dark bluish-to-brown patch on the face of an adult.

# Melanocytic tumours arising in congenital naevi

## Melanoma arising in giant congenital naevus

Massi G.
Bastian B.C.
LeBoit P.E.
Prieto V.G.
Xu X.

### Definition

Melanoma arising in giant congenital naevus is a potentially deadly form of melanoma that can develop in a giant (or garment/bathing suit) congenital naevus. In prepubescent patients, the epicentre of the lesion is intradermal or subcutaneous. In adults, most melanomas arising in congenital naevus arise at the junction, as do most melanomas arising in acquired naevi.

### ICD-O code

8761/3

### Synonym

Melanoma in large or garment-like congenital naevus

### Epidemiology

The lifetime risk of melanoma arising in giant congenital naevus is estimated at 2–5%. Most melanomas appear during the first 5 years of life {1982,2754,2888}. Garment/bathing suit naevi have a 10–15% chance of developing melanoma at some point in the patient's lifetime. The coincidental presence of meningeal involvement is an additional risk factor; melanoma develops in the CNS in one third of cases {1893}. The risk of melanoma may be overstated in the literature, because at the time of some earlier diagnoses, proliferating nodules (which can simulate melanoma histopathologically) may have been interpreted as melanomas.

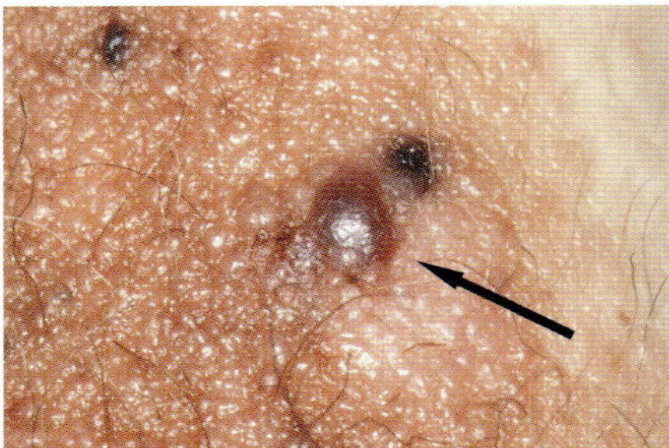

**Fig. 2.94** Melanoma arising in giant congenital naevus presenting as reddish brown nodule (arrow).

### Etiology

*NRAS* p.Q61 mutation is reported frequently, whereas *BRAF* mutation or fusion is infrequent {613,1378,1595,2286}.

### Localization

The scalp and back are commonly involved sites.

### Clinical features

Melanomas arising in this setting typically appear as rapidly growing nodules or plaques, which frequently ulcerate. The colour and texture are patently different from those of the congenital naevus in the background. Synchronous lymph node metastatic disease is a frequent finding at presentation.

### Histopathology

The intradermal melanoma in children often has obvious malignant features. There are three main histological patterns: epithelioid cells with hyperchromatic nuclei and visible nucleoli; small cells resembling Ewing sarcoma; and large epithelioid cells with central, prominent nucleoli (spitzoid). Mitotic figures are frequent. There may be necrosis. There is occasional heterologous differentiation (smooth or striated muscle, neural tissue, and adipocytes).

### Differential diagnosis

The most important differential diagnosis is proliferative nodules in congenital melanocytic naevus (which are much more prevalent than are bona fide melanomas). Features indicating melanoma are marked pleomorphism and sharp circumscription with an expansive pattern. Mitotic figures can occur in proliferative nodules, but atypical forms are a clue to malignancy. In very young children, the distinction can be difficult. Immunohistochemistry and FISH are not contributory

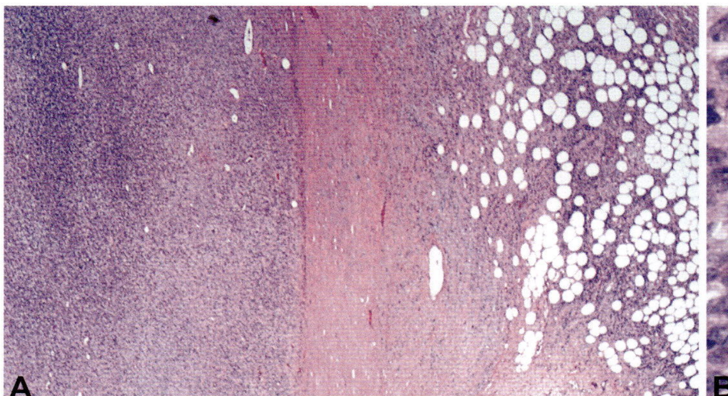


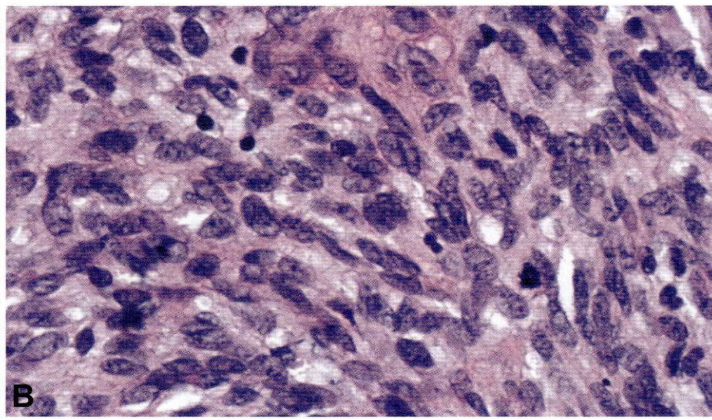


**Fig. 2.95** Melanoma arising in giant congenital naevus. **A** There is a sharp border between the naevus in the background and the melanoma. **B** An undifferentiated spindle cell neoplasm is one possible presentation of melanoma arising in giant congenital naevus; mitoses are abundant. Note the chaotic arrangement of the nuclei.

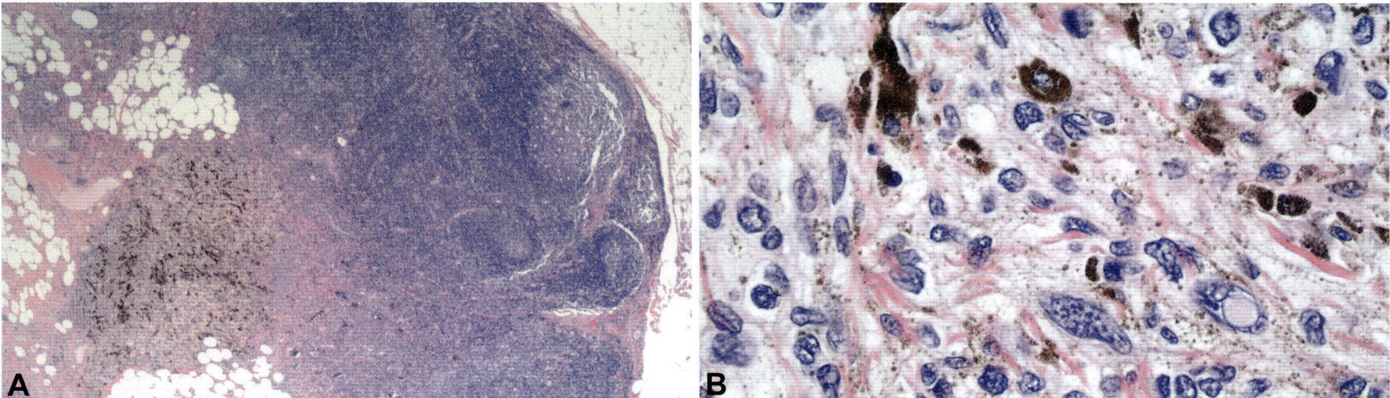


**Fig. 2.96** Melanoma arising in giant congenital naevus. **A** Lymph node metastasis is a very frequent synchronous finding with the cutaneous melanoma. **B** At high magnification, a striking nuclear and cellular pleomorphism is evident; note the contrast between the cellular phenotype and the cutaneous lesion.

to the diagnosis {2734}. The levels of H3K27me3 (a chromatin mark important in gene regulation) and 5-hydroxymethylcytosine are relatively low in melanomas arising in congenital naevi, but not in proliferative nodules {345,2016}. Comparative genomic hybridization can help to distinguish melanomas from benign proliferative nodules. Mass spectrometry has also been reported to be helpful in this distinction {1507}.

## Genetic profile

Comparative genomic hybridization typically shows copy-number changes such as gains and losses of arms or segments of chromosomes, whereas proliferating nodules typically harbour copy-number changes involving entire chromosomes {172}. Analysis of genome-wide copy-number changes is recommended to improve diagnostic accuracy and to guide management in challenging cases {1377}. An exceptional case with metastatic spread from a lesion with only whole chromosome copy changes was recently reported {1621}.

## Prognosis and predictive factors

The prognosis of melanoma in the dermal portion of a congenital naevus is poor. This may reflect the fact that such lesions are not detected early, and they typically have a high tumour thickness/volume by the time they are noticed.

# Congenital melanocytic naevus

Massi G.
Bastian B.C.
LeBoit P.E.
Prieto V.G.
Xu X.

## Definition

Congenital melanocytic naevus is a benign melanocytic neoplasia present at birth or appearing in the first year of life (late or tardive congenital naevus). Some forms of blue naevi can also be congenital; those are discussed in the section *Blue naevus and cellular blue naevus* (p. 126).

## ICD-O code

8761/0

## Synonym

Congenital naevocytic naevus

## Epidemiology

About 1% of newborns have a small congenital melanocytic naevus. Large congenital melanocytic naevus has a frequency of 5–15 cases per 100 000 births; giant (garment) congenital naevus has a frequency of 5 cases per 100 000 births.

## Localization

Congenital melanocytic naevus can occur anywhere on the body.

## Clinical features

In adults, congenital melanocytic naevi are categorized as small (< 1.5 cm), intermediate (1.5–20 cm and typically amenable to surgical resection), or giant (> 20 cm or unresectable). Small congenital melanocytic naevi typically present as symmetrical, oval or round, brown to black, well-circumscribed macules or plaques that are homogeneous in texture and often have prominent terminal hairs. Large naevi localized on the scalp and back, in particular those with satellite naevi, can involve the CNS (a condition called neurocutaneous melanosis) {52}.

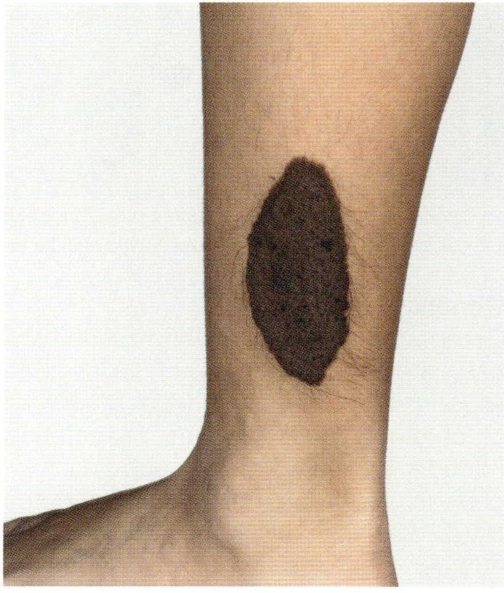

**Fig. 2.97** Congenital melanocytic naevus. A broad plaque lesion, which in this instance is generally uniformly pigmented brown; this lesion is intermediate in terms of size.

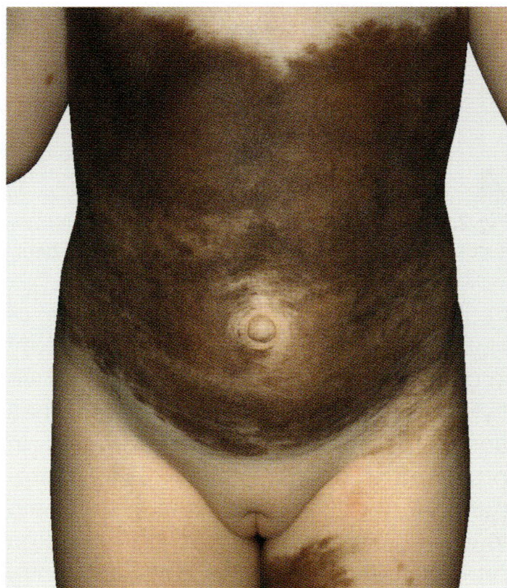

**Fig. 2.98** Giant congenital naevus. This pigmented lesion, which was present at birth, covers a large area of skin; such lesions are sometimes referred to as garment naevi; note the smaller satellite lesion on the thigh.

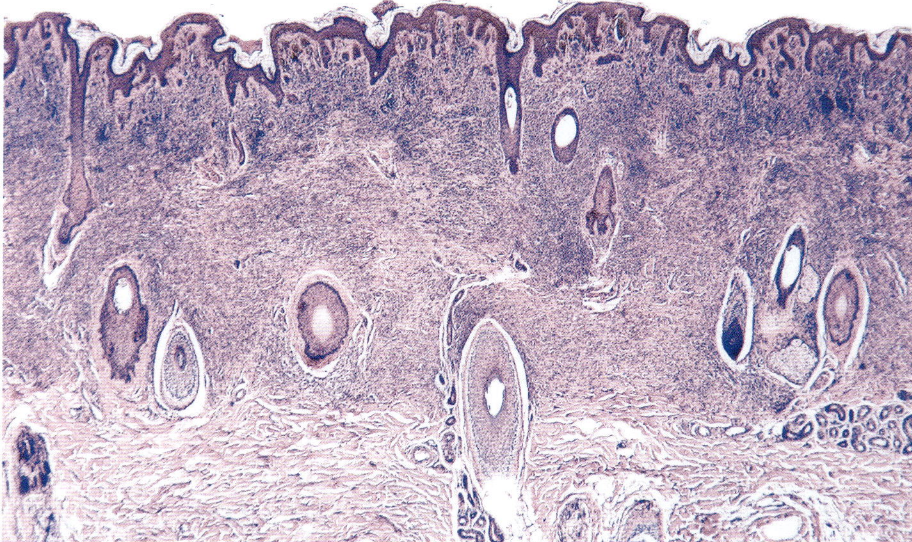

**Fig. 2.99** Congenital melanocytic naevus. Note the depth of the dermal component and the concentration of cells around skin adnexa.

## Histopathology

Congenital melanocytic naevi typically differ from common acquired naevi in that they are larger in diameter and they involve the reticular dermis or subcutis, with splaying of naevus cells between collagen bundles and with naevus cells in close proximity to (or within) dermal appendages and neurovascular bundles. In infants, there may be striking pagetoid migration and confluence of the intraepidermal nests in the centre of the lesions. Cells in the dermis may evolve from large epithelioid type A naevus cells (often arranged in nests in the upper dermis to small lymphocyte-like type B cells to spindled type C cells, which often show signs of Schwannian differentiation, such as wavy fibre bundles, serpentine nuclei, and structures mimicking sensory nerve end organs, and a lesser tendency to nesting.

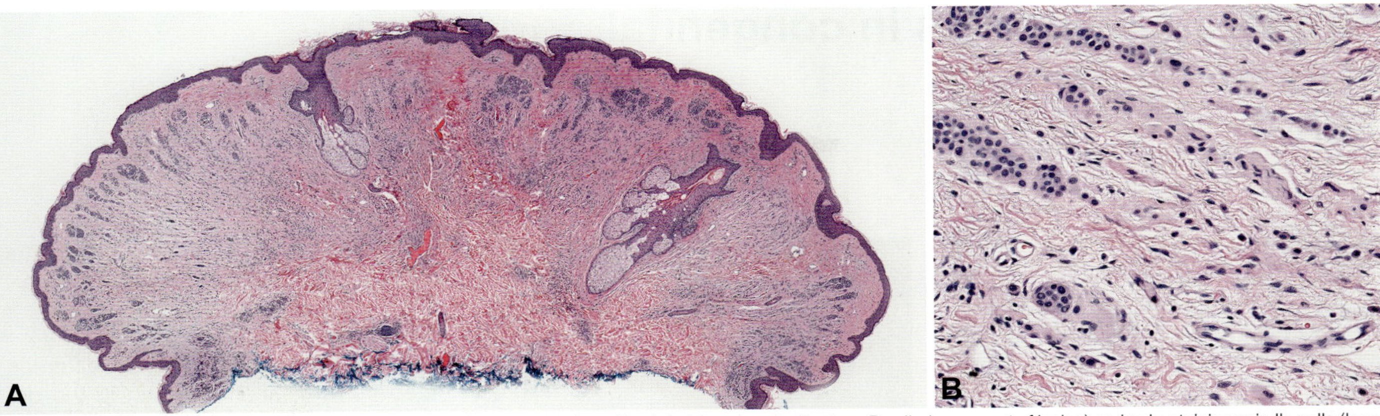

**Fig. 2.100** Neurotized dermal naevus. **A** Dome-shaped lesion composed mostly of dark lymphocyte-like type B cells (upper part of lesion) and pale-staining spindle cells (lower part of lesion). **B** Higher magnification shows greater detail of naevus with lymphocyte-like type B cells and spindled type C cells. The type C cells mimic neural structures, exhibiting Schwannian differentiation.

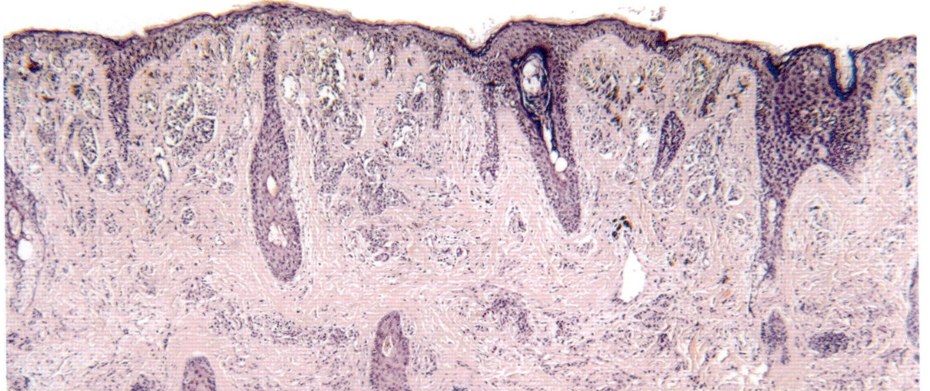
**Fig. 2.101** Congenital melanocytic naevus with junctional atypia. A congenital melanocytic naevus is present in the dermis and at the junction.

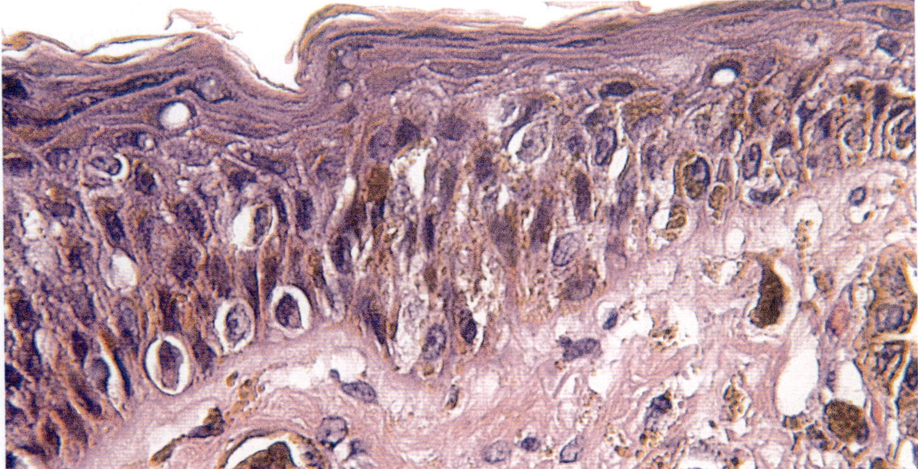
**Fig. 2.102** Congenital melanocytic naevus with junctional atypia. In the uppermost part of the lesion, cells are homogeneous and typical.

## Differential diagnosis

Congenital melanocytic naevi with an atypical junctional proliferation of melanocytes may simulate melanoma in situ, but such areas are typically restricted to the centre of the lesion and may be reactive. Cases with increased cellularity can be difficult to distinguish from naevoid melanoma. Deep (so-called peripheral) mitotic figures in clusters or atypical configuration are the most important distinctive features. Additional clues favouring melanoma are sheet-like growth, nuclear hyperchromatism, and pleomorphism {116,303,2522}.

## Genetic profile

The majority (~90%) of large congenital melanocytic naevi harbour *NRAS* mutations but no *BRAF* mutations {180}.

## Prognosis and predictive factors

Congenital melanocytic naevi are benign lesions.

# Proliferative nodules in congenital melanocytic naevus

Massi G.
Bastian B.C.
LeBoit P.E.
Prieto V.G.
Xu X.

## Definition
Proliferative nodules in congenital melanocytic naevus can be considered new naevi developed inside the dermal component of a congenital melanocytic naevus. They can be present at birth or develop later in life. Eventually, they become smaller and regress.

## ICD-O code 8762/1

## Synonyms
Expansive and cellular nodules; atypical proliferative nodules

## Epidemiology
Proliferative nodules are considered rare events.

## Localization
They have a strong predilection for congenital melanocytic naevi on the trunk.

## Clinical features
The proliferative nodules typically strongly contrast with the congenital melanocytic naevus in the background, and are occasionally ulcerated. There is no convincing evidence that bona fide proliferative nodules evolve into melanoma.

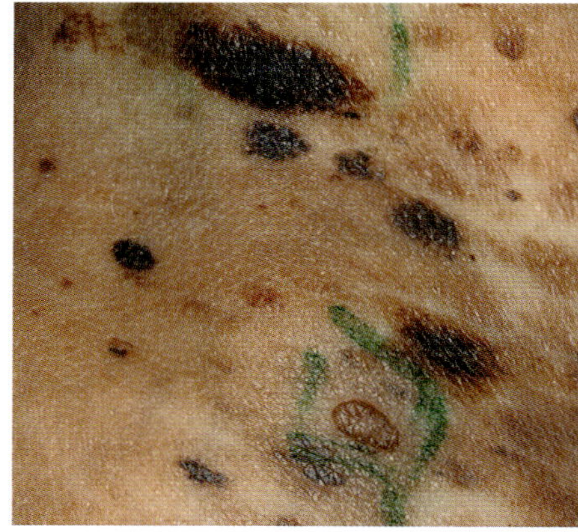

**Fig. 2.103** Proliferative nodule in a giant congenital naevus. In this symmetrical nodule there is a mammillated surface similar to that of a naevus. Other, smaller papules are also present.

## Histopathology
The cells are epithelioid, spindled, or small (so-called melanoblasts). Rarely, nodules have the features of a mesenchymal neoplasm. The cells in some nodules blend with those of the background naevus; in others, there is sharp demarcation. In very young patients (aged < 1 year) there may be striking cytological atypia and high cellularity. A subgroup of lesions, called atypical proliferative nodules, have striking atypia, sharp circumscription, and pushing borders; these typically occur in young children.

## Differential diagnosis
Proliferative nodules must be differentiated from melanoma arising in the dermal portion of a congenital melanocytic naevus. The main criteria that favour melanoma are an expansive pattern, necrosis, and obvious cytological atypia (e.g. pleomorphism, nuclear gigantism and hyperchromasia, numerous mitotic figures, and atypical shape) {1900}.

## Genetic profile
In proliferative nodules, comparative genomic hybridization typically reveals copy-number changes involving whole chromosomes. In contrast, melanomas arising in congenital melanocytic naevus are characterized by multiple gains and losses of large portions of chromosomes. The background naevus is devoid of these chromosomal alterations {172,179,2888}.

## Prognosis and predictive factors
Proliferative nodules are almost invariably reported as benign, even in cases with atypical cytological features.

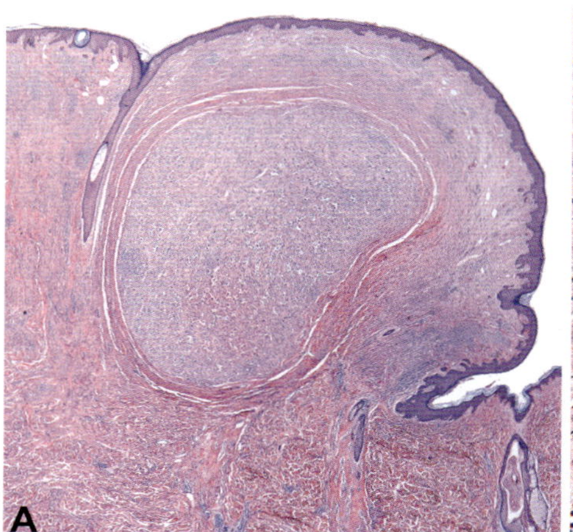


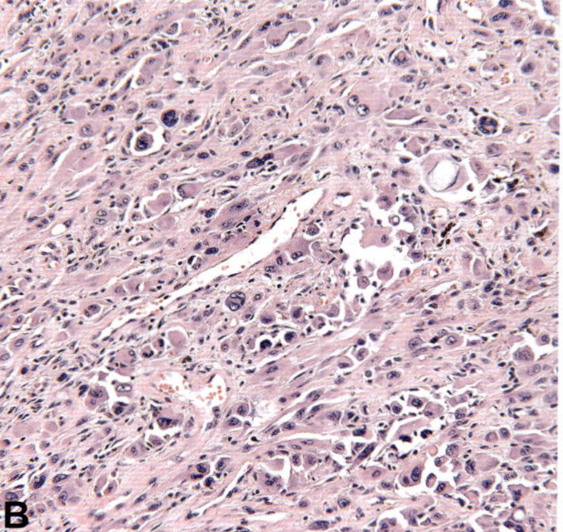


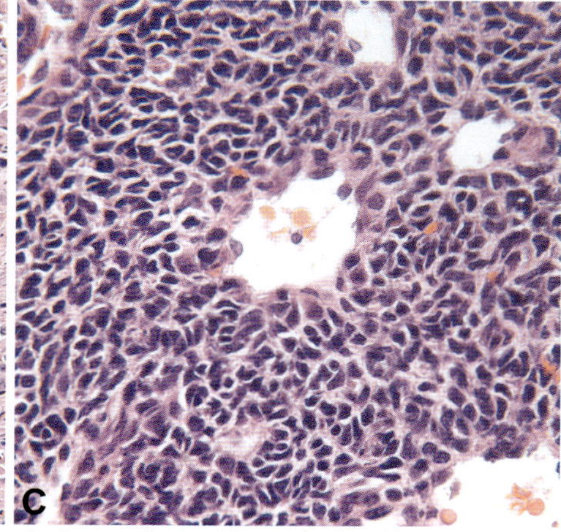


**Fig. 2.104** Proliferative nodule in a congenital naevus. **A** Proliferative nodule with atypical features. The nodule is sharply circumscribed and there is no blend between the cells of the nodule and those of the naevus. **B** Proliferative nodule with atypical features. Cytologically, the nodule has desmoplastic Spitz naevus–like features. **C** Proliferative nodule in a congenital naevus. Melanocytes are small and achromic. The presence of large vessels is reminiscent of a haemangiopericytoma.

# Ocular melanocytic tumours

## Uveal melanoma

Coupland S.
Folberg R.
Kivelä T.
Prieto V.G.

### Definition

Uveal melanoma is a malignant tumour arising from melanocytes in the iris, ciliary body, or choroid. A full description of this tumour is provided in the *WHO classification of tumours of the eye* volume {948A}.

### ICD-O codes

| | |
|---|---|
| Epithelioid cell melanoma | 8771/3 |
| Spindle cell melanoma, type A | 8773/3 |
| Spindle cell melanoma, type B | 8774/3 |

### Synonyms

Iris melanoma; ciliary body melanoma; choroidal melanoma; intraocular melanoma

### Epidemiology

Uveal melanoma is most common in White populations, with an incidence of 2–8 million cases per year, increasing with latitude {2745,2893}. Presentation usually occurs in adulthood, at a median age of about 60 years. There is no sex predilection {571}.

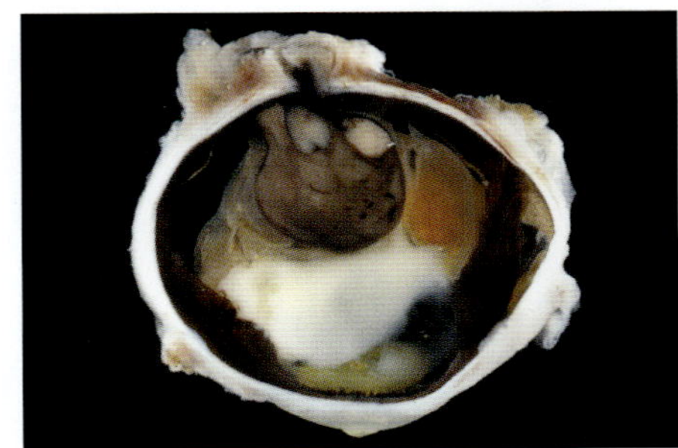

**Fig. 2.105** Uveal melanoma.

### Etiology

Risk factors include uveal naevi {707, 1385,2449}, congenital ocular melanocytosis {2448}, and *BAP1* tumour predisposition syndrome {374,2448,2828}.

### Localization

Approximately 90% of uveal melanomas develop in the choroid; the other 10% arise in the ciliary body or iris {2745,2893}.

### Clinical features

Most patients present with visual symptoms. Uveal melanomas vary in pigmentation and typically occur as dome-shaped or mushroom-shaped tumours. Choroidal melanomas cause retinal pigment epithelium disruption, lipofuscin accumulation, and serous retinal detachment. Necrotic tumours may cause painful uveitis and/or glaucoma. Extrascleral spread can occur along and within vortex veins and along small nerves into the orbit or subconjunctivally. Optic nerve invasion is seen in 5–6% of cases {1565,1566}.

### Histopathology

Uveal melanomas are composed of spindle and/or epithelioid cells with mitotic figures, occasionally with necrotic foci. Most tumours show scattered lymphocytic infiltrates and pigment-laden macrophages. Tumour cells variably express melanocytic markers and may show nuclear BAP1 protein loss, a finding associated with poor prognosis {1268}.

### Differential diagnosis

The differential diagnosis includes naevus, melanocytoma, choroidal metastasis, choroidal haemangioma, adenoma of the retinal pigment epithelium, and congenital hypertrophy of the retinal pigment epithelium.

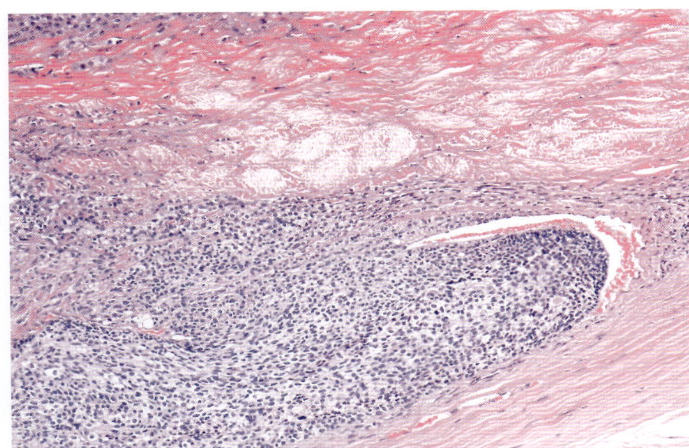

**Fig. 2.106** Choroidal melanoma. Note the infiltration of tumour into an intrascleral emissary channel.

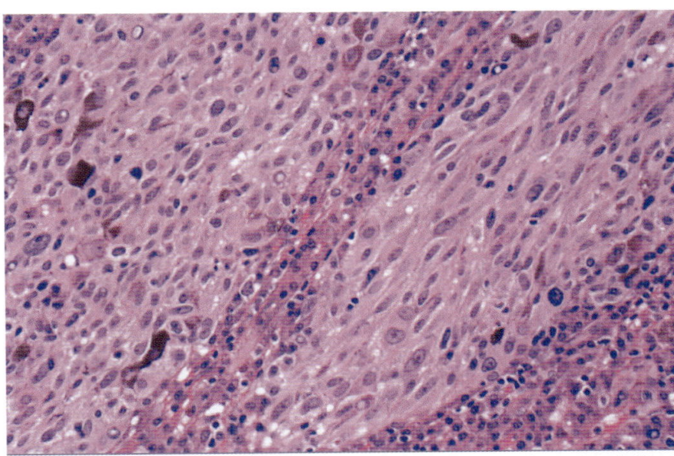

**Fig. 2.107** Choroidal melanoma, spindle cell type. This melanoma features an infiltrate of lymphocytes and scattered melanophages.

### Histogenesis

Most cases develop de novo, but uveal naevi can sometimes transform into melanoma {707,1385,2449}.

### Genetic profile

Uveal melanomas lack the most typical cutaneous melanoma–associated mutations (of *BRAF*, *NRAS*, and *NF1*) and are instead characterized by a different set of oncogenic or loss-of-function mutations, including mutations in *GNA11*, *GNAQ*, *BAP1*, *EIF1AX*, *SF3B1*, *PLCB4*, and *CYSLTR2* {1009,2699,2700,2860}, resembling melanomas arising in blue naevi in these attributes. Chromosome 3 and 8 status also strongly correlates with clinical outcome {570,2198,2375}.

### Genetic susceptibility

Uveal melanoma is associated with *BAP1* tumour predisposition syndrome and dysplastic naevus syndrome.

### Prognosis and predictive factors

More than 50% of patients develop haematogenous metastases, usually involving the liver {570,1453}. Poor prognostic factors include large tumour size, ciliary body involvement, extraocular spread, epithelioid cytomorphology, high mitotic count, large nucleoli, abundant tumour-infiltrating macrophages, specific extracellular matrix patterns (vasculogenic mimicry), microvessel density, loss of nuclear BAP1 expression, chromosome 3 loss, chromosome 8q gain, lack of chromosome 6p gain, the class 2 gene expression profile, and *BAP1* mutation {570, 802, 1268, 1644, 1834, 1950, 2198, 2860}.

# Conjunctival melanoma

Coupland S.
Folberg R.
Prieto V.G.
Zembowicz A.

## Definition
Conjunctival melanoma is an invasive malignant melanocytic neoplasm. Histologically malignant conjunctival melanocytic proliferations confined to the epithelium are often diagnosed as conjunctival primary acquired melanosis with atypia rather than melanoma in situ.

## ICD-O code
Melanoma NOS 8730/3

## Synonym
Invasive conjunctival melanoma

## Epidemiology
Conjunctival melanoma accounts for 5% of all ocular melanoma cases, with an estimated incidence of 0.7 cases per 1 million person-years {2646}. It is most common in older White individuals (with peak incidence in the seventh decade of life). There is no sex predilection {568,1137,2668}.

## Etiology
The increased occurrence in sun-exposed areas and genetic profile of conjunctival melanoma suggest a role of ultraviolet (UV) radiation and cumulative sun damage (CSD) {568,1137,2668}.

## Localization
Most conjunctival melanomas develop in the bulbar conjunctiva {2410}.

## Clinical features
Conjunctival melanoma can arise de novo, in association with a precursor naevus or (most commonly – in 50% of cases) in association with primary acquired melanosis with atypia. It presents as a pigmented papule or nodule with an irregular shape and size. Pigmentation can vary and change over time. The presence of feeder vessels is very characteristic. Some tumours can be amelanotic.

## Histopathology
The histological features of conjunctival melanoma are identical to those of invasive melanoma in the skin or mucosa {2929}. All histological variants of melanoma are represented. An intraepithelial component can be nested, lentiginous, or (rarely) absent. It can extend well beyond the invasive component and can involve the skin and/or minor lacrimal glands. Induction of conjunctival cysts typical for naevi is exceptionally rare. The subepithelial component shows stromal invasion by nests or sheets of atypical melanocytes. Melanoma cells can show the entire spectrum of cytomorphology encountered in melanoma elsewhere, ranging from small naevoid cells to highly atypical pleomorphic melanocytes with spindle or epithelioid cytomorphology. Nuclei can be hyperchromatic with inconspicuous nucleoli or vesicular with prominent nucleoli. Mitotic activity can usually be seen in larger tumours. A residual naevus may be present. Conjunctival melanoma expresses melanocytic markers such as S100 protein, SOX10, melan-A (MART1), MITF, and HMB45 antigen.

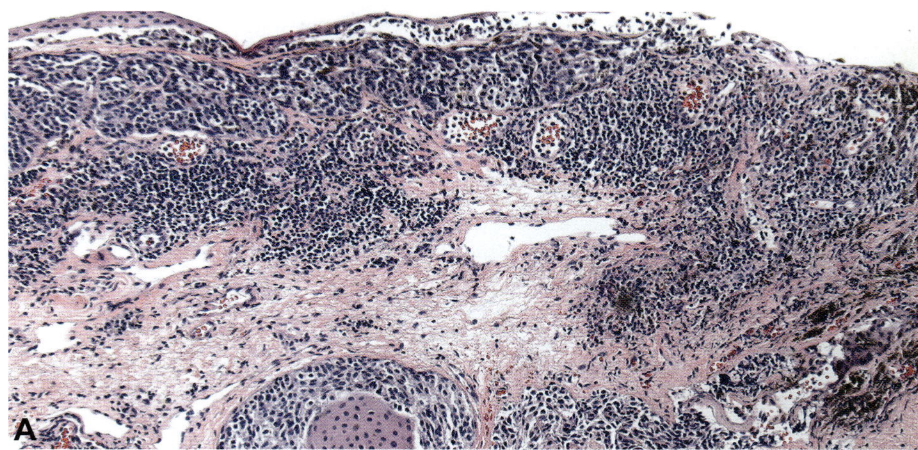


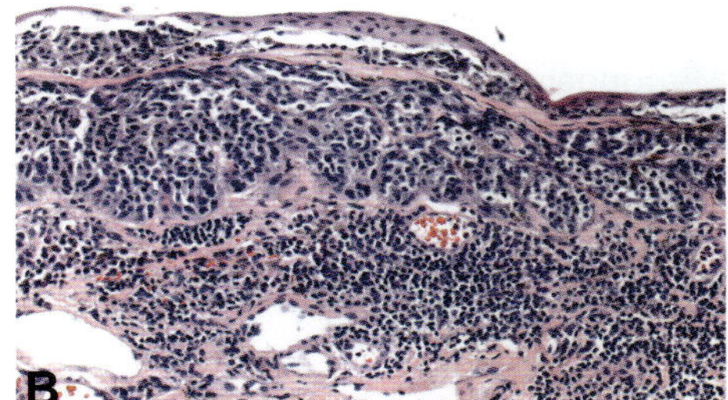


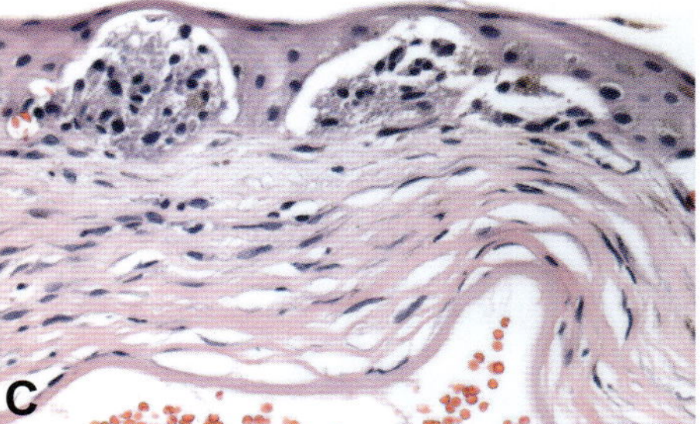


**Fig. 2.108** Conjunctival melanoma. **A** Extensive junctional involvement of minor lacrimal glands and stromal invasion by melanoma cells. **B** Superficial stromal invasion by nest of atypical melanocytes. **C** Extension of the junctional component into corneal epithelium.

## Differential diagnosis
Histological overdiagnosis of conjunctival naevus as melanoma can be avoided by keeping in mind that conjunctival naevi can show worrying architectural patterns such as lateral extension beyond the subepithelial component, large size and irregular shape of junctional nests, pagetoid growth, and confluence at the base {2929}. Rapidly growing conjunctival naevi in children and adolescents can induce brisk lymphocytic activity and show mitotic activity {468,2604,2910}. The most diagnostic features of conjunctival melanoma are cellular and nuclear pleomorphism of spindled or epithelioid cells, frequent mitoses, and destructive infiltration of anatomical structures such

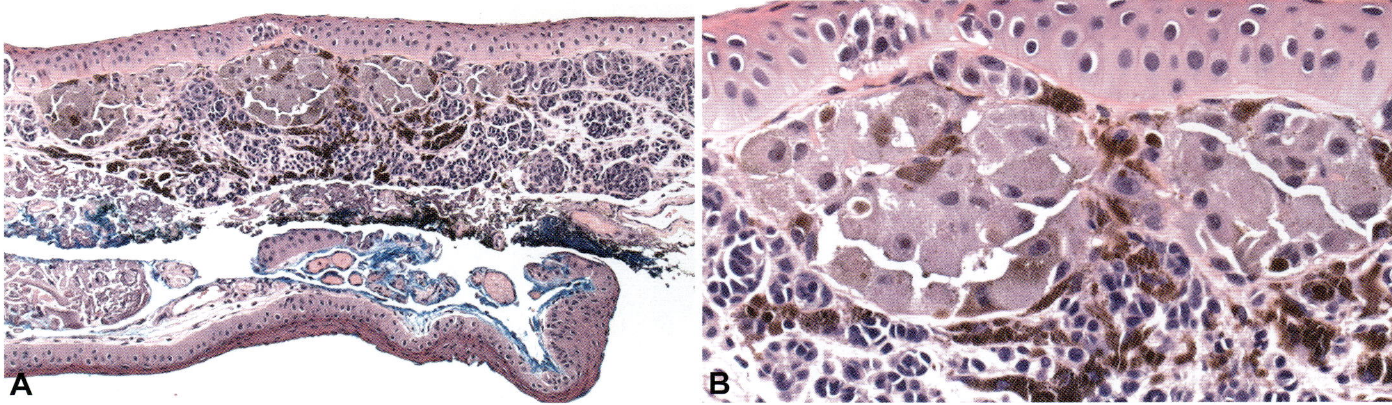


**Fig. 2.109** Conjunctival melanoma. **A** Relatively well-circumscribed tumour with naevoid architecture and an area of severe epithelioid cell atypia. **B** Invasive nests of naevoid melanoma showing severely atypical epithelioid melanocytes with marked pleomorphism and abundant cytoplasm with dusty pigmentation.

as the cornea, ocular adnexa, and skeletal muscle {1209}.

## Histogenesis

Conjunctival melanoma can occur de novo. In 50–70% of cases, conjunctival melanoma supervenes in primary acquired melanosis with atypia {804} or a naevus.

## Genetic profile

Conjunctival melanoma is genetically diverse. About 40% of conjunctival melanomas show BRAF p.V600 mutations typical of melanomas in skin with a low degree of CSD (low-CSD melanomas). However, other melanomas harbour mutations in *NRAS* and *KIT*, suggesting that some conjunctival melanomas are genetically related to high-CSD and mucosal melanomas. Like in cutaneous melanoma, *TERT* mutations are frequent {185,937,939,1483,1493}.

## Prognosis and predictive factors

The 10-year survival rate with conjunctival melanoma is 70–75% {708,1986,2410}. Conjunctival melanoma can metastasize to regional lymph nodes and distant sites {2410}. Adverse prognostic indicators include involvement of the palpebral conjunctiva, local tumour recurrence, multifocal tumours, extensive intraepithelial disease, increased tumour thickness, epithelioid morphology, high mitotic count, lymphatic invasion, and sentinel lymph node positivity {708,1986,2410}.

# Conjunctival melanocytic intraepithelial neoplasia/ primary acquired melanosis

Cree I.A.
Zembowicz A.

## Definition

Conjunctival primary acquired melanosis (PAM) with atypia is a macular pigmented conjunctival melanocytic proliferation showing cytological atypia and/or a substantial increase in cellularity. Clinically similar lesions devoid of melanocytic atypia are referred to as conjunctival PAM without atypia {804}.

## ICD-O code

Conjunctival primary acquired melanosis with atypia/melanoma in situ 8720/2

## Synonyms

Conjunctival melanocytic intraepithelial neoplasia (C-MIN score of 2–4); conjunctival melanoma in situ

## Epidemiology

PAM with atypia accounts for 11% of conjunctival melanocytic proliferations. It is most common among older White individuals, but can occur at any age and in all races {2411}. There is no sex predilection.

## Etiology

PAM with atypia has a higher incidence in the bulbar conjunctiva, which is exposed to ultraviolet (UV) radiation {2898}.

## Localization

Most lesions develop in the bulbar conjunctiva close to the limbus {804,2411}.

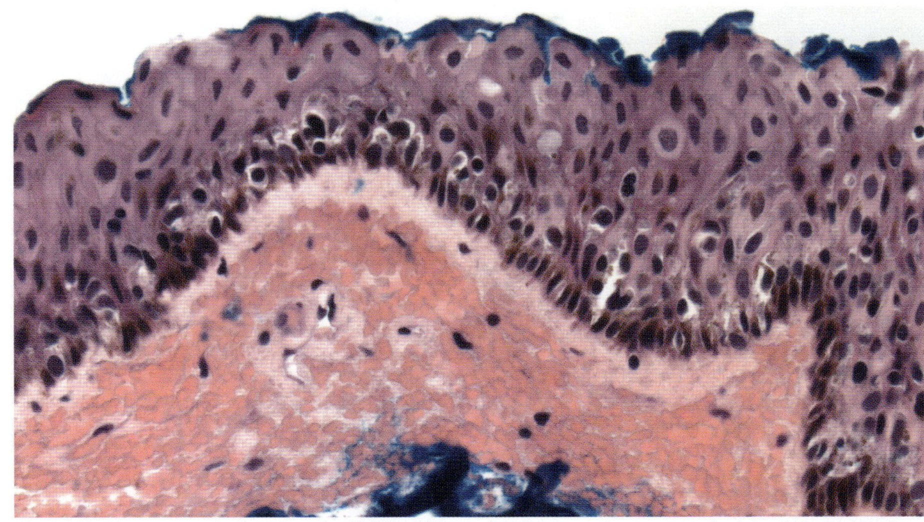

**Fig. 2.110** Primary acquired melanosis (PAM) with atypia. An example composed of lentiginous junctional proliferation limited to the base of the epithelium of small to medium-sized melanocytes with hyperchromatic nuclei and scant cytoplasm. This is a lesion from the low end of the spectrum of atypia encountered in PAM with atypia.

## Clinical features

"Conjunctival melanosis" is a clinical term used for diffuse macular pigmented conjunctival lesions that are not melanocytic naevi. When melanosis is not congenital or secondary to a known cause (i.e. Addison disease or postinflammatory hyperpigmentation), it is called PAM. Clinically, it is impossible to reliably distinguish between PAM caused by increased activation of normal melanocytes (PAM without atypia) and PAM caused by proliferation of premalignant or malignant melanocytes (PAM with atypia). Compared with junctional conjunctival naevus, which is usually well circumscribed, PAM is larger, and it has an irregular shape and coloration. It is often multifocal, involving multiple clock hours of the bulbar conjunctiva {2411}. Bilateral involvement can occur. Pigmentation can change over time and even disappear {2411}.

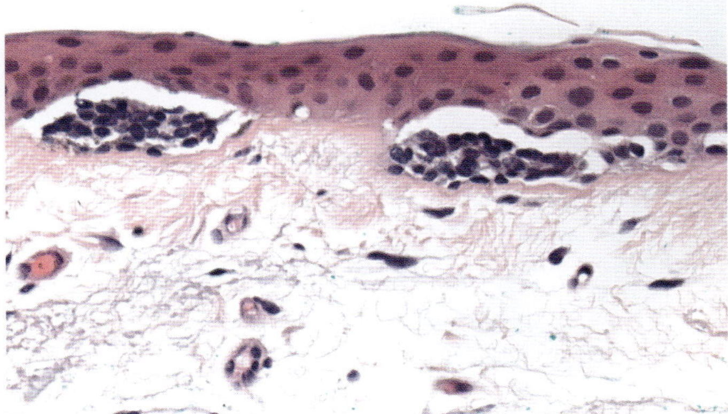

**Fig. 2.111** Primary acquired melanosis (PAM) with atypia. An area with nested proliferation of small to medium-sized melanocytes with hyperchromatic nuclei and scant cytoplasm.

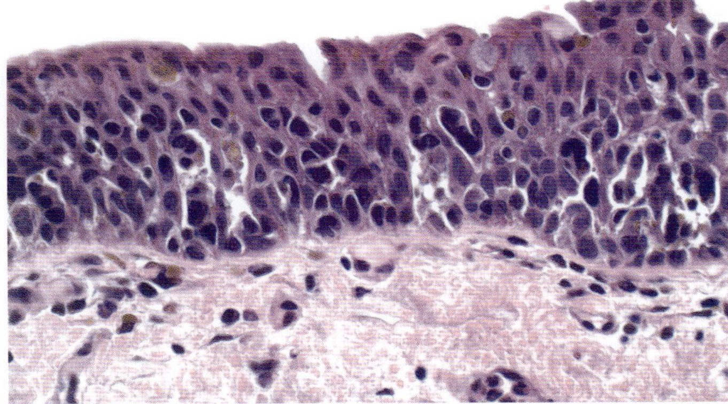

**Fig. 2.112** Primary acquired melanosis with atypia. Lentiginous junctional proliferation of medium-sized to large melanocytes. Nuclei are hyperchromatic but some cells have epithelioid morphology with abundant cytoplasm. Multinucleated cells are also present.

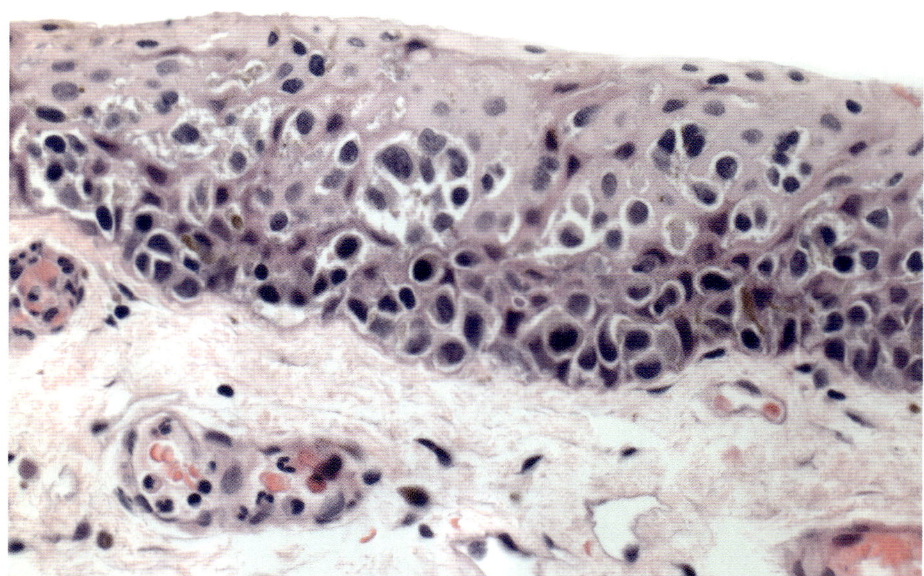

**Fig. 2.113** Conjunctival primary acquired melanosis with atypia. A lentiginous junctional proliferation of medium-sized to large epithelioid melanocytes with abundant cytoplasm, prominent nesting, and a pagetoid growth pattern. Such a lesion could be considered to constitute melanoma in situ.

### Histopathology

The key microscopic feature in PAM with atypia is the presence of intraepithelial melanocytes with cytological atypia and/or increased cellularity {804,1349,2929}. The spectrum of cytological features ranges from small melanocytes with nuclear hyperchromasia and scant cytoplasm to severely atypical large pleomorphic epithelioid cells with ample cytoplasm and prominent eosinophilic nucleoli. The criteria for grading cytological atypia in PAM as mild, moderate, or severe are similar to those used in the skin and other mucosal sites {804,1651}. Architecturally, PAM with atypia can show various patterns, including basilar single-cell hyperplasia, basilar nesting, intraepithelial nests, pagetoid proliferation of single cells, and a confluent growth pattern at the epithelial–stromal junction {804}.

Alternative terminology for PAM, based on a scoring system evaluating architectural features (i.e. horizontal and vertical spread) and cytological atypia of conjunctival melanocytic intraepithelial neoplasia (C-MIN) has been proposed {569}. In this system, a C-MIN score of 1 corresponds to PAM without atypia, a score of 2–4 corresponds to PAM with atypia, and a score of ≥ 5 equates to melanoma in situ. It has been proposed that PAM with atypia associated with a high-risk cytological phenotype (i.e. epithelioid cell morphology) {2530} and lesions with a C-MIN score of ≥ 5 {1349} should be reported as melanoma in situ, to indicate the higher probability of concomitant or subsequent invasive melanoma {568}.

### Differential diagnosis

PAM without atypia (conjunctival hypermelanosis) shows conjunctival epithelial pigmentation associated with a minimal increase in the number of small melanocytes scattered along the base of the epithelium. Junctional conjunctival naevus is mostly nested, whereas a lentiginous pattern predominates in PAM with atypia. Histological differentiation between junctional naevus and PAM can be very difficult and may require clinical information (i.e. patient age). Naevi are small and well circumscribed, whereas PAM with atypia is larger and irregular in shape and pigmentation. Any lesion with features of PAM with atypia that is associated with an atypical subepithelial component and is not a naevus should be reclassified as melanoma. Rarely, pigmented ocular surface squamous neoplasia can mimic PAM with atypia {2409}.

### Genetic profile

*TERT* promoter mutations, typical of the progression of melanocytic neoplasms to melanoma in situ, were found in 2 of 25 cases of PAM with atypia {1427}. *GNAQ* and *GNA11* mutations are absent {651}.

### Prognosis and predictive factors

PAM is a precursor of 50–70% of all conjunctival melanomas {1349}. Epithelioid cell morphology in PAM with cytological atypia is associated with an increased risk of progression to melanoma {804,2530,2929}. PAM with atypia composed solely of hyperchromatic melanocytes with scant cytoplasm and nuclei devoid of discernible nucleoli is less likely to be associated with invasive melanoma than is PAM with atypia composed of epithelioid cells {2530}. Complex melanocytic hyperplasia, nesting, and pagetoid spread have also been used (together with the Ki-67 proliferation index) to correlate histology with risk of recurrence and progression {1651}.

# Conjunctival naevus

Cree I.A.
Zembowicz A.

## Definition
Conjunctival naevus is a benign melanocytic conjunctival neoplasm. The histological subtypes of conjunctival naevi correspond to those of their cutaneous counterparts and melanocytic naevi occurring at other mucosal sites {803,1465,2929}.

## ICD-O code 8720/0

## Synonyms
The variants of common acquired conjunctival naevus include junctional conjunctival naevus, compound conjunctival naevus, and stromal conjunctival naevus. Rapidly proliferating naevi in children and adolescents are often referred to as juvenile (inflammatory) conjunctival naevi. Special variants of benign melanocytic proliferations, such as Spitz naevus, combined naevus, blue naevus, deep penetrating naevus, and pigmented epithelioid melanocytoma, can also occur in the conjunctiva.

## Epidemiology
Conjunctival naevi are rare lesions that can occur at any age. Most are acquired, but they sometimes present at birth. Junctional naevi are most common in children and adolescents {877,2408,2929}. Compound and subepithelial naevi have mean ages of occurrence of 21 years and 46 years, respectively {53,877,2408,2929}.

## Etiology
Conjunctival naevi arise in areas exposed to ultraviolet (UV) radiation {2898}.

## Localization
Most acquired conjunctival naevi are localized to the peribulbar juxtalimbal conjunctiva, caruncle, and plica semilunaris {803,877,2408}.

## Clinical features
Conjunctival melanocytic naevi present as well-circumscribed, macular or papular pigmented lesions {877,2408}. Rarely, they can be amelanotic. Clinical signs favouring conjunctival naevus over melanoma include the presence of epithelial inclusion cysts {53,2408}, a lack of involvement of the cornea {2929}, and the absence of feeder vessels {53,2408,2929}. Conjunctival naevi in children and adolescents can display rapid growth.

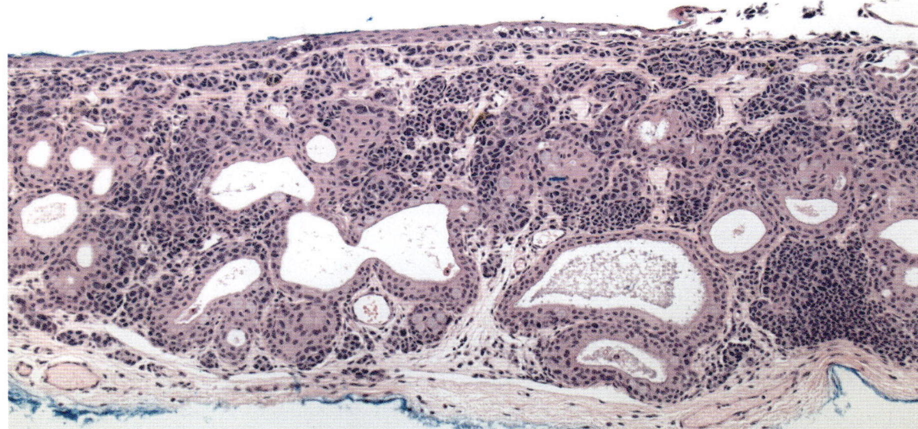

**Fig. 2.114** Compound conjunctival naevus. Prominent induction of conjunctival cysts is common in conjunctival naevi.

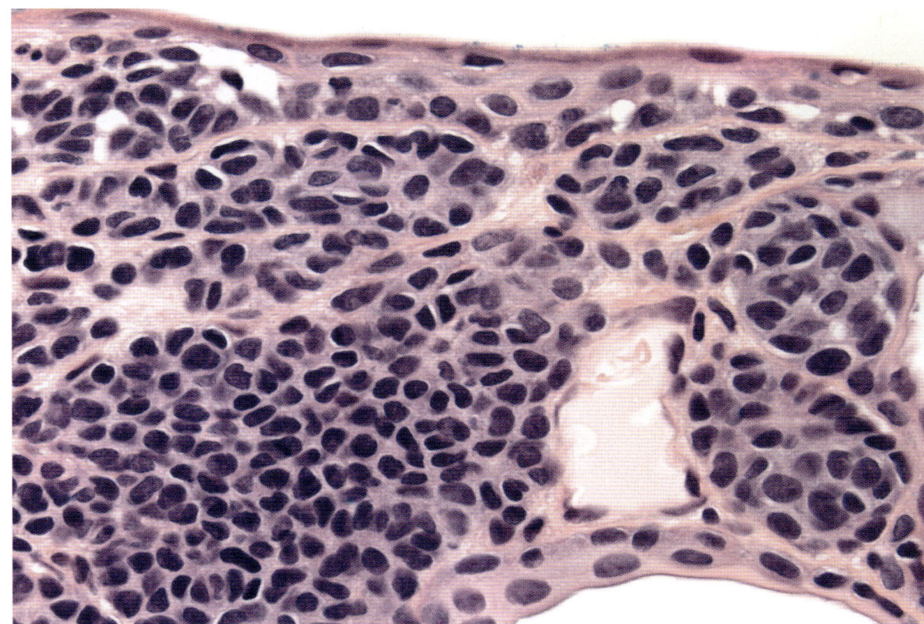

**Fig. 2.115** Compound conjunctival naevus. Bland cytological features.

## Histopathology
The histopathology of the various subtypes of conjunctival naevus is discussed in greater detail in the corresponding chapters of the *WHO classification of tumours of the eye* volume {948A}. Junctional, compound, and stromal naevi are recognized, mimicking those in skin and representing maturation. The microscopic features of common acquired conjunctival subepithelial naevus and special naevus types (e.g. Spitz, blue, and deep penetrating naevi) are essentially identical to

those of their cutaneous counterparts. In contrast to the epidermis, the conjunctival epithelium can be only 3–5 cells thick in some areas and lacks strong desmosomes. Therefore, junctional and compound conjunctival naevi often produce worrying architectural patterns, such as horizontal extension of the junctional component far beyond the subepithelial component, large and irregularly shaped nests, a pagetoid growth pattern, and confluence of melanocytic proliferation at the epithelial–subepithelial junction {803,2604,2910,2929}. This is particularly common in cases arising in children and young adults. Combined naevi with clonal epithelioid type A and/or a deep penetrating component are common. Involvement of superficially located palpebral skeletal muscle by naevus cells should not be interpreted as evidence of an invasive growth pattern. The subepithelial component in rapidly growing lesions may show limited maturation with depth. Paradoxically, the subepithelial melanocytes in juvenile conjunctival naevi may be larger than the junctional melanocytes, giving impression of reverse maturation {2604}. Unlike in the skin, the diagnosis of conjunctival naevi with worrying architectural patterns should rely more on cytology than on architecture.

## Differential diagnosis

Bland cytological features, rather than architecture, must be relied upon for the differential diagnosis between conjunctival naevi and melanoma. Helpful diagnostic features distinguishing conjunctival naevi from melanoma are the induction of epithelial cysts and sparing of the cornea {468,2929}. Conjunctival naevi occurring in children and adolescents often display an inflammatory host response and increased size of melanocytes, which can have small but prominent basophilic or (rarely) eosinophilic nucleoli {2604,2910}. Mitotic activity is usually absent in conjunctival naevi, but a rare mitosis can be observed in proliferating lesions, most commonly in children and adolescents. Sporadic pleomorphism of individual cells is rarely present. The differential diagnosis between junctional naevus and primary acquired melanosis requires clinicopathological correlation, including age, duration, size, and site of occurrence {803,2929}.

## Histogenesis

Conjunctival naevus arises from neural crest–derived melanocytes {803}.

## Genetic profile

Some conjunctival naevi harbour *BRAF* c.1799T>A (p.V600E) mutation {905}. There is no evidence of *GNAQ* mutations {651}.

## Genetic susceptibility

Acquired conjunctival naevi have been described in patients with dysplastic naevus syndrome or a family history of cutaneous melanoma {1465,2408}.

## Prognosis and predictive factors

The prognosis is excellent. Progression to melanoma is extremely rare {803,2408}.

# Nodular, naevoid, and metastatic melanomas

## Nodular melanoma

Cochran A.J.
Bastian B.C.
Elder D.E.

### Definition

Most invasive and tumorigenic primary cutaneous melanomas arise from a pre-existing radial-growth-phase (RGP) proliferation of atypical melanocytes in the epidermis and superficial dermis in the overlying and/or flanking skin. A minority lack a contiguous epidermal component and are described as primary melanoma without an RGP, or more commonly as nodular melanoma {491}.

Nodular melanomas are by definition tumorigenic, and thus in the vertical growth phase (VGP; see *Melanocytic tumours: Introduction*, p. 66); they likely share features with the VGP tumours that arise in a background of RGP of various subtypes. Metastatic melanomas are also purely tumorigenic and may share similar but distinguishable features {2458}.

### ICD-O code

8721/3

### Synonyms

Rapidly growing melanoma (subset) {1574}; primary melanoma without a radial growth phase

### Epidemiology

The epidemiology is likely heterogeneous, paralleling that of the RGP-derived melanomas {1054} (see the relevant sections). The prevalence seems to be increased among older men {2404}.

### Etiology

The etiology is heterogeneous, paralleling that of RGP melanomas.

### Localization

The distribution in the skin is widespread and parallels that of other melanomas.

### Clinical features

Nodular melanomas present as clinically and histologically nodular tumours that range widely in pigmentation, from very dark, heavily melanized variants to hypomelanotic and amelanotic variants that can present considerable diagnostic difficulty for the clinician and microscopist because of a lack of diagnostic features of the RGP (e.g. pagetoid scatter and lentiginous proliferation in the epidermis); this can result in delayed diagnosis {486,954}.

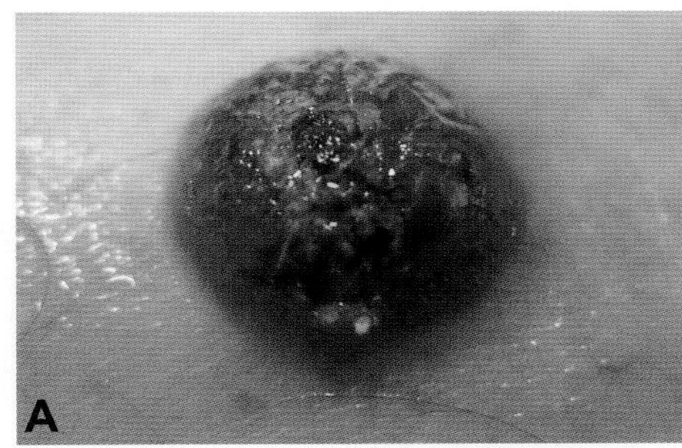


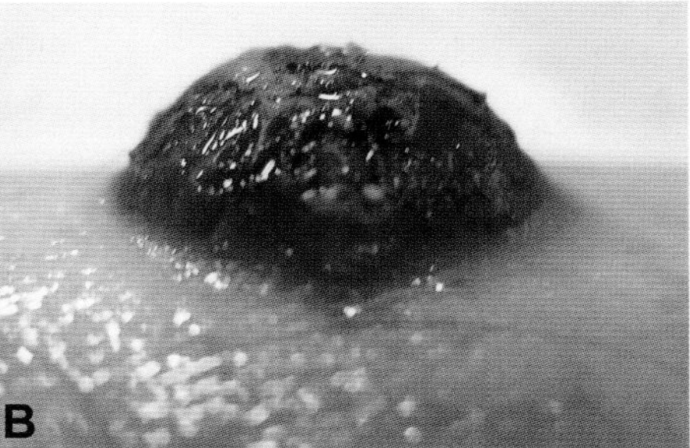


**Fig. 2.116** Nodular melanoma. **A** A bulky nodular tumour in sun-damaged skin. **B** The side view emphasizes the elevation of the tumour above the background skin; there is no adjacent radial-growth-phase/in situ component.

### Histopathology

Histologically, nodular melanomas consist of an invasive and tumorigenic component in the dermis, often with overlying junctional melanoma cells that are usually nested, possibly associated with epidermal ulceration and coterminous with the dermal component. There is often a collarette {2458}. A tumorigenic VGP is minimally defined as a cluster of cells in the dermis that is larger than the largest intraepidermal cluster, but most nodular melanoma nodules are much larger than this. Some of the tumours have a polypoid configuration, but this pattern has no prognostic significance when standard prognostic factors are controlled for (see below). The epidermis adjacent to the tumour is anatomically normal, without markedly increased numbers of melanocytes. Ascension of single melanoma cells through the overlying epidermis in a pagetoid pattern is unusual. It is likely that some or all of these tumours have had an RGP that was limited in extent, and with lesional progression became incorporated into the nodular tumour or underwent spontaneous regression. True nodular melanoma can sometimes be distinguished from primary melanomas in which the entire epidermal component has undergone spontaneous regression, as well as from primary dermal melanoma {397}, and should also be distinguished from epidermotropic metastases (see *Metastatic melanoma*, p. 150). Epidermis that has been the site of regression of RGP melanoma is usually underlain by a zone of variably vascular fibrosis in which pigment-containing macrophages and free melanin may be identified.

The melanoma cells of the dermal component are most often epithelioid, but fusiform and/or mixed cytology is also encountered. Tumour cytology can be uniform throughout the invasive component or can vary widely between separate adjacent domains, forming a patchwork or so-called clonal pattern. Clonality may be associated with peritumoural and intratumoural lymphocytic infiltration, which may vary widely in density and extent of tumour mass penetration, in populations of tumour cells that differ in morphology, and in mitotic rate and pigmentation. Plasma cells may be prominent in the infiltrate {2458}. The cytology of the invasive melanoma cells may vary with depth of invasion, with more-superficial tumour cells being larger than those that are more deeply located. This is a potentially misleading

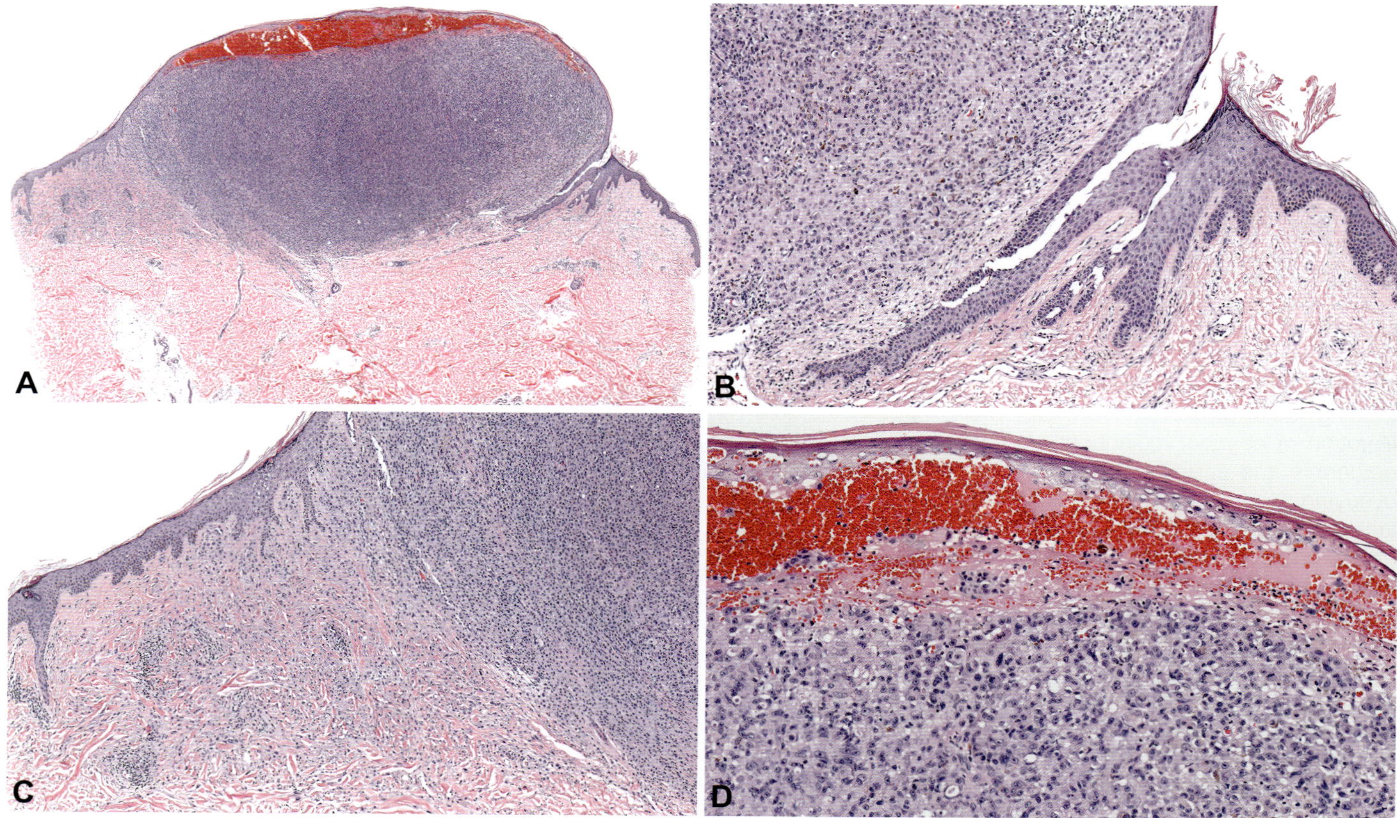


**Fig. 2.117** Nodular melanoma. **A** Discrete nodular tumour in the skin. **B** Adjacent to the tumour nodule, there is an epidermal collarette, and there is no adjacent intraepidermal or microinvasive radial-growth-phase component. **C** On the other side of the nodule, there is a dermal naevus, extending into the reticular dermis in a so-called congenital pattern, providing supportive evidence that the tumour is primary at this site. **D** The tumour is composed of large epithelioid cells with large nuclei, irregular nuclear membranes, clumped chromatin, and prominent nucleoli; there are frequent mitoses. In the single field shown here, the appearance is indistinguishable from that of a tumorigenic melanoma arising in association with a radial growth phase, or from that of a metastasis to this site.

characteristic, reminiscent of the more commonly encountered naevoid maturation in naevi and in naevoid melanomas.

## Differential diagnosis

Tumours that express no or limited melanin can present considerable diagnostic difficulty, and must be distinguished from squamous cell carcinomas, appendageal tumours, sarcomas, and cutaneous lymphomas. Detection of limited melanin can be facilitated by a silver stain for melanin, but the immunohistochemical detection of epitopes associated with melanocyte-derived cells (e.g. melan-A, HMB45 antigen, tyrosinase, S100 protein, and SOX10), and the absence of keratinocyte-derived cells (e.g. cytokeratins recognized by AE1/AE3), and lymphoid cells (CD3, leukocyte common antigen, and other markers as indicated) is usually sufficient to establish the diagnosis of a melanocytic tumour {397}. Electron microscopy is less commonly used now, but the presence of (pre)melanosomes remains powerful evidence of melanocytic histogenesis.

## Histogenesis

Unlike other melanomas, nodular melanomas progress to the VGP without an appreciable antecedent RGP. Possible explanations include that nodular melanomas acquire the genetic alterations required for invasive melanoma to form in rapid succession or in altered sequential order, so that the barriers that keep partially transformed tumour from deep invasion are overrun early or even before the proliferation-inducing alterations are acquired.

## Genetic profile

Although there are few directly pertinent studies on nodular melanoma {934}, the mutation patterns overlap with those of other melanoma subtypes that present with RGP components, including superficial spreading melanoma, lentigo maligna melanoma, acral melanoma, and mucosal melanomas, as discussed in other sections of this volume. It is therefore likely that nodular melanomas represent accelerated evolutionary trajectories of these subtypes, rather than a subtype with a distinct genomic profile.

## Genetic susceptibility

The genetic susceptibility likely parallels that of the melanomas with an RGP.

## Prognosis and predictive factors

Standard prognosticators, in particular tumour thickness, Clark level of invasion, and extent of ulceration, have the same value as in other melanomas {490,679} (see *Melanocytic tumours: Introduction*, p. 66).

# Naevoid melanoma

Cook M.G.
Gerami P.
Kossard S.
van den Oord J.

## Definition

Naevoid melanomas are subtypes of melanoma that resemble in general architecture (and to some extent in cytology) the main variants of common intradermal and compound melanocytic naevi.

## ICD-O code 8720/3

## Synonyms

There are many synonyms and variants, including papillomatous, non-papillomatous, small cell, and verrucous naevoid melanomas, as well as melanoma showing paradoxical maturation.

## Epidemiology

Because definitions of naevoid melanoma vary, precise estimates of incidence have not been established. It seems that the papillomatous form is very uncommon, whereas the form maturing to a small cell dermal component is slightly less uncommon.

Both forms occur in a wide age range. In a European Organisation for Research and Treatment of Cancer (EORTC) study, the mean patient age for the papillomatous form was 40 years (range: 16–89 years) and for the maturing naevoid type, 56 years (range: 16–89 years) {522}. There was no clear sex predominance.

## Etiology

The etiology is not substantially different from that of other melanomas. The site distribution suggests that ultraviolet (UV) radiation exposure may play a part in some cases, but it is unknown what initiates the naevoid type of differentiation. The naevoid component in the maturing type shows some features of senescence immunohistochemically.

## Localization

The papillomatous form occurs predominantly on the head and neck and the limbs in the EORTC study, but is more widely distributed in other reports {256,2348,2930}. The maturing naevoid form occurs most commonly on the limbs and trunk but is seen in most areas.

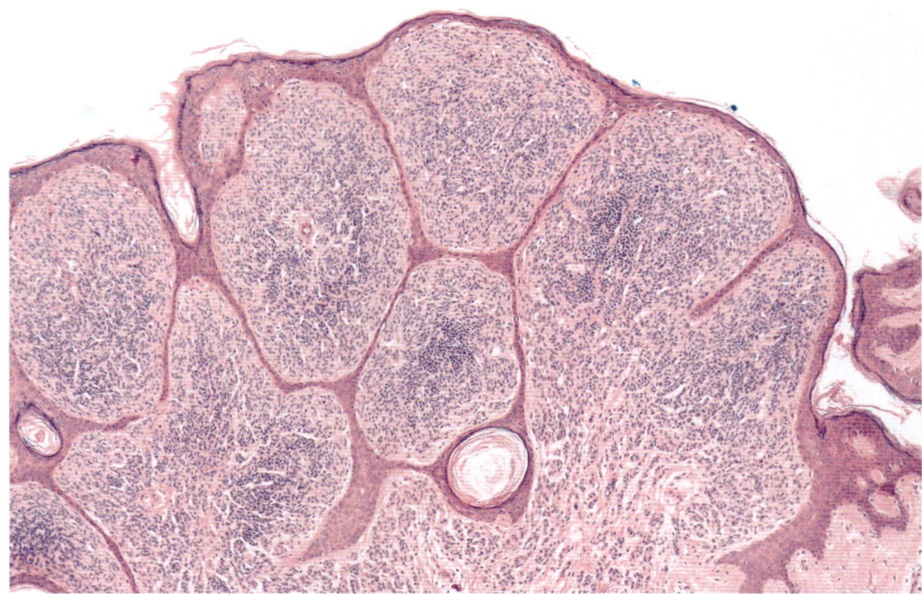

**Fig. 2.118** Papillomatous naevoid melanoma with exophytic growth and segmentation by epidermal strands.

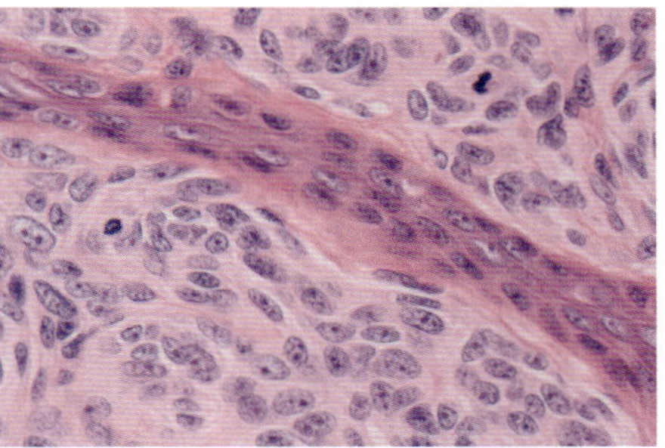

**Fig. 2.119** Papillomatous naevoid melanoma. The epidermal extension is not associated with junctional proliferation; the adjacent melanocytes include many mitoses.

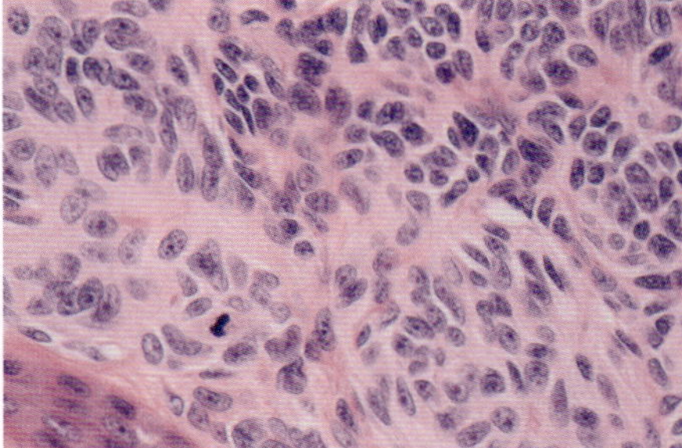

**Fig. 2.120** Papillomatous naevoid melanoma. The melanocytes in the centre of a compartment (upper right) show hyperchromatic angulated nuclei with scant cytoplasm.

## Clinical features

The papillomatous form has an appearance very similar to that of a raised nodular intradermal naevus; it usually has moderate pigment and a small macular component. It is sometimes only recognized as a recurrent tumour following excision of what was thought to be a benign naevus. The maturing small cell variant resembles a dysplastic compound naevus.

## Histopathology

The papillomatous variant of naevoid melanoma has been terms verrucous pseudonaevoid {256} and papillomatous {1681}, and it occurs as an exophytic nodule covered by intact but often attenuated epidermis. It is usually characterized by long, thin, interconnecting epidermal strands separating the melanocytic component into compartments. The melanocytes have crowded hyperchromatic nuclei with scant cytoplasm. Mitoses are always evident, often in a broad rim of melanocytes at the periphery of the compartments. There is only a minor junctional component, so the low-power appearance is that of an intradermal naevus. In cases where an additional

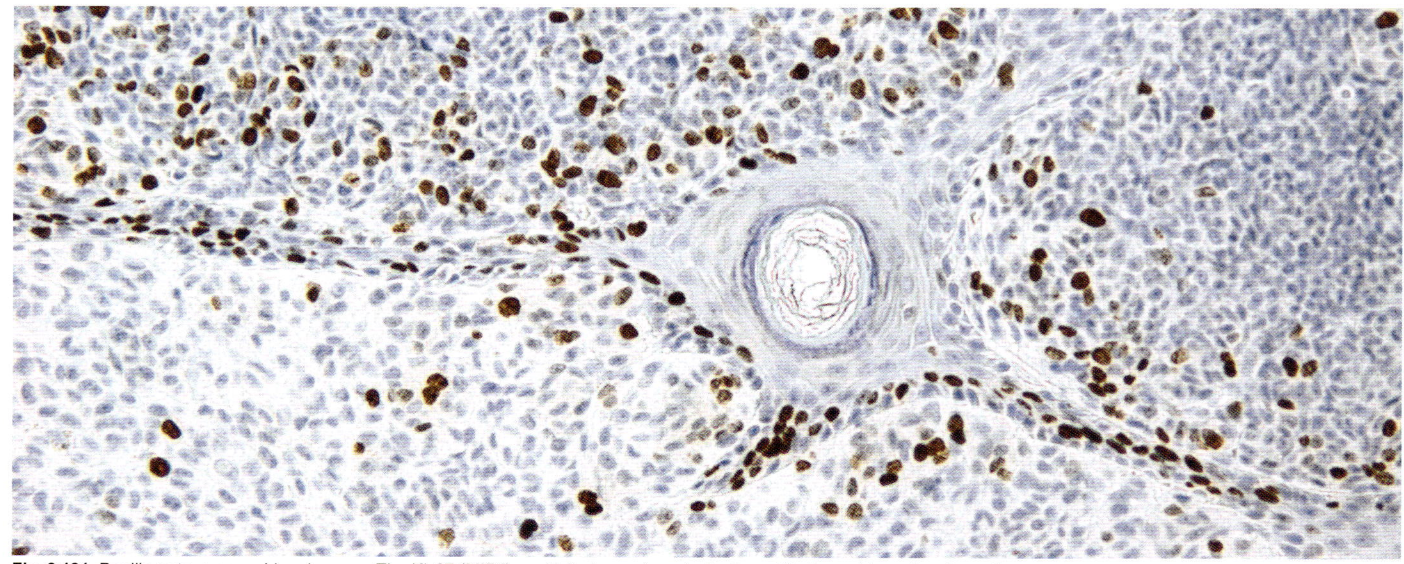
**Fig. 2.121** Papillomatous naevoid melanoma. The Ki-67 (MIB1) positivity is most marked adjacent to the epidermal prolongations.

true benign naevus is present, the contrast is clear.
Some authors have described naevoid melanoma as one entity with variation in histology {633}; others have considered the maturing naevoid melanoma to be a separate form, variously termed non-papillomatous melanoma {1681}, small cell naevoid melanoma {257,1435}, and melanoma with paradoxical maturation {2256}. The superficial component is sufficiently disordered and atypical to qualify as invasive melanoma, but it merges with small (but still atypical) melanocytes in the mid- to deep papillary dermis or the superficial reticular dermis. Maturing naevoid melanomas are usually thin (< 1 mm), but can occasionally reach 2 mm in thickness. The small hyperchromatic naevoid cells are usually arranged in nests without individual surrounding stroma, but with abundant dense fibrosis between the nests. The nests tend to become larger with depth.

## Differential diagnosis

The differential diagnosis of papillomatous naevoid melanoma includes exophytic intradermal naevus. The distinction depends on the subtle atypia and proliferative features. The alternative to a maturing naevoid melanoma is a dysplastic compound naevus, but the crowded atypical small round cells are characteristic of the dermal component and distinct from benign naevus cells, although lesions with similar histopathological findings have been described as sclerosing naevi with pseudomelanomatous features {726,1395}.
An infiltrative small cell melanoma has been described {1435} occurring in association with atypical lentiginous lesions, and this case seems very similar to some of the cases described by others {257,522,2256}.
Other naevi, such as Spitz naevus and deep penetrating naevus, are distinctly different and are covered elsewhere.
Early nodular melanoma may be indistinguishable from papillomatous naevoid melanoma.

## Histogenesis

Papillomatous naevoid melanoma appears to arise from superficial dermal melanocytes in polypoid intradermal

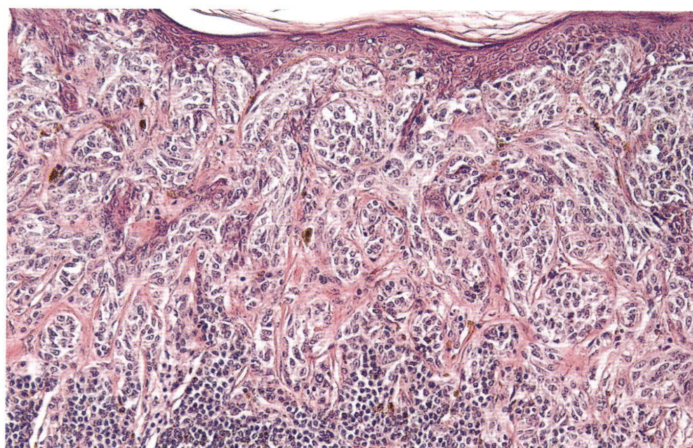
**Fig. 2.122** Maturing naevoid melanoma. Atypical-looking melanocytes change in the superficial dermis to small round naevoid cells.

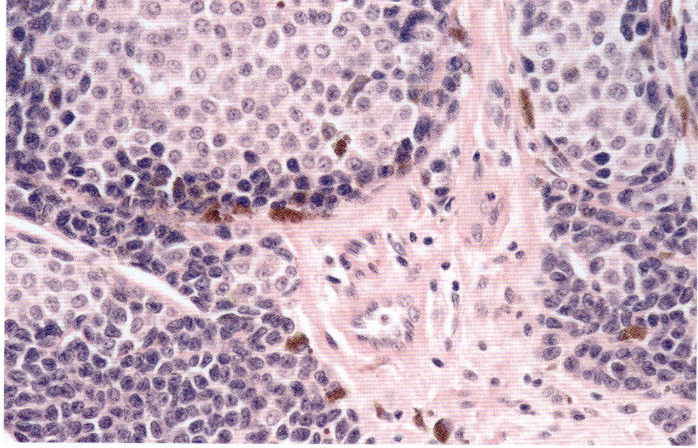
**Fig. 2.123** Maturing naevoid melanoma. Large epithelioid melanocytes in sheets merge with small melanocytes with scant cytoplasm but still atypical hyperchromatic nuclei.

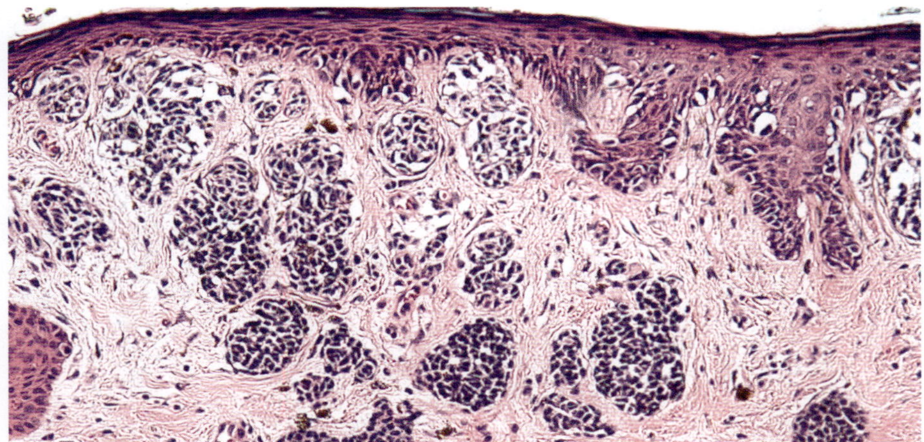

**Fig. 2.124** Maturing naevoid melanoma. A disorderly junctional proliferation of melanocytes shows gradual change in the superficial dermis to atypical small naevoid cells arranged in large irregular nests.

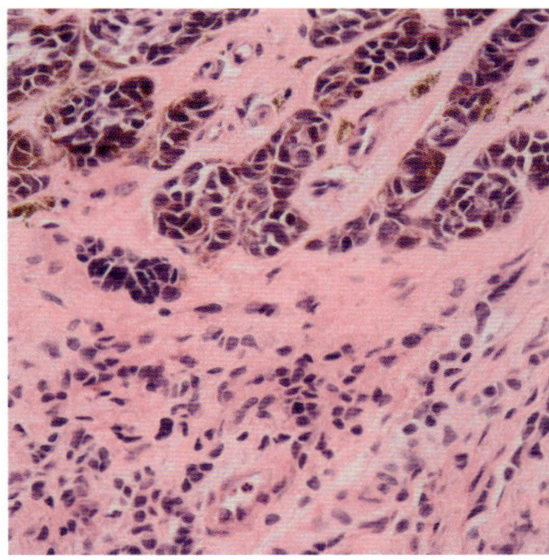

**Fig. 2.125** Maturing naevoid melanoma. Nests of small atypical hyperchromatic melanocytes adjacent to naevus cells with smaller nuclei and abundant stroma.

naevi. Occasionally, pre-existing true naevus cells can be seen adjacent to the atypical cells, supporting this assumption. The overall configuration of the lesion shows similarities to that of a small or early nodular melanoma.

Maturing naevoid melanoma has a junctional component indistinguishable from the intraepidermal component of superficial spreading melanoma or lentiginous melanoma, and is not usually prominently pagetoid.

The arrangement of the dermal component suggests it is derived from the superficial atypical component {257,2256}. The tumours tend to be nested, without the fine collagenous background of an intradermal naevus. When a dermal element of a true naevus is seen subjacent to the maturing naevoid melanoma, it is obviously different. These features suggest that these melanomas begin to invade the dermis before changing their characteristics to those of a less-aggressive form. Whether this is inherent in the tumour or a response to the microenvironment is unclear.

## Genetic profile

Of the few cases assessed by Cook et al. {522}, all 3 of the 3 papillomatous naevoid melanomas showed *NRAS* mutation; of the 8 cases of maturing naevoid melanoma, 2 showed *BRAF* mutations, 4 showed *NRAS* mutation, and 2 showed neither.

## Prognosis and predictive factors

In papillomatous naevoid melanoma, the thickness and mitotic count appear to be predictive. The survival is said to be similar to that of other forms of melanoma. In some studies, 33% of patients experienced recurrence or metastasis {522}. A similar metastatic rate (37.5%) was observed in another study {2930}, but those investigators reported a local recurrence rate of 75%.

According to recent preliminary studies, maturing small cell melanoma appears to be much less likely to metastasize, and therefore shows no decrease in survival. No metastases have been seen so far in a series of 79 cases {522}. This finding may be partially explained by the tumours' mean thickness (measured to the depth of the atypical small cell component) being < 1 mm, which in turn is probably related to the characteristic pseudomaturation.

It has been noted that naevoid melanomas referred to as being of small cell type may be associated with good survival {257,1435}. In these cases, recognition of the pattern simulating maturation resulting in a small cell (but still atypical) dermal component appears to be the main predictor of good survival. Therefore, if these suppositions are confirmed, it may be appropriate to regard this variant of naevoid melanoma as a melanocytic neoplasm of low malignant potential, even though some examples are > 0.8 mm thick; the apparent heterogeneity of these melanomas makes this difficult to assess. In some series, the group of naevoid melanomas as a whole was found to have behaviour similar to that of other melanomas {2889}.

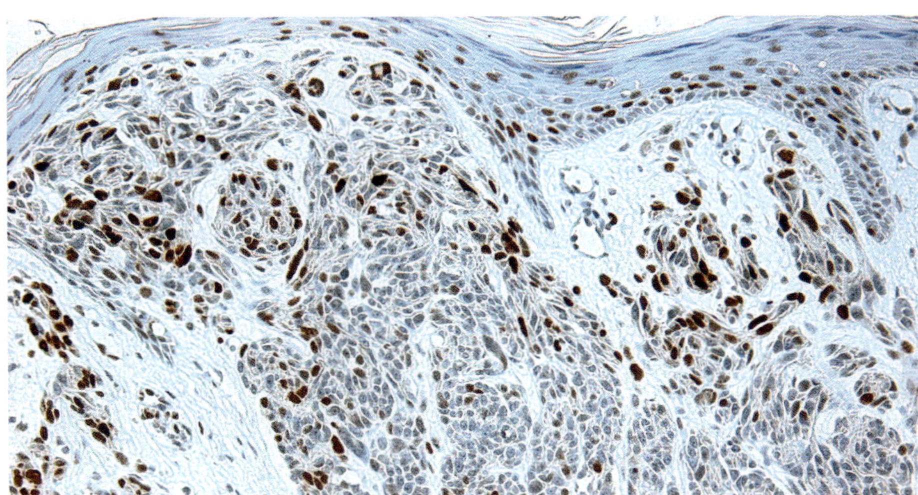

**Fig. 2.126** Maturing naevoid melanoma. Staining for p21 shows positivity in the superficial dermal component, diminishing more deeply.

# Metastatic melanoma

Cochran A.J.
Elder D.E.
Lowe L.
Heenan P.J.
Messina J.
Mihic-Probst D.
Shea C.

## Definition

Metastatic melanoma is a secondary tumour derived from a primary melanoma. Here we consider mainly cutaneous metastases, which must be distinguished from primary melanomas.

## ICD-O code 8720/6

## Epidemiology

The epidemiology is that of the primary tumour.

## Localization

The skin is the most common site of melanoma metastasis (affected in 56% of cases), with metastases arising from local, regional, or distant extension via cutaneous lymphatic spread, haematogenous spread, perivascular migration (angiotropism), or perineural routes {148,2328}. In one study, 8.3% of patients presented with cutaneous metastasis as the only manifestation of disease {2073}. In the largest recent study, the leg was most commonly affected (accounting for 18% of cases), followed by the scalp (15%), arm (13%), and face (7%) {2073}.

## Clinical features

The majority (92%) of cases present as a solitary, pigmented dermal nodule {2073}. Zosteriform, blue naevus–like, erysipelas-like, sclerodermiform, and purpuric lesions have been described {2319,2327}.

Cutaneous metastases close to (i.e. within 2 cm of) the primary site are called satellite metastases. Melanoma deposits that are located >2 cm from the primary site but have not reached ipsilateral regional lymph nodes are called in-transit metastases.

## Histopathology

The classic pattern is a well-circumscribed unencapsulated dermal nodule (which may extend into the subcutis), most frequently composed of epithelioid cells, with little to no inflammatory infiltrate {2849}. Surrounding fibrosis is often noted. Epidermotropism is seen in

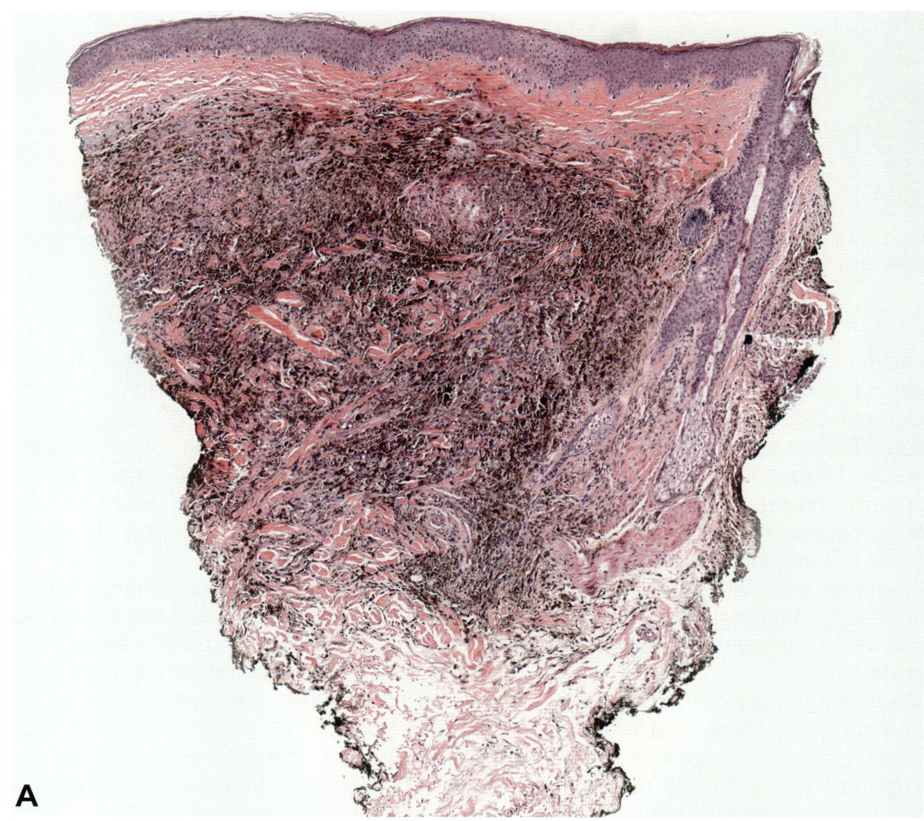

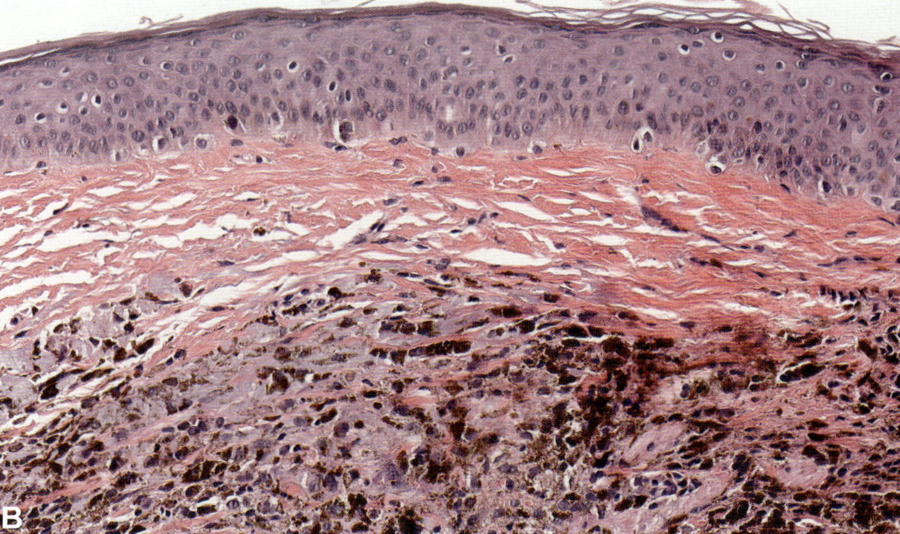

**Fig. 2.127** Metastatic melanoma. **A** There is a cellular tumour in the dermis; in this example, the metastasis is heavily pigmented, but these lesions are often essentially amelanotic. **B** Higher magnification shows that the tumour is composed of uniformly atypical melanocytes (many containing pigment) admixed with pigmented melanophages. The lack of involvement of the epidermis is an important distinguishing feature from primary nodular melanoma.

as many as 5% of cases. Angiolymphatic invasion is seen in about 5%.

The histology and cytology of most melanoma metastases are identical or closely similar to those of the primary tumour. It is useful to review available primary tumour pathology or consider the relevant pathology report. In some metastases, there may be variation of cytology from the primary tumour, affecting the entire tumour or in a patchwork (clonal) pattern. The tumour should be scrutinized for fine cytoplasmic melanin granules (i.e. single melanosomes that indicate melanogenesis within the cell, an almost unique attribute of cells of melanocytic lineage) and coarser aggregated melanin granules (more characteristic of melanophages). Melanophages aggregate in locations likely to contain melanogenic tumour cells. Silver stains may facilitate the detection of minute quantities of free and cellular melanin; however, for the most part immunohistochemistry is currently used for the identification of melanocytic differentiation.

The melanocytic origin of a metastatic tumour can be readily confirmed immunohistochemically {2849} with staining for S100 protein, melan-A (MART1), HMB45 antigen, tyrosinase, and/or SOX10. S100 staining is highly sensitive (positive in virtually 100% of melanomas) but is not specific for melanocytic lineage; there is cross-reaction with nerves, paracortical dendritic cells, capsular naevi, and fat cells. Melan-A and HMB45 antigen are more specific, but are negative in as many as 15% of metastatic melanoma cells. Tyrosinase is highly sensitive, but may also be detected in Schwann cells. SOX10 is also highly sensitive {497} and is of particular value in distinguishing melanoma cells from melanophages. In naevoid cases, assessment of proliferative activity with Ki-67 staining is recommended. Melanoma cells may also be identifiable by the detection of premelanosomes and melanosomes using electron microscopy. Staining for PDL1 may be indicated to assess potential susceptibility to immune checkpoint blockade therapy {579,1267}.

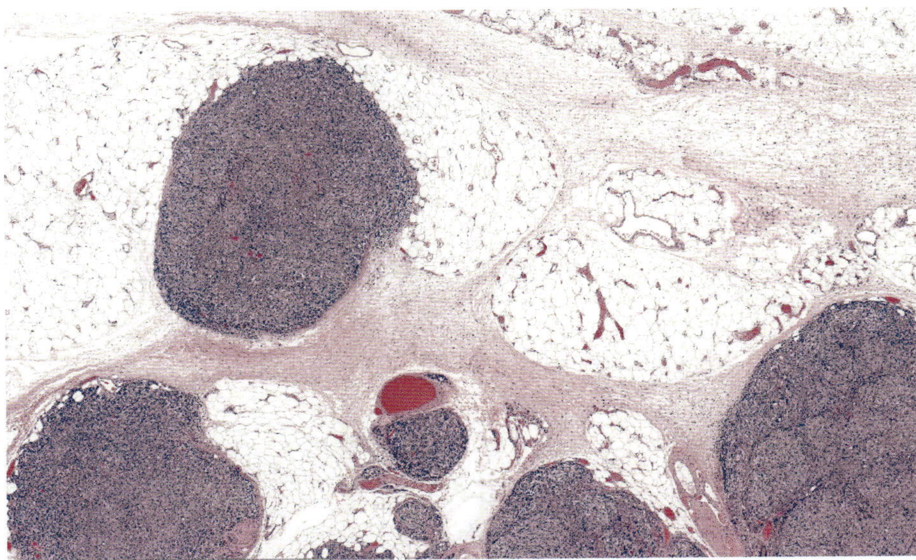

**Fig. 2.128** Metastatic melanoma in subcutis. There are multiple nodules of tumour in the subcutaneous fat.

### Differential diagnosis

Clinical history is of paramount importance for the diagnosis of cutaneous metastatic melanoma, and is necessary to exclude primary melanoma that has lost its junctional component because of trauma or prior biopsy, as well as primary dermal melanoma. Primary dermal melanoma is a subtype of melanoma characterized by a well-circumscribed dermal-based tumour with no epidermal involvement, but with a prognosis similar to that of primary melanoma. Immunohistochemically, primary dermal melanoma has lower levels of staining for p53, Ki-67, and cyclin D1 than do metastatic melanoma and primary nodular melanoma {397}.

In epidermotropic cutaneous metastatic melanoma, the finding of a dermal component broader than the junctional component and the absence of adnexal involvement are helpful in excluding a primary melanoma {2811}. Conversely, the presence of an accompanying benign naevus may help establish a diagnosis of primary melanoma. Metastases of small cell melanoma or metastases with a small diameter may resemble cutaneous naevi. The presence of sheet-like growth, disturbance of surrounding stroma, mitotic activity, and elevated N:C ratio (so-called pseudomaturation) are clues to the diagnosis of metastatic melanoma. Rarely, metastases of spindle cell melanoma can mimic blue naevi, but will demonstrate rare atypical epithelioid cells, a perivascular lymphocytic infiltrate, and mitotic activity {340,2821}.

Cutaneous metastases can occur at all anatomical sites, including the scar or graft at the primary excision site; true

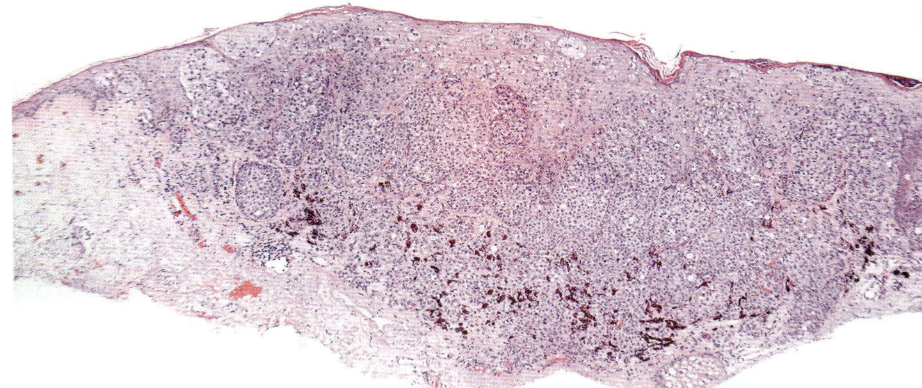

**Fig. 2.129** Epidermotropic metastatic melanoma. There is a dermal tumour composed of uniformly atypical cells; immunohistochemistry may be required to confirm melanocytic differentiation. There is involvement of the epidermis above (and also to a limited extent adjacent to) the tumour. Adjacent involvement is unusual in this condition, and this lesion can be distinguished from a primary melanoma only by the history that this lesion is one of multiple metastases from a known primary tumour.

local recurrence due to incompletely excised primary melanoma (persistent melanoma) can also occur at the primary site. The distinction between these two entities, which is essential to the understanding of the effects of different margins of excision on survival and so-called local recurrence of melanoma, depends on their identification according to their distinctive histological features and review of the primary excision specimen. Local metastases have the same histological features as cutaneous satellites, in-transit metastases, and distant cutaneous metastases, whereas persistent melanoma has the features of the primary melanoma {2899A}.

## Genetic profile

Metastatic melanoma is characterized by a wide range of mutations, mostly consistent with an ultraviolet (UV) radiation signature. The most important of these from a clinical perspective are mutations in the driver oncogenes.

These mutations are often studied with next-generation sequencing in an effort to detect mutations that may be associated with oncoproteins that are targetable by inhibitor molecule therapy {1267}. The most common of these are activating driver mutations of *BRAF* and *NRAS*. Metastases derived from melanoma arising in blue naevus or ocular melanoma may have mutations of *GNAQ* or *GNA11*. Rare metastases of spitzoid melanoma could have fusion genes characteristic of these conditions. Mucosal melanomas tend to have *NRAS* and also *KIT* mutations. Acral melanomas tend to have increased copy numbers and/or mutations of *CCND1*, and some have *KIT* (or other) driver mutations. Many metastases are found to be apparently wildtype when studied with next-generation sequencing targeted panels, indicating that their driver oncogenes have yet to be discovered.

## Genetic susceptibility

The genetic susceptibility is that related to the various primary tumour pathways.

## Prognosis and predictive factors

Locoregional cutaneous metastases, especially those on the lower limbs, are amenable to regional therapies such as isolated limb perfusion, and thus have a better prognosis than do disseminated cutaneous metastases from angiolymphatic spread. In general, the management is similar to that of metastases elsewhere, except that local resection may more often be feasible when disease is confined to the skin {2849}.

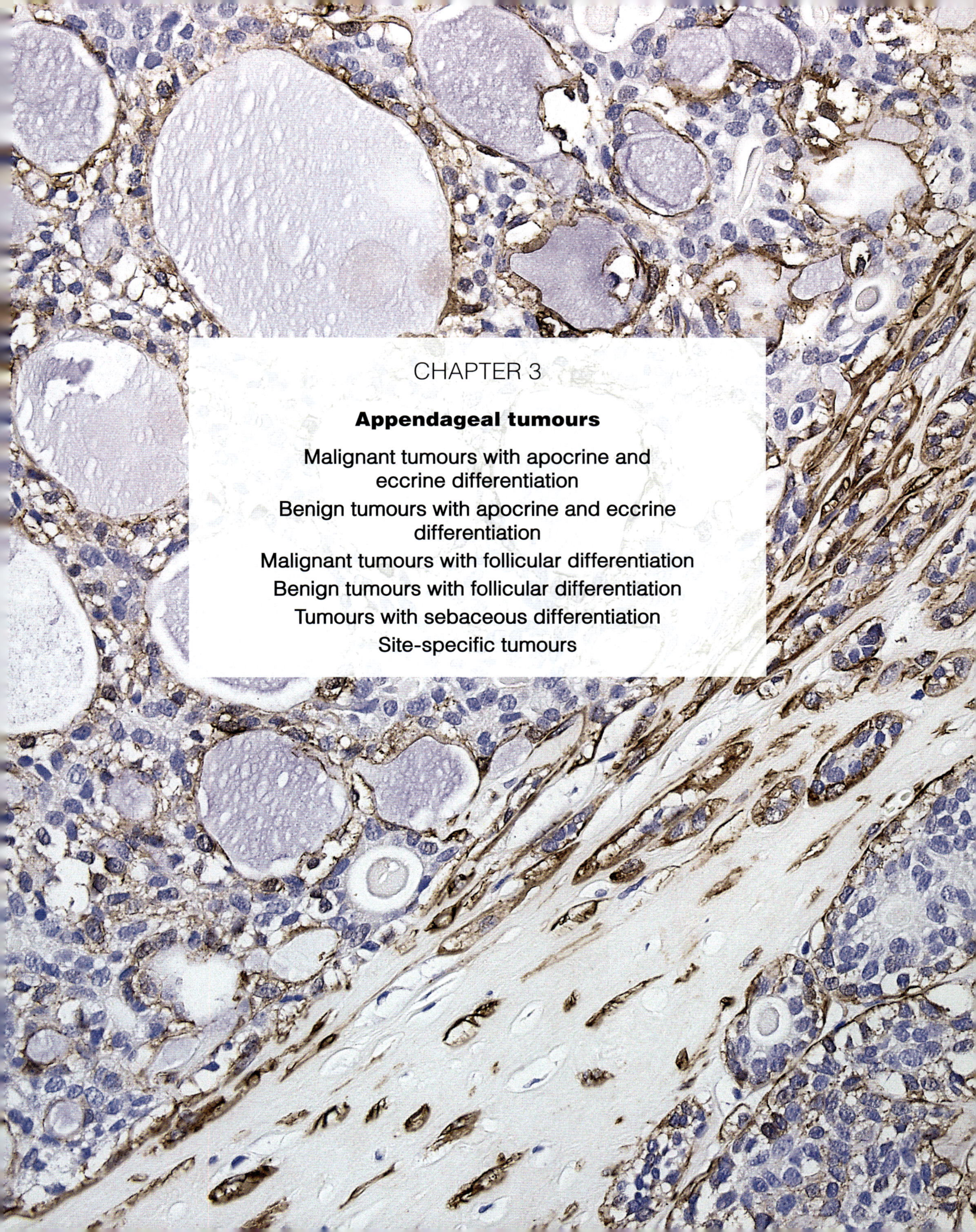

CHAPTER 3

# Appendageal tumours

Malignant tumours with apocrine and eccrine differentiation

Benign tumours with apocrine and eccrine differentiation

Malignant tumours with follicular differentiation

Benign tumours with follicular differentiation

Tumours with sebaceous differentiation

Site-specific tumours

# Appendageal tumours: Introduction

Massi D.
Cree I.A.
Elder D.E.
Kazakov D.V.
Scolyer R.A.

Cutaneous adnexal tumours are a wide and heterogeneous group of neoplasms that differentiate towards one or more of the skin appendages or recapitulate events occurring during embryo development. They include tumours with predominant apocrine, eccrine, follicular, sebaceous, and multilineage differentiation; in this volume, we also consider entities that are site-specific and derive from specific anatomical structures, such as the glands of Moll and anogenital mammary-like glands. Although many lesions show remarkable variability in histological appearance, there is considerable morphological overlap between entities, reflecting the marked plasticity characteristic of cutaneous adnexal neoplasms. Some adnexal tumours have extracutaneous counterparts, typically in the salivary glands and breast, but most of these lesions are unique to the skin. Benign tumours are far more common than their malignant counterparts, and can occur at any age {1184}. Adnexal carcinomas are rare, but their incidence is increasing, in part in association with ageing populations {348,1650,2498}. They are more frequent in men than in women, and in non-Hispanic White population than in other racial groups {254}.

Adnexal neoplasms may constitute cutaneous markers of a wide range of hereditary syndromes; therefore, a correct diagnosis is essential to alert the clinician to the possibility of these conditions. Syndromic cases of cutaneous adnexal neoplasms are usually multiple and are nearly identical histopathologically to their sporadic counterparts. However, certain microscopic features in some neoplasms may be indicative of a syndromic association. A large proportion of syndromes associated with cutaneous adnexal lesions have an autosomal dominant pattern of inheritance, and these syndromes are usually associated with tumour suppressor genes. Except in the syndromic setting and a few additional sporadic entities with identified genetic alterations, not much is known about the etiology or pathogenesis of adnexal tumours. Ultraviolet (UV) radiation exposure and immunosuppression have been proposed as possible triggering factors {1015}, and some neoplasms express putative follicular stem cell markers {1639,2118}, suggesting development from pluripotent stem cells. Nonetheless, their origin is still the subject of debate and investigation.

Cutaneous adnexal tumours have a peculiar clinical presentation; they can occur as solitary lesions or with multiple papules, nodules, and plaques {376,1090}. Some lesions have a distinctive clinical appearance (e.g. syringoma), making clinical diagnosis straightforward, but in most cases diagnosis is possible only on the basis of microscopic investigation. Carcinomas commonly arise de novo, but some have a benign component indicating progression from a pre-existing benign lesion. Certain lesions may be associated with skin adnexal tumours; for example, sebaceous naevus is a hamartoma in which trichoblastoma is the most common neoplasm to develop {1165}. The diagnosis of cutaneous adnexal tumours is sometimes complicated by their ability to produce cysts or because pigmented variants have been reported. The growth rate and resulting symptoms can vary greatly, with lesions ranging from completely asymptomatic to very painful. Features such as asymmetry, irregular borders, colour variation, erosion, and ulceration may suggest a malignant tumour, but some benign neoplasms also exhibit these traits. Colour, lobulation, and variable induration can be clues in narrowing down the clinical diagnosis {2914}. Dermoscopy does not reveal pathognomonic features; the most commonly described presentation being an atypical or polymorphous vascular pattern {2387}. Immunohistochemistry has limited value in the diagnosis of appendageal tumours but may be useful in particular situations. Because of these considerations, it is common to experience uncertainty in deciding whether a particular tumour is benign or malignant; in such cases, it is appropriate to give a descriptive diagnosis, such as "atypical skin adnexal tumour" or "skin adnexal tumour of uncertain malignant potential", along with a differential diagnosis and a recommendation for complete excision and consideration of follow-up. Overall, the most common location is the head and neck region, where cutaneous adnexal tumours can mimic skin cancers arising on sun-exposed areas. For adnexal carcinomas, extensive clinical evaluation is necessary, to exclude metastasis from elsewhere.

Malignant skin appendageal tumours can be locally aggressive and can affect deep extradermal structures. They spread by local dissemination. Once lymphatic and/or blood vascular vessels have been invaded, there may be involvement of regional lymph nodes or (in a minority of cases) primary haematogenous dissemination {118,1673}. A treatment algorithm for invasive cutaneous adnexal carcinomas has not yet been developed {146}. In most cases, adnexal carcinomas diagnosed at a localized stage and treated by wide surgical excision with clear margins have an indolent course, with an excellent prognosis. Conversely, patients with metastatic disease have a poor prognosis {254,2498}. The role of lymph node staging remains to be determined.

# Malignant tumours with apocrine and eccrine differentiation

## Adnexal adenocarcinoma not otherwise specified

Massi D.
Prieto V.G.
Cree I.A.
Elder D.E.
Scolyer R.A.
Singh R.

### Definition
Adnexal adenocarcinoma not otherwise specified (NOS) is a primary carcinoma of the skin with ductal/glandular differentiation but lacking specific histological features that would allow further classification. The primary importance of this entity is its similarity to adenocarcinomas metastatic to the skin {1638,1879}.

### ICD-O code
8390/3

### Synonyms
Sweat gland carcinoma; sweat duct carcinoma; eccrine carcinoma; high-grade eccrine syringomatous carcinoma

### Localization
Adnexal adenocarcinoma can involve any site, but occurs most commonly in the head and neck (in particular the cheek), followed by the trunk {829}.

### Clinical features
It usually presents as a solitary nodule or plaque of variable size and colour, which may be longstanding and slow-growing.

### Histopathology
The lesions are asymmetrical, poorly circumscribed, and infiltrative. They often involve the full thickness of the dermis and extend into the subcutaneous and deeper tissues. Tumour cells are arranged in tubules, cords, and nests, with ductal/glandular structures devoid of an obvious myoepithelial cell layer. There may be solid areas. Tumour cells exhibit abundant eosinophilic or granular cytoplasm and pleomorphic nuclei, occasionally with numerous mitotic figures. There may be squamous differentiation. Lumina may contain homogeneous eosinophilic material, foamy histiocytes, and necrotic debris {2310}. Before a diagnosis of primary adenocarcinoma of the skin is established, the possibility of cutaneous metastasis from a visceral adenocarcinoma should be ruled out through histological, immunohistochemical, and clinicopathological correlation.

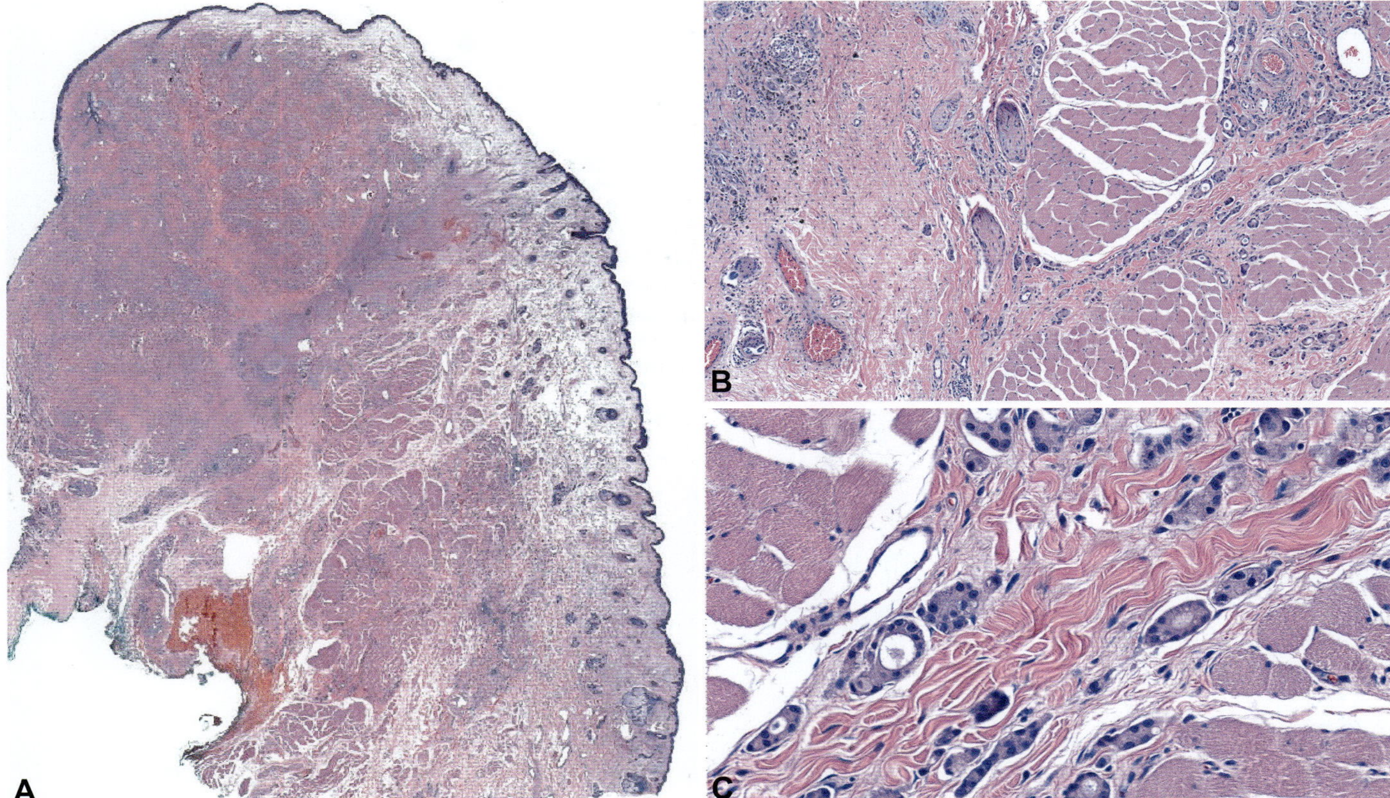


**Fig. 3.01** Adnexal adenocarcinoma. **A** Low-power view of a large, deeply invasive lesion involving most of the eyelid. **B** Deep invasion involving skeletal muscle. **C** Ducts and glands with high-grade atypia, infiltrating among skeletal muscle fibres.

The ductal structures are highlighted by staining for EMA (epithelial membrane antigen) and CEA. p63 and p40 are at least focally expressed in adnexal adenocarcinoma. CK5/6, CK7, calretinin, and podoplanin (recognized by D2-40) may also be expressed {1192,1527,1557,1638, 2074,2119}.

### Differential diagnosis

Microcystic adnexal carcinoma has a superficial component with keratin-filled (follicular) cysts, as well as a deeper glandular component that has less atypia than is seen in adnexal adenocarcinoma. Apocrine carcinoma shows glandular and ductal structures, with cytologically malignant cells showing decapitation secretion. Basal cell carcinoma with eccrine differentiation shows obvious basal cell carcinoma (i.e. basaloid cells with peripheral palisading, clefting, and myxoid stroma) and focal ductal differentiation. Squamoid eccrine ductal carcinoma shows malignant squamous epithelium in the superficial regions, occasionally resembling squamous cell carcinoma in situ {2689}.

Distinguishing primary from metastatic cutaneous adenocarcinoma often presents a diagnostic conundrum. Adnexal adenocarcinoma NOS may resemble skin metastasis, typically from the breast, lung, gastrointestinal tract, kidney, or ovary {2319,2365}. Internal malignancies tend to metastasize to the skin of the region (i.e. lung carcinomas to the skin of the trunk; gastrointestinal, genitourinary, and gynaecological carcinomas to the skin of the abdomen – in particular the umbilicus). On histology, the combination of epidermal involvement and absence of multifocality or lymphovascular invasion favours primary adenocarcinoma rather than metastasis {574}.

### Prognosis and predictive factors

Adnexal adenocarcinoma NOS can recur and metastasize {2543}.

# Microcystic adnexal carcinoma

Kazakov D.V.
Argenyi Z.B.
Brenn T.
Calonje E.
Mehregan D.A.
Mehregan D.R.
Requena L.
Sangüeza O.P.
Santa Cruz D.J.
Scolyer R.A.
Zembowicz A.

## Definition

Microcystic adnexal carcinoma (MAC) is a locally infiltrative adnexal carcinoma that microscopically shows malignant architectural features but bland cytology {909}.

## ICD-O code

8407/3

## Synonyms

Sclerosing sweat duct carcinoma; syringomatoid carcinoma; eccrine epithelioma; malignant syringoma {527,1717,2160}

## Epidemiology

There is no sex predilection. Patients are usually affected in their fifth or sixth decade of life, but the reported age range is wide (11–90 years). The neoplasm predominantly affects White populations and is rare in Black populations {461,2037}.

## Etiology

The etiology is unknown. A previous history of radiation therapy has been reported in association with some tumours.

## Localization

The central face, including the upper lip and nasolabial fold, is preferentially involved; the cheek, chin, and periorbital area are less commonly involved. Extrafacial lesions are rare {1940}.

## Clinical features

Most cases present as a firm or hard plaque, with an average diameter of 2 cm; less commonly, they can present as a poorly defined area of induration, a small nodule, or a cyst-like tumour. Ulceration is unusual. Exceptionally, pain, numbness, and a burning sensation have been reported, probably associated with perineural invasion.

## Histopathology

MAC is an infiltrative neoplasm that involves the dermis and often extends to underlying tissues, commonly showing horizontal stratified zonation. It is composed of various proportions of cornifying cysts with compact or laminated keratinous material, usually distributed in the upper part of the lesion; solid nests, strands, and columns of small monomorphous epithelial cells in the midzone; and duct-like structures composed of two layers of small cuboidal cells (empty or filled with eosinophilic material) in the lower part. Perineural or muscle invasion is common, but there is usually no pleomorphism or necrosis, and mitoses are rare or absent. The stroma is sclerotic, hyalinized, and paucicellular, and may contain foci of granulomatous inflammation induced by the rupture of calcified cysts. Focal clear cell change is common. Less common features include other types of adnexal differentiation (i.e. follicular or sebaceous), the occurrence of metaplastic bone (which should not be confused with bone invasion), and conspicuous single-file cell infiltration resulting in a resemblance to metastatic lobular carcinoma of the breast {250,1322,2156}. The immunoprofile is not specific. The neoplasm stains for various cytokeratins (e.g. CK14, CK5, CK1, CK10, and CK6), any of which may help to identify subtle invasion; expression of PHLDA1 is variable. Ductal differentiation can be highlighted by staining for EMA (epithelial membrane antigen) or CEA {829,2817}.

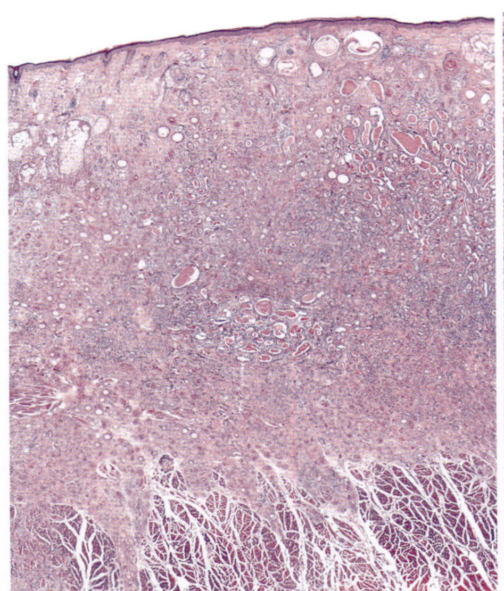

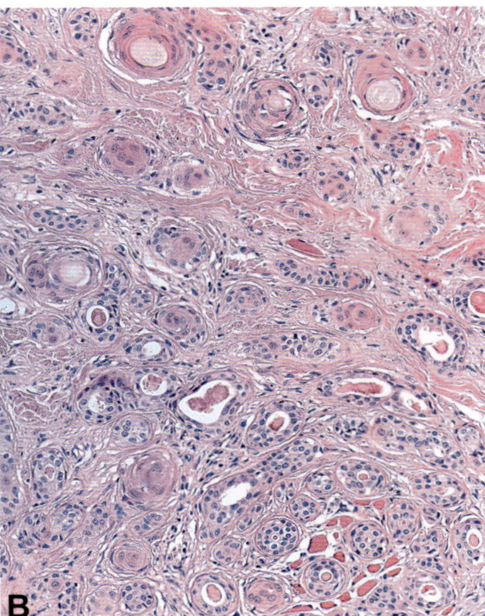

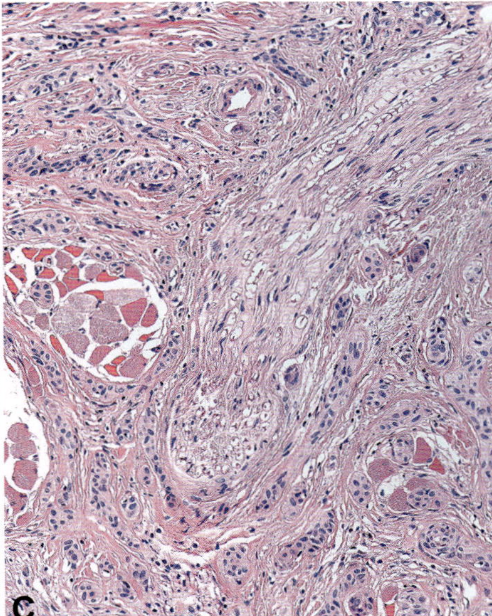


**Fig. 3.02** Microcystic adnexal carcinoma. **A** The infiltrative neoplasm involves the dermis and extends to underlying tissues. **B** The tumour is composed of cornifying cysts with compact or laminated keratinous material, solid nests, strands, and duct-like structures. **C** Perineural invasion is a common feature.

GCDFP15 and BerEP4 are consistently negative.

## Differential diagnosis

The diagnosis of MAC is usually straightforward but may be difficult or even impossible in small and superficial biopsies in which deep extension and an infiltrative edge cannot be identified. The clear distinction of MAC from its mimics is not possible in some cases, even with the adjunct of immunohistochemistry {231,1092,2467,2661,2817}. The tadpole-like structures sometimes seen in MAC may be reminiscent of syringoma, but syringoma is a more superficial neoplasm that often {1306} presents as numerous papules, whereas MAC is a solitary lesion usually occurring in older subjects. However, in small biopsies syringoma with a sclerotic stroma can be indistinguishable from MAC. Lesions virtually indistinguishable from MAC are seen in a rare and poorly defined condition, probably related to Nicolau–Balus syndrome (characterized by atrophoderma vermiculata and multiple syringomas), that clinically presents with bilateral plaque-like lesions on the cheeks, forehead, and arms during childhood. Despite their histological similarity to MAC, these lesions have a benign course {2339}. Desmoplastic trichoepithelioma (also called columnar trichoblastoma) is usually limited to the upper to mid-dermis and is composed of cords of basaloid cells with rims of collagen bundles around neoplastic cells, featuring a typical central depression (a dell). Desmoplastic trichoepithelioma (columnar trichoblastoma) is positive for CK20 (Merkel cells) and androgen receptor, whereas MAC is usually negative for these markers {713}. Sclerosing/morphoeic basal cell carcinoma is distinguished from MAC by its positive immunoreaction for BerEP4 {1443}. Conspicuous infundibulocystic structures may be encountered in benign adnexal neoplasms (e.g. trichoadenoma and sebaceoma) and may closely resemble the superficial portion of MAC; for such cases, re-excision and examination of the whole lesion is needed {800}. Syringomatous adenoma of the nipple is microscopically identical to MAC, but the clinical context permits the correct diagnosis {2232}.

## Histogenesis

Dual sweat duct and follicular differentiation was originally proposed {909, 1288,1901,2817}. Supporting evidence for follicular differentiation is the presence within MAC of germ-like structures with associated follicular papilla, clear cells associated with trichohyaline granules, and bluish-grey corneocytes and cornified material resembling shadow cells {1314,1515}. The rare presence of mature sebocytes and sebaceous ducts indicates the potential differentiation of MAC along the lines of the folliculoapocrine–sebaceous unit {85,1515,2104}.

## Prognosis and predictive factors

The tumours are locally aggressive and capable of involving deep underlying tissue, including bone. When incompletely excised, MAC is associated with frequent recurrence, but regional lymph node and distant metastases are rare {137,461,826,841,1865,2473}.

# Porocarcinoma

Kazakov D.V.
Argenyi Z.B.
Brenn T.
Calonje E.
Mehregan D.A.
Mehregan D.R.
Requena L.
Sangüeza O.P.
Santa Cruz D.J.
Scolyer R.A.
Zembowicz A.

## Definition

Porocarcinoma is the malignant counterpart of poroma; it is composed of poroid and cuticular cells and shows signs of malignancy. Porocarcinoma evolves from a pre-existing poroma in some cases, but it can also develop de novo.

## ICD-O codes

| | |
|---|---|
| Porocarcinoma | 8409/3 |
| Porocarcinoma in situ | 8409/2 |

## Synonyms

Malignant eccrine poroma; malignant hidroacanthoma simplex

## Epidemiology

In one large series, the incidence of porocarcinoma was 18 cases in 450 000 consecutive skin biopsy specimens (0.004%). Demographic data vary greatly in the literature, with the reported sex predilection ranging from a female-to-male ratio of 2:1 {2203}, to none, to a male bias {2474}.

## Localization

The most common site is the lower limbs, followed by the trunk, head, and upper limbs {2075,2163,2203,2706}.

## Clinical features

Porocarcinoma presents as an ulcerated nodule or tumour and is rarely pigmented. Sudden rapid growth, ulceration, and bleeding of a longstanding pre-existing poroma may also be observed. In large series, the mean age has varied from 61.5 to 73 years (range: 12–91 years).

## Histopathology

Porocarcinoma in situ is confined to the epidermis and usually shows the pattern of classic poroma in which there are cytological features of malignancy, including nuclear pleomorphism, nuclear hyperchromasia, and atypical mitoses {145,947,1189,2067}. About 10% of all porocarcinomas are in situ lesions {2203}. Invasive porocarcinoma, which is more common, additionally displays an intradermal proliferation with infiltrative borders and atypical cytological features that vary from moderate to frankly anaplastic. Perineural and intravascular invasion, necrosis en masse, and ductal differentiation are variable features. In some invasive tumours, an intraepidermal or intradermal benign residuum is seen instead of an intraepidermal in situ component. Rare features include clear cell change, focal squamous cell differentiation, sarcomatoid (metaplastic) transformation, intratumoural melanin deposits, melanocytic colonization, and focal sebaceous differentiation {901,1318,1641,2171}.

Porocarcinoma has no specific immunoprofile. Ductal differentiation, including abortive attempts in the form of intracytoplasmic lumina, can be highlighted by staining for EMA (epithelial membrane antigen) or CEA {496}.

## Differential diagnosis

Porocarcinomas with low-grade atypia can be very difficult to distinguish from poroma in which enlarged, slightly to moderately atypical p53-positive cuticular cells are a feature {2584}. In such cases, the diagnosis of porocarcinoma is made on the basis of an invasive

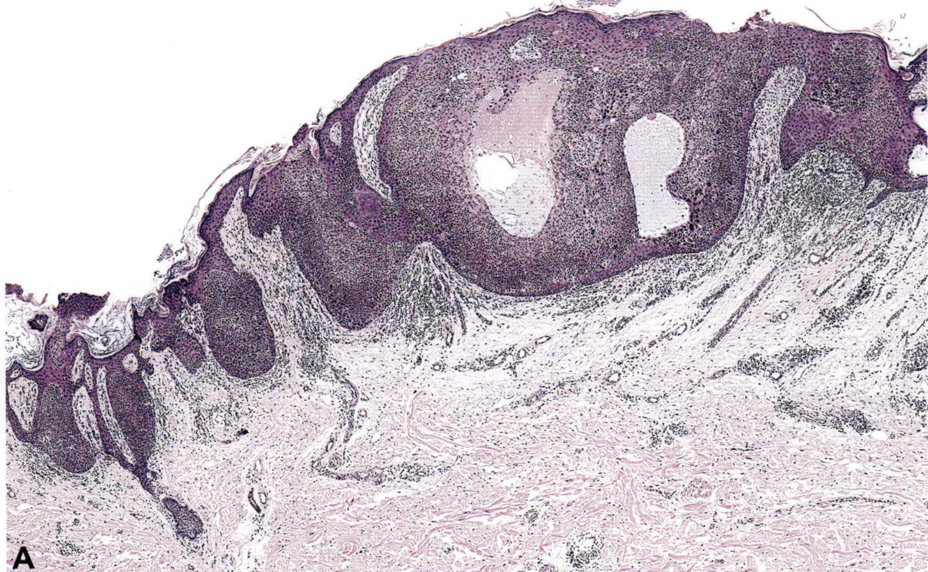


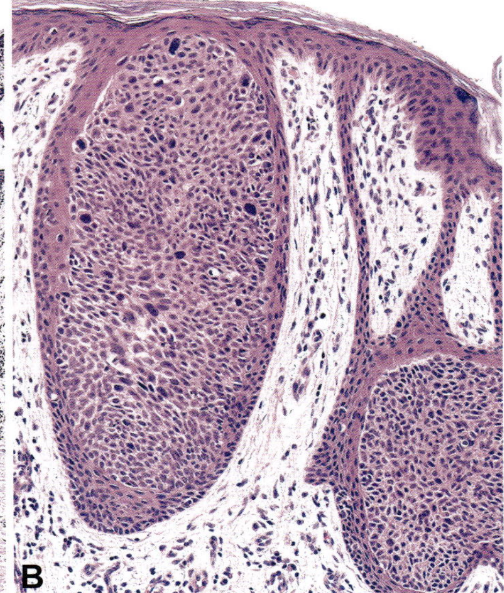


**Fig. 3.03** Porocarcinoma. **A,B** Porocarcinoma in situ is confined to the epidermis and is composed of poroid cells showing nuclear pleomorphism, nuclear hyperchromasia, and atypical mitoses.

architectural pattern. Poorly differentiated porocarcinoma may be difficult to identify because the typical composition of poroid cells and cuticular cells is often no longer recognizable. Single-cell necrosis in other neoplasms may result in pseudoductal structures that can mimic porocarcinoma. In such cases, the distinction can be made using staining for CEA and EMA, which highlights true ductal differentiation. Porocarcinoma manifests a variety of features (squamous cell areas, clear cells, etc.), making its histopathological presentation quite variable. Identifying a parent lesion (i.e. a pre-existing poroma or porocarcinoma in situ, squamous cell carcinoma in situ, etc.) is the best way to avoid misinterpretation in such cases.

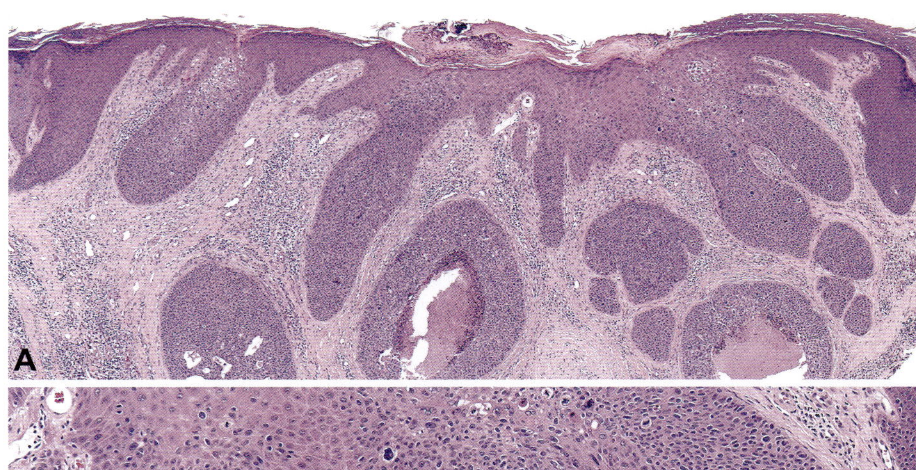

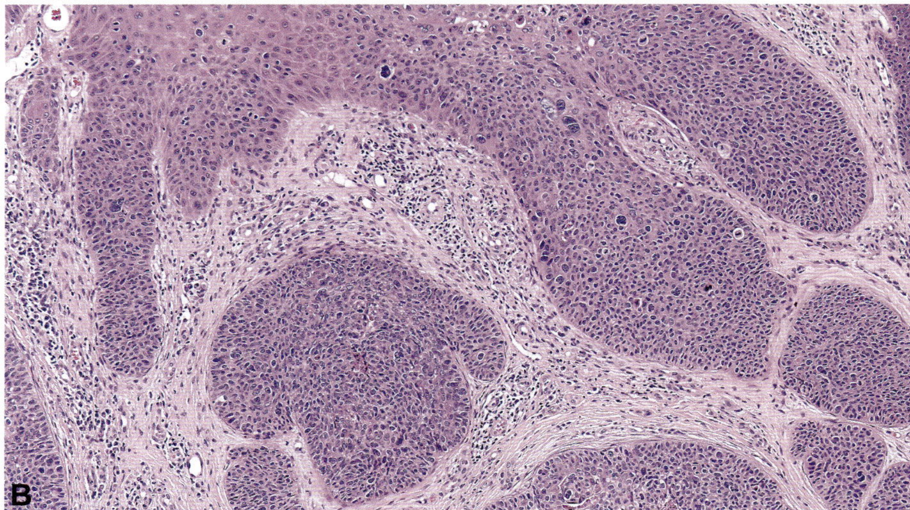

**Fig. 3.04** Porocarcinoma. **A** An invasive porocarcinoma displays, in addition to the in situ lesion, an intradermal proliferation with infiltrative borders and atypical cytological features. **B** Higher magnification.

## Prognosis and predictive factors

A meta-analysis of 105 published cases showed both local recurrence and regional metastatic rates to be approximately 20% and the distant metastatic rate to be 12% {2474}. However, no distinction between in situ and malignant lesions was made {2474}. In another study, of 54 invasive lesions, 9 (17%) recurred locally, 10 (19%) metastasized to regional lymph nodes, and 6 (11%) metastasized to distant sites and/or caused the death of the patient. High mitotic index and lymphovascular invasion are strongly predictive of death. High mitotic index also correlates with lymph node involvement. The gross size of the tumour has no significant relationship to prognosis, but tumour depth > 7 mm predicts death or lymph node involvement. An infiltrative (vs pushing) tumour margin has been found to be associated with an increased local recurrence rate {2203}.

# Malignant neoplasms arising from spiradenoma, cylindroma, or spiradenocylindroma

Kazakov D.V.
Argenyi Z.B.
Brenn T.
Calonje E.
Mehregan D.A.
Mehregan D.R.
Requena L.
Sangüeza O.P.
Santa Cruz D.J.
Scolyer R.A.
Zembowicz A.

## Definition

Malignant neoplasms arising from spiradenoma, cylindroma, or spiradenocylindroma are rare sweat gland carcinomas whose diagnosis depends on the recognition of a pre-existing benign spiradenoma, cylindroma, or spiradenocylindroma. These carcinomas can be divided into morphologically low-grade and high-grade tumours, with the malignant component showing a wide morphological spectrum. The morphological features correlate with outcome, and aggressive behaviour may be associated with high-grade tumours.

## ICD-O code 8403/3

## Synonyms

Spiradenocarcinoma; cylindrocarcinoma; spiradenocylindrocarcinoma
Other synonyms add the terms "malignant" or "carcinoma ex" to the name of the parent benign neoplasm (e.g. "malignant cylindroma" and "carcinoma ex spiradenoma").

## Epidemiology

Adults are affected (median age: 63.5 years), with no significant sex bias {562,928,1333,2690}.

## Localization

The anatomical distribution is wide, with a predilection for the head and neck area {562,928,1333,2690}.

## Clinical features

The tumours usually present as large nodules, several centimetres in size (median: 4 cm). In some cases, recent rapid growth is seen in a longstanding lesion {562,928,1333,2690}. The lesions typically occur as sporadic solitary neoplasms or as a component of Brooke–Spiegler syndrome, an inherited autosomal dominant disease characterized by the development of multiple adnexal cutaneous neoplasms (most commonly spiradenoma, cylindroma, spiradenocylindroma, and trichoepithelioma). In the syndromic setting, large, rapidly growing, bleeding or ulcerated tumours occur in a background of multiple smaller pre-existing benign neoplasms {948,1333,2574}.

## Histopathology

The tumours are large and multinodular, involving dermis and subcutis. A pre-existing benign spiradenoma, cylindroma, or hybrid spiradenocylindroma is at least focally present, with gradual or abrupt transition. Morphologically low-grade tumours are easily mistaken for spiradenoma or cylindroma. Loss of the dual cell population, cytological atypia, increased mitotic activity, and loss of intratumoural lymphocytes are evident upon careful examination. Other clues include infiltrative growth with neoplastic aggregates located far away from the main bulb of the tumour and less-conspicuous basement membrane surrounding neoplastic aggregates (in malignant tumours evolving from cylindroma). The microscopic appearances of the malignant component are quite variable. They include the basal cell adenocarcinoma–like, low-grade (BCAC-LG) pattern; the basal cell adenocarcinoma–like, high-grade (BCAC-HG) pattern; invasive adenocarcinoma NOS; and sarcomatoid (metaplastic) carcinoma. The BCAC-LG and BCAC-HG patterns resemble salivary gland basal cell adenocarcinoma, low-grade and high-grade, respectively. The BCAC-LG pattern is characterized by infiltrative areas composed of small to medium-sized basaloid cells with mild to moderate nuclear pleomorphism and increased mitotic activity. Lesions manifesting the BCAC-HG pattern are composed of medium-sized to large pleomorphic basaloid cells with numerous

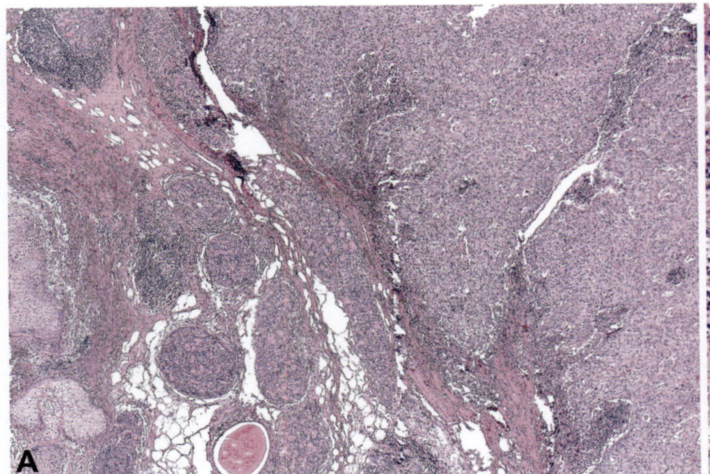


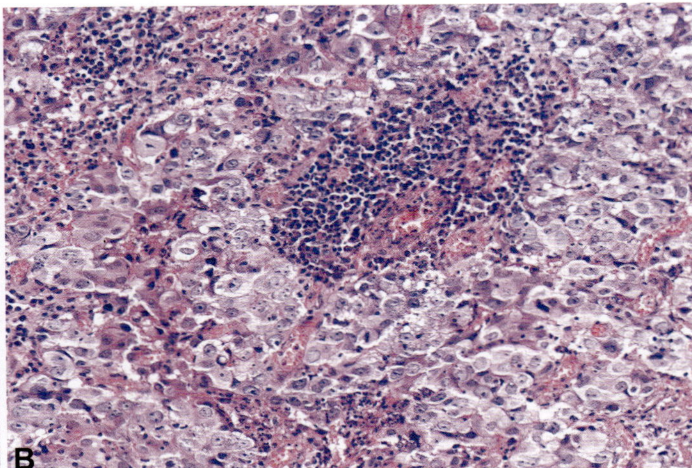


**Fig. 3.05** High-grade basal cell adenocarcinoma arising in a pre-existing spiradenoma. **A** A residuum of spiradenoma can be seen at the lower left. **A,B** The malignant portion is composed of medium-sized to large pleomorphic basaloid cells with numerous atypical mitotic figures and necrotic cells, presenting as confluent sheets and nodules with an infiltrative growth pattern (basal cell adenocarcinoma–like pattern, high-grade).

atypical mitotic figures and necrotic cells, presenting as confluent sheets and nodules with an infiltrative growth pattern. Invasive adenocarcinoma NOS is characterized by infiltrative sheets of large pleomorphic cells with ample pale to eosinophilic cytoplasm, sometimes displaying poorly developed glands with apocrine secretion. These gland-like structures are devoid of a peripheral myoepithelial cell layer. Sarcomatoid (metaplastic) carcinoma is a biphasic lesion, with epithelial and sarcomatoid malignant components. The epithelial component manifests varying combinations of the BCAC-HG and BCAC-LG patterns, or invasive adenocarcinoma NOS. Areas of squamous cell carcinoma may also be found. The appearances of the sarcomatoid component include unspecified pleomorphic sarcoma; spindle cell sarcoma; low-grade or high-grade chondrosarcoma; and tumours with osteosarcomatous, rhabdomyosarcomatous, and leiomyosarcomatous differentiation, sometimes occurring conjointly.

Immunohistochemically, the tumours express cytokeratins, and ductal differentiation is highlighted by staining for EMA (epithelial membrane antigen) and CEA. Although staining for MYB is seen in benign spiradenoma, cylindroma, and spiradenocylindroma, MYB expression is lost in the malignant counterparts. The Ki-67 (MIB1) proliferation index may be increased in the malignant areas, and there is variable expression of p53 {1309,2042,2690}.

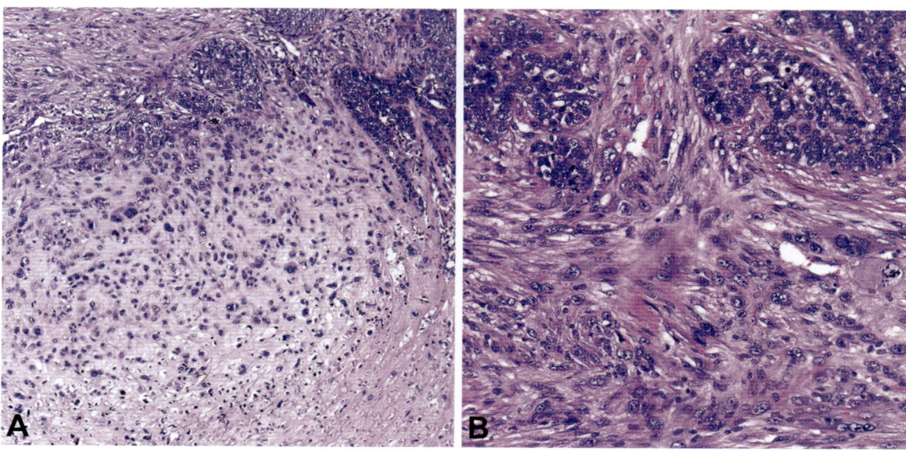

**Fig. 3.07** Several malignant patterns, including sarcomatoid carcinoma, in a pre-existing spiradenoma. **A,B** Note the transition from the atypical basaloid component to a sarcomatoid component.

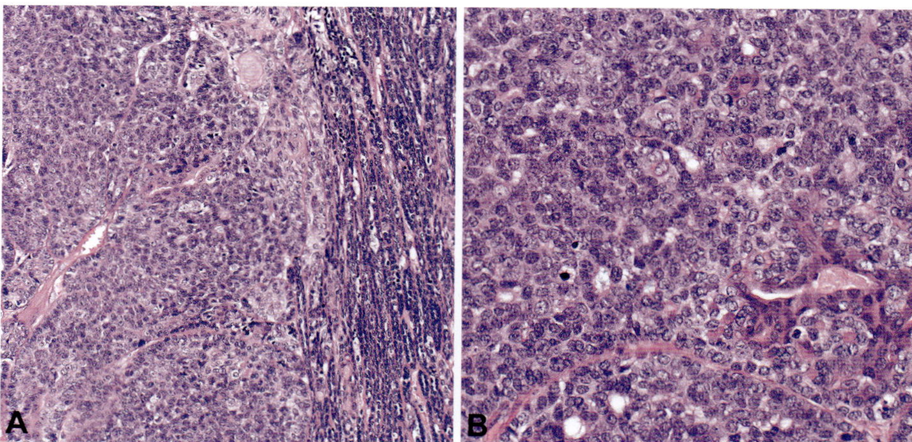

**Fig. 3.08** Malignant neoplasm arising in pre-existing spiradenoma. **A** The transition between the benign parent lesion and the evolving malignant neoplasm. **B** Higher magnification shows that the low-grade malignant area is characterized by loss of the dual cell differentiation, mild to moderate cytological atypia with nuclear crowding, and mitotic activity.

## Differential diagnosis

Rare spiradenomas focally display an atypical adenomatous/adenomyoepitheliomatous component, which may be a precursor adenocarcinoma in situ, but this component is not sufficient to qualify the neoplasm as malignant {1255,1320}. Rare variants of HPV-induced basaloid (cloacogenic) squamous cell carcinoma in the perianal area must be considered in the differential diagnosis {452,1258}.

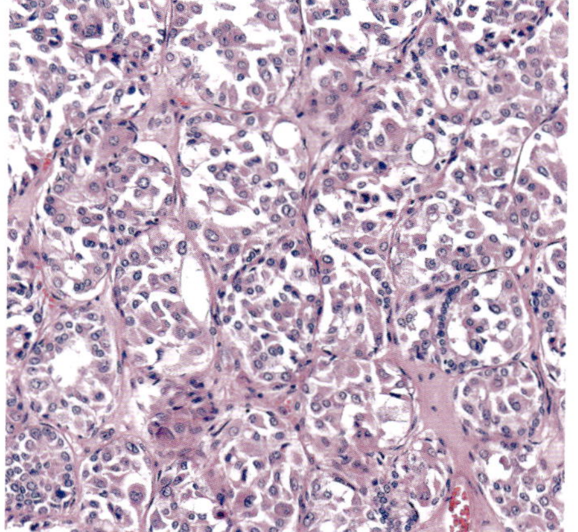

**Fig. 3.06** Invasive adenocarcinoma NOS arising from pre-existing spiradenoma exhibiting highly atypical cells arranged in an alveolar pattern with occasional lumina.

## Histogenesis

The tumours show sweat gland differentiation.

## Genetic profile

Little is known about the genetics of these tumours. Despite immunoexpression of p53, *TP53* mutations appear to be rare. *CYLD* mutations appear to be limited to tumours arising in the setting of Brooke–Spiegler syndrome {1298}.

## Genetic susceptibility

The tumours may arise in the setting of Brooke–Spiegler syndrome {1298}.

## Prognosis and predictive factors

Morphologically low-grade tumours have potential for local recurrence and can (rarely) extend into the underlying bone (on the scalp). Metastatic disease and mortality have only been reported with morphologically high-grade tumours. The behaviour of sarcomatoid (metaplastic) carcinomas appears to be favourable.

# Malignant mixed tumour

Kazakov D.V.
Argenyi Z.B.
Brenn T.
Calonje E.
Mehregan D.A.
Mehregan D.R.
Requena L.
Sangüeza O.P.
Santa Cruz D.J.
Scolyer R.A.
Zembowicz A.

### Definition

As strictly defined, the diagnosis of cutaneous malignant mixed tumour should only be made when a neoplasm has a clearly identifiable pre-existing benign component. However, in most reports published to date, this diagnosis was instead based on the biphasic (so-called mixed) appearance of a neoplasm in the absence of a recognizable pre-existing benign mixed tumour. In some cases, the benign neoplasm may have been completely overgrown by the evolving malignant neoplasm, but it is likely that tumours of different lineage have also been included in these reports. Cutaneous malignant mixed tumour as strictly defined is an extremely rare neoplasm {866,1190,1596, 1760,2142,2298,2367,2438,2655}.

### ICD-O code

8940/3

### Synonyms

Malignant chondroid syringoma; malignant apocrine mixed tumour

### Epidemiology

This neoplasm predominantly occurs in the elderly, with no sex predilection.

### Localization

The anatomical distribution is wide, with no specific site predilection.

### Clinical features

The neoplasms occur as a solitary nodule or tumour and may reach a large size (as large as 10 cm). There is sometimes a history of sudden rapid growth. Multiple cutaneous lesions have been reported in rare patients who presented with metastatic disease {866}.

### Histopathology

A pre-existing benign mixed tumour (usually an apocrine mixed tumour) in association with a malignant component is a prerequisite for the diagnosis of malignant mixed tumour. The remnants of the benign neoplasm are either juxtaposed with the malignant tissue or blend gradually with it. The malignant component shows heterogeneity from case to case and can display the following patterns: adenocarcinoma (apocrine), myoepithelial carcinoma, carcinoma NOS, and sarcomatoid (metaplastic) carcinoma. Adenocarcinoma is composed of sheets of tumour cells arranged in nodules, with glands and papillary structures in which apocrine secretion can be identified. In the absence of convincing apocrine features, the malignant component may be referred to as a carcinoma NOS. Myoepithelial carcinoma is usually diagnosed in lesions in which the pre-existing apocrine mixed tumour displays prominent myoepithelial cell differentiation (i.e. hyaline cell–rich tumours). Like the benign residual tumour cells, the malignant myoepithelial cells have eccentric nuclei and abundant eosinophilic hyaline cytoplasm, but display marked pleomorphism, atypical mitoses, and (sometimes) vascular involvement. Sarcomatoid (metaplastic) carcinoma is characterized by a gradual transition from a carcinomatous element to sarcomatoid tissue, which has the appearance of pleomorphic or spindle cell sarcoma NOS or of chondrosarcoma {866,1322,2367}.

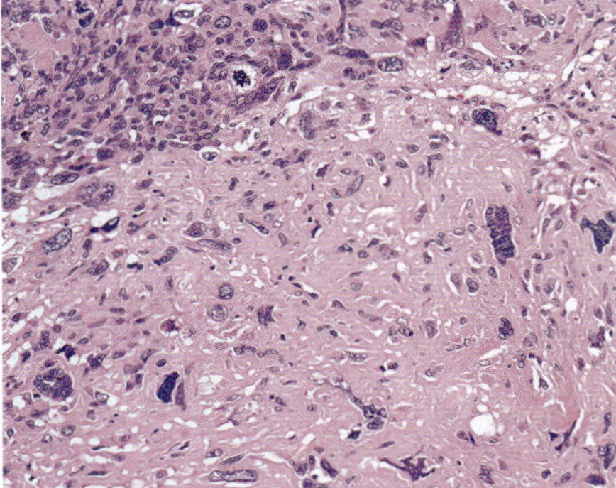

**Fig. 3.10** Malignant mixed tumour. In this example, the malignant component has a sarcomatous appearance.

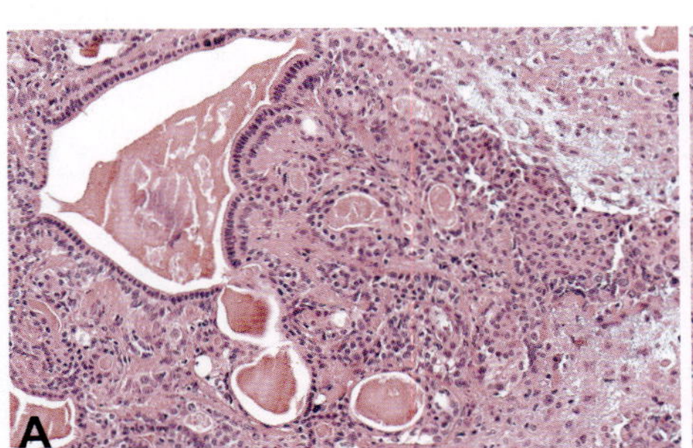

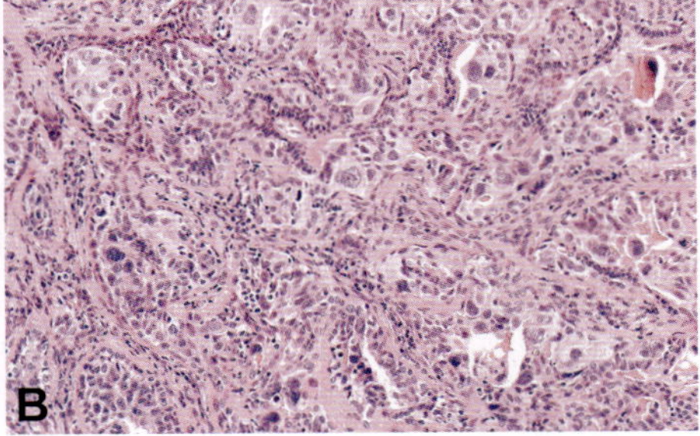

**Fig. 3.09** Malignant mixed tumour. **A** This part of the neoplasm exhibits features of apocrine mixed tumour (the pre-existing lesion). **B** There is transformation to adenocarcinoma. Note the atypical cells in the tubular areas.

### Differential diagnosis

Approximately 10% of cases of benign apocrine mixed tumour show focal atypical cytological features, including enlarged hyperchromatic cells and multinucleated bizarre cells, which are mainly seen in the areas with squamous cell metaplasia, among hyaline cells, or in foci of oxyphilic metaplasia {1299,1305}. However, most of these lesions manifest benign architectural features and follow a benign course. An important diagnostic pitfall is the presence of intravascular tumour deposits in an otherwise benign apocrine mixed tumour, which occurs in 1–2% of the neoplasms {1315}. An origin in another anatomical structure should be considered for tumours developing in skin overlying salivary glands, orbital tumours, and external auditory meatus tumours.

### Histogenesis

Although some apparent cases show no evidence of a benign residuum, it is disputed whether these tumours can occur de novo {2156}.

### Prognosis and predictive factors

There have been reports of recurrences and metastases to lymph nodes and distant sites in cases fulfilling the strict definition given above.

# Hidradenocarcinoma

Kazakov D.V.
Argenyi Z.B.
Brenn T.
Calonje E.
Mehregan D.A.
Mehregan D.R.
Requena L.
Sangüeza O.P.
Santa Cruz D.J.
Scolyer R.A.
Zembowicz A.

## Definition

Hidradenocarcinoma is a rare adnexal neoplasm constituting the malignant counterpart of hidradenoma, a residuum of which can be detected in some cases. Tumours in which no benign residuum is seen may have occurred de novo, or the carcinoma might have overgrown the benign parent lesion.

## ICD-O code 8402/3

## Synonyms

Clear cell eccrine hidradenocarcinoma; clear cell hidradenocarcinoma; malignant clear cell acrospiroma; mucoepidermoid carcinoma; apocrine hidradenocarcinoma; malignant eccrine acrospiroma

## Epidemiology

There is a slight male predominance, with most patients in the fifth to seventh decade of life.

## Localization

There is a slight predilection for the head and neck, but the anatomical distribution is wide.

## Clinical features

Hidradenocarcinoma is a solitary tumour varying in size from 1 cm to 6 cm. Rare patients with metastatic disease present with multiple cutaneous lesions. The reported duration of the symptoms is 1–40 years. The very rapid growth of some longstanding neoplasms is consistent with the malignant transformation of a pre-existing hidradenoma.

## Histopathology

Hidradenocarcinoma is composed of the same cell types as in hidradenoma, including clear cells, squamoid cells, oncocytic cells, mucinous cells, eosinophilic polygonal cells, and transitional elements in variable proportions, usually with a predominance of clear cells or squamoid cells. The malignant cells show nuclear pleomorphism, increased mitotic activity, an infiltrative growth pattern, necrosis, and perineural and lymphovascular invasion. Both low-grade and high-grade tumours are recognized, and some neoplasms contain frankly anaplastic areas. In about one third of cases, a residuum of a benign hidradenoma is observed. However, in low-grade cases, the pre-existing hidradenoma can be difficult to recognize, because cytologically bland areas blend imperceptibly with the atypical cells. The stroma is often sclerotic and hyalinized; foci of desmoplastic stromal reaction, as well as clefts between the aggregates of the neoplastic cells and the stroma, are common {1312,1336,2543,2852}. An example of apocrine hidradenocarcinoma with mucinous cells showing intraepidermal pagetoid spread of neoplastic cells has been reported {2761}.

CEA and EMA (epithelial membrane antigen) decorate the luminal borders of ductal structures. Overexpression of ERBB2 (HER2) has occasionally been documented and has not been associated with *ERBB2* gene amplification as demonstrated by FISH {1312,1878,1887}. Ki-67 and p53 have been evaluated for their value in distinguishing between hidradenoma and hidradenocarcinoma, with inconclusive results. However, the pre-existing benign hidradenoma is always p53-negative, a feature that can be useful as an aid to diagnosis {1396,1878,1887,1989}.

## Differential diagnosis

Low-grade neoplasms must be distinguished from benign hidradenoma, in which scattered mild cellular atypia can be found. The term "atypical hidradenoma" is as yet incompletely defined

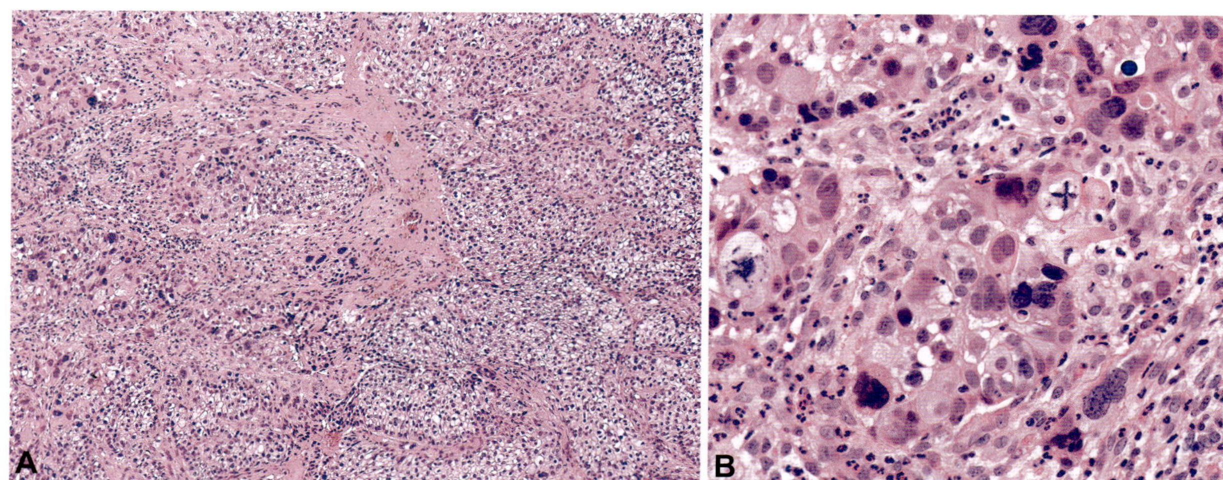

**Fig. 3.11** High-grade hidradenocarcinoma. **A,B** This neoplasm has a predominance of relatively bland clear cells admixed with highly pleomorphic, sometimes multinucleated bizarre cells exhibiting abnormal mitotic figures.

{1887}. A particular diagnostic pitfall is posed by cases of histologically benign hidradenomas with lymphatic involvement or evidence of a tumour in a regional lymph node diagnosed simultaneously with the cutaneous primary. Because follow-up of such cases has not revealed any adverse outcomes, it has been suggested that these tumours constitute so-called benign metastases. However, longer follow-up of more cases is needed to prove or disprove this theory {2505}. For clear cell–predominant cases, the differential diagnosis includes metastatic clear cell renal cell carcinoma, which is usually richly vascularized (often with so-called blood lakes or intratumoural haemorrhage) and typically coexpresses vimentin, PAX8, and carbonic anhydrase {51,1322}.

## Histogenesis

The histogenesis is unknown. Both apocrine and eccrine lineage have been proposed.

## Genetic profile

The t(11;19) translocation involving the genes *CRTC1* (previously called *MECT1*) and *MAML2* has been identified in hidradenocarcinoma, but this finding is significantly less common than in hidradenoma, in which about 50% of cases harbour the translocation {191,1312,1477,2841}. Less than 20% of hidradenocarcinomas harbour a mutation in *TP53* {1312}.

## Prognosis and predictive factors

The available data are limited and vary across studies. The aggressive course (with distant metastasis to skin, lymph nodes, bones, and lungs) and poor prognosis found in some studies {1396,2489} have not been supported by others {1312,1887}. Metastatic disease has been documented in both low-grade and high-grade tumours {1312}.

# Mucinous carcinoma

Kazakov D.V.
Argenyi Z.B.
Brenn T.
Calonje E.
Mehregan D.A.
Mehregan D.R.
Requena L.
Sangüeza O.P.
Santa Cruz D.J.
Scolyer R.A.
Zembowicz A.

## Definition

Mucinous carcinoma of the skin is a rare adnexal carcinoma histopathologically identical to homologous lesions in the breast. Some tumours that are solid, have a minimal mucinous component, and express neuroendocrine markers are best diagnosed as endocrine mucin-producing sweat gland carcinoma, which is considered by some authors to be a precursor entity {2927}.

## ICD-O code 8480/3

## Synonyms

Colloid carcinoma; gelatinous carcinoma

## Epidemiology

To date, < 350 cases have been reported. A systematic review of 159 published cases found that 122 (~77%) of the patients were White, 20 (~13%) were Asian, and 16 (~10%) were Black {1269}. There is no sex predominance, and the majority of patients are elderly (mean age: 63–65 years) {298,299,1329}.

## Localization

The most commonly reported location is the periorbital area (i.e. the eyelid or brow; accounting for 50% of cases), followed by non-periorbital areas of the face or neck (20% of cases) and the scalp (17% of cases) {1269}. Other localizations are rare. For rare neoplasms occurring in the anogenital area, an origin from anogenital mammary-like glands has been proposed {484}.

## Clinical features

Primary cutaneous mucinous carcinoma presents as a solitary, slow-growing nodule or cyst-like lesion that is flesh-coloured, blue, or erythematous and 0.5–8 cm in size, with most cases measuring 1.5–2 cm.

## Histopathology

The stereotypical presentation is that of neoplastic cells arranged in nests, strands, or individual units floating in lakes of extracellular mucin, sometimes separated by variably thin fibrous septa. The histopathological spectrum of primary cutaneous mucinous carcinoma is wide, and analogous to that seen in its mammary counterparts, with at least two distinguishable variants: a more common pure tumour in which extracellular mucin constitutes > 90% and a rare mixed form in which there is an invasive ductal component in addition to the mucinous element {1329,2874}. The floating neoplastic epithelial cells are usually relatively monomorphous, although some tumours may show substantial nuclear pleomorphism. Mitoses are generally scarce. An essential feature, which should be looked for, is an in situ component; it is detected in most cases (60–70%) and defines the neoplasm as primary cutaneous. In situ lesions usually constitute the minor moiety, and they include (using mammary pathology terminology) ductal hyperplasia, atypical ductal hyperplasia, and ductal carcinoma in situ (cribriform, micropapillary, papillary, and solid), occurring individually or (more rarely) in combination.

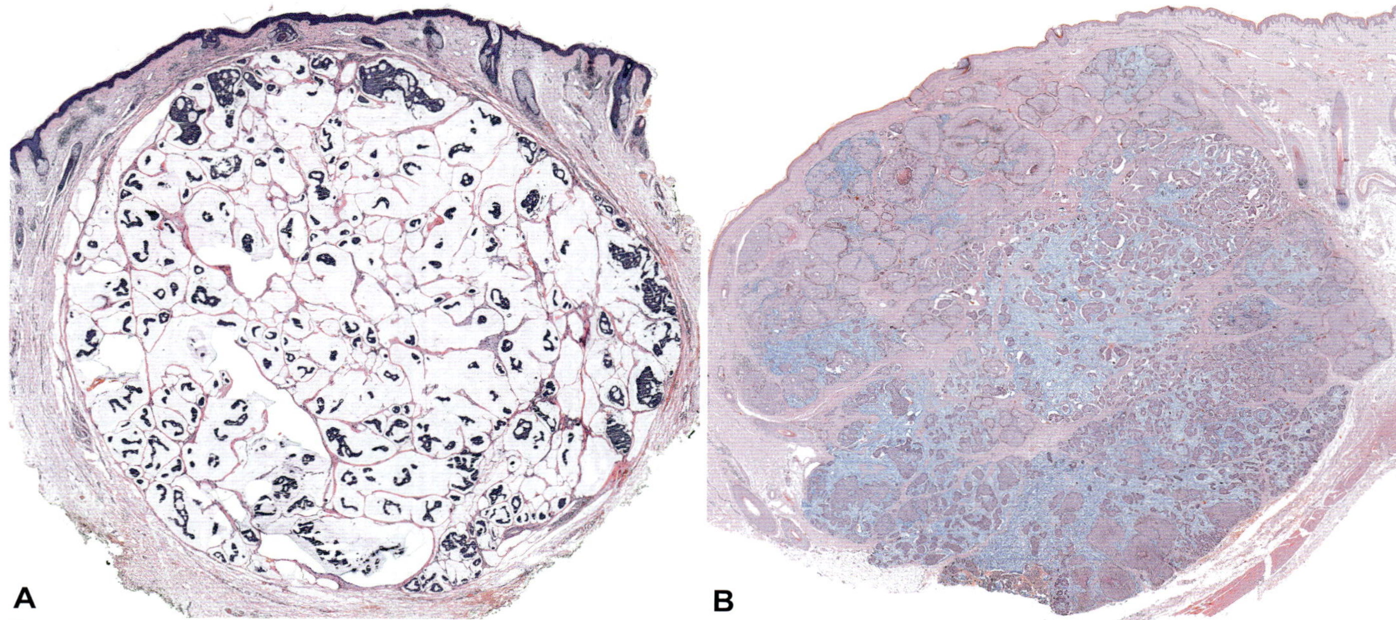


**Fig. 3.12** Mucinous carcinoma. **A** Neoplastic cells are arranged in nests, strands, or individual units floating in lakes of extracellular mucin, separated by variably thin fibrous septa. In this lesion, extracellular mucin constitutes > 90% (the pure type of mucinous carcinoma). **B** There is an invasive ductal component in addition to the mucinous component (the mixed type of mucinous carcinoma).

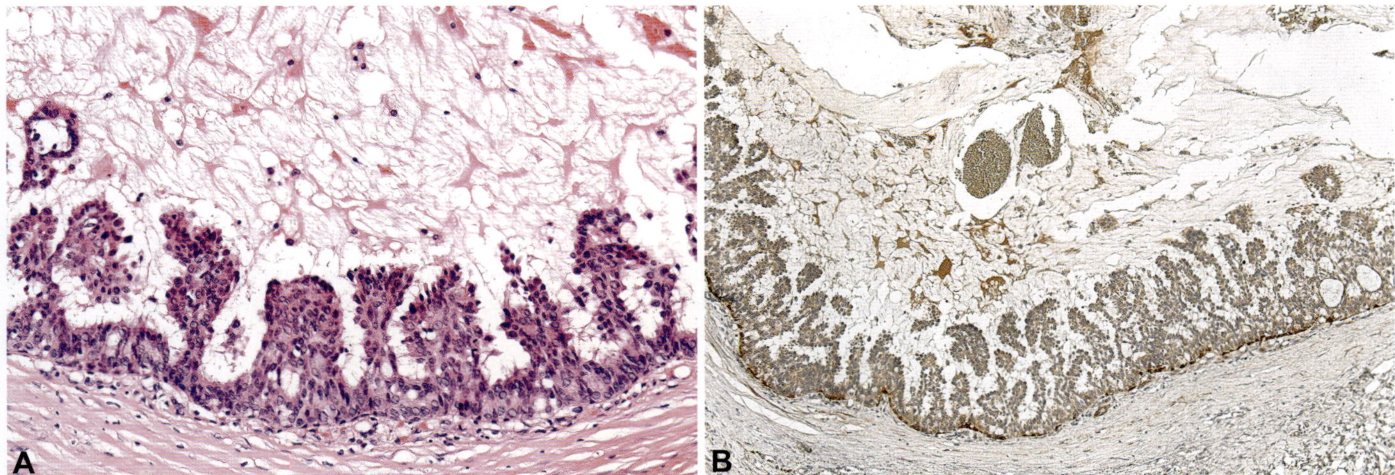


**Fig. 3.13** Mucinous carcinoma. An in situ component in mucinous carcinoma of the skin is a strong indicator of primary cutaneous origin; in situ lesions range from various types of ductal hyperplasia to ductal carcinoma in situ. **A** The in situ component corresponds to ductal carcinoma in situ of micropapillary type. **B** Staining for calponin highlights preserved basal/myoepithelial cells in the ductal carcinoma in situ.

Immunohistochemically, the in situ component may be highlighted by staining for myoepithelial markers (including p63 and calponin). The epithelial neoplastic cells express low-molecular-weight cytokeratins, EMA (epithelial membrane antigen), CEA, E-cadherin, and GCDFP15. Estrogen receptor and progesterone receptor are expressed in most cases. The typical CK7+/CK20− phenotype can sometimes be useful in the differential diagnosis with metastatic lesions. Neuroendocrine differentiation can be encountered in cutaneous mucinous carcinomas of both pure and mixed types, without a prominent solid component.

## Differential diagnosis

Because histologically identical neoplasms can occur in other organs, primary cutaneous mucinous carcinoma must be differentiated from a metastasis or direct invasion from an underlying extracutaneous neoplasm {1981}. The presence of an in situ component qualifies the tumour as primary cutaneous; however, its absence does not necessarily imply an extracutaneous origin, because disrupted myoepithelial cells may no longer be identifiable during disease progression {1329,2120}. For such cases, a full clinical work-up is needed to establish the origin. Potential pitfalls related to in situ lesions include mammary carcinoma originating from an intradermal lactiferous duct (which could be indistinguishable from a primary cutaneous lesion) and the misinterpretation of normal-looking pre-existing ducts and glands as an in situ lesion. Localization of the tumour on the chest wall and axilla is a strong indicator of mammary origin, whereas microscopic identification of dirty necrosis (derangement of cells resulting in cellular debris) and goblet cell differentiation is a clue to intestinal origin. Rare cases of primary mucinous carcinoma with numerous signet-ring cells, lesions associated with extramammary Paget disease, and lesions in which the mucinous component is scant also pose particular pitfalls. For lesions in which the mucinous component is scant, serial sections or other blocks may reveal the typical mucinous appearance {1329}.

## Histogenesis

Although electron microscopic studies have suggested an eccrine lineage, about 50% of cases exhibit apocrine secretion, supporting apocrine differentiation.

## Genetic profile

The gene encoding ERBB2 (HER2) was not found to have been amplified in the few tumours in which it has been investigated.

## Prognosis and predictive factors

Primary cutaneous mucinous carcinoma has a propensity to recur, but the recurrence rate is lower after surgery with intraoperative evaluation of surgical margins (i.e. either Mohs surgery or excision with frozen section control) {1269,1977}. Tumours located on the trunk tend to have a worse outcome than those on the head and neck; however, some trunk lesions involve the axilla, raising the possibility of a misdiagnosed breast primary. Increased rates of recurrence and metastasis have been associated with White race, younger age at presentation, and large tumour size (> 1.5 cm) {1269}.

# Endocrine mucin-producing sweat gland carcinoma

Zembowicz A.
Argenyi Z.B.
Brenn T.
Calonje E.
Mehregan D.A.
Mehregan D.R.
Requena L.
Sangüeza O.P.
Santa Cruz D.J.
Scolyer R.A.

## Definition

Endocrine mucin-producing sweat gland carcinoma is a low-grade neuroendocrine neoplasm and the cutaneous analogue of solid papillary adenocarcinoma of the breast. It shows a striking predilection for the eyelid and periorbital skin. In at least some cases, endocrine mucin-producing sweat gland carcinoma is a precursor of mucinous carcinoma {2927}.

## ICD-O code 8509/3

## Epidemiology

Endocrine mucin-producing sweat gland carcinoma is a rare tumour with a predilection for older individuals (i.e. in the sixth and seventh decades of life). Women are affected more frequently than men {2927}.

## Localization

Most endocrine mucin-producing sweat gland carcinomas arise on the eyelids and periorbital skin. However, occurrence in an extrafacial location has also been reported {2657}.

## Clinical features

Endocrine mucin-producing sweat gland carcinoma presents as a slow-growing skin-coloured or bluish nodule or papule. Some lesions give the clinical impression of a cyst. Multiple tumours in the same patient have been described {2927}.

## Histopathology

Endocrine mucin-producing sweat gland carcinoma grows as well-demarcated expansile nodules with cystic, solid, papillary, or cribriform architecture. Papillary projections are associated with fibrovascular cores. The tumour cells are small to intermediate-sized, polygonal to round ductal cells with amphophilic or bluish cytoplasm and round to oval nuclei with very fine chromatin and inconspicuous nucleoli. Small amounts of intracellular and extracellular mucin can be demonstrated by mucicarmine staining {793,2927}. Mitotic activity is low. The Ki-67 proliferation index is < 5–10%. Tumour necrosis is not observed. An origin of carcinoma in situ within dilated eccrine ducts lined by benign ductal epithelium with myoepithelial cells can be demonstrated in many cases. Larger expansile nodules usually lack the myoepithelial cell layer consistent with carcinoma with pushing invasion. The presence of extracellular pools of stromal

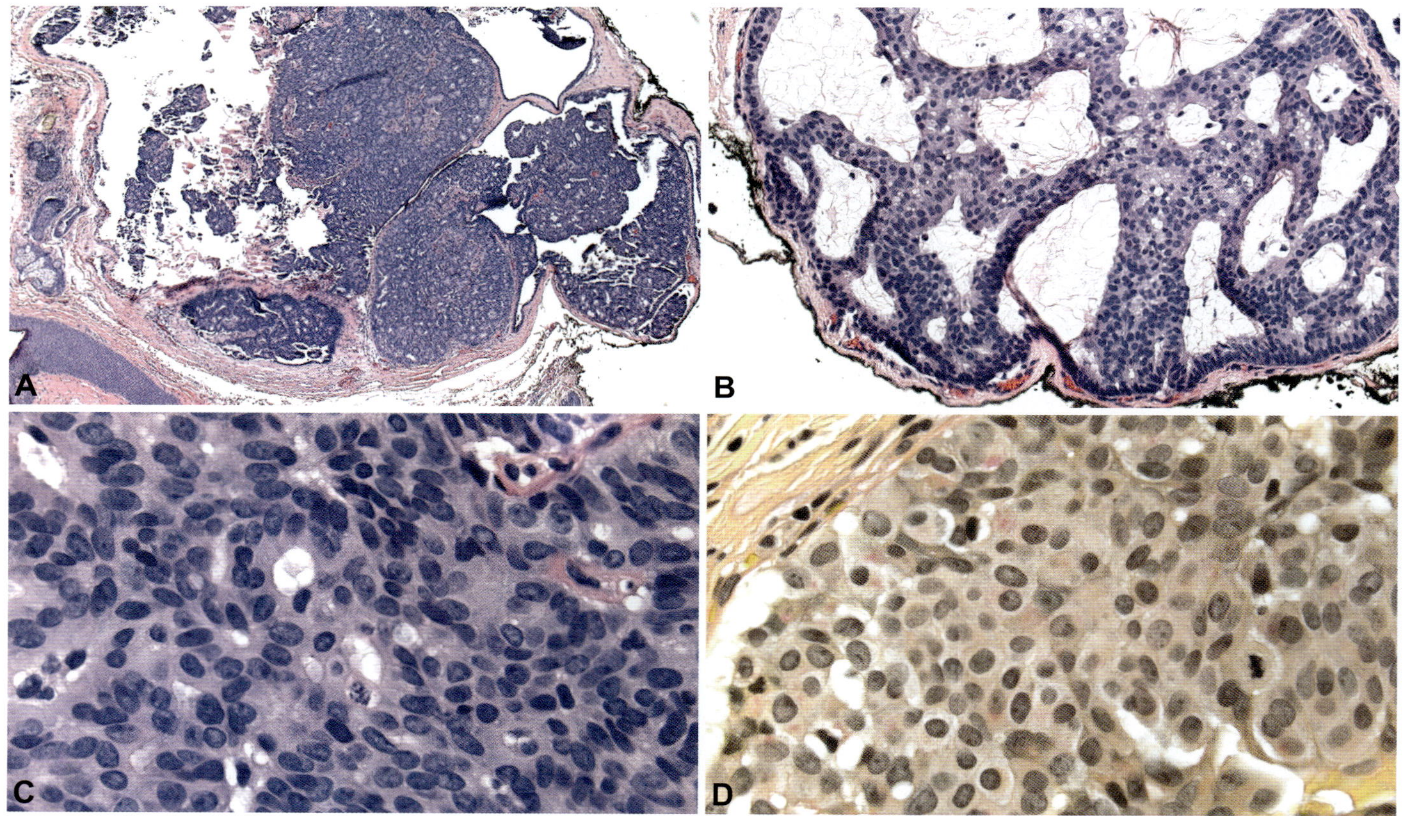


**Fig. 3.14** Endocrine mucin-producing sweat gland carcinoma. **A** Well-demarcated nodule with solid, papillary, and cystic growth patterns. **B** An area of cribriform architecture. **C** Intermediate-sized ductal cells with amphophilic cytoplasm and fine chromatin. **D** Intracellular and intercellular mucin is highlighted by mucicarmine staining.

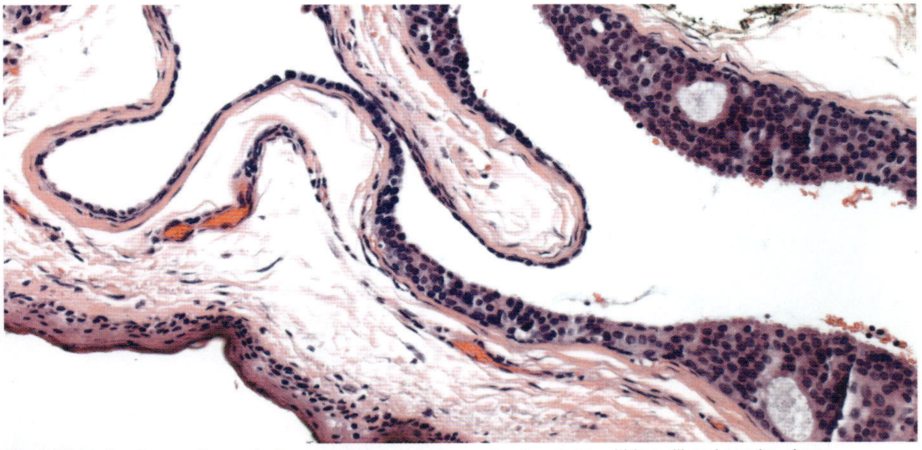

Fig. 3.15 Endocrine mucin-producing sweat gland carcinoma in situ arising within a dilated eccrine duct.

mucin and/or infiltrating tumour glands and nests indicates progression to mucinous adenocarcinoma. Immunohistochemically, endocrine mucin-producing sweat gland carcinoma is positive for CK7, CK8, CK18, AE1/AE3, CAM5.2, EMA (epithelial membrane antigen), GCDFP15, WT1, estrogen receptor, and progesterone receptor {11,754,2430,2927}. The intensity of expression of neuroendocrine markers (chromogranin and synaptophysin) varies. Staining can be weak and focal or even absent in a small biopsy. Myoepithelial markers help identify areas of carcinoma in situ lined by myoepithelial cells, but are usually negative in larger nodules {2927}.

## Differential diagnosis

The histological differential diagnosis of endocrine mucin-producing sweat gland carcinoma includes hidradenoma, hidrocystoma with papillary ductal hyperplasia, apocrine adenoma, and apocrine adenocarcinoma. Hybrid lesions containing mucinous adenocarcinoma should be diagnosed as mucinous adenocarcinoma.

## Histogenesis

Endocrine mucin-producing sweat gland carcinoma arises in eccrine ducts.

## Prognosis and predictive factors

In the absence of mucinous adenocarcinoma, endocrine mucin-producing sweat gland carcinoma has an excellent prognosis after excision with clear margins, but the tumour can recur {685,1412}. Metastases of endocrine mucin-producing sweat gland carcinoma have not been documented.

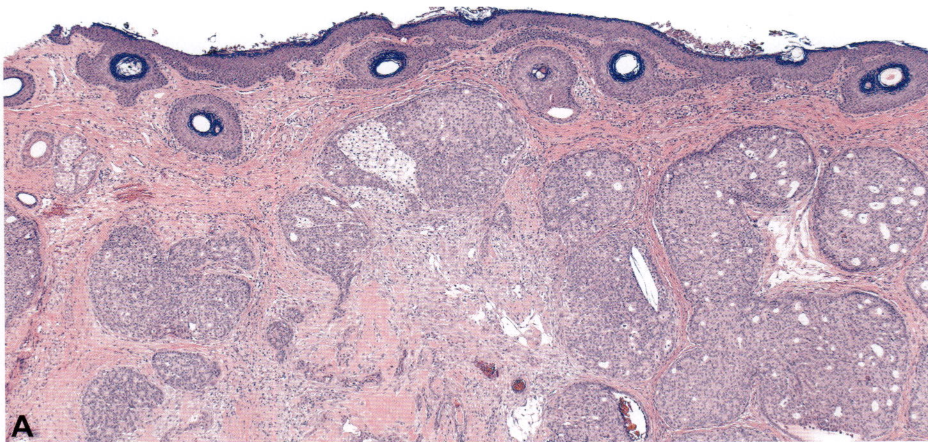


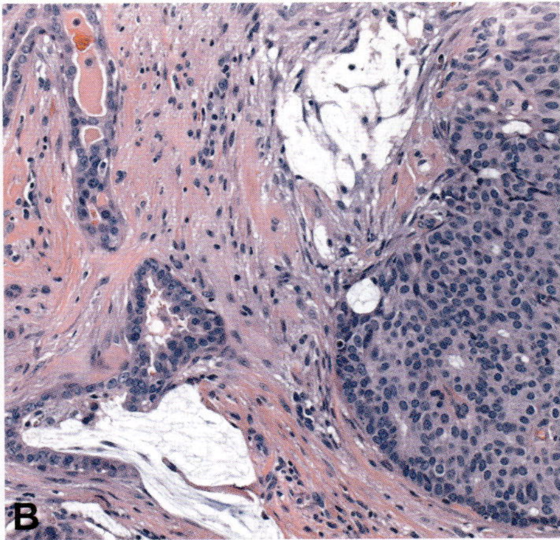


Fig. 3.16 Endocrine mucin-producing sweat gland carcinoma. **A** A focus of early mucinous adenocarcinoma arising in an endocrine mucin-producing sweat gland carcinoma. **B** Higher magnification reveals the presence of stromal mucin and glands, indicating progression to mucinous adenocarcinoma.

# Digital papillary adenocarcinoma

Kazakov D.V.
Argenyi Z.B.
Brenn T.
Calonje E.
Mehregan D.A.
Mehregan D.R.
Requena L.
Sangüeza O.P.
Santa Cruz D.J.
Scolyer R.A.
Zembowicz A.

### Definition
Digital papillary adenocarcinoma is a malignant adnexal tumour with a marked predilection for acral sites. Historically, both aggressive digital papillary adenomas and digital adenocarcinomas were recognized, but cases originally classified as aggressive digital papillary adenoma later developed metastases {1282}; therefore, the term "adenoma" has now been abandoned in this setting, and all such lesions are classified as digital papillary adenocarcinoma.

### ICD-O code 8408/3

### Synonyms
Aggressive digital papillary adenoma and adenocarcinoma; digital papillary carcinoma

### Epidemiology
The patient age at presentation is 14–83 years (average: 52 years), with a male preponderance {655,2527}.

### Etiology
A history of antecedent trauma has been reported by some patients {655}.

### Localization
The fingers, toes, and adjacent skin of the palms and soles are affected. The hands are more commonly involved (accounting for >80% of cases) than the feet.

### Clinical features
The neoplasm presents as a slow-growing, asymptomatic, deeply seated nodule in most cases, measuring an average of 1.7 cm (range: 0.4–4.3 cm). The reported duration of symptoms prior to excision is between 2 months and 15 years. The tumour can sometimes be clinically confused with a ganglion or a cyst. Ulceration is rare. Pain may occur if the neoplasm involves the underlying bone, joint, or nerves. Rarely, patients present with metastatic disease.

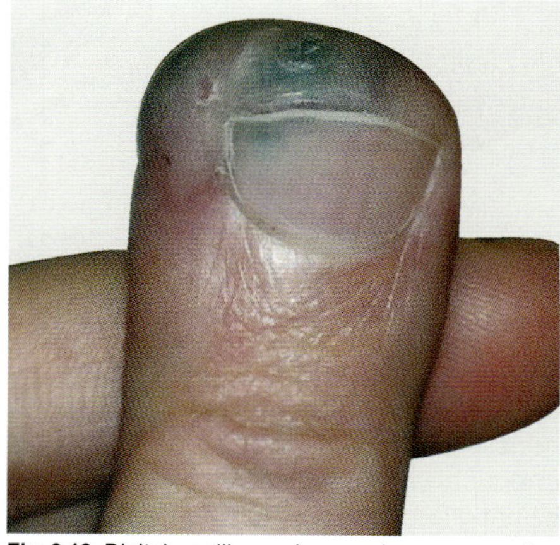

**Fig. 3.18** Digital papillary adenocarcinoma presenting as an asymmetrical deep-seated nodule.

### Histopathology
Digital papillary adenocarcinoma is usually a multinodular, poorly or well-circumscribed lesion located within the dermis and often the subcutaneous tissue, without a connection to the epidermis. A mixture of solid, cystic, and papillary growth patterns is usually seen. In the areas with papillary structures, both true papillae with a supportive fibrous core and pseudopapillae lacking a core protruding into or lying free within the cystic spaces may be seen. A typical feature is the presence of fused back-to-back glands lined by cuboidal to low columnar epithelial cells, occasionally showing apocrine secretion. At the periphery of the glands, basal/myoepithelial cells can sometimes be recognized. In rare cases, all tumour lobules and nests are associated with a peripheral layer of myoepithelial cells consistent with an adenocarcinoma in situ {1322,2527}. In invasive areas, myoepithelial cells are absent, suggesting an adenocarcinoma in situ–invasive adenocarcinoma sequence. Cytological atypia is mild to moderate in most cases; high-grade lesions are less

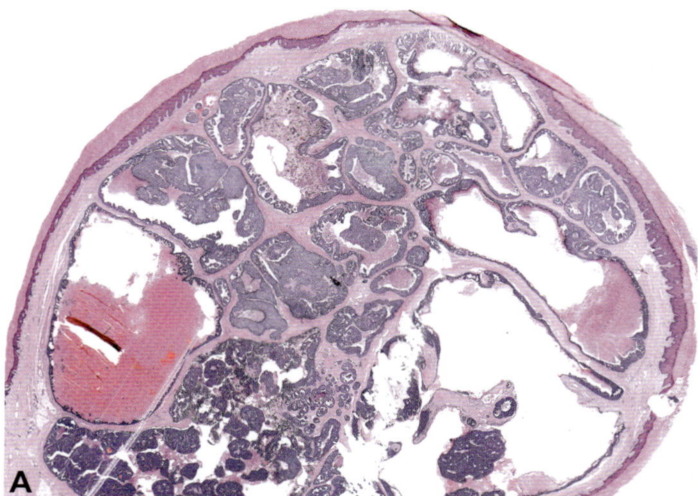

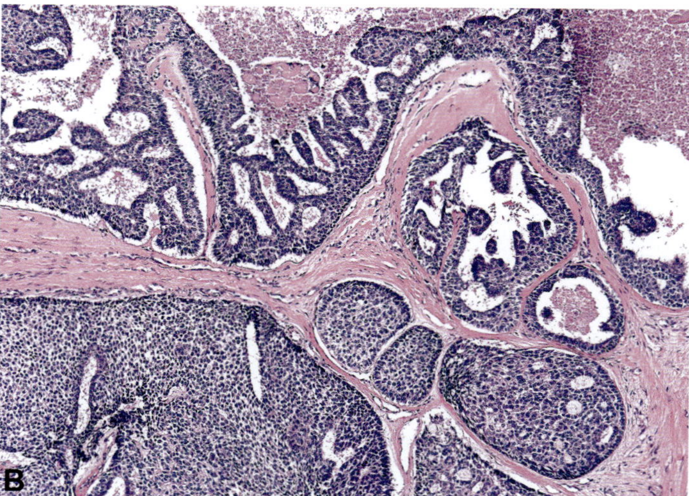

**Fig. 3.17** Digital papillary adenocarcinoma. **A,B** Multinodular, poorly circumscribed neoplasm exhibiting solid, cystic, and papillary areas.

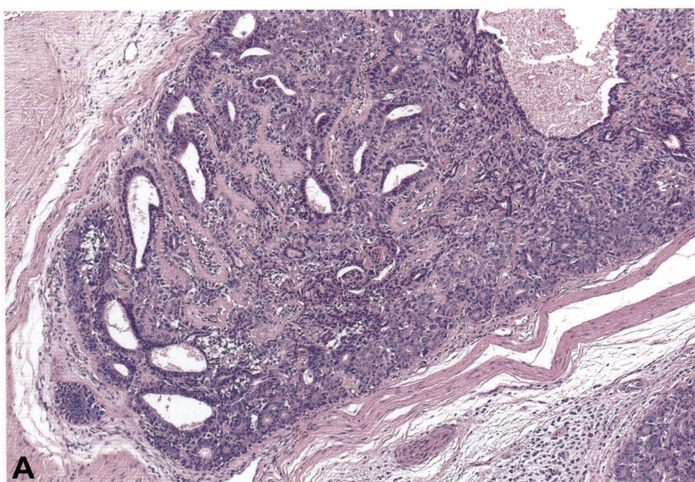
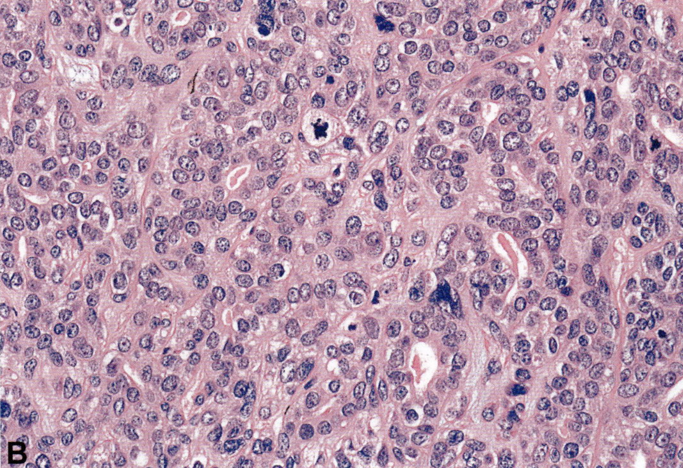

**Fig. 3.19** Digital papillary adenocarcinoma. **A** Glandular structures can be prominent. **B** Note the nuclear pleomorphism and mitotic figures.

common. The mitotic rate is extremely variable {655,2527,2527}. In a subset of cases, more solid areas dominate, and as many as 20% of these neoplasms are essentially solid, with areas of necrosis. Squamous metaplasia and focal clear cell change may be present. The stroma is paucicellular, hyalinized, and (rarely) myxomatous. Involvement of lymphatic vessels is uncommon {198,2527}.

Immunohistochemically, the tumour cells are diffusely positive for pancytokeratin and CK7. Staining for EMA (epithelial membrane antigen) and CEA highlights the glands and luminal borders of the papillae. Immunostaining for S100 protein is variable in both luminal cells and myoepithelial cells. The myoepithelial cells stain for SMA, calponin, p63, and (focally) podoplanin (recognized by D2-40) {1322,2265,2527}.

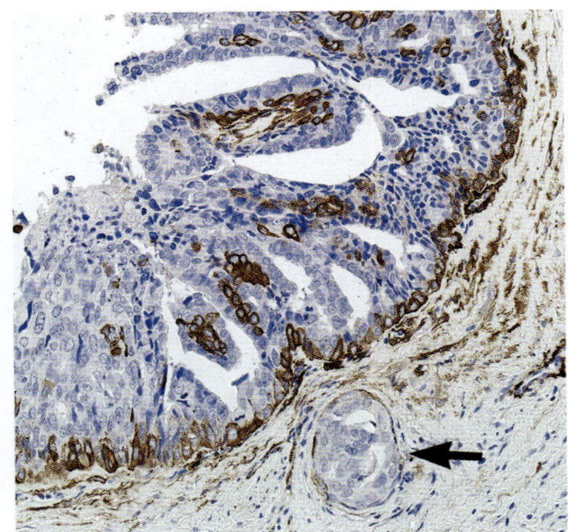

**Fig. 3.20** Digital papillary adenocarcinoma. Staining for α-SMA reveals a myoepithelial cell layer around glands and its absence around an invasive focus (arrow).

## Differential diagnosis

When partial biopsies of acral lesions show papillary changes, complete excision is recommended {1814}.

Tubular papillary adenoma is a neoplasm in which micropapillary or (rarely) true papillary projections are seen, but the tumour is usually well circumscribed and lacks solid areas and back-to-back glands {1302,2156}.

A particular pitfall occurs in superficial small biopsies in acral locations showing large unilocular or multilocular intradermal cystic spaces lined by a double layer of epithelial cells with micropapillae lacking cellular atypia or necrosis, closely resembling apocrine hidrocystoma or cystadenoma. It is important to remember that true acral apocrine hidrocystomas and cystadenomas are exceedingly rare {2311}.

The rare cases of hidradenoma and hidradenocarcinoma that feature glandular differentiation and areas of micropapillary growth can be difficult to distinguish from digital papillary adenocarcinoma, especially in limited biopsy specimens {1322}. However, these tumours have different cytological components, often combining clear cells, epidermoid (squamoid) cells, mucinous cells, and some transitional cellular forms. The lack of an outer myoepithelial cell layer in the glandular areas is a clue to the possibility of hidradenoma, a diagnosis which should be made with great circumspection in this site.

## Histogenesis

The decapitation secretion of apocrine type seen in some neoplasms may indicate apocrine differentiation; however, ultrastructural studies have demonstrated three types of neoplastic cells: clear cells, dark cells, and myoepithelial cells, with the presence of dense granules in the luminal border of some dark cells, leading to the conclusion that digital papillary adenocarcinoma is an eccrine tumour {1282}. The predilection of this neoplasm for acral sites, where eccrine glands are abundant, also supports an eccrine lineage.

## Genetic profile

A study of 9 cases revealed a single case with a BRAF p.V600E mutation; other oncogenic mutations (i.e. of *EGFR*, *PIK3CA*, *KRAS*, *NRAS*, *HRAS*, and *MET*) were not identified {198}.

## Prognosis and predictive factors

The reported rates of local recurrence and metastasis are 5–21% and 26–50%, respectively {655,2527}. Complete excision, or a partial amputation of the affected digit, considerably decreases the risk of recurrence and metastasis {2527}. The most common site of metastasis is the lung, followed by the lymph nodes. Metastases have been reported to develop as long as 20 years after excision of the primary neoplasm {2527}. Half of the patients with metastatic disease died in one series {655}. Histopathological features appear not to be predictive of metastatic potential {2527}.

# Adenoid cystic carcinoma

Kazakov D.V.
Argenyi Z.B.
Brenn T.
Calonje E.
Mehregan D.A.
Mehregan D.R.
Requena L.
Sangüeza O.P.
Santa Cruz D.J.
Scolyer R.A.
Zembowicz A.

## Definition

Adenoid cystic carcinoma (ACC) of the skin is a rare malignant neoplasm histologically identical to homonymous tumours in the salivary gland, respiratory tract, ear, lacrimal gland, ceruminous gland, Bartholin gland, and breast {19,211,1052,1610}.

## ICD-O code 8200/3

## Epidemiology

An incidence rate of 0.23 cases per 1 million person-years has been reported {643}. This neoplasm generally affects middle-aged to elderly individuals (average age: ~60 years). There is a slight female predilection, with a female-to-male ratio of 1.5:1.

## Localization

The most common location is the scalp (affected in ~30% of cases), followed by the trunk (in particular the chest wall) and abdomen, which are affected in about 25% of cases. Other locations are rare {2819}.

## Clinical features

ACC presents as a solitary nodule averaging 3 cm in size (range: 0.5–8 cm), often present for several years prior to diagnosis. Pain and hyperaesthesia have rarely been reported {525}.

## Histopathology

ACCs are characterized by a mixture of cribriform, tubular, and solid patterns forming variably shaped nodules in the dermis and/or subcutis. The essential diagnostic feature is the coexistence of true small bilayered ducts and pseudocysts. The true ductal structures are usually sparse, have small round lumina, and are composed of inner epithelial cells with uniform round nuclei (sometimes with small nucleoli) surrounded by an outer layer of basal/myoepithelial cells. Intraluminal secretion can be seen. The pseudocystic structures are usually larger than ducts, and they contain abundant basophilic mucinous material that stains positively with Alcian blue at pH 2.5 and/or hyalinized eosinophilic material that gives a positive periodic acid–Schiff (PAS) reaction. The pseudocysts are often surrounded on the luminal edge by a thin layer of hyalinized connective tissue. The solid areas are composed of small basaloid cells with hyperchromatic, slightly angulated nuclei and scant cytoplasm. Mitotic activity is typically low in ACC, and cellular pleomorphism is usually not a feature, although rare cases with high-grade atypia have been reported {2128}. Perineural invasion is a common feature, whereas intraneural invasion is rare. The stroma is hyalinized and paucicellular. Occasional tumours display myxoid change, and fibrosis may be seen.

Immunohistochemically, the neoplastic cells show diffuse cytoplasmic positivity for broad-spectrum keratins, CAM5.2, and CK7. Staining with CK5/6 and D2-40 is variable. The basaloid and myoepithelial cells display nuclear staining for SOX10. EMA (epithelial membrane antigen), CEA, and CK15 label the luminal cells surrounding the true ducts. The myoepithelial component is highlighted by staining for SMA, p63, and calponin. The pattern of staining for vimentin is similar to that for p63. Most tumours express MYB, and all tumours are positive for KIT (CD117) {714,1918}.

## Differential diagnosis

Cutaneous secretory carcinoma consists of back-to-back tubules and microcysts with conspicuous intraluminal secretions and shows a distinctive positivity for S100 protein, mammaglobin, STAT5A, and NTRK3 {253}. Adenoid basal cell carcinoma is distinguished from ACC by its lack of true ductal structures with

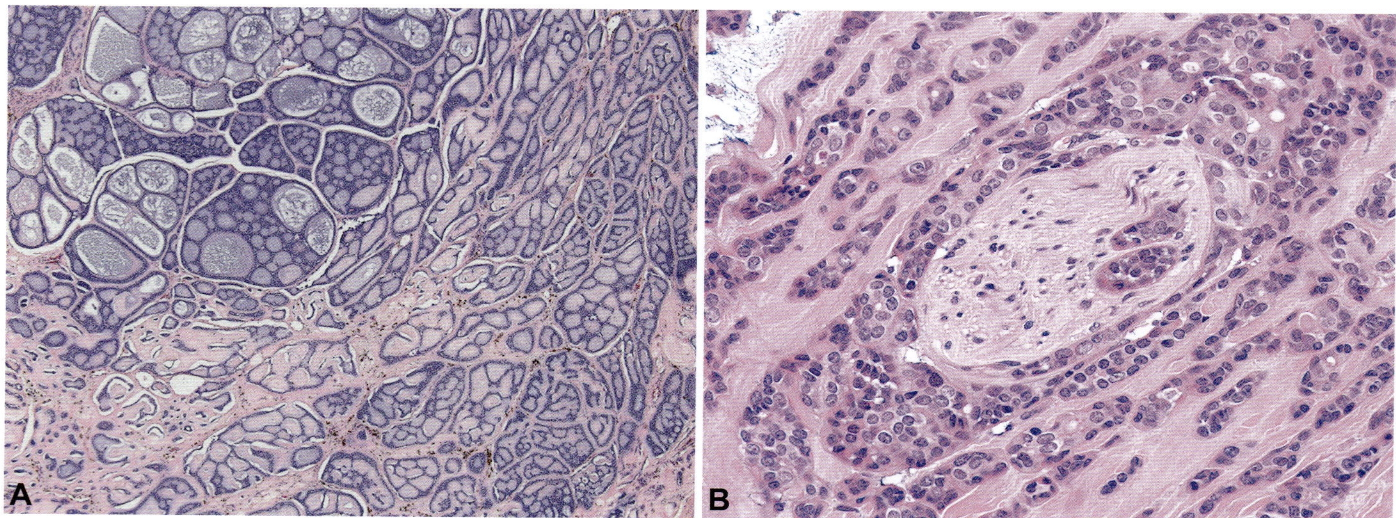

Fig. 3.21 Adenoid cystic carcinoma. The cribriform pattern (**A**) and perineural or intraneural invasion (**B**).

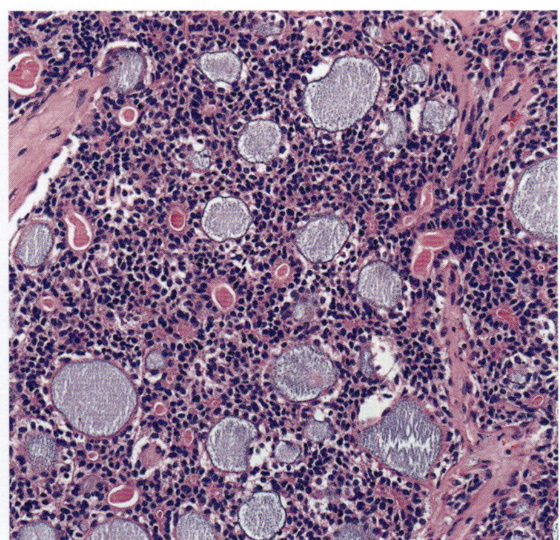

**Fig. 3.22** Adenoid cystic carcinoma. The essential diagnostic feature is the coexistence of true small bilayered ducts and pseudocysts.

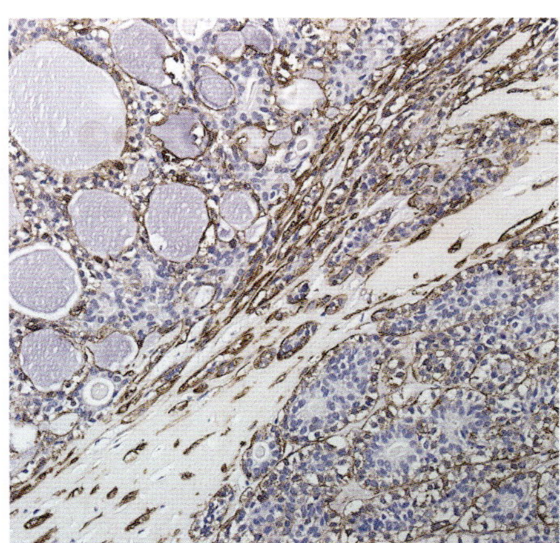

**Fig. 3.23** Adenoid cystic carcinoma. Areas with myoepithelial differentiation stain positively for α-SMA.

myoepithelial cells, the presence of peripheral palisading of neoplastic cells and retraction artefact (often associated with stromal mucin), and at least focal areas of conventional basal cell carcinoma {2819}. Cribriform carcinoma is composed of more eosinophilic cells, lacks myoepithelial cells, and focally manifests solid areas and peculiar thin thread-like intraluminal bridging strands {1323,2264}. Rare cases of spiradenoma and spiradenocylindroma display areas resembling ACC by virtue of a cribriform pattern; homogeneous, eosinophilic, or granular basophilic material; and/or ductal structures with a recognizable peripheral myoepithelial cell layer. The proportion of the ACC-like pattern varies from 5% to 30% of the tumour volume; therefore, the identification of typical areas of spiradenoma/cylindroma, as well as the absence of nuclear pleomorphism, perineural growth, and increased mitotic activity, facilitates the recognition of this spiradenoma/spiradenocylindroma variant {2040}. MYB immunoexpression alone does not equate with the diagnosis of ACC; other adnexal tumours have also been found to significantly express MYB {714}.

## Histogenesis

The eccrine or apocrine origin of this tumour remains disputed.

## Genetic profile

About 60% of ACCs harbour *MYB* gene activations, either through *MYB* chromosomal abnormalities or (less commonly) by *MYB-NFIB* fusion {2100}. The *MYB-NFIB* fusion oncogene, which results from the recurrent chromosomal translocation t(6;9)(q22-23;p23-24), activates the transcription of genes involved in cell-cycle control, DNA repair, and apoptosis. The t(6;9) translocation appears to be tumour-type–specific; it has been identified in ACCs arising in various anatomical locations {1918}.

## Prognosis and predictive factors

ACC of the skin has a propensity for local recurrence, which has been reported to occur in >50% of cases {2368}. Rare cases metastasizing to regional lymph nodes or distant sites (lung, pleura, or liver) have been reported {434}. Lesions located in the vulva may behave more aggressively, but larger studies are needed to validate this supposition. No statistically significant association has been found between tumour grade and local recurrence {2128}.

# Apocrine carcinoma

Kazakov D.V.
Argenyi Z.B.
Brenn T.
Calonje E.
Mehregan D.A.
Mehregan D.R.
Requena L.
Sangüeza O.P.
Santa Cruz D.J.
Scolyer R.A.
Zembowicz A.

## Definition

Apocrine carcinoma is a rare cutaneous adnexal neoplasm that manifests unequivocal signs of apocrine secretion (i.e. decapitation secretion and/or cytoplasmic zymogen granules) and lacks the defining microscopic features of other well-defined lesions with apocrine differentiation (e.g. syringocystadenocarcinoma papilliferum or mucinous carcinoma). It is not associated with and does not evolve from any pre-existing well-defined benign neoplasm (e.g. apocrine mixed tumour, cylindroma, or spiradenoma), and it is not associated with a specific glandular origin (e.g. the glands of Moll, ceruminous glands, or anogenital mammary-like glands). It has an association with apocrine glands via either direct transition from apparently intact apocrine units or evolution from various in situ precursor lesions {1322}.

## ICD-O code 8401/3

## Synonyms

Apocrine adenocarcinoma;
apocrine gland carcinoma

## Epidemiology

Apocrine carcinoma predominantly affects adults in their fifth or sixth decade of life, with no sex or race predilection.

## Localization

The axilla is the most commonly involved site; the distribution generally parallels the normal distribution of apocrine glands {424,1806,1907,2783}. Bilateral lesions are extremely rare {1907}. Other reported locations include the scalp and extremities {2001}.

## Clinical features

The neoplasm occurs as a solitary nodule or multinodular mass ≥ 2 cm in size. Ulceration and haemorrhage may be present. The lesions usually grow slowly and have often been present for a long time before the diagnosis {2204,2783}.

## Histopathology

The neoplasm is usually an asymmetrical, unencapsulated lesion with jagged or pushing borders, involving the dermis and subcutaneous tissue. Papillary, tubular, and solid are the most common growth patterns, which usually indicate an invasive component. The neoplastic cells have abundant eosinophilic cytoplasm, which may be granular and sometimes partly vacuolated. Small lumina or intracytoplasmic vacuoles resulting from abortive ductal differentiation may be present, but decapitation secretion is usually less conspicuous than in an associated in situ component. There is variable nuclear pleomorphism and mitotic activity. Perineural invasion and intravascular involvement may rarely be seen. The in situ component, if present, displays different ductal proliferations, analogous to those in mammary pathology (i.e. typical ductal hyperplasia, atypical ductal hyperplasia, and ductal carcinoma in situ with various patterns). In some tumours, only an invasive component is evident, suggesting either that an in situ lesion has become overgrown by the invasive tumour mass or that the whole neoplasm developed de novo {1048,1322,2204,2798}.

Rare reported features include conspicuous signet-ring or histiocytoid cells in the invasive component identical to those seen in periorbital signet-ring cell/histiocytoid carcinoma, as well as other variations {1460,2161,2204,2919}.

Immunohistochemically, the tumour cells express cytokeratins (including CK7), are usually positive for GCDFP15, and are variably positive for CEA {2001}. S100 protein, EMA (epithelial membrane

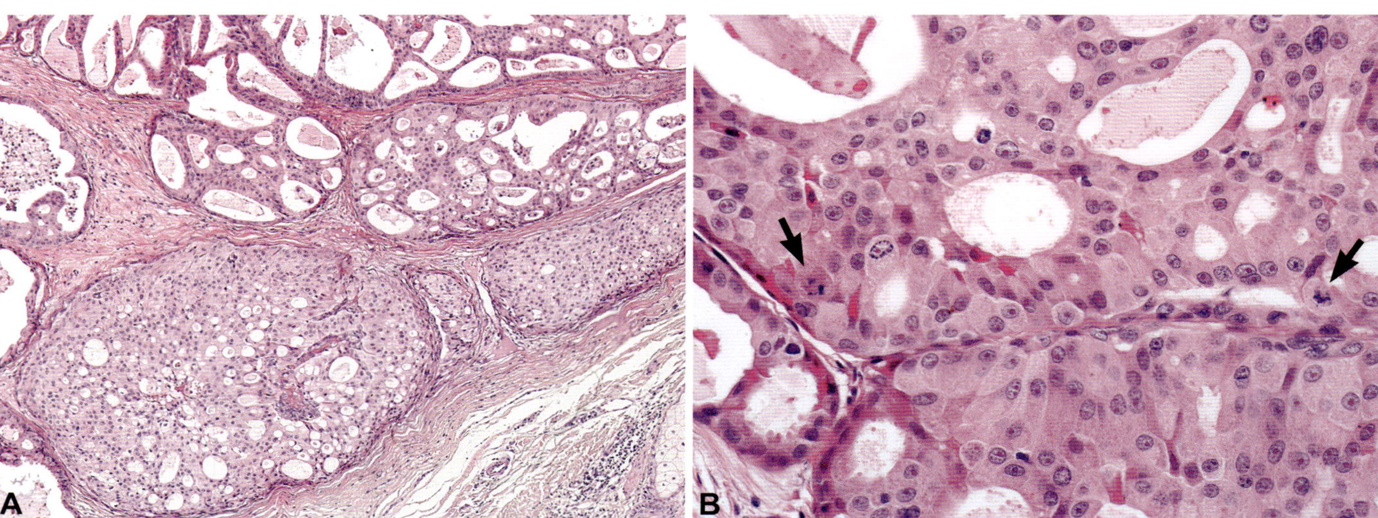


**Fig. 3.24** Apocrine carcinoma. **A,B** Part of this tumour constitutes ductal carcinoma in situ; it has a cribriform appearance, with atypical epithelial cells showing abnormal mitotic figures (arrows) and intact peripheral basal/myoepithelial cells. Focal apocrine secretion is evident.

antigen), estrogen receptor (ER), progesterone receptor (PR), and androgen receptor (AR) are variably expressed. An in situ component is best identified by an intact peripheral basal/myoepithelial cell layer {2204}.

## Differential diagnosis

Mammary ductal carcinoma metastatic to the skin, or involving it by contiguous extension in axillary lesions, can be difficult or even impossible to distinguish from primary cutaneous apocrine carcinoma. However, in situ precursor lesions or evidence of transition from pre-existing apocrine glands, if present, identify the neoplasm as a primary cutaneous tumour. Immunohistochemistry can also be helpful; EGFR (HER1), podoplanin (recognized by D2-40), and p63 are more frequently expressed in primary tumours than in metastatic adenocarcinomas. A panel of several antibodies may have some utility in the distinction; metastatic breast carcinoma is adipophilin+, ER−, PR−, ERBB2 (HER2)+, CK5/6+/− (weak), and mammaglobin+/− (weak), whereas primary apocrine carcinoma is adipophilin−, ER+, PR+/−, ERBB2 (HER2)−, CK5/6+/− (strong and diffuse), and mammaglobin+/− (strong and diffuse). However, full clinical investigation remains the gold standard {2068}. Axillary tumours with histiocytoid cells must be distinguished from invasive lobular carcinoma located in the axillary tail of the mammary gland or ectopic mammary tissue. Malignant tumours essentially representing apocrine carcinoma have been reported to arise from pre-existing benign lesions including spiradenoma, apocrine mixed tumour, and naevus sebaceus of Jadassohn {1324,1333,1581}. Carcinomas with apocrine secretions occurring in the anogenital areas usually represent lesions of anogenital mammary-like glands {751,1301,1327}.

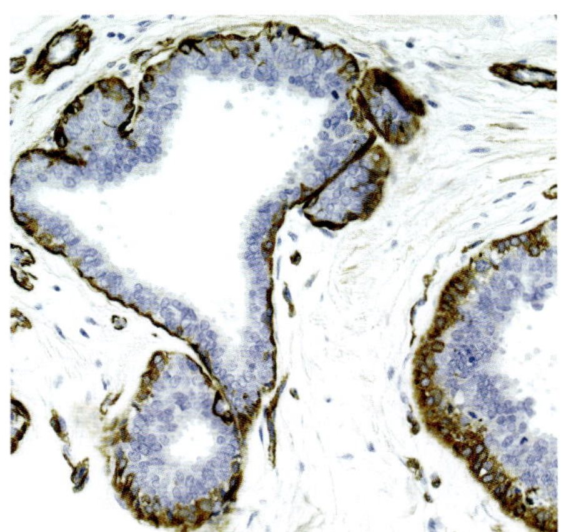

**Fig. 3.25** In situ component in apocrine carcinoma. Staining for α-SMA reveals a myoepithelial cell layer around atypical glands.

## Histogenesis

The finding of an in situ ductal component in apocrine carcinoma suggests that the neoplasm is best compared to invasive breast carcinoma of no special type (also known as invasive mammary ductal carcinoma).

## Genetic profile

ER mRNA has been demonstrated by RT-PCR in some cases, including cases that were immunonegative for ER {293}.

## Prognosis and predictive factors

Apocrine carcinoma metastasizes to regional lymph nodes in about 40% of cases, and less commonly to visceral organs. In one study, 24% of the patients died of metastatic tumour {2204}. It has been proposed that invasive apocrine carcinomas be classified according to the modified Bloom–Richardson grading system for breast carcinomas (also called the Nottingham system) {2204}. This system grades tumours on the basis of three criteria: mitotic rate (number of mitoses/$mm^2$), degree of pleomorphism (mild, moderate, or severe), and tubule formation. A score of 1, 2, or 3 is assigned for each criterion, and the three scores are combined to give an overall tumour grade of 1, 2, or 3. Statistically significant differences in survival have been found with grade 3 versus grade 1–2 tumours. No significant association with survival has been found with any of the other variables studied, including sex, age, anatomical site, tumour size, morphological pattern (solid, tubular, or tubulopapillary), immunohistochemical profile, and hormone receptor expression {2204}.

# Squamoid eccrine ductal carcinoma

Brenn T.
Argenyi Z.B.
Calonje E.
Mehregan D.A.
Mehregan D.R.
Requena L.
Sangüeza O.P.
Santa Cruz D.J.
Scolyer R.A.
Zembowicz A.

## Definition

Squamoid eccrine ductal carcinoma is a biphasic malignant tumour showing squamous and ductal differentiation. It likely constitutes a distinct variant of adenosquamous carcinoma.

## ICD-O code 8560/3

## Synonym

Adenosquamous carcinoma of the skin

## Epidemiology

With only about 60 cases reported, these tumours appear to be rare, but are likely under-recognized {2689}. They present in sun-damaged skin of elderly (median age: 80 years) White individuals, with a male predominance {829,831,2689,2851}.

## Etiology

Ultraviolet (UV) radiation–induced damage and immunosuppression may play a role {829}.

## Localization

The head and neck area is typically affected. Other anatomical sites, including the limbs and trunk, are rarely involved {829,831,2689,2851}.

## Clinical features

The tumours present as large nodules and plaques (as large as a few centimetres) {829,831,2689,2851}.

## Histopathology

Squamoid eccrine ductal carcinoma is a poorly marginated and frequently ulcerated dermal-based neoplasm with diffusely infiltrative margins and frequent invasion of subcutis. The median tumour thickness is 4.3 mm (range: 1.5–18 mm), and the tumour has a biphasic appearance. In the superficial aspects, the tumour is composed of lobules and nests with overt squamous differentiation and multifocal epidermal connection, closely resembling well-differentiated to moderately differentiated squamous cell carcinoma. In the deeper areas, the tumour is characterized by a diffusely infiltrative growth pattern of irregular cords and strands of cuboidal cells with prominent cytological atypia, nuclear pleomorphism, and ductal differentiation in a desmoplastic stroma. Perineural infiltration is relatively common. Lymphovascular invasion and tumour necrosis may be additional findings.

Immunohistochemically, the tumour cells express cytokeratins, and ductal differentiation can be confirmed by staining for EMA (epithelial membrane antigen) and CEA {1397,2689}.

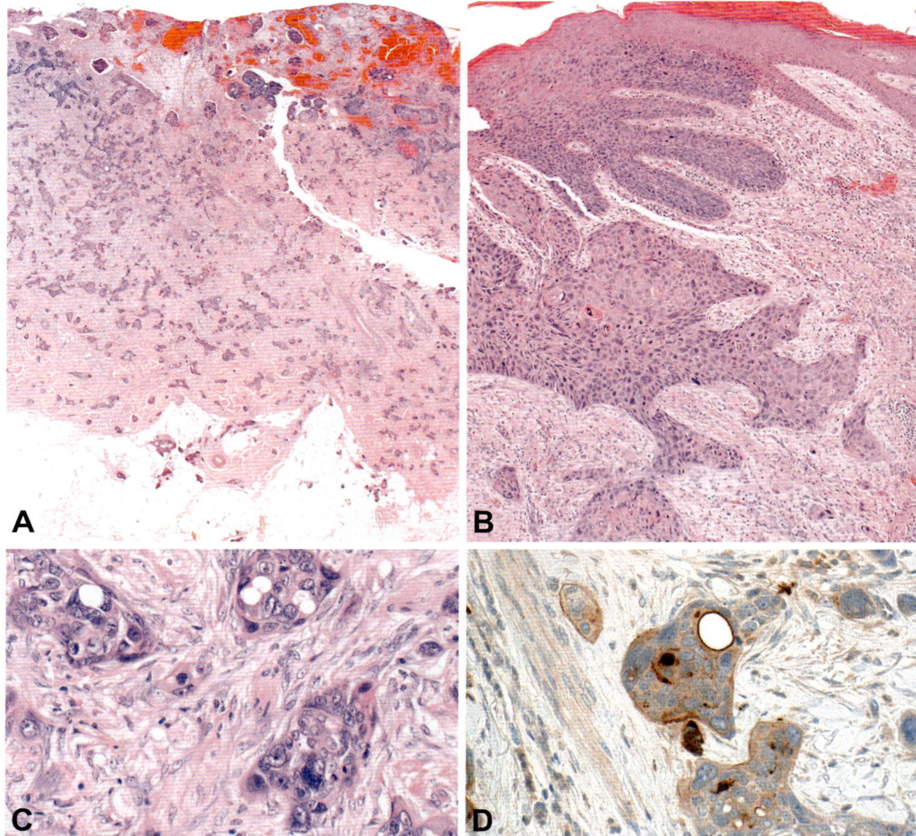

**Fig. 3.26** Squamoid eccrine ductal carcinoma. **A** This ulcerated dermal-based tumour is poorly circumscribed, with infiltrative margins and invasion of subcutis. **B** Superficially, the features are indistinguishable from those of invasive squamous cell carcinoma; an epidermal connection is present. **C** In the deeper aspects, higher magnification highlights the nuclear pleomorphism of the cuboidal tumour cells and the ductal differentiation; mitotic activity is easily identified. **D** Ductal differentiation is highlighted by immunostaining for CEA.

## Differential diagnosis

On superficial biopsies, squamoid eccrine ductal carcinoma may be indistinguishable from invasive squamous cell carcinoma, if the deeper-seated ductal component is not represented in the biopsy. This may be one reason for the under-recognition of this entity. However, this distinction is of little clinical consequence, because the prognosis and treatment recommendations are similar. Similarly, porocarcinoma may show squamous differentiation. It lacks the zonation, and the tumour cells show poroid features. The presence of a pre-existing poroma is helpful. The behaviour and treatment are similar to those of squamoid eccrine carcinoma. Microcystic adnexal carcinoma shows follicular and ductal differentiation, with a zonation similar to that seen in squamoid eccrine carcinoma. It is cytologically bland, lacks prominent cytological atypia, and does not show areas resembling outright squamous cell carcinoma.

### Histogenesis

The tumours display features of both squamous cell carcinoma and ductal carcinoma.

### Prognosis and predictive factors

Despite complete surgical excision, local recurrence rates are high (25%), and there is a 13% chance of regional lymph node metastasis. However, distant metastasis and disease-related mortality are rare, occurring in only 3% of cases {2689}. Adverse prognostic factors have not been comprehensively studied but may include subcutaneous tissue invasion, perineural invasion, and lymphovascular invasion.

# Syringocystadenocarcinoma papilliferum

Kazakov D.V.
Argenyi Z.B.
Brenn T.
Calonje E.
Mehregan D.A.
Mehregan D.R.
Requena L.
Sangüeza O.P.
Santa Cruz D.J.
Scolyer R.A.
Zembowicz A.

### Definition

Syringocystadenocarcinoma papilliferum is a rare adnexal neoplasm evolving (in most cases) from a pre-existing syringocystadenoma papilliferum, usually in the setting of naevus sebaceus of Jadassohn {267,1308,1324,2156}.

### ICD-O code 8406/3

### Epidemiology

Syringocystadenocarcinoma papilliferum is extremely rare, with <40 reported cases {267,1308,1324,2156}.

### Localization

Because syringocystadenocarcinoma papilliferum usually evolves from a pre-existing syringocystadenoma papilliferum (a common secondary tumour in naevus sebaceus of Jadassohn), the most common location is the head and neck area, in particular the scalp {1324,2156,2396}.

### Clinical features

The lesion appears clinically as a nodule, inflammatory plaque, or tumour (sometimes ulcerated), 2–6 cm in size. It is sometimes associated with a sebaceous naevus {1322,1984,2156}.

### Histopathology

In most cases, the tumour shows the overall papillary architecture of syringocystadenoma papilliferum (or direct transition from syringocystadenoma papilliferum can be seen), with areas exhibiting nuclear and cellular atypia, abnormal mitotic figures, loss of polarity, and a focal disorderly proliferation of the neoplastic cells, resulting in solid areas and/or cribriform structures. In situ tumours are associated with an intact myoepithelial cell layer. The invasive adenocarcinomatous component usually appears as a well- or moderately differentiated

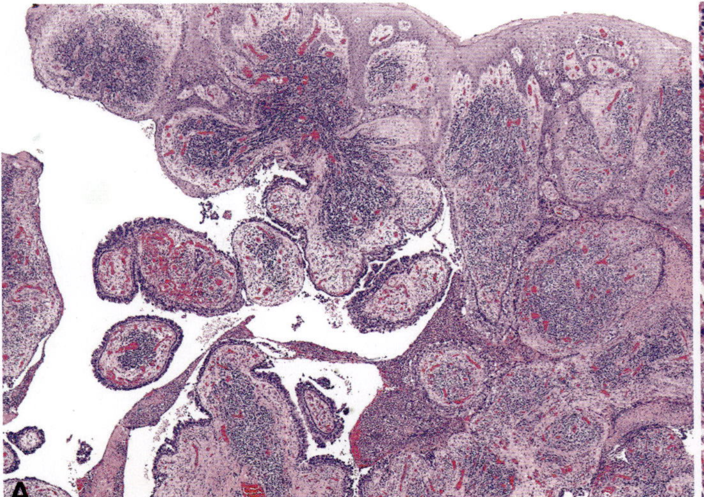


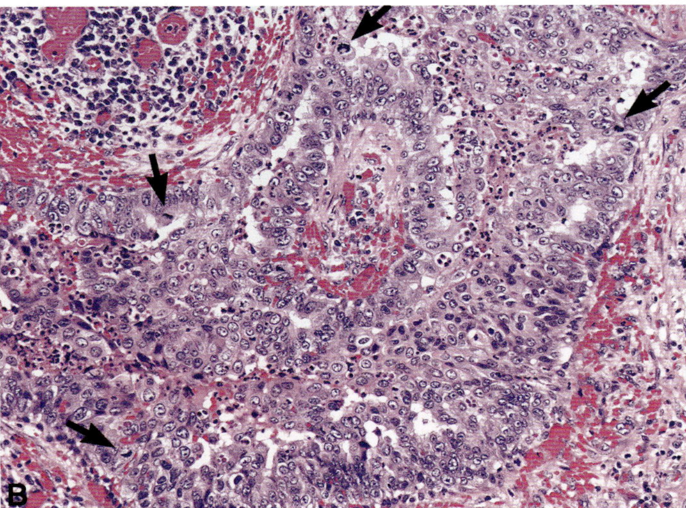


**Fig. 3.27** Syringocystadenocarcinoma papilliferum. **A** The tumour shows the overall papillary architecture. **B** There are areas exhibiting nuclear and cellular atypia, abnormal mitotic figures (arrows), loss of polarity, and a focal disorderly proliferation of the neoplastic cells. The atypical epithelium is delineated from the adjacent dermis by an intact basal/myoepithelial cell layer, qualifying this tumour as syringocystadenocarcinoma papilliferum in situ.

adenocarcinoma; rarely, an intradermal proliferation of small ductal structures composed of a single cell layer involving the full thickness of the dermis or sarcomatoid (metaplastic) carcinoma is seen {1147,1322,1984,2652}. Intravascular invasion is extremely rare {1984}. Other rare appearances of the invasive component include well- to moderately differentiated squamous cell carcinoma (seen in the immediate vicinity of or occurring as an abrupt transition from the glandular epithelium, and perhaps related to a field effect or metaplastic change), lesions resembling lymphoepithelioma-like carcinoma, and tumours with a basaloid component {1324,2932}. Other findings include various ductal changes in the intradermal component and pagetoid spread of the neoplastic cells within the adjacent/overlying epidermis, hair follicles, or both {447,1324,2845}. Features of a pre-existing sebaceous naevus or other secondary neoplasm occurring in the naevus can sometimes be recognized {1308,1324,1984}.

Immunohistochemically, the in situ component can be highlighted by staining for myoepithelial cell markers. The epithelial cells, in both the pre-existing benign lesion and the carcinoma (including areas with pagetoid spread), stain for CK7 and CAM5.2 {2845}.

### Differential diagnosis

Areas of hyperplasia of luminal cells with mild architectural disorder, nuclear crowding, and formation of solid or cribriform areas may sometimes be seen in otherwise benign syringocystadenoma papilliferum, but unless unequivocal cytological atypia and abnormal mitotic figures are present, such lesions should not be diagnosed as syringocystadenocarcinoma papilliferum (in situ) {399}. Rare cases of syringocystadenoma papilliferum associated with florid pseudocarcinomatous hyperplasia in the overlying or adjacent epidermis or adnexal epithelium should be distinguished from syringocystadenocarcinoma papilliferum in which an invasive component is represented by a well-differentiated squamous cell carcinoma {1539}. Pagetoid spread of the neoplastic cells in syringocystadenocarcinoma papilliferum should not be misinterpreted as extramammary Paget disease, especially in small specimens. Clinicopathological correlation is essential in such cases {1322,1419}.

### Histogenesis

Syringocystadenocarcinoma papilliferum is a tumour with apocrine differentiation {2156}.

### Prognosis and predictive factors

Surgical excision appears to be sufficient to prevent recurrence or metastasis. Metastatic disease has been reported in 4 cases, but it is unclear whether all of these tumours are genuine examples {105,1984}.

# Secretory carcinoma

Kazakov D.V.
Argenyi Z.B.
Brenn T.
Calonje E.
Mehregan D.A.
Mehregan D.R.
Requena L.
Sangüeza O.P.
Santa Cruz D.J.
Scolyer R.A.
Zembowicz A.

## Definition

Secretory carcinoma is a rare adnexal carcinoma that is histopathologically identical to homologous lesions in the salivary gland and breast {253,1322,2459}.

## ICD-O code 8502/3

## Synonyms

Primary cutaneous mammary analogue secretory carcinoma; mammary-type secretory carcinoma of the skin

## Epidemiology

Secretory carcinoma is a rare and probably under-recognized neoplasm, with <20 cases reported. There is no sex preponderance. The reported age range is wide: 22–71 years {69,253,291,1310,1322}.

## Localization

In approximately half of the reported cases, the tumours were located in the axilla. Rare sites are the face (including the lips), trunk, and limbs {50,253,433,1322,1444}.

## Clinical features

The neoplasm presents as a solitary nodule of about 1 cm {253}.

## Histopathology

The neoplasm usually manifests as intradermal, circumscribed, unencapsulated nodules composed of bland neoplastic cells arranged in microcystic, tubular, and solid growth patterns, with characteristic abundant secretion within the microcystic and tubular spaces. Cells in the tubular areas may have a cuboidal appearance. Necrosis, perineural invasion, and lymphovascular involvement are not seen. The mitotic rate is low. Immunohistochemically, the neoplastic cells are diffusely positive for S100 protein, mammaglobin, and STAT5A, and they are variably positive for NTRK3 {253}.

## Differential diagnosis

Primary cutaneous secretory carcinoma appears identical to its extracutaneous counterparts; therefore, clinical correlation is essential to distinguish it from a metastasis from a breast or salivary gland primary. The presence of prominent intraluminal secretions sometimes resembling thyroid colloid may occasionally raise the possibility of a metastasis from a thyroid carcinoma, but secretory carcinoma is negative for TTF1. Of note, there are thyroid gland neoplasms histologically resembling secretory carcinoma, as well as tumours with different morphology but harbouring the *ETV6-NTRK3* translocation {637,2041}. Cribriform carcinoma of the skin composed of solid areas punctuated by small round spaces arranged in a cribriform pattern may occasionally resemble a secretory carcinoma, in particular when abundant eosinophilic secretion that gives a homogeneous positive periodic acid–Schiff (PAS) reaction is evident in the lumina of the cystic and tubular spaces. However, in cribriform carcinoma, the cells in the tubular areas are not cuboidal, the glands are not distributed back-to-back, and all tumours are

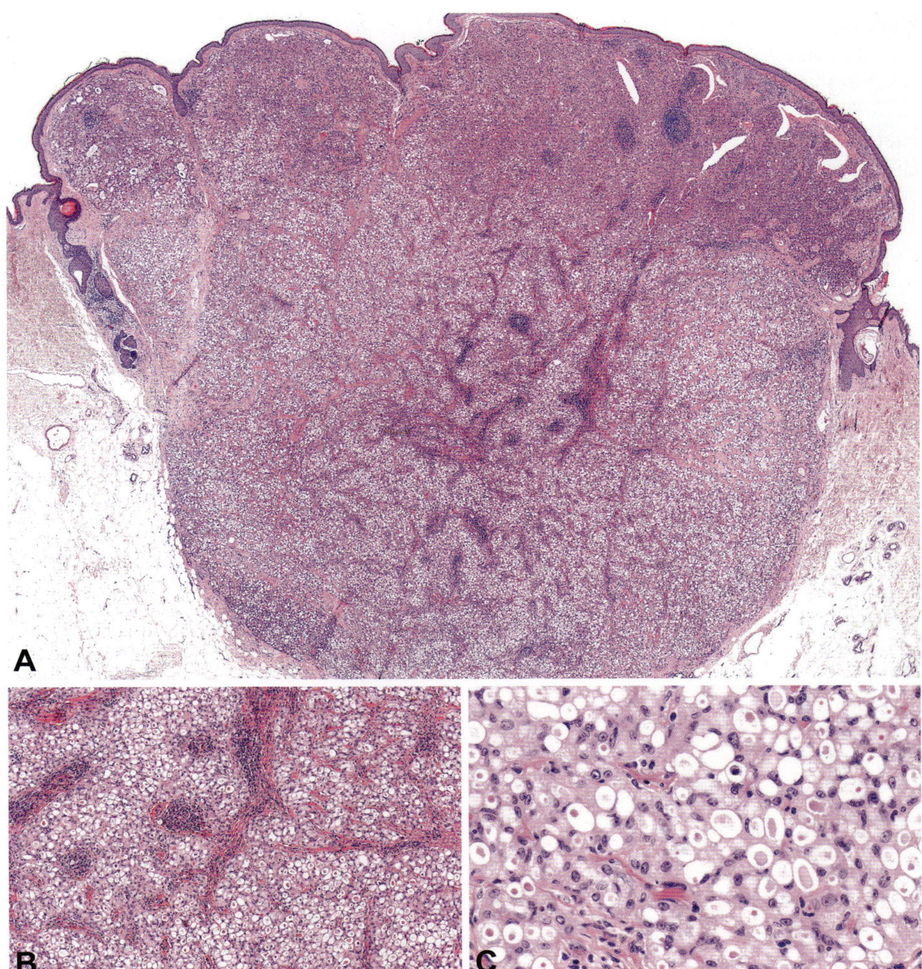

**Fig. 3.28** Secretory carcinoma. **A** The neoplasm usually occurs as an intradermal circumscribed nodule. **B,C** The tumour is composed of bland neoplastic cells arranged in microcystic, tubular, and solid growth patterns, with characteristic abundant secretion within the microcystic and tubular spaces.

characterized by peculiar thin thread-like intraluminal bridging strands resembling those seen in adenomatoid tumours of the urogenital tract {1076,1323}. Adenoid cystic carcinoma manifests a cribriform pattern, but the presence of true ductal structures with limited secretions, pseudolumina filled with mucin or homogeneous basophilic and eosinophilic material, and basaloid tumour cells are distinguishing features {2128}.

### Histogenesis

Because of the localization in the axilla and lips, a relationship with mammary tissue (ectopic) and salivary glands (minor) has been suggested. However, the lack of direct connection to (and lack of residua of) mammary tissue or salivary glands argues against this theory {253}.

### Genetic profile

Similar to homonymous neoplasms of the breast and salivary glands, a subset of cutaneous secretory carcinoma is associated with the characteristic balanced t(12;15)(p13;q25) *ETV6-NTRK3* translocation, but the frequency of this feature appears be lower than in extracutaneous homologues {253}.

### Prognosis and predictive factors

Secretory carcinoma has an apparently indolent disease course, but studies with long follow-up are limited.

# Cribriform carcinoma

Kazakov D.V.
Argenyi Z.B.
Brenn T.
Calonje E.
Mehregan D.A.
Mehregan D.R.
Requena L.
Sangüeza O.P.
Santa Cruz D.J.
Scolyer R.A.
Zembowicz A.

### Definition

Cribriform carcinoma is an indolent adnexal tumour of presumed apocrine lineage. Although this tumour was originally reported as a carcinoma, its malignant potential is uncertain {376,799}.

### ICD-O code 8201/3

### Synonyms

Primary cutaneous cribriform carcinoma; solid-cribriform carcinoma

### Epidemiology

Cribriform carcinoma is a rare neoplasm. The female-to-male ratio is 2:1, and the reported age range is 20–77 years, with a median patient age of 47 years {101,1322,2156,2264}.

### Localization

The site of predilection is the lower extremities, affected in >80% of cases. The head and neck area and other sites are rarely involved {101,2264}.

### Clinical features

Cribriform carcinoma manifests as a solitary skin-coloured nodule of 1–3 cm in diameter, often having a firm consistency on palpation. The duration of symptoms

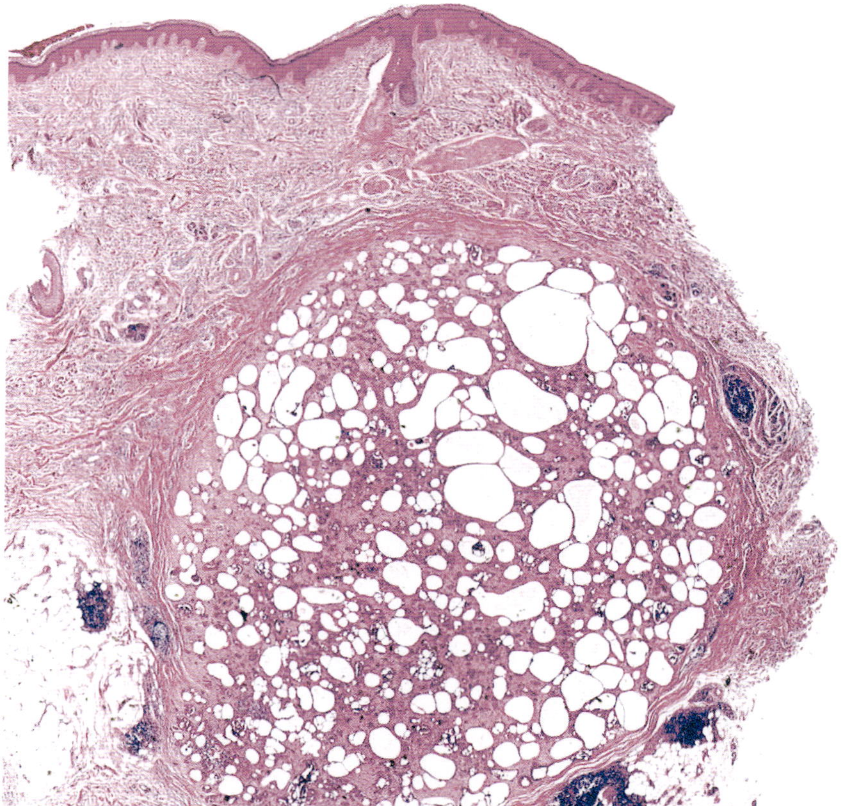

**Fig. 3.29** Cribriform carcinoma. An example with pronounced cribriform architecture. Note the lymphoid aggregates at the periphery of the neoplasm and the layer of compressed fibrous tissue.

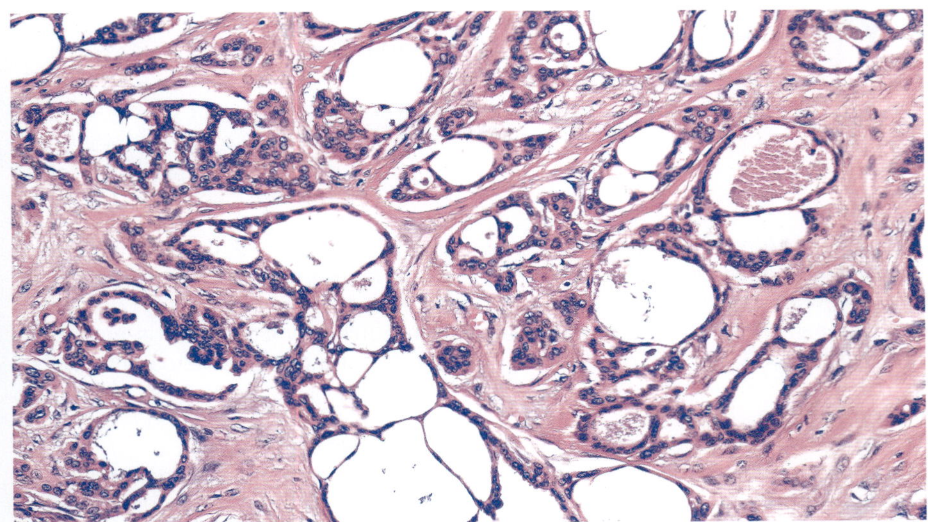

**Fig. 3.30** Cribriform carcinoma. Note the thin thread-like intraluminal bridges.

ranges from several months to several years {101,1322,2264}.

## Histopathology

The neoplasm is usually located within the dermis, sometimes extending into the subcutaneous fat, without apparent connection to the epidermis or adnexa. Most tumours are well circumscribed, although the borders are occasionally jagged and there may be small satellite-like aggregates of tumour cells seemingly separated from the main lesion. The neoplasm is composed of multiple interconnected solid nests of epithelial cells with round or oval, hyperchromatic, slightly pleomorphic nuclei; inconspicuous or absent nucleoli; granular chromatin; and scant eosinophilic cytoplasm. In addition to the solid areas, there are also small round lumina that are either empty or filled with eosinophilic substance that gives a homogeneous positive periodic acid–Schiff (PAS) reaction, giving rise to a cribriform pattern. The ratio of solid to cribriform areas varies both within a given neoplasm and among tumours. Larger ductal spaces (sometimes with decapitation secretion), intraluminal micropapillary projections, and thin thread-like intraluminal bridging strands are common features. Mitotic figures, especially atypical ones, are rare. Individual necrotic cells or foci of necrosis can be evident focally. The small satellite-like aggregates, composed of a single cell to 3–4 cells, usually display more-pronounced pleomorphism and nuclear hyperchromasia than does the main tumour bulk, but perineural or lymphovascular invasion is not a feature. The stroma is scant and fibrotic, often containing nodular lymphoid aggregates at the periphery of the neoplasm {1322,1323,2264}.

The neoplastic cells are positive for various cytokeratins (MNF116, AE1/AE3, CAM5.2, and CK7) and BerEP4, and variably positive for KIT. Staining for CEA and EMA (epithelial membrane antigen) highlights the ductal component. CK20, GCDFP15, estrogen receptor, and progesterone receptor are negative. Immunoreactivity for S100 protein and p63 is variable. No myoepithelial cell component is identified by staining for α-SMA, MSA, or calponin, which is an important differential diagnostic feature {101,2264}.

## Differential diagnosis

Adenoid cystic carcinoma manifests a cribriform pattern but is composed of basaloid epithelial cells disposed around pseudolumina (pseudocysts) filled with mucin or eosinophilic or basophilic material. In addition to pseudocystic structures, there are small true ducts with myoepithelial cell differentiation. These dual-type lumina are never seen in cribriform carcinoma; neither are the deposits of basement membrane material and perineural invasion typical of adenoid cystic carcinoma {2128}. Cutaneous secretory carcinoma also shows cribriform areas but consists of back-to-back proliferations of tubules and microcysts with conspicuous intraluminal secretions. Coexpression of S100 protein, mammaglobin, STAT5A, and NTRK3 helps to distinguish the neoplasm from cribriform carcinoma {253}. Rare cases of tubular adenoma may show overlap with cribriform carcinoma, but the presence of basal/myoepithelial cells in tubular adenoma distinguishes it {101}.

## Histogenesis

The histogenesis is unknown. Because of evidence of apocrine secretion in some cases, the neoplasm is considered to be apocrine.

## Genetic susceptibility

No hereditary syndromes, susceptibility genes, or SNPs have been reported to date.

## Prognosis and predictive factors

Cribriform carcinoma is an indolent neoplasm of uncertain malignant potential, with no cases of recurrent or metastatic disease reported to date {376,799}. A few cases have been reported to persist at the site secondary to incomplete excision {101}.

# Signet-ring cell/histiocytoid carcinoma

Kazakov D.V.
Brenn T.
Kutzner H.
Requena L.
Sangüeza O.P.

## Definition
Signet-ring cell/histiocytoid carcinoma is a rare aggressive adnexal neoplasm preferentially affecting the eyelid and histopathologically resembling a metastatic lobular carcinoma of the breast and/or some adenocarcinomas arising in the gastrointestinal tract {2161}.

## ICD-O code 8490/3

## Epidemiology
Signet-ring cell/histiocytoid carcinoma is a rare neoplasm, with <40 cases reported. The tumour mainly affects males, with a male-to-female ratio of about 4:1 {2161}.

## Localization
Most tumours involve the eyelids; identical neoplasms have rarely been reported in the axilla {2161}.

## Clinical features
Eyelid lesions present with diffuse thickening of the involved lid, covered by normal or erythematous skin; they are often misinterpreted as inflammatory disorders, which can delay the correct diagnosis and worsen the prognosis. Extension into the adjacent eyelid results in a monocle appearance. A case with involvement of both eyes (a binocle presentation) has also been described {218}. The reported age range is 42–87 years, with a median patient age of 66 years {2161}.

## Histopathology
The epidermis is usually spared. There is a diffuse infiltration of the dermis by sheets or cords of single rows of cells arranged interstitially between collagen bundles. The cells have eccentric nuclei displaced by vacuolated cytoplasm (in the signet-ring cell variant) or exhibit eosinophilic granular cytoplasm (in the histiocytoid variant). Both cell types can be found in a single lesion, but one type usually predominates.

Immunohistochemically, the neoplastic cells express high-molecular-weight and low-molecular-weight pancytokeratins, CK7, E-cadherin, CEA, EMA (epithelial membrane antigen), GCDFP15, and human milk fat globule {2161}.

## Differential diagnosis
Metastatic lobular carcinoma of the breast and adenocarcinomas with a signet-ring cell morphology originating from the gastrointestinal tract are the main differential diagnoses. Immunohistochemistry (i.e. lack of CK5/6, CDX2, and ERBB2 expression) can be helpful in some cases, but careful clinicopathological correlation with a full clinical work-up is mandatory to rule out a primary internal malignancy {2161}.

## Histogenesis
Apocrine differentiation and origin from the glands of Moll are discussed on the basis of the location and immunophenotype {1198,2161}.

## Prognosis and predictive factors
This is an aggressive neoplasm (often persisting after incomplete surgical excision) with the potential to involve the adjacent eyelid and orbit. In one third of the reported cases, the patient developed regional lymph node or distant metastasis. Axillary lesions appear to be less aggressive; only metastasis to the adjacent lymph nodes has been reported {360,1460,2161}.

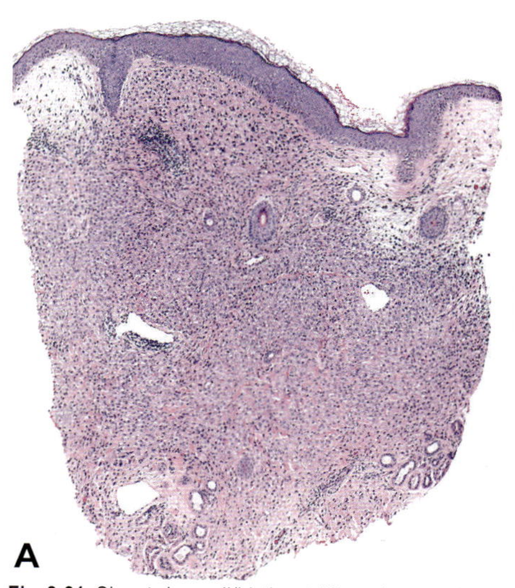


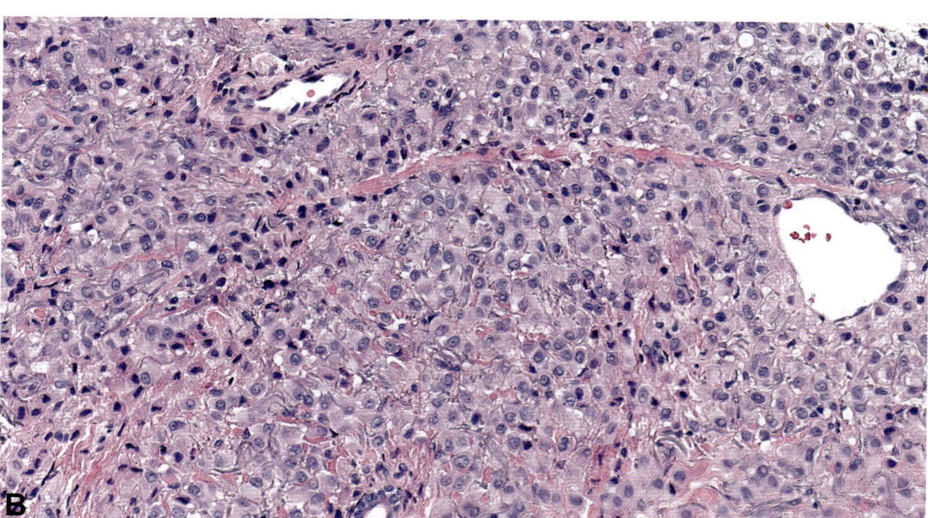


**Fig. 3.31** Signet-ring cell/histiocytoid carcinoma. **A** The neoplasm involves the whole dermis. **B** It is composed of sheets of large so-called histiocytoid cells with abundant cytoplasm; some cells contain intracytoplasmic vacuoles.

# Benign tumours with apocrine and eccrine differentiation

## Hidrocystoma/cystadenoma

Sangüeza O.P.
Cassarino D.S.
Glusac E.J.
Kazakov D.V.
Requena L.
Swanson P.E.
Vassallo C.

### Definition
Hidrocystoma/cystadenoma constitutes a spectrum of benign cystic lesions of predominantly ductal sweat gland origin, with architecture ranging from simple cystic (hidrocystoma) to more complex (cystadenoma).

### ICD-O code
8404/0

### Synonyms
Apocrine gland cyst;
apocrine cystadenoma;
eccrine ductal cyst

### Epidemiology
Hidrocystoma affects middle-aged adults of both sexes {2166}.

### Etiology
Hidrocystomas usually increase in size during the summer or after exposure to heat; they decrease in size or disappear in winter.

### Localization
Most hidrocystomas occur on the eyelids, but they can also affect the ears, vulva, and fingers.

### Clinical features
Hidrocystomas are solitary, asymptomatic lesions, usually located on the face and often bluish in colour. They are typically 0.5–1 cm, but can reach 7 cm in size. The lesions are cystic and often translucent. Multiple lesions (Robinson-type hidrocystomas) are rare {739}. Schöpf–Schulz–Passarge syndrome, a form of ectodermal dysplasia, is associated with multiple hidrocystomas at the edges of the eyelids {810}. Multiple hidrocystomas may also be associated with bilateral keratoconus, oesophageal papillomas, and hiatal hernias in patients with Goltz syndrome {2906}. Occasionally, multiple hidrocystomas of the face have been reported in patients with Graves disease {1368}.

### Histopathology
Hidrocystomas typically present as round to oval single cystic lesions, but they can also present as multiple cysts. These structures are lined by columnar epithelium, often showing decapitation secretion, surrounded by myoepithelial cells and a basement membrane. Mucin may be present in the columnar cells. Most cases contain abundant mucin in the lumen, but the content is sometimes homogeneous and eosinophilic. Accumulation of secretion material can compress and flatten the epithelium without evidence of apocrine secretion.

In some cases, hidrocystomas have papillary-like epithelial projections or more-complex architecture that may be described as cystadenoma.

Immunohistochemically, hidrocystomas are positive for EMA (epithelial membrane antigen) and CEA in luminal cells; the myoepithelial elements are immunoreactive for S100 protein. Other markers found in hidrocystomas include GCDFP15, as well as various keratins in a pattern similar to that seen in the secretory portion of the eccrine glands {2166}.

### Differential diagnosis
The differential diagnosis includes lacrimal gland cysts.

### Histogenesis
Most hidrocystomas result from obstruction of the duct, but some may be neoplastic. Most appear to be of apocrine origin, but some may be eccrine.

### Prognosis and predictive factors
Hidrocystomas are benign lesions.

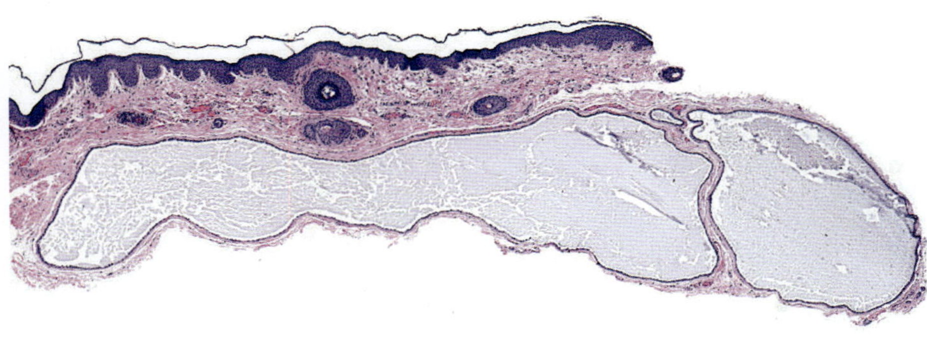


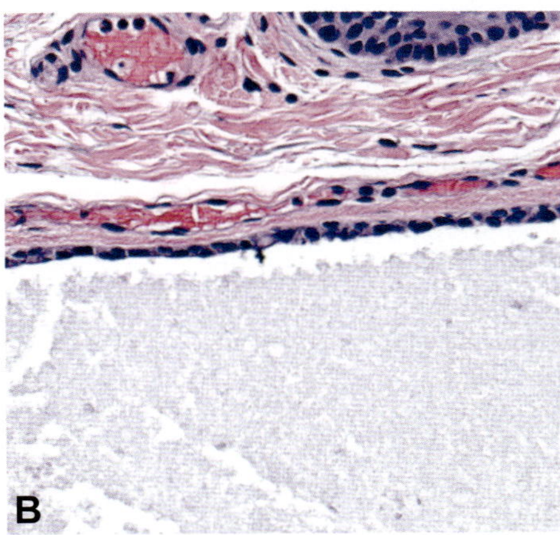


**Fig. 3.32** Hidrocystoma. **A** The lesion is composed of several cystic spaces, containing a bluish material. **B** Detail of the cuboidal epithelium.

# Syringoma

Sangüeza O.P.
Cassarino D.S.
Glusac E.J.
Kazakov D.V.
Requena L.
Swanson P.E.
Vassallo C.

## Definition

Syringoma is a small benign sweat gland tumour.

## ICD-O code 8407/0

## Epidemiology

Syringomas most commonly affect elderly women, but the eruptive variant is most common in young women {2478}. Clear cell syringoma, which is more common in people with diabetes, is histopathologically characterized by ducts and solid aggregates of epithelial cells with optically clear cytoplasm.

## Localization

Most syringomas arise in the lower eyelids and periorbital area {1063}. Eruptive lesions tend to occur on the neck, chest, axillae, pubic area, umbilicus, and genital region.

## Clinical features

Syringoma presents as skin-coloured or slightly yellow smooth papules.

Eruptive syringoma presents as several scattered, small papules (mostly on the anterior chest wall and flexural areas of the limbs), which may coalesce to form plaques {1520}. They can have a linear and one-sided distribution. Vulvar syringomas are usually pruritic {2585}.

Multiple syringomas may resemble milia cysts. When the lesions are pigmented, they may simulate urticaria pigmentosa or confluent and reticulated papillomatosis of Gougerot–Carteaud.

## Histopathology

Syringomas are well-circumscribed lesions typically affecting the upper half of the dermis; occasionally they can extend into the deep dermis or even the subcutis. Syringoma has two components: epithelial cells forming ducts, cords, tubules, and cysts, and a homogeneous and sclerotic stroma. The lumina of the ductal and tubular structures are lined by a double layer of cuboidal cells, sometimes containing a granular basophilic material. The ducts often show characteristic extensions resembling a tadpole tail. Solid collections of epithelial cells are also observed, often containing multiple confluent cytoplasmic vacuoles. Small cysts are often present, filled with basket-weave, basophilic, and orthokeratotic keratin and lined by squamous epithelium. The stroma consists of thick bundles of compact and sclerotic collagen. In eruptive syringoma, the stroma is less prominent.

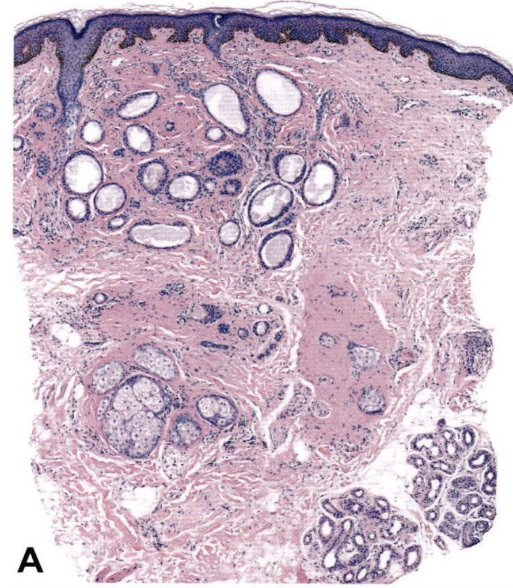


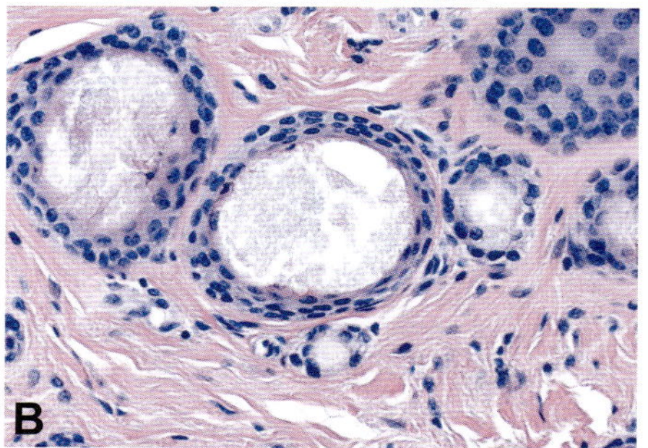


**Fig. 3.33** Syringoma. **A** Scanning magnification shows several cystic spaces embedded in a sclerotic stroma. **B** Detail of the cystic spaces.

## Differential diagnosis

In superficial biopsies, the differential diagnosis includes microcystic adnexal carcinoma, sclerosing/morphoeic basal cell carcinoma, and desmoplastic trichoepithelioma/columnar trichoblastoma, from which distinction may be impossible without complete removal and clinicopathological correlation. Ductal proliferations in cicatricial alopecia, alopecia areata, and prurigo nodularis may resemble syringoma; however, in such cases, the stroma is different. Eruptive hamartomas of clear cells of the eccrine duct (or so-called clear cell metaplasia of the eccrine duct) resemble clear cell syringomas {2444}, but these lesions affect only the excretory ducts of pre-existing eccrine glands.

## Histogenesis

Syringomas resemble the ductal portion of the eccrine gland.

## Genetic profile

Syringomas of the eyelids are common in patients with Down syndrome {2343}, and they have also been described in patients with hyperthyroidism, Ehlers–Danlos syndromes, Marfan syndrome, and Nicolau–Balus syndrome {657}. In familial forms, multiple syringomas affect several family members.

## Prognosis and predictive factors

Syringomas are benign lesions.

# Poroma

Sangüeza O.P.
Cassarino D.S.
Glusac E.J.
Kazakov D.V.
Requena L.
Swanson P.E.
Vassallo C.

## Definition

Poromas are benign neoplasms with differentiation towards the intradermal portion of the sweat apparatus. They can be wholly intraepidermal (hidroacanthoma simplex), wholly intradermal (dermal duct tumour and poroid hidradenoma), or juxtaepidermal (both epidermal and dermal) in distribution.

## ICD-O code 8409/0

## Synonym

Acrospiroma

## Epidemiology

The age of presentation is 60–80 years.

## Localization

Intraepidermal poroma commonly involves the extremities, but it can affect other sites. About 65% of classic poromas involve the palms or soles. Intradermal poroma commonly involves the head and neck region.

## Clinical features

Classic poromas typically present as a solitary sessile or pedunculated papule or an asymptomatic nodule ranging from 2 mm to 2 cm in size, but they can also be cup-shaped, papillomatous, or wart-like. The colour of the lesion varies from red to the normal skin colour. Pigmentation has also been described {2839}. Multiple poromas have been described after radiotherapy or allogenic bone marrow transplantation and immunosuppression {1000}.

## Histopathology

All poromas are composed of poroid and cuticular cells. Poroid cells have a rounded or oval nucleus and scant cytoplasm. Cuticular cells have ample eosinophilic cytoplasm and a central nucleus, sometimes with moderate atypia. Ductal differentiation is seen in the form of small intracytoplasmic vacuoles or the formation of authentic intracellular ductal structures. Additional findings include areas of necrosis, cystic areas, foci of keratinization, pale cells, dendritic melanocytes, melanin pigment, and keratohyaline granules. Superficially traumatized lesions may show focal cytological atypia and increased mitotic activity.

Hidroacanthoma simplex is mainly intraepidermal. Classic poromas include cords and aggregates of poroid cells that connect with the epidermis in the superficial dermis. Dermal duct tumour is composed of small nodules of similar cells scattered within the upper dermis without connection with the epidermis. Poroid hidradenomas have either single or several nodules with solid and cystic areas {1691}. The stroma surrounding poromas is often richly vascular and may resemble granulation tissue.

Apocrine and eccrine poromas are similar. However, apocrine poromas may connect to follicular structures {2905}. Focal decapitation secretion, sebocytes, and focal follicular germinative differentiation may also be seen {2023}.

CEA staining highlights the luminal border of ductal structures; EMA (epithelial membrane antigen) decorates the neoplastic cells {1911}.

## Differential diagnosis

Clonal-type seborrhoeic keratosis can be confused with hidroacanthoma simplex, but the ductal structures and two populations of cells in hidroacanthoma simplex facilitates correct diagnosis. Hidradenomas are composed mainly of cells with pale cytoplasm, whereas poromas include both poroid and cuticular cells.

## Histogenesis

Poromas can be either eccrine or apocrine {2167}.

## Genetic susceptibility

Some poromas show loss of heterozygosity in the *APC* gene, but the significance of this genetic anomaly is uncertain {1164}.

## Prognosis and predictive factors

Poromas are benign neoplasms.

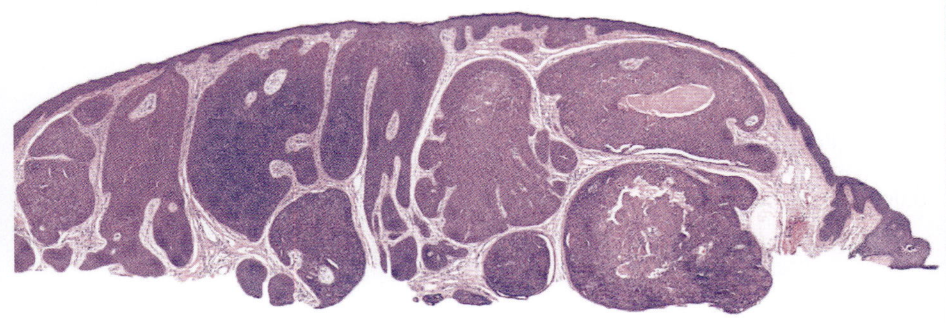


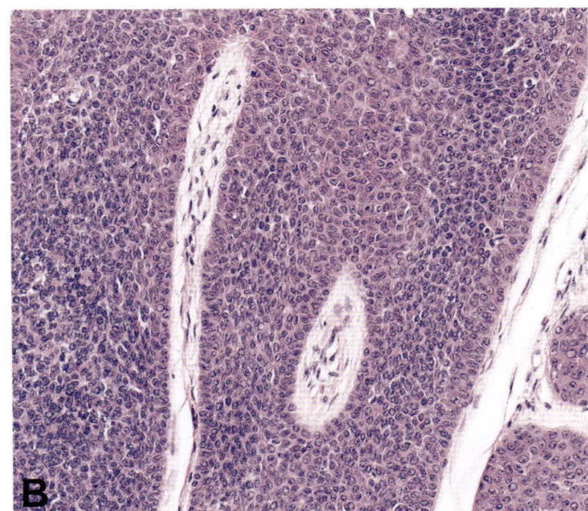


**Fig. 3.34** Poroma. **A** Well-circumscribed lesion composed of collections of basaloid cells and small areas of necrosis. **B** Detail of the poroid cells in the lower part of the picture. There are a few cuticular cells in the upper part of the field; small ductal structures are also present.

# Syringofibroadenoma

Sangüeza O.P.
Cassarino D.S.
Glusac E.J.
Kazakov D.V.
Requena L.
Swanson P.E.
Vassallo C.

## Definition

Syringofibroadenoma is characterized by a proliferation of cords and strands of epithelial cells with ductal differentiation.

## ICD-O code 8392/0

## Synonyms

Acrosyringeal naevus; eccrine syringofibroadenomatous hyperplasia

## Epidemiology

Syringofibroadenoma affects older patients, with an average age of 60 years.

## Etiology

In most non-syndromic settings, it is considered to be a reactive process.

## Localization

It involves mainly the lower extremities and exceptionally the nails {816}.

## Clinical features

Solitary syringofibroadenomas have variable morphology. Multiple lesions (eccrine syringofibroadenomatosis) present as small papules or plaques of >5 cm, which in some cases have a linear distribution. The surface is usually hyperkeratotic and often shows features of chronic lymphoedema. Rare associations include Schöpf–Schulz–Passarge syndrome and Clouston syndrome {810,2501}.

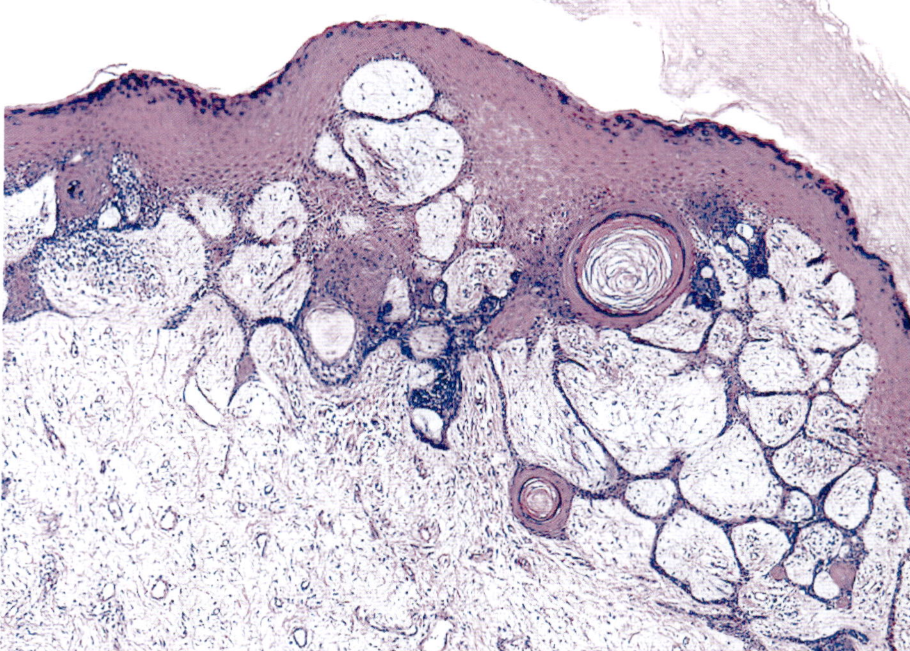

**Fig. 3.35** Syringofibroadenoma. Cords of epithelial cells in a fenestrating pattern, anastomosing with each other; the stroma is oedematous, with loose collagen.

## Histopathology

Syringofibroadenoma presents with ductal epithelial hyperplasia in a fenestrating pattern, oriented perpendicularly to the surface of the skin. The cords of epithelium are interconnected. Numerous ductal structures are present. The stroma shows loose fibrillary collagen containing abundant mucin and a lymphoplasmacytic infiltrate. Venules and thick-walled capillaries are abundant. In some syringofibroadenomas, the ductal cells give a positive periodic acid–Schiff (PAS) reaction and stain positively with colloidal iron {816}.

Immunohistochemical studies have demonstrated the presence of CEA, EMA (epithelial membrane antigen), and filaggrin in the lumina of the small ducts, as well as a pattern of cytokeratin expression similar to that seen in the distal portion of the eccrine duct {2168}.

## Differential diagnosis

Poromas contain more solid areas and different stroma. Fibroepithelial basal cell carcinoma shows a reticular proliferation of epithelial cells; however, focally there is stromal retraction and nuclear palisading, as well as primitive follicular germinative buds.

## Histogenesis

Eccrine syringofibroadenomas are reactive hyperplasias {2173}.

## Prognosis and predictive factors

Syringofibroadenoma is a benign condition.

# Hidradenoma

Sangüeza O.P.
Cassarino D.S.
Glusac E.J.
Kazakov D.V.
Requena L.
Swanson P.E.
Vassallo C.

## Definition

Hidradenoma is a benign solid and cystic sweat gland neoplasm with focal ductal and glandular differentiation.

## ICD-O code 8402/0

## Synonyms

Clear cell hidradenoma; solid cystic hidradenoma; nodular hidradenoma; eccrine acrospiroma; clear cell myoepithelioma

## Epidemiology

Hidradenoma can affect people of any age, both male and female {642}.

## Localization

The anatomical distribution is wide, with a predilection for the trunk and limbs.

## Clinical features

Hidradenoma is an asymptomatic, solitary, firm nodule, usually < 2–3 cm in diameter, although it can be > 10 cm {1158}. Occasionally, lesions may be ulcerated {2362}.

## Histopathology

Hidradenomas are well-circumscribed dermal neoplasms that may extend into the subcutaneous tissue. Most hidradenomas are solid lobular proliferations, but some contain large cystic spaces filled with homogeneous eosinophilic material. The majority of hidradenomas are composed of pale or clear cells (hence the synonym "clear cell hidradenoma"). However, other cell types, including polygonal, mucinous, squamoid, oxyphilic/oncocytic, and epidermoid cells, can also be present. The proportion of various cell types and their combinations vary from case to case. The characteristic cytoplasmic clarity is due to abundant intracellular glycogen. The nuclei are small, round, and usually eccentrically located. In some examples of hidradenoma, polygonal and epidermoid cells are the most prominent component. Mucinous cells usually appear in small groups and can be recognized by the presence of ample granular bluish cytoplasm. When polygonal cells with ample eosinophilic cytoplasm predominate, hidradenomas have an appearance reminiscent of oncocytoma {2245}. Squamoid cells have abundant eosinophilic cytoplasm and are separated by well-defined intercellular bridges; some may keratinize individually and appear as dyskeratotic keratinocytes. Areas of ductal and glandular differentiation are usually present even in solid neoplasms. These structures are lined by cuboidal cells that elaborate an eosinophilic luminal cuticle. In some cases, glandular structures lined by columnar cells with evidence of secretion by decapitation in the luminal border are also seen. Myoepithelial cells are not present in ductal or glandular structures of apocrine hidradenoma. The stroma in apocrine hidradenoma is characteristically sclerotic, separating epithelial islands; in lesions of long evolution, this sclerosis may be very marked, leaving only small aggregates of neoplastic cells. Focal cytological atypia can be encountered.

Immunostaining for EMA (epithelial membrane antigen) and CEA highlights ductal differentiation.

## Differential diagnosis

Poroid hidradenoma has two cell types (poroid and cuticular), both of which are very different from the cells of apocrine hidradenoma. In poroid hidradenoma, tubular structures are only seen in the areas of cuticular cells. Like other poromas, poroid hidradenoma frequently shows areas of necrosis en masse. Trichilemmomas consist of pale or clear cells showing signs of trichilemmal differentiation; they often expand the follicular infundibulum and exhibit peripheral palisading surrounded by a thick and prominent basement membrane. In contrast, apocrine hidradenoma can connect with pre-existing infundibular structures,

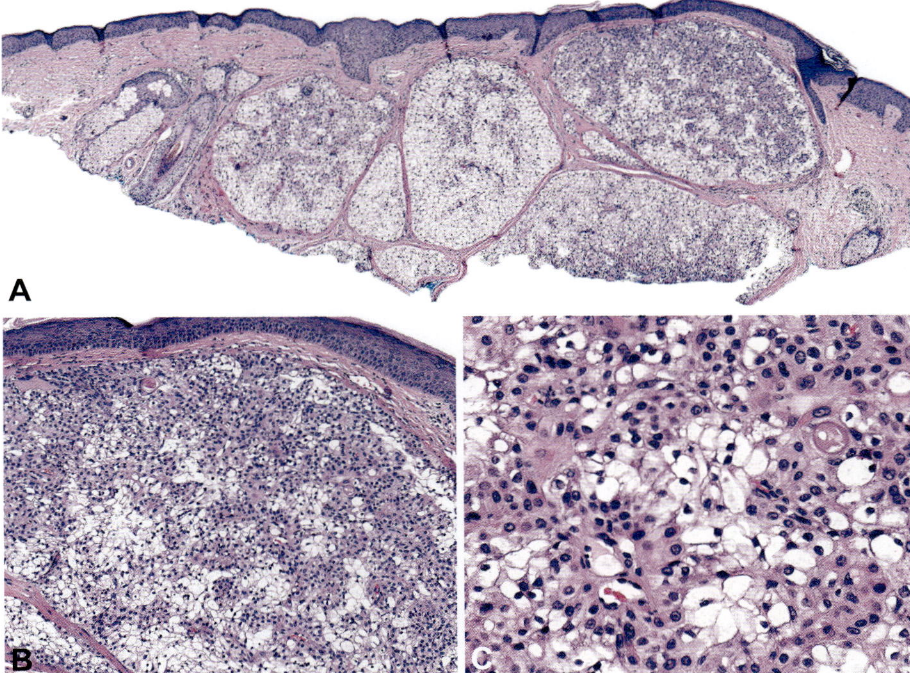

**Fig. 3.36** Hidradenoma. **A** Well-circumscribed nodules with a predominance of clear cells. **B** Clear cells admixed with cells with an eosinophilic cytoplasm and central nuclei. **C** There are areas with squamoid differentiation and a few ducts.

but the neoplastic epithelial islands form solid aggregates in the dermis and subcutis. Apocrine hidradenomas with a predominantly solid pattern must be distinguished from glomus tumour that shows SMA positivity {1044}. Apocrine hidradenoma must also be distinguished from a cutaneous metastasis of renal carcinoma, which is characterized by an abundant blood supply, numerous atypical mitoses and areas of necrosis of both individual and groups of neoplastic cells, and extracellular blood lakes. A combination of PAX8 and CAIX staining may be used to solve the differential diagnosis.

## Genetic profile

Hidradenomas harbour a t(11;19) translocation, which results in the fusion of *CRTC1* (previously called *MECT1*) at 19p13.1 with *MAML2* at 11q21. The *CRTC1-MAML2* fusion gene is not exclusive to apocrine hidradenoma; it has also been identified in salivary gland mucoepidermoid carcinoma. This translocation leads to aberrant activation of downstream cAMP/CREB signalling genes {672,2841}.

## Prognosis and predictive factors

Hidradenoma is a benign neoplasm. Exceptional cases of benign-looking hidradenomas may present with lymphatic invasion or single regional lymph node deposits. Limited follow-up suggests that this is a benign phenomenon {2505}.

# Spiradenoma

Sangüeza O.P.
Cassarino D.S.
Glusac E.J.
Kazakov D.V.
Requena L.
Swanson P.E.
Vassallo C.

## Definition

Spiradenoma is a (multi)nodular solid benign sweat gland neoplasm showing substantial morphological overlap with cylindroma.

## ICD-O code

8403/0

## Synonyms

Spiroma; eccrine spiradenoma; cystic epithelioma of the sweat glands

## Etiology

Multiple spiradenomas, which are inherited in an autosomal dominant pattern, are often associated with multiple trichoepitheliomas, cylindromas, and tumours of the parotid gland, an association known as Brooke–Spiegler syndrome {339}.

## Localization

Spiradenomas most commonly occur on the face or upper part of the trunk.

## Clinical features

Spiradenomas are rare neoplasms that usually appear in adulthood, although congenital cases have been described {2347}. Most spiradenomas are solitary subcutaneous nodules; however, multiple lesions can occur in both syndromic and sporadic settings, sometimes in a linear distribution. Pain is a common clinical feature associated with spiradenoma {1652}. The cause of pain is unknown, although various theories have been proposed, including the contraction of myoepithelial cells and an abnormal distribution of sensory nerves inside the neoplasm.

## Histopathology

Spiradenomas consist of single or several round nodules of basaloid cells with smooth borders. They are centred in the dermis and occasionally extend into subcutaneous tissue. The stroma is oedematous, with numerous dilated blood and lymph vessels. The lesion is often populated by numerous lymphocytes. Spiradenomas are composed of two types of cells: light (or clear) and dark. The clear cells tend to occupy the centre of the neoplastic nodules, and the dark cells form the peripheral layer. Ductal structures are frequently seen inside the solid areas of spiradenoma. Rarely, true adenomatous or adenomyoepitheliomatous areas may be seen {1320}. Basement membrane material can be seen in the form of a thick basement membrane surrounding the islets of tumour cells or in the form of round deposits inside the aggregates, although these deposits of basement membrane are not as abundant as they are in cylindromas. Perineural growth has been exceptionally reported {1605}. Cystic degeneration can resemble tumour necrosis.

## Differential diagnosis

Rare histopathological findings in spiradenoma include prominent cystic change from which immature basaloid cells emanate in a fenestrated pattern, which can simulate trichoblastoma. Some cases show features overlapping those of cylindroma, emphasizing the close relationship between these tumours. Rarely, the lesions focally resemble adenoid cystic carcinoma {2040}.

## Genetic profile

Brooke–Spiegler syndrome, which is inherited in an autosomal dominant pattern, is characterized by spiradenomas associated with multiple trichoepitheliomas, cylindromas, and tumours of the parotid gland. The gene responsible for this syndrome, *CYLD*, is located at 16q12.1 and shows sequence mutations or loss of heterozygosity at 16q typical of a tumour suppressor gene.

## Prognosis and predictive factors

Spiradenoma is a benign neoplasm.

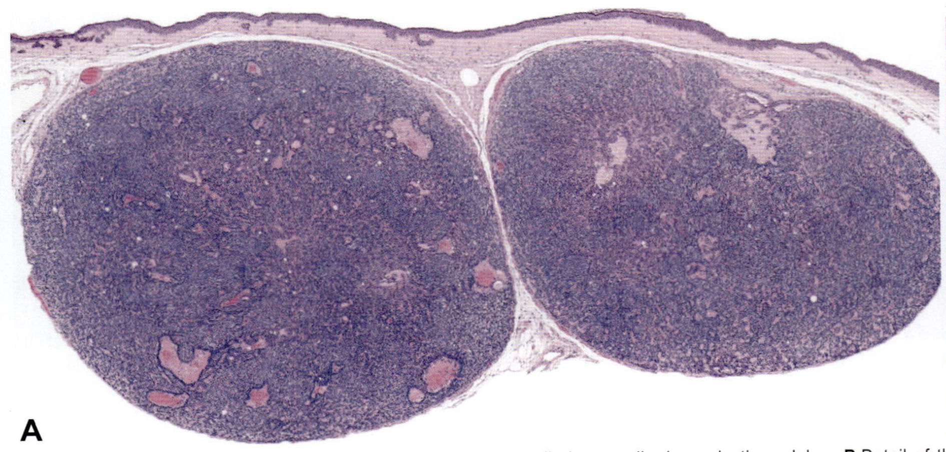


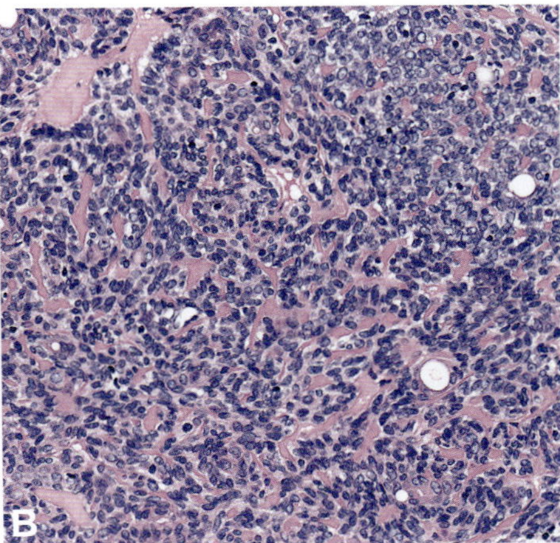


**Fig. 3.37** Spiradenoma. **A** Scanning magnification shows two well-circumscribed neoplastic nodules. **B** Detail of the basaloid cells and the basement membrane material; numerous ductal structures are present.

# Cylindroma

Sangüeza O.P.
Cassarino D.S.
Glusac E.J.
Kazakov D.V.
Requena L.
Swanson P.E.
Vassallo C.

## Definition
Cylindroma is a benign adnexal neoplasm with a mosaic microscopic pattern. Cylindroma commonly occurs as a hybrid with spiradenoma, a phenomenon that has been referred to as cylindrospiradenoma or spiradenocylindroma.

## ICD-O code
8200/0

## Synonyms
Cylindrospiradenoma; spiradenocylindroma

## Epidemiology
Cylindromas can be solitary or multiple. They can arise sporadically or as part of Brooke–Spiegler syndrome (BSS). There is no sex predilection.

## Etiology
The etiology is unknown. Multiple cylindromas are seen in patients with BSS, an inherited autosomal dominant disease characterized by the development of multiple adnexal cutaneous neoplasms, most commonly spiradenoma, cylindroma, spiradenocylindroma, and trichoepithelioma {1298}. The gene implicated in the pathogenesis of BSS is *CYLD*, a tumour suppressor gene located at 16q12.1 {284}. Germline *CYLD* mutations are found in about 80–85% of patients with the classic BSS phenotype. Loss of heterozygosity at 16q has also been found in sporadic cylindromas and spiradenomas.

## Localization
Cylindroma most commonly affects the head and neck, but it is also found on the trunk and extremities.

## Clinical features
Cylindromas are typically smooth, dome-shaped, hairless, reddish-brown papules or nodules. Multiple cylindromas located on the scalp have historically been referred to as turban tumours.

## Histopathology
Cylindroma is a symmetrical, well-circumscribed lesion. It consists of multiple aggregates of basaloid cells disposed in a jigsaw-puzzle arrangement and surrounded by a prominent basement membrane that gives a positive periodic acid–Schiff (PAS) reaction. Two types of cells form the epithelial collections: small basaloid and larger pale cells. There are also ductal structures. Many neoplasms show findings of both spiradenoma and cylindroma in the same lesion (spiradenocylindroma) {2521}.

## Differential diagnosis
Adenoid cystic carcinoma with prominent jigsaw-puzzle arrangement can enter the differential diagnosis, as can rare examples of basal cell carcinoma in which a thick basement membrane surrounds the aggregates of basaloid cells {674,2128}.

## Genetic profile
Several genetic studies have identified mutations of the tumour suppressor gene *CYLD* in patients with BSS {242,948}.

## Prognosis and predictive factors
Cylindroma is a benign neoplasm.

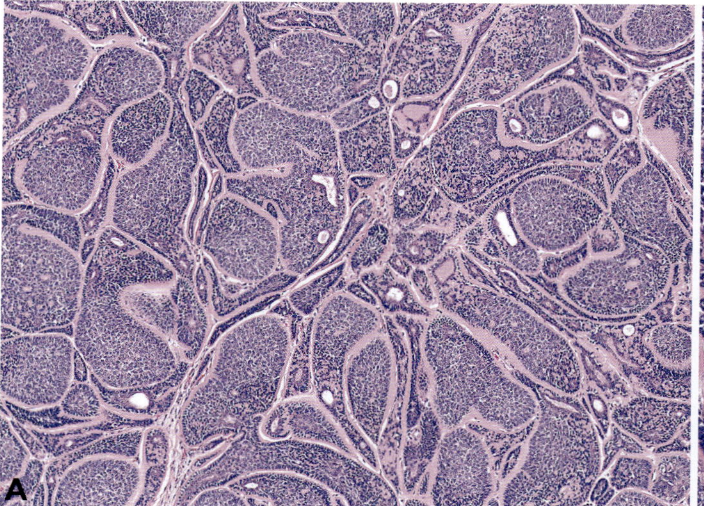


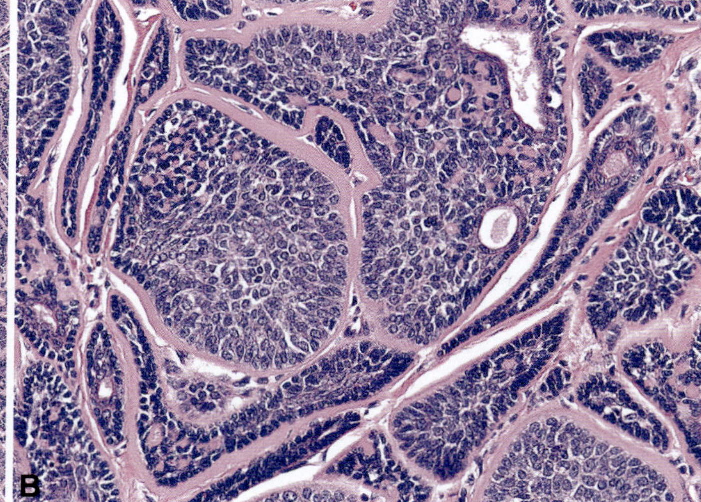


**Fig. 3.38** Cylindroma. **A** The epithelial collections are composed of two types of cells: there is a peripheral layer of small basaloid cells in a palisade arrangement and larger cells with pale cytoplasm in the centre. **B** Higher magnification of the cells and areas with ductal differentiation.

# Tubular adenoma

Sangüeza O.P.
Cassarino D.S.
Glusac E.J.
Kazakov D.V.
Requena L.
Swanson P.E.
Vassallo C.

## Definition

Tubular adenoma is a benign dermal neoplasm composed of tubules and glandular structures with or without papillae.

## ICD-O code

8211/0

## Synonyms

Tubular papillary adenoma; papillary eccrine adenoma; tubular apocrine adenoma

## Epidemiology

Tubular adenoma most frequently occurs in middle-aged women {2591}.

## Localization

It is most common in skin of the lower limbs, but can also affect the face and scalp.

## Clinical features

The lesions present as asymptomatic, single, round, well-circumscribed nodules with a smooth surface. In some cases, they show a papillated surface and can be ulcerated. Their size ranges from < 1 cm to 7 cm, although most cases are < 2 cm.

## Histopathology

Tubular adenomas are well-circumscribed dermal neoplasms that may extend into the subcutis. They have an overall lobular architecture and are typically encased by a fibrous stroma. The lobules consist of multiple irregularly shaped tubular structures that have a double- to several-layered epithelial lining. The peripheral epithelial layer consists of cuboidal to flattened (myoepithelial) cells, and the luminal layer consists of columnar cells that sometimes demonstrate decapitation secretion. In some tubules, papillary cellular extensions that are devoid of stroma project into the lumina. Cellular debris and eosinophilic granular material are found within some lumina {1487}. The neoplasm lacks cytological atypia and mitotic activity. Overlying epidermal hyperplasia may be present. In cases that occur in conjunction with syringocystadenoma papilliferum {77,2627}, the tubular adenoma component is typically present underlying the syringocystadenoma component.

The luminal cells of the tubules are positive for CEA and EMA (epithelial membrane antigen), whereas the outer cell layer is typically reactive for myoepithelial markers {2165}. A focal lack of myoepithelial cells can be seen in areas with prominent squamous metaplasia or intraluminal secretions.

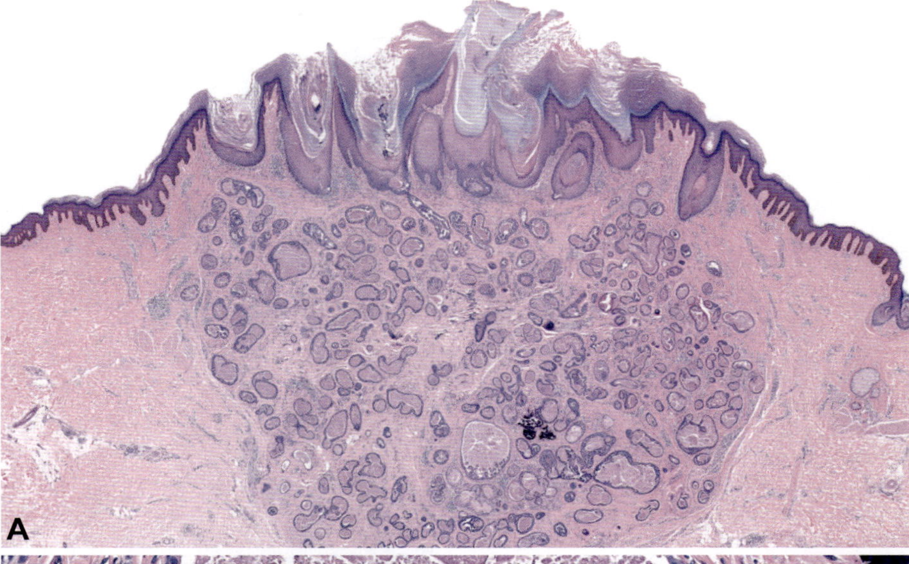


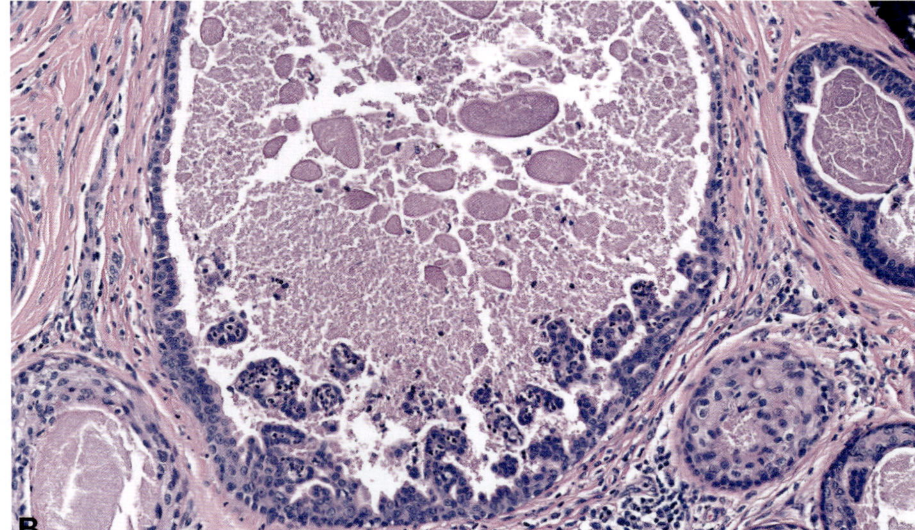


**Fig. 3.39** Tubular papillary adenoma. **A** Well-circumscribed neoplasm composed of tubules and cystic structures in the dermis. **B** Papillary projections with signs of secretion by decapitation and a focus of necrosis.

## Differential diagnosis

Tubular adenoma and syringocystadenoma papilliferum are probably variants of the same neoplasm {1302}.

## Prognosis and predictive factors

Tubular adenoma is a benign neoplasm.

# Syringocystadenoma papilliferum

Sangüeza O.P.
Cassarino D.S.
Glusac E.J.
Kazakov D.V.
Requena L.
Swanson P.E.
Vassallo C.

## Definition

Syringocystadenoma papilliferum (SCAP) is a benign apocrine neoplasm that presents either as an isolated lesion or in association with naevus sebaceus of Jadassohn.

## ICD-O code

8406/0

## Epidemiology

The tumours are more common in females than in males, with a wide age range.

## Localization

About 90% of cases are located on the head and neck, including the eyelids {1236} and external auditory canal {1844}. Less commonly, they may involve the mammary region {1925} and lower extremities.

## Clinical features

Most lesions appear as a solitary papule or nodule. Less frequently, they present as multiple grouped, oozing, crusted papules or nodules forming a plaque or horn. Many cases are associated with naevus sebaceus of Jadassohn.

## Histopathology

SCAP is an endophytic crateriform lesion, connected focally to the epidermis/hair follicle and composed of two layers of cells forming dilated papillary and cystic structures. The luminal cells are columnar with rounded or oval nuclei near the basal pole of the cell and abundant eosinophilic cytoplasm with decapitation secretion. Mucinous metaplasia may be observed. The outer layer consists of basal/myoepithelial cells. The overlying squamous epithelium often displays prominent hyperplasia. The epidermis surrounding SCAP is often papillomatous or wart-like, particularly in cases associated with naevus sebaceus of Jadassohn. The stroma contains numerous plasma cells.

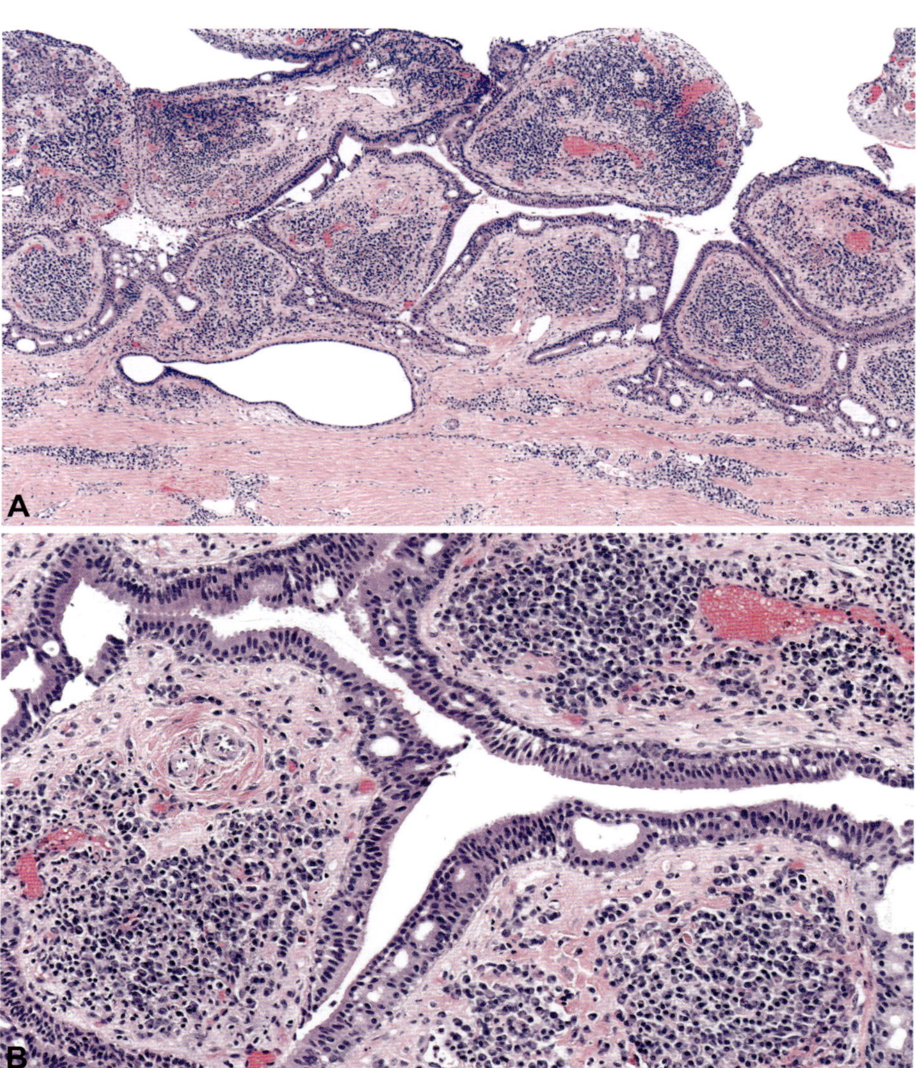

**Fig. 3.40** Syringocystadenoma papilliferum. **A** The lesion has numerous papillary projections lined by two or more rows of apocrine epithelium. **B** High-power view.

## Differential diagnosis

The histopathological differential diagnosis of SCAP includes hidradenoma papilliferum and nipple adenoma {1421}. Hidradenoma papilliferum has papillary formations similar to those of SCAP, and the epithelial cells lining these structures also show evidence of secretion by decapitation. However, hidradenoma papilliferum is not connected to the epidermis, lacks plasma cells, and is localized in the vulva {2509}. Proliferation of tubular structures is more prominent in adenoma of the nipple, connections with follicular infundibula are less obvious, and there are no plasma cells.

## Prognosis and predictive factors

SCAP is a benign neoplasm.

# Mixed tumour

Sangüeza O.P.
Cassarino D.S.
Glusac E.J.
Kazakov D.V.
Requena L.
Swanson P.E.
Vassallo C.

## Definition

Mixed tumour is a benign sweat gland neoplasm composed of epithelial, myoepithelial, and mesenchymal elements; it is the cutaneous analogue of pleomorphic adenoma.

## ICD-O code

8940/0

## Synonym

Chondroid syringoma

## Epidemiology

Mixed tumour is most common in middle-aged men. The reported age range is 10–96 years (median: 53.5 years) {1299}.

## Localization

These tumours often involve the scalp and face, but can also affect the external ear canal, eyelids, hands, and arms. The trunk and genital region are rarely involved.

## Clinical features

Mixed tumours are solitary (rarely multiple), well-circumscribed nodules with a smooth surface. They are typically 0.5–3.0 cm, but can be as large as 12 cm. Tumours with an osteocartilaginous component may be firm {2169}.

## Histopathology

Mixed tumour has two variants: eccrine and apocrine. Apocrine cases present as a well-circumscribed lesion with three components: epithelial, myoepithelial, and mesenchymal (i.e. mucinous, chondroid, osseous, adipocytic, or fibrotic). The epithelial component is composed of elongated branched tubules and cystic spaces. These epithelial structures are lined by two cell layers; the peripheral layer is composed of cuboidal myoepithelial cells, and the inner layer is formed by columnar cells. The luminal cell layer may exhibit secretion by decapitation. Cystic areas often contain homogeneous eosinophilic material. Solid aggregates of epithelial cells, as well as isolated polygonal and plasmacytoid epithelial cells, may be also seen. Tumours with a prominent myoepithelial component may show focal cytological atypia; such cases have been called hyaline cell–rich mixed tumour {265,1305}. Follicular and/or sebaceous differentiation can be present {2875}.

The eccrine variant of mixed tumour is less common. It is composed of numerous non-branching, round ductal elements lined by a single layer of cuboidal cells embedded in a predominantly myxoid or chondromyxoid stroma. Small solid epithelial aggregates may be seen. Unusual findings include cribriform areas, clear cell changes, hyaline cells, pseudorosette-like structures, prominent osseous metaplasia, and striking intracytoplasmic vacuolization of the neoplastic cells resulting in physaliphorous-like cells {1313}.

## Differential diagnosis

Myoepithelioma is a related entity distinguished by the lack of ductal structures. When the mesenchymal component is prominent, the differential diagnosis of mixed tumour includes chondroma, but chondromas do not contain epithelial cells.

## Histogenesis

Pluripotent cells are probably the source of glandular and myoepithelial cells {2169}.

## Genetic profile

*PLAG1* {131} and *EWSR1* {795} are rearranged in cutaneous mixed tumours.

## Prognosis and predictive factors

These are benign neoplasms that grow slowly, but over the course of years they can reach several centimetres in size.

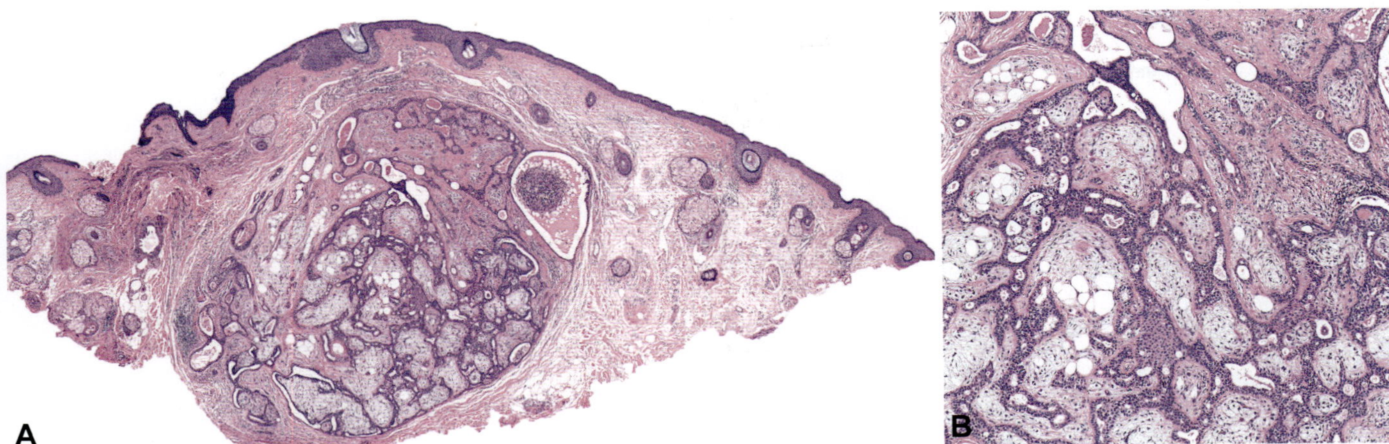


**Fig. 3.41** Apocrine mixed tumour of the skin. **A** Scanning magnification shows a well-circumscribed neoplasm with two components: epithelial and mesenchymal. **B** The epithelial component is composed of numerous branching tubules embedded in a myxoid stroma.

# Myoepithelioma

Hornick J.L.
Fisher C.
LeBoit P.E.

## Definition
Cutaneous myoepithelioma is composed exclusively of myoepithelial cells, similar to its salivary gland and soft tissue counterparts. Syncytial myoepithelioma is a distinct cutaneous variant. Although considered soft tissue neoplasms, myoepitheliomas are morphologically similar to cutaneous mixed tumour, and they are therefore discussed with adnexal neoplasms.

## ICD-O code 8982/0

## Epidemiology
Myoepithelioma usually arises in adults, with peak incidence in the third through fifth decades and a male-to-female ratio of 3:1 {1122,1230,1470,1768}.

## Etiology
Myoepithelioma is sporadic.

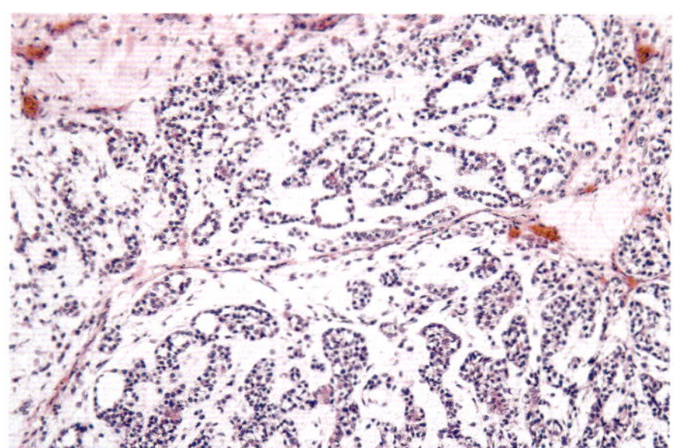

**Fig. 3.42** Cutaneous myoepithelioma. The tumour is composed of uniform epithelioid cells showing a trabecular and nested growth pattern, within a prominent myxoid stroma.

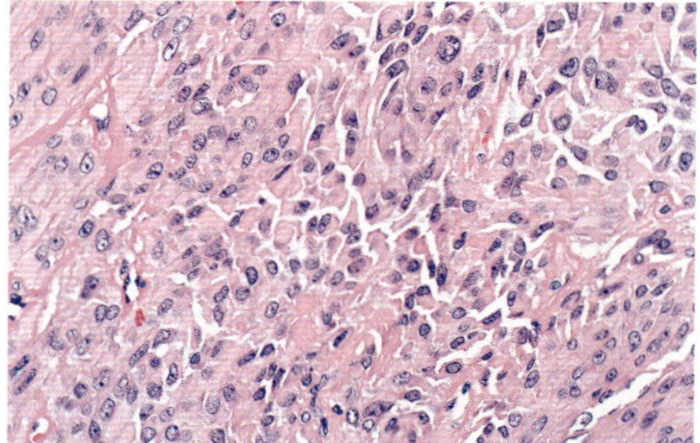

**Fig. 3.43** Cutaneous myoepithelioma. Some myoepitheliomas are dominated by plasmacytoid (hyaline) cells.

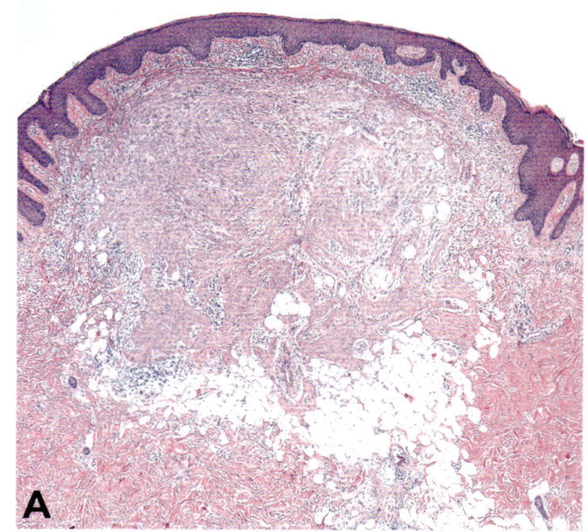


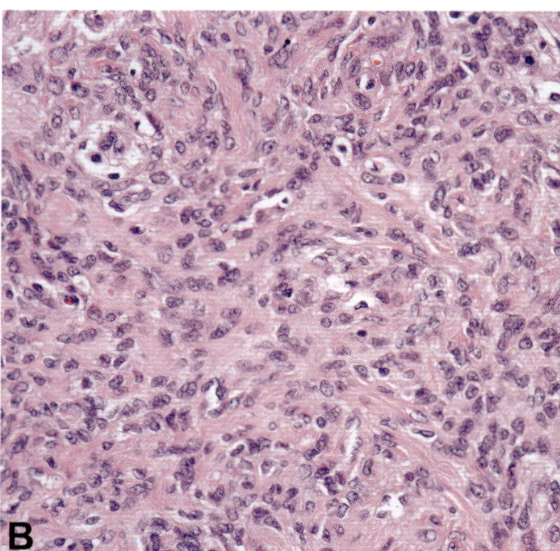


**Fig. 3.44** Cutaneous syncytial myoepithelioma. **A** This distinctive, often exophytic variant shows a sheet-like growth pattern; note the adipocytic metaplasia in the deep aspect of the tumour. **B** The histiocytoid to short spindle cells contain abundant, palely eosinophilic, syncytial cytoplasm.

## Localization
Cutaneous myoepithelioma shows a wide anatomical distribution, with a predilection for the extremities {1230,1750}.

## Clinical features
Cutaneous myoepithelioma presents as a painless, slow-growing papule or nodule {1122,1230,1750}.

## Histopathology
Cutaneous myoepitheliomas are well-circumscribed, occasionally with an epidermal collarette. Some tumours are lobulated and composed of a trabecular or nested arrangement of epithelioid, spindled, plasmacytoid, or clear cells, usually within a myxoid or hyalinized stroma, with areas of solid, sheet-like growth {1122,1750}. Extension into the subcutis may be seen. The exceptionally rare myoepithelial carcinomas often show marked atypia and a high mitotic rate; the minimal criteria for malignancy have not been established in the skin {828,1122,1750}. Cutaneous syncytial myoepitheliomas (accounting for 50% of cases) are composed of sheets of histiocytoid to short spindle cells with palely eosinophilic cytoplasm; one third show adipocytic metaplasia, whereas chondroid differentiation is rare {1230}. Cutaneous myoepitheliomas are consistently positive for EMA (epithelial membrane antigen) and S100 protein. Expression of keratins, GFAP, SOX10, p63, and SMA is variable {1122,1750,1768}. Syncytial myoepitheliomas are usually negative for keratins {1230}.

## Differential diagnosis
The differential diagnosis includes cutaneous mixed tumour, epithelioid schwannoma, ossifying fibromyxoid tumour, and extraskeletal myxoid chondrosarcoma. For syncytial cases, epithelioid fibrous histiocytoma and spitzoid melanocytic tumours can also enter the differential.

## Genetic profile
About 80% of all syncytial myoepitheliomas harbour *EWSR1* rearrangements, with unknown fusion partners {1230}. *EWSR1* rearrangements are less common in other cutaneous myoepitheliomas {795}. Similar translocations have not been demonstrated in cutaneous mixed tumour.

## Prognosis and predictive factors
Cutaneous myoepitheliomas are benign and rarely recur {1122,1230,1768}. Myoepithelial carcinomas may metastasize and follow an aggressive course {828}.

# Malignant tumours with follicular differentiation

## Pilomatrical carcinoma

Requena L.
Crowson A.N.
Kaddu S.
Kazakov D.V.
Michal M.

### Definition

Pilomatrical carcinoma is an adnexal carcinoma with matrical differentiation.

### ICD-O code 8110/3

### Synonyms

Malignant pilomatricoma; matrical carcinoma; matrix carcinoma; pilomatrix carcinoma

### Epidemiology

Pilomatrical carcinoma is an uncommon neoplasm {1073}. Most cases develop in middle-aged or elderly individuals.

### Localization

The site of predilection is the face, although examples in other locations have also been reported.

### Clinical features

Pilomatrical carcinoma presents as a solitary, often ulcerated nodule.

### Histopathology

Pilomatrical carcinoma appears as a poorly circumscribed and asymmetrical neoplasm involving the deep dermis, subcutaneous tissue, and even skeletal muscle and fascia. The lesion is composed of solid aggregates of immature basaloid cells. Neoplastic matrical cells show scant cytoplasm, a vesicular nucleus, and a prominent nucleolus, with numerous mitoses. Although shadow cells are less abundant in pilomatrical carcinoma than in pilomatricoma, they are very characteristic of the diagnosis {2325}. In some cases, inner root sheath differentiation (including trichohyaline granules and nests of bluish-grey cornified material) can be seen. More frequently, the neoplasm shows cystic spaces containing keratin and detritus material between the aggregates of matrical cells, resulting from necrosis en masse. Uncommon histopathological findings in pilomatrical carcinoma include desmoplastic stroma and vascular, lymphatic, and perineural involvement by neoplastic cells.

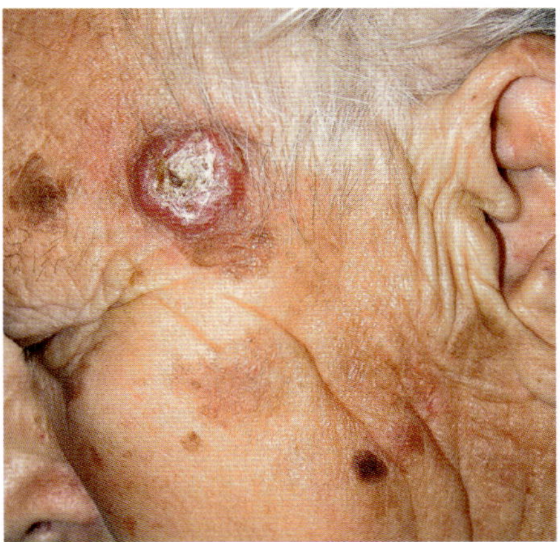

**Fig. 3.45** Pilomatrical carcinoma presenting as an ulcerated nodule on the left temple of an elderly man.

Immunohistochemically, pilomatrical carcinomas show both nuclear and cytoplasmic staining for β-catenin in the basaloid matrical cells; BerEP4 is negative {1041}.

### Differential diagnosis

The histopathological differential diagnosis of pilomatrical carcinoma includes pilomatricoma and basal cell carcinoma with matrical differentiation. Pilomatricoma is a benign cystic neoplasm that appears as a symmetrical, well-circumscribed lesion with regular and smooth borders; it usually does not show any areas of necrosis en masse or the cytological atypia seen in pilomatrical carcinoma. Pilomatricoma often exhibits numerous mitotic figures, but this is not a discriminating feature. Basal cell carcinoma with matrical differentiation is a neoplasm with all the architectural and cytological features of a basal cell carcinoma, plus collections of shadow cells in some areas; rarely, areas with matrical differentiation dominate and show certain cytological atypia {1476}.

### Genetic profile

In the few cases of pilomatrical carcinoma that have been cytogenetically analysed, mutations in the gene encoding β-catenin (*CTNNB1*) were found {1325}.

### Prognosis and predictive factors

There have been reports of pilomatrical carcinomas developing regional lymph node or visceral metastasis, and of patients dying as a consequence of the tumour {300,1786,1904}. Recurrence is a risk factor for metastasis {1073}.

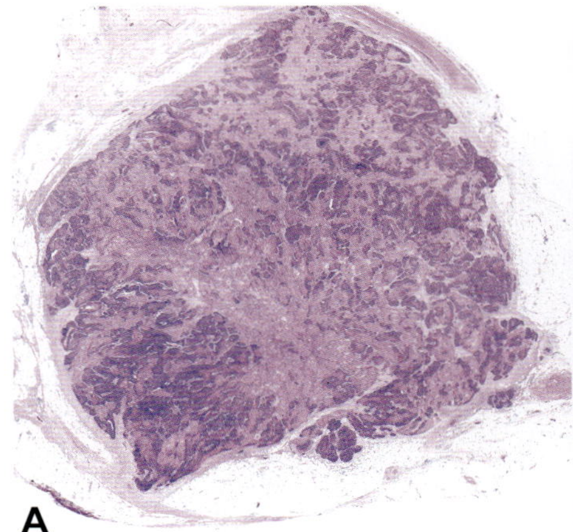

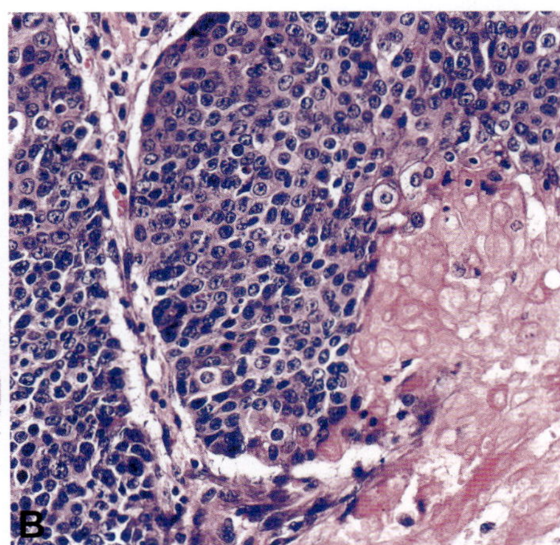

**Fig. 3.46** Pilomatrical carcinoma. **A** A scanning view showing a well-circumscribed nodule. **B** Higher magnification reveals pleomorphic matrical cells that keratinized, resulting in shadow cells.

# Proliferating trichilemmal tumour

Requena L.
Crowson A.N.
Kaddu S.
Kazakov D.V.
Michal M.

## Definition

Proliferating trichilemmal tumour (PTT) is a solid-cystic neoplasm with predominant outer root sheath differentiation at the isthmus. This entity encompasses a morphological spectrum including benign, atypical (intermediate), and rare malignant lesions.

## ICD-O code

8103/1

## Synonyms

Proliferating trichilemmal cyst; proliferating trichilemmal cystic carcinoma; proliferating tricholemmal tumour

## Epidemiology

This neoplasm most commonly occurs in women aged > 40 years.

## Etiology

The etiology is unknown. Some cases originate from a pre-existing trichilemmal cyst.

## Localization

The neoplasm is located on the scalp in > 90% of cases.

## Clinical features

PTT usually appears as a solitary, slow-growing, exophytic lesion, 2–25 cm in size. Some lesions show rapid growth.

## Histopathology

PTT spans a morphological continuum. At one end of the spectrum, it appears as a well-circumscribed solid and cystic neoplasm that involves the dermis and sometimes extends to the subcutaneous tissue. In addition to the typical features of a trichilemmal (pilar) cyst, this tumour shows prominent epithelial infoldings into the cyst lumen. The epithelium shows peripheral palisading of small basaloid cells arranged along a thick vitreous membrane, differentiating towards large keratinocytes with ample eosinophilic cytoplasm and abrupt keratinization without a granular layer. Often, areas of calcification and abundant cholesterol crystals can be seen within the compact eosinophilic keratin. The neoplastic cells are monomorphous, without significant cytological atypia and with only rare mitoses {1218,1923}.

At the other end of the morphological spectrum are neoplasms with malignant features such as invasive growth extending beyond the confines of the cyst wall coupled with nuclear pleomorphism and high mitotic activity. These areas may be indistinguishable from squamous cell carcinoma (SCC).

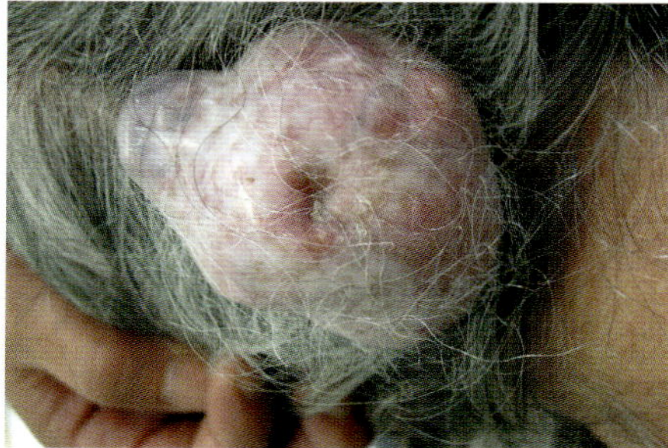

**Fig. 3.48** Large proliferating trichilemmal tumour on the scalp of an elderly woman.

## Differential diagnosis

The histopathological differential diagnosis of PTT includes ruptured trichilemmal cyst, giant trichilemmal horn, SCC, and the proliferating variant of epidermal (infundibular) cyst. Ruptured trichilemmal cysts may show irregular aggregates of keratinocytes with trichilemmal keratinization, but they lack the solid multilobular structure that characterizes PTT. Giant cutaneous trichilemmal horns consist of a mixture of squamous epithelial cells and trichilemmal keratinized debris.

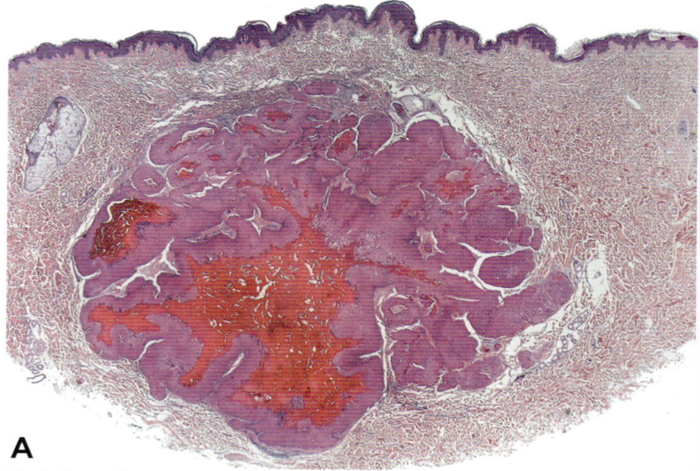

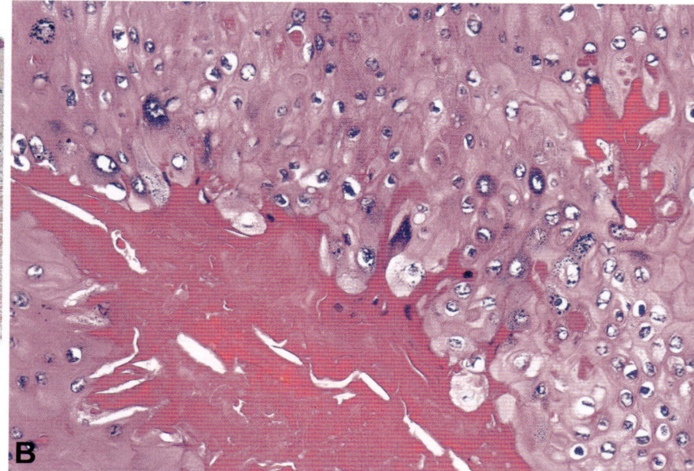

**Fig. 3.47** Proliferating trichilemmal tumour. **A** At scanning magnification, the tumour appears as a well-circumscribed dermal nodule. **B** At higher magnification, trichilemmal keratinization is evident: there are several layers of large and eosinophilic keratinocytes showing keratinization, without a granular layer, resulting in an eosinophilic, compact, orthokeratotic keratin.

In some cases, the base of the horn is directly connected with an underlying trichilemmal cyst of the scalp. Mitoses are common, but atypical mitoses are not observed. The nuclei of the squamous cells is monomorphous, without hyperchromasia or atypia {1764}. Uncommonly, SCC may show a cystic configuration, but the nuclear atypia of the neoplastic cells of SCC is more marked. There is no authentic trichilemmal differentiation in the neoplastic aggregates of SCC. The so-called proliferating variant of epidermal (infundibular) cyst {2324} consists of cystic structures lined by the infundibular epithelium and containing basket-weave, basophilic, and orthokeratotic keratin. It has been reported that there is degeneration into SCC in 20% of cases {2324}.

## Genetic profile

*TP53* mutation and loss of heterozygosity at 17p have been found in the malignant areas of malignant PTT, whereas the benign areas were found to have retained chromosome arm 17p {2562}. *CTNNB1* mutations do not seem to play a role in the histogenesis of this neoplasm {1325}.

## Prognosis and predictive factors

Most reported cases have shown benign biological behaviour. In rare instances, malignant transformation may occur in a pre-existing PTT, with the development of distant metastases {975,1696,1987,2800}.

# Trichoblastic carcinoma/carcinosarcoma

Requena L.
Crowson A.N.
Kaddu S.
Kazakov D.V.
Michal M.

## Definition

Trichoblastic carcinoma is a biphasic malignant neoplasm with dual differentiation towards the specialized follicular stroma (like that of trichoblastoma) and germinative follicular cells, which can be strikingly atypical. The term "trichoblastic carcinoma" is no longer used as a synonym for basal cell carcinoma.

Trichoblastic carcinosarcoma is a rare biphasic follicular neoplasm consisting of a malignant epithelial component resembling follicular germinative cells closely associated with a malignant stromal component differentiating towards specific follicular mesenchyme {1316,1322}.

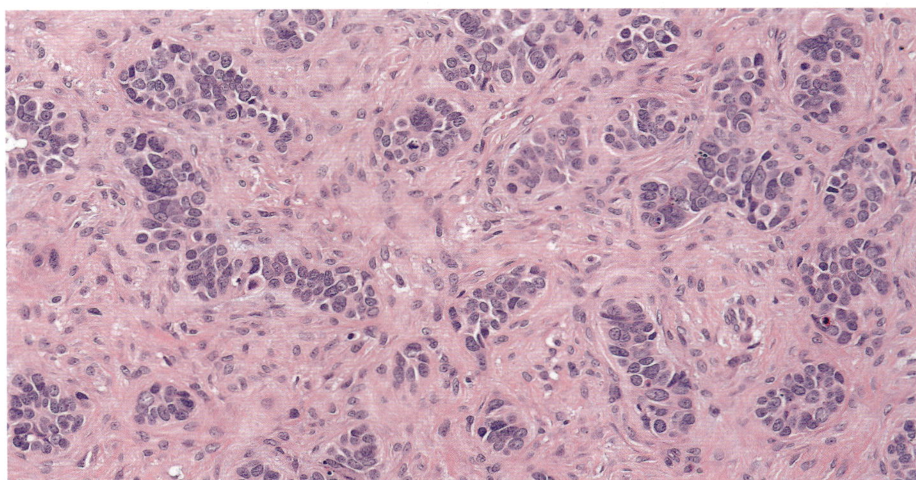

**Fig. 3.49** Trichoblastic carcinoma. This entity resembles a trichoblastoma because of its epithelial basaloid (follicular germinative) cell nodules associated with abundant specific follicular stroma, but unlike in trichoblastoma, there is cellular atypia in the epithelial component and atypical mitotic figures.

## ICD-O code 8100/3

## Synonym

Malignant trichoblastoma

## Epidemiology

Both neoplasms are very rare and probably under-recognized.

## Localization

The reported lesions have occurred in the head and neck and the trunk.

## Clinical features

These neoplasms appear to affect elderly patients and present as a solitary nodule.

## Histopathology

Trichoblastic carcinoma is composed of a stromal component identical to that of trichoblastoma and a basaloid component that shows moderate to severe atypia. In trichoblastic carcinosarcoma, both the epithelial and the mesenchymal components are malignant, with pleomorphic cells, abnormal mitotic figures, crowding, and hyperchromasia. Each epithelial nodule is intimately associated with the stroma, which recapitulates specific follicular mesenchyme by virtue of papilla-like aggregations that are often aligned across a broad front resembling so-called continuous papillae. Despite their close association throughout the tumour, the epithelial and stromal cells are sharply separated, with no gradual transition between the two elements; this is an important feature distinguishing this neoplasm from sarcomatoid (metaplastic) basal cell carcinoma.

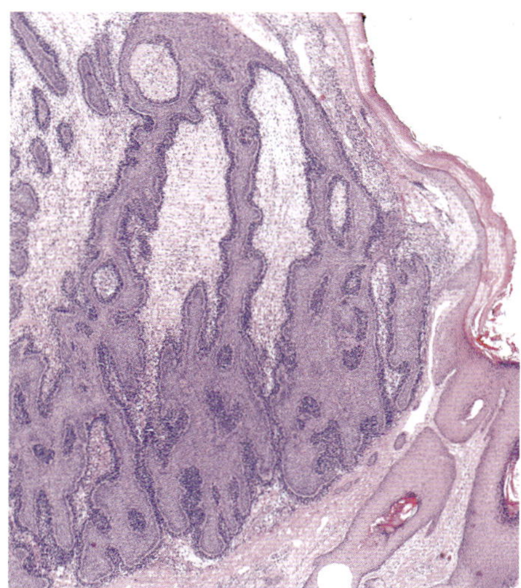

**Fig. 3.50** Trichoblastic carcinosarcoma. The tumour is composed of epithelial and stromal components with distinctive appearances.

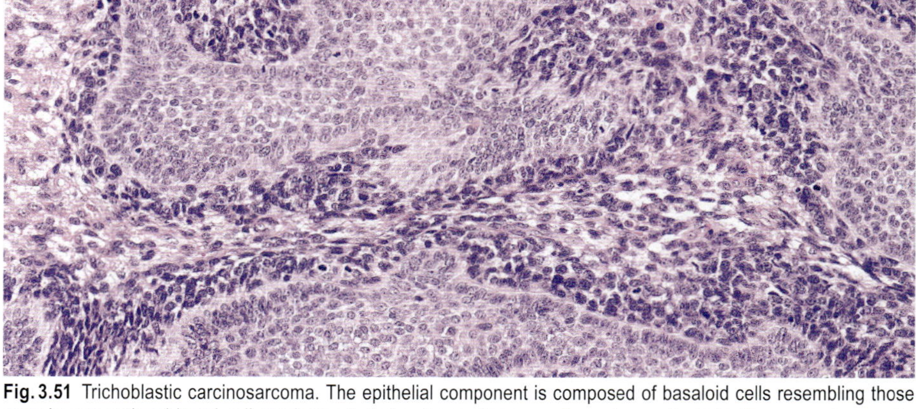

**Fig. 3.51** Trichoblastic carcinosarcoma. The epithelial component is composed of basaloid cells resembling those seen in conventional basal cell carcinoma but showing nuclear crowding, abnormal mitotic figures, and necrosis; germ-like structures are present focally. The epithelial component is intimately associated with the stroma, which recapitulates specific follicular mesenchyme by virtue of its papilla-like aggregations but is composed of clearly atypical cells with numerous abnormal mitotic figures, crowding, and hyperchromasia.

## Differential diagnosis

Trichoblastic carcinoma is distinguished from trichoblastoma by atypia in the epithelial component. Basal cell carcinoma lacks the specialized follicular stroma and is composed of basaloid epithelial cells that are less atypical than those seen in trichoblastic carcinoma/carcinosarcoma. In basal cell carcinoma with sarcomatoid differentiation, the transition between the epithelial and mesenchymal components is gradual, and the mesenchymal component appears as pleomorphic sarcoma rather than resembling follicular papillae {1332}. Trichoblastic carcinoma should be differentiated from benign plaque-like trichoblastomas that occur around the mouth and frequently involve the underlying skeletal muscle, which is a normal constituent of the deep dermis in this area {64,705}.

## Prognosis and predictive factors

Reported cases have shown indolent biological behaviour after complete removal. The term "trichoblastic carcinoma" has been used by some authors for various tumours occurring as a result of malignant transformation of a pre-existing trichoblastoma, and some of these tumours have demonstrated an aggressive clinical course {1379,1529,2147}.

# Trichilemmal carcinoma

Rongioletti F.
Luzar B.
Calonje E.
Crowson A.N.
Kaddu S.
Michal M.

## Definition

Trichilemmal carcinoma is a malignant adnexal neoplasm with outer root sheath differentiation. By this definition, trichilemmal carcinoma is the malignant counterpart of trichilemmoma. The concept of trichilemmal carcinoma, as originally proposed by Headington in 1976 {1051}, is debated, and some authors consider it to be a clear cell variant of squamous cell carcinoma {567}.

## ICD-O code 8102/3

## Synonyms

Tricholemmal carcinoma; trichilemmomal carcinoma

## Epidemiology

Trichilemmal carcinoma has a predilection for elderly individuals. The majority of cases occur between the seventh and ninth decades of life, with no sex predominance {857}.

## Etiology

The pathogenesis seems to be related to actinic damage, long-term low-dose X-irradiation, and malignant transformation of trichilemmoma. Total loss of the tumour suppressor gene *TP53* may contribute to the development of trichilemmal carcinoma {2562}.

## Localization

Trichilemmal carcinoma involves sun-exposed areas, most commonly the face, scalp, and neck, and less frequently the back of the hands.

## Clinical features

Trichilemmal carcinoma presents as an erythematous, tan, or flesh-coloured papule; a keratotic nodule; or an indurated plaque. They are frequently ulcerated. Trichilemmal carcinoma may arise in patients exposed to chronic actinic damage, receiving radiotherapy treatment with long latency periods, or affected by xeroderma pigmentosum. It can also occur in solid-organ transplant recipients. Presentation with multiple tumours and occurrence in Black patients has been reported. Unlike trichilemmoma, trichilemmal carcinoma is not associated with Cowden syndrome {1281,1656,1656}.

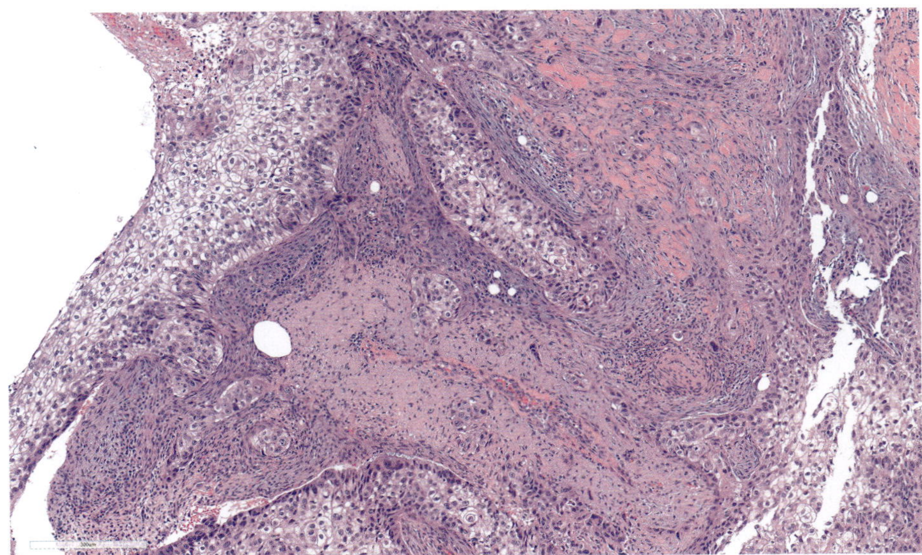

**Fig. 3.52** Trichilemmal carcinoma. High-power view showing the vacuolated cytoplasm and the irregular shape of the nests, with stromal invasion.

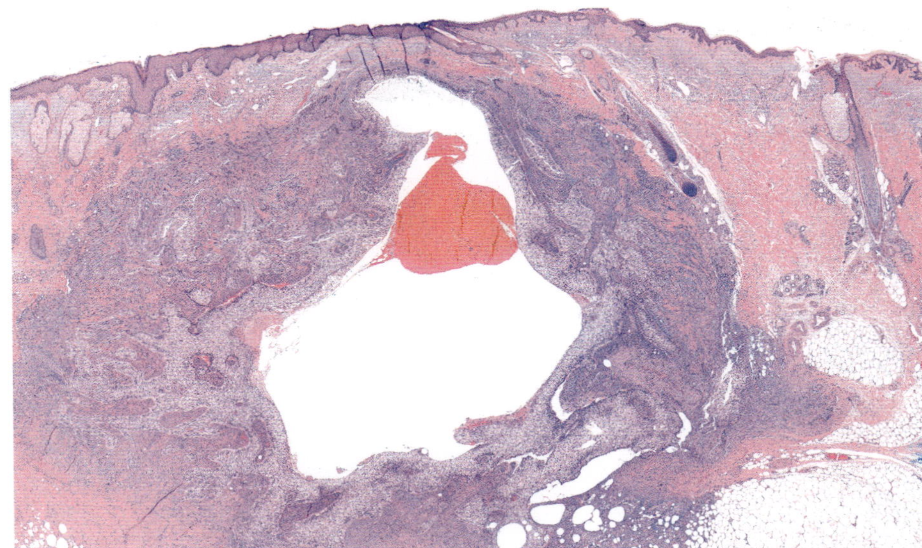

**Fig. 3.53** Trichilemmal carcinoma. Low-power view showing a poorly circumscribed infiltrative lesion with a central cystic area.

## Histopathology

Trichilemmal carcinoma is characterized by a proliferation of tumoural lobules (composed of large atypical cells with clear cytoplasm) with a sharply defined border and pushing margins continuous with the epidermis or pilosebaceous structures. The tumour cells give a positive periodic acid–Schiff (PAS) reaction, and there are prominent nucleoli, frequent mitoses, and foci of trichilemmal keratinization. At the periphery of the lobules, the keratinocytes show palisading and are surrounded by a prominent connective tissue sheath. The tumour is more commonly associated with an invasive component centred on a pilosebaceous unit and may show pagetoid spread in the overlying epidermis. The tumour cells are strongly positive for p53 and focally positive for CD34 (My10), which is a marker of differentiation from the outer root sheath. They are occasionally positive for EMA (epithelial membrane antigen). Trichilemmal carcinoma also expresses CK1, CK10, CK14, and CK17, suggesting that it differentiates towards follicular infundibulum {857,1466,2151,2225}.

### Differential diagnosis

The main differential diagnosis of trichilemmal carcinoma is clear cell squamous cell carcinoma, although these tumours are considered by some authors to be the same entity {567}. Squamous cell carcinoma with clear cells lacks trichilemmal keratinization or lobular proliferation. Trichilemmal carcinoma must be distinguished from other skin cancers with clear cell changes. The identification of ductal differentiation with CEA and EMA staining is useful for differentiating hidradenocarcinoma from trichilemmal carcinoma. Desmoplastic benign trichilemmoma may exhibit an infiltrative growth pattern but lacks pleomorphism and mitoses. Malignant proliferating trichilemmal tumour, which is often confused with trichilemmal carcinoma, demonstrates extensive areas of necrosis, abrupt keratinization, minimal pleomorphism, low mitotic activity, and foci resembling a trichilemmal cyst. Proliferating trichilemmal tumour is regarded as a distinct clinicopathological entity. Sebaceous carcinoma is distinguished by the presence of multiple intracytoplasmic lipid-rich vacuoles indenting the nucleus {2151}.

### Histogenesis

Trichilemmal carcinoma is thought to derive from adnexal keratinocytes with outer root sheath (trichilemmal) differentiation.

### Prognosis and predictive factors

Trichilemmal carcinoma is a carcinoma of low-grade malignancy with good prognosis that exceptionally can metastasize {1086,1393,2475,2937}. Tumour-free margins are a necessity because of the potential for local invasion and recurrence. Prognostic factors in trichilemmal carcinoma are limited to lymph node status and surgical margins {2475}.

# Benign tumours with follicular differentiation

## Trichoblastoma

Kutzner H.
Kaddu S.
Kanitakis J.
Kazakov D.V.
Schulz T.
Singh R.

### Definition

Trichoblastoma is a benign biphasic neoplasm with dual differentiation towards follicular germinative epithelium and specific follicular stroma. On the basis of their architectural features, trichoblastomas can be grouped into various types, including large nodular, small nodular, adamantinoid (lymphadenoma), retiform, and racemiform variants. Conventional and desmoplastic trichoepithelioma have also been referred to as cribriform and columnar trichoblastoma, respectively {243,1326,1331,1546}.

Most cases are sporadic, but multiple lesions are usually associated with Brooke–Spiegler syndrome or its phenotypical variant multiple familial trichoepithelioma, in which trichoepithelioma predominates {243,1326,1331,1546}.

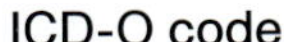

### ICD-O code 8100/0

### Synonyms

Trichoblastic fibroma; immature trichoepithelioma; cutaneous lymphadenoma

### Epidemiology

Sporadic tumours typically occur in the fifth or sixth decade, whereas syndromic lesions usually develop around puberty.

### Localization

The head and neck area are predilection sites for all trichoblastoma variants.

### Clinical features

Sporadic lesions are typically solitary, asymptomatic, skin-coloured or reddish, and 0.5–3 cm in size. Large nodular trichoblastoma is often associated with sebaceous naevus and appears pigmented. Syndromic tumours appear as bilateral, small (0.2–1 cm), discrete and/or confluent skin-coloured papules and nodules on the face, preferentially involving the nasolabial folds.

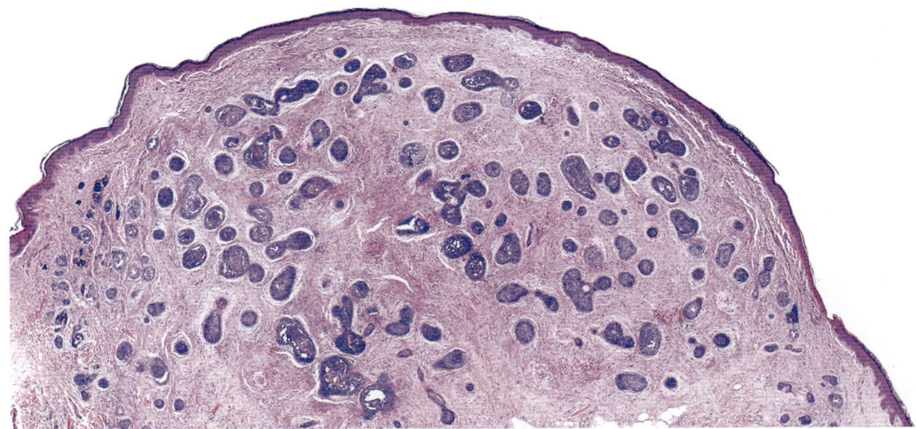

**Fig. 3.54** Trichoblastoma. Multinodular arrangement, with prominent stroma.

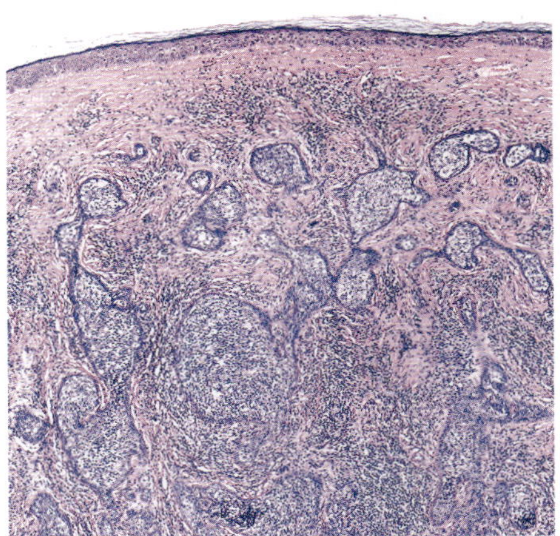

**Fig. 3.55** Trichoblastoma. The adamantinoid variant (also called cutaneous lymphadenoma).

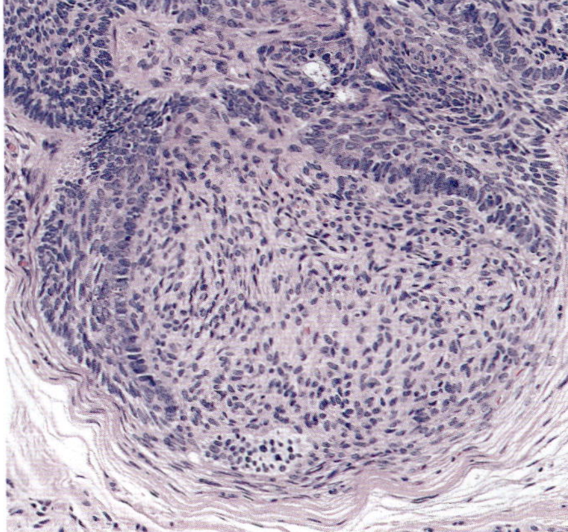

**Fig. 3.56** Trichoblastoma. A papillary mesenchymal body in close contact with basaloid epithelia.

### Histopathology

All trichoblastoma variants are usually well-circumscribed, non-ulcerated neoplasms confined to the dermis, rarely involving the subcutis. Occasionally, trichoblastoma can be shelled out or shows a multinodular arrangement, with the formation of distinct fibroepithelial units, usually separated by clefts. Tumours are composed of uniform basaloid cells with scant cytoplasm associated with a stromal component that resembles specific follicular mesenchyme, including follicular papillae (mesenchymal cell aggregations, also known as papillary mesenchymal bodies) and the perifollicular sheath (delicate fibrillary collagen bundles and numerous spindled fibroblasts). This type of stroma is less conspicuous in adamantinoid and large nodular trichoblastomas, as well as in desmoplastic trichoepithelioma (also called columnar trichoblastoma). In conventional trichoepithelioma (also called cribriform trichoblastoma), the predominant arrangement of the epithelial elements is cribriform (sieve-like), although the so-called racemiform pattern (cellular

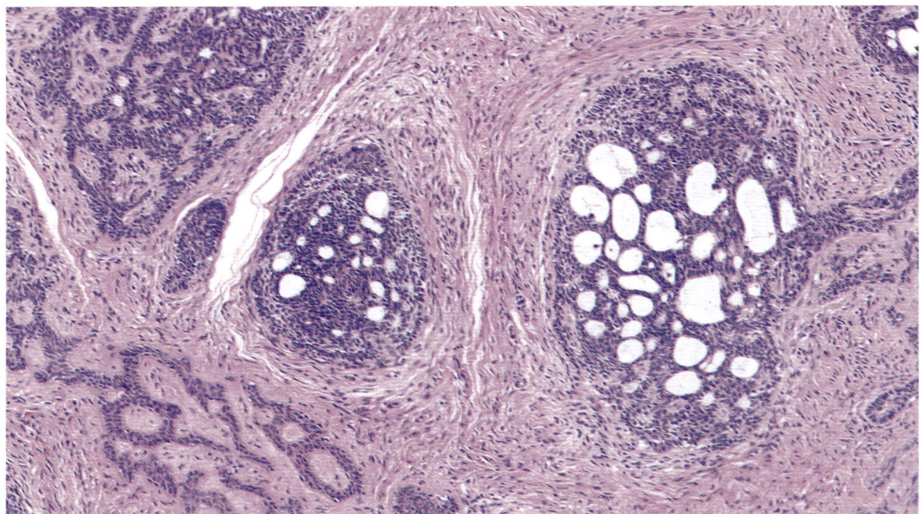

**Fig. 3.57** Trichoblastoma. A retiform tumour pattern, with prominent stroma.

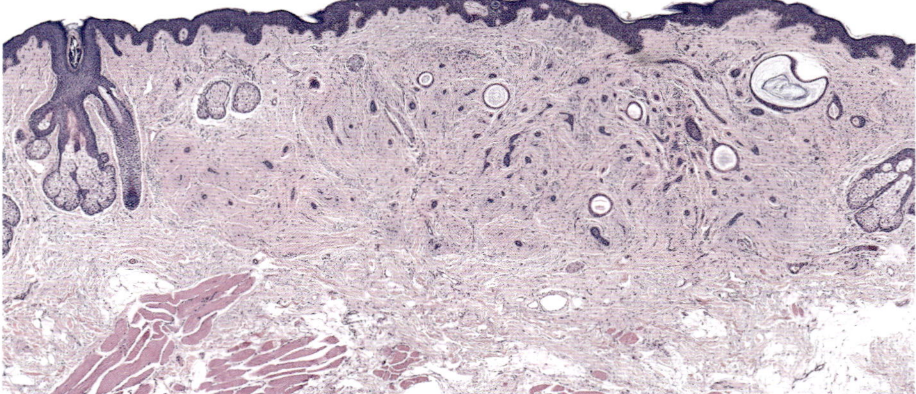

**Fig. 3.58** Desmoplastic trichoepithelioma (also called columnar trichoblastoma). The low-power view shows a well-demarcated, discrete dermal lesion. There are narrow cords of compact epithelial cells and keratinous microcysts in a background of dense and collagenous sclerotic stroma.

aggregations resembling clusters of grapes) and retiform structures (cords and columns of neoplastic cells in a net-like pattern) are also often seen, suggesting that all may represent various stages in growth or are seen in different planes of section. Several discrete or confluent large nodules, often with melanin deposits, are seen in large nodular trichoblastoma. In the small nodular variant, the stroma may dominate over small epithelial aggregates of follicular germinative cells. Adamantinoid trichoblastoma is composed of epithelial cell nodules with peripherally located palisaded basaloid cells and centrally located pale larger cells with vesicular nuclei, prominent nucleoli, and abundant faintly eosinophilic or amphophilic cytoplasm admixed with numerous small lymphocytes and occasional large multinucleated cells resembling Reed–Sternberg cells.

Desmoplastic trichoepithelioma (columnar trichoblastoma) is usually located in the upper reticular dermis and is composed of basaloid cells arranged in short cords, thin columns, and small nests. It is enveloped by bundles of collagen; rudimentary follicular papillae are rarely seen {18,232,1322,1854,2211,2309}.

Histopathological features variably encountered in trichoblastomas include advanced follicular differentiation (i.e. a second population of epithelial cells with abundant eosinophilic to clear cytoplasm, likely representing differentiation towards the upper part of the outer root sheath or isthmus, infundibulocystic structures, etc.), clear cell change (likely recapitulating outer root sheath at the bulb/stem), focal sebaceous differentiation, focal ductal differentiation, melanocytic colonization, melanocytic hyperplasia overlying the tumours or an association with a melanocytic naevus (seen in 10–15% of desmoplastic trichoepitheliomas/columnar trichoblastomas), epithelial multinucleated cells, and various stroma alterations (e.g. amyloid deposits, lipomatous metaplasia, and prominent myxoid change) {63,949,1321,1322,2309}.

Immunohistochemically, the epithelial cells are positive for BerEP4 {1467,1724,1939,2079}. Data on the presence of CK20-positive Merkel cells in trichoblastoma are somewhat conflicting: although some studies have found a consistent presence of Merkel cells, there are also cases completely devoid of Merkel cells. When present, ductal structures stain positively for EMA (epithelial membrane antigen) and CEA {1030,1031,1724,2355}.

## Differential diagnosis

Basal cell carcinoma is distinguished by its lack of a specialized follicular stroma. Microcystic adnexal carcinoma shows an infiltrative growth pattern and is negative for BerEP4, but distinction on superficial biopsies may be impossible.

## Histogenesis

Trichoblastomas are believed to manifest dual differentiation towards both the follicular germinative epithelium and the specific follicular mesenchyme, thus recapitulating events seen in the embryo and in postnatal anagen hair follicles.

## Genetic profile

Mutations (and polymorphisms) in *CTNNB1* (encoding β-catenin), *HRAS*, and *PTCH1* have been found in a minority of sporadic tumours {981,1325,2402}.

## Genetic susceptibility

Syndromic cases (occurring in the settings of multiple familial trichoepithelioma and Brooke–Spiegler syndrome) are associated with germline mutations in *CYLD*. Somatic mutations identified in the syndromic tumours are either loss of heterozygosity or sequence change {284,948,1331,2445}.

## Prognosis and predictive factors

Trichoblastomas are benign neoplasms. Malignant transformation is rare and is seen rarely in syndromic cases, in which basal cell carcinoma can develop within the background of pre-existing benign lesions {1330}.

# Pilomatricoma

Kutzner H.
Kaddu S.
Kanitakis J.
Kazakov D.V.
Schulz T.

## Definition

Pilomatricoma is a benign cutaneous adnexal tumour differentiating towards the matrix and the hair cortex.

## ICD-O code

8110/0

## Synonyms

Pilomatrixoma;
calcifying epithelioma of Malherbe

## Epidemiology

Pilomatricoma is common, accounting for about 1% of all pathologically diagnosed benign skin lesions {961}. It is the most common non-melanocytic cutaneous tumour excised in children {1591}. It can occur at any age (reported patient age range: 3 months to 93 years), but nearly half of all cases are diagnosed during the first two decades of life {961}. Most studies have noted a modest female predominance {1040,1929,2361}.

## Localization

The predominant location is the head and neck region (affected in 50% of cases), followed by the extremities (upper: 25% of cases, lower: 10% of cases) and the trunk (15% of cases) {961}.

## Clinical features

Pilomatricomas present as firm or hard, dermal or hypodermal, slow-growing, usually asymptomatic, solitary nodules measuring 1–3 cm {1072}. The overlying skin may look normal, show red or bluish discolouration, or be anetodermic or bullous/lymphangiectatic {1554,1804}. Giant and perforating forms exist {368,1804}. As many as 5% of patients have multiple pilomatricomas, usually in association with genetic syndromes (see below).

## Histopathology

Pilomatricomas consist of one or several dermal nodules, sometimes extending to the hypodermis. They are made of cells with a variable appearance. The peripheral cells are monomorphous, small, deeply basophilic, and mitotically active, with indistinct borders. Peripheral cells keratinize towards the so-called shadow (or ghost or mummified) cells, found towards the centre of the nodules; these are cells with distinct borders, an eosinophilic cytoplasm, and an empty space where the nucleus was once located. The transition occurs via an intermediate zone of cells with a small, pyknotic, basophilic nucleus and pale cytoplasm. The ratio of basophilic cells to shadow cells decreases with increasing age/maturation of the lesion. Pilomatricomas are sometimes cystic (most commonly those associated with Gardner syndrome). Calcification and ossification occur in old lesions, accounting for their stone-hard consistency. The surrounding dermis is fibrotic and often contains a foreign-body granulomatous infiltration. Pathological variants include pigmented and proliferating pilomatricoma (consisting predominantly of mitotically active basaloid cells). Pilomatricoma (basaloid) cells express β-catenin {1188,1554}.

## Differential diagnosis

Pilomatricoma should be differentiated from other pilar tumours that may show (focally) matrical differentiation (i.e. basal cell carcinoma, trichoblastoma, and melanocytic matricoma) and from its malignant counterpart, pilomatrical carcinoma. Pathological features favouring pilomatrical carcinoma include poor circumscription, an asymmetrical silhouette, frequent atypical mitoses, and lymphovascular invasion {1073}.

## Genetic profile

Most pilomatricomas harbour activating mutations in the exon 3 of the gene

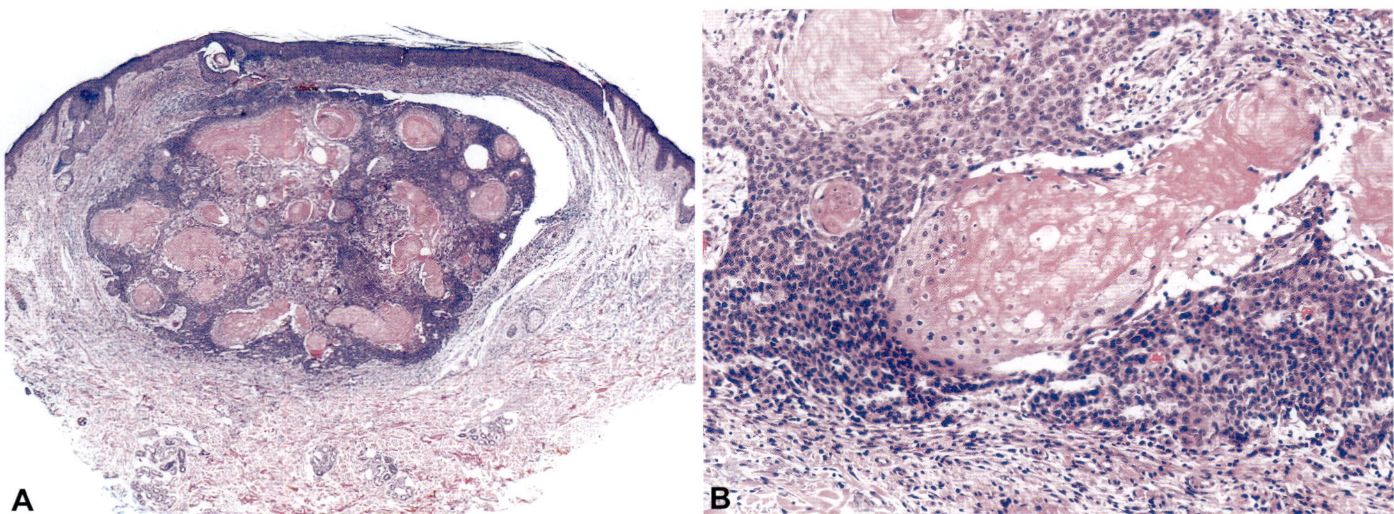


**Fig. 3.59** Pilomatricoma. **A** A circumscribed basophilic tumour with prominent cornification. **B** Gradual transition from germinative cells to cornified cells via shadow cells with pale cytoplasm and clumped nuclei.

encoding β-catenin (*CTNNB1*); the 92 kDa protein encoded by this gene is involved in cell–cell adhesion and in the WNT signalling pathway, which regulates cell proliferation, differentiation, and survival {1442}. Basaloid cells often harbour trisomy of chromosome 18, which carries the antiapoptotic *BCL2* gene, suggesting that the BCL2 oncoprotein may play a role in the growth and differentiation of pilomatricoma {28}.

### Genetic susceptibility

The vast majority of cases are sporadic; however, pilomatricomas can also be familial {1072} or multiple {634}, often in the setting of complex genetic syndromes such as myotonic dystrophy, Gardner syndrome, Turner syndrome, Rubinstein–Taybi syndrome, Goldenhar syndrome, Kabuki syndrome, Sotos syndrome, trisomy 9, and *DICER1* syndrome.

### Prognosis and predictive factors

Pilomatricomas are benign tumours. Rarely, they may recur, most commonly when incompletely excised {961,1040}.

# Trichilemmoma

Kutzner H.
Kaddu S.
Kanitakis J.
Kazakov D.V.
Schulz T.

### Definition

Trichilemmoma is a benign epithelial proliferation associated with the hair follicle infundibulum and showing trichilemmal differentiation. Multiple trichilemmomas occur in the setting of Cowden syndrome.

### ICD-O code

8102/0

### Synonym

Tricholemmoma

### Epidemiology

This is a relatively common cutaneous proliferation that develops predominantly in adults {324}. Multiple trichilemmomas are one of the cutaneous manifestations of Cowden syndrome {323,325,2059}.

### Localization

The tumours occur mostly on the head and neck, most commonly in the centrofacial area {324}.

### Clinical features

Trichilemmoma is usually a solitary lesion, either dome-shaped or wart-like. The tumours are small, typically ≤ 8 mm. Multiple trichilemmomas are almost invariably associated with Cowden syndrome {2500,2502}.

### Histopathology

Trichilemmoma typically presents as a superficial exo-endophytic epithelial proliferation, usually in association with one or more pre-existing hair follicles. There is marked digitated to bulbous thickening of the follicular infundibulum, with superficial hypergranulosis and hyperkeratosis. Trichilemmomas are often surrounded by a reactive epidermal collarette {324}.

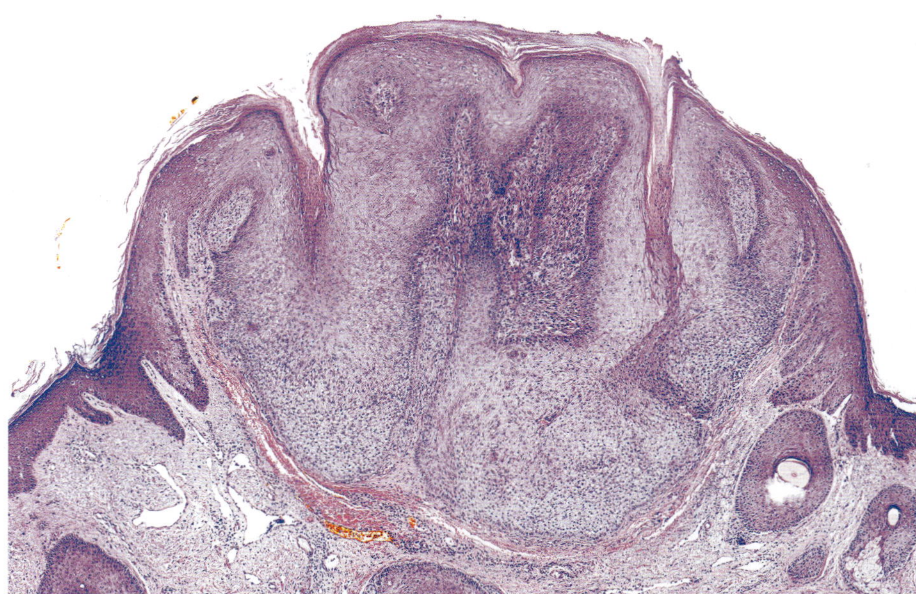

**Fig. 3.60** Trichilemmoma. Scanning magnification shows an exo-endophytic epithelial tumour with a wart-like silhouette.

The key diagnostic feature of trichilemmoma is at least focal trichilemmal differentiation of keratinocytes, reminiscent of cells of the outer root sheath (the trichilemma) of the lower hair follicle. These monomorphic cells are pale and clear. Central foci of infundibular keratinization, squamous eddies, and microcysts are occasional findings. There are no mitoses. At the periphery of the lobules, the pale cells are columnar and arranged in a palisade, bordered by a rim of hyaline deposits, recapitulating the prominent basement membrane of the lower hair follicle.

There is sometimes exaggerated deposition of basement membrane–like material, resulting in desmoplastic-looking stroma with embedded small irregular epithelial strands of cells with minimal evidence of trichilemmal differentiation, simulating an invasive carcinoma

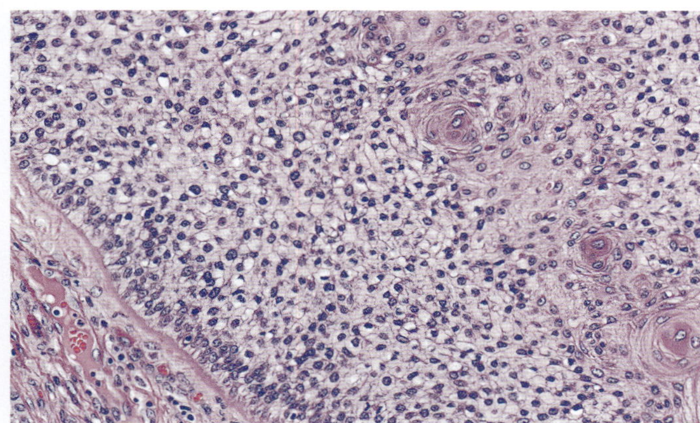

**Fig. 3.61** Trichilemmoma. There is characteristic trichilemmal (clear cell) differentiation, which is a key diagnostic criterion. There is also palisaded epithelial arrangement at the outer margin with prominent basement membrane, as well as occasional squamous eddies representing spiralling ducts within the follicular epithelium.

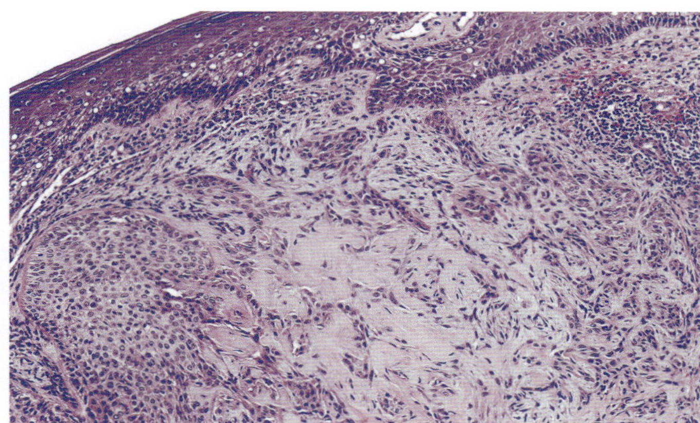

**Fig. 3.62** Desmoplastic trichilemmoma. Irregular epithelial nests and strands embedded in a desmoplastic stroma.

{1156,2590}. The term "desmoplastic trichilemmoma" has been coined for such lesions {1156}.

PTEN expression may be lost, more commonly in lesions from patients with Cowden syndrome {43}. Both conventional and desmoplastic trichilemmomas commonly express p16 and CD34 {1079,2576}.

## Differential diagnosis

The main differential diagnosis is basal cell carcinoma with trichilemmal differentiation. The surface of trichilemmoma may be indistinguishable from verruca vulgaris, and inverted follicular keratosis displays numerous squamous eddies and no thickening of basement membrane {17,2185}.

## Genetic profile

Solitary trichilemmomas do not have any genetic associations. Multiple trichilemmomas are a major diagnostic criterion for Cowden syndrome, which is part of the *PTEN* hamartoma tumour syndrome spectrum {323,2059}.

## Prognosis and predictive factors

Trichilemmoma is benign.

# Trichofolliculoma

Kutzner H.
Kaddu S.
Kanitakis J.
Kazakov D.V.
Schulz T.

## Definition

Trichofolliculoma is a rare cystic neoplasm with panfollicular differentiation, consisting of a central, dilated hair follicle from which several smaller secondary follicles radiate into the surrounding dermis
.

## ICD-O code 8101/0

## Epidemiology

Trichofolliculoma is rare. It has a slight male predominance and a predilection for middle-aged adults {1790,2221}. Congenital cases exist {2221}.

## Localization

The vast majority of trichofolliculomas develop on the face {1790,2221}. Rare locations include the genitalia {2036}, lip, and upper limbs {467}.

## Clinical features

Trichofolliculoma presents as a skin-coloured, dome-shaped papule or nodule measuring an average of 7 mm. A characteristic feature is the presence of a central pore with a tuft of thin (white) vellus hairs {2221}. Trichofolliculomas may rarely be multiple {467}.

## Histopathology

There is a central, dilated, vertically oriented hair follicle opening to the skin surface by an ostium corresponding to the pore seen macroscopically. From this follicle, several smaller secondary (and occasionally tertiary), more or less mature or abortive follicles radiate to the surrounding dermis, showing differentiation towards the inferior hair follicle segment. The central follicle contains keratinous material and occasional hair shafts. Sebaceous glands may be associated with the hair follicles, and in some tumours they constitute the dominant element (sebaceous trichofolliculoma). Incidental focal acantholytic dyskeratosis has been reported {264}. Morphological variations have been reported according to the age of the lesion, because the (secondary) hair follicles may undergo the phases of the hair cycle {1790}. The lesion is embedded in a fibrocytic connective tissue sheath.

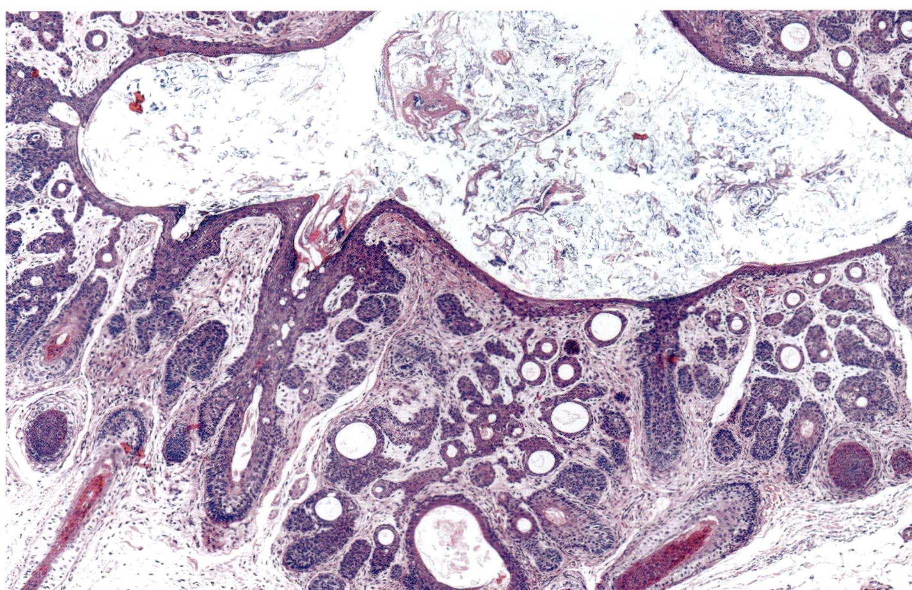

**Fig. 3.63** Trichofolliculoma. Incompletely formed and immature/abortive hair follicles with partial cystic differentiation.

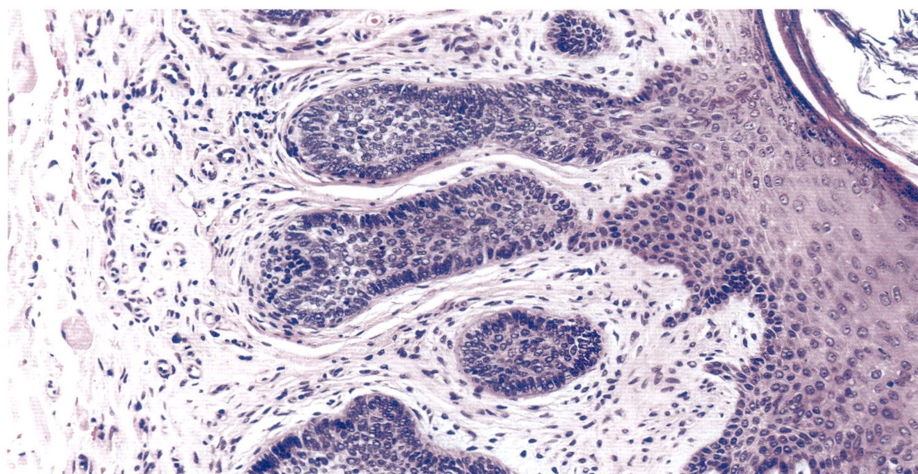

**Fig. 3.64** Trichofolliculoma. Hair bulbs and hair papillae are typical of abortive hair follicles.

## Differential diagnosis

Folliculocystic sebaceous hamartoma, which consists of a central dilated cystic infundibular structure to which sebaceous glands connect, is considered by some to be a late-stage trichofolliculoma, but this theory has recently been challenged {1790}.

## Histogenesis

Signalling pathways involving bone morphogenetic proteins and PYGO2 are associated with the experimental development of trichofolliculoma-like proliferations {2532}.

## Prognosis and predictive factors

Trichofolliculoma is a benign lesion with exceptional recurrences {902,2221}.

# Pilar sheath acanthoma

Kutzner H.
Kaddu S.
Kanitakis J.
Kazakov D.V.
Schulz T.

## Definition

Pilar sheath acanthoma is a benign follicular adnexal neoplasm characterized mainly by differentiation towards infundibular and isthmic epithelium of a normal hair follicle.

## ICD-O

8104/0

## Synonym

Infundibuloisthmicoma

## Epidemiology

Pilar sheath acanthoma is rare. It typically develops in middle-aged and elderly individuals (age range: 30–76 years), with no sex predilection.

## Clinical features

Pilar sheath acanthoma presents as a solitary 0.5–1 cm papule or nodule with a central keratin-plugged depression. The face (upper lip and central facial region) is the most commonly affected site {240,473,1731,2472,2681}.

## Histopathology

The tumour is an endophytic dermal lesion. The upper portion (infundibular component) is characterized by a large, central cystic, keratin-filled crater representing contiguous dilated infundibula, and is connected to the epidermis. The lower portion consists of numerous lobules of pink keratinocytes (isthmic cells) radiating centrifugally from the base of the infundibular component. The lobules display a focal palisade arrangement and a thin rim of fibrous tissue. Additional findings may include whorls of cornified cells and signs of sebaceous ductal and apocrine differentiation.

## Differential diagnosis

The differential diagnosis includes dilated pore (of Winer), trichofolliculoma, and fibrofolliculoma/trichodiscoma.

## Prognosis and predictive factors

Pilar sheath acanthoma is a benign neoplasm.

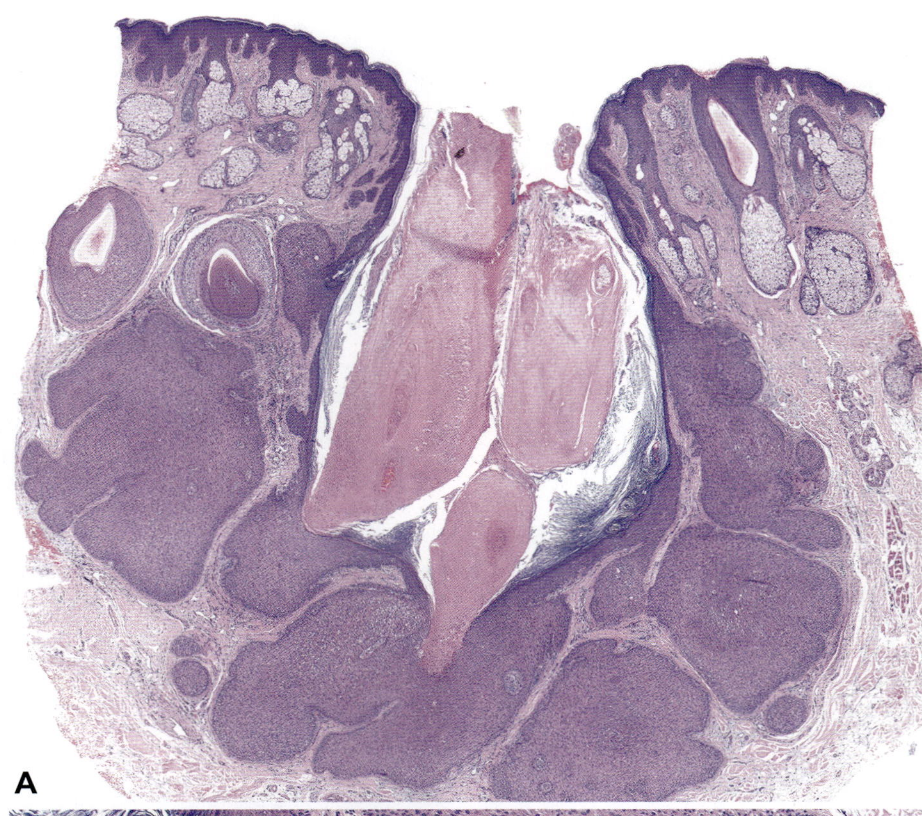


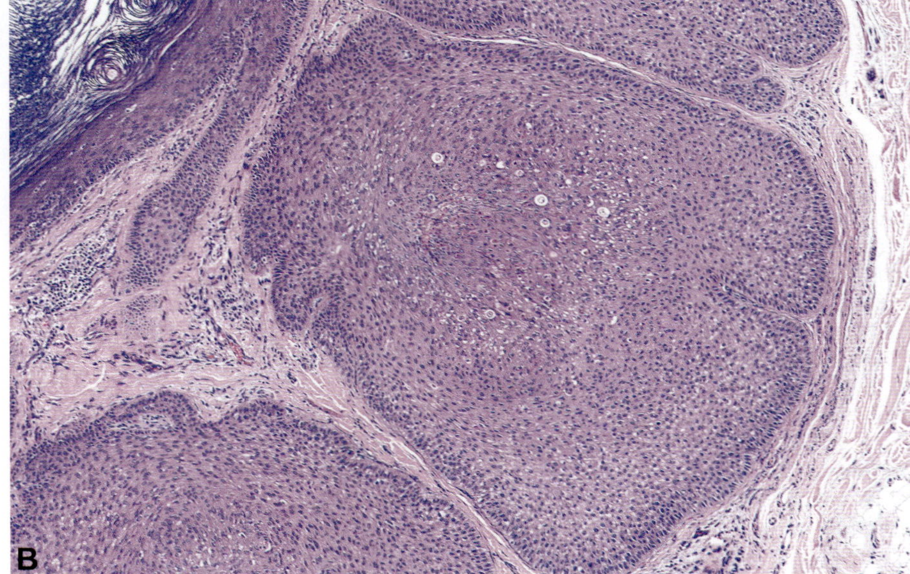


**Fig. 3.65** Pilar sheath acanthoma. **A** A well-circumscribed cystic tumour with an upper portion consisting of a widely dilated infundibulum filled with cornified cells and a lower portion showing lobules of cells with isthmic differentiation. **B** Lobules of keratinocytes (isthmic cells) radiate from the base of the infundibular component.

# Tumour of the follicular infundibulum

Kutzner H.
Kaddu S.
Kanitakis J.
Kazakov D.V.
Schulz T.

## Definition

Tumour of the follicular infundibulum is a rare adnexal follicular proliferation with predominantly isthmic differentiation {1730}.

## ICD-O

8104/0

## Synonyms

Infundibular tumour; tumour of the follicular isthmus; infundibuloma {1434}

## Epidemiology

These tumours have a relative frequency of 3–17 cases per 100 000 skin biopsies {4}. There is no sex predominance {4}.

## Localization

This lesion typically occurs on the face.

## Clinical features

Tumour of the follicular infundibulum typically occurs as a single, small (0.3–1 cm) papule or plaque, or (rarely) as several or multiple (from a dozen to hundreds) hypopigmented macules or papules. It usually presents in adults aged 60–70 years {1118,1415}.

## Histopathology

The lesion is a plate-like, superficial, horizontal proliferation of pale isthmic cells with abundant eosinophilic cytoplasm and small oval or round monomorphous nuclei. The cells emanate from the epidermis, are sometimes contiguous with follicular infundibula, and grow as strands in a fenestrated pattern. The base is usually smooth and focally exhibits basophilic palisaded cells. Focal sebaceous ductal differentiation can be encountered. The stroma is scant and fibrotic; no cytological atypia or clefts between the epithelial component and the stroma are seen.

## Differential diagnosis

Superficial basal cell carcinoma shows peripheral clefts and cytological atypia.

## Prognosis and predictive factors

Tumour of the follicular infundibulum is a benign lesion.

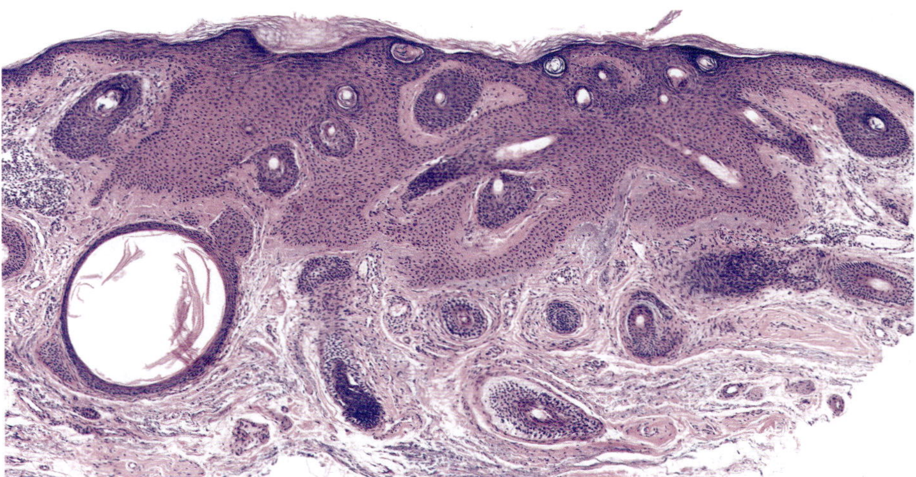

**Fig. 3.66** Tumour of the follicular infundibulum. Thin, streamer-like strands of pale epithelia emanating from the epidermis.

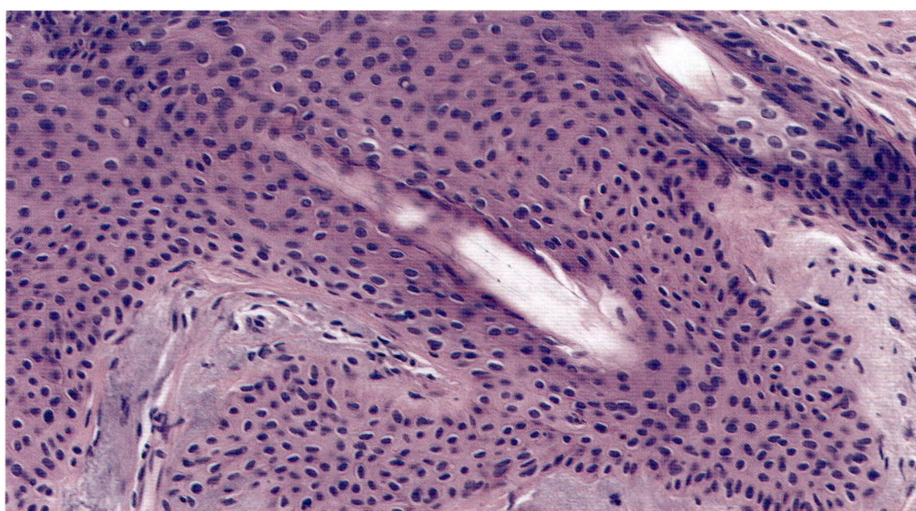

**Fig. 3.67** Tumour of the follicular infundibulum. Tumour cells emanate from the epidermis and grow as strands in a fenestrated pattern.

# Melanocytic matricoma

Kutzner H.
Kaddu S.
Kanitakis J.
Kazakov D.V.
Schulz T.

## Definition

Melanocytic matricoma is a pilar tumour recapitulating the bulb of the anagen hair follicle, with numerous intratumoural, pigmented, dendritic melanocytes.

## ICD-O 8110/0

## Epidemiology

Melanocytic matricoma is rare, with only about 22 cases reported {380}. The tumour typically affects elderly men, with a male-to-female ratio of 3:1.

## Localization

The most common location is the head and neck, followed by the trunk and the limbs.

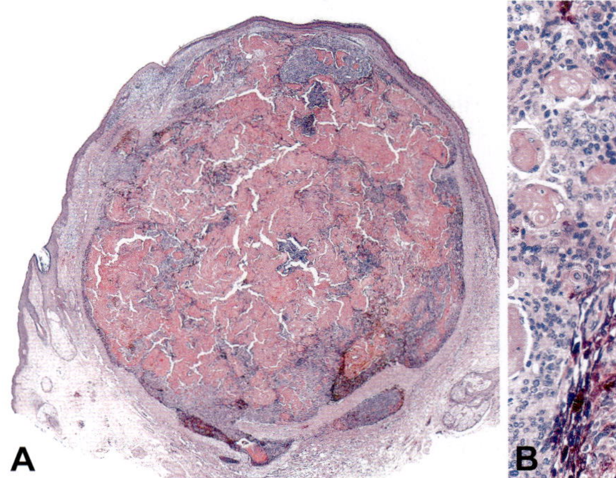

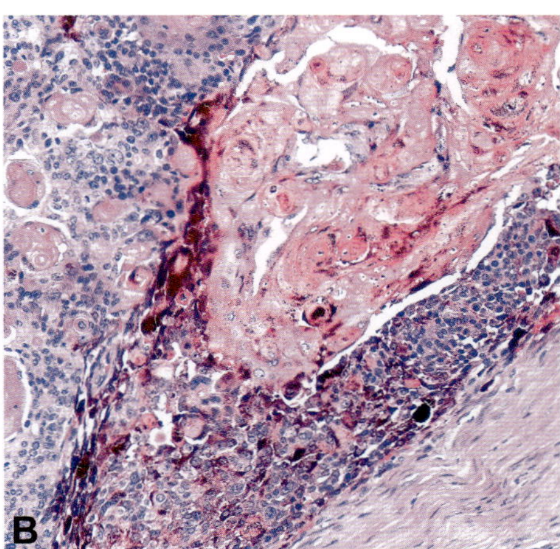

**Fig. 3.68** Melanocytic matricoma. **A** The sharply circumscribed tumour is composed of basophilic germinative hair matrix cells. **B** Pigmented dendritic melanocytes among germinative epithelia.

## Clinical features

Melanocytic matricoma manifests as a small, pigmented, purple or brownish-black papule or nodule. It may be ulcerated/crusted and painful {2572}.

## Histopathology

Melanocytic matricoma presents as a solid, well-circumscribed dermal tumour composed of aggregations of basophilic germinative, mitotically active, hair matrix cells with scant cytoplasm and prominent nucleoli. The tumour masses contain melanin deposits and pigmented, dendritic melanocytes. A few shadow cells usually exist, either isolated or in small groups. With rare exceptions {1191}, there is no connection with the epidermis or hair follicles. Rare tumours contain atypical melanocytes {161} or epithelial cells {87}. The matrical cells express PHLDA1 and (nuclear) β-catenin, but not BerEP4 {175,2477,2572}. Intratumoural melanocytes express S100 protein, HMB45 antigen (gp100), and melan-A {161,2572}.

## Differential diagnosis

The differential diagnosis includes pigmented pilomatricoma/pilomatrical carcinoma and basal cell carcinoma with matrical differentiation.

## Prognosis and predictive factors

Melanocytic matricoma is benign. Cases with more-prominent melanocytic and matrical atypia have sometimes been reported as malignant melanocytic matricoma {87}, but their clinical behaviour has not been well characterized.

# Spindle cell–predominant trichodiscoma

Kutzner H.
Kaddu S.
Kanitakis J.
Kazakov D.V.
Schulz T.

## Definition
Spindle cell–predominant trichodiscoma (SCPT) is a hamartomatous tumour of the follicular unit. It differentiates towards the mantle region of the hair follicle (mantleoma) {1256,1792,1792}.

## ICD-O code 8391/0

## Synonym
Neurofollicular hamartoma (obsolete)

## Epidemiology
SCPT is rare. It occurs equally commonly in men and women, usually not before the third decade of life {1473}.

## Localization
These tumours occur predominantly on the nose, and rarely in the perinasal area.

## Clinical features
SCPT typically presents as a solitary, protuberant, usually dome-shaped, skin-coloured, and smooth-surfaced 10 mm papule. Clinically, it may be mistaken for a basal cell carcinoma, naevus, cyst, or fibroma {1473}.

## Histopathology
SCPT is a symmetrical tumour composed of hyperplastic mitt-like sebaceous lobules on both sides, and an abundant central mucinous stroma with fascicular and haphazard proliferation of fibrocytes showing elongated, slightly wavy nuclei and tapering cytoplasm {1473}. Discrete lipomatous metaplasia is a common feature. Morphological variants with focal palisaded schwannoma-like arrangement of stromal cells {1256} or with hyperchromatic pleomorphic fibrocytes (symplastic SCPT) are rare {177}. SCPT is positive for CD34 and negative for S100 protein.

## Differential diagnosis
The differential diagnosis includes fibrofolliculoma, dermal spindle cell lipoma, and neurofibroma. Banal trichodiscomas are much smaller. A morphological variant of SCPT with few entrapped S100-positive nerves was previously known as neurofollicular hamartoma {1924,2306}.

## Histogenesis
Fibrofolliculoma and SCPT are hamartomas representing opposite ends of the mantleoma spectrum. SCPT is the late-stage lesion of this spectrum, showing mature sebaceous lobules surrounding an exaggerated stroma reminiscent of the peri-isthmic connective tissue.

## Genetic profile
The genetic profile is unknown. There is no association with Birt–Hogg–Dubé syndrome.

## Prognosis and predictive factors
This is a benign hamartoma. There have been no reported recurrences.

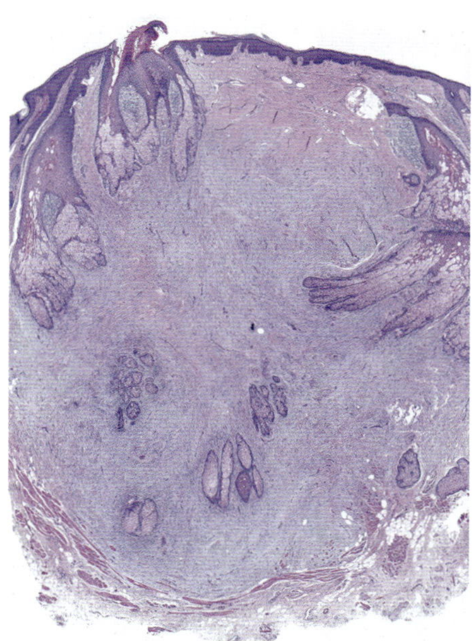

**Fig. 3.69** Spindle cell–predominant trichodiscoma. Characteristic mitt-like hyperplastic sebaceous glands on either side of a slightly myxoid cellular spindle cell proliferation.

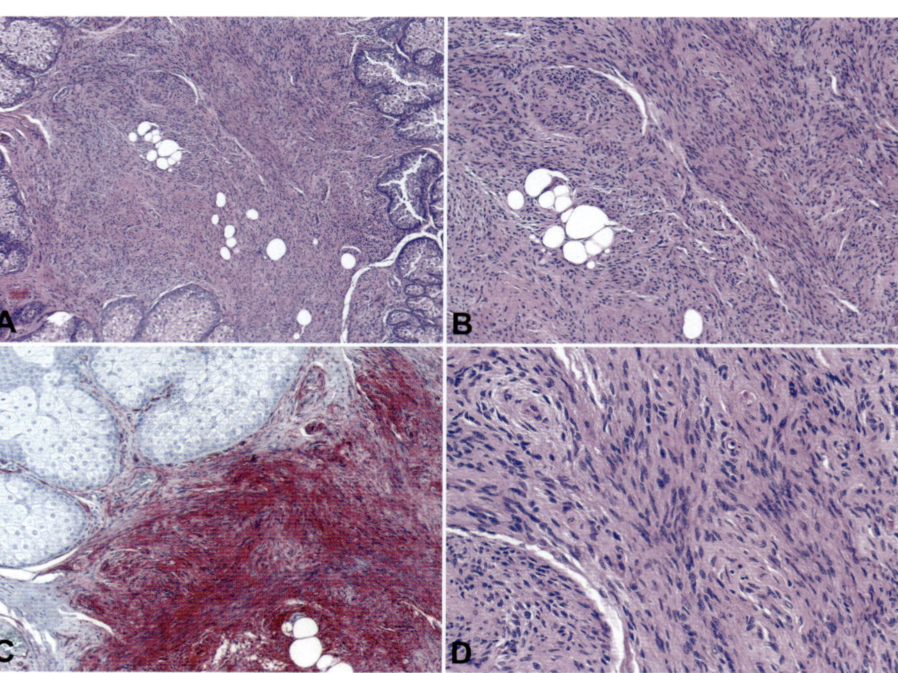


**Fig. 3.70** Spindle cell–predominant trichodiscoma. Strands and small fascicles of CD34-positive spindled fibroblasts and a few entrapped fat cells.

# Tumours with sebaceous differentiation

## Sebaceous carcinoma

Wick M.R.
Cree I.A.
Kazakov D.V.
Lazar A.J.
Michal M.
Sangüeza O.P.
Singh R.
Wood B.A.
Zembowicz A.

### Definition

Sebaceous carcinoma is a malignant neoplasm demonstrating sebocytic differentiation.

### ICD-O code 8410/3

### Synonym

Meibomian gland carcinoma (for eyelid tumours)

### Epidemiology

Sebaceous carcinoma usually arises in middle-aged or elderly adults, with no race or sex predilection. The median age at diagnosis is 73 years. The estimated incidence (per 1 million person-years) is approximately 2 cases in White populations, 1 case among Asians and Pacific Islanders, and 0.5 cases in Black populations {578}. Tumours of the eyelids may occur as a complication of prior radiotherapy {1132}. A minority (approximately 25%) of individuals with this tumour have Muir–Torre syndrome, but eyelid lesions have almost no association with the condition {3,238,1635,2395}.

### Localization

Sebaceous carcinoma can occur in any site. However, it has a predisposition for the skin of the head and neck, in particular periocular locations.

### Clinical features

Sebaceous carcinomas present as painless tan-pink or yellowish nodular lesions, as large as several centimetres in greatest dimension; some become ulcerated. In the ocular adnexae, they may be mistaken clinically for chalazions, blepharitis, cicatricial (mucous membrane) pemphigoid, or conjunctivitis {638,892,2846}. Extraocular sebaceous carcinomas are most commonly encountered in the skin of the head and neck, followed by that of the trunk, genitals, and extremities. Rare cases occur in the mouth, salivary gland, lung, and breast {999,1958,2542}. Sebaceous carcinoma may arise in sebaceous naevi {1308}, and it occasionally occurs in immunocompromised individuals {1170}.

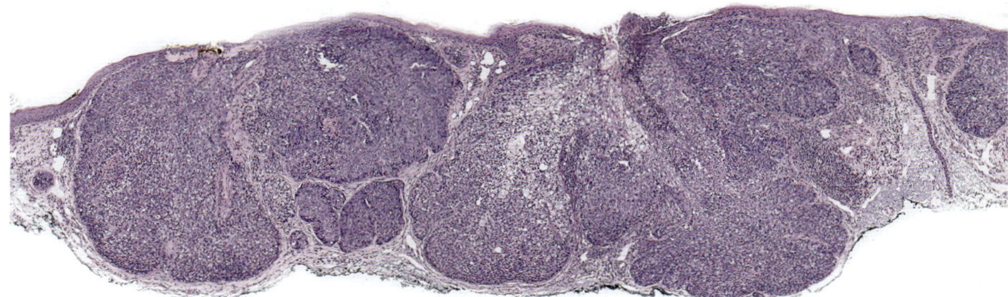

**Fig.3.71** Sebaceous carcinoma. Proliferation of neoplastic cells with sebaceous differentiation, showing multivesicular cytoplasmic clearing; focal squamoid differentiation is evident.

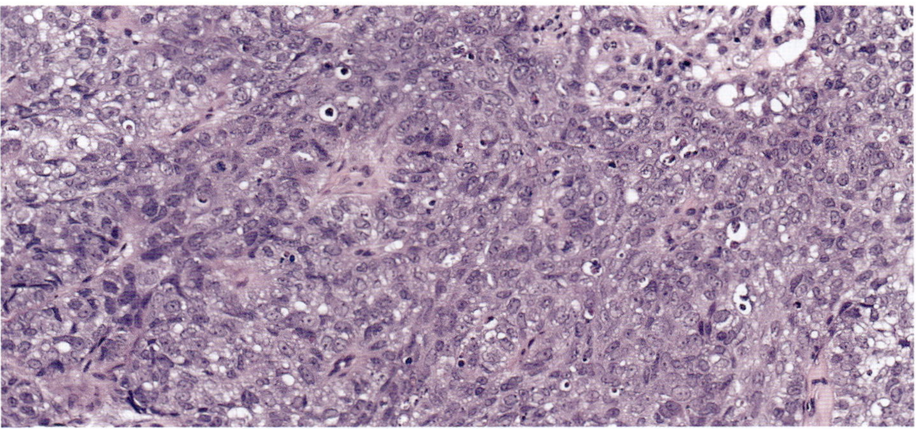

**Fig. 3.72** Sebaceous carcinoma. Bubbly cytoplasmic vacuolization, pleomorphism, and mitotic activity are evident.

### Histopathology

Sebocytic differentiation, typified by multivesicular cytoplasmic clearing, and frequently with nuclear scalloping, is the sine qua non for sebaceous neoplasms, including sebaceous carcinoma. It must be distinguished from simple cytoplasmic clarity, a microscopic change that is relatively common in cutaneous neoplasms of several other lineages {2534}. Sebaceous carcinomas typically show lobules of variably atypical polygonal cells, with a fibrovascular stroma. Central portions of the tumour cell nests may be necrotic, yielding a comedo growth pattern. The cells of well-differentiated neoplasms show abundant cytoplasm and oval vesicular nuclei with distinct nucleoli; mitotic figures are variable in number. More poorly differentiated sebaceous carcinomas show high N:C ratios, nuclear pleomorphism, prominent nucleoli, brisk mitotic activity (sometimes with atypical forms), and amphophilic or basophilic cytoplasm. Intracellular vacuoles are sometimes not readily apparent in more poorly differentiated lesions. In poorly differentiated tumours arising in the eyelid, bubbly cytoplasm may be the only evidence of sebaceous differentiation. In such cases, squared-off nuclei are a helpful clue {315}.

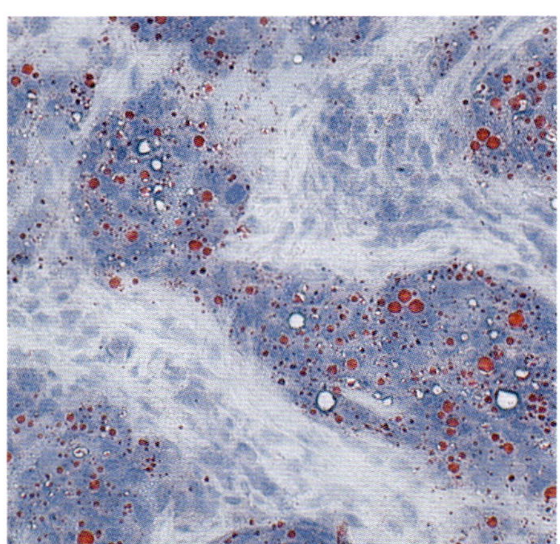

**Fig. 3.73** Sebaceous carcinoma. Oil Red O staining highlights the presence of lipid vacuoles.

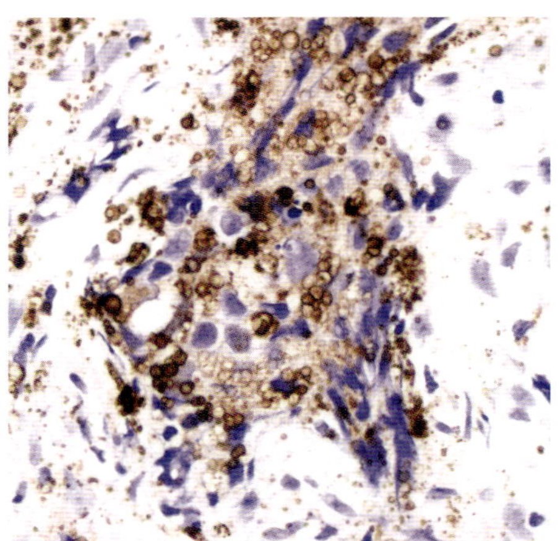

**Fig. 3.74** Sebaceous carcinoma. Immunostaining for adipophilin highlights the intracytoplasmic vacuoles.

A histological grading system based on growth patterns has been proposed for sebaceous carcinomas. Tumours with well-demarcated, roughly equally sized cellular lobules are grade I; those with an admixture of well-defined nests with infiltrative profiles or confluent cell groups are grade II; and those with highly invasive growth or a medullary sheet-like pattern are grade III {2135}. There is some evidence that grading correlates with prognosis {704}.

An intraepithelial component, resembling squamous carcinoma in situ or extramammary Paget disease, is seen in 60% of cases involving the eyelid and 40% of cases involving the conjunctiva {2031}. Involvement or complete replacement of pre-existing pilosebaceous units is common. These two findings are helpful clues to the diagnosis. Intraepidermal growth is less common at extraocular sites. Occasional examples of so-called sebaceous carcinoma in situ involving the epidermis (but not the sebaceous glands) have been reported {114,1319}. A small number of extraocular sebaceous carcinomas associated with apparently genuine squamous dysplasia (actinic keratosis and squamous cell carcinoma in situ) have also been documented {76,76,1187}.

Variants of sebaceous carcinoma may mimic other cutaneous tumours {2846}. Basaloid sebaceous carcinoma consists of small cells with scant cytoplasm, and often shows nuclear palisading at the periphery of cellular nests. It commonly manifests a grade III growth pattern, and overtly sebocytic elements are sparse and difficult to identify. Squamoid sebaceous carcinoma shows prominent squamous metaplasia, often with keratin pearl formation; some examples may also demonstrate spindle cell areas, yielding a sarcomatoid appearance. Other examples of sebaceous carcinoma may demonstrate a pseudoneuroendocrine rippled organoid growth pattern, focally resembling the pattern of carcinoid tumours {1317,1475}, and cases with myoepithelial differentiation have been documented {2425}. A form of sebaceous carcinoma that additionally manifests partial apocrine differentiation has been described using the term "seboapocrine carcinoma" {1307}.

Sebaceous carcinoma shows immunoreactivity for pankeratin, EMA (epithelial membrane antigen), p40, and p63 {78,1961}. EMA labelling may enhance the cytoplasmic vacuolization of the tumour cells in this neoplasm, as may immunostaining for adipophilin and other proteins in the perilipin family {1961}. Positivity for CD10, DOG1, KIT (CD117), and factor XIIIa has also been reported in sebaceous carcinoma {919,1552}.

## Differential diagnosis

A high index of suspicion for sebaceous carcinoma is required when examining basaloid, squamoid, and clear cell tumours in periocular locations. The differential diagnosis includes sebaceoma, balloon cell melanoma, clear cell squamous cell carcinoma, basal cell carcinoma, Merkel cell carcinoma, and metastatic clear cell carcinomas from visceral organs.

## Histogenesis

Sebaceous carcinoma demonstrates differentiation towards cutaneous sebocytes.

## Genetic susceptibility

The absence of immunoreactivity in sebaceous carcinoma for various DNA mismatch repair gene products, including MLH1, MSH2, MSH6, and PMS2, has been found to have a possible relationship to Muir–Torre syndrome {3,238,1234,1635,1811,2395}. However, a newly described rare autosomal recessive form of Muir–Torre syndrome lacks all aberrations in the expression of mismatch repair gene products {1234}.

In a group of sebaceous tumours of various histotypes studied with next-generation sequencing technology, mutations were found in *TP53*, *CDKN2A*, *EGFR*, *CTNNB1*, and *KRAS*; abnormalities in *TP53* were most common {1035}.

## Prognosis and predictive factors

Both eyelid and extraocular sebaceous carcinomas have a 30–40% risk of local tumour recurrence, a 20–25% risk of distant metastasis, and a 10–30% risk of tumour-related mortality {578,1828}. Approximately 70% of all patients with sebaceous carcinoma survive for ≥ 5 years after diagnosis {578}.

# Sebaceous adenoma

Wick M.R.
Cree I.A.
Kazakov D.V.
Lazar A.J.
Michal M.
Wood B.A.
Zembowicz A.
Sangüeza O.P.

## Definition

Sebaceous adenoma is a benign neoplasm composed mostly of fully differentiated sebocytes, admixed with basaloid epithelial cells.

## ICD-O code 8410/0

## Epidemiology

Sebaceous adenomas are principally seen as solitary lesions in people aged >40 years {2259}. They are usually located in sun-damaged skin of the head and neck area. Rarely, patients may have multiple lesions, which should raise the possibility of Muir–Torre syndrome {2258}.

## Localization

Sebaceous adenoma is principally seen in the skin of the head and neck.

## Clinical features

Sebaceous adenoma is a relatively small, nondescript, yellowish-tan nodule {2609}.

## Histopathology

This well-circumscribed neoplasm is composed of small lobular aggregates of mature sebocytes, with a variable rim of basaloid cells, recapitulating normal sebaceous glands {1706}. The vacuolated sebocytes predominate over the basaloid cells, and may be the only elements present in some lesions. Sebaceous adenoma is often connected to the overlying epidermis, which may be covered by keratin and cellular debris.

## Differential diagnosis

The principal differential diagnosis for sebaceous adenoma is sebaceous hyperplasia, in which sebaceous lobules are arranged around a central follicle that is connected to the epidermis, but sebaceous hyperplasia shows a clear-cut association between the proliferating sebaceous lobules and the central hair follicle, whereas sebaceous adenoma does not. Sebaceoma is another benign nodular lesion composed of a more equal admixture of basaloid epithelial cells and small groups of vacuolated sebocytes {282}. Considerable morphological overlap may exist between sebaceous adenoma and sebaceoma {2271}.

## Genetic susceptibility

The absence of immunoreactivity in sebaceous adenoma for various DNA mismatch repair gene products, including MLH1, MSH2, MSH6, and PMS2, has been found to have a possible relationship to Muir–Torre syndrome {3,238,1234,1635,1811,2395}. However, a newly described rare autosomal recessive form of Muir–Torre syndrome lacks all aberrations in the expression of mismatch repair gene products {1234}.

In a group of sebaceous tumours of various histotypes studied with next-generation sequencing technology, mutations were found in *TP53*, *CDKN2A*, *EGFR*, *CTNNB1*, and *KRAS*; abnormalities in *TP53* were most common {1035}.

## Prognosis and predictive factors

Sebaceous adenoma is a benign lesion, and simple excision is curative. However, the subset of patients with this tumour who have Muir–Torre syndrome may experience morbidity and mortality from associated visceral malignancies {1234}.

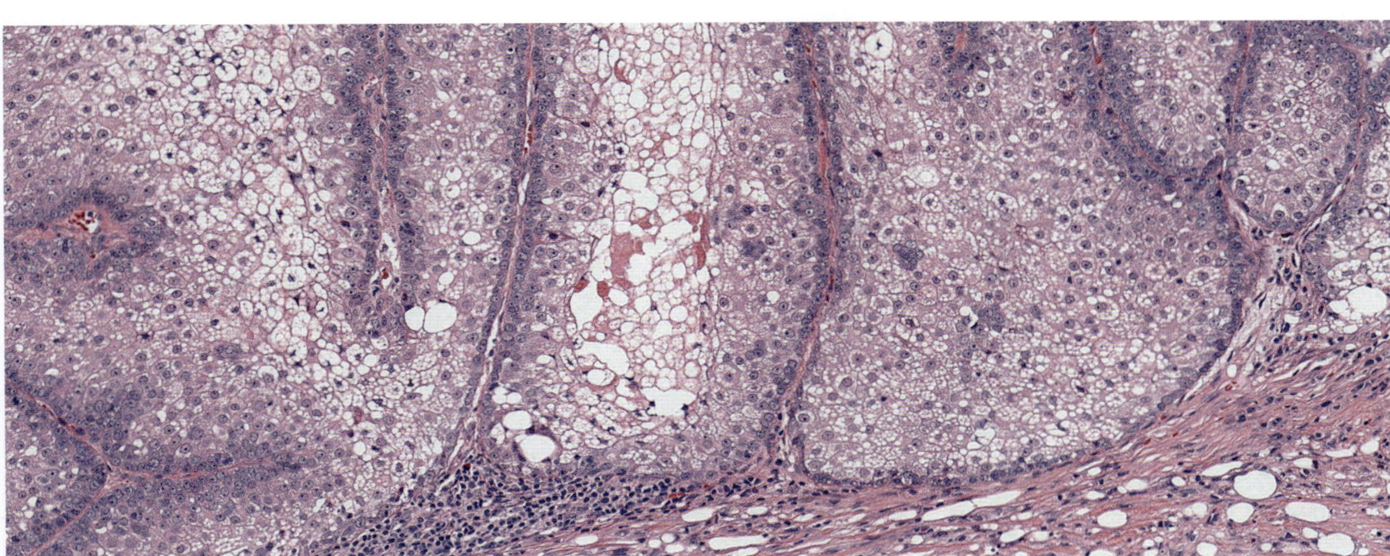

**Fig. 3.75** Sebaceous adenoma. A well-circumscribed lobulated proliferation of sebocytes with admixed basaloid cells; sebocytes are predominant; minimal cytological atypia is present.

# Sebaceoma

Wick M.R.
Cree I.A.
Kazakov D.V.
Lazar A.J.
Michal M.
Sangüeza O.P.
Singh R.
Wood B.A.
Zembowicz A.

## Definition

Sebaceoma is a benign adnexal neoplasm showing sebaceous differentiation. It is characterized by multiple rounded cellular lobules and microcystic spaces, and is predominantly composed of immature sebocytes admixed with occasional mature sebocytes {1793}.

## ICD-O code 8410/0

## Synonym

Sebaceous epithelioma

## Epidemiology

Sebaceomas are rare sebaceous lesions that may be associated with Muir–Torre syndrome {1794}. The mean age at diagnosis is 70 years {2656}. These tumours have a predilection for females {1793,2656}.

## Localization

Sebaceomas occur principally on the face and scalp, with only rare cases on the truncal skin or extremities {233,632,2656}.

## Clinical features

Sebaceomas are solitary yellowish-tan to orange papules {2656}. They may arise in a pre-existing sebaceous naevus {429,1871}, and lesions that are associated with Muir–Torre syndrome may be multifocal {1794}.

## Histopathology

Sebaceoma is composed of well-circumscribed cellular lobules of various sizes; it is centred in the reticular dermis. This neoplasm may contain duct-like structures and cystic areas containing holocrine secretions; only rarely do they connect with the overlying epidermis {798}. Eosinophilic cuticular material often lines the ducts and cysts, as seen in normal sebaceous ducts. Cytologically, this tumour consists mostly of small, monomorphic basaloid cells with bland nuclear features, admixed with haphazardly distributed mature sebaceous cells {282,2656}. The sebaceous cells have abundant vacuolated cytoplasm, ovoid nuclei, and scalloped nuclear membranes. Mitoses may be common in the immature component, but atypical mitotic figures and necrosis are not expected. The surrounding dermis consists of dense eosinophilic connective tissue. Cleft-like spaces are not seen between the neoplastic lobules and the stroma. A variety of growth patterns has been described in sebaceoma, sometimes even within the same neoplasm {429}. They include reticulated (rippled), cribriform, and glandular configurations {75,282,1317}.

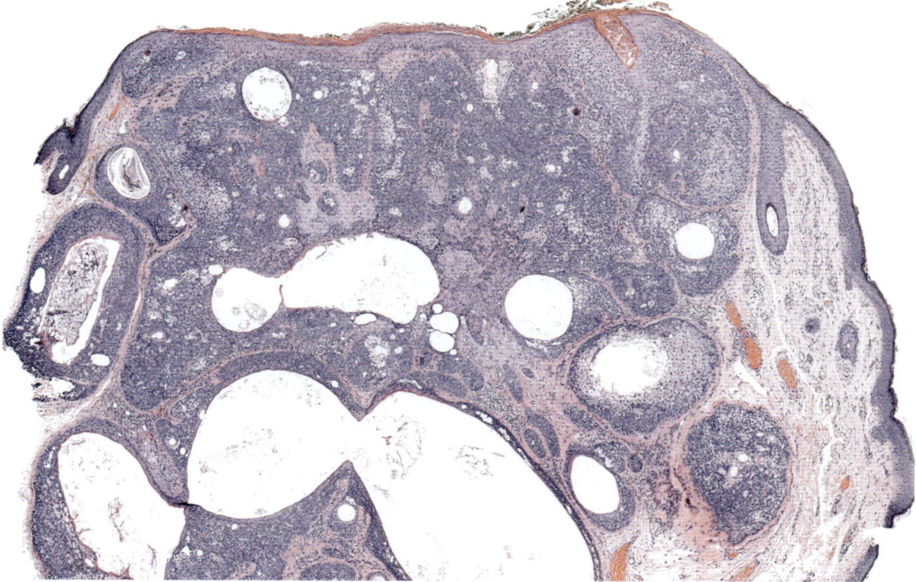

**Fig.3.76** Sebaceoma. Low-power view showing a nodular proliferation of sebaceous and basaloid cells.

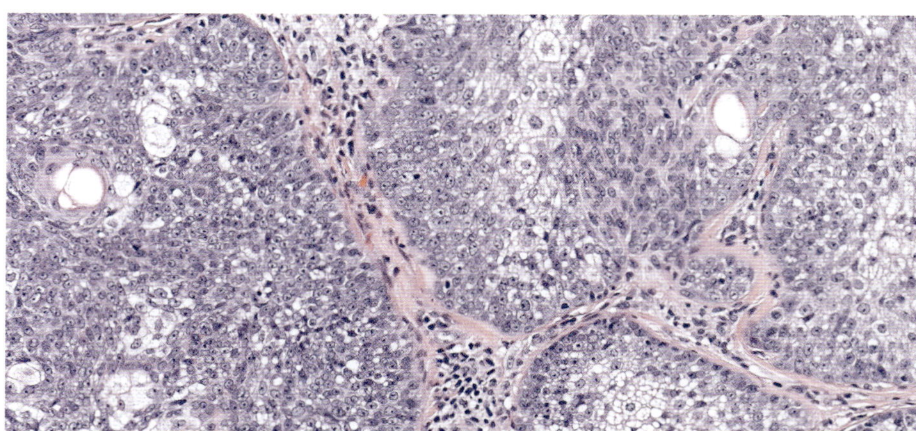

**Fig.3.77** Sebaceoma. There is a predominance of basaloid cells; minimal cytological atypia may be seen.

## Differential diagnosis

Sebaceous carcinoma and adenoma are the most common differential diagnoses. In superficial biopsies, BerEP4 negativity helps in the distinction from basal cell carcinoma {732}.

## Genetic susceptibility

The absence of immunoreactivity in

sebaceoma for various DNA mismatch repair gene products, including MLH1, MSH2, MSH6, and PMS2, has been found to have a possible relationship to Muir–Torre syndrome {3,238,1234,1635,1811,2395}. However, a newly described rare autosomal recessive form of Muir–Torre syndrome lacks all aberrations in the expression of mismatch repair gene products {1234}.

In a group of sebaceous tumours of various histotypes studied with next-generation sequencing technology, mutations were found in *TP53*, *CDKN2A*, *EGFR*, *CTNNB1*, and *KRAS*; abnormalities in *TP53* were most common {1035}.

## Prognosis and predictive factors

Sebaceoma is a benign neoplasm that is typically cured by simple excision {75,282,1793,2656}. Anecdotal examples have been reported that underwent malignant transformation to the histological pattern of a sebaceous carcinoma {1797,2773}. Patients who have associated Muir–Torre syndrome are at risk for the development of internal malignancies {1794}.

# Site-specific tumours

## Mammary Paget disease

Kacerovska D.
Prieto V.G.

### Definition

Mammary Paget disease (MPD) is a neoplastic lesion composed of malignant epithelial cells within the epidermis of the nipple and areola. In > 95% of cases, there is an underlying breast carcinoma.

### ICD-O code 8540/3

### Synonyms

Paget disease of breast;
Paget disease of the nipple

### Epidemiology

MPD accounts for 1–4% of all breast carcinomas. It almost exclusively affects women; < 1% of reported cases occurred in men. The age range is 26–88 years. About 10–28% of cases are incidental findings in the nipple in mastectomy specimens, with no clinically apparent lesion {1095}.

### Etiology

Most cases are associated with an underlying mammary carcinoma.

### Localization

MPD involves the nipple and areola; in advanced cases, it may extend to the adjacent skin. One breast is typically involved, but there may be both synchronous and metachronous involvement {1095}. A supernumerary nipple (or ectopic breast tissue adjacent to a supernumerary nipple) can also very rarely be involved {1297}.

### Clinical features

There is an eczematous scaly or crusted lesion confined to the nipple or areola, sometimes associated with ulceration or inversion of the nipple and discharge.

### Histopathology

The neoplastic cells (Paget cells) have abundant weakly eosinophilic or pale-staining cytoplasm and large vesicular nuclei. They are scattered in the epidermis (pagetoid spread) in the form of solitary units, clusters, or (rarely) acinar/glandular structures. Skin adnexae can also be involved. Paget cells contain intracellular mucin in 40% of cases, and they may contain melanin due to phagocytosis (a possible diagnostic pitfall {2039}). The epidermis is often hyperkeratotic and acanthotic, especially in longstanding lesions. An underlying carcinoma (most commonly a high-grade invasive carcinoma) may be present in the specimen.

Paget cells usually have an immunoprofile identical to that of the underlying carcinoma. They express low-molecular-weight cytokeratins (CAM5.2), CK7, human milk fat globule, and mammary-type apomucin EMA (epithelial membrane antigen). As many as 90% of cases are positive for ERBB2 (HER2). Approximately half of the cases express GCDFP15. There is variable positivity for polyclonal CEA. Androgen receptor has been found in most cases; estrogen receptor and/or progesterone receptor are present in approximately 10–30% of cases {1095}. Paget cells are negative for CK20. Rare cases fail to express CK7, but typically still express GATA3 {1965}.

### Differential diagnosis

Clinically, MPD must be distinguished from eczema and nipple adenoma. The histological differential diagnosis includes spongiotic dermatoses, candidiasis/dermatophytes, squamous cell carcinoma in situ (Bowen disease), and superficial spreading melanoma. In some cases, hyperplasia of Toker cells,

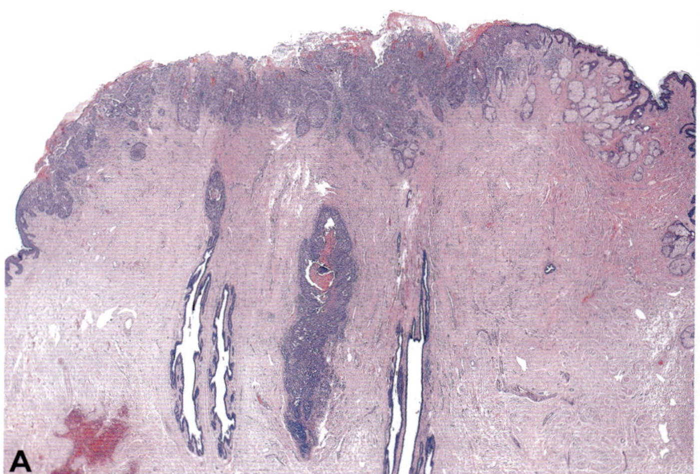


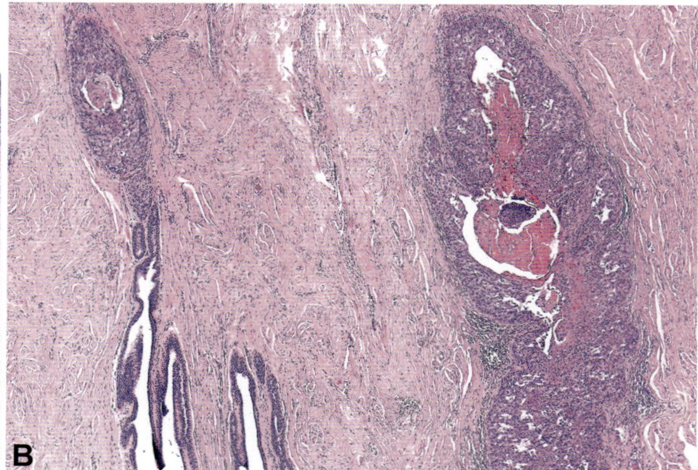


**Fig. 3.78** Mammary Paget disease. **A** A low-power view of ductal carcinoma in situ associated with Paget disease. **B** Higher-power view showing a comedo growth pattern.

a normal component of the nipple, may present a diagnostic dilemma {621,1297}.

### Histogenesis

More than 95% of cases are associated with an underlying mammary cancer representing a retrograde extension of the breast carcinoma into the epidermis in a contiguous fashion through spread along the lactiferous ducts {1095}. Cases without underlying carcinoma have been postulated to originate from Toker cells, a hypothesis supported by the observation of rare cases in which the Paget cells are genetically different from the neoplastic cells forming an underlying breast carcinoma {1826}.

### Prognosis and predictive factors

The prognosis of MPD is determined by the features of the associated mammary carcinoma and the stage of the disease. The 5-year overall survival rates are 94–98% and 73–93% in the presence of ductal carcinoma in situ and invasive carcinoma, respectively {2435}.

# Extramammary Paget disease

Kacerovska D.
Prieto V.G.
Singh R.

### Definition

Extramammary Paget disease (EMPD) is a rare adenocarcinoma histopathologically characterized by a predominant intraepithelial growth of neoplastic cells originating in the skin (primary EMPD) or representing intraepithelial spread of an underlying visceral carcinoma (secondary EMPD).

### ICD-O code

8542/3

### Synonym

Paget disease

### Epidemiology

EMPD accounts for about 1% of all neoplasms in the anogenital area. It mostly occurs in White postmenopausal women, with the median age of about 70–75 years. Men are affected less often.

### Etiology

The inciting factors for primary EMPD are unknown, but secondary EMPD represents skin involvement from an underlying carcinoma originating from the lower gastrointestinal tract (distal colon or rectum) or urinary tract (urinary bladder or prostate).

### Localization

The labium majus is the most common site, followed by the labium minus and clitoris. The perineum, perianal area, scrotum, penis, lower abdomen, and inguinal folds can also be affected. Outside the anogenital region, EMPD is very rare.

### Clinical features

The most common presentation is a relatively well-demarcated flat or slightly elevated, scaly, oozing, erythematous patch or plaque accompanied by pruritus or burning. The lesions often resemble eczema. Rare forms include lesions with hyper- or hypopigmentation and multicentric lesions (i.e. genital lesions associated with unilateral or bilateral axillary involvement, occurring synchronously or metachronously).

### Histopathology

The intraepithelial neoplastic cells (Paget cells) have vesicular nuclei with prominent nucleoli and abundant basophilic to amphophilic cytoplasm. They are predominantly distributed in a solitary fashion, or may form well-demarcated solid nests or gland-like structures. Involvement of adnexae, especially of hair follicles and eccrine ducts, is seen in most cases {1423}. Occasionally, single cells, nodules, glands, and strands/solid sheets can be found in the dermis; this is considered to constitute invasion or microinvasion (i.e. stromal invasion to a depth of ≤ 1.0 mm below the basement membrane) {2426,2436}. However, this definition of invasion cannot be applied to cases associated with an underlying adenocarcinoma of mammary type with a ductal in situ component {1424}. Other (less common) morphological changes include mammary-type changes in anogenital mammary-like glands, various proliferative epidermal changes, areas resembling syringocystadenocarcinoma papilliferum in situ, syringoma-like structures, melanin pigment within the cytoplasm of the neoplastic cells simulating a melanocytic lesion, signet-ring cell morphology, and association with another distinct vulvar lesion {1327,1417,1419,2039}. Paget cells usually stain positively with mucicarmine and Alcian blue, and give a diastase-resistant positive periodic acid–Schiff (PAS) reaction. Immunohistochemically, the neoplastic cells in primary EMPD are consistently CK7-positive and CAM5.2-positive, and they often express CEA, GCDFP15, ERBB2 (HER2/neu), CA125, and androgen receptor {2600}.

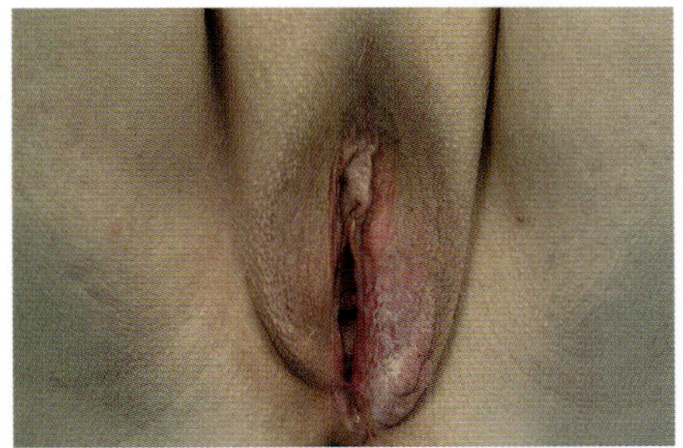

**Fig. 3.79** Extramammary Paget disease. Clinical presentation in the anogenital area, involving the left labium majus.

### Differential diagnosis

The most important issue is distinction

between primary and secondary EMPD. Dirty necrosis in glandular structures and coexpression of CK20 and CDX2 by the Paget cells suggest a colorectal origin. Uroplakin III expression is typical for urothelial carcinoma, whereas coexpression of prostate-specific antigen and NKX3-1 indicates an underlying prostatic carcinoma.

Potential mimics of EMPD are vulvar Toker cells, vulvar and penile analogues of cervical stratified mucin-producing intraepithelial lesion {1709,1767}, high-grade squamous intraepithelial lesion, melanoma, pagetoid dyskeratosis, and clear cell papulosis. In addition to immunohistochemistry, clinicopathological correlation is essential for correct diagnosis.

## Histogenesis

The histogenesis of primary EMPD is unknown.

## Genetic profile

*ERBB2* gene amplification is rare {551}. Mutations in genes encoding the PI3K/AKT cascade have been found to significantly correlate with *CDH1* hypermethylation {1279,1422}. A study using comparative genomic hybridization revealed amplification at chromosomes Xcent-q21 and 19, and loss at 10q24-qter {1531}.

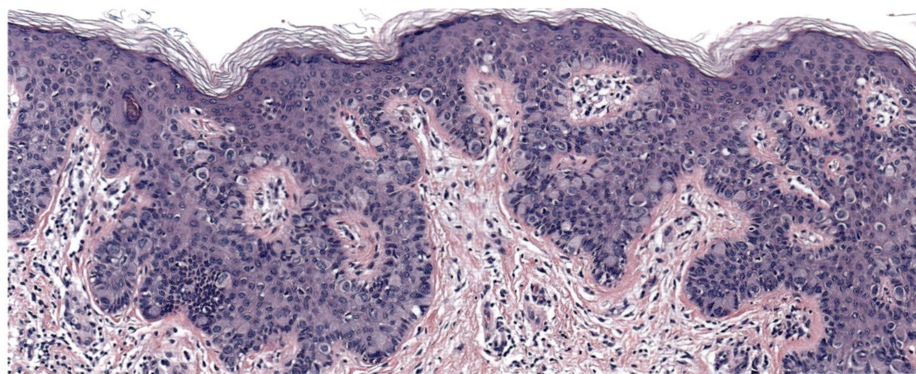

**Fig. 3.80** Extramammary Paget disease. Intraepidermal proliferation of predominantly single cells with admixed nests throughout the epidermis. Individual cells are large, with ample amphophilic cytoplasm, a large nucleus, and prominent nucleoli.

## Prognosis and predictive factors

Data related to primary EMPD show that the prognosis, in particular for non-recurrent cases and those with no invasive component, is generally good. The mortality rate in these cases is not significantly different from that in the general matched population. However, EMPD has a recurrence rate of 12–58%. This may be related to positive surgical margins, multicentricity, and skip areas {1322}. Primary EMPD with an invasive component is significantly associated with both lymph node metastasis and worse prognosis {2436}. Cases with mutant *PIK3CA* and *AKT1* often appear to be invasive {1279,1422}. The prognosis of secondary EMPD depends on the underlying malignancy.

# Adenocarcinoma of anogenital mammary-like glands

Kacerovska D.
Prieto V.G.

## Definition
Adenocarcinoma of anogenital mammary-like glands (AGMLGs) is a relatively heterogeneous group of malignant neoplasms that are presumed to arise from AGMLGs and that have morphological features very similar, if not identical, to those of homologous mammary carcinomas.

## ICD-O code 8500/3

## Synonym
Adenocarcinoma of the vulva with breast carcinoma features

## Epidemiology
These malignant neoplasms typically occur in multiparous women aged ≥ 60 years.

## Localization
The most commonly affected site is the labium majus.

## Clinical features
A solitary nodule is seen in most cases {1327,2600}.

## Histopathology
The most common type of adenocarcinoma of AGMLGs is adenocarcinoma identical to invasive ductal carcinoma as defined in breast pathology. Rare lesions exhibit features of lobular carcinoma, carcinoma with mixed ductal and lobular features, or tubulolobular carcinoma; all such lesions have features similar to those of their mammary counterparts, including immunopositivity for E-cadherin in ductal lesions {7,751,1301,2643}.

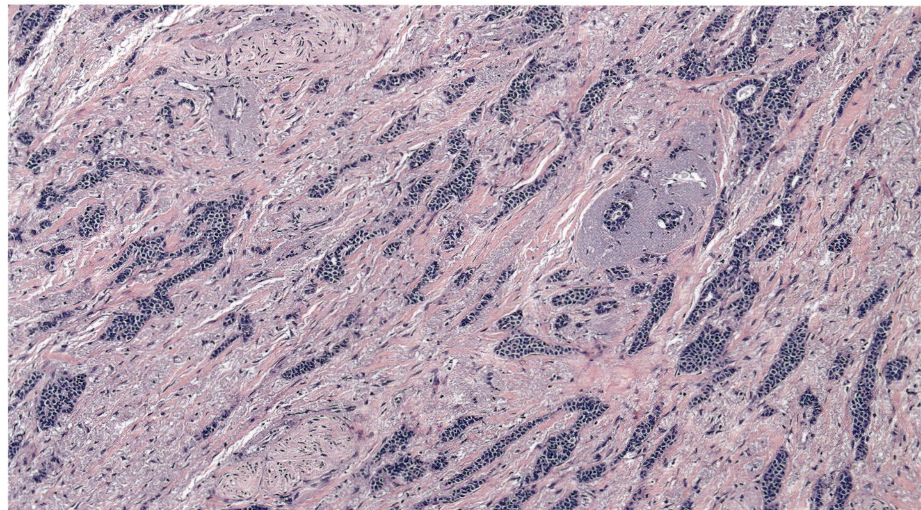

**Fig. 3.81** Adenocarcinoma of mammary-like glands of the vulva. Mammary-type tubulolobular carcinoma with areas of both tubular formation and a single-file pattern, resembling an invasive lobular carcinoma. Note the stromal and periductal elastosis.

## Differential diagnosis
A primary anogenital tumour can be distinguished from metastatic breast carcinoma by identification of an in situ component and/or clinical investigation.

## Histogenesis
These tumours probably originate in AGMLGs, given their marked similarity to homologous mammary carcinomas, the presence of AGMLGs in the vicinity of the lesions, and transitions between the benign residuum and the carcinoma in some cases.

## Genetic profile
Mutations in genes encoding the PI3K/AKT cascade have been found in rare cases {1422}.

## Prognosis and predictive factors
As a group, adenocarcinomas of AGMLGs seem to be locally aggressive. They are associated with lymph node metastasis in approximately 60% of cases, but the clinical course has not been well characterized for specific histopathological variants, because of their rarity {1322,1327}.

# Hidradenoma papilliferum

Sangüeza O.P.
Cassarino D.S.
Glusac E.J.
Kazakov D.V.
Requena L.
Swanson P.E.
Vassallo C.

## Definition

Hidradenoma papilliferum is a benign apocrine neoplasm that typically affects the vulva and presumably arises from anogenital mammary-like glands.

## ICD-O code 8405/0

## Synonyms

Papillary cystadenoma; papillary hidradenoma

## Epidemiology

Hidradenoma papilliferum almost exclusively affects women aged 20–89 years {2711}. It is extremely rare in children {2744}. Hidradenoma papilliferum is mainly identified in White populations; it is rare in Black populations.

## Localization

Most cases arise in the anogenital skin of adult women, most commonly on the labium majus.

## Clinical features

Hidradenoma papilliferum is typically a small solitary skin-coloured papule or nodule with a cystic appearance. The lesion is well circumscribed and mobile. The overlying epidermis is usually normal {2164}.

## Histopathology

At scanning magnification, hidradenoma papilliferum appears as a well-circumscribed cystic or solid neoplasm. Within the cystic cavity, there are numerous and prominent papillary, maze-like projections. The papillae consist of a central axis of connective tissue lined by two layers of tumour cells: peripheral cuboidal myoepithelial cells and luminal columnar cells with decapitation secretion. The stroma supporting the neoplasm is composed of fibrous tissue that is separated from the surrounding dermis by retraction clefts. Remnants of anogenital mammary-like glands can be seen {1421}. In solid areas with oncocytic metaplasia, there may be mild nuclear atypia {1447}.

## Differential diagnosis

Unlike syringocystadenoma papilliferum, hidradenoma papilliferum is usually not connected to pre-existing follicular infundibula, and it lacks plasma cells in the stroma.

## Histogenesis

Hidradenoma papilliferum is associated with anogenital mammary-like glands {2691}.

## Genetic susceptibility

Mutations in *AKT1* and *PIK3CA* have been identified {1422,1426,1558}.

## Prognosis and predictive factors

Hidradenoma papilliferum is a benign neoplasm.

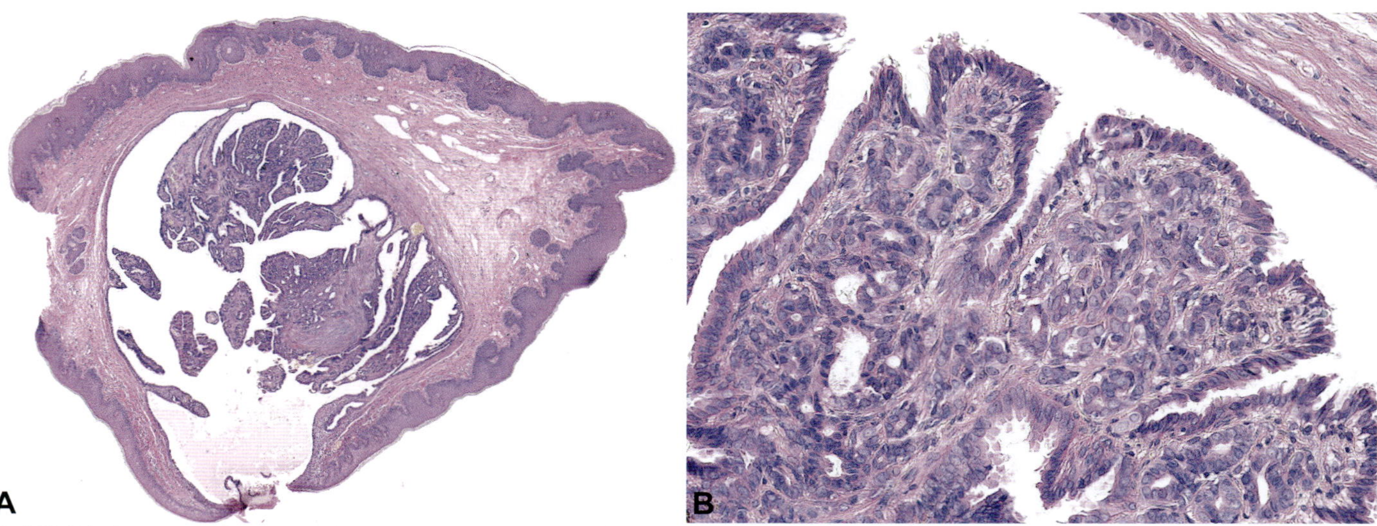


**Fig. 3.82** Hidradenoma papilliferum. **A** Well-circumscribed cystic neoplasm with prominent papillary projections. **B** The double epithelial lining consists of a peripheral layer of cuboidal myoepithelial cells and a luminal layer of columnar cells, many of which exhibit decapitation secretion.

# Fibroadenoma and phyllodes tumour of anogenital mammary-like glands

Kazakov D.V.
Konstantinova A.M.

## Definition

Fibroadenoma and phyllodes tumour of anogenital mammary-like glands are biphasic fibroepithelial neoplasms composed of an epithelial glandular component and a predominant stromal component; they are microscopically identical to their mammary homologues {1327,1328}.

## ICD-O codes

| | |
|---|---|
| Fibroadenoma of anogenital mammary-like glands | 9010/0 |
| Phyllodes tumour of anogenital mammary-like glands | 9020/0 |

## Epidemiology

Both tumours are extremely rare, with < 60 cases reported to date. Most patients are female {1047,1328}.

## Localization

Most cases occur in the vulva and perianal area {1303}. Rare patients also present with mammary fibroadenoma, similar lesions in the axilla {1047}, and bilateral anogenital tumours {109,336,1042}.

## Clinical features

Fibroadenoma and phyllodes tumour occur as solitary nodules measuring 0.8–6 cm (mean size: 3 cm). In the reported cases, the age at diagnosis is 20–69 years (mean: 39 years) {390,1328}.

## Histopathology

Fibroadenoma is a well-circumscribed neoplasm composed of round or elongated, often branching and anastomosing glandular structures surrounded by usually paucicellular stroma containing bland spindled or stellate cells, showing low or practically no mitotic activity. When the glandular lumina maintain round or oval configurations, the image is that of a pericanalicular growth pattern, whereas abundant stroma compressing the glandular elements into slit-like structures produces the so-called intracanalicular pattern. The distinction between the two patterns has no practical connotations, and some neoplasms show a combination of both.

Phyllodes tumour shows a growth pattern with leaf-like projections into glandular lumina. The stroma is usually hypercellular, typically with periglandular condensation; cellularity commonly varies within a given neoplasm {479,880,1303,1328}. Three categories are delineated: benign, low-grade, and high-grade; the grade is defined by stromal atypia. Most vulvar phyllodes tumours are either benign or low-grade; high-grade phyllodes tumour is exceptionally rare {832,2587}.

Rare features in these tumours include mammary-type ductal lesions (with columnar cell change, usual ductal hyperplasia, and florid ductal hyperplasia), hyperplasia of myoepithelial cells, pseudoangiomatous stromal hyperplasia (PASH), various types of metaplasia in the glandular component and stroma, and lactation-like changes {390,1303,1328,2727}.

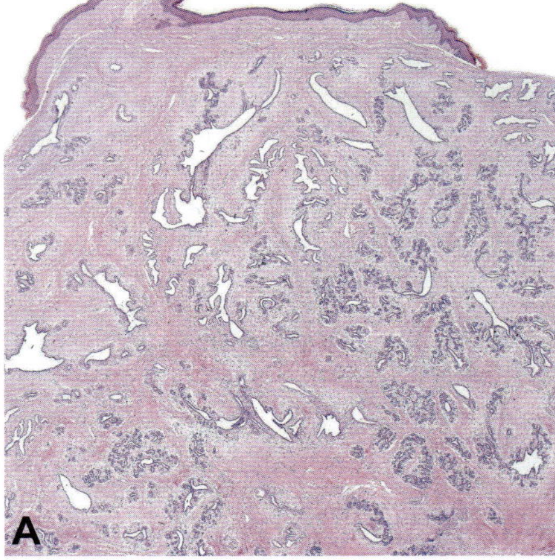

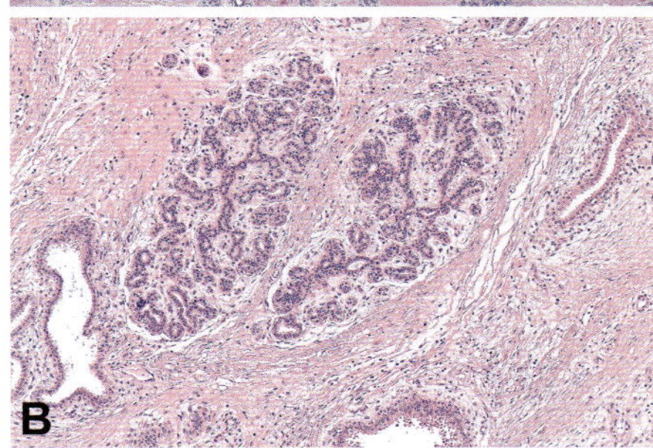

**Fig. 3.84** Fibroadenoma of anogenital mammary-like glands. **A** The biphasic neoplasm is composed of elongated, branching, and anastomosing glandular structures surrounded by paucicellular stroma; the glandular lumina maintain round to oval configurations (a pericanalicular growth pattern). **B** Higher magnification.

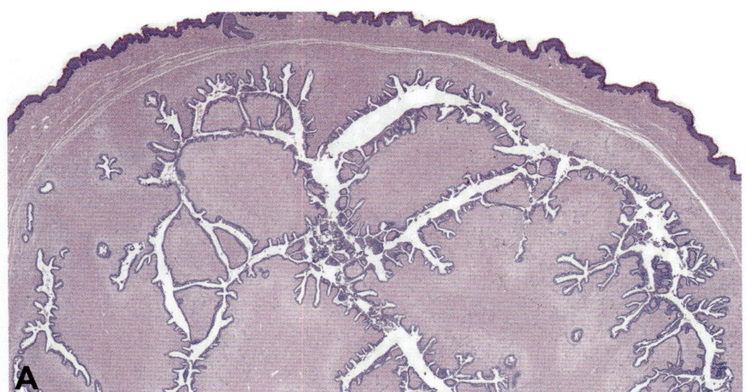

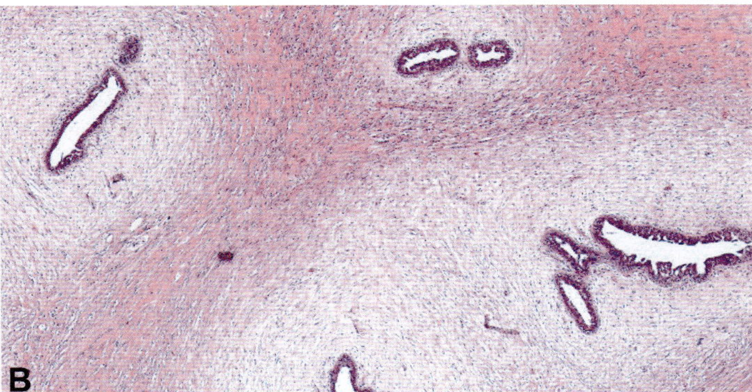

**Fig. 3.83** Phyllodes tumour of anogenital mammary-like glands. **A** Benign tumour with a leaf-like growth pattern and stromal hypercellularity. **B** Note the classic periglandular condensation of the stroma.

Immunohistochemically, the epithelial component stains for epithelial markers, estrogen receptor, and progesterone receptor, whereas ERBB2 (HER2) is negative. Stromal cells, including those in PASH areas, are positive for vimentin and CD34 and variably positive for actins {880,1303,2454,2727}. Vascular markers are negative in PASH {1303}.

### Differential diagnosis

Fibroadenoma and benign phyllodes tumour manifest overlapping features; in some cases, distinguishing between them can be difficult. Generally, phyllodes tumours have more-cellular stroma (with variation within a lesion), less-regular outlines, and leaf-like projections. Focal connection to the epidermal surface with numerous plasma cells may resemble syringocystadenoma papilliferum. Fibroepithelial foci resembling fibroadenoma may rarely be found in other complex lesions of anogenital mammary-like glands {1311,2723,2797}. Fibrocystic disease and other lesions with prominent ductal hyperplasia may be differential diagnoses in a limited specimen {1304,1311,1418}. Lactation-like change (secretory hyperplasia), with large cells having hyperchromatic nuclei must not be confused with malignancy; the presence of intracytoplasmic vacuoles and intraluminal secretion is the clue to the diagnosis. PASH (open, slit-like, anastomosing channels devoid of erythrocytes and lined by discontinuous, often attenuated, inconspicuous cells without atypia or mitotic activity) should be distinguished from low-grade angiosarcoma, which, in contrast to the bland cytology of PASH, exhibits at least mild nuclear pleomorphism and immunopositivity for vascular markers.

### Histogenesis

The tumours are thought to arise from anogenital mammary-like glands {1420,1425,2691}.

### Genetic profile

One study identified *AKT1* and *MET* mutations in fibroadenoma and *ABL1* and *TP53* mutations in low-grade phyllodes tumour {1426}.

### Prognosis and predictive factors

Most cases are benign. Local recurrence can occur in phyllodes tumours {1328}.

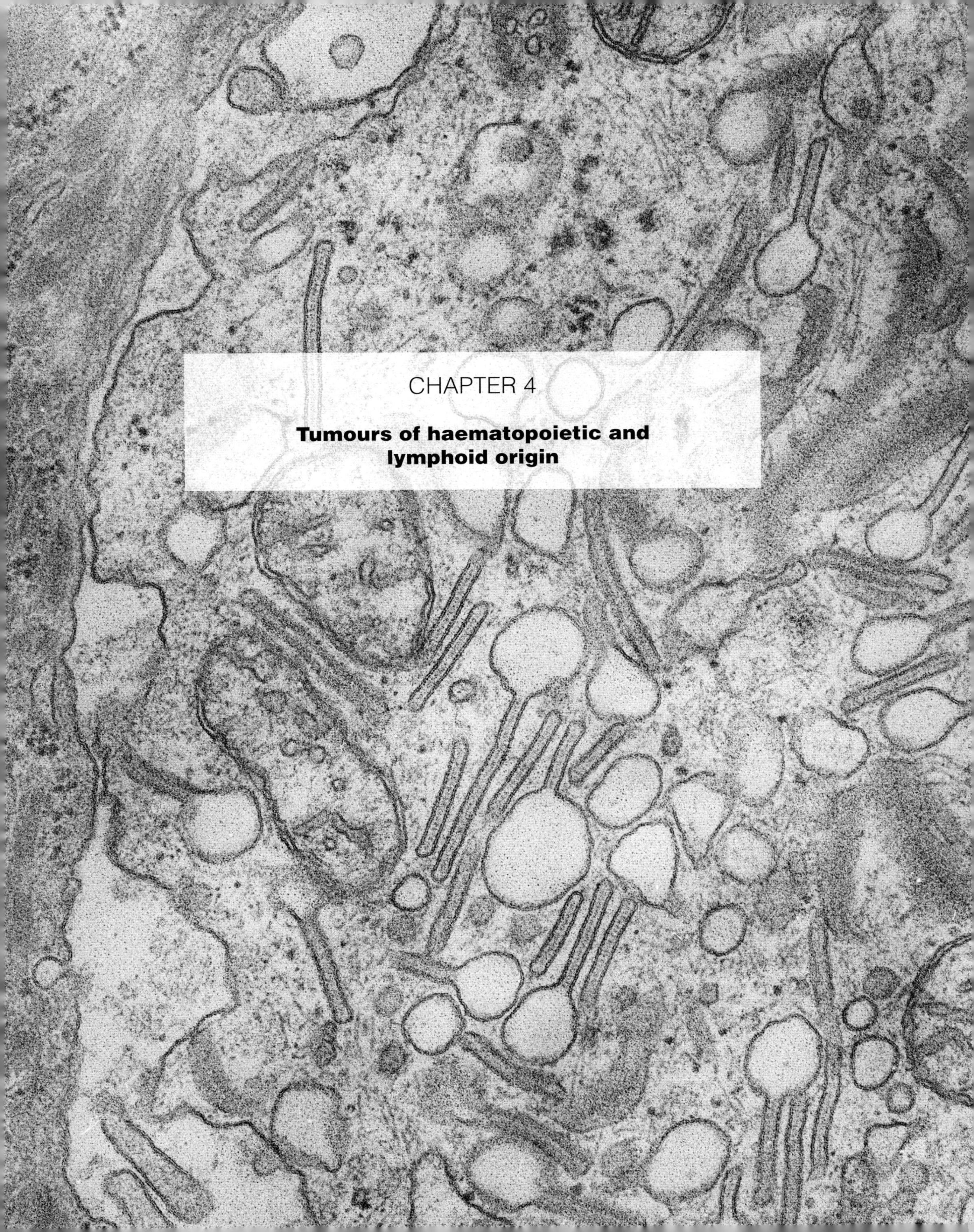

CHAPTER 4

# Tumours of haematopoietic and lymphoid origin

# Tumours of haematopoietic and lymphoid origin: Introduction

Willemze R.
Berti E.
Facchetti F.
Kempf W.
Jaffe E.S.

This chapter on tumours of haematopoietic and lymphoid origin describes primary cutaneous lymphomas and systemic leukaemias/lymphomas that commonly involve the skin secondarily, as well as histiocytic and dendritic cell neoplasms and cutaneous mastocytosis. Primary cutaneous lymphomas are defined as non-Hodgkin lymphomas presenting in the skin with no evidence of extracutaneous disease at the time of diagnosis {2832}; classic mycosis fungoides presenting with concurrent skin and lymph node involvement, as well as Sézary syndrome, which has peripheral blood involvement by definition, are included in this category. Not included in this category are cases of intravascular large B-cell lymphoma and B-lymphoblastic lymphoma first presenting in the skin; these are instead considered to be manifestations of systemic disease and should be treated accordingly, even the rare cases in which initial staging is still negative. Similarly, some lymphomas (e.g. plasmablastic lymphoma) commonly present in extranodal sites, including the skin; but because the features of cases presenting in the skin are similar to those in other extranodal sites, these cases are not considered to constitute primary cutaneous lymphoma.

Primary cutaneous lymphomas include a heterogeneous group of cutaneous T-cell lymphomas (CTCLs) and cutaneous B-cell lymphomas (CBCLs). In the Western Hemisphere, CTCLs constitute approximately 75–80% of all primary cutaneous lymphomas, with CBCLs accounting for the other 20–25% {2832}. However, different distributions are seen in other parts of the world. For example, EBV-associated NK/T-cell lymphomas are more prevalent in south-eastern Asia than in the Western Hemisphere, and CBCLs are much less common.

A major advantage when diagnosing cutaneous lymphomas (vs lymphomas arising at other sites) is that they are visible to the naked eye and can easily be biopsied. This provides the unique opportunity to correlate clinical appearance and clinical behaviour with the histological, immunophenotypic, and genetic features of these conditions. Clinicopathological correlation is often essential in making a definite diagnosis. For example, in cases with a diffuse dermal infiltrate of large CD30+ T cells histologically, clinical examination is necessary to differentiate between primary cutaneous anaplastic large cell lymphoma (generally presenting as a solitary tumour or a few localized tumours), lymphomatoid papulosis with recurrent self-healing papules, and transformed mycosis fungoides (characterized by prior or concurrent patches and plaques). Over the past three decades, clinicopathological correlation has contributed significantly to the diagnosis and classification of primary cutaneous lymphomas; it has resulted in the recognition of new types of CTCLs other than mycosis fungoides and Sézary syndrome, as well as new types of CBCLs. These more newly recognized types of CTCL and CBCL have been found to have highly characteristic clinical and histological features. They often have a completely different clinical behaviour and prognosis than do morphologically similar nodal lymphomas, and require different treatment {2834}. Primary cutaneous lymphomas have therefore been included as distinct entities in recent lymphoma classifications. They were initially covered in a separate classification specifically for primary cutaneous lymphomas, published by the European Organisation for Research and Treatment of Cancer (EORTC) {2834}. Then, following the 2005 WHO-EORTC consensus classification {2832}, included in the 3rd edition of the WHO classification of skin tumours in 2006 {1514A}, they were incorporated into the 2008 *WHO classification of tumours of haematopoietic and lymphoid tissues* {2546} and its 2017 revision {2545}. The cutaneous lymphoma entity names and definitions of the updated WHO-EORTC classification in this 4th edition are for the most part identical to those used in the 2017 revision of the WHO haematopoietic tumours classification. However, in the latter classification primary cutaneous marginal zone lymphoma is not listed as a separate entity, but included in the broad category of extranodal marginal zone lymphomas of mucosa-associated lymphoid tissue (MALT lymphoma), notwithstanding differences in histology, genetic profile and clinical behaviour. Interestingly, recent studies have described the existence of two subsets of primary cutaneous marginal zone lymphoma {2544}. Heavy chain class-switched cases, which are characterized by expression of immunoglobulin G (or IgG), a high number of T cells, and no expression of CXCR3, are the more common form of primary cutaneous marginal zone lymphoma, and are considered by some authors to constitute a clonal chronic cutaneous lymphoproliferative disorder rather than overt lymphoma {2544}. Non–class-switched cases, which express IgM and CXCR3 and present with large sheets of B cells, are uncommon; they share many features with MALT lymphomas at other extranodal sites and are more likely to have extracutaneous disease.

Compared to the WHO-EORTC classification included in the 2006 3rd edition of the WHO classification for skin tumours, some new entities have been added, while the terminology of some other entities has been modified. In addition to the classic variants of lymphomatoid papulosis (lymphomatoid papulosis types A, B, and C), several new subtypes have been described in recent years, including lymphomatoid papulosis type D (simulating primary cutaneous CD8+ aggressive epidermotropic cytotoxic T-cell lymphoma), lymphomatoid papulosis type E (simulating angioinvasive/angiodestructive lymphomas), and lymphomatoid papulosis with *DUSP22-IRF4* rearrangement (a subtype with chromosomal rearrangements of 6p25.3 similar to those found in ~25% of primary cutaneous anaplastic large cell lymphomas) {1340}. Recognition of these various lymphomatoid papulosis subtypes is important in order to avoid misdiagnosis of other, often more

**Table 4.01** Characteristic clinical and immunophenotypic features of various types of cutaneous T-cell lymphomas

| Disease | Clinical features | T-cell phenotype | Cytotoxic proteins | CD56 | Major lineage | EBV |
|---|---|---|---|---|---|---|
| Mycosis fungoides | Patches and plaques; (ulcerating) tumours in advanced stages | CD3+, CD4+, CD8− | − | − | αβ T-cell | − |
| C-ALCL | Solitary or localized nodules or tumours | CD3+, CD4+, CD8−, CD30+ | + | − | αβ T-cell | − |
| SPTCL | Subcutaneous nodules and plaques | CD3+, CD4−, CD8+ | + | − | αβ T-cell | − |
| Extranodal NK/T-cell lymphoma | (Ulcerating) plaques and tumours | CD3+, CD4−, CD8−, surface CD3− | + | + | NK-cell | + |
| PCGD-TCL | Ulcerating plaques and tumours | CD3+, CD4−, CD8−/+ | + | + | γδ T-cell | − |
| CD8+ AECTCL | Diffuse eruptive papules, nodules, and tumours | CD3+, CD4−, CD8+ | + | − | αβ T-cell | − |
| Primary cutaneous acral CD8+ T-cell lymphoma | Solitary papule or nodule at an acral site (ear, nose) | CD3+, CD4−, CD8+ | +/−[a] | − | αβ T-cell | − |
| Primary cutaneous CD4+ small/medium T-cell LPD | Solitary plaque or nodule on the face, neck, or upper trunk | CD3+, CD4+, CD8−, PD1+ | − | − | αβ T-cell | − |

C-ALCL, cutaneous anaplastic large cell lymphoma; CD8+ AECTCL, primary cutaneous CD8+ aggressive epidermotropic cytotoxic T-cell lymphoma; LPD, lymphoproliferative disorder; PCGD-TCL, primary cutaneous γδ T-cell lymphoma; SPTCL, subcutaneous panniculitis-like T-cell lymphoma.

[a] Primary cutaneous acral CD8+ T-cell lymphoma expresses a non-activated cytotoxic phenotype, positive for TIA1, but negative for other cytotoxic proteins.

aggressive types of CTCL, but the subtypes themselves have no therapeutic or prognostic implications.

Two new provisional entities in the current classification are EBV-positive mucocutaneous ulcer and primary cutaneous acral CD8+ T-cell lymphoma. EBV-positive mucocutaneous ulcer affects patients with age-related and iatrogenic immunosuppression or HIV infection, and is clinically characterized by sharply circumscribed ulcers at mucocutaneous sites and a self-limited, indolent course {641}. Primary cutaneous acral CD8+ T-cell lymphoma, originally designated "indolent CD8+ lymphoid proliferation of the ear", is a rare cutaneous tumour characterized by skin infiltration of clonal atypical medium-sized CD8+ cytotoxic lymphocytes and preferential involvement of acral sites (in particular the ears) {2046}. Although the prognosis is generally excellent, staging is not recommended for typical cases, and aggressive therapies are not required, the term "lymphoma" (rather than "lymphoproliferative disorder") is preferred for this entity mainly because of its cytological atypia. In contrast, the name for "primary cutaneous CD4+ small/medium T-cell lymphoma" has been updated to "primary cutaneous CD4+ small/medium T-cell lymphoproliferative disorder", because of its indolent clinical behaviour and its clinicopathological similarities to the cutaneous pseudo-T-cell lymphomas with a nodular growth pattern described in the past {419}.

This 4th edition volume contains a new section on cutaneous manifestations of chronic active EBV infection, which includes hydroa vacciniforme–like lymphoproliferative disorder and severe mosquito bite allergy. The term "hydroa vacciniforme–like lymphoproliferative disorder" encompasses all of the various manifestations of the EBV-associated hydroa vacciniforme–like skin lesions, including classic hydroa vacciniforme, severe or systemic hydroa vacciniforme, and hydroa vacciniforme–like lymphoma {2545}. Both hydroa vacciniforme–like lymphoproliferative disorder, which is primarily derived from T cells, and severe mosquito bite allergy, which is more often derived from NK cells, present primarily in children and are associated with a risk of progression to systemic EBV-associated NK/T-cell lymphoma.

In the section on histiocytic and dendritic cell neoplasms, Erdheim–Chester disease is recognized as a new entity, separate from the other members of the juvenile xanthogranuloma family. An introduction to this heterogeneous group of diseases has been added.

In recent years, genome-wide genetic studies have contributed to a better understanding of the molecular pathways involved in the pathogenesis of the various types of cutaneous lymphoma, which has resulted in the identification of additional diagnostic and prognostic criteria and new potential therapeutic targets. Although genetic markers are becoming increasingly important, the integration of histological, immunophenotypic, genetic, and (in particular for cutaneous lymphomas) clinical data remains essential for accurate diagnosis. In recent decades, collaboration between pathologists, dermatologists, haematologists and radiation oncologists has been crucial for defining new entities and classifications, and it is also the best guarantee for further progress in the diagnosis and treatment of patients with cutaneous lymphoma.

# Mycosis fungoides

Cerroni L.
Sander C.A.
Smoller B.R.
Willemze R.

## Definition

Mycosis fungoides is an epidermotropic, primary cutaneous T-cell lymphoma of small to medium-sized T lymphocytes with cerebriform nuclei. The term "mycosis fungoides" should only be used for classic cases, characterized by the evolution of patches, plaques, and tumours and variants with a similar clinical course. Folliculotropic mycosis fungoides, granulomatous slack skin, and pagetoid reticulosis have distinctive clinicopathological features and are discussed separately as distinct variants.

## ICD-O code 9700/3

## Epidemiology

Mycosis fungoides is the most common type of cutaneous T-cell lymphoma, and it accounts for almost 50% of all primary cutaneous lymphomas {2832}. Most patients are adults/elderly, but the disease can also occur in children and adolescents {261,780}. The male-to-female ratio is 2:1 {2832}. The worldwide incidence is about 5–6 cases per 1 million person-years, with marked regional variation {1431}. The incidence is higher in Black populations {1082}.

## Etiology

The etiology of mycosis fungoides remains unknown. Genetic predisposition may play a role in some cases. Associations with long-term exposure to various allergens and associations with chronic skin disorders have also been suggested as possible etiological factors. No convincing link to viral infections has yet been demonstrated. Mycosis fungoides has been observed in solid-organ transplant recipients, suggesting that immunosuppression may contribute to the development of the disease.

## Localization

As a rule, the disease is limited to the skin. It has variable distribution and a protracted duration. Extracutaneous dissemination may occur in advanced stages, mainly to lymph nodes, liver, spleen, lungs, and blood {586}. Involvement of the bone marrow is rare {2832}.

## Clinical features

Mycosis fungoides has an indolent clinical course, with slow progression (over years or sometimes decades) from patches to more-infiltrated plaques and eventually tumours. In early stages, the lesions are often confined to sun-protected areas. Patients with tumour-stage mycosis fungoides characteristically show a combination of patches, plaques, and tumours, which often show ulceration {2832}. Uncommonly, patients present with or develop an erythrodermic stage of disease that lacks the haematological criteria for Sézary syndrome. In addition to the clinicopathological variants discussed separately, several other clinical and/or histopathological variants of the disease have been described (e.g. hypopigmented mycosis fungoides) {406}.

The exact nosology of so-called parapsoriasis and its relationship to mycosis fungoides are unclear {407}. Although progression of parapsoriasis to more-advanced stages of mycosis fungoides can occur, most patients experience an indolent course with remissions and

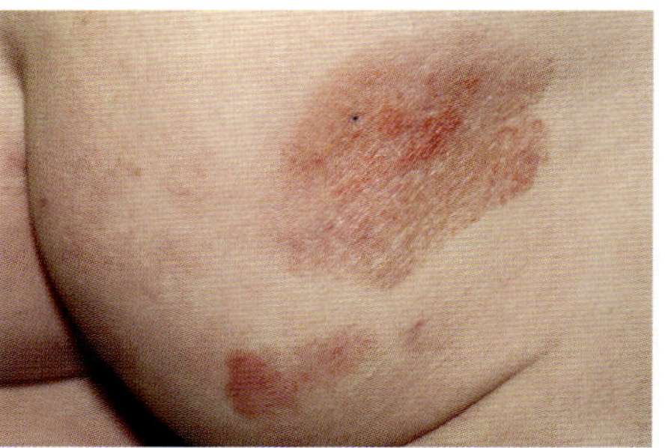

**Fig. 4.01** Mycosis fungoides. Localized patch / thin plaques on the buttock, covering < 10% of the body surface (stage IA).

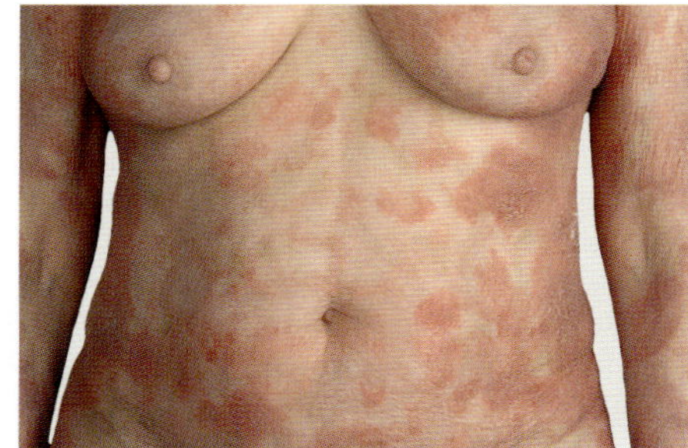

**Fig. 4.02** Mycosis fungoides. Generalized patches and plaques (stage IB).

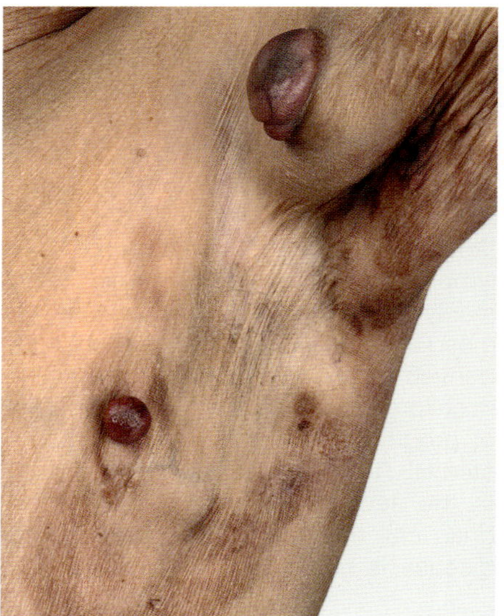

**Fig. 4.03** Mycosis fungoides. Tumours arising in the proximity of or within pre-existing patches (stage II).

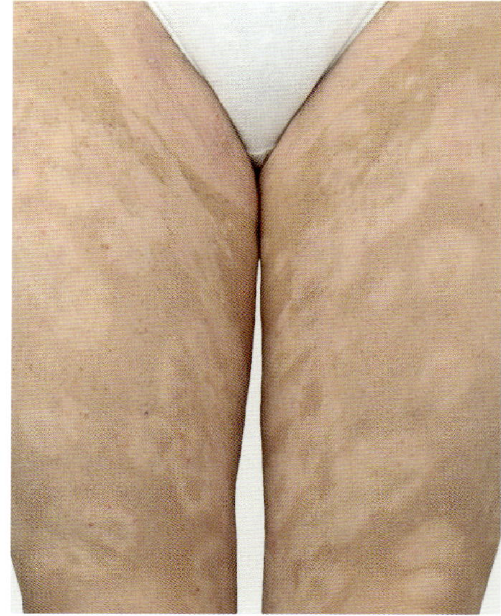

**Fig. 4.04** Hypopigmented mycosis fungoides. Hypopigmented patches with focal erythematous areas on both legs.

**Table 4.02** Staging of mycosis fungoides and Sézary syndrome according to the International Society for Cutaneous Lymphomas (ISCL) and the cutaneous lymphoma task force of the European Organisation for Research and Treatment of Cancer (EORTC) {1946}

| TNMB stages | |
|---|---|
| **Skin** | |
| $T_1$ | Limited patches,* papules, and/or plaques† covering < 10% of the skin surface. May further stratify into $T_{1a}$ (patch only) vs $T_{1b}$ (plaque ± patch). |
| $T_2$ | Patches, papules or plaques covering ≥ 10% of the skin surface. May further stratify into $T_{2a}$ (patch only) vs $T_{2b}$ (plaque ± patch). |
| $T_3$ | One or more tumors‡ (≥ 1-cm diameter) |
| $T_4$ | Confluence of erythema covering ≥ 80% body surface area |
| **Node** | |
| $N_0$ | No clinically abnormal peripheral lymph nodes§; biopsy not required |
| $N_1$ | Clinically abnormal peripheral lymph nodes; histopathology Dutch grade 1 or NCI $LN_{0-2}$ |
| $N_{1a}$ | Clone negative# |
| $N_{1b}$ | Clone positive# |
| $N_2$ | Clinically abnormal peripheral lymph nodes; histopathology Dutch grade 2 or NCI $LN_3$ |
| $N_{2a}$ | Clone negative# |
| $N_{2b}$ | Clone positive# |
| $N_3$ | Clinically abnormal peripheral lymph nodes; histopathology Dutch grades 3-4 or NCI $LN_4$; clone positive or negative |
| $N_X$ | Clinically abnormal peripheral lymph nodes; no histologic confirmation |
| **Visceral** | |
| $M_0$ | No visceral organ involvement |
| $M_1$ | Visceral involvement (must have pathology confirmation¶ and organ involved should be specified) |
| **Blood** | |
| B0 | Absence of significant blood involvement: ≤ 5% of peripheral blood lymphocytes are atypical (Sézary) cells‖ |
| $B_{0a}$ | Clone negative# |
| $B_{0b}$ | Clone positive# |
| B1 | Low blood tumor burden: > 5% of peripheral blood lymphocytes are atypical (Sézary) cells but does not meet the criteria of $B_2$ |
| $B_{1a}$ | Clone negative# |
| $B_{1b}$ | Clone positive# |
| B2 | High blood tumor burden: ≥ 1000/μL Sézary cells‖ with positive clone# |

| Stage | | | | |
|---|---|---|---|---|
| IA | T1 | N0 | M0 | B0, B1 |
| IB | T2 | N0 | M0 | B0, B1 |
| II | T1, T2 | N1, N2 | M0 | B0, B1 |
| IIB | T3 | N0, N1, N2 | M0 | B0, B1 |
| III | T4 | N0, N1, N2 | M0 | B0, B1 |
| IIIA | T4 | N0, N1, N2 | M0 | B0 |
| IIIB | T4 | N0, N1, N2 | M0 | B1 |
| IVA1 | Any T | N0, N1, N2 | M0 | B2 |
| IVA2 | Any T | N3 | M0 | Any B |
| IVB | Any T | N0, N1, N2, N3 | M1 | Any B |

* For skin, patch indicates any size skin lesion without significant elevation or induration. Presence/absence of hypo- or hyperpigmentation, scale, crusting, and/or poikiloderma should be noted.

† For skin, plaque indicates any size skin lesion that is elevated or indurated. Presence or absence of scale, crusting, and/or poikiloderma should be noted. Histologic features such as folliculotropism or large-cell transformation (> 25% large cells), CD30+ or CD30−, and clinical features such as ulceration are important to document.

‡ For skin, tumor indicates at least one 1-cm diameter solid or nodular lesion with evidence of depth and/or vertical growth. Note total number of lesions, total volume of lesions, largest size lesion, and region of body involved. Also note if histologic evidence of large-cell transformation has occurred. Phenotyping for CD30 is encouraged.

§ For node, abnormal peripheral lymph node(s) indicates any palpable peripheral node that on physical examination is firm, irregular, clustered, fixed or 1.5 cm or larger in diameter. Node groups examined on physical examination include cervical, supraclavicular, epitrochlear, axillary, and inguinal. Central nodes, which are not generally amenable to pathologic assessment, are not currently considered in the nodal classification unless used to establish N3 histopathologically.

¶ For viscera, spleen and liver may be diagnosed by imaging criteria.

‖ For blood, Sézary cells are defined as lymphocytes with hyperconvoluted cerebriform nuclei. If Sézary cells are not able to be used to determine tumor burden for B2, then one of the following modified ISCL criteria along with a positive clonal rearrangement of the TCR may be used instead: (1) expanded CD4+ or CD3+ cells with CD4/CD8 ratio of 10 or more, (2) expanded CD4+ cells with abnormal immunophenotype including loss of CD7 or CD26.

# A T-cell clone is defined by PCR or Southern blot analysis of the T-cell receptor gene.

**NCI, US National Cancer Institute; TCR, T-cell receptor; TNMB, tumour, node, metastasis, blood.**

Fig. 4.05 Early mycosis fungoides. Band-like lymphoid infiltrates with epidermotropic lymphocytes and several Pautrier microabscesses.

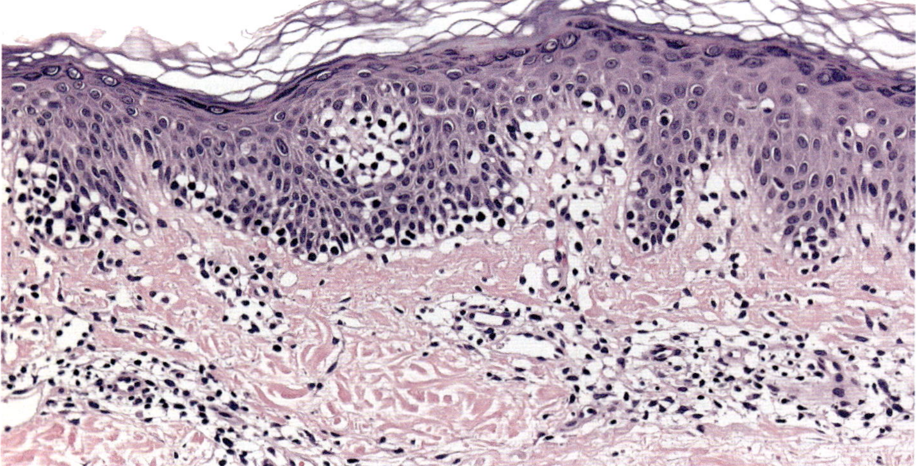

Fig. 4.06 Early mycosis fungoides. Epidermotropic lymphocytes aligned along the basal layer (basilar epidermotropism).

relapses, and management should be non-aggressive.

## Histopathology

The histology of the skin lesions varies with the stage of the disease. Early patch lesions show superficial band-like or lichenoid infiltrates, mainly consisting of lymphocytes and histiocytes. Atypical cells with small to medium-sized, highly indented (cerebriform) nuclei are few and mostly confined to the epidermis, where they characteristically colonize the epidermal basal layer, often as haloed cells, either singly or in a linear distribution {1687}. In typical plaques, epidermotropism is more pronounced. The presence of intraepidermal collections of atypical cells (Pautrier microabscesses) is a highly characteristic feature, but is seen in only a minority of cases {1687}. On occasion, mycosis fungoides may present with a granulomatous reaction; such cases have been termed granulomatous mycosis fungoides {1347}. With progression to the tumour stage, the dermal infiltrates become more diffuse, and epidermotropism may be lost. The tumour cells increase in number and size, showing variable proportions of small, medium-sized, and large cerebriform cells with pleomorphic or blastoid nuclei {2832}. Histological transformation, defined by >25% large lymphoid cells in the dermal infiltrates, may occur mainly, but not exclusively in the tumour stage {413,1264,2733}. These large cells can be positive or negative for CD30.

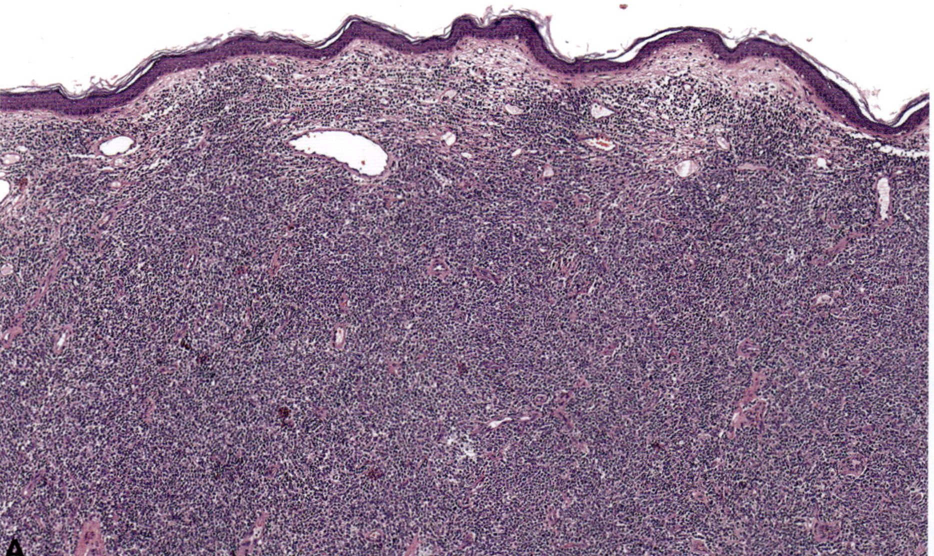


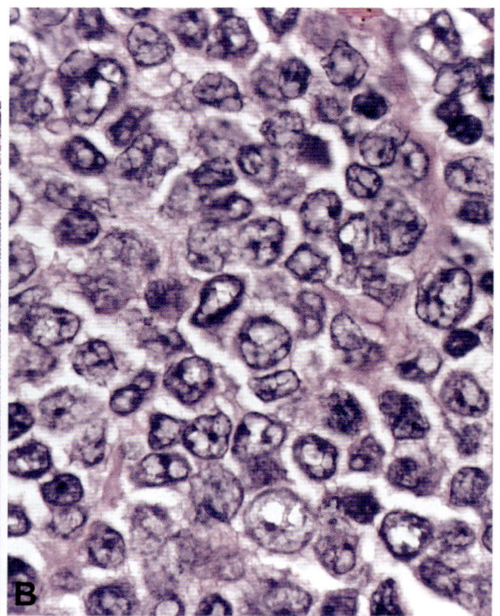


Fig. 4.07 Advanced mycosis fungoides. **A** A tumoural lesion with sheets of lymphocytes in the dermis without epidermotropism. **B** Detail of large, atypical lymphocytes.

Enlarged lymph nodes from patients with mycosis fungoides frequently show dermatopathic lymphadenopathy, with paracortical expansion due to the presence of large numbers of histiocytes and interdigitating cells with abundant, pale cytoplasm. The staging system for mycosis fungoides and Sézary syndrome proposed by the International Society for Cutaneous Lymphomas (ISCL) and the European Organisation for Research and Treatment of Cancer (EORTC) includes three categories for clinically abnormal lymph nodes (> 1.5 cm), reflecting no involvement (N1); early involvement, with no architectural effacement (N2); and overt involvement, with partial or complete architectural effacement (N3) {1946}; see Table 4.02, p. 227. Recognition of the early infiltrates, which can be difficult, can be facilitated by T-cell receptor (TCR) analysis {1946}. N3 lymph nodes may simulate peripheral T-cell lymphoma NOS or Hodgkin lymphoma.

The typical phenotype is positivity for CD2, CD3, TCRβ chain, CD5, and CD4 and negativity for CD8 and TCRγ chain. Cases with a cytotoxic phenotype (i.e. positive for CD8 and/or TCRγ chain) are well recognized {1685,2214}. Such cases have the same clinical behaviour and prognosis as CD4+ cases, and should not be considered a separate entity {1685}. A CD8+ phenotype has been reported more commonly in paediatric mycosis fungoides. Cutaneous lymphocyte antigen (CLA), associated with lymphocyte homing to the skin, is expressed in most cases. Lack of CD7 expression is frequent in all stages of the disease. Other alterations in the expression of T-cell antigens may be seen, but mainly occur in the advanced (tumour) stages. Partial expression of CD30 by neoplastic cells may be found in all stages, in particular in plaques and tumours. Cytotoxic granule proteins are uncommonly expressed in the early patch/plaque lesions, but may be positive in neoplastic cells in more-advanced lesions {2736}. A T follicular helper (TFH) phenotype has been found in a proportion of cases of both early and advanced mycosis fungoides {1567}.

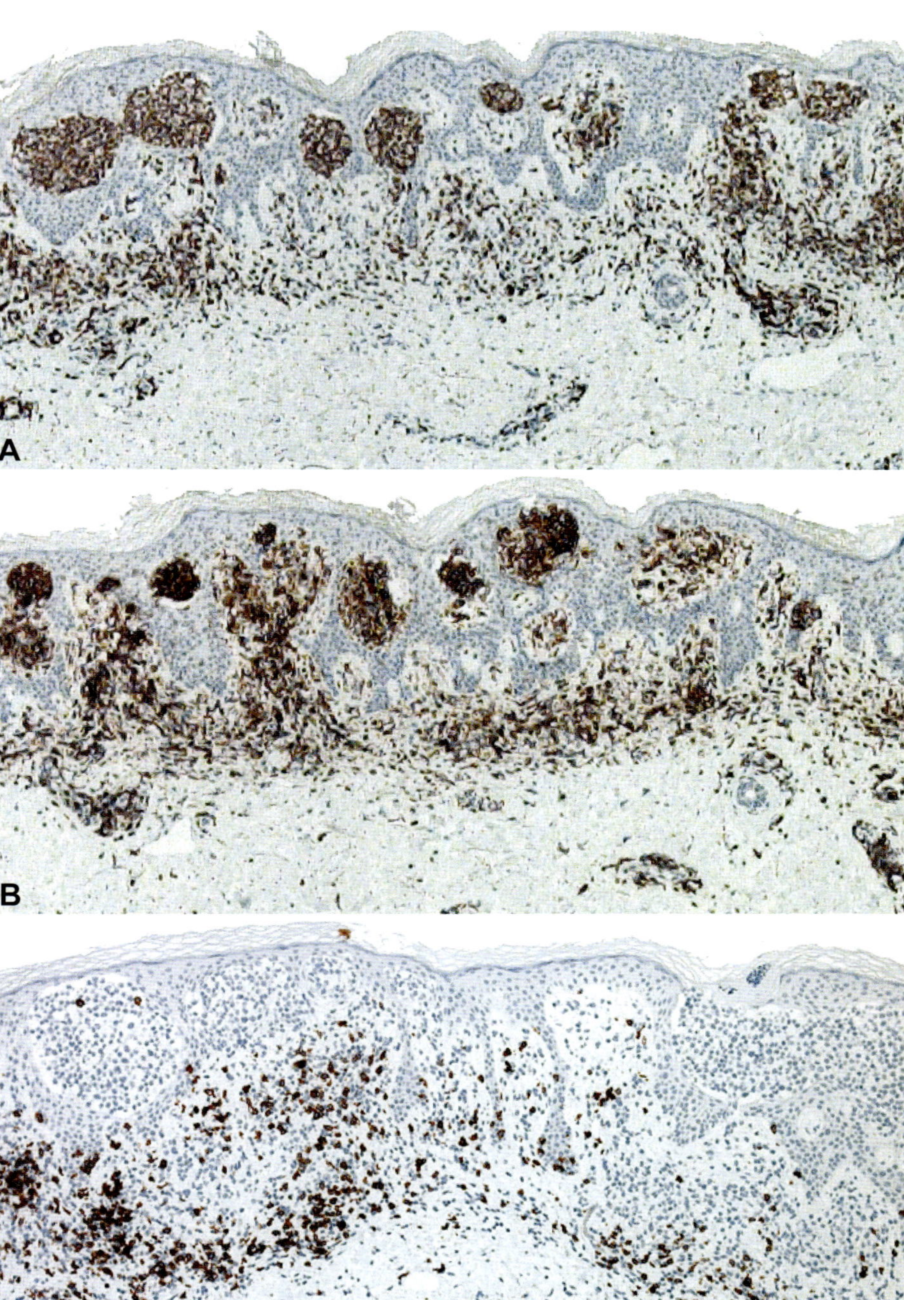

**Fig. 4.08** Early mycosis fungoides. The lymphocytes are positive for CD3 (**A**) and CD4 (**B**), and negative for CD8 (**C**).

### Differential diagnosis

Mycosis fungoides must be distinguished from other epidermotropic lymphomas, in particular primary cutaneous γδ T-cell lymphoma and primary cutaneous CD8+ aggressive epidermotropic cytotoxic T-cell lymphoma. Epidermotropic infiltrates may also be observed in other primary and secondary cutaneous T-cell lymphomas, and in lymphomatoid papulosis. Mycosis fungoides must also be distinguished from several benign inflammatory conditions that can show similar features clinically and/or histopathologically (e.g. actinic reticuloid and lichen planus–like keratosis). Synthesis of clinicopathological and phenotypic features is sufficient for a precise classification in the vast majority of cases.

### Histogenesis

The postulated normal counterparts are skin-homing mature T cells (mostly CD4-positive).

### Genetic profile

When sufficiently sensitive techniques are used, e.g. the BIOMED-2 protocols or next generation sequencing (NGS), TR genes are found to be clonally rearranged in the majority of cases {2083}. Complex karyotypes are present in many patients, in particular in the advanced stages. Somatic copy-number variants constitute the vast majority of all driver mutations, including mutations in multiple components of the TCR signalling pathway, genes that drive T helper 2 (Th2) cell differentiation, genes that facilitate escape from TGF-β–mediated growth suppression, and genes that confer resistance to TNFRSF-mediated apoptosis {471,2639,2695}. Activating *JAK3* mutations, observed in a recent study, may be targeted by specific drugs {1713}. A minority of patients show point mutations and genomic gains of the gene encoding TNFRSF1B (also known as TNFR2) {2677}. Constitutive activation of *STAT3* and inactivation of *CDKN2A* (*P16INK4a*) and *PTEN* have been identified and may be associated with disease progression {2333}.

### Prognosis and predictive factors

The single most important prognostic factor in mycosis fungoides is the extent of cutaneous and extracutaneous disease, as reflected in the clinical stage. Patients with limited disease generally have an excellent prognosis, with survival similar to that in the general population {24,2112,2705}. Large Pautrier microabscesses and dermal atypical lymphocytes in early lesions have been associated with progression to advanced stage {2752}. In the advanced stages, prognosis is poor, in particular for patients with skin tumours and/or extracutaneous dissemination {209,2705}. Absence of complete remission after initial treatment, age > 60 years, and an elevated lactate dehydrogenase level are adverse prognostic parameters {24,623,2331}, as is histological transformation with > 25% blast cells {106,413,2331}.

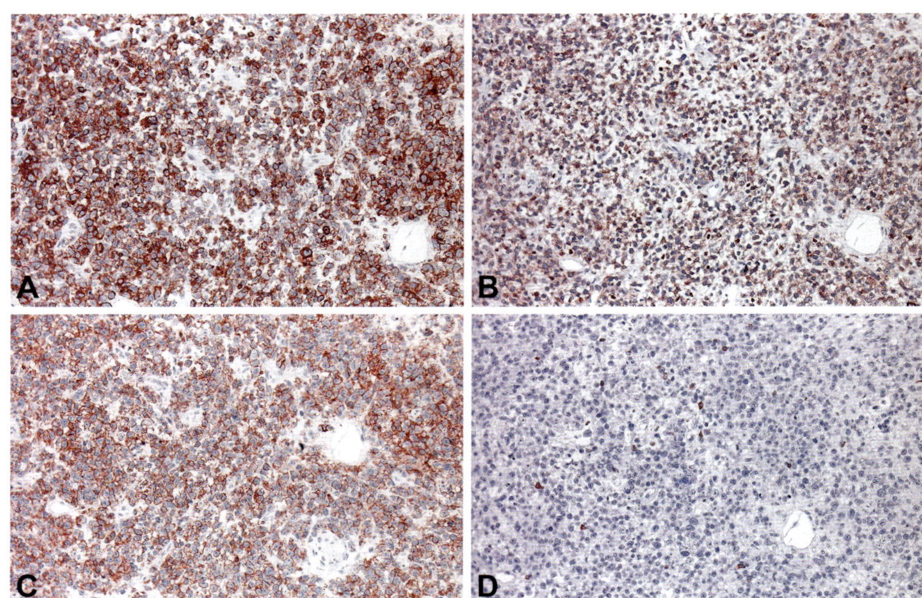


**Fig. 4.09** Advanced mycosis fungoides. Neoplastic lymphocytes show positivity for CD2 (**A**), CD3 (**B**), and CD4 (**C**), as well as loss of CD5 expression (**D**).

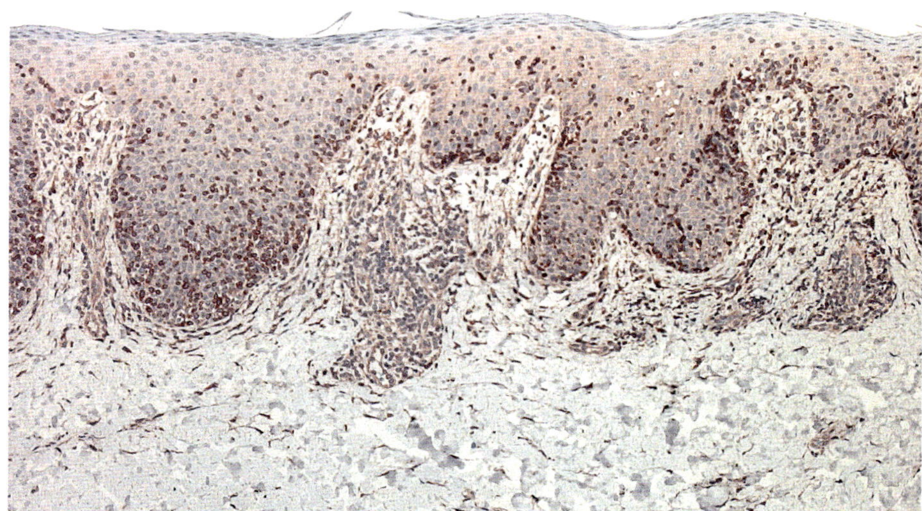

**Fig. 4.10** Cytotoxic mycosis fungoides. Staining for T-cell receptor γ chain highlights a superficial, epidermotropic infiltrate with a cytotoxic γδ phenotype.

# Variants of mycosis fungoides

Cerroni L.
Hodak E.
Kempf W.
Pincus L.B.
Smoller B.R.
Willemze R.

In addition to the classic (Alibert–Bazin) type of mycosis fungoides, many clinical and histological variants have been reported. Clinical variants, such as bullous, hyperpigmented, and hypopigmented mycosis fungoides, have clinical behaviour similar to that of classic mycosis fungoides; they are therefore not considered separately. In contrast, folliculotropic mycosis fungoides, granulomatous slack skin, and pagetoid reticulosis have distinctive clinicopathological features and different prognoses, and are considered separately in the following sections.

## *Folliculotropic mycosis fungoides*

### Definition

Folliculotropic mycosis fungoides is a variant of mycosis fungoides characterized by folliculotropic infiltrates, often with sparing of the epidermis, and by skin lesions that are located preferentially on the head and neck area and are frequently associated with alopecia. It should be noted that focal involvement of the hair follicles by neoplastic lymphocytes can also be observed in patients with otherwise conventional mycosis fungoides.

### ICD-O code 9700/3

### Synonyms

Pilotropic mycosis fungoides; follicular mycosis fungoides

### Epidemiology

Folliculotropic mycosis fungoides occurs in adults (and rarely in children) of both sexes.

### Localization

In early stages, folliculotropic mycosis fungoides is confined to the skin. The lesions preferentially involve the head and neck area, but the entire skin can be affected. Alopecia of the eyebrows (as a result of destruction of the hair follicles) is a characteristic finding.

### Clinical features

Folliculotropic mycosis fungoides presents clinically with grouped follicular patches, papules, and plaques that are frequently associated with alopecia {2704}. Solitary lesions may be seen {1801}. Tiny keratotic spines may protrude from affected follicles, conferring the lesion a resemblance to lichen spinulosus. In some cases, several grouped comedones and/or small infundibular cysts surrounded and infiltrated by neoplastic lymphocytes can be seen; such cases are called mycosis fungoides with eruptive cysts and comedones. Secondary bacterial infection is much more frequent in folliculotropic mycosis fungoides than in other variants.

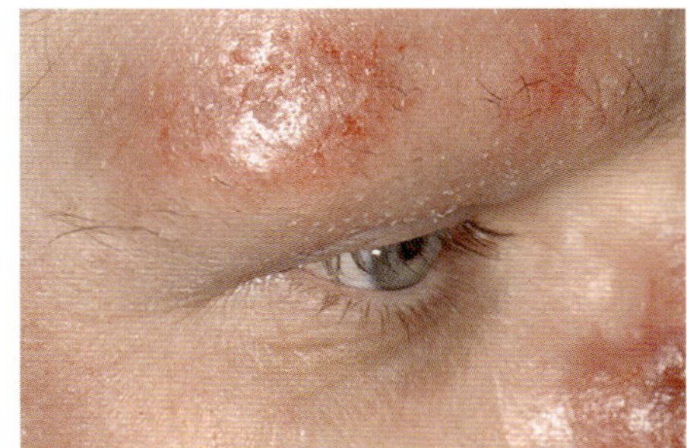

**Fig. 4.11** Folliculotropic mycosis fungoides. Erythematous lesions with subsequent alopecia of the eyebrow.

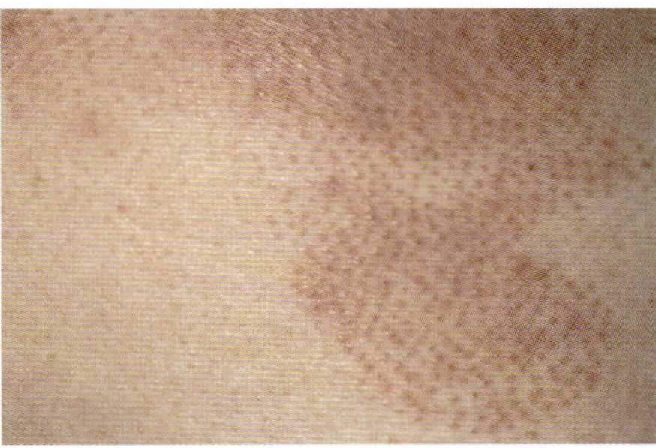

**Fig. 4.12** Folliculotropic mycosis fungoides. Confluent erythematous patches with prominent involvement of many hair follicles.

### Histopathology

Folliculotropic mycosis fungoides is characterized by the presence of perifollicular

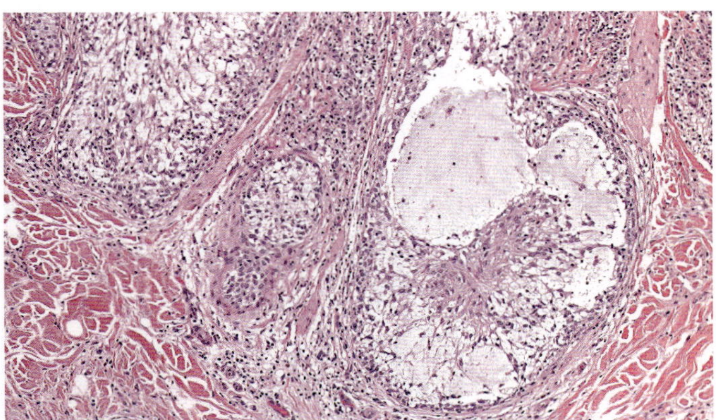

**Fig. 4.13** Folliculotropic mycosis fungoides. Hyperplastic follicles with prominent mucin deposition, surrounded and infiltrated by lymphocytes.

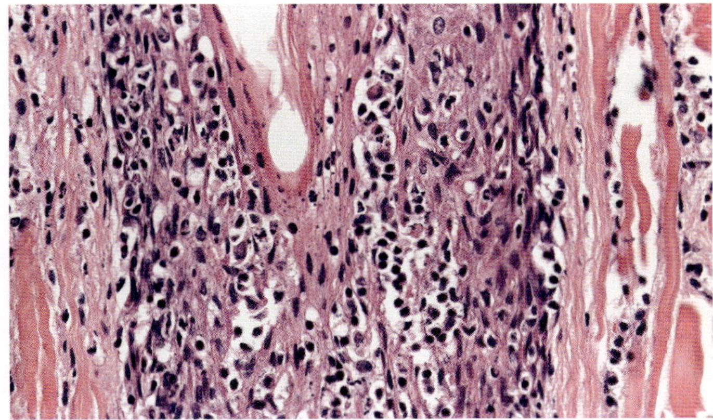

**Fig. 4.14** Folliculotropic mycosis fungoides. Intraepithelial lymphocytes in a case characterized by absence of mucin deposition within the follicle.

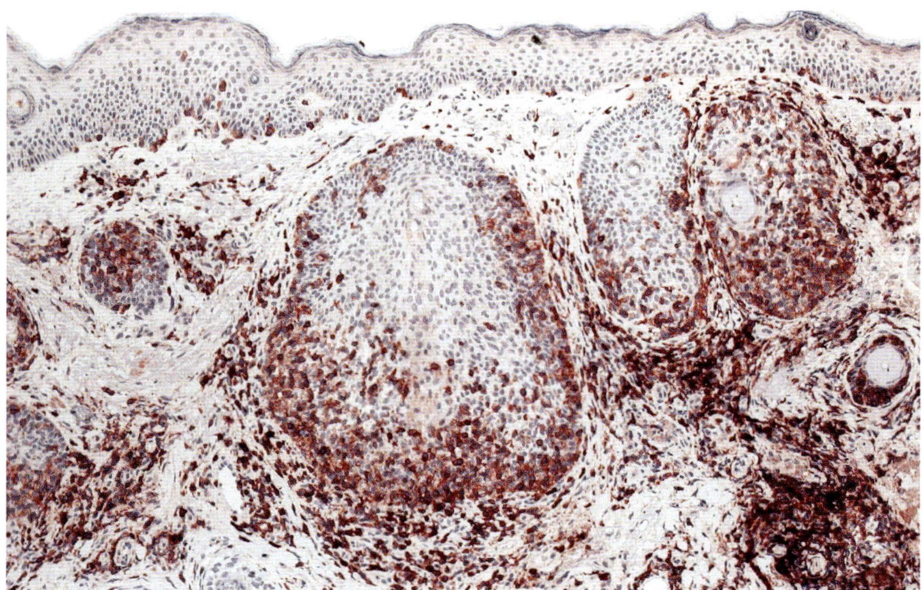

**Fig. 4.15** Folliculotropic mycosis fungoides. CD3 staining highlights intrafollicular lymphocytes; note the absence of histopathological features of mycosis fungoides within the epidermis.

infiltrates, with variable infiltration of the follicular epithelium by neoplastic CD4+ T lymphocytes {411}. The epidermis between the affected hair follicles is often spared. Many cases show mucinous degeneration of the hair follicles (follicular mucinosis), but mucin deposition can also be absent {2704}. Eosinophils are present in most cases, and may occasionally be a prominent feature. Folliculotropic mycosis fungoides has features overlapping with those of syringotropic mycosis fungoides, and features of both variants can sometimes be seen in a single lesion; such cases are called adnexotropic mycosis fungoides {2061}.

### Differential diagnosis

The differentiation of folliculotropic mycosis fungoides from benign follicular mucinosis is an ongoing source of debate. Patients with solitary lesions of follicular mucinosis (usually children or adolescents with a single lesion on the face) have an excellent prognosis and according to current evidence should not be diagnosed with folliculotropic mycosis fungoides.

### Histogenesis

The postulated normal counterparts are skin-homing mature, typically CD4+ T-cells.

### Genetic profile

TR genes are clonally rearranged in the majority of cases.

### Prognosis and predictive factors

The prognosis of folliculotropic mycosis fungoides has been the subject of several studies with conflicting results. Earlier reports suggested a worse prognosis compared with conventional mycosis fungoides {2704}, but more-recent studies have shown that early lesions of folliculotropic mycosis fungoides have a prognosis similar to that of corresponding stages of mycosis fungoides {1097,2709}. Nonetheless, because of the deep localization of the neoplastic infiltrate, folliculotropic mycosis fungoides is less accessible for skin-targeted therapies, and management of the condition remains challenging {2710}.

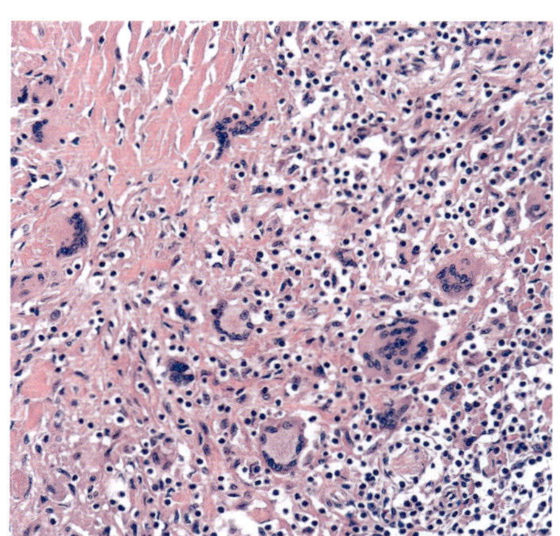

**Fig. 4.16** Granulomatous slack skin. Diffuse lymphoid infiltrate, throughout the entire dermis, with scattered multinucleated giant cells.

## Granulomatous slack skin

### Definition

Granulomatous slack skin (GSS) is an extremely rare variant of mycosis fungoides characterized by the development of bulky, pendulous skin folds.

### ICD-O code 9700/3

### Epidemiology

GSS is exceedingly rare. Both sexes are affected. Most patients are adults, but onset in children has been reported. Most reported cases of GSS have been associated with mycosis fungoides {1513}, but in some cases the disease was concomitant with Hodgkin lymphoma.

### Localization

The disease is usually limited to the skin and confined to flexural areas (i.e. the axillae and groins). Involvement of a regional lymph node by the same clone of T lymphocytes has been reported {201}.

### Clinical features

In the early stages, GSS is indistinguishable from conventional mycosis fungoides. The diagnosis can be made only once bulky, pendulous skin folds develop, conferring an appearance similar to that resulting from cutis laxa. The overlying skin is erythematous and atrophic, similar to what can be observed in mycosis fungoides.

### Histopathology

Histologically, GSS is characterized by a granulomatous infiltrate within the dermis and subcutaneous tissues {1347,

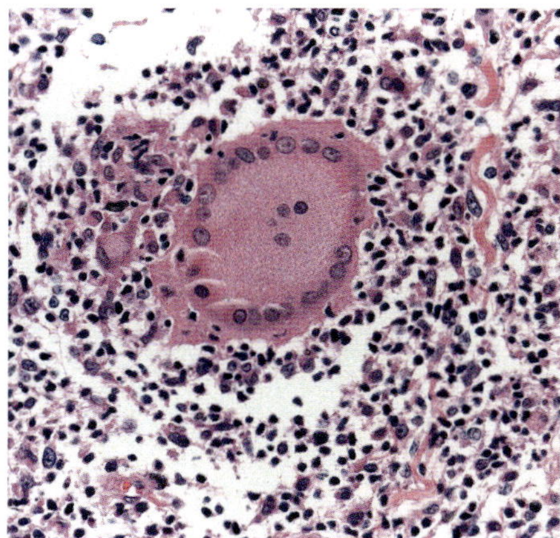

**Fig. 4.17** Granulomatous slack skin. A diffuse lymphoid infiltrate with a histiocytic giant cell.

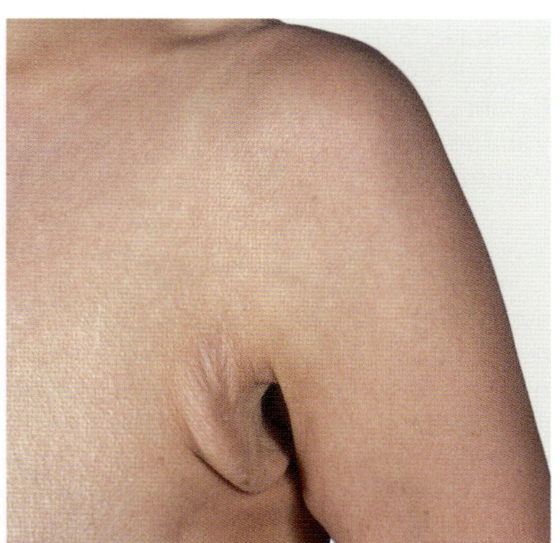

**Fig. 4.18** Granulomatous slack skin. Pendulous skin with a wrinkled, slightly erythematous surface in the left axilla.

1513,2388}. The infiltrate is composed of clonal CD4+ T cells admixed with abundant macrophages. Elastophagocytosis and focal loss of elastic fibres are common. A characteristic finding is multinucleated giant cells with many nuclei. The granulomatous infiltrate in GSS is usually diffuse and involves the subcutaneous tissues, in contrast to the patchy dermal granulomas conventional granulomatous mycosis fungoides. However, in many cases it can be impossible to distinguish GSS from conventional granulomatous mycosis fungoides histopathologically, and differentiation instead relies on the key clinical features {1347}.

### Histogenesis

The postulated normal counterpart is a skin-homing mature CD4+ T cell.

### Genetic profile

TR genes are clonally rearranged in the majority of cases. A t(3;9)(q12;p24) translocation has been reported in one case {1167}.

### Prognosis and predictive factors

GSS is characterized by an indolent and slowly progressive clinical course, but it responds poorly to conventional treatments {1513}. Surgical excision of the bulky, pendulous skin has been performed in some cases, but recurrence over time is typical.

## *Pagetoid reticulosis*

### Definition

Pagetoid reticulosis is a localized variant of mycosis fungoides characterized by patches and plaques with an intraepidermal proliferation of neoplastic T cells {985}. The term "pagetoid reticulosis" should only be used for localized (Woringer–Kolopp type) disease and not for disseminated (Ketron–Goodman type) disease, because most disseminated cases should instead be classified as primary cutaneous CD8+ aggressive epidermotropic cytotoxic T-cell lymphoma or cutaneous $\gamma\delta$ T-cell lymphoma {2832}.

### ICD-O code 9700/3

### Synonyms

Solitary mycosis fungoides;
Woringer–Kolopp disease

### Epidemiology

Pagetoid reticulosis is very rare.
Both sexes are affected, and the disease can occur in both children and adults.

### Localization

Pagetoid reticulosis is confined to the skin and occurs mostly on acral sites, in particular the hands and feet.

### Clinical features

Pagetoid reticulosis is characterized clinically by the presence of slow-growing, psoriasiform, scaly or crusty patches or plaques. Small lesions with a verrucous appearance may sometimes be mistaken for viral warts.

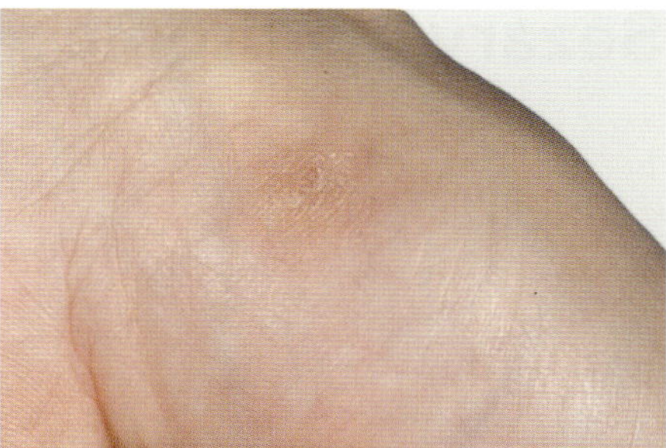

**Fig. 4.19** Pagetoid reticulosis. A solitary, small plaque on the wrist.

### Histopathology

Biopsy specimens reveal a dense intraepidermal proliferation of neoplastic T cells. The intraepidermal distribution of the cells resembles that seen in Paget disease (thus the designation "pagetoid"). The atypical cells have medium-sized or large cerebriform nuclei, and either a CD4–/CD8+ phenotype or (less commonly) a CD4+/CD8– or CD4–/CD8– phenotype. CD30 is often expressed.

### Histogenesis

The postulated normal counterpart is a skin-homing mature T cell.

### Genetic profile

TR genes are clonally rearranged in the majority of cases.

### Prognosis and predictive factors

The prognosis is excellent. Unlike with classic mycosis fungoides, extracutaneous dissemination or disease-related deaths have never been reported in association with pagetoid reticulosis {2832}.

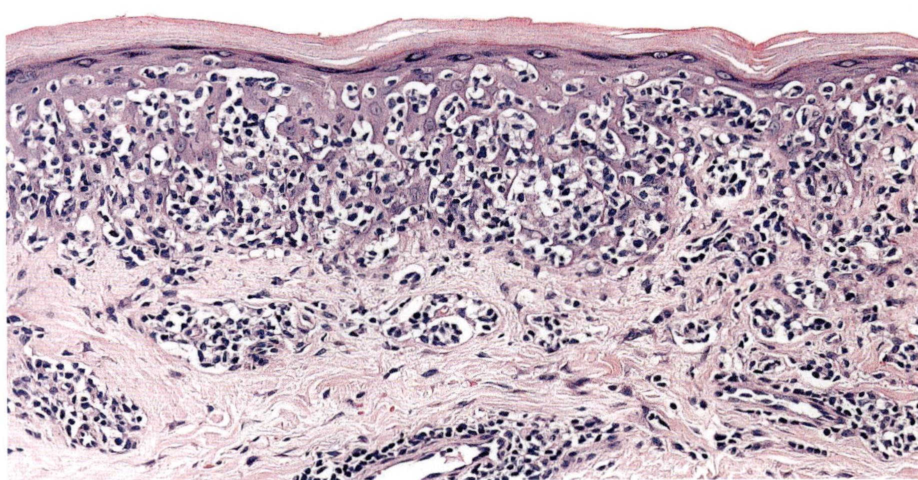

**Fig. 4.20** Pagetoid reticulosis. The epidermis is infiltrated by numerous lymphocytes, with a pagetoid pattern.

# Sézary syndrome

Whittaker S.J.
Cerroni L.
Ortonne N.
Vermeer M.H.
Willemze R.

## Definition

Sézary syndrome is defined by the triad of erythroderma; generalized lymphadenopathy; and the presence of clonally related neoplastic T cells with cerebriform nuclei (Sézary cells) in the skin, lymph nodes, and peripheral blood. In addition, one or more of the following criteria are also required: an absolute Sézary cell count ≥1000/μL, an expanded CD4+ T-cell population resulting in a CD4:CD8 ratio of ≥10, and loss of one or more T-cell antigens. A CD4+:CD7– ratio of ≥30 and/or a CD4+:CD26– ratio of ≥40 are accepted alternative diagnostic criteria {219,1876,2476}. Sézary syndrome and mycosis fungoides are closely related neoplasms, but they are considered separate entities on the basis of differences in clinical behaviour and cell of origin {2832}.

## ICD-O code

9701/3

## Epidemiology

This is a rare disease, accounting for <5% of all cutaneous T-cell lymphomas {2832}. It occurs in adults (typically aged >60 years) and has a male predominance.

## Localization

As a leukaemia, Sézary syndrome is by definition a generalized disease. In the advanced stages, any visceral organ can be involved, but the most common sites of involvement are the oropharynx, lungs, and CNS. Bone marrow involvement is variable.

## Clinical features

Patients present with erythroderma and generalized lymphadenopathy. Other features are pruritus, alopecia, ectropion, palmar and/or plantar hyperkeratosis, and onychodystrophy. Rarely, Sézary syndrome patients present with only generalized pruritus {1062}. An increased prevalence of secondary cutaneous and systemic malignancies has been reported in Sézary syndrome; this is attributed to immunoparesis associated with the skewing of the normal T-cell repertoire and the loss of normal circulating CD4+ cells {1142}.

## Histopathology

The histological features of Sézary syndrome can be similar to those of mycosis fungoides; however, the cellular infiltrates in Sézary syndrome are more often monotonous, and epidermotropism is sometimes absent. The dermal lymphocytic infiltrate is often perivascular. In as many as one third of biopsies from patients with otherwise classic Sézary syndrome, the histological picture may be nonspecific {2653}. Involved lymph nodes characteristically show a dense, monotonous infiltrate of Sézary cells, with effacement of the normal lymph node architecture {2340}. Bone marrow may be involved, but infiltrates are often sparse and mainly interstitial {2439}.

The neoplastic T cells have a CD3+, CD4+, CD8– phenotype, with variable loss of T-cell antigens such as CD7, CD26, and CD2 {1390}. PD1 (CD279) is expressed by neoplastic cells in the skin and blood in almost all cases {418}. Sézary cells express cutaneous lymphocyte antigen (CLA) and the skin-homing receptor CCR4, as well as CCR7 {779}. The NK cell markers CD158k (KIR3DL2) and NKp46 may also be expressed {1954,1955}.

## Differential diagnosis

Sézary syndrome must be distinguished from erythrodermic inflammatory dermatoses and other haematological malignancies presenting with erythroderma.

## Histogenesis

The normal counterparts of Sézary cells are circulating central memory T cells (CD27+, CD45RA–, CD45RO+); whereas the tumour cells of mycosis fungoides derive from skin-resident memory T cells {361}.

## Genetic profile

TR genes are clonally rearranged {2083,2814,2815}. A characteristic gene expression signature consists of overexpression of *PLS3*, *DNM3*, *TWIST1*, and *EPHA4* and underexpression of *STAT4* {987,1286,2703}. Recurrent balanced chromosomal translocations have not been detected in Sézary syndrome, but complex numerical and structural alterations (similar to those seen in mycosis fungoides) are common {173,369,1659}, including losses of 1p, 6q, and 10q and gains of 8q, with isochromosome 17q as a recurrent feature of Sézary syndrome {2738}.

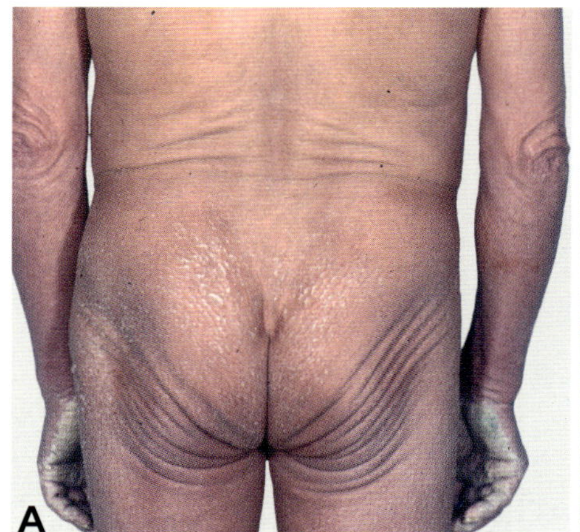


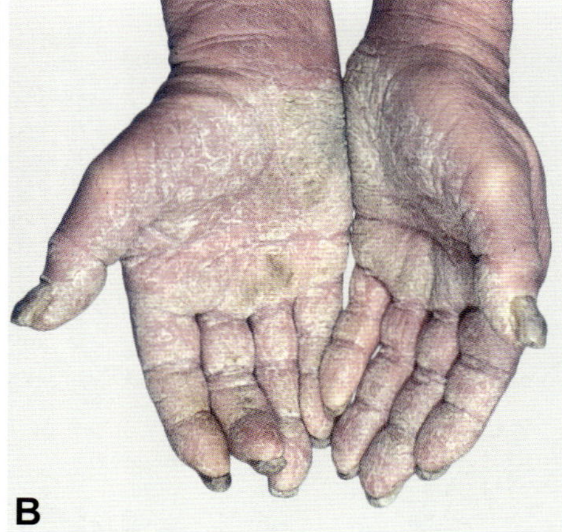


**Fig. 4.21** Sézary syndrome. **A,B** Generalized skin involvement (erythroderma) with palmar hyperkeratosis and onychodystrophy.

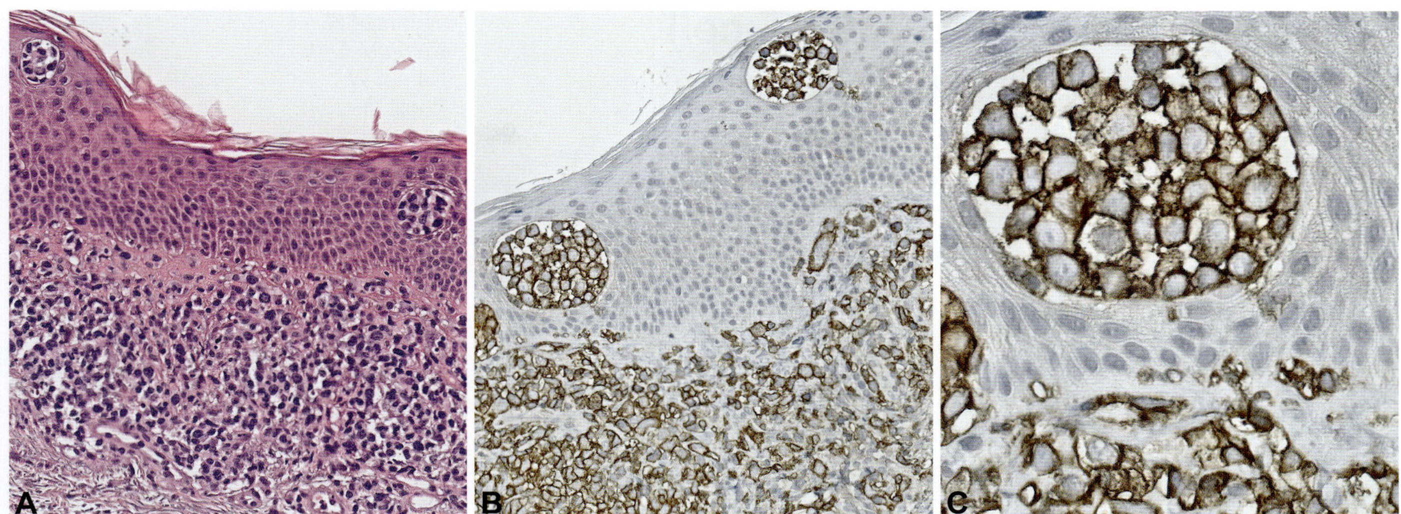

**Fig. 4.22** Sézary syndrome. **A** Band-like infiltrate of atypical lymphoid cells in superficial dermis, with formation of Pautrier microabscesses. **B** Strong expression of PD1 (CD279) by the atypical T cells. **C** Higher magnification of PD1 (CD279) staining.

High-throughput sequencing has revealed a heterogeneous pattern of gene mutations and focal copy-number variants, some of which have also been detected in other mature T-cell malignancies. There appears to be selection for deregulation of genome maintenance, T-cell homeostasis, cell survival, and epigenetic processes {471,557,1355,2093,2677,2714,2777,2862}. Loss-of-function mutations affecting *POT1* and *ATM* may contribute to genomic instability. Frequent inactivating mutations of *TP53* and deletions of *CDKN2A* (*P16INK4a*) {2332} likely contribute to impaired cell senescence. Recurrent gain-of-function mutations affecting genes involved in T-cell receptor signalling, including *PLCG1*, *CD28*, *CARD11*, and *TNFRSF1B*, as well as *ZEB1* deletions, may explain constitutive activation of NF-κB in Sézary syndrome. Other recurrent activating mutations include *CCR4* and *RHOA* mutations, as seen in other mature T-cell lymphomas. The constitutive activation of STAT3 in Sézary syndrome may be explained by both single-nucleotide mutations and copy-number variants affecting genes encoding members of the JAK/STAT pathway {557,2862}. Recurrent loss-of-function aberrations also target epigenetic modifiers (including *ARID1A*) in 40% of Sézary syndrome cases, as well as chromatin-modifying genes such as *ASXL3*, *DNMT3A*, *TET1*, and *TET2*. Genes involved in the FAS-dependent apoptotic pathway are commonly inactivated by hypermethylation {1243}.

### Prognosis and predictive factors

Sézary syndrome is an aggressive disease, with a median survival of 32 months and a 5-year overall survival rate of 10–30%, depending on stage {2832}. Most patients die of opportunistic infections. The degree of peripheral blood involvement at diagnosis may have an impact on prognosis {2753}, but the prognostic relevance of bone marrow involvement is unknown.

# Primary cutaneous CD30+ T-cell lymphoproliferative disorders

Willemze R.
Kadin M.E.
Kempf W.
Paulli M.

## *Introduction*

Primary cutaneous CD30+ T-cell lymphoproliferative disorders are the second most common group of cutaneous T-cell lymphomas, accounting for approximately 30% of cases. This group includes lymphomatoid papulosis, primary cutaneous anaplastic large cell lymphoma, and borderline cases.

Lymphomatoid papulosis and cutaneous anaplastic large cell lymphoma have overlapping clinical, histological, and phenotypic features and form a spectrum of disease {2832}. The clinical appearance and course are used as decisive criteria for the definitive diagnosis and choice of treatment. The term "borderline" refers to cases in which, despite careful clinicopathological correlation, a definite distinction between lymphomatoid papulosis and cutaneous anaplastic large cell lymphoma cannot be made. However, clinical examination during follow-up will generally reveal the correct diagnosis {194}.

## *Lymphomatoid papulosis*

### Definition

Lymphomatoid papulosis (LyP) is a chronic skin disease with recurrent, self-healing lesions; it usually follows a benign clinical course, but has histological features suggesting a (CD30+) cutaneous T-cell lymphoma.

### ICD-O code 9718/1

### Epidemiology

LyP most often occurs in adults (median age: 45 years), but children can also be affected. The male-to-female ratio is between 2:1 and 3:1 {194,597,1573,2697}.

### Etiology

The cause is unknown. A viral etiology has been suggested, but tests for HTLV-1, EBV, herpes simplex virus types 1 and 2, HHV6, HHV7, and HHV8 have been consistently negative {1266,1341,2835}.

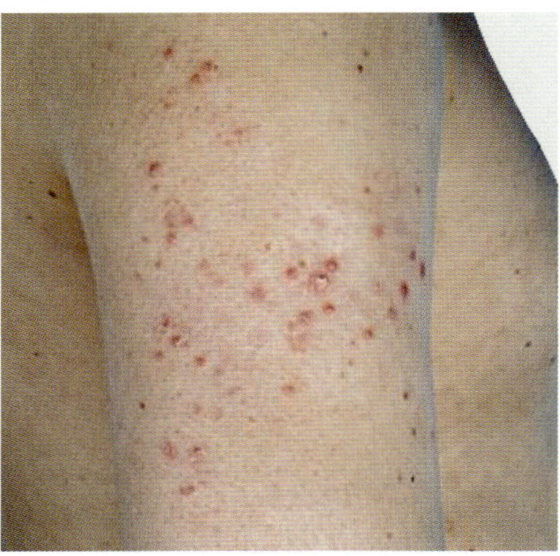

**Fig. 4.23** Lymphomatoid papulosis. Grouped papules in various stages of evolution.

### Localization

LyP is a skin-limited disease that most frequently affects the trunk and extremities {194}. In very rare cases, concurrent oral mucosal lesions may be present.

### Clinical features

LyP is characterized by the presence of papular, papulonecrotic, and/or nodular skin lesions. Characteristically, skin lesions in various stages of evolution coexist {194,597}. The number of lesions ranges from several to more than a hundred. Individual lesions disappear within 3–12 weeks, and may leave behind superficial scars. The duration of disease ranges from several months to decades. In as many as 20% of patients, LyP may be preceded by, associated with, or followed by another type of lymphoma, most commonly mycosis fungoides, cutaneous anaplastic large cell lymphoma, Hodgkin lymphoma, or Hodgkin lymphoma mimics {194,597,662,670,1339,1573,2774}.

### Histopathology

The histological picture of LyP is extremely variable, and in part correlates with the age of the biopsied skin lesion. Several histological subtypes of LyP have been described.

*LyP type A* (>80% of cases) is characterized by scattered or small clusters of large, atypical, and sometimes multinucleated or Reed–Sternberg–like CD30+ cells intermingled with numerous inflammatory cells, including small lymphocytes, neutrophils, and/or eosinophils {194,670}.

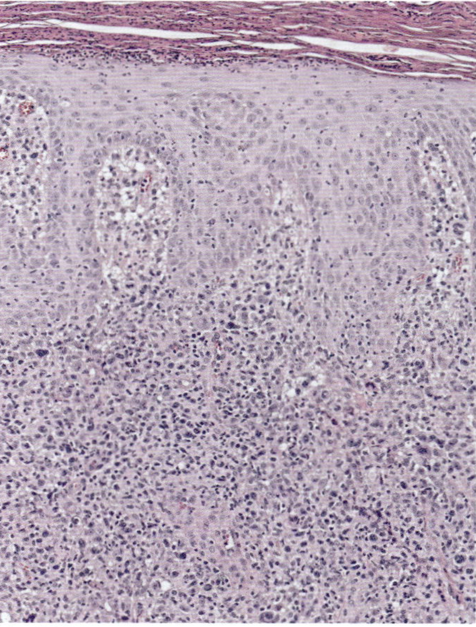

**Fig. 4.24** Lymphomatoid papulosis type A. Mixed inflammatory infiltrate with scattered large atypical cells.

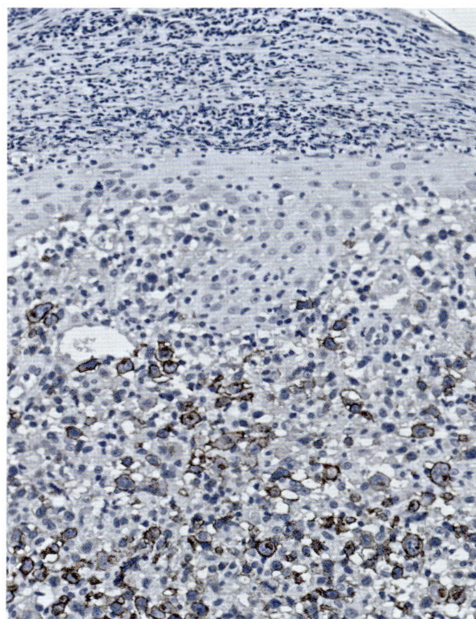

**Fig. 4.25** Lymphomatoid papulosis type A. Inflammatory infiltrate with scattered large atypical CD30+ cells.

*LyP type B* (< 5% of cases) is characterized by a predominantly epidermotropic infiltrate of small atypical CD30+ or CD30− cells with cerebriform nuclei, histologically simulating early-stage (plaque-stage) mycosis fungoides {194,670}

*LyP type C* (~10% of cases) is characterized by a monotonous population or cohesive sheets of large CD30+ T cells with relatively few admixed inflammatory cells, very similar to cutaneous anaplastic large cell lymphoma {194,670}.

*LyP type D* (< 5% of cases) is characterized by a strongly epidermotropic, sometimes pagetoid infiltrate of atypical small to medium-sized CD8+, CD30+ pleomorphic T cells, mimicking primary cutaneous CD8+ aggressive epidermotropic cytotoxic T-cell lymphoma {2276}. Some cases may have a γδ T-cell phenotype {2214}.

*LyP type E* (< 5% of cases) is characterized by angiocentric and angiodestructive infiltrates of small to medium-sized CD30+ and in most cases CD8+ pleomorphic T cells {1346}. Vascular occlusion, haemorrhage, extensive necrosis, and ulceration may be present. Clinically, patients present with a few papulonodular lesions that rapidly ulcerate and evolve into large necrotic eschar-like lesions.

*LyP with DUSP22-IRF4 rearrangement* (< 5% of cases) is characterized by chromosomal rearrangements involving the *DUSP22-IRF4* locus at 6p25.3 {1285}. The affected patients are older adults and often present with localized skin lesions. Histologically, the skin lesions show extensive epidermotropism by weakly CD30+ small to medium-sized T cells with cerebriform nuclei and strongly CD30+ medium-sized to large blast cells in the dermis, simulating transformed mycosis fungoides.

Other rare histological subtypes have also been described, including folliculotropic, syringotropic, and granulomatous variants {670,1342}. Different types of LyP may occur in distinct but concurrent lesions, and a single LyP lesion may show histological features of multiple LyP subtypes. Recognition of the various LyP subtypes is important in order to avoid misdiagnosis of other, often more aggressive types of cutaneous T-cell lymphoma (see Table 4.03), but the subtypes themselves have no therapeutic or prognostic implications.

The large atypical cells in LyP type A and type C lesions have the same

**Table 4.03** Histological subtypes and differential diagnosis of lymphomatoid papulosis (LyP) {2545}

| Histological subtype (relative frequency) | Predominant phenotype | Main differential diagnoses |
|---|---|---|
| LyP type A (> 80%) | CD4+, CD8− | Cutaneous anaplastic large cell lymphoma, tumour-stage mycosis fungoides, and Hodgkin lymphoma |
| LyP type B (< 5%) | CD4+, CD8− | Early-stage (plaque-stage) mycosis fungoides |
| LyP type C (~10%) | CD4+, CD8− | Cutaneous anaplastic large cell lymphoma and transformed (CD30+) mycosis fungoides |
| LyP type D (< 5%) | CD4−, CD8+ | Primary cutaneous CD8+ aggressive epidermotropic cytotoxic T-cell lymphoma |
| LyP type E (< 5%) | CD4−, CD8+ | Extranodal NK/T-cell lymphoma |
| LyP with *DUSP22-IRF4* rearrangement (< 5%) | CD4−, CD8+ or CD4−, CD8− | Transformed mycosis fungoides |

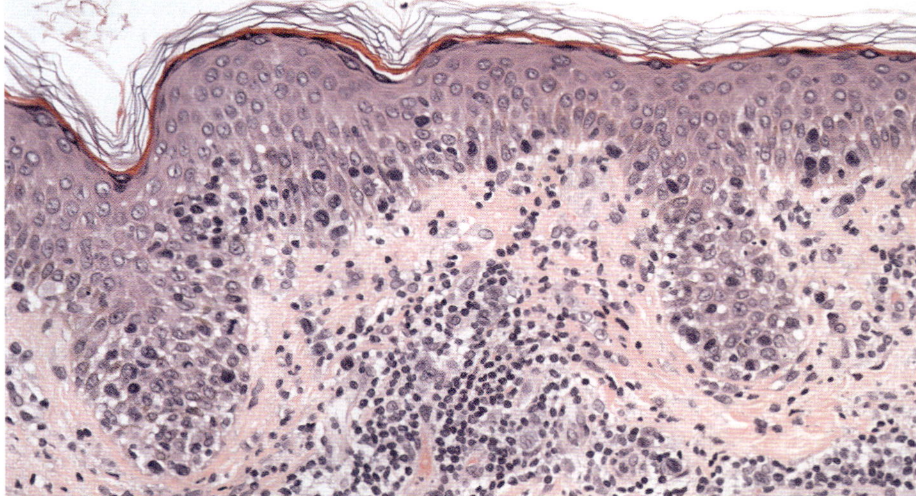

**Fig. 4.26** Lymphomatoid papulosis type B. An epidermotropic lymphocytic infiltrate mimicking early-stage mycosis fungoides; the atypical intraepidermal T cells have a CD4+, CD30+ T-cell phenotype.

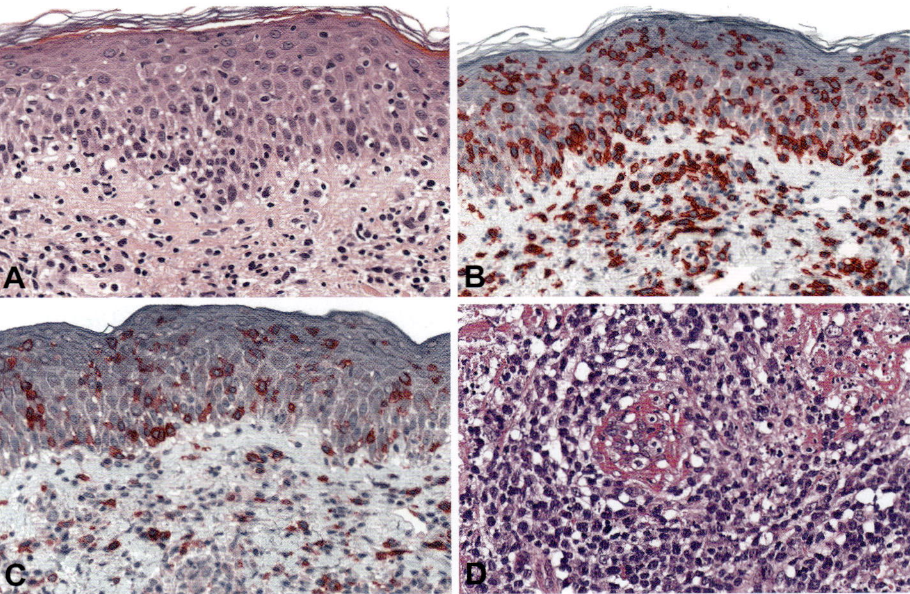


**Fig. 4.27** **A** Lymphomatoid papulosis type D. An epidermotropic infiltrate of small to medium-sized atypical lymphocytes, which express CD8 (**B**) and CD30 (**C**). **D** Lymphomatoid papulosis type E. Extensive angiocentric and angiodestructive infiltration by medium-sized to large atypical lymphocytes.

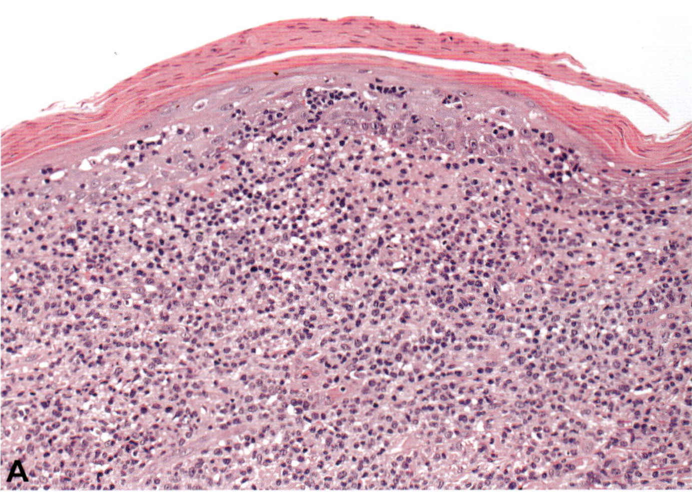
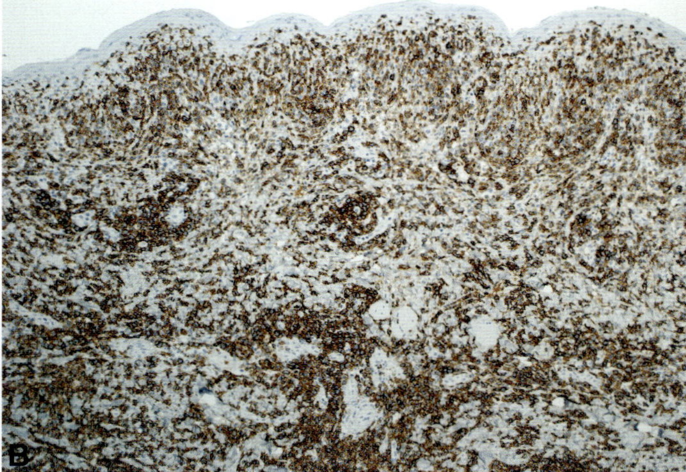

**Fig. 4.28** Lymphomatoid papulosis with *DUSP22-IRF4* rearrangement. **A** Intraepidermal mycosis fungoides–like small cells and dermal large blastic cells. **B** CD30 staining is diffusely positive and is stronger in dermal cells with blastic cytology.

immunophenotype as the tumour cells in cutaneous anaplastic large cell lymphoma. The atypical cells are predominantly CD4+ in LyP types A–C, CD8+ in LyP types D and E, and either CD8+ or double-negative for CD4 and CD8 in LyP with *DUSP22-IRF4* rearrangement. Expression of CD56 has been sporadically reported {195,785}.

### Differential diagnosis

Because of its wide spectrum of histological presentations, LyP must be differentiated from various types of cutaneous and nodal lymphomas (see Table 4.03, p. 237). Clinicopathological correlation is essential to differentiate LyP not only from these lymphomas, but also from a wide variety of infectious and inflammatory skin diseases that can contain substantial numbers of CD30+ cells {963,1338}.

### Histogenesis

The postulated normal counterpart is an activated skin-homing T lymphocyte.

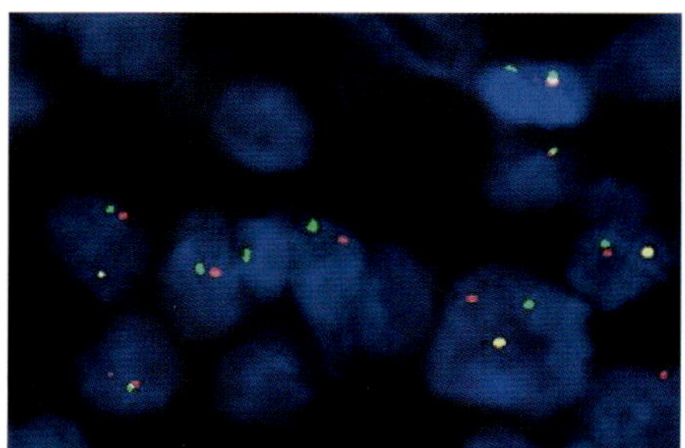

**Fig. 4.29** Lymphomatoid papulosis with *DUSP22-IRF4* rearrangement. Break-apart FISH shows *DUSP22* translocation.

### Genetic profile

Clonally rearranged TR genes have been detected in 40–60% of LyP lesions {474,583,587,935}, and identical rearrangements have been demonstrated in associated lymphomas {474,583,587}. No consistent cytogenetic abnormalities have been described. The t(2;5)(p23;q35) translocation is not found in LyP {600}. Rearrangements involving the *DUSP22-IRF4* locus at 6p25.3 are found in a small subset of LyP cases {1285,2755}.

### Prognosis and predictive factors

The vast majority of LyP cases have an excellent prognosis. Although patients with LyP have an increased risk of developing another form of cutaneous or nodal lymphoma, the reported mortality rates due to associated lymphomas are low {194,597,2822}. Because of the risk of developing a second lymphoma, long-term follow-up is recommended {1348}.

## *Primary cutaneous anaplastic large cell lymphoma*

### Definition

Primary cutaneous anaplastic large cell lymphoma (C-ALCL) is composed of large cells with an anaplastic, pleomorphic, or immunoblastic cytomorphology, with most of the tumour cells (> 75%) expressing CD30 {2832}.

### ICD-O code

9718/3

### Epidemiology

C-ALCL is the second most common type of cutaneous T-cell lymphoma {2832}. The median age is 60 years. Children are sporadically affected. The male-to-female ratio is between 2:1 and 3:1 {194}.

### Localization

This is a skin-limited disease with no clear predilection site {210,2856}.

### Clinical features

Most patients present with solitary or localized nodules or tumours, and sometimes papules, which often show ulceration {194,1573}. Multifocal lesions are seen in about 20% of cases. The skin lesions may show partial or complete spontaneous regression, as seen in lymphomatoid papulosis. These lymphomas frequently relapse in the skin. Extracutaneous dissemination occurs in approximately 10% of cases, and mainly involves the regional lymph nodes {194}.

### Histopathology

Histology shows diffuse infiltrates with cohesive sheets of large CD30+ tumour cells. Epidermotropism may be present, and is particularly marked in cases with *DUSP22-IRF4* rearrangement {1948}. In most cases, the tumour cells have the characteristic morphology of anaplastic cells, with round, oval, or irregularly shaped nuclei; prominent eosinophilic nucleoli; and abundant cytoplasm {2832}. Less commonly (in 20–25% of cases), they have a non-anaplastic (i.e. a pleomorphic or immunoblastic) appearance {194,1686,2012}. Reactive lymphocytes are often present at the periphery of the lesions. Ulcerating lesions may show a lymphomatoid papulosis–like histology, with an abundant inflammatory infiltrate of reactive T cells, histiocytes, eosinophils, and neutrophils, and relatively few CD30+ cells. In such cases, epidermal hyperplasia may be prominent. The inflammatory background is especially prominent in the rare neutrophil-rich (pyogenic) and eosinophil-rich variant {333}. Rare cases of intralymphatic and intravascular C-ALCL have been reported {2295,2776}.

The neoplastic cells show an activated CD4+ T-cell phenotype, with variable loss of CD2, CD5, CD7, and CD3 and frequent expression of cytotoxic proteins (granzyme B, TIA1, and perforin) {194,280,1458}. Some cases may have a CD4−/CD8+ or CD4+/CD8+ T-cell phenotype {1683}. CD30 is by definition expressed by a majority (> 75%) of the neoplastic cells {2832}. Unlike systemic anaplastic large cell lymphomas, most C-ALCLs express cutaneous lymphocyte antigen (CLA), but do not express EMA (epithelial membrane antigen) or ALK {585,600,2593}. CD15 is expressed in approximately 40% of cases, and staining for IRF4 (MUM1) is positive in almost all cases {208,2787}. Coexpression of CD56 is observed in rare cases, but does not appear to be associated with an unfavourable prognosis {1884}.

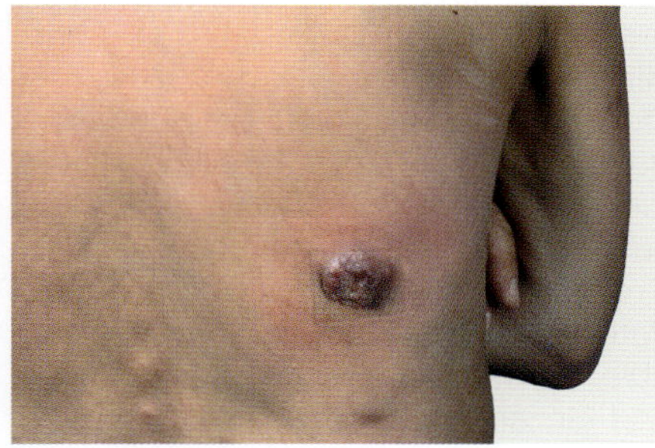

**Fig. 4.30** Primary cutaneous anaplastic large cell lymphoma presenting with a solitary tumour on the back.

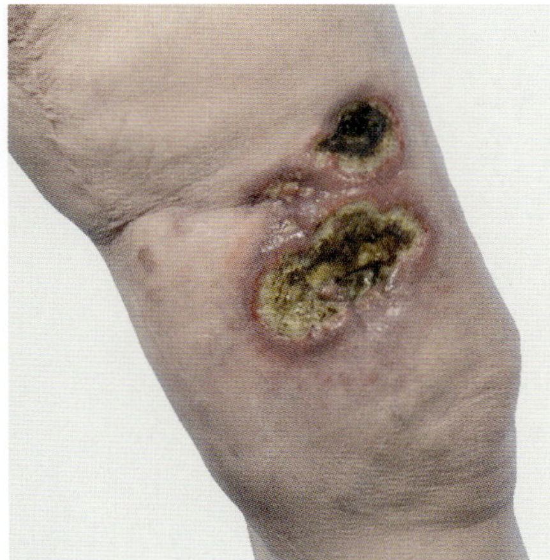

**Fig. 4.31** Primary cutaneous anaplastic large cell lymphoma presenting with large ulcerating tumours on the left leg.

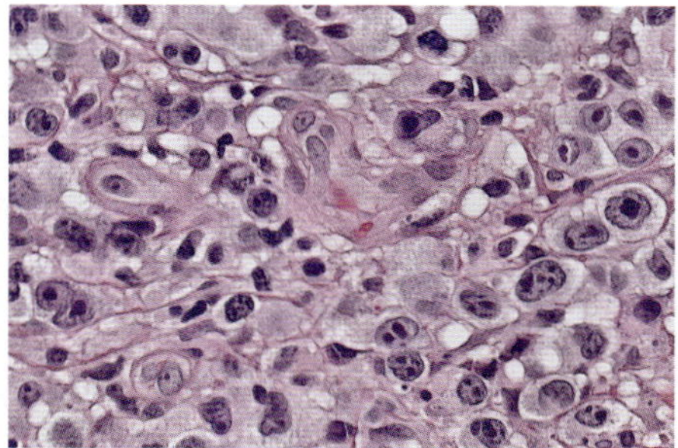

**Fig. 4.32** Primary cutaneous anaplastic large cell lymphoma. Confluent sheets of large cells with anaplastic morphology.

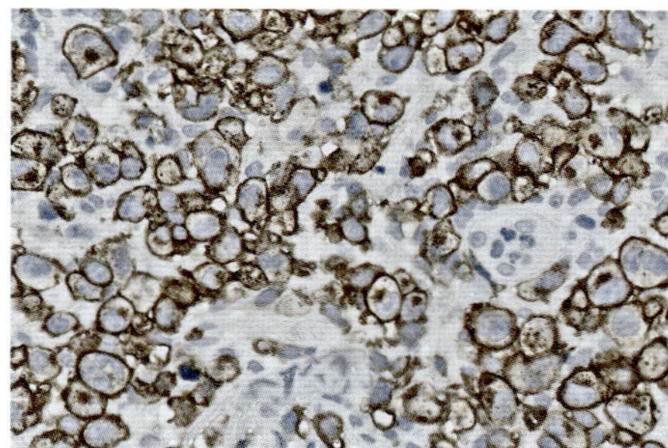

**Fig. 4.33** Cutaneous anaplastic large cell lymphoma. Cohesive sheets of CD30+ anaplastic cells.

## Differential diagnosis

Patients diagnosed with C-ALCL should not have clinical evidence or history of mycosis fungoides; in such cases, the diagnosis of mycosis fungoides with large cell transformation (which can be positive or negative for CD30) is more likely {209}. Primary C-ALCL must also be distinguished from systemic anaplastic large cell lymphoma with cutaneous involvement, which is a separate disease with different cytogenetics, clinical features, and outcome {2867}.

## Histogenesis

The postulated normal counterpart is an activated skin-homing T lymphocyte.

## Genetic profile

Clonal rearrangement of the TR genes is detected in most cases {1618}. However, T-cell receptor proteins are often not expressed {269}. Unlike systemic anaplastic large cell lymphomas, the vast majority of C-ALCLs dos not carry translocations involving the *ALK* gene at chromosome 2 {600}. However, unusual cases of ALK-positive C-ALCL, including cases showing strong nuclear and cytoplasmic staining characteristic of the t(2;5) chromosomal translocation and cases expressing cytoplasmic ALK protein (indicative of a variant translocation), have been reported in children and adults {111,1265,1956,2116}. Many of these cases had an excellent prognosis. Rearrangements of the *DUSP22-IRF4* locus at 6p25.3 are found in approximately 25% of C-ALCL cases and in a small subset of lymphomatoid papulosis cases {2053,2755}. Rearrangements of the *TP63* gene on chromosome 3q28 are associated with poor survival in ALK-negative systemic anaplastic large cell lymphoma, but are not or only rarely found in C-ALCL {2351,2721}. Frequent chromosomal aberrations, found in almost half of all cases, are gains of 7q31 and losses at 6q16-21 and 13q34 {1481,2696}. Unlike in tumour-stage mycosis fungoides and peripheral T-cell lymphoma NOS, loss of 9p21.3 (harbouring the tumour suppressor gene *CDKN2A*) is rarely observed in C-ALCL {1903}. A novel recurrent *NPM1-TYK2* gene fusion, resulting in constitutive STAT signalling, has been described in both C-ALCL and lymphomatoid papulosis {2728}. *TYK2* breaks were found in 15% of primary cutaneous CD30+ T-cell lymphoproliferative disorders. Gene expression profiling has revealed high expression of the skin-homing chemokine receptor genes *CCR10* and *CCR8* in C-ALCL, which may explain these lymphomas' affinity for the skin and low tendency to disseminate to extracutaneous sites {2696}.

## Prognosis and predictive factors

The prognosis is usually favourable, with a 10-year disease-related survival rate of approximately 90% {194,1573}. Patients presenting with multifocal skin lesions and patients with involvement of regional lymph nodes have a prognosis similar to that of patients with only skin lesions {194}. Patients presenting with extensive skin lesions on the legs, or in the setting of immunodeficiency, have a reduced survival rate {210,1573,2370,2856}.

# Cutaneous adult T-cell leukaemia/lymphoma

Tokura Y.
Iwatsuki K.
Jaffe E.S.

## Definition

Adult T-cell leukaemia/lymphoma (ATLL) is a malignancy of mature CD4+ T cells caused by human T-cell leukaemia virus type 1 (HTLV-1) {2420}.

## ICD-O code 9827/3

## Epidemiology

ATLL is endemic in some regions of the world, in particular south-western Japan, the Caribbean islands, South America, sub-Saharan Africa, and localized areas of the Islamic Republic of Iran and of Melanesia {2102,2322}. The number of HTLV-1 carriers worldwide has been estimated to be 15–20 million {2102}. After > 20 years of viral persistence, approximately 5% of carriers develop HTLV-1–associated disease (i.e. ATLL, HTLV-1–associated myelopathy/tropical spastic paraparesis, and uveitis). The three main routes of HTLV-1 transmission are breast-feeding, sexual intercourse, and blood transfusion {2322}.

## Etiology

HTLV-1 proviral DNA is monoclonally integrated in the malignant T cells. HTLV-1 encodes the transcriptional activator Tax, which can transform T cells by increasing the expression of a unique set of cellular genes involved in T-cell proliferation {1091}.

## Clinical features

On the basis of organ involvement and severity, ATLL is divided into four clinical subtypes: acute, chronic, lymphoma-type, and smouldering {2420}. Cutaneous involvement is seen in as many as 50% of cases. ATLL eruptions can be categorized as patch-type (accounting for 6.7% of cases), plaque-type (26.9%), multipapular (19.3%), nodulotumoural (38.7%), erythrodermic (4.2%), or purpuric (4.2%) {2330}. In smouldering ATLL, skin involvement may be the primary clinical manifestation of disease, with minimal leukaemic involvement and no lymphadenopathy or other sites of disease. Other cutaneous manifestations of HTLV-1 infection include childhood infective dermatitis {883,1480} and lichenoid dermatitis {2622}.

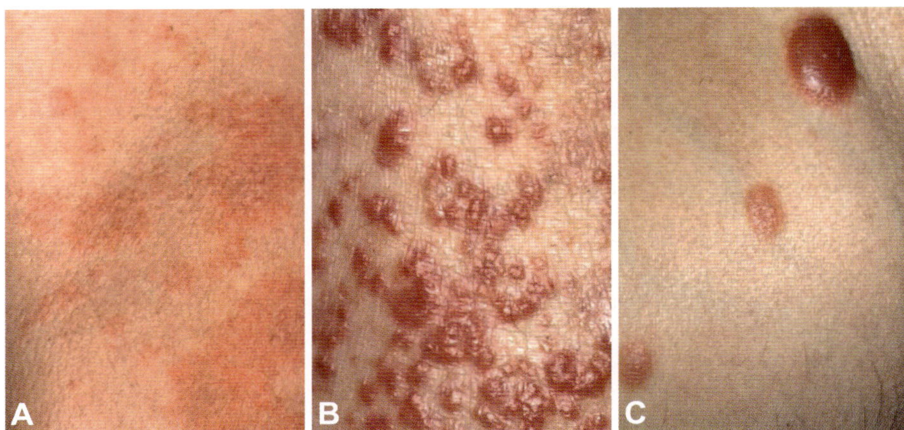


**Fig. 4.34** Adult T-cell leukaemia/lymphoma. Macroscopic findings of cutaneous lesions have been classified as erythema (**A**), papules (**B**), and nodules (**C**).

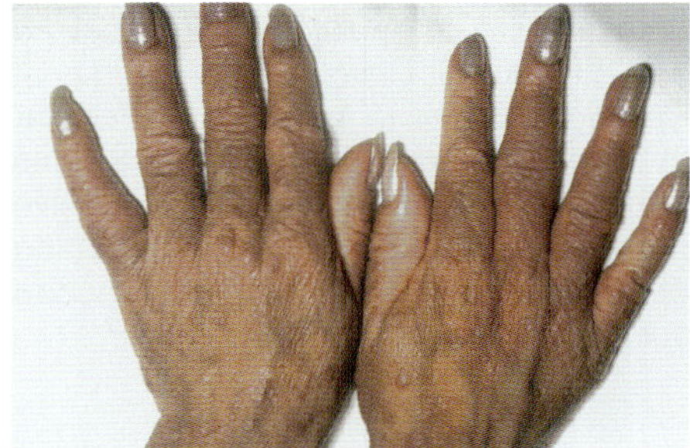

**Fig. 4.35** Adult T-cell leukaemia/lymphoma, smouldering variant. Diffuse exfoliative skin rash.

## Histopathology

Individual skin lesions exhibit various degrees of tumour cell infiltration from the epidermis to subcutaneous tissue. Epidermotropism of the malignant T cells is present in most cases, and Pautrier microabscesses (indistinguishable from those of mycosis fungoides and Sézary syndrome) are often seen

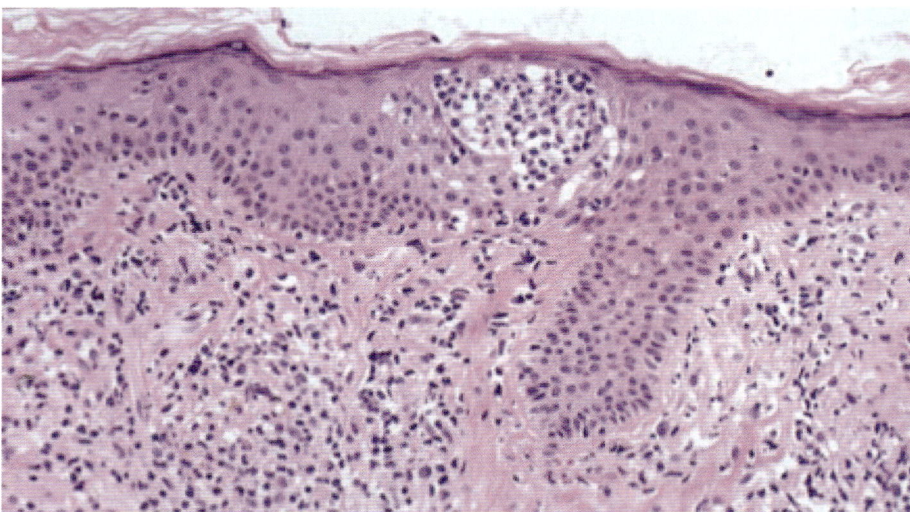

**Fig. 4.36** Adult T-cell leukaemia/lymphoma. An erythematous macule showing infiltration of atypical lymphocytes in the upper dermis, with Pautrier microabscess.

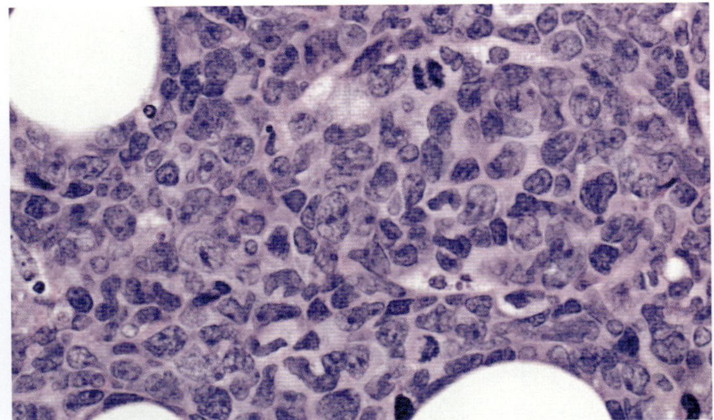

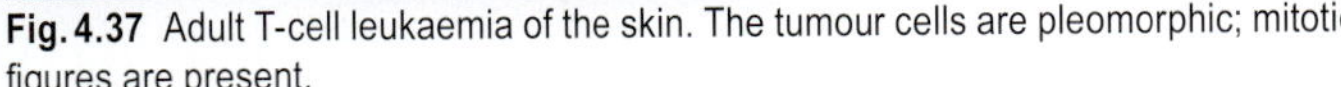

**Fig. 4.37** Adult T-cell leukaemia of the skin. The tumour cells are pleomorphic; mitotic figures are present.

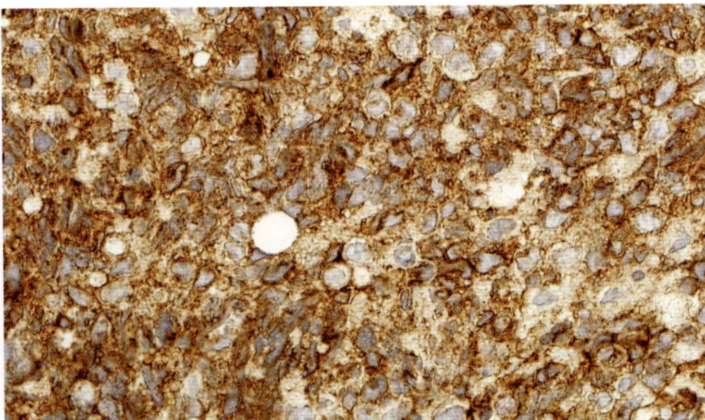

**Fig. 4.38** Adult T-cell leukaemia. The tumour cells are positive for CD25.

{2420}. The cells have medium-sized to large pleomorphic nuclei and occasionally show mitoses. Nuclear irregularity may be marked, with polylobated flower cells often seen in the blood and tissues. Eosinophils may be intermingled with lymphocytes.

The malignant T cells are positive for CD3, CD4, CD25, CD45RO, and CCR4 {2417}, but negative for CD7, CD8, CD19, and CD20. The large transformed cells may be positive for CD30.

## Genetic profile

TR genes are clonally rearranged {1624}. Neoplastic cells show monoclonal integration of HTLV-1 (no clonal integration is present in healthy carriers) {2666}. Tax, a critical non-structural protein encoded by the HTLV-1 pX region, activates a variety of cellular genes and plays a central role in leukaemogenesis {2029}. Enhancement of CREB phosphorylation by the virus also appears to play a role in leukaemogenesis {1369}. *CCR4* mutations can be detected by whole-transcriptome sequencing in about one quarter of cases, and are associated with gain of function {1867}. HTLV-1 bZIP factor (HBZ) has also been found to affect multiple pathways involved in tumorigenesis {2933}. Almost all cases of ATLL have clonal chromosome numerical and structural abnormalities, but none of the abnormalities are specific.

## Prognosis and predictive factors

The major prognostic factors are clinical subtype, patient age, performance status, and serum calcium and lactate dehydrogenase levels {1292,1293}. The acute and lymphoma-type subtypes are associated with survival times ranging from 2 weeks to >1 year. The chronic and smouldering subtypes have a more protracted clinical course, but progress to an acute phase in approximately 25% of patients.

# Subcutaneous panniculitis-like T-cell lymphoma

Jaffe E.S.
Willemze R.
Cerroni L.
Guitart J.

## Definition

Subcutaneous panniculitis-like T-cell lymphoma (SPTCL) is a cytotoxic T-cell lymphoma that preferentially infiltrates subcutaneous tissue. It is composed of atypical lymphoid cells of varying size, typically with prominent apoptotic activity and associated fat necrosis. Cases expressing $\gamma\delta$ T-cell receptor are excluded; such cases are instead classified as primary cutaneous $\gamma\delta$ T-cell lymphoma.

## ICD-O code 9708/3

## Epidemiology

SPTCL is a rare form of lymphoma, accounting for < 1% of all non-Hodgkin lymphoma cases. It is slightly more common in females than in males and has a broad patient age range {1457}. Approximately 20% of patients are aged < 20 years (median patient age: 35 years) {2833}, and the disease can also present in infancy {1159}. As many as 20% of patients may have associated autoimmune disease, most commonly systemic lupus erythematosus {2833}. The differential diagnosis with lupus panniculitis may be challenging.

## Etiology

Autoimmune disease may play a role in some cases. The lesions may show features overlapping with those of lupus panniculitis, and a diagnosis of systemic lupus erythematosus has been documented in some cases {1630,1688}. In some patients, the early lesions can closely mimic lobular panniculitis. It is unclear whether benign lobular panniculitis precedes the development of SPTCL in patients without systemic lupus erythematosus. EBV is absent {1457}.

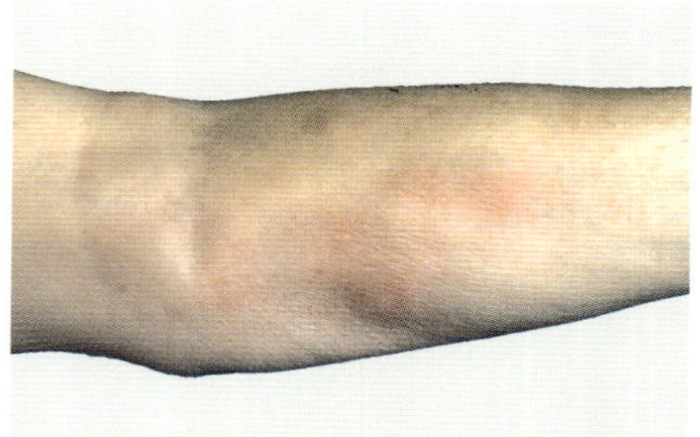

**Fig. 4.39** Subcutaneous panniculitis-like T-cell lymphoma. Multiple subcutaneous nodules are common on the extremities. The overlying epidermis may show mild to moderate erythema.

## Localization

Patients present with multiple subcutaneous nodules or plaques, usually in the absence of other extracutaneous sites of disease. The most common sites of localization are the extremities and trunk. The nodules range from 5 mm to several centimetres in diameter. Larger nodules may become necrotic, but ulceration is rare {1457,2833}. It is rare for patients to present with only a single skin lesion.

## Clinical features

The clinical symptoms are primarily related to the subcutaneous nodules. Systemic symptoms are reported by as many as 50% of patients. Laboratory abnormalities (e.g. cytopenias and elevated liver function tests) are common, and a frank haemophagocytic syndrome is seen in 15–20% of cases {911,2833}, leading to hepatosplenomegaly in affected patients {1457}. Lymphadenopathy is usually absent. PET and/or CT findings are essential for determining the extent of disease.

## Histopathology

The infiltrate involves the fat lobules, usually with sparing of septa. The overlying dermis and epidermis are typically uninvolved. The neoplastic cell size varies from case to case, but is relatively consistent in any given case. The neoplastic cells have pleomorphic nuclei with pale cytoplasm. A helpful diagnostic feature is the rimming of the neoplastic cells surrounding individual fat cells. Admixed reactive histiocytes are frequently present, in particular in areas of fat infiltration and destruction. The histiocytes are frequently vacuolated, due to ingested lipid material. Typically, there is an absence of other inflammatory cells, including plasma cells and plasmacytoid dendritic cells, which are both common in lupus panniculitis {1457,1689}. Vascular invasion is seen in some cases, and necrosis and karyorrhexis are common {1457,2833}. Although cutaneous $\gamma\delta$ T-cell lymphomas sometimes show panniculitis-like features, such lymphomas commonly involve the dermis and epidermis and may show epidermal ulceration.

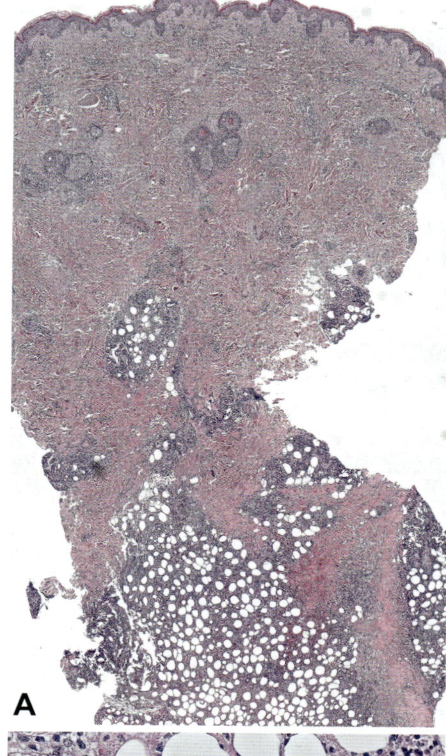

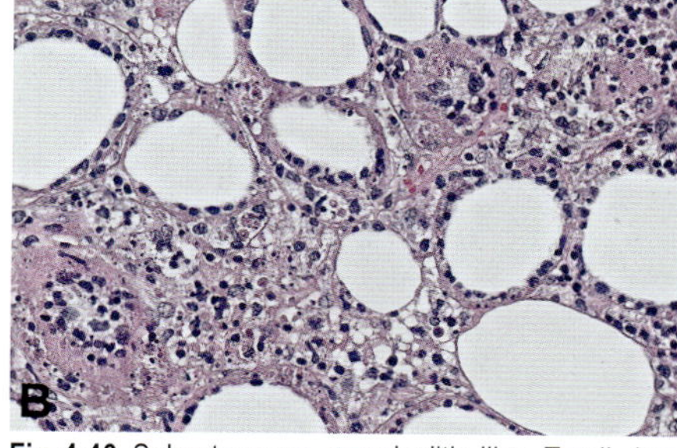

**Fig. 4.40** Subcutaneous panniculitis-like T-cell lymphoma. **A** The infiltrate involves the subcutaneous tissue and spares the overlying dermis and epidermis. **B** Atypical cells rim fat spaces; macrophages are increased in number and contain apoptotic debris.

The neoplastic cells have a mature, usually CD8+ αβ T-cell phenotype, with expression of cytotoxic proteins including granzyme B, perforin, and TIA1 {1457,2288,2833}. The T cells express αβ T-cell receptor and are negative for γδ T-cell receptor and CD56, facilitating the distinction from primary cutaneous γδ T-cell lymphoma {2628,2833}. CD123 is generally negative, whereas in lupus profundus it frequently highlights clusters of plasmacytoid dendritic cells {276}.

## Histogenesis

The normal counterpart is a mature cytotoxic αβ T-cell.

## Genetic profile

The neoplastic cells show rearrangement of TR genes and are negative for EBV sequences. Highly recurrent genetic aberrations have not been reported, but the mutations encountered involve several pathways, including the JAK/STAT pathway and the PI3K/AKT/mTOR pathway. Mutations in several epigenetic modifiers have also been reported {1555}.

## Prognosis and predictive factors

Dissemination to lymph nodes and other organs is rare {911,2288,2833}. The median 5-year overall survival rate is 80%; however, prognosis is poor when a haemophagocytic syndrome is present {911,1689,1957,2833}. Traditionally, combination chemotherapy has been administered, but more-recent studies suggest that more-conservative immunosuppressive regimens (e.g. ciclosporin and prednisone) may be effective {955,1240,1861,2665,2833}. The distinction from cutaneous γδ T-cell lymphoma is important, because SPTCL has a much better prognosis {2629,2833}.

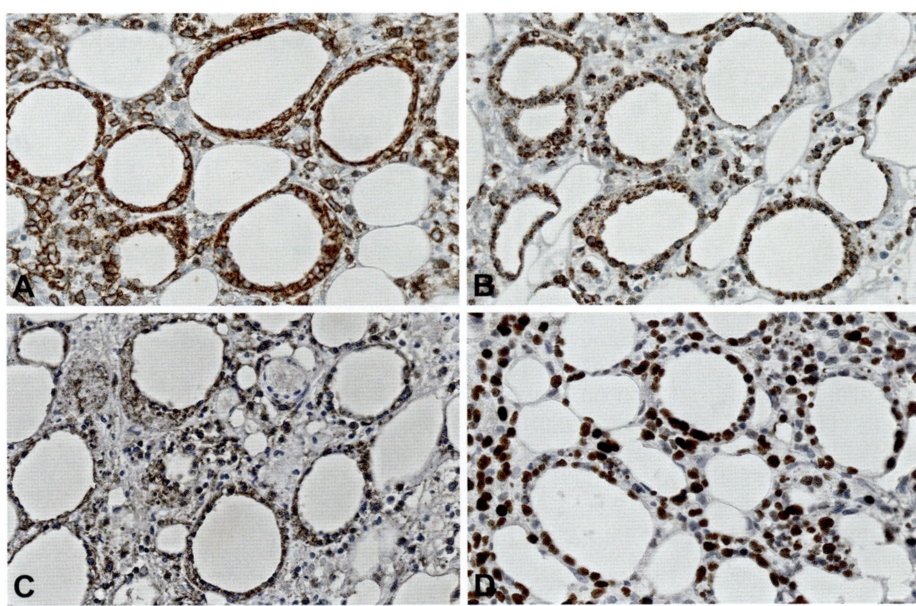


**Fig. 4.41** Subcutaneous panniculitis-like T-cell lymphoma. **A** Atypical cells, which are positive for CD8, rim fat spaces. **B** The cells are positive for TIA1. **C** βF1 is also positive. **D** Ki-67 (MIB1) staining reveals a high proliferation rate in the atypical cells.

# Cutaneous manifestations of chronic active EBV infection

Quintanilla-Martinez L.
Iwatsuki K.
Ko Y.-H.

## Definition
Cutaneous manifestations of chronic active EBV infection include hydroa vacciniforme–like lymphoproliferative disorder (HV-like LPD) and severe mosquito bite allergy. Both conditions present primarily in children and are associated with a risk of progression to systemic EBV-associated NK/T-cell lymphoma. HV-like LPD is primarily derived from T cells, whereas severe mosquito bite allergy is more often of NK-cell origin.

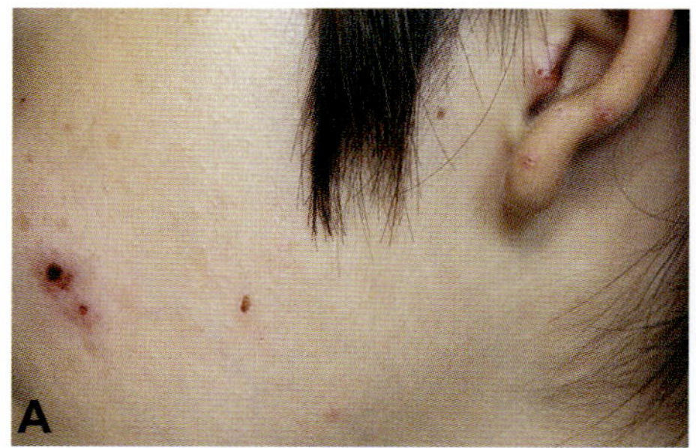
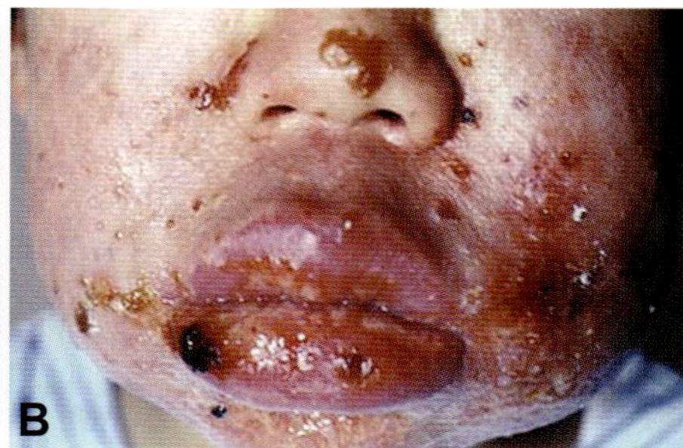

**Fig. 4.42** Hydroa vacciniforme–like lymphoproliferative disorder. **A** Sun-exposed areas of the face and ear lobes exhibit a papulovesicular eruption, with crusts. **B** Extensive skin lesions on the face. There is oedema and erythema of the lips and cheeks, with multiple vesicles and crusts.

## ICD-O code
Hydroa vacciniforme–like lymphoproliferative disorder 9725/1

## Synonym
The term "HV-like LPD" encompasses all of the various manifestations of the EBV-associated hydroa vacciniforme–like skin lesions, including classic hydroa vacciniforme, severe or systemic hydroa vacciniforme, and hydroa vacciniforme–like lymphoma {906,971,1197,1805,2481}.

## Epidemiology
These disorders are seen mainly in children and adolescents from Asia {464,748,1195,1196,2871}, and in indigenous populations of Central America {636}, South America {163,2213,2305}, and Mexico {1625,2117}. The mean age at diagnosis is 6–8 years (range: 1–18 years). HV-like LPD shows a slight male predilection, with a male-to-female ratio of 2.3:1. Cutaneous manifestations of chronic active EBV infection are rare in adults {464,1915,1916,2305}.

## Etiology
The etiology is unknown. Genetic predisposition might play a major role.

## Localization
HV-like LPD typically affects the skin of the face, the dorsal surface of the hands, and the ear lobes, but in advanced stages it can be generalized {2117}. Severe mosquito bite allergy can involve any cutaneous site.

## Clinical features
HV-like LPD is characterized by a papulovesicular eruption that typically proceeds to ulceration and scarring. The clinical presentation and the severity of the skin lesions vary among patients, with a broad spectrum. Some cases have a very indolent course, with localized skin lesions in sun-exposed areas and no systemic symptoms (classic hydroa vacciniforme). Spontaneous remissions and clearing after photoprotection occur, but most cases have a long clinical course,

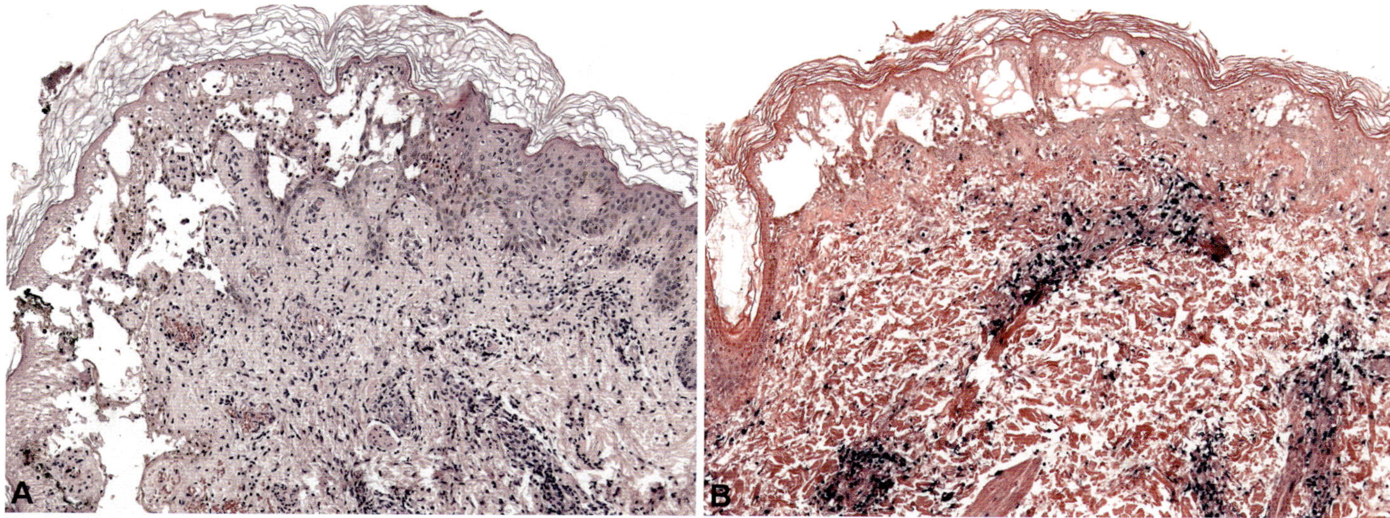

**Fig. 4.43** Hydroa vacciniforme–like lymphoproliferative disorder. **A** A skin biopsy with intraepidermal bullae and a subtle infiltrate in the upper dermis surrounding adnexae and blood vessels. **B** The lymphoid cells are EBV-positive, as demonstrated by in situ hybridization for EBV-encoded small RNA (EBER).

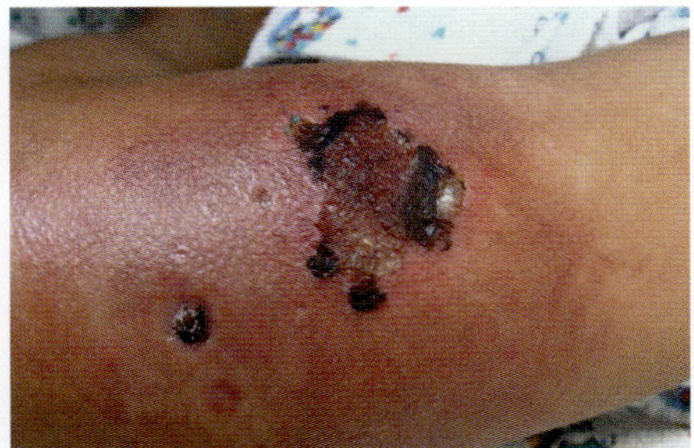

**Fig. 4.44** Severe mosquito bite allergy. The upper arm shows severe oedema and erythema, with necrosis and a haemorrhagic crust after a mosquito bite.

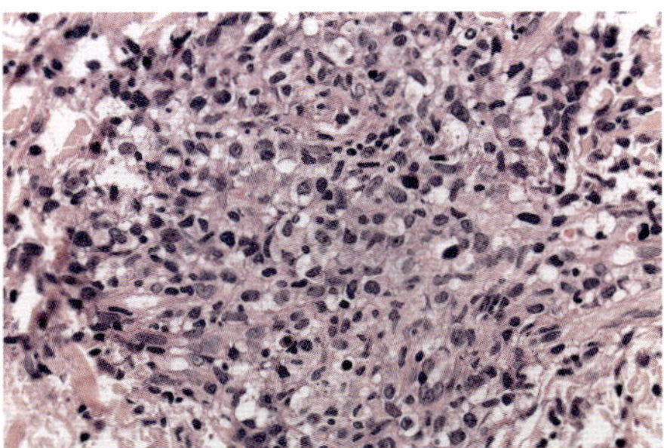

**Fig. 4.45** Severe mosquito bite allergy. The infiltrate is polymorphic but mainly composed of large cells with bland nuclei, inconspicuous nucleoli, and abundant pale cytoplasm. In situ hybridization for EBV-encoded small RNA (EBER) was positive in most cells (not shown).

with remissions and recurrences, and may ultimately progress to more-severe disease {465}. There is also seasonal variation, with increased frequency of recurrences in spring and summer. In more-severe cases (in particular late in the course of the disease), systemic symptoms such as fever, wasting, lymphadenopathy, and hepatosplenomegaly may be present in addition to extensive skin lesions {1196,1371,2117,2305}. A rare clinical presentation with primarily periorbital swelling has been reported in children in the Plurinational State of Bolivia {2072}. Some patients develop hypersensitivity to mosquito bites {1085,2117}. Skin lesions at the site of the mosquito bite typically show erythema and bullae that subsequently become necrotic and ulcerated. The lesions eventually heal, with scarring. Systemic symptoms can be present in both forms of cutaneous chronic active EBV infection.

## Histopathology

The characteristic histological feature of hydroa vacciniforme is epidermal reticular degeneration leading to intraepidermal spongiotic vesiculation. The lymphoid infiltrate predominates in the dermis and may also extend deep into the subcutaneous tissue. The infiltrate is mainly located around adnexae and blood vessels, often with angiodestructive features. The intensity of the infiltrate and atypia of the lymphocytes varies. The neoplastic cells are generally small to medium-sized, without substantial atypia.

The cells have a cytotoxic T-cell phenotype. Most cases are CD8-positive; a few are CD4-positive. Some cases show an NK-cell phenotype with expression of CD56 {1371,2117,2213}. Clonal expansion of γδ T cells has been documented in the peripheral blood in most cases {1085,1371,2757}, but such expansion is rare in the infiltrating lymphocytes in the skin {1625,2117,2757}. CCR4 is expressed in the γδ T cells {1276}. CD30 is often expressed in the infiltrating EBV-positive T cells. LMP1 is usually negative {2117}.

In severe mosquito bite allergy, the skin at the site of the bite exhibits epidermal necrosis and ulceration. The dermis shows oedema, with a polymorphic infiltrate that extends from the dermis to subcutaneous tissue. Polymorphonuclear leukocytes and eosinophils with admixed nuclear debris, as well as extravasated red blood cells, are common.

## Histogenesis

The postulated normal counterpart of HV-like LPD is a skin-homing cytotoxic T cell or NK cell. Both γδ T cell response and cytotoxic T lymphocyte response have been proposed to play a central role in the formation of hydroa vacciniforme–like eruptions {1296,2876}. In severe mosquito bite allergy, the cells are activated NK cells.

## Genetic profile

Most cases of HV-like LPD have clonal rearrangements of the TR genes {1371,2117}. In situ hybridization for EBV-encoded small RNA (EBER) is positive, but the number of positive cells varies from case to case. LMP1 is negative immunohistochemically, but it can be detected in the peripheral blood by PCR in most cases, indicating type II EBV latency {1194}. In both HV-like LPD and severe mosquito bite allergy, EBV is clonal as determined by terminal repeat analysis.

## Genetic susceptibility

The observed racial predisposition indicates a genetic defect in the host response to EBV.

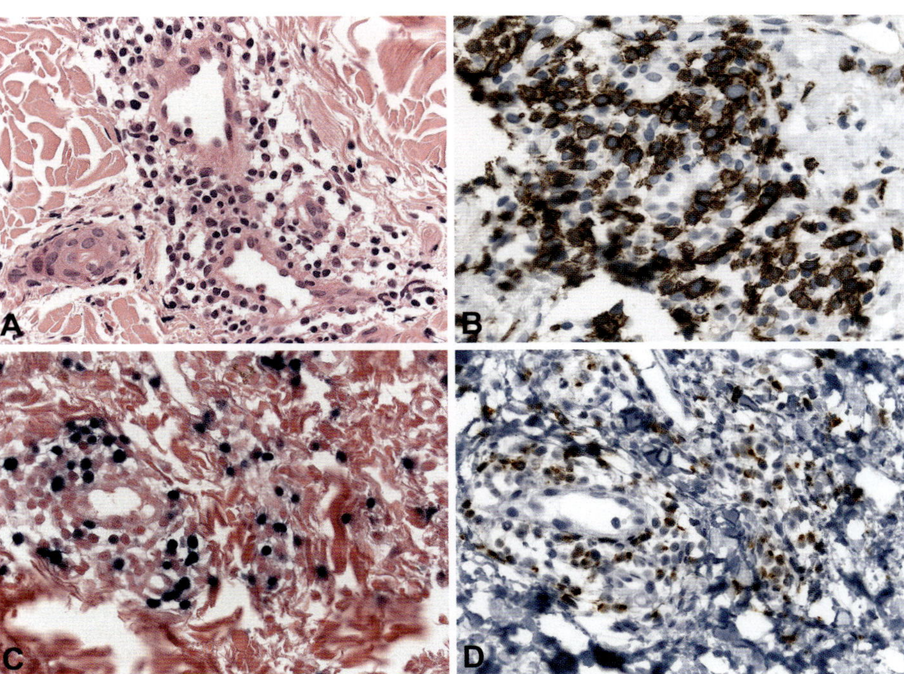

**Fig. 4.46** Hydroa vacciniforme–like lymphoproliferative disorder. **A** The neoplastic cells are predominantly small, without atypia. **B** CD8 is positive in the majority of the infiltrating cells. **C** Many of the lymphoid cells are EBV-positive, as demonstrated by in situ hybridization for EBV-encoded small RNA (EBER). **D** The infiltrating cells are TIA1-positive.

## Prognosis and predictive factors

The clinical course of HV-like LPD is variable; patients may have recurrent skin lesions for as long as 10–15 years before progression to systemic involvement or development of a systemic lymphoma occurs. With systemic spread, the clinical course is much more aggressive. There is no association between eventual progression to systemic disease or development of a systemic lymphoma and factors such as T-cell clonality, proportion of EBV-positive cells, or density of the infiltrate. Disease onset after the age of 9 years and expression of the EBV-encoded transcript BZLF1 in skin lesions have been associated with poor prognosis. No standard treatment recommendation has been established. The disease is resistant to conventional chemotherapy, and treated patients have often died of infectious complications. In indolent cases, a conservative approach is recommended; in more-advanced cases, haematopoietic stem cell transplantation has been performed as a curative therapy {1371,1805,2117}.

Severe mosquito bite allergy has a long clinical course, and patients have an increased risk of developing haemophagocytic syndrome and/or aggressive NK-cell leukaemia after 2–17 years (median: 12 years). Rare cases with chromosomal aberrations have a higher risk of progression {1371,2621}.

# Extranodal NK/T-cell lymphoma, nasal type

Chan J.K.C.
Ko Y.-H.

## Definition

Extranodal NK/T-cell lymphoma, nasal type, is a predominantly extranodal lymphoma of NK cells or cytotoxic T cells, characterized by vascular damage and destruction, prominent necrosis, a cytotoxic phenotype, and association with EBV. The skin is the second most common site of involvement (after the upper aerodigestive tract).

## ICD-O code 9719/3

## Epidemiology

Overall, extranodal NK/T-cell lymphoma is uncommon. It is more prevalent among Asians and in indigenous populations of Mexico, Central America, and South America {952}. It occurs most often in adults, with a male predominance {427,2561}.

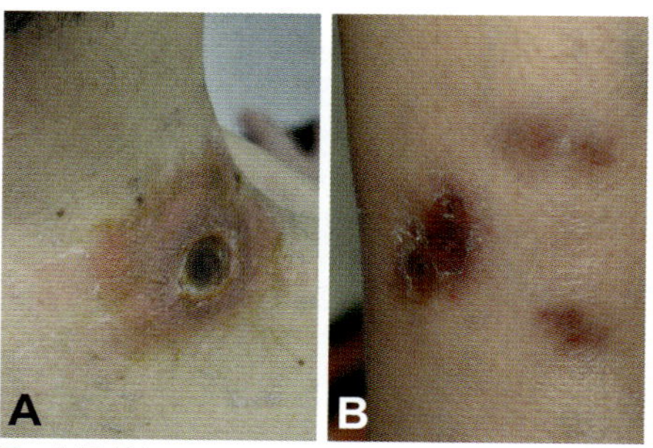

Fig. 4.47 Primary cutaneous extranodal NK/T-cell lymphoma, nasal type. **A** Nodule with necrosis and ulceration. **B** Macular lesion with scaling.

## Etiology

The very strong association with EBV, irrespective of racial origin, indicates a pathogenic role of the virus.

## Localization

More than one cutaneous region is typically involved, most commonly the trunk and extremities {427,1536,1840,2561,2899}. There may also be simultaneous or subsequent involvement of extracutaneous sites, most commonly the nose and upper respiratory tract.

## Clinical features

Cutaneous involvement can take the form of nodules (with or without ulceration), cellulitis or abscess-like swellings, and erythematous to purpuric patches {1536}. Systemic symptoms such as fever, malaise, and weight loss can be present. Some cases may be complicated by haemophagocytic syndrome.

## Histopathology

The skin shows a dermal lymphoid infiltrate that is diffuse or predominantly perivascular and periadnexal, variably accompanied by subcutaneous involvement. Angioinvasion and necrosis are common. Epidermotropism or pseudoepitheliomatous hyperplasia can be present. The lymphoid cells exhibit a broad cytological spectrum, ranging from small to

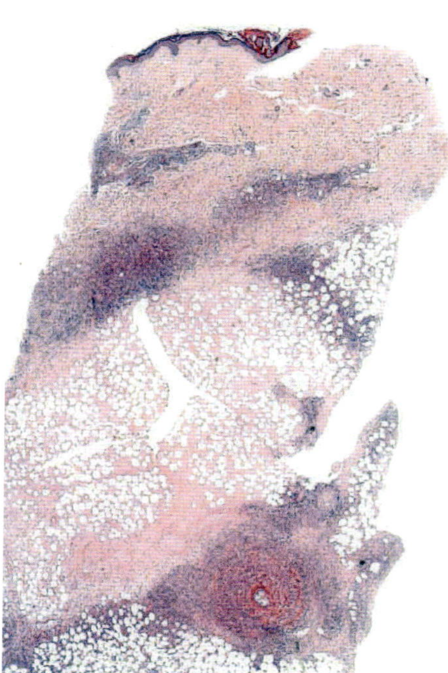

Fig. 4.48 Primary cutaneous extranodal NK/T-cell lymphoma, nasal type. The skin shows perivascular and periadnexal lymphomatous infiltration in the dermis, together with interstitial infiltration of the subcutis and extensive necrosis. A blood vessel in the subcutis is infiltrated by lymphoma cells.

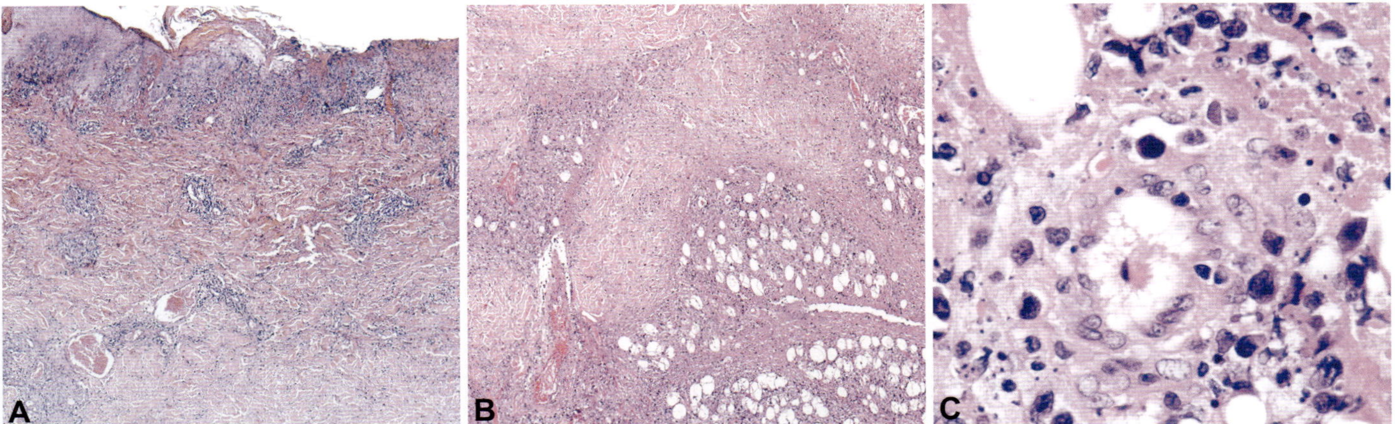

**Fig. 4.49** Primary cutaneous extranodal NK/T-cell lymphoma, nasal type. **A** The skin shows dermal infiltration by abnormal lymphoid cells, accompanied by ulceration. **B** The subcutis is also infiltrated, and vascular damage is evident at the left of the field. **C** The lymphoma cells are medium-sized, with irregularly folded nuclei; apoptosis and necrosis are evident.

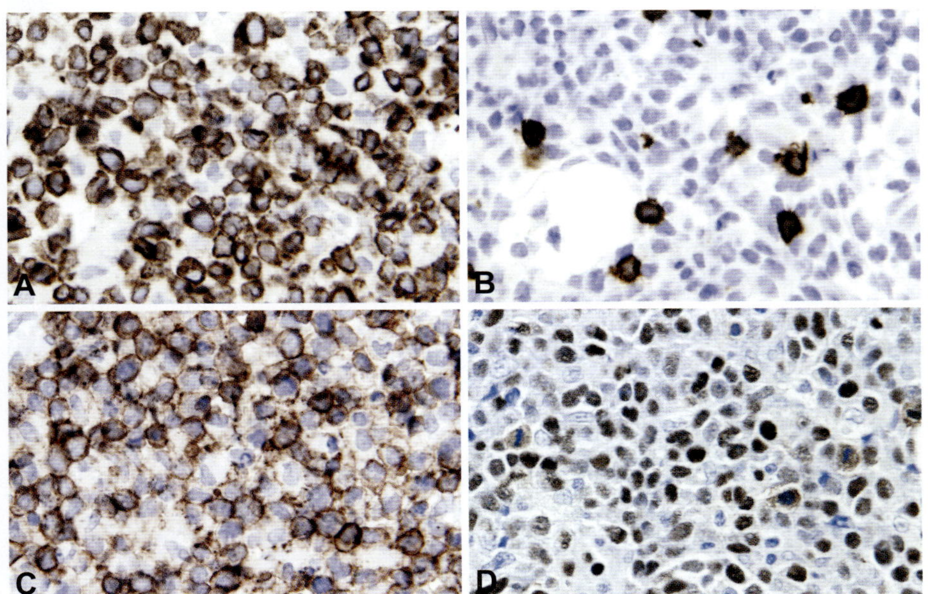

**Fig. 4.50** Primary cutaneous extranodal NK/T-cell lymphoma, nasal type. Most commonly, cases are CD3-positive (**A**), CD5-negative (**B**), CD56-positive (**C**), and EBV-positive, as demonstrated by in situ hybridization for EBV-encoded small RNA (EBER) (**D**).

large cells, with medium-sized cells being most common; they often show irregular nuclear folding, moderately dense chromatin, and pale cytoplasm. Rare cases of intravascular NK/T-cell lymphoma have been reported {412,1943}.

Most commonly, the cells are positive for CD3ε, cytotoxic markers, and CD56 (although some cases can be CD56-negative) and negative for surface CD3, CD4, CD8, CD5, and T-cell receptor. The cells are usually of NK-cell lineage, but some cases may express αβ or γδ T-cell receptor, indicating a T-cell lineage. CD30 is positive in approximately 60% of cases {2561}. LMP1 is often negative, whereas in situ hybridization for EBV-encoded small RNA (EBER) is positive.

### Histogenesis

The postulated normal counterpart is an activated NK cell or, less commonly, a cytotoxic T-cell

### Genetic profile

TR genes are usually in germline configuration, but may be clonally rearranged in a proportion of cases.

### Prognosis and predictive factors

Cutaneous extranodal NK/T-cell lymphoma is highly aggressive {113}, with a 5-year overall survival rate of 26% {1537,2561} and a median overall survival of 12–15 months {32,1840}. The prognosis is better for patients with localized disease {32} and particularly poor for patients with generalized skin lesions and extracutaneous involvement {1840,2899}.

# Primary cutaneous peripheral T-cell lymphomas, rare subtypes

Berti E.
Willemze R.
Guitart J.
Jaffe E.S.
Kempf W.
Petrella T.
Robson A.
Cerroni L.
Torres-Cabala C.A.

## Introduction

Primary cutaneous peripheral T-cell lymphoma NOS is a diagnosis of exclusion; the term refers to a heterogeneous group of cutaneous T-cell lymphomas that do not fit into one of the well-defined subtypes of mature T-cell leukaemias/lymphomas. On the basis of characteristic clinicopathological and prognostic features, three subtypes of cutaneous T-cell lymphoma were defined and included as provisional entities in the joint WHO–European Organisation for Research and Treatment of Cancer (WHO-EORTC) classification for cutaneous lymphomas {2832}, and they were subsequently included as rare subtypes of primary cutaneous peripheral T-cell lymphoma in the 2008 *WHO classification of tumours of haematopoietic and lymphoid tissues* {2546}: primary cutaneous γδ T-cell lymphoma, primary cutaneous CD8+ aggressive epidermotropic cytotoxic T-cell lymphoma, and primary cutaneous CD4+ small/medium T-cell lymphoma (recently renamed primary cutaneous CD4+ small/medium T-cell lymphoproliferative disorder). The last two entities are still considered to be provisional here in the 4th edition *WHO classification of skin tumours* volume, as is a fourth subtype, which was first added as a provisional entity in the 2017 revision of the WHO haematopoietic and lymphoid tumours classification {2545}: primary cutaneous acral CD8+ T-cell lymphoma {2547}. For cases that still do not fit into any of the well-defined types of cutaneous T-cell lymphoma (including the rare and provisional subtypes), the term "primary cutaneous peripheral T-cell lymphoma NOS" is retained. Such cases generally have a poor prognosis, and the distinction between primary and secondary cutaneous involvement seems to be less important within this category.

## Primary cutaneous gamma-delta T-cell lymphoma

### Definition

Primary cutaneous γδ T-cell lymphoma (PCGD-TCL) is a lymphoma composed of a clonal proliferation of mature, activated γδ T cells with a cytotoxic phenotype. This group includes cases previously called subcutaneous panniculitis-like T-cell lymphoma with a γδ phenotype. γδ T-cell lymphomas presenting primarily in mucosal sites (formerly called mucocutaneous γδ T-cell lymphomas) are likely unrelated conditions constituting other site-dependent peripheral T-cell lymphoma entities {99,850,2548}. γδ T-cell receptor (TCR) may also be expressed by rare cases of otherwise classic mycosis fungoides and lymphomatoid papulosis, which have the same indolent clinical course as cases with an αβ T-cell phenotype {1674,1685,2214}. Such cases should be diagnosed as mycosis fungoides or lymphomatoid papulosis, irrespective of TCRγ chain expression {2545}.

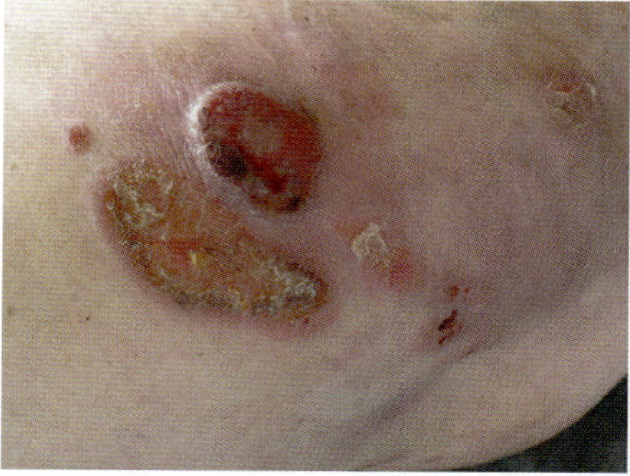

**Fig. 4.51** Primary cutaneous γδ T-cell lymphoma. A large plaque with a deep ulcerated nodulotumoural lesion on the left leg.

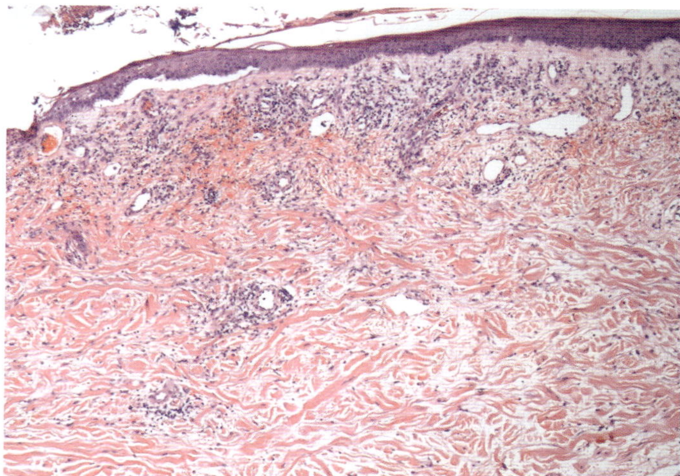

**Fig. 4.52** Primary cutaneous γδ T-cell lymphoma. A skin section showing a superficial infiltrate of neoplastic cells involving superficial dermis and epidermis.

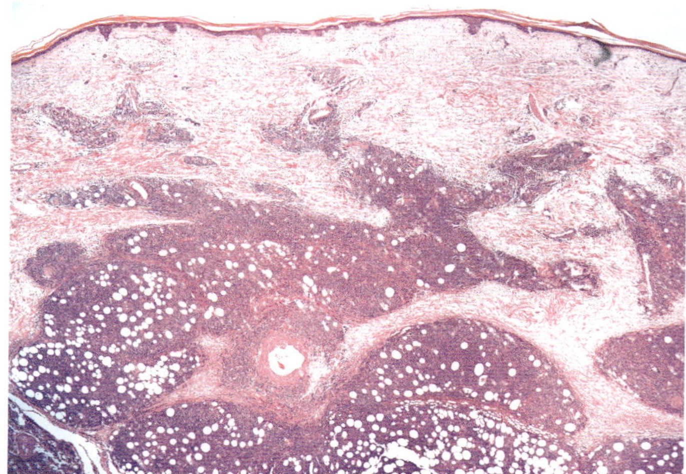

**Fig. 4.53** Primary cutaneous γδ T-cell lymphoma. A skin section showing a deep multinodular infiltrate of neoplastic cells involving perivascular areas and adipose tissue.

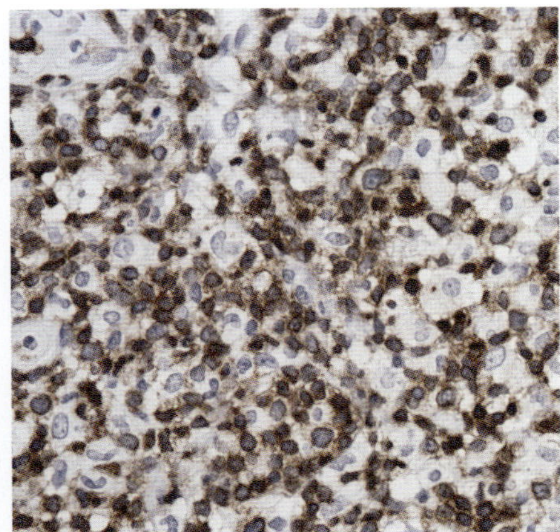

**Fig. 4.54** Primary cutaneous γδ T-cell lymphoma. Immunoexpression of T-cell receptor γ chain.

## ICD-O code 9726/3

### Epidemiology

PCGD-TCLs are rare, accounting for approximately 1% of all cutaneous T-cell lymphomas {2629,2832,2833}. Most cases occur in adults. There is no sex predilection.

### Localization

PCGD-TCLs often present with generalized skin lesions, preferentially affecting the extremities.

### Clinical features

The clinical presentation is variable. The disease may be predominantly epidermotropic and present with patches and/or plaques. Some patients may present with deep dermal or subcutaneous tumours, with or without epidermal necrosis and ulceration {226,2629,2833}. The lesions are most often present on the extremities, but other sites can also be affected {2629,2833}. Dissemination to mucosal and other extranodal sites is frequently observed, but involvement of lymph nodes, spleen, and/or bone marrow is uncommon. A haemophagocytic syndrome is common, especially in patients with panniculitis-like tumours {2629,2833}. Most patient experience B symptoms, including fever, night sweats, and weight loss. PET and/or CT findings are essential for determining the extent of disease.

### Histopathology

PCGD-TCL has three major histological patterns: epidermotropic, dermal, and subcutaneous. Multiple histological patterns are often present in the same patient, either in different biopsies or within a single specimen {226,2629,2833}. Epidermal infiltration may occur, from mild epidermotropism to marked pagetoid reticulosis–like infiltration {226}. Subcutaneous cases may show rimming of fat cells similar to that seen in subcutaneous panniculitis-like T-cell lymphoma of αβ T-cell origin, but such cases usually show dermal and/or epidermal involvement in addition {2629,2833}. The neoplastic cells are generally medium-sized to large, with coarsely clumped chromatin {2629}. Large blastic cells with vesicular nuclei and prominent nucleoli are infrequent. Apoptosis and necrosis are common, often occurring with angioinvasion {2629,2833}.

The tumour cells express γδ TCR and are negative for αβ TCR. They have a CD3+, CD2+, CD5−, CD7+/−, CD56+ phenotype, with strong expression of cytotoxic proteins, including granzyme B, perforin, and TIA1 {1205,2288,2629,2833}. Most cases lack both CD4 and CD8, although CD8 may be expressed in some cases {2629,2833}. Coexpression of αβ and γδ TCR has been reported {862,2214}.

### Histogenesis

PCGD-TCL is derived from mature and activated cytotoxic γδ T cells of the innate immune system.

### Genetic profile

The cells show clonal rearrangement of the TRG and TRD genes. TRB may be rearranged or deleted, but is not expressed. PCGD-TCLs usually express Vδ2, consistent with the prevalence of Vδ2γ T cells residing in the skin {2244}. EBV is negative {99,2548,2629}. Like other tumours of γδ T-cell origin, some cases have activating mutations in *STAT5B* and (rarely) *STAT3*.

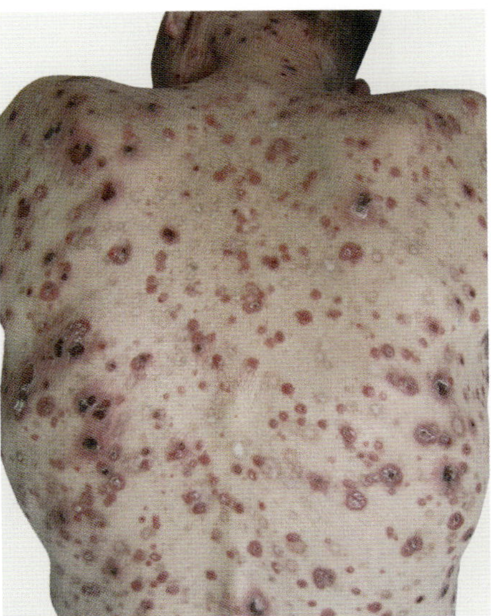

**Fig. 4.55** Primary cutaneous CD8+ aggressive epidermotropic cytotoxic T-cell lymphoma. Lesions are often haemorrhagic; they are diffuse and associated with epidermal ulceration.

### Prognosis and predictive factors

PCGD-TCL is an aggressive lymphoma, with a median survival of approximately 12 months {2629,2833}. Patients with subcutaneous fat involvement tend to have a more unfavourable prognosis than do those with epidermal or dermal disease only {2629}. However, cases with an indolent clinical course have been reported {111,689,965,2116}.

# Primary cutaneous CD8+ aggressive epidermotropic cytotoxic T-cell lymphoma

### Definition

Primary cutaneous CD8+ aggressive epidermotropic cytotoxic T-cell lymphoma is a cutaneous T-cell lymphoma (CTCL) characterized by proliferation of epidermotropic CD8+ cytotoxic T cells and aggressive clinical behaviour. Differentiation from other CTCLs with a CD8+ cytotoxic T-cell phenotype is based on clinical presentation, clinical behaviour, and specific histological features, such as marked epidermotropism with epidermal necrosis. This is a provisional entity in the current classification.

## ICD-O code 9709/3

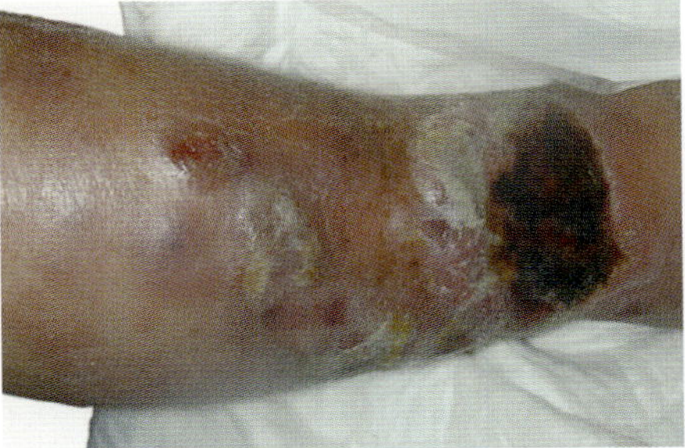

**Fig. 4.56** Primary cutaneous CD8+ aggressive epidermotropic cytotoxic T-cell lymphoma. A large localized nodulotumoural lesion on the leg, showing ulceration and epidermal necrosis.

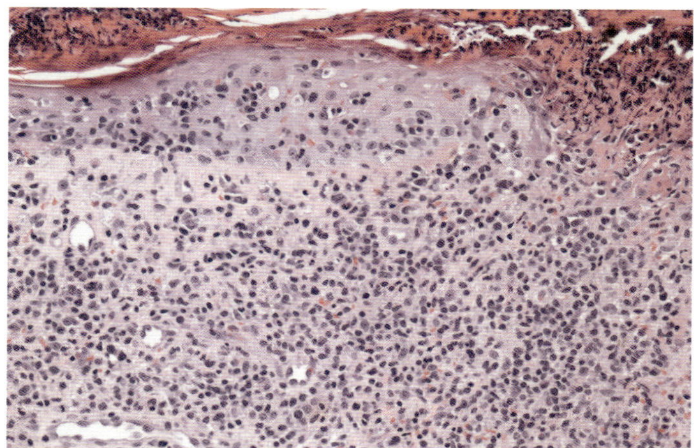

**Fig. 4.57** Primary cutaneous CD8+ aggressive epidermotropic cytotoxic T-cell lymphoma. The atypical pleomorphic medium to large cell lymphoid infiltrate occupies the superficial dermis, extending to the epidermis in a pagetoid fashion and leading to epidermal necrosis.

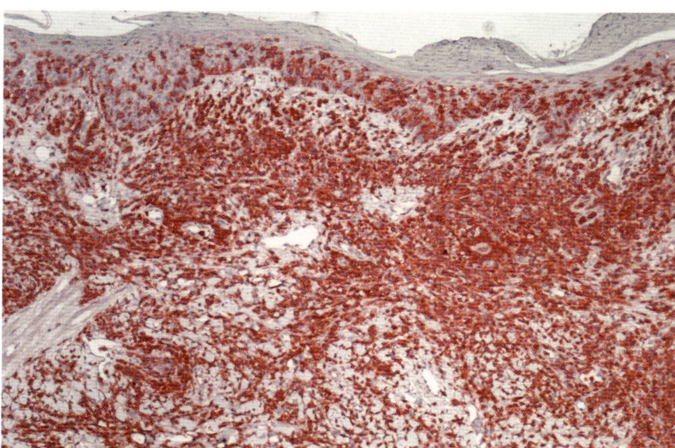

**Fig. 4.58** Primary cutaneous CD8+ aggressive epidermotropic cytotoxic T-cell lymphoma. CD8 staining highlights the epidermotropic neoplastic cells.

### Epidemiology

This is a rare disease, accounting for < 1% of all CTCLs {26,228,2832}. It occurs mainly in adults. There are no predisposing factors.

### Localization

Patients present with generalized or localized skin lesions. The oral mucosa or perimucosal skin may be involved.

### Clinical features

Clinically, these lymphomas are characterized by localized ulcerated nodules, tumours, and plaques or (more commonly) by diffuse eruptive papules, nodules, and tumours showing central ulceration and necrosis {228,2202,2313}. Some patients may have a prodrome of chronic patches prior to the development of aggressive ulcerative lesions {962A}. These lymphomas may disseminate to visceral sites (e.g. the lung, testes, and CNS), but lymph nodes are usually spared {228,1675,2116,2202}.

### Histopathology

The histological appearance varies from a lichenoid pattern with marked pagetoid epidermotropism to deeper, less epidermotropic infiltrates. The epidermis may be spongiotic (with blister formation), necrotic, or ulcerated {26,228,2202}. Syringotropism and folliculotropism are commonly observed, but angiocentricity is rarely seen {1684,2202}. The tumour cells are small/medium or medium/large, with pleomorphic cytomorphology {228}. The tumour cells are positive for αβ T-cell receptor, CD3, CD8, granzyme B, perforin, TIA1, and CD45RA, with a high Ki-67 proliferation index. Most cases lack CD2, CD5, and CD30, with variable expression of CD7 {26,196,228,1684,2116,2202,2313}. Rare cases with a null (CD4−/CD8−) cytotoxic phenotype have the same clinically aggressive presentation {2202}. Primary cutaneous CD8+ aggressive epidermotropic cytotoxic T-cell lymphoma may be indistinguishable from lymphomatoid papulosis type D, which is characterized by self-healing papules and nodules, with spontaneous resolution {2276}. Clinical information is important to differentiate this entity from other CD8+ CTCLs (e.g. CD8+ mycosis fungoides {2116}), particularly cases showing protracted, nonspecific cutaneous lesions {2202}.

### Histogenesis

The postulated normal counterpart is a skin-homing cytotoxic αβ T cell.

### Genetic profile

The neoplastic T cells show clonal TR gene rearrangements. EBV is negative {196,1684,2202}.

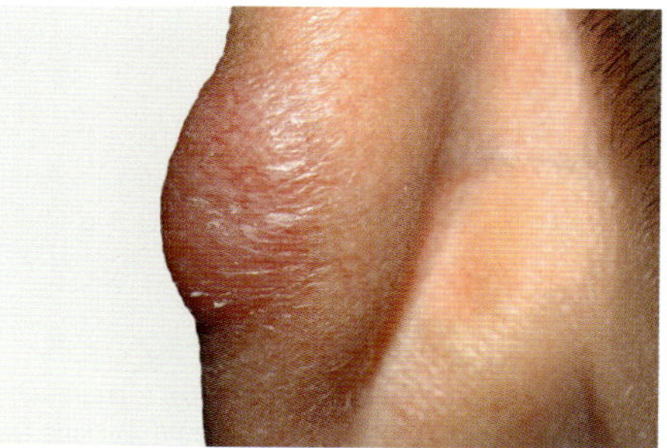

**Fig. 4.59** Primary cutaneous acral CD8+ T-cell lymphoma presenting as erythematous tumour of the left helix.

### Prognosis and predictive factors

These lymphomas have an aggressive course (median survival: 12 months) {2202}. There is no difference in survival between cases with small cell versus large cell morphology {196}, or between cases with localized versus diffuse lesions {2202}.

## *Primary cutaneous acral CD8+ T-cell lymphoma*

### Definition

Primary cutaneous acral CD8+ T-cell lymphoma is a rare cutaneous tumour characterized by skin infiltration of clonal atypical medium-sized CD8+ cytotoxic lymphocytes, preferential involvement of acral sites (in particular the ears), and good prognosis {2046}. This is a provisional entity in the current classification.

### ICD-O code 9709/3

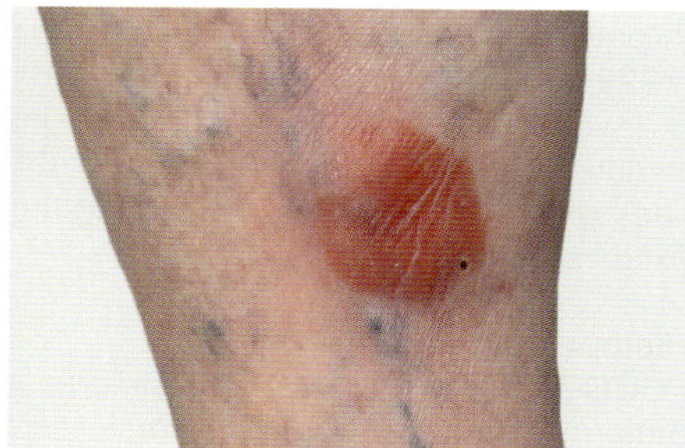

**Fig. 4.60** Primary cutaneous acral CD8+ T-cell lymphoma. A reddish nodule on the lower leg.

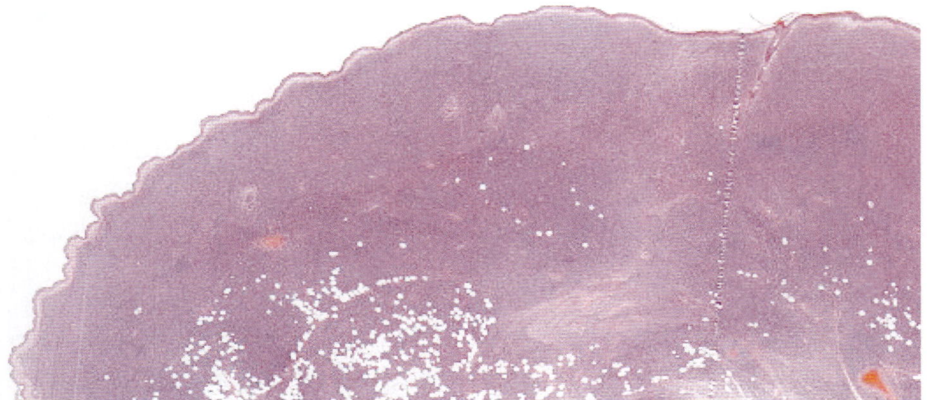

**Fig. 4.61** Primary cutaneous acral CD8+ T-cell lymphoma. A dense lymphoid infiltrate of the helix involving the dermis and the fat tissue; there is sparing of the cartilage and the epidermis (with a subepidermal grenz zone).

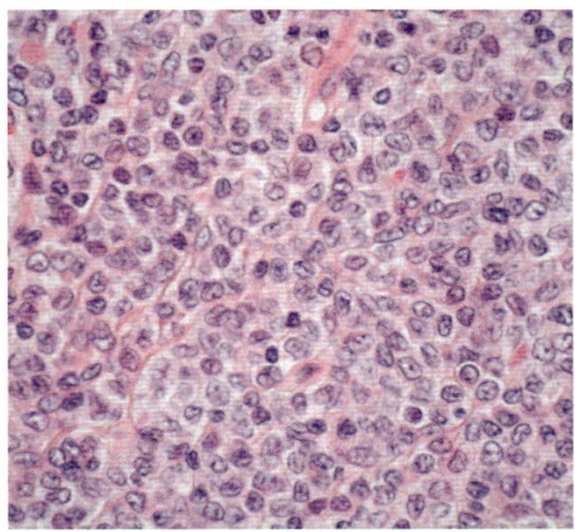

**Fig. 4.62** Primary cutaneous acral CD8+ T-cell lymphoma. At high power, the infiltrate is monomorphic and composed of atypical lymphoid cells, with some nuclear irregularity and fine chromatin.

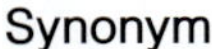

## Synonym

Indolent CD8+ lymphoid proliferation of the ear

## Epidemiology

The disease affects adults; no paediatric cases have been reported. The median age is 56 years, and there is a male predominance, with a male-to-female ratio of 1.7:1 {1391}.

## Etiology

A local trigger agent may be suspected, but no infectious or toxic candidate has yet been identified.

## Localization

The predominant sites are the ears (generally the helix or the conch, but rarely the lobe), nose, and lower limbs.

## Clinical features

The lesions are most often solitary reddish papules or nodules measuring between several millimetres and 3–4 cm, with a history of slow growth over several weeks or months. The most common sites are the ears (affected in 61% of cases), nose (in 22%), and lower limbs (in 8%). Other skin sites have been reported anecdotally (e.g. the eyelids, hands, shoulders, and trunk) {933,984,1344}. Occasionally, the lesions are multiple {933} and can be bilateral, in particular on the ears {203,349,2046} and feet {2843}. Local recurrence after treatment is possible. Recurrence may occur at other cutaneous sites {229,933,1553,2844}.

## Histopathology

The tumours are composed of a monotonous dermal proliferation of atypical medium-sized lymphocytes with irregular and frequently folded nuclei and small nucleoli {2046}. Mitoses and apoptotic figures are absent or very rare. Reactive B-cell lymphoid aggregates of follicles may be seen within the atypical infiltrate. Plasma cells, histiocytes, neutrophils, and eosinophils are absent or very rare. The epidermis is most often spared, separated from the infiltrate by a grenz zone. Occasionally, minimal epidermotropism (including Pautrier microabscess) may be seen {349,933}. Skin appendages are always spared, and angiotropism, angiodestruction, and necrosis are never seen. The proliferation frequently involves the underlying subcutis.

The tumour cells express CD3, CD8, TIA1, CD99, and αβ T-cell receptor. CD4 is always negative. CD2, CD5, and CD7 are regularly positive, but one or more of these markers can be lost or only weakly positive. Granzyme B and perforin are generally negative. CD56, CD57, CD30, and TdT are always negative, as are the T follicular helper (TFH) cell markers (i.e. CD10, BCL6, PD1, and CXCL13) {933}. CD68 is frequently positive, displaying

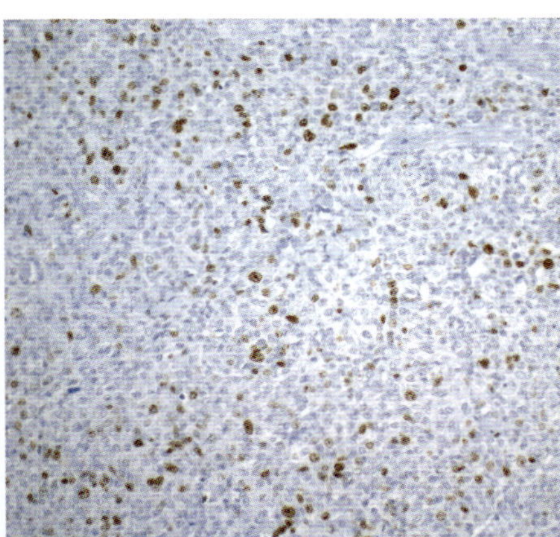

**Fig. 4.63** Primary cutaneous acral CD8+ T-cell lymphoma. Ki-67 immunostaining reveals < 10% positive cells.

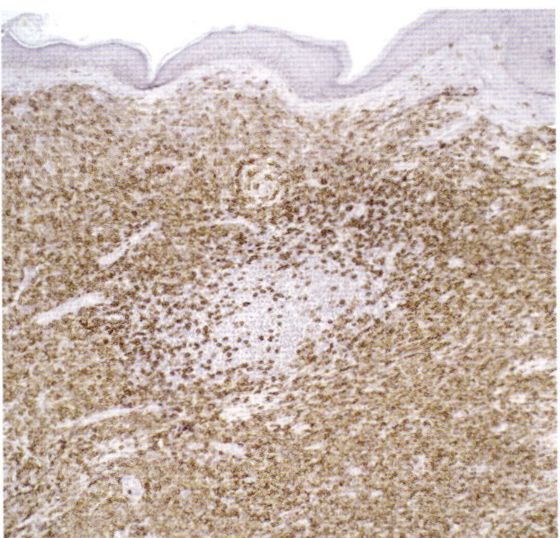

**Fig. 4.64** Primary cutaneous acral CD8+ T-cell lymphoma. Diffuse immunopositivity for CD8; an unstained nodule corresponds to a reactive B-cell aggregate.

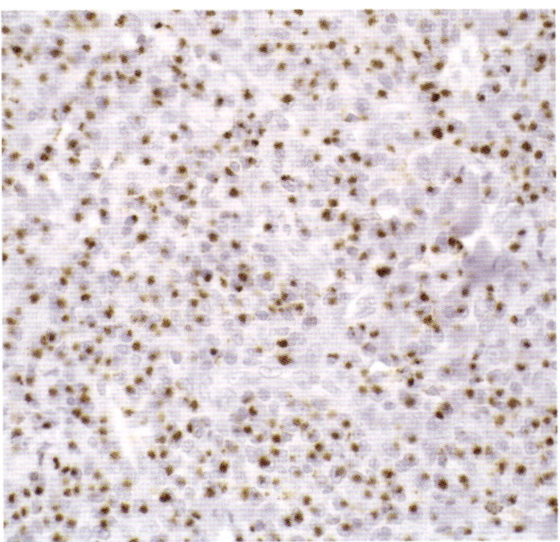

**Fig. 4.65** Primary cutaneous acral CD8+ T-cell lymphoma. Diffuse immunopositivity for TIA1 in large cytoplasmic dots.

(as does TIA1) Golgi-like or dot-like staining {2844}. The Ki-67 proliferation index is typically low (< 10%), although a few cases with a high proliferation index have been reported {2550}. When the proliferation rate is > 50%, other CD8+ cutaneous lymphomas should be considered. Staining for B-cell markers (CD20 and CD79a) may reveal reactive B-cell aggregates or follicles. LMP1 and EBV-encoded small RNA (EBER) are always negative.

### Histogenesis

The postulated normal counterpart is a skin-homing CD8+ T cell. However, cases very similar in terms of morphology, phenotype, and clinical outcome have also been recently described in the gastrointestinal tract {2033} and genital tract {2554}, suggesting a new lymphoma entity arising from tissue-resident CD8+ memory T cells.

### Genetic profile

The neoplastic T cells show clonal TR gene rearrangements. Specific genetic abnormalities have not yet been described.

### Prognosis and predictive factors

The tumour has a very good prognosis. Complete remission after surgical excision or radiotherapy is the rule. Local relapses or recurrences at other skin sites may occur, but dissemination to extracutaneous sites has been reported in only a single case {229}. For typical cases, staging is not recommended, and chemotherapy is not required. It is important to recognize this disease in order to avoid overtreatment.

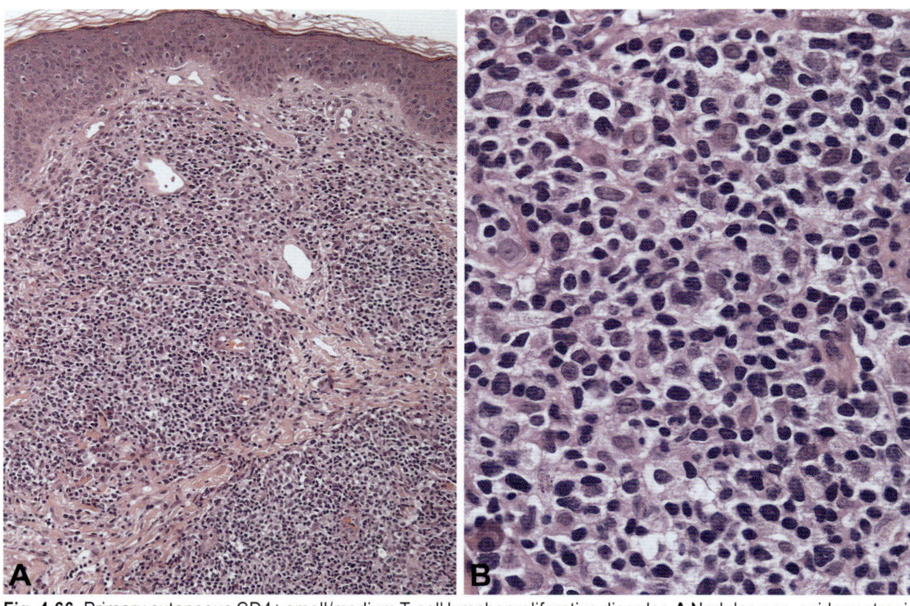

**Fig. 4.66** Primary cutaneous CD4+ small/medium T-cell lymphoproliferative disorder. **A** Nodular, non-epidermotropic infiltrate throughout the entire dermis. **B** Detail of the atypical infiltrate, showing a predominance of small/medium pleomorphic T cells.

## *Primary cutaneous CD4+ small/medium T-cell lymphoproliferative disorder*

### Definition

Primary cutaneous CD4+ small/medium T-cell lymphoproliferative disorder is a provisional entity characterized by a predominance of small to medium-sized CD4+ pleomorphic T cells, presentation with a solitary skin lesion, and no evidence of the patches or plaques that are typical of mycosis fungoides. Cases have the same clinicopathological features and benign clinical course as cutaneous pseudo-T-cell lymphomas with a nodular growth pattern {202,419,2116}; therefore, the term "lymphoproliferative disorder" (rather than "lymphoma") is preferred. Rare cases presenting with widespread skin lesions, large rapidly growing tumours, > 30% large pleomorphic T cells, and/or a high proliferation rate do not belong to this group {849,943}. Such cases usually have more-aggressive clinical behaviour and are better classified as peripheral T-cell lymphoma NOS.

### ICD-O code 9709/1

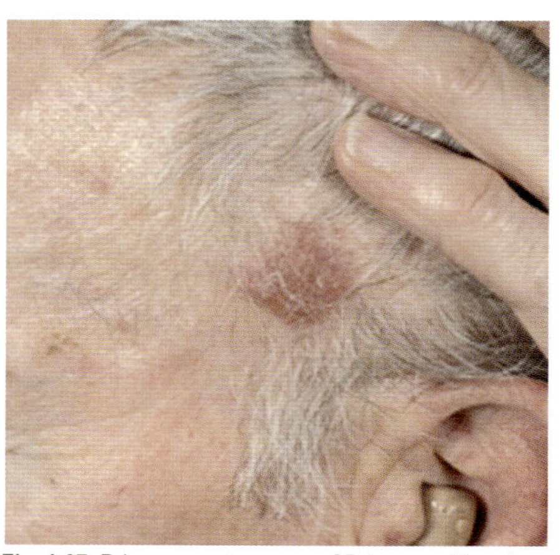

**Fig. 4.67** Primary cutaneous CD4+ small/medium T-cell lymphoproliferative disorder. A solitary tumour on the left temple.

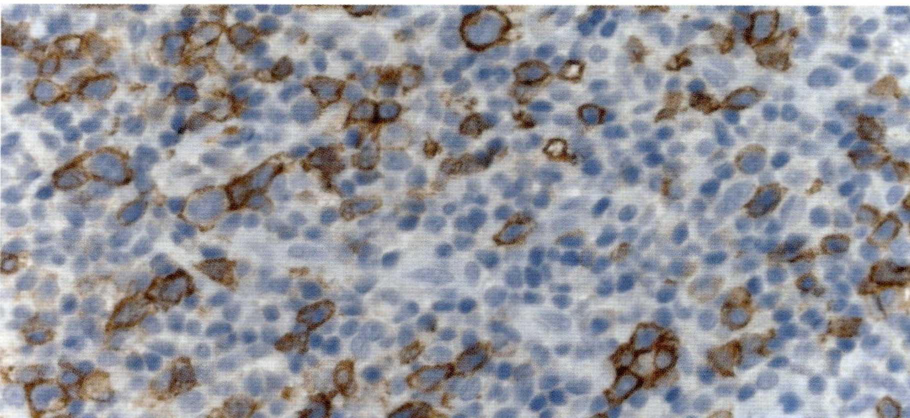

**Fig. 4.68** Primary cutaneous CD4+ small/medium T-cell lymphoproliferative disorder. Expression of PD1 by atypical T cells partly arranged in clusters.

## Synonym

Primary cutaneous CD4+ small/medium T-cell lymphoma (no longer used)

## Epidemiology

This is a rare disease, accounting for about 2% of all cutaneous T-cell lymphomas {2832}.

## Localization

Patients usually present with a solitary plaque or nodule, most commonly on the face, neck, or upper trunk {202,419,849,1210}.

## Clinical features

Clinical presentation with a solitary skin lesion is the sole manifestation of disease. In rare cases, multiple lesions are present {202,419}. By definition, patches typical of mycosis fungoides are absent.

## Histopathology

These lymphomas show dense, diffuse, or nodular infiltrates within the dermis, with a tendency to infiltrate the subcutis. Epidermotropism may be present focally, but if epidermotropism is conspicuous, a diagnosis of mycosis fungoides should be considered. There is a predominance of small/medium pleomorphic T cells {196,202,419,849}. Large pleomorphic cells, if present, account for only a small proportion (< 30%) of the infiltrate {197}. Almost all cases show a considerable admixture with small reactive CD8+ T cells, B cells, plasma cells, and histiocytes (including multinucleated giant cells) {202,419,2209}.

By definition, these proliferations have a CD3+, CD4+, CD8–, CD30– phenotype. CD7 is sometimes negative, but loss of other pan–T-cell antigens is uncommon {202,419,943,2209}. A variable proportion of atypical CD4+ T cells, often scattered or forming small clusters, express PD1 (CD279), ICOS, BCL6, and CXCL13, suggesting derivation from T follicular helper (TFH) cells {230,419,2209}. CD10 is usually negative. The Ki-67 proliferation index is generally low (typically ~5% and at most 20%).

## Histogenesis

The postulated normal counterpart is a skin-homing CD4+ T cell with TFH cell characteristics.

## Genetic profile

TR genes are clonally rearranged in most cases {419,2209}. Specific genetic abnormalities have not been described {230}. EBV is negative.

## Prognosis and predictive factors

The prognosis is excellent. Preferred treatment modalities include intralesional steroids, surgical excision, and radiotherapy {202,419,943}. Spontaneous remission after biopsy has been reported {419,943,1210}. Local recurrence is rare.

# Secondary cutaneous involvement in T-cell lymphomas and leukaemias

Feldman A.
Gaulard P.
Pileri S.A.
Willemze R.

## Introduction

The skin is a relatively common extranodal site of involvement in systemic T-cell lymphomas and leukaemias. Morphological, phenotypic, and in some cases genetic features are helpful in classifying these lesions correctly; however, clinical correlation is of paramount importance in distinguishing primary cutaneous T-cell neoplasms from secondary cutaneous involvement by a systemic process. The entities most likely to involve the skin secondarily are discussed below or in their respective sections.

## Systemic anaplastic large cell lymphoma

Systemic anaplastic large cell lymphoma typically presents with adenopathy and is often associated with extranodal disease, including involvement of skin and/or subcutis in about 20% of cases {2326}. Skin lesions are often generalized and may manifest as papules, nodules, or (ulcerating) tumours; they may be present at diagnosis or can develop during disease progression {194}. Distinguishing between skin lesions in systemic anaplastic large cell lymphoma and primary cutaneous anaplastic large cell lymphoma is important because of differences in management and clinical outcome {194}. Features favouring a diagnosis of cutaneous anaplastic large cell lymphoma include presentation with solitary or localized skin lesions, expression of cutaneous lymphocyte antigen (CLA), negative staining for EMA (epithelial membrane antigen), lack of t(2;5), and negative staining for ALK {585,600,2593}. However, recent studies have identified a small subgroup of ALK-positive anaplastic large cell lymphomas presenting exclusively with cutaneous disease, which may have an excellent prognosis {1956} (see *Primary cutaneous anaplastic large cell lymphoma*, p. 238).

### ICD-O codes

| | |
|---|---|
| Systemic anaplastic large cell lymphoma, ALK-positive | 9714/3 |
| Systemic anaplastic large cell lymphoma, ALK-negative | 9715/3 |

## Angioimmunoblastic T-cell lymphoma

### Definition

Angioimmunoblastic T-cell lymphoma (AITL) is a neoplasm of mature T follicular helper (TFH) cell origin. It accounts for up to 35% of all peripheral T-cell lymphomas etc. and 1–2% of all non-Hodgkin lymphomas {111,743,1500A,2254}.

### ICD-O code 9705/3

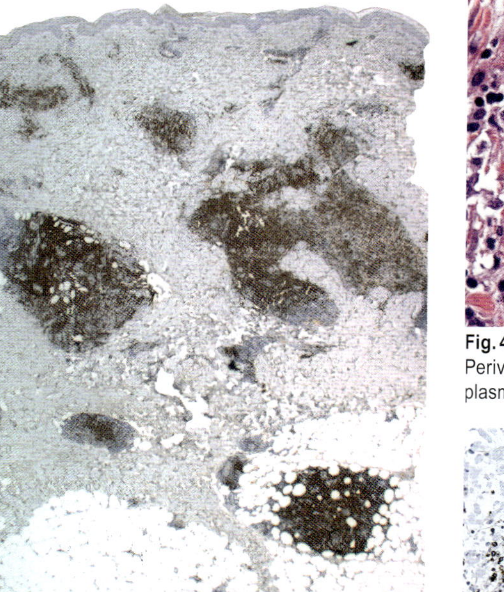

**Fig. 4.69** Cutaneous involvement by angioimmunoblastic T-cell lymphoma. Immunostaining for PD1 highlights the neoplastic infiltrates.

### Epidemiology

Most patients are older adults, with males and females equally affected.

### Clinical features

Patients typically present with lymphadenopathy, hepatosplenomegaly, systemic symptoms, and hypergammaglobulinaemia. Cutaneous manifestations are present in about 50% of cases. A generalized maculopapular rash is the most common skin finding, but a wide variety of appearances have been reported; tumour nodules may occur late in the disease {278}. Rarely, cutaneous lesions are the first manifestation of AITL {2526}.

### Histopathology

Skin biopsies typically reveal a perivascular infiltrate of small to medium-sized lymphocytes with variable cytological atypia and admixed eosinophils, plasma

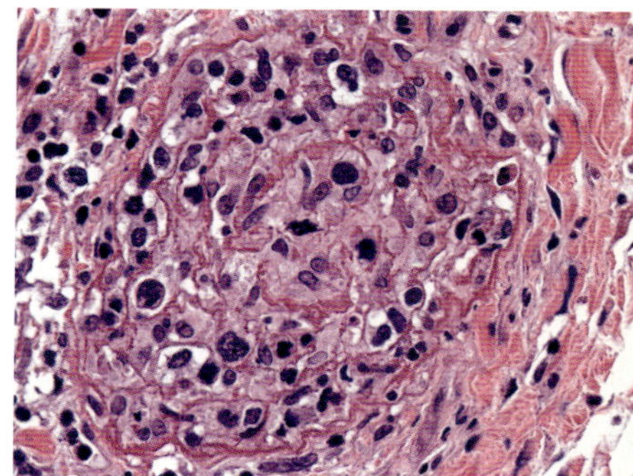

**Fig. 4.70** Angioimmunoblastic T-cell lymphoma. Perivascular atypical lymphoid cells with clear cytoplasm.

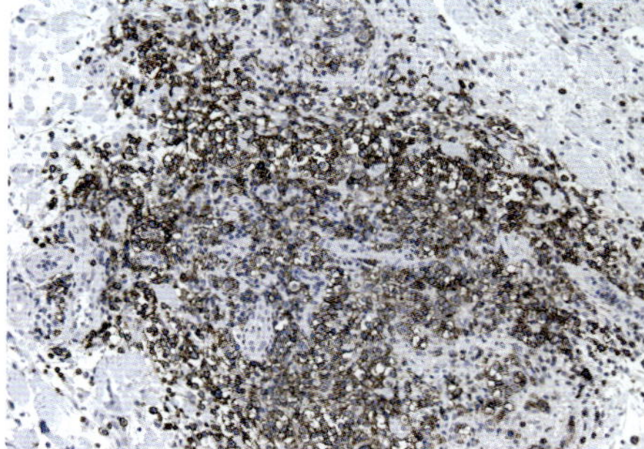

**Fig. 4.71** Angioimmunoblastic T-cell lymphoma. PD1 (CD279) is positive in atypical cells.

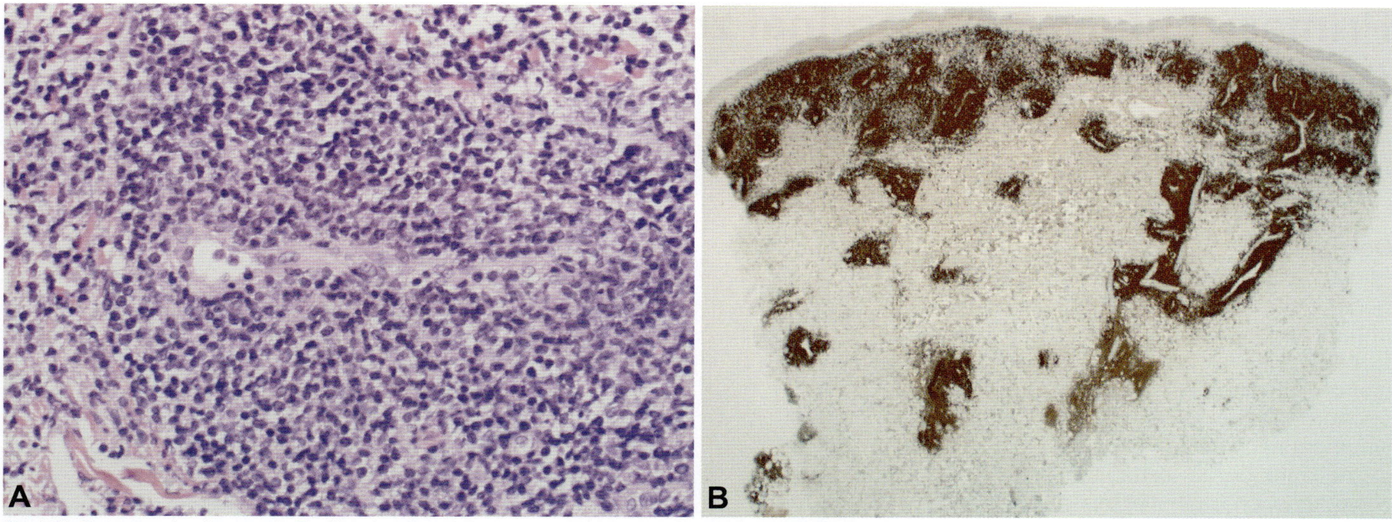


**Fig. 4.72** Cutaneous involvement by T-cell prolymphocytic leukaemia. **A** Perivascular lymphocytic infiltrate in the dermis. **B** Immunostaining for TCL1A highlights the neoplastic infiltrate.

cells, and/or histiocytes. Early lesions may be indistinguishable from inflammatory conditions, whereas nodular lesions typically have an overtly lymphomatous appearance. Most of the lymphocytes are CD4+ T cells; positivity for TFH cell markers (e.g. PD1 [CD279], ICOS, CD10, BCL6, and CXCL13) is helpful in distinguishing AITL from reactive lesions {278,1516}. EBV-positive B cells may be present {1516,1530,2878}.

### Genetic profile

A clonal T-cell population may be demonstrable in skin biopsies {278,1667}. *RHOA* c.50G>T (p.G17V) and IDH2 p.R172K/S mutations have been reported {1516}.

### Prognosis and predictive factors

AITL generally has a poor prognosis, with a 5-year overall survival rate of 33% {595A,743}.

## *T-cell prolymphocytic leukaemia*

### Definition

T-cell prolymphocytic leukaemia is a neoplasm of mature T lymphocytes that generally involves the peripheral blood, bone marrow, liver, spleen, and lymph nodes.

### ICD-O code 9834/3

### Epidemiology

Most patients are older adults, with a median age of 63 years {1208}.

### Clinical features

Patients typically present with hepatosplenomegaly, lymphadenopathy, and a peripheral blood lymphocytosis with anaemia and thrombocytopenia. Skin involvement is seen in about 30% of cases, often at initial presentation {1135, 1631,1649,1702}. The most common skin findings are localized erythema, nodules, and erythroderma, which may mimic Sézary syndrome clinically.

### Histopathology

Skin biopsies typically reveal perivascular or diffuse infiltrates of small to medium-sized lymphocytes in the dermis, without epidermotropism. The neoplastic cells usually express CD2, CD3, CD7, TCL1A, and CD52, which can be targeted therapeutically {1208,2019}. The phenotype may be CD4+/CD8− (seen in 60% of cases), CD4+/CD8+ (in 21%), or CD4−/CD8+ (in 13%) {1702}. Coexpression of CD4 and CD8 is helpful diagnostically, and expression of TCL1 on T cells is especially helpful.

### Genetic profile

Clonal TR gene rearrangements may be detected in skin biopsies {1631}. TRA/*TCL1A* translocations may facilitate diagnosis and can be detected by FISH; some cases have an alternative, TRA/*MTCP1* translocation {1138}.

### Prognosis and predictive factors

T-cell prolymphocytic leukaemia generally has a poor prognosis, with a median overall survival of 19 months {1208}.

# Primary cutaneous marginal zone (MALT) lymphoma

Kempf W.
Duncan L.M.
Swerdlow S.H.
Willemze R.

## Definition

Primary cutaneous marginal zone lymphoma (PCMZL) is an indolent lymphoma composed of neoplastic small B cells, plasma cells, and a variable number of reactive T cells. In the 2017 revision of the WHO classification of lymphoid neoplasms PCMZL is included in the category of extranodal marginal zone lymphoma of mucosa-associated lymphoid tissue (MALT lymphoma) {2547}. Cases previously referred to as immunocytoma, cutaneous follicular hyperplasia with monotypic plasma cells, and primary cutaneous plasmacytoma are now considered to be PCMZLs {1300,2190,2345,2832}.

## ICD-O code 9699/3

## Epidemiology

PCMZL accounts for 30–40% of all primary cutaneous B-cell lymphomas overall, and it is the most common form of cutaneous B-cell lymphoma in children and adolescents {910,1343,1802,2381}. PCMZL most commonly affects adults in the fifth and sixth decades of life, with a male preponderance {873,1101}.

## Etiology

PCMZL may develop as a result of chronic antigenic stimulation by antigens inserted intradermally, such as tattoo pigments, vaccines, and tick-borne bacteria (*Borrelia* sp.) {311,2191}. An association with *Borrelia burgdorferi* infection has been found in areas endemic for the species in Europe, but not in the USA or Asia {415,915,2563,2859}.

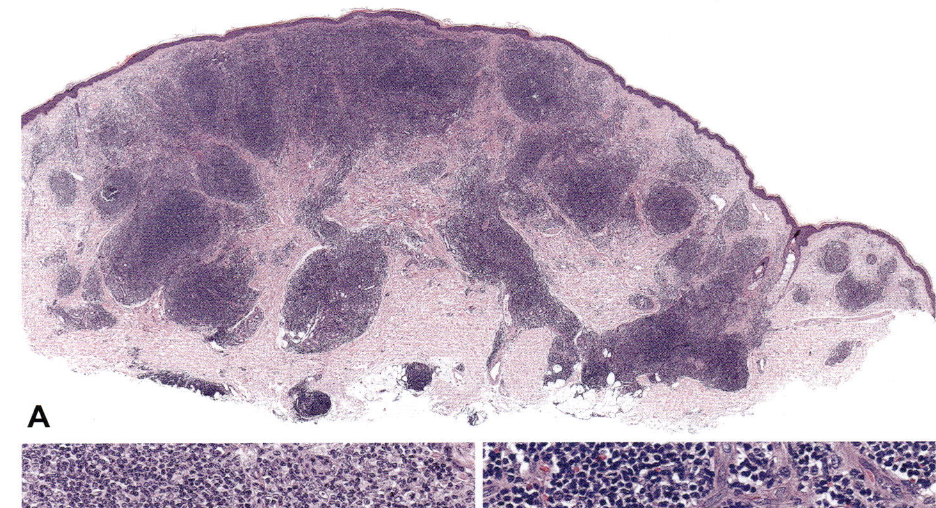



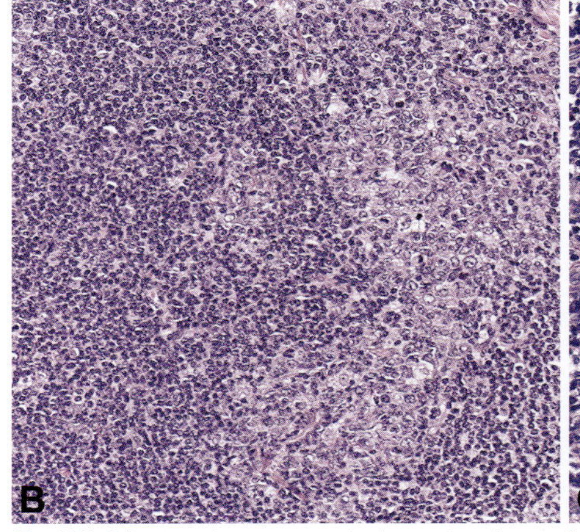



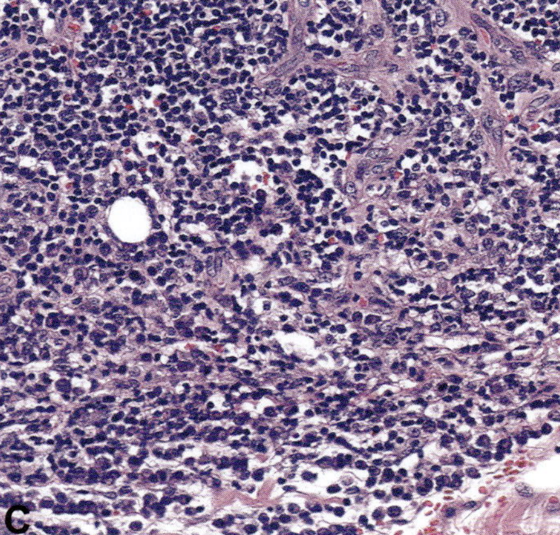



**Fig. 4.74** Primary cutaneous marginal zone lymphoma. **A** Nodular infiltrates of small lymphocytes and germinal centres. **B** Infiltrate of small lymphocytes surrounding reactive germinal centres. **C** Plasma cells at the periphery of the infiltrates.

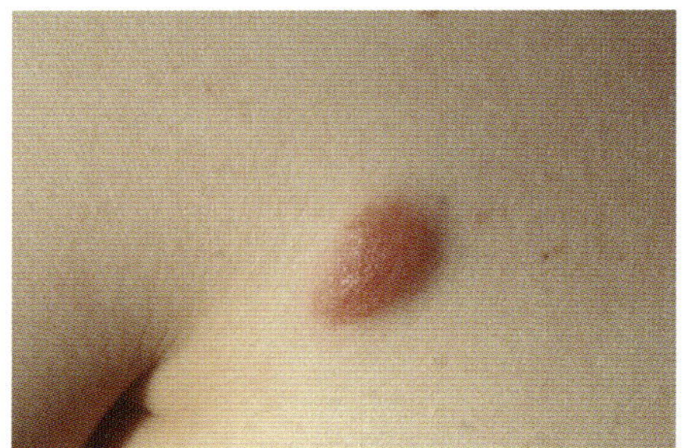

**Fig. 4.73** Primary cutaneous marginal zone lymphoma. Erythematous nodule on the upper back.

## Localization

PCMZL is preferentially localized on the trunk and upper arms {910,1101,2381}.

## Clinical features

PCMZL typically presents with multifocal and sometimes solitary red or violaceous plaques or nodules {664,874,910,1101,2384}. The lesions may wax and wane and can undergo spontaneous regression {760,2544}. The development of anetoderma in spontaneously regressing lesions has been reported {1096,2544,2720}. In a recent study, PCMZL was associated with high incidence rates of gastrointestinal disorders and autoimmune diseases {962}.

## Histopathology

PCMZL shows a dense dermal multinodular infiltrate of small lymphocytes, plasma cells, and follicles with reactive germinal centres {136,873,910,2544}. The plasma cells are typically located at the periphery of the infiltrate and in the subepidermal compartment. In most cases, the small B cells have a lymphoplasmacytoid morphology. A predominance of monocytoid B cells and the expression of IgM should raise suspicion for a secondary cutaneous MALT

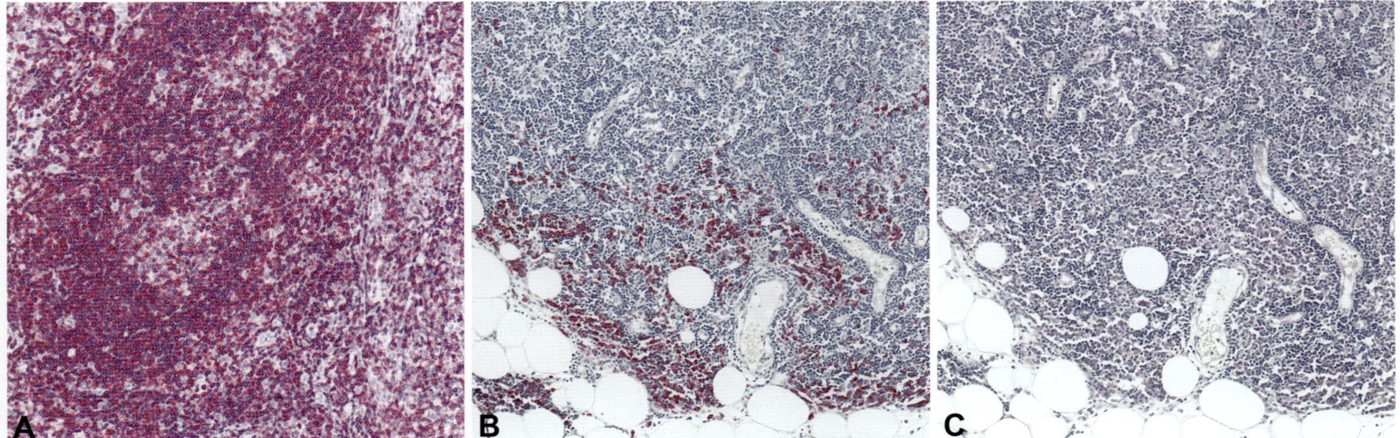

**Fig. 4.75** Primary cutaneous marginal zone lymphoma. **A** BCL2 is positive in neoplastic cells and negative in residual germinal centre. **B** Monotypic expression of immunoglobulin κ light chain. **C** Absence of expression of immunoglobulin λ light chain.

lymphoma {664}. Transformation to large B-cell lymphoma is very rare {1632}.

The neoplastic B cells express B-cell markers including CD19, CD20, and CD79a. They are also BCL2-positive, but negative for CD5, CD10, BCL6, and cyclin D1 (see Table 4.04). The reactive germinal centres contain BCL6+ and BCL2– cells and are supported by networks of CD21+ follicular dendritic cells. The plasma cells show monotypic expression of immunoglobulin light chains in most cases. Reactive T cells may be prominent. Clusters of CD123+ plasmacytoid dendritic cells and convergence of CD1a+ dendritic cells around lymphoid nodules are typically seen in the periphery of the infiltrates {921,1469}. Some cases (up to 39%) of PCMZL with plasmacytic differentiation are IgG4-positive; this finding is not associated with signs of a systemic IgG4-related disorder {310,598}.

Two subsets of PCMZL have been identified: the more common heavy chain class-switched form is characterized by expression of IgG, IgA, or IgE; a high number of T cells; and no expression of CXCR3, whereas the much less common non–class-switched form expresses IgM and CXCR3 and presents with large sheets of B cells {664,2708}. The class-switched cases are considered by some authors to constitute clonal chronic cutaneous lymphoproliferative disorder rather than overt lymphoma {664,2544}.

**Table 4.04** Differential diagnostic markers in cutaneous small B-cell lymphoproliferations (most-typical phenotypes). From: Jaffe ES et al. Hematopathology, 2nd edition. Elsevier: 2016 {1204}

| | CD20 and CD79a | BCL6 | BCL2 | CD10 | CD5 | Cyclin D1 |
|---|---|---|---|---|---|---|
| Cutaneous lymphoid hyperplasia (reactive germinal centres) | + | + | – | + | – | – |
| PCMZL | + | – | + | – | – | – |
| PCFCL | + | + | –/+ | –/+ | – | – |
| Secondary cutaneous follicular lymphoma | + | + | + | + | – | – |
| Mantle cell lymphoma | + | – | + | – | + | + |
| CLL/SLL | + | – | + | – | + | – |

CLL/SLL, chronic lymphocytic leukaemia/small lymphocytic lymphoma; PCFCL, primary cutaneous follicle centre lymphoma; PCMZL, primary cutaneous marginal zone lymphoma.

## Histogenesis

The postulated normal counterpart is a post–germinal centre B lymphocyte with plasmacytic differentiation.

## Genetic profile

A B-cell clone can be detected by BIOMED-2 PCR assay in the majority of PCMZLs {1825}. Occasionally, different clones can be detected at different sites and at different points during disease evolution {760,834}. The IGH/*MALT1* translocation (t14;18)(q32;q21) is uncommonly found {1970,2519,2520,2855}. IGH/*BCL2* translocation and other translocations involving IGH, *BCL10*, *MALT1*, *BCL2*, and *BIRC3* are absent or only very rarely associated with PCMZL {843,2353}. Methylation of *DAPK1* and *CDKN2A* (*P16INK4a*) is common {2563}. PCMZL does not have *MYD88* c.818T>C (p.L265P) mutations {309}.

## Prognosis and predictive factors

The prognosis is favourable, with a 5-year disease-specific survival rate of >98%. Recurrences are common. Extracutaneous spread occurs rarely (in only ~4% of patients) and is more frequently observed in longstanding multifocal disease, in the non–class-switched form, and in cases with transformation {664,874,2384}.

# Primary cutaneous follicle centre lymphoma

Willemze R.
Santucci M.
Swerdlow S.H.
Vergier B.

## Definition

Primary cutaneous follicle centre lymphoma (PCFCL) is a tumour of neoplastic follicle centre cells, including centrocytes and variable numbers of centroblasts, that has a follicular, follicular and diffuse, or diffuse growth pattern and generally presents on the head or trunk {2547,2832}. Irrespective of site, nearly all lymphomas with a diffuse growth pattern and a monotonous proliferation of centroblasts and immunoblasts are classified as primary cutaneous diffuse large B-cell lymphoma, leg type {2547,2832}. Cases with a secondary cutaneous follicular lymphoma can have a very similar clinical presentation, so staging is important in order to rule out systemic disease {1360}.

## ICD-O code

9597/3

## Epidemiology

PCFCL accounts for approximately 50% of all primary cutaneous B-cell lymphoma cases. It mainly affects middle-aged adults, with a male-to-female ratio of approximately 1.5:1 {997,2381,2940}.

## Localization

PCFCL characteristically presents with solitary or localized skin lesions on the scalp, forehead, or trunk. Approximately 5% of cases present with skin lesions on the legs, and 15% present with multifocal skin lesions {1403,2381,2940}.

## Clinical features

Patients present with firm, erythematous to violaceous non-ulcerating plaques, nodules, or tumours of variable size. Particularly on the trunk, tumours may be surrounded by erythematous papules and by slightly infiltrated (sometimes figurate) plaques, which may also precede the development of tumorous lesions by months or years {225,2312,2834}. A small minority of cases present with multifocal skin lesions {923,2381}. Cutaneous relapses occur in about 30% of cases, but dissemination to extracutaneous sites is uncommon (occurring in ~10% of cases) {2381,2940}.

## Histopathology

PCFCL shows perivascular and periadnexal to diffuse infiltrates, with sparing of the epidermis. The infiltrates have a follicular, follicular and diffuse, or diffuse growth pattern {332,2312,2834}. Cases with a follicular growth pattern show nodular infiltrates throughout the

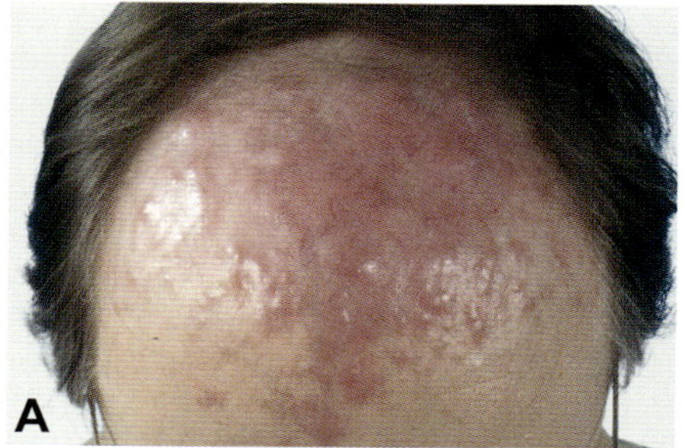

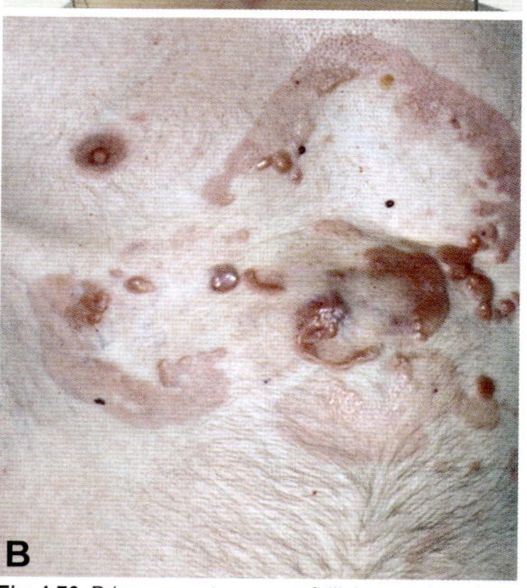

**Fig. 4.76** Primary cutaneous follicle centre lymphoma. **A** Characteristic clinical presentation on the scalp. **B** Characteristic clinical presentation with localized skin lesions on the chest.

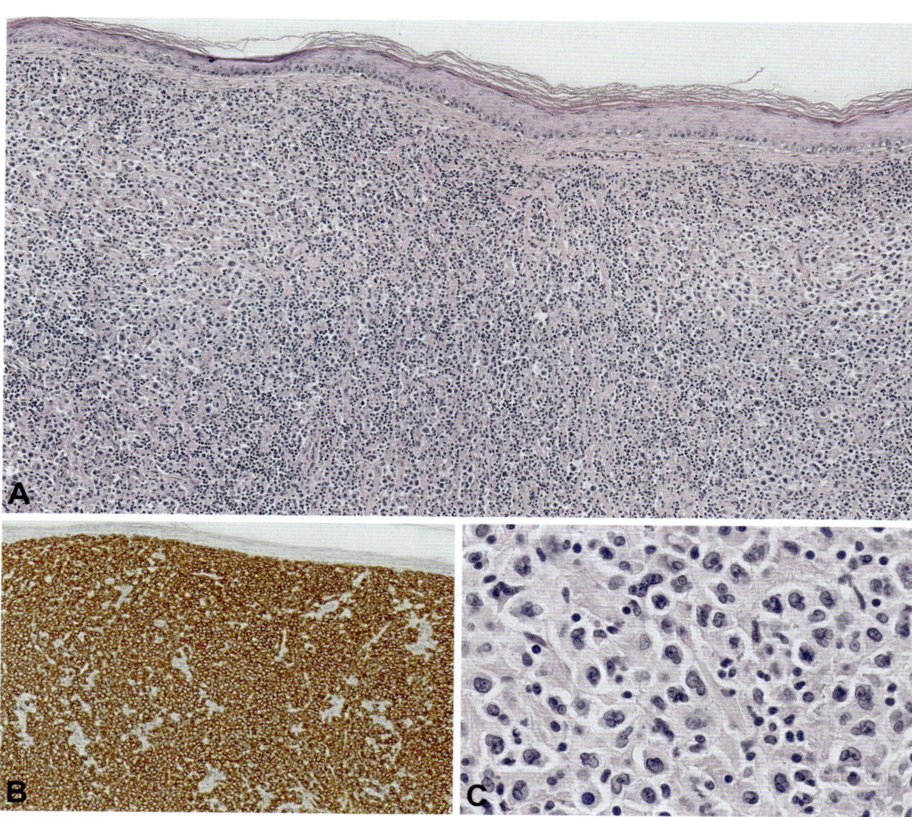

**Fig. 4.77** Primary cutaneous follicle centre lymphoma with a diffuse growth pattern. **A** Diffuse, non-epidermotropic infiltrate. **B** Diffuse infiltrate of CD20-positive B cells. **C** Higher magnification shows that the cellular infiltrate contains many multilobated cells.

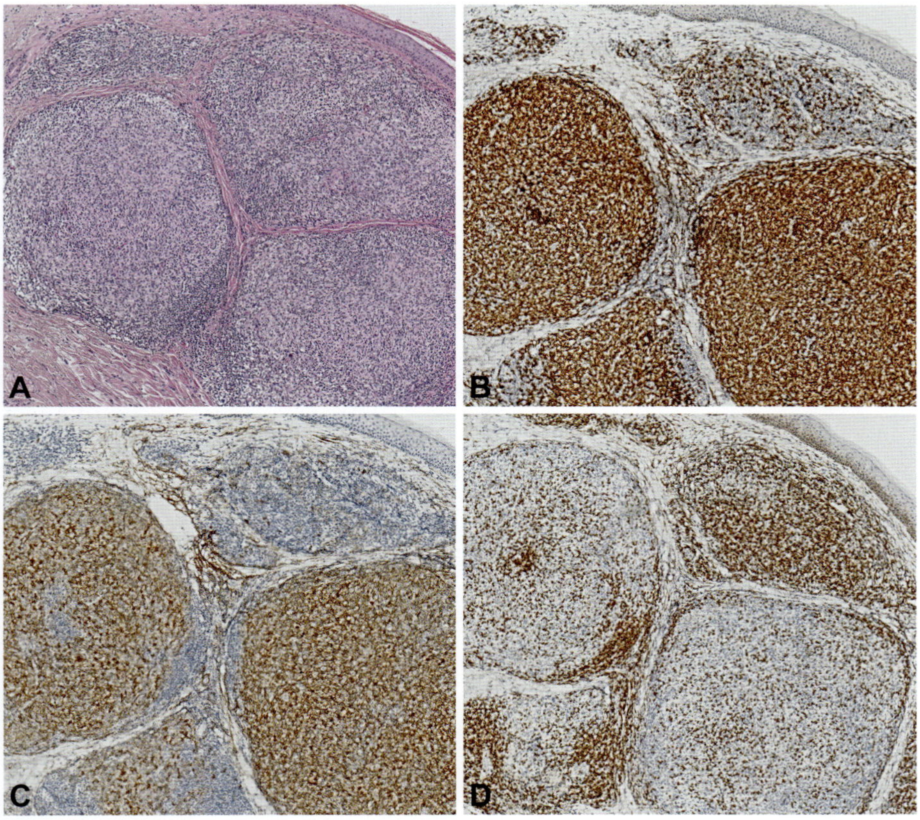

**Fig. 4.78** Primary cutaneous follicle centre lymphoma with a follicular growth pattern. **A** Low-power view (H&E). **B** Positive staining for CD79a. **C** Positive staining for CD10. **D** Intrafollicular neoplastic B cells are negative for BCL2.

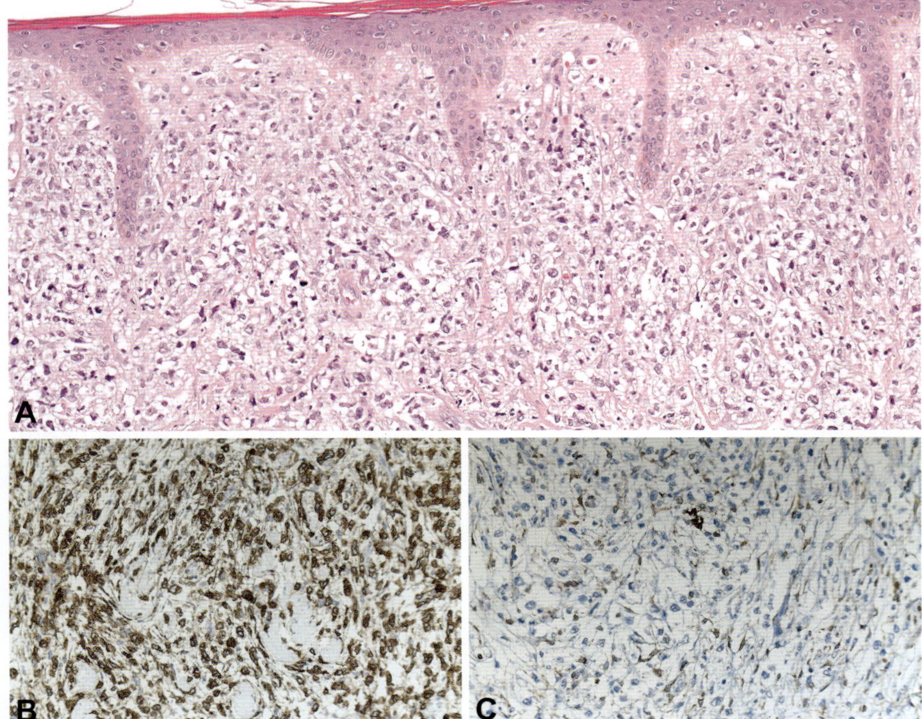

**Fig. 4.79** Primary cutaneous follicle centre lymphoma (spindle-shaped). **A** Diffuse proliferation of centrocytes with a spindle cell morphology. **B** The tumour cells express CD79a. **C** The neoplastic B cells are negative for BCL2.

entire dermis, often extending into the subcutis. Unlike in cutaneous follicular hyperplasias, the follicles in PCFCL are often poorly defined, show a monotonous proliferation of BCL6+ follicle centre cells enmeshed in a meshwork of CD21+/CD35+ follicular dendritic cells, lack tingible-body macrophages, generally have an attenuated or absent mantle zone, and have a low proliferation rate {408,916}. Reactive T cells may be numerous, and a prominent stromal component is usually present.

Cases with a diffuse growth pattern usually show a monotonous population of large centrocytes, some of which may have a multilobated appearance, and variable numbers of admixed centroblasts {225,923,2312,2834}. In rare cases, the large centrocytes can be spindle-shaped {410,914}. In some cases, foci of CD21+/CD35+ follicular dendritic cells may still be present; in other cases, they may be totally absent {966}. The proliferation rate in these diffuse PCFCLs is generally high. The neoplastic cells express CD20 and CD79a, but are usually immunoglobulin-negative. PCFCLs consistently express BCL6. CD10 may be positive in cases with a follicular growth pattern, but is generally negative in cases with a diffuse growth pattern {595,1403,1789,2381}. Most cases show either no BCL2 staining in the neoplastic B cells or only faint staining (weaker than in admixed T cells) in only a minority of the neoplastic cells {408,459,1403,2381}. However, several studies have found BCL2 expression in a substantial proportion of PCFCLs with at least a partially follicular growth pattern {30,917,1789,2051}. Notwithstanding such reports, strong expression of both BCL2 and CD10 by the neoplastic B cells should always raise suspicion for a nodal follicular lymphoma involving the skin secondarily {1100}. Staining for IRF4 (MUM1) and FOXP1 is negative in most cases; CD5 and CD43 are always negative {1403,2381}.

## Histogenesis

The postulated normal counterpart is a mature germinal centre B lymphocyte.

## Genetic profile

Clonally rearranged IG genes, with somatic hypermutation, are present {1,834,865,1825}. In many studies, PCFCL, including cases with a follicular growth pattern, did not show (or only rarely showed) *BCL2* rearrangements {184,966,2051,2732}. However, other studies have reported *BCL2* rearrangements (demonstrated by PCR and/or FISH) in about 10–40% of cases with a follicular growth pattern, as well as in some completely diffuse cases {1360,1789,2051,2551}. PCFCLs show the gene expression profile of germinal centre–like large B-cell lymphomas, and often show amplification of *REL* {1,629,1099}. Deletion of chromosome 14q32.33 has been reported {629}. Unlike in primary cutaneous diffuse large B-cell lymphoma, leg type, *MYD88* c.818T>C (p.L265P) mutation and inactivation of the *CDKN2A* and *CDKN2B* gene loci on chromosome 9p21.3 by deletion or promoter hypermethylation are not (or are only rarely) found in PCFCL {629,1738}.

### Prognosis and predictive factors

Irrespective of the growth pattern (follicular and/or diffuse), the number of blast cells, the presence of t(14;18) and/or BCL2 expression, or the presence of either localized or multifocal skin disease, PCFCLs have an excellent prognosis, with a 5-year survival rate of >95% {923,2312,2381,2940}. PCFCLs presenting on the leg are reported to have a less favourable prognosis {1403,2381}. In patients with localized or few scattered lesions, local radiotherapy is the preferred treatment {997,2381}. Cutaneous relapses, which occur in about 30% of cases, do not indicate progressive disease. Systemic therapy is only required for patients with very extensive cutaneous disease, extremely thick skin tumours, or extracutaneous disease.

# Primary cutaneous diffuse large B-cell lymphoma, leg type

Willemze R.
Battistella M.
Duncan L.M.
Vergier B.

### Definition

Primary cutaneous diffuse large B-cell lymphoma, leg type (PCLBCL-LT) is a primary cutaneous diffuse large B-cell lymphoma (DLBCL) composed exclusively of centroblasts and immunoblasts, most commonly arising in the leg.

### ICD-O code 9680/3

### Epidemiology

PCLBCL-LT accounts for 4% of all primary cutaneous lymphomas and 20% of primary cutaneous B-cell lymphomas {2832}. It typically occurs in elderly people, and is more common in women, with a female-to-male ratio between 3:1 and 4:1. The median age is in the eighth decade of life {2737}.

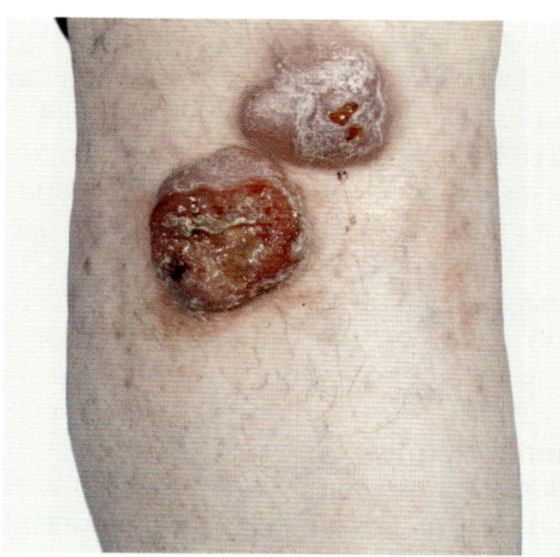

**Fig. 4.80** Primary cutaneous diffuse large B-cell lymphoma, leg type. Typical clinical presentation with tumours on the leg.

### Localization

These lymphomas preferentially affect the lower legs, but 10–15% of cases arise at other sites {1403,2381,2940}.

### Clinical features

PCLBCL-LT presents with red or bluish-red, often rapidly growing tumours on one or both of the lower legs {923,1403,2381,2940}. These lymphomas frequently disseminate to extracutaneous sites.

### Histopathology

PCLBCL-LT consists of a monotonous, diffuse, non-epidermotropic infiltrate of confluent sheets of centroblasts and immunoblasts {923,2737}. Mitotic figures are frequent. Small B cells and CD21+/CD35+ follicular dendritic cell meshworks are absent. Reactive T cells are relatively few and are often confined to perivascular areas.

The neoplastic B cells express monotypic immunoglobulin, CD20, and CD79a. Unlike primary cutaneous follicle centre lymphomas (PCFCLs), PCLBCL-LTs usually strongly express BCL2, IRF4 (MUM1), FOXP1, MYC, and cytoplasmic IgM, with coexpression of IgD in 50% of cases {609,917,926,1100,1403,1405}. However, approximately 10% of cases do not express BCL2 or IRF4 (MUM1) {1403,2381}. The proliferation rate is high. BCL6 is expressed by most cases (but may be dim), whereas CD10 staining is negative {1100}.

### Differential diagnosis

PCLBCL-LT should be differentiated from PCFCLs with a diffuse growth pattern, other rare types of cutaneous DLBCL, iatrogenic immunodeficiency–associated lymphoproliferative disorders (which can develop in patients taking methotrexate or other immunosuppressive drugs), and secondary cutaneous DLBCL. Features that support a diagnosis of PCFCL include numerous admixed T cells; follicular dendritic cell meshworks; negative staining for BCL2, IRF4 (MUM1), MYC, and cytoplasmic IgM; and the characteristic clinical presentation with localized skin lesions on the head or trunk. The very rare cases that do not meet the diagnostic

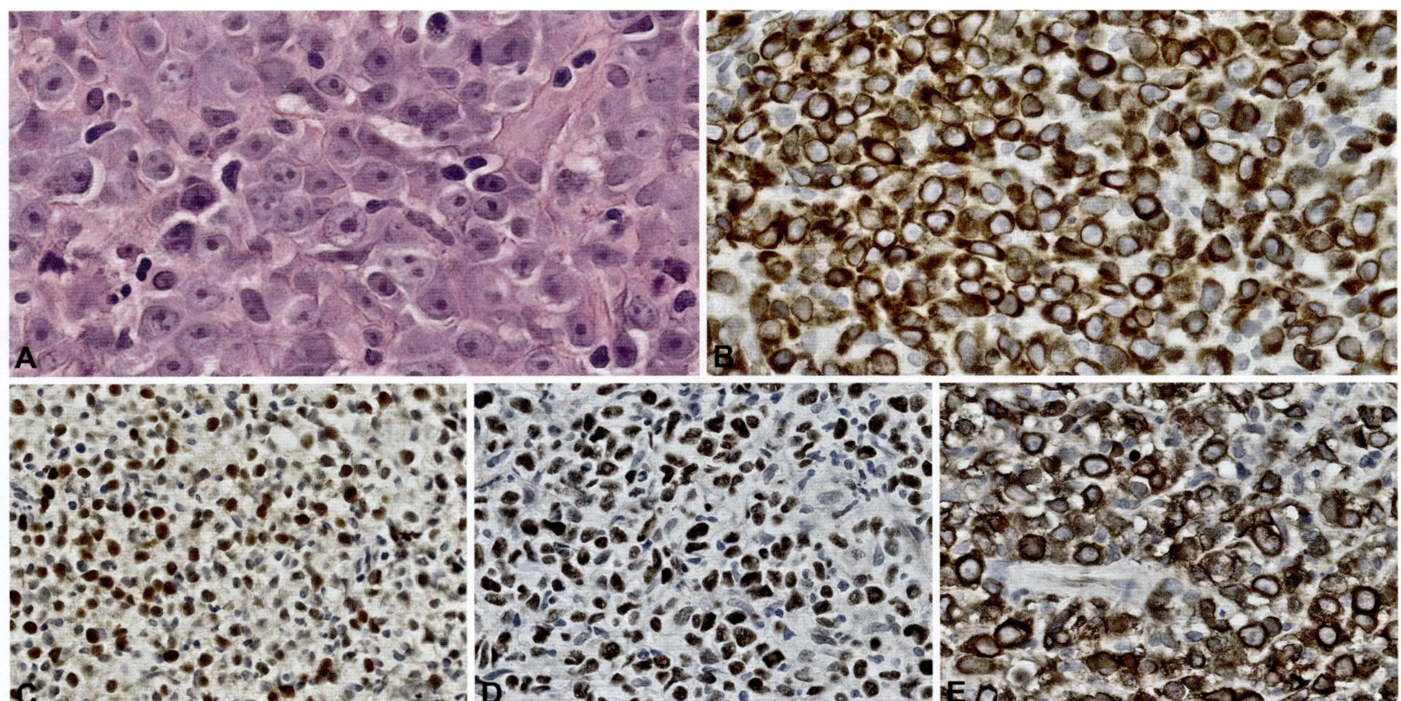

**Fig. 4.81** Primary cutaneous diffuse large B-cell lymphoma, leg type. **A** Cohesive sheets of large transformed cells with prominent nucleoli. The neoplastic cells show strong cytoplasmic staining for BCL2 (**B**), nuclear staining for IRF4 (MUM1) (**C**) and MYC (**D**), and strong cytoplasmic staining for IgM (**E**).

criteria for either PCLBCL-LT or PCFCL should be diagnosed as primary cutaneous DLBCL-NOS. The skin can also be the primary site of presentation for some histological variants of DLBCL, such as plasmablastic lymphoma and T-cell/histiocyte-rich large B-cell lymphoma {518,1902,2370,2742}. Such cases generally show (or soon develop) systemic disease and are not considered primary cutaneous lymphoma. Plasmablastic lymphomas are seen almost exclusively in the setting of HIV infection or other immunodeficiencies, and they typically involve mucosal sites {518,1902,2370}. It is important to distinguish PCLBCL-LT from iatrogenic immunodeficiency–associated lymphoproliferative disorders (including EBV-positive mucocutaneous ulcer), because these lymphoproliferative disorders may regress after reduction or withdrawal of immunosuppressive therapy {1404,2194}. In all cases, staging is necessary in order to distinguish PCLBCL-LT from secondary cutaneous DLBCL.

## Histogenesis

The postulated normal counterparts are peripheral B cells of post-germinal centre origin.

## Genetic profile

PCLBCL-LT has many genetic similarities to DLBCLs arising at other sites, but it has marked differences from PCFCL with a diffuse proliferation of large B cells. PCLBCL-LT has the gene expression profile of activated B-cell–like DLBCLs {1099}. Interphase FISH analysis commonly reveals translocations involving the *MYC*, *BCL6*, and IGH genes in PCLBCL-LT {991}. In one study using array comparative genomic hybridization and FISH analyses, high-level DNA amplifications of 18q21.31-21.33, including the *BCL2* and *MALT1* loci, were detected in 67% of cases {629}. Amplification of *BCL2* may explain the strong BCL2 expression in these cases, particularly given that t(14;18) translocation is not found in these lymphomas {629,992}. Loss of the *CDKN2A* and *CDKN2B* gene loci on chromosome 9p21.3 (by either gene deletion or promoter methylation) has been reported in as many as 67% of PCLBCL-LT cases, and correlates with an adverse prognosis {629,2382}. *MYD88* c.818T>C (p.L265P) mutations (found in 60–76% of cases), as well as mutations in genes encoding various components of the B-cell receptor signalling pathway, including *CARD11* (mutated in 10% of cases), *CD79B* (in 20%), and *TNFAIP3* (encoding TNFAIP3 [A20]; mutated in 40% of cases), strongly suggest constitutive NF-κB activation in PCLBCL-LT {1406,2050,2052}. In contrast, *MYD88* c.818T>C (p.L265P) mutations have not been detected in PCFCL with a diffuse proliferation of large B cells {1738}. The similarities in gene expression profile and cytogenetic alterations (including translocations and NF-κB–activating mutations) underscore that PCLBCL-LT may constitute the cutaneous counterpart of activated B-cell–like DLBCL {2052}.

## Prognosis and predictive factors

Some studies have reported a 5-year survival rate of approximately 50% {923,924,2737}; however, more-recent studies report a significantly better clinical outcome for patients when rituximab is added to a multiagent (i.e. CHOP or CHOP-like) chemotherapy regimen {925,997}. Multiple skin lesions at diagnosis, inactivation of *CDKN2A* (by either deletion or promoter hypermethylation), and *MYD88* c.818T>C (p.L265P) mutation have been reported to be associated with an inferior prognosis {629,923,924,2049,2381,2382}.

# Intravascular large B-cell lymphoma

Nakamura S.
Campo E.
Ponzoni M.

## Definition

Intravascular large B-cell lymphoma is a rare disease characterized by exclusively extranodal multiorgan involvement and the proliferation of lymphoma cells within the lumina of blood vessels (in particular capillaries, and with the exception of larger arteries and veins), without an obvious extravascular tumour mass. The skin is most commonly affected, with diverse dermatological manifestations.

## ICD-O code 9712/3

## Epidemiology

The median patient age at diagnosis is in the seventh decade, and there is no sex predilection. The frequency and clinical presentation differ depending on the geographical origin of the patient {326,765,1852,2086,2087,2126,2414}.

## Localization

This lymphoma is widely disseminated in extranodal sites and can present in virtually any organ, including apparently "normal" skin devoid of any obvious macroscopic abnormality, with sparing of lymph nodes. Sometimes lymphomatous cells may colonize the vessels of pre-existing cutaneous haemangiomas {2085}.

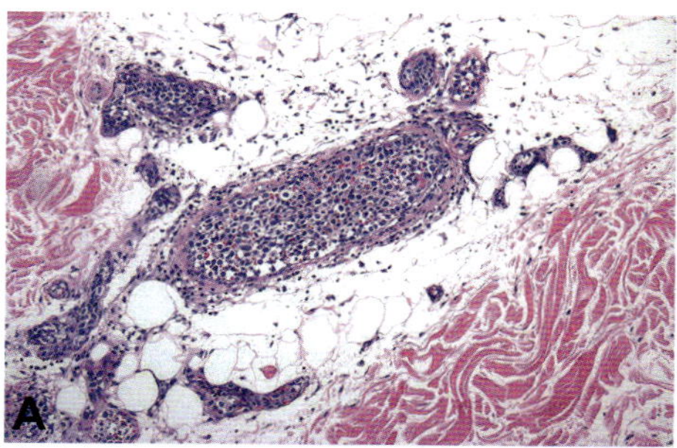


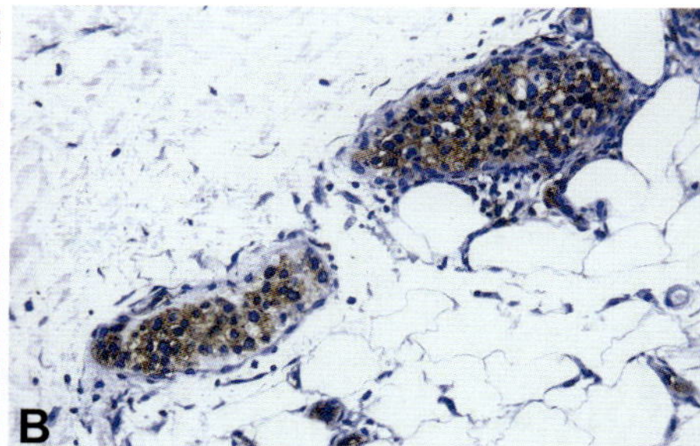


**Fig. 4.84** Intravascular large B-cell lymphoma. **A** In this random skin biopsy (including subcutaneous fat tissue), dilated vessels are filled with densely packed large neoplastic lymphoid cells. **B** The tumour cells are highlighted by immunostaining for CD20.

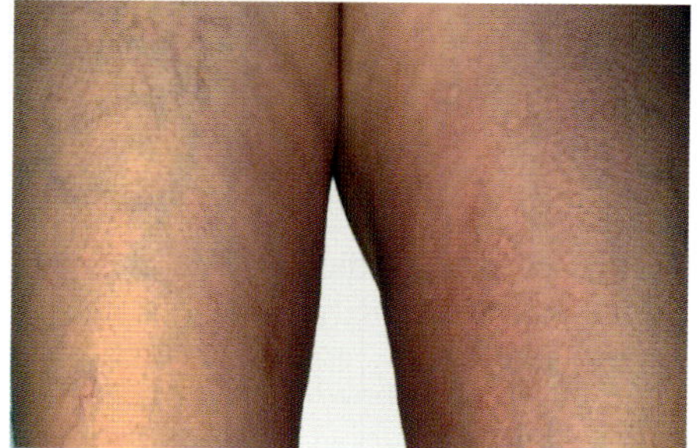

**Fig. 4.82** Intravascular large B-cell lymphoma. Involvement of the cutis, with livedoid erythema.

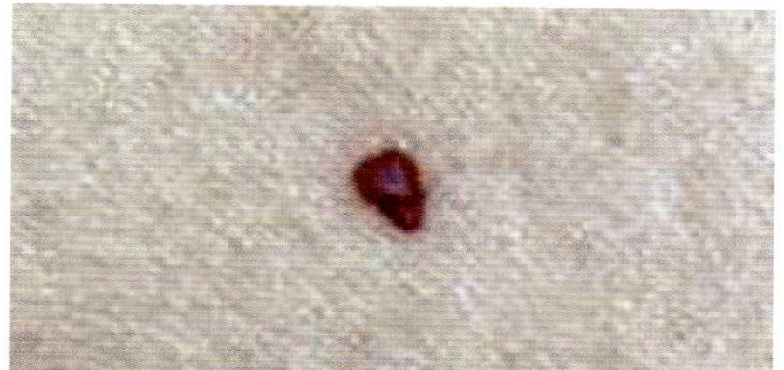

**Fig. 4.83** Intravascular large B-cell lymphoma. A senile haemangioma colonized by lymphoma cells.

## Clinical features

Two major clinical patterns are recognized: a so-called classic form (mostly present in western countries), which predominantly involves the skin and nervous system, and a haemophagocytic syndrome–associated form, originally documented as an Asian variant, in which patients present with multiorgan failure and peripheral blood cytopenias {326,765,1852,2086,2087,2414}. The cutaneous variant is a distinct form in which the tumour cells are confined to the skin at the time of diagnosis; it predominantly affects females and is more frequently encountered in the Western Hemisphere (where the cutaneous variant accounts for 24% of all cases) than in Asia (where it account for only 3%) {2087}. Skin lesions usually occur as erythematous macules, livid plaques, and ulcerated nodules on the upper arms, legs, abdomen, and inframammary area. Telangiectasias, oedema, and pain are often concomitant, simulating inflammatory skin diseases. Random deep biopsies of normal-looking skin (with the inclusion of subcutaneous fat tissue being mandatory) are helpful for definitive diagnosis {20,107,882,1386,1510,1698,2078}.

## Histopathology

Even in the haemophagocytic syndrome–associated form, the tumour cells often spare the dermis and are present in the subcutaneous tissue even when there is no skin eruption. They are large, have prominent nucleoli and frequent mitotic figures, and are confined to the lumina of small or intermediate vessels; minimal extravascular involvement may occur.

The tumour cells express B-cell–associated antigens. CD5 and CD10 expression is seen in 38% and 13% of cases, respectively. Most cases are positive for IRF4 (MUM1), indicative of a non–germinal centre B-cell subtype. The observed intravascular trapping of neoplastic cells might result from defects in homing receptors and adhesion molecules {767,2085,2416}.

## Histogenesis

The postulated normal counterpart is a post–follicle centre transformed B cell.

## Genetic profile

Clonal IG gene rearrangement has been detected, but few recurrent karyotypic abnormalities have been described {2414,2415}. Segmental tandem triplication of *KMT2A* (*MLL*) has been reported {604}. These lymphomas show high prevalence of *MYD88* L265P mutations and *CD79B* Y196 mutations {2531A}.

## Prognosis and predictive factors

Intravascular large B-cell lymphoma generally has a poor prognosis, but the cutaneous variant is associated with better survival {2414}. Rituximab-containing chemotherapies significantly improve outcome {764,766,2414,2415}.

# EBV-positive mucocutaneous ulcer

Jaffe E.S.
Dojcinov S.

## Definition

EBV-positive mucocutaneous ulcer affects patients with age-related or iatrogenic immunosuppression or HIV infection. Histologically, it contains Hodgkin-like, EBV-positive B cells in a mixed inflammatory background. It usually follows a self-limited, indolent course {641}. This is a provisional entity in the current classification.

## ICD-O code 9680/1

## Epidemiology

EBV-positive mucocutaneous ulcer occurs in the setting of defective surveillance for EBV, including due to advanced age, iatrogenic immunosuppression for autoimmune diseases (e.g. with methotrexate, azathioprine, ciclosporin, or TNF inhibitors), solid-organ transplantation, and HIV infection {331,1027,1889}. The median age at presentation is > 70 years (with a slight male preponderance), but iatrogenically immunosuppressed patients tend to be younger.

## Etiology

There is a strong association with EBV infection, resulting from defective immunosurveillance {641}. Reduced T-cell repertoire and functionality likely play a pathogenetic role, at least in elderly individuals {640}. EBV-positive mucocutaneous ulcer often involves sites with pre-existing inflammatory lesions due to a variety of unrelated causes {1456}.

## Localization

EBV-positive mucocutaneous ulcers are ulcerated lesions in the oropharyngeal mucosa (tonsils, tongue, buccal mucosa, and palate), skin, and gastrointestinal tract {331,640,641}. Evidence of bone marrow or systemic involvement should prompt consideration of other EBV-associated lymphomas {1883}.

## Clinical features

EBV-positive mucocutaneous ulcers are sharply circumscribed, isolated, indurated ulcers. Patients are without symptoms apart from those related to the ulcer or predisposing conditions.

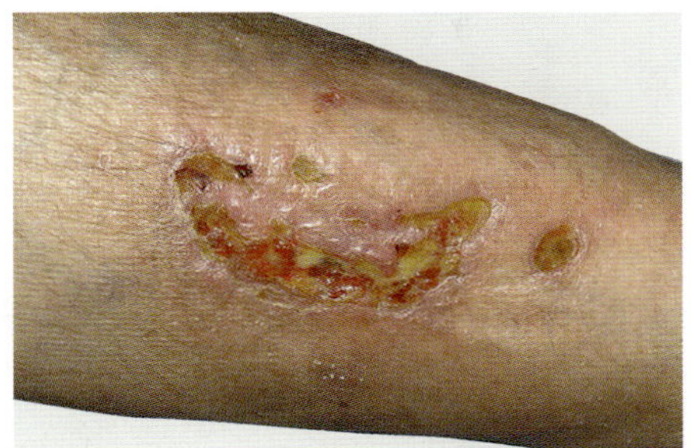

**Fig. 4.85** EBV-positive mucocutaneous ulcer. This lesion presented in a 75-year-old man on long-term azathioprine and prednisolone therapy for autoimmune haemolytic anaemia. The lesion developed on the lower leg, a site of chronic venous stasis. It rapidly enlarged following local trauma. Following reduction of immunosuppression, the lesion healed over a period of 9 weeks.

## Histopathology

The infiltrate underlying the ulcer is a polymorphic mixture of plasma cells, lymphocytes, histiocytes, and eosinophils, with scattered large transformed atypical immunoblasts with Hodgkin/Reed–Sternberg–like morphology. Focal necrosis can be present in addition to surface ulceration {640,641}. Histological distinction from classic Hodgkin lymphoma may be difficult; the diagnosis of classic Hodgkin lymphoma in the skin or mucosa should be rendered with extreme caution.

The large transformed cells are at least partially positive for CD20, but also express PAX5 and OCT2 and have a non-germinal centre (IRF4 [MUM1]+, CD10−, BCL6−) phenotype. CD30 is positive and CD15 is coexpressed in about half of all cases. LMP1 is typically coexpressed with EBV-encoded small RNA (EBER) in the cells with Hodgkin/Reed–Sternberg–like morphology. The background T lymphocytes are a mixture of CD4+ and CD8+ cells, with a distinctive rim at the base of the lesion.

## Differential diagnosis

The differential diagnosis includes polymorphic post-transplant lymphoproliferative disorder and EBV-positive diffuse large B-cell lymphoma NOS. Post-transplant lymphoproliferative disorder is generally not associated with cutaneous ulceration. EBV-positive diffuse large B-cell lymphoma rarely occurs as an isolated cutaneous or mucosal lesion.

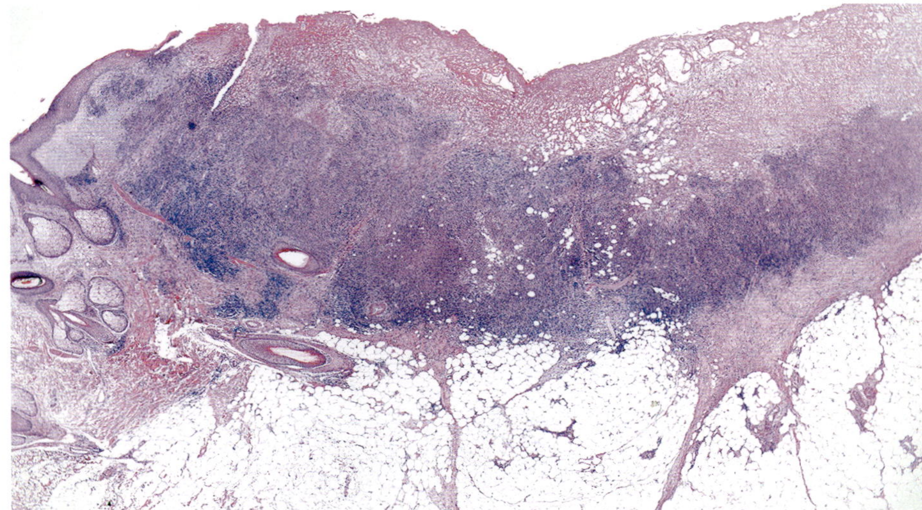

**Fig. 4.86** EBV-positive mucocutaneous ulcer. This lesion presented on the cheek of a 79-year-old man with no other risk factors; the skin surface is ulcerated and sharply demarcated from the adjacent epidermis; the dermis contains a dense, polymorphous infiltrate. A band of reactive lymphocytes lies at the base.

## Histogenesis

The postulated normal counterpart is an EBV-transformed post-germinal centre B cell.

## Genetic profile

Less than 50% of EBV-positive mucocutaneous ulcers show clonal IG gene rearrangements. A restricted (oligoclonal) T-cell repertoire is common, reflecting diminished T-cell response {620,640,641}.

## Prognosis and predictive factors

EBV-positive mucocutaneous ulcer follows a benign course, with nearly all reported cases responding to a reduction of immunosuppression without additional chemotherapy or radiotherapy. The outcome appears to be superior to that associated with other forms of post-transplant lymphoproliferative disorder {112,1712,2549,2873}.

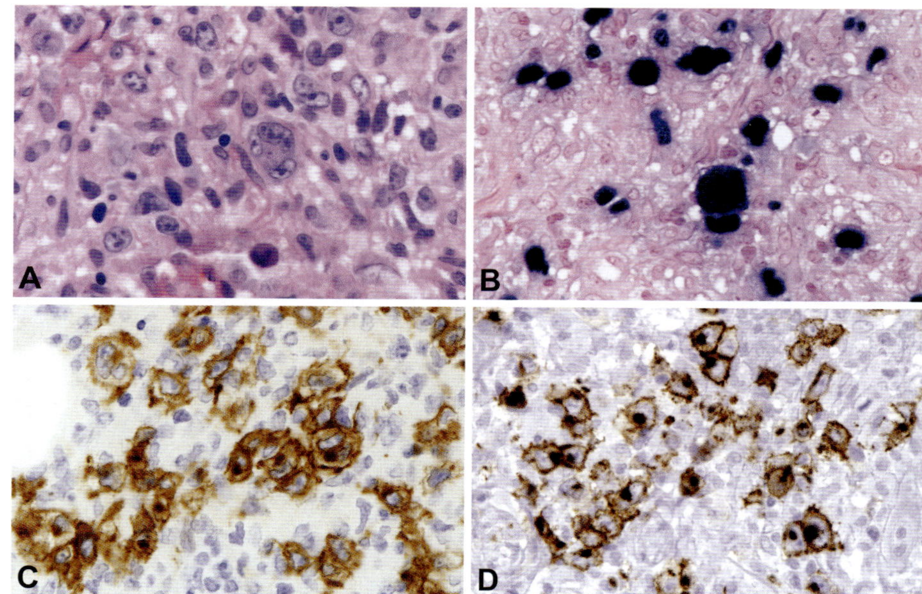

**Fig. 4.87** EBV-positive mucocutaneous ulcer, presenting in the skin of the right arm of a 75-year-old woman. **A** The infiltrate contains large Hodgkin/Reed–Sternberg–like (HRS-like) cells in a background of reactive histiocytes and lymphocytes. **B** The atypical lymphoid cells are positive for EBV, as demonstrated by in situ hybridization for EBV-encoded small RNA (EBER). **C** The atypical HRS-like cells are immunopositive for CD30 and also for CD15 (**D**).

# Lymphomatoid granulomatosis

Pittaluga S.
Jaffe E.S.

## Definition

Lymphomatoid granulomatosis is an angiocentric and angiodestructive lymphoproliferative disease involving extranodal sites; it is composed of EBV-positive B cells admixed with a predominance of reactive T cells. The skin is the most common extrapulmonary site of involvement.

## ICD-O codes

| Lymphomatoid granulomatosis | |
|---|---|
| Grade 1–2 | 9766/1 |
| Grade 3 | 9766/3 |

## Epidemiology

Lymphomatoid granulomatosis is rare. It usually presents in adults, with a male-to-female ratio of > 2:1 {1294,2480}.

## Etiology

With careful analysis, reduced immune function can usually be identified {2482,2837}. Some cases may be associated with underlying immunodeficiency {960,1008}.

## Localization

The skin (affected in 25–50% of cases) is the most common site of involvement apart from the lung, but cutaneous involvement is rarely (if ever) seen in the absence of pulmonary disease. The extremities and trunk are the most common locations {186,382,1105,1206,1294, 1295,1723,2480}.

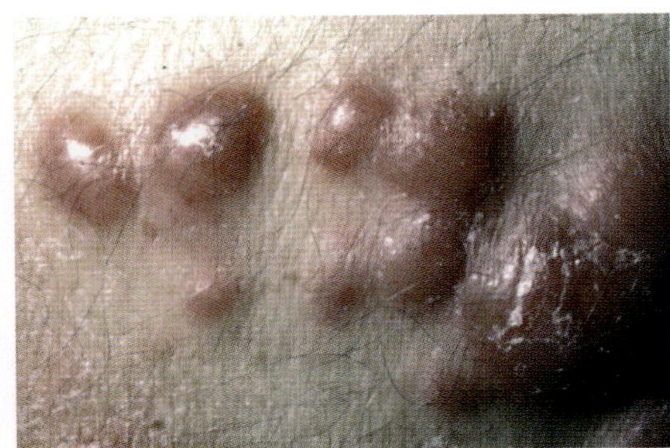

Fig. 4.88 Lymphomatoid granulomatosis. The larger nodules may show ulceration.
Adapted with permission from: Beaty MW et al. (2001) Am J Surg Pathol. 25:1111-20. Wolters Kluwer.

## Clinical features

Patients usually present with pulmonary symptoms {1206,1295,2480}. The skin lesions consist of multiple erythematous papules and/or subcutaneous nodules. Necrosis and ulceration are usually associated with larger nodules. Indurated plaques, lichen sclerosus–like lesions, and alopecia are less commonly seen {186,1212}. Cutaneous lesions rarely precede pulmonary disease; they are seen either at diagnosis (in 30% of cases) or later in the disease course {186}. Other sites of involvement include the brain, kidney, and liver. The lymph nodes and spleen are spared {1206,1294,1295,1433,2480}.

## Histopathology

Most cutaneous lesions show a lymphohistiocytic infiltration of the subcutaneous fat, with or without dermal involvement. Lymphocytic vasculitis is frequent, and fibrinoid necrosis may be present {2599}. Well-formed granulomas are usually absent, but a granulomatous reaction may be secondary to fat necrosis. EBV-positive B cells are often present in the lung, but they are generally rare to absent in the skin {186}. CD3+/CD4+ T cells predominate in these lesions. Grading is usually performed at the primary site of presentation (nearly always the lung).

## Histogenesis

The postulated normal counterpart is a mature B lymphocyte, transformed by EBV.

## Genetic profile

Clonal IG gene rearrangement is more often found in higher-grade lesions, most commonly grade 3. Clonal IG gene rearrangement is nearly always absent in the skin {2480}.

## Genetic susceptibility

Genetic susceptibility is associated with a variety of primary immunodeficiencies, such as Wiskott–Aldrich syndrome and X-linked lymphoproliferative syndrome.

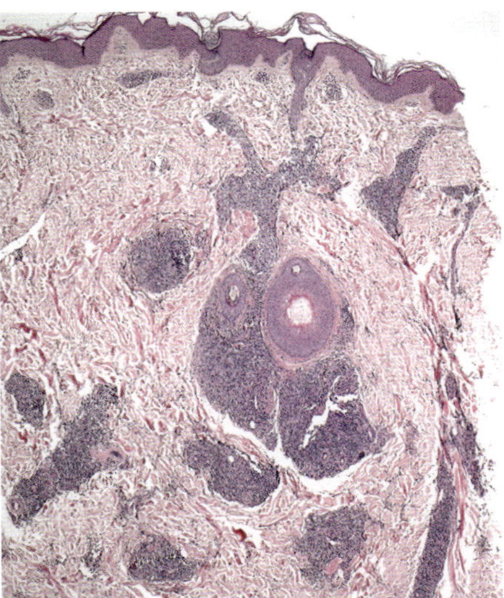

Fig. 4.89 Lymphomatoid granulomatosis. Histological features include a perivascular dermal infiltrate. Adapted with permission from: Beaty MW et al. (2001) Am J Surg Pathol. 25:1111-20. Wolters Kluwer.

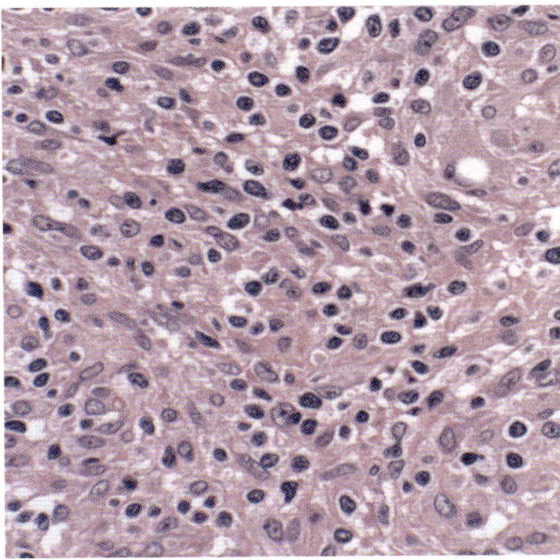

Fig. 4.90 Cutaneous lymphomatoid granulomatosis. Granulomatous panniculitis is a common histological pattern.

## Prognosis and predictive factors

The natural history of lymphomatoid granulomatosis is variable. In some patients, it may follow a waxing and waning clinical course, with spontaneous remissions. However, in most patients it is more aggressive {2231,2837,2837}. The most common cause of death is progressive pulmonary involvement. Skin lesions may appear without evidence of relapse at other sites {186,2837}.

# Cutaneous involvement in primarily extracutaneous B-cell lymphomas and leukaemias

Ferry J.A.
Jansen P.M.
Swerdlow S.H.

## Introduction

In addition to the various types of primary cutaneous B-cell lymphoma, the skin can also be involved secondarily by primarily systemic B-cell lymphomas and leukaemias. Published reports on secondary cutaneous B-cell lymphoma are scarce, and detailed information on clinical presentation, prognosis, and relative frequency is lacking. Additionally, the skin may be the primary site of presentation for some histological variants of lymphoma that are not unique to the skin, such as diffuse large B-cell lymphoma NOS and plasmablastic lymphoma. Plasmablastic lymphoma frequently involves a variety of extranodal mucosal, and sometimes cutaneous sites {518,2370}. Distinguishing between primary and secondary cutaneous B-cell lymphoma is important, because of differences in management and outcome.

Differences between primary cutaneous marginal zone lymphoma; primary cutaneous follicle centre lymphoma; and primary cutaneous diffuse large B-cell lymphoma, leg type, and their nodal counterparts involving the skin secondarily are discussed in the respective sections. Herein, the characteristics of skin localizations of mantle cell lymphoma, Burkitt lymphoma, and chronic lymphocytic leukaemia/small lymphocytic lymphoma (CLL/SLL) are discussed.

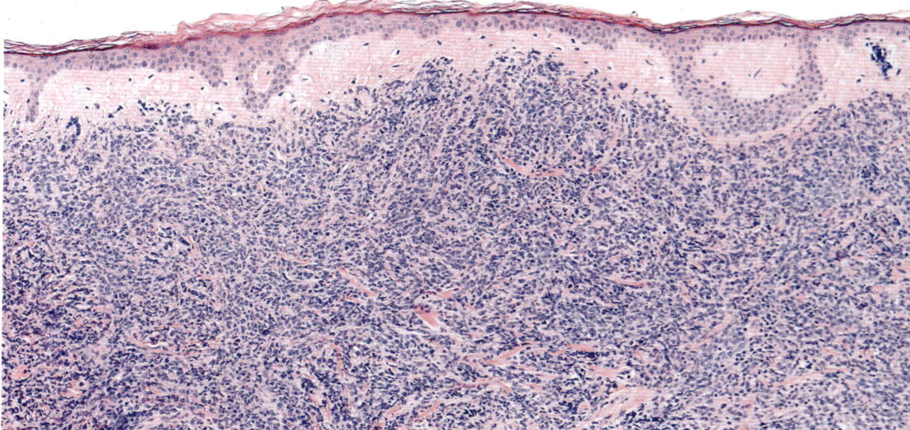

**Fig. 4.91** Mantle cell lymphoma (blastoid variant), involving skin. The patient was diagnosed with mantle cell lymphoma 6 years earlier, and had received aggressive therapy including bone marrow transplant. The patient relapsed with widespread disease, and died within 1 week of this skin biopsy being performed. The dermis is filled with a diffuse proliferation of blastoid cells; a grenz zone separates the infiltrate from the epidermis.

## Mantle cell lymphoma

### Definition
Mantle cell lymphoma is a B-cell neoplasm composed of monotonous, small to medium-sized cells. *CCND1* translocation is present in > 95% of cases.

### ICD-O code
9673/3

### Epidemiology
The skin is involved in 1–12% of mantle cell lymphoma cases {129,2293,2793}. Cutaneous mantle cell lymphoma affects older adults (median age: > 60 years), and the male-to-female ratio is about 3:1 {366,1134,2793}.

### Localization
The lesions, which are usually multiple, involve the trunk, lower extremities, head, and (infrequently) upper extremities {996,1186,2379,2793}.

### Clinical features
Mantle cell lymphoma can involve the skin at presentation or relapse, typically with widespread extracutaneous disease {129,366,2379,2793}. Primary cutaneous presentation of mantle cell lymphoma is rare {417,711,996,2379}. The lesions are nodules, infiltrated plaques, macules, or papules {366,1186,2379,2793}.

### Histopathology
Mantle cell lymphoma produces a nodular, diffuse, or perivascular/periadnexal infiltrate in the dermis (and sometimes the subcutis), with epidermal sparing {366}. Classic mantle cell lymphoma shows small to medium-sized lymphoid cells with dark, irregular nuclei, inconspicuous nucleoli, and scant cytoplasm. The blastoid variant, which is common among cutaneous cases, shows medium-sized cells with dispersed chromatin, frequent mitoses {366,417,711,2379}, and a Ki-67 proliferation index > 40% {2793}. The pleomorphic variant has larger, pleomorphic nuclei {996}.

Mantle cell lymphoma is typically positive for CD20, CD5, BCL2, and cyclin D1; SOX11 is positive in about 90% of cases. CD10, BCL6, and CD23 are usually negative {1134,1821,2379,2793}. Occasionally, cases can be CD5-negative {366,1186,1821,2379}, CD10-positive {417,2793}, or CD23-positive {89,2293}.

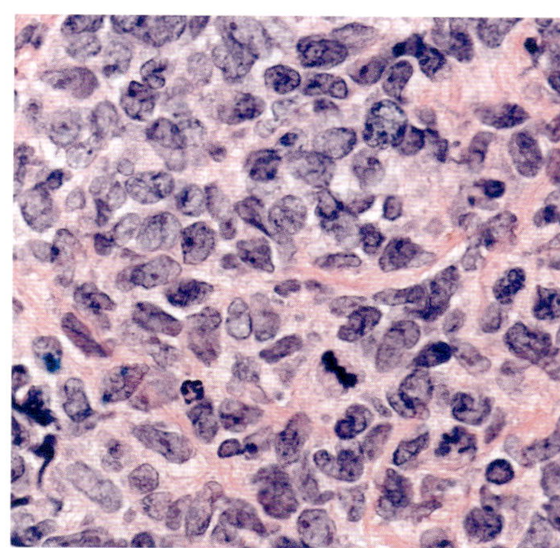

**Fig. 4.92** Mantle cell lymphoma (blastoid variant). The neoplastic cells are mitotically active, medium-sized atypical cells with oval and irregular nuclei, finely dispersed chromatin, occasional small nucleoli, and scant cytoplasm.

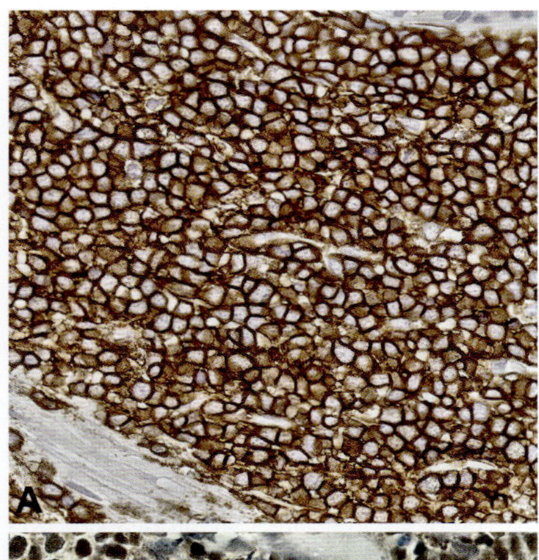


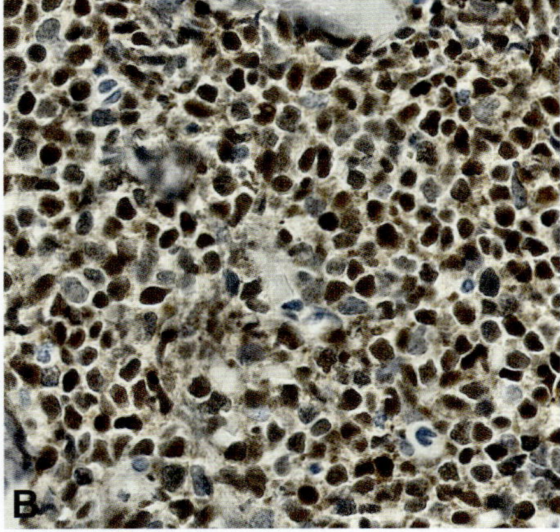


**Fig. 4.93** Mantle cell lymphoma showing strong immunostaining for CD20 (**A**) and cyclin D1 (**B**).

Infrequently, cyclin D1 or SOX11 can be negative {1134}.

### Histogenesis
The postulated normal counterpart is an inner follicle mantle B cell.

### Genetic profile
The t(11;14)(q13;q32) translocation, resulting in IGH/*CCND1* fusion, is characteristic {711,996,2379}. Common secondary changes include deletion and/or mutation of *ATM* and *TP53*, deletion of *CDKN2A* {2249}, and abnormalities of *MYC* {2890}.

### Prognosis and predictive factors
In general, the prognosis of mantle cell lymphoma is worse with older age, aggressive variants (blastoid and pleomorphic mantle cell lymphoma), a high proliferation index, a high-risk designation according to the Mantle Cell Lymphoma International Prognostic Index (MIPI), and increasing number of genetic alterations {89,129,2249,2293}.

## Burkitt lymphoma

### Definition
Burkitt lymphoma is a highly aggressive B-cell lymphoma with a germinal centre immunophenotype, typically with IG-*MYC* translocation. Skin involvement is extremely rare.

### ICD-O code 9687/3

### Epidemiology
Cutaneous Burkitt lymphoma occurs in the setting of HIV infection {531,2215}, as well as in individuals who are otherwise healthy. Only 2% of HIV-positive patients with Burkitt lymphoma have cutaneous involvement {596}. Nearly all patients with cutaneous Burkitt lymphoma are male, and adults are affected more commonly than children {125,531,899,2215}.

### Etiology
A subset of cases are related to immunodeficiency.

### Localization
The disease is often widespread {596,899,1202,2215}; it tends to involve the trunk and/or head {531,596}.

### Clinical features
Cutaneous involvement can be seen at presentation {531,899,2215} or relapse {125,899}, with subcutaneous nodules {125,596,899,2215} or (less often) macules, papules {596}, or large plaques {1202}, typically along with extracutaneous disease. The lesions are usually multiple and widespread, suggesting haematogenous dissemination {596,899}. The skin can be involved via extension from underlying lymphoma {125,596}.

### Histopathology
A diffuse infiltrate of medium-sized, monotonous lymphoid cells with round nuclei, finely clumped chromatin, multiple medium-sized basophilic nucleoli, and deeply basophilic cytoplasm involves the dermis and/or subcutis, sparing the epidermis. Mitoses are numerous. Interspersed apoptotic debris is often abundant. Tingible-body macrophages typically impart a so-called starry-sky appearance {125,596,721,899}. The neoplastic cells are positive for CD20, CD10, BCL6, and MYC and negative for BCL2 and TdT. EBV, as demonstrated by in situ hybridization for EBV-encoded small RNA (EBER), can be positive or negative, and the Ki-67 proliferation index is nearly 100%.

### Histogenesis
The postulated normal counterpart is a germinal centre B cell.

### Genetic profile
Translocation involving *MYC* and *IGH*, or less often *IGK* or *IGL*, is characteristic, with few other abnormalities. Translocations of *BCL2* and *BCL6* are absent.

### Prognosis and predictive factors
With appropriate therapy, the prognosis is good. Disseminated cutaneous involvement appears to be an unfavourable prognostic factor {596}.

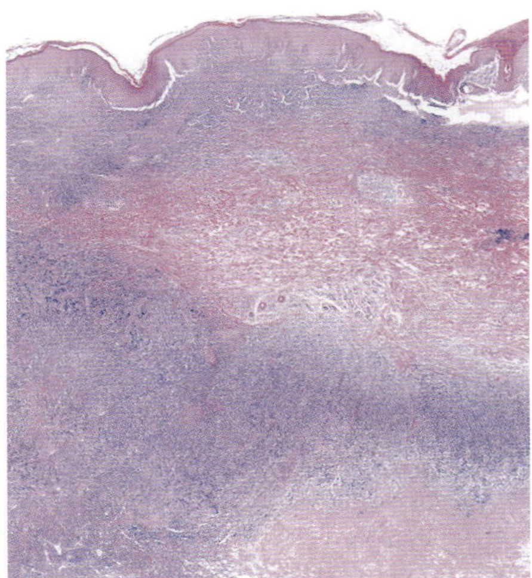

**Fig. 4.94** Burkitt lymphoma involving the skin and subcutaneous tissue. This low-power view shows a dense, diffuse infiltrate of lymphoid cells with foci of necrosis.

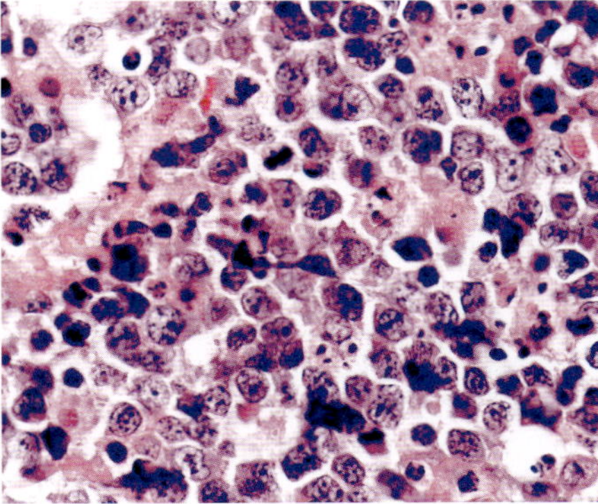

**Fig. 4.95** Burkitt lymphoma. High magnification with oil immersion shows that the infiltrate consists of medium-sized lymphoid cells with round to oval (occasionally irregular) nuclei, granular chromatin, and small nucleoli, with a few admixed tingible-body macrophages. The tumour cells were CD20+, CD10+, BCL6+, and BCL2−, with a very high proliferation index and with *MYC* translocation demonstrated by FISH.

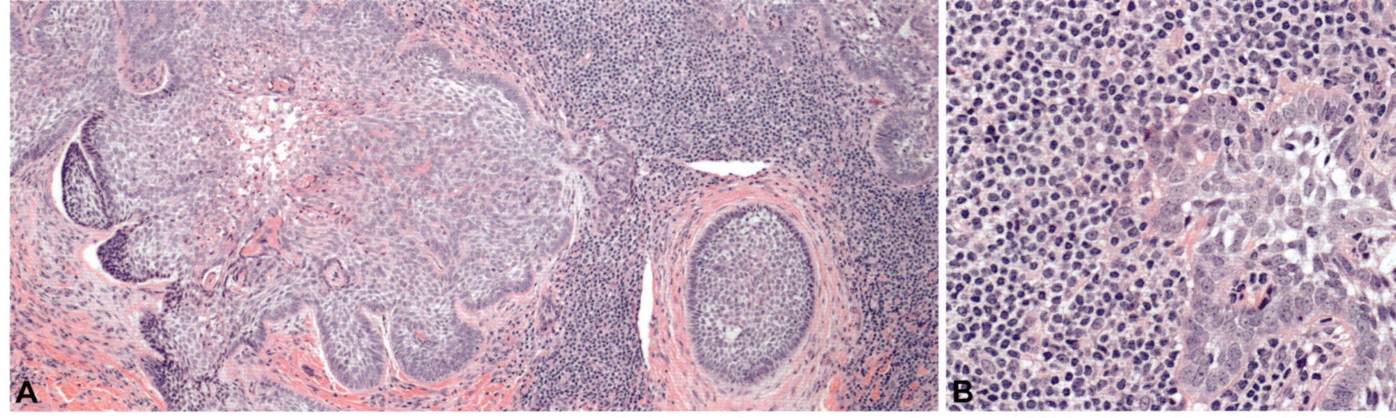

**Fig. 4.96** Chronic lymphocytic leukaemia/small lymphocytic lymphoma (CLL/SLL) involving the skin, with basal cell carcinoma (BCC), in a 75-year-old man with a history of CLL/SLL. **A** Dense lymphocytic infiltrate adjacent to foci of BCC. **B** Monotonous infiltrate of small lymphocytes surrounds a nest of BCC.

## Chronic lymphocytic leukaemia/small lymphocytic lymphoma

### Definition

Chronic lymphocytic leukaemia (CLL) is a small B-cell neoplasm characterized by ≥ 5 × $10^9$/L clonal B cells with a distinctive immunophenotype (typically CD20dim+, CD5+, CD23+, immunoglobulin light chain dim+) in the peripheral blood. Cases with extramedullary involvement and fewer clonal B cells in the blood are classified as small lymphocytic lymphoma. Cases with fewer circulating clonal B cells than in CLL, but without the extramedullary involvement characteristic of small lymphocytic lymphoma are classified as monoclonal B-cell lymphocytosis {420,2547}.

### ICD-O code

9823/3

### Epidemiology

CLL is the most common leukaemia among adults in the Western Hemisphere {420}. The skin is the most common extramedullary, extranodal site {2137}. Patients are middle-aged and older adults, with a median age at diagnosis in the seventh decade of life {414,1134,1262}. The male-to-female ratio is between 1.5:1 and 2:1 {414,1134,1262}.

### Etiology

In some cases, CLL cells may be recruited to the skin to participate in immunological reactions {414,2939}.

### Localization

Cutaneous lesions can be single, aggregated but localized, or generalized {414,2195}.

### Clinical features

Skin involvement by CLL usually occurs in patients already known to have CLL {414,1134,2137}, but in some cases, CLL is first detected in the skin {1353,1703,2071,2768}. The lesions are erythematous papules, plaques, nodules, or large tumours {414,1550,2071}. CLL may involve sites of herpes simplex virus or varicella zoster virus infection {414,1006,2939}, sites of other infections

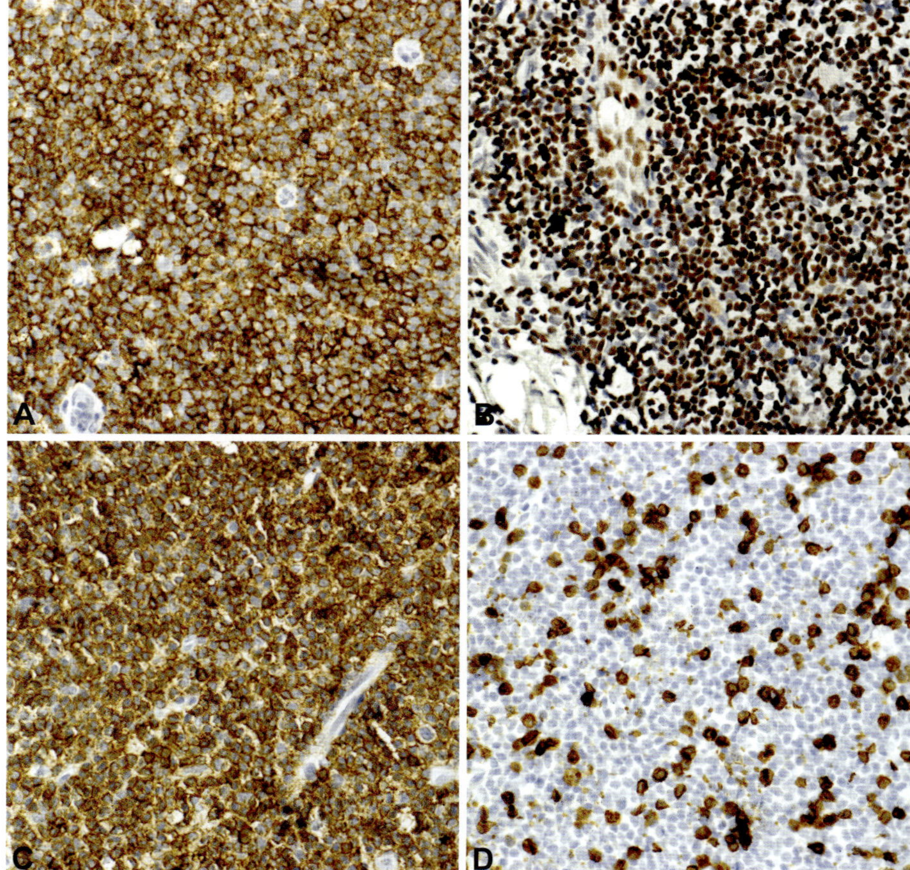

**Fig. 4.97** CLL/SLL involving skin. Immunostains show a predominance of CD20+ B cells (**A**) with co-expression of LEF1 (**B**) and CD5 (**C**). CD3+ T cells are a small minority (**D**).

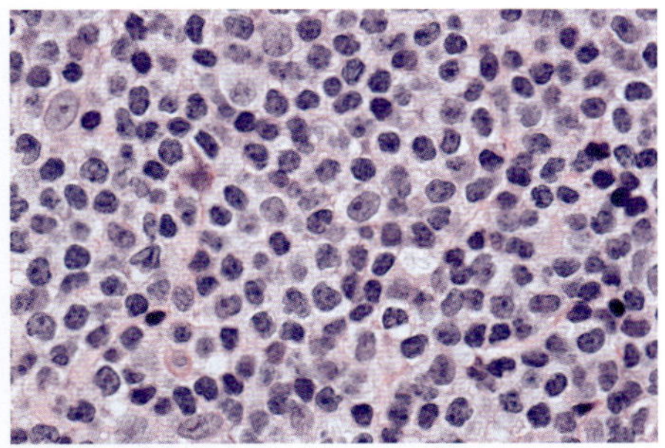

**Fig. 4.98** Chronic lymphocytic leukaemia/small lymphocytic lymphoma involving the skin. Most of the neoplastic cells are small lymphocytes with round to slightly irregular nuclei and scant pale cytoplasm. There are also infrequent prolymphocytes with larger oval nuclei and distinct nucleoli (at the centre of the field).

{1345,2071,2195}, foci of trauma {2071}, or stroma surrounding epithelial malignancies {1556,2768}.

## Histopathology

CLL/small lymphocytic lymphoma takes the form of a perivascular/periadnexal, nodular, diffuse, or (rarely) band-like infiltrate of small, monotonous lymphocytes in the dermis with extension to the subcutis {414,1262,2071}. Proliferation centres are uncommon {414,2939}. A variable number of T cells, occasionally eosinophils, and uncommonly granulomas are present in the infiltrate, in particular if another disease process is also present {414}.

The neoplastic cells typically have a CD20+, CD5+, CD23+, CD43+, CD10–, LEF1+, cyclin D1–, SOX11– phenotype {512,1134,1373,1550}.

Rarely, the skin is the site of transformation of CLL to diffuse large B-cell lymphoma (Richter syndrome) {414,656,1392}.

## Histogenesis

The postulated normal counterpart is a mature, antigen-experienced B cell.

## Genetic profile

IG genes are clonally rearranged {2575,2939}. Cytogenetic {639} and molecular genetic abnormalities {956} are variable. Information about cutaneous cases is limited.

## Genetic susceptibility

Individuals who have a family member with CLL are at a higher risk of developing the disease themselves {2461}.

## Prognosis and predictive factors

Adverse prognostic factors include older age, male sex, higher stage, worse Eastern Cooperative Oncology Group (ECOG) performance status, del(17p), del(11q), unmutated *IGHV*, and Richter syndrome {414,639,656,2048}. Skin involvement may not be an adverse prognostic factor {414,512,2127}.

# T-lymphoblastic and B-lymphoblastic leukaemia/lymphoma

Berti E.
Venkataraman G.

## Definition

Lymphoblastic leukaemia/lymphoma arises from immature/precursor lymphoid cells of T or B lineage. It presents in the bone marrow, peripheral blood, and/or solid tissues. Because of their common origin from precursor lymphoid cells and their similar clinical presentations, T-lymphoblastic leukaemia/lymphoma (T-ALL/LBL) and B-lymphoblastic leukaemia/lymphoma (B-ALL/LBL) are discussed here together.

## ICD-O codes

| | |
|---|---|
| T-lymphoblastic leukaemia/ lymphoma | 9837/3 |
| B-lymphoblastic leukaemia/ lymphoma | 9811/3 |

## Epidemiology

These entities, which are very uncommon, occur more frequently in children than in adults {2300}. In the paediatric population, 1.8% of all leukaemias involve the skin. B-ALL/LBL is more common than T-ALL/LBL {462,1780,2301}.

## Clinical features

Cutaneous manifestations usually occur simultaneously with nodal, extranodal, and blood involvement and present as solitary or multiple nodules. B-ALL/LBL often shows a solitary lesion in the head and neck region {262,1538}.

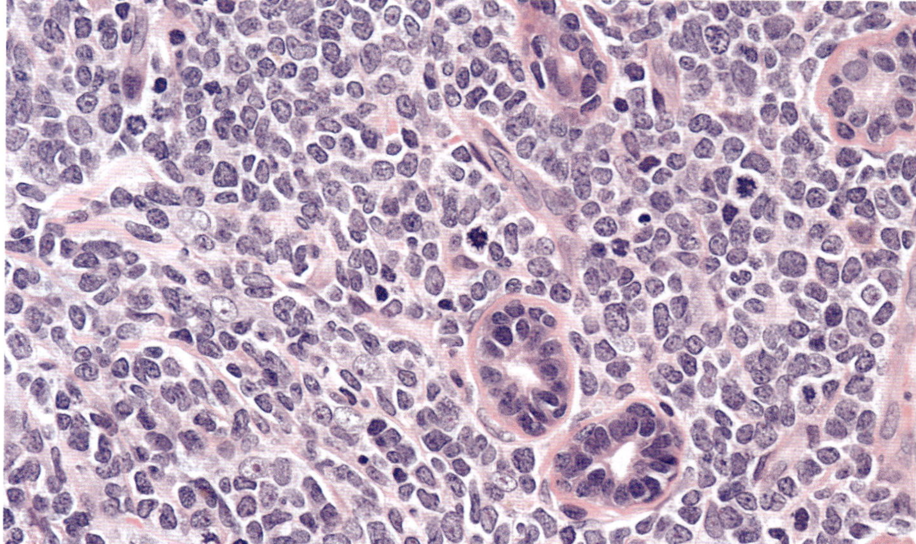

**Fig. 4.100** T-lymphoblastic leukaemia/lymphoma. Skin section showing a diffuse infiltrate of medium-sized to large lymphoblasts.

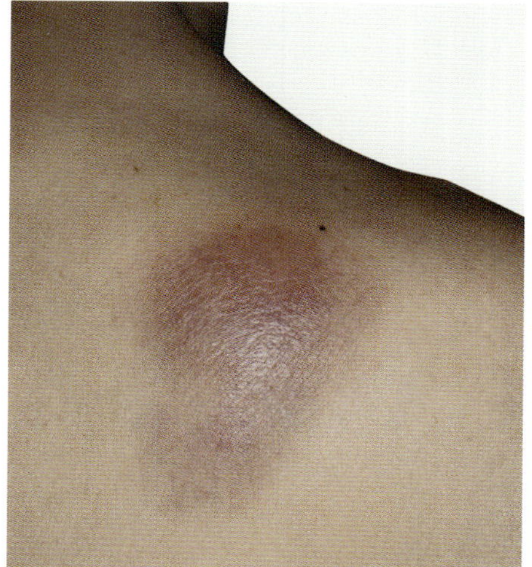

**Fig. 4.99** T-lymphoblastic leukaemia/lymphoma. A large nodular ecchymotic/purpuric lesion on the right shoulder.

## Histopathology

Both entities show a dense, monotonous dermal infiltrate of small to medium-sized blastic cells. The blasts spare the upper dermis and surround appendages, dissecting collagen fibres. Mitoses and apoptotic debris are associated with a high proliferation rate. Tumour-infiltrating lymphocytes are rare.

In T-ALL/LBL, CD34, TdT, and CD99 are positive. Cytoplasmic CD3 is expressed prior to surface CD3. T-cell markers, which are expressed according to the maturational stage, include CD1a, CD2, CD4, CD8, CD5, and CD7. Some cases variably express CD13, CD33, KIT (CD117), CD10, and/or CD79a {520,537,2064}.

In B-ALL/LBL, CD19, CD79a, CD22, TdT, CD10, CD24, and PAX5 are frequently expressed {327}. CD20 is usually negative. Cytoplasmic immunoglobulin heavy chain μ is expressed prior to IG light chain gene rearrangement and the expression of surface immunoglobulin.

## Histogenesis

The postulated normal counterpart is a precursor T or B lymphoblast.

## Genetic profile

IG and TR gene rearrangements are present in all cases of B-ALL/LBL and T-ALL/LBL, respectively. Cross-lineage rearrangements (i.e. clonal TR rearrangement in B-ALL/LBL) are frequent {2553}. Genetic studies have identified high-risk subgroups of *BCR-ABL1*–like B-lymphoblastic leukaemia and early T-cell precursor lymphoblastic leukaemia {537,1175}.

## Prognosis and predictive factors

Lymphoblastic leukaemias/lymphomas are aggressive diseases; however, they can be cured, in particular in children, with appropriate systemic multiagent chemotherapy. Clinical outcomes are largely determined by the phenotype and underlying genetic abnormalities.

# Blastic plasmacytoid dendritic cell neoplasm

Petrella T.
Facchetti F.
Pileri S.A.

## Definition

Blastic plasmacytoid dendritic cell neoplasm (BPDCN) is an aggressive tumour derived from the precursor of plasmacytoid dendritic cells (PDCs), characterized by high skin tropism and a tendency for bone marrow and leukaemic dissemination {855,2044}.

## ICD-O code 9727/3

## Epidemiology

This is a rare neoplasm, with no known race predilection. The male-to-female ratio is 3.3:1. Most patients are elderly, with a mean/median age at diagnosis of 61–67 years, but BPDCN can occur at any age, including in childhood {777,1070,1201}.

## Etiology

There are currently no clues to the etiology of BPDCN, but the association of some cases with myelodysplastic syndrome may suggest a related pathogenesis. There is no association with EBV.

## Localization

The disease tends to involve multiple sites, but the strongest predilection is for the skin (affected in 64–100% of cases), followed by the bone marrow, peripheral blood, and lymph nodes {1070,1672,2043}.

## Clinical features

Three types of skin presentation are most commonly observed: isolated (single or few) purplish-red tumours (seen in two thirds of cases); isolated (single or few) bruise-like papules; and disseminated purplish tumours, papules, and/or macules {535,1250}. Isolated tumours preferentially arise on the head and lower limbs and can be > 10 cm in diameter. The isolated bruise-like papule type is clinically very challenging. The disseminated type is the most characteristic. In some patients with leukaemic presentation and no skin involvement, the diagnosis is made on the basis of peripheral blood or bone marrow analysis. Regional lymphadenopathy at presentation is common (seen in 20% of cases). Peripheral blood and bone marrow involvement can be minimal at presentation, but invariably develops with progression of disease. Oral mucosal infiltration may be seen. Cytopenias (in particular thrombocytopenia) can be present at diagnosis {777,1070}. Following initial response to chemotherapy, relapses invariably occur, involving the skin alone or along with other sites. In most cases, a fulminant leukaemic phase ultimately develops {777}. About 10–20% of cases of BPDCN are associated with or develop into other myeloid neoplasms: chronic myelomonocytic leukaemia (most frequently), myelodysplastic syndrome, or acute myeloid leukaemia {1070,1354,2043,2747}. BPDCN must be distinguished from mature PDC proliferation, which can also present with skin manifestations {577,2045,2739,2747}.

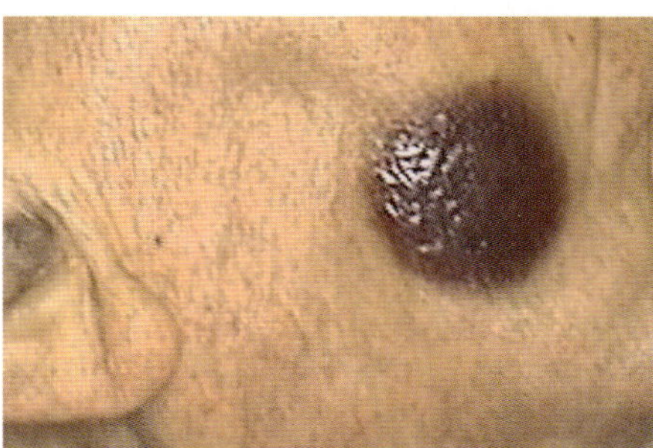

**Fig. 4.101** Blastic plasmacytoid dendritic cell neoplasm. Solitary purplish-red tumour on the right cheek.

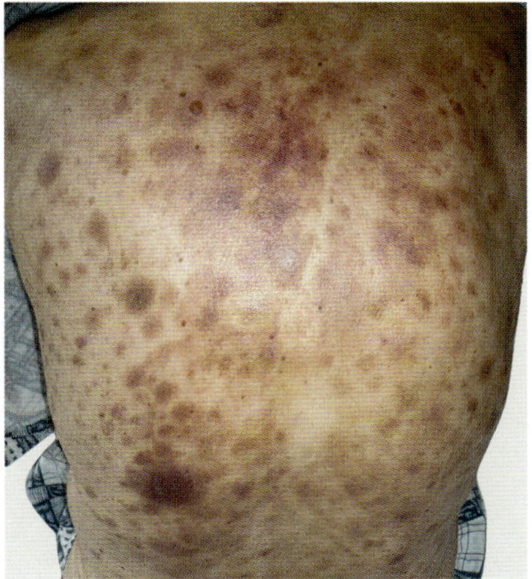

**Fig. 4.102** Blastic plasmacytoid dendritic cell neoplasm. Disseminated erythematous, brownish, or violaceous plaques and tumours.

## Histopathology

BPDCN is characterized by a dermal infiltrate of medium-sized blast cells {535,1070,1249,2044}. The nuclei have an irregular contour, fine chromatin, and one to several small nucleoli. The cytoplasm is usually scant and appears greyish-blue and agranular when Giemsa-stained. Mitoses are variable in number. Angioinvasion and necrosis are absent.

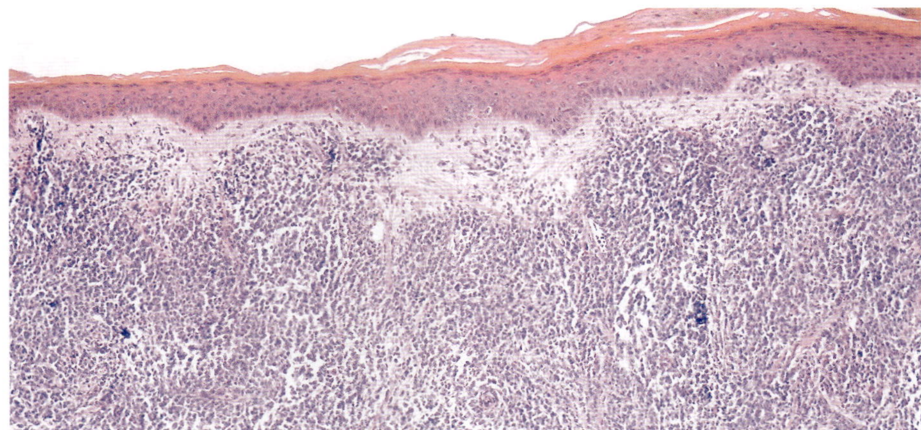

**Fig. 4.103** Blastic plasmacytoid dendritic cell neoplasm. Low-magnification view of a skin biopsy showing dense and diffuse monomorphous infiltration of the dermis, separated from the epidermis by a grenz zone.

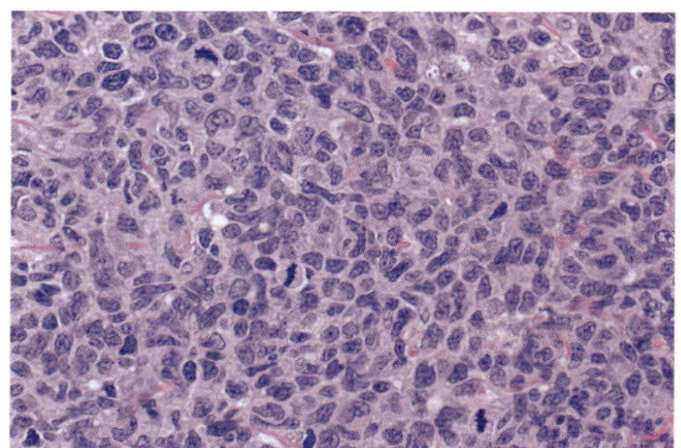

**Fig. 4.104** Blastic plasmacytoid dendritic cell neoplasm. A high-magnification view of an H&E-stained skin biopsy showing medium-sized cells with slightly irregular nuclei, small nucleoli, and scant cytoplasm; a few mitoses are present.

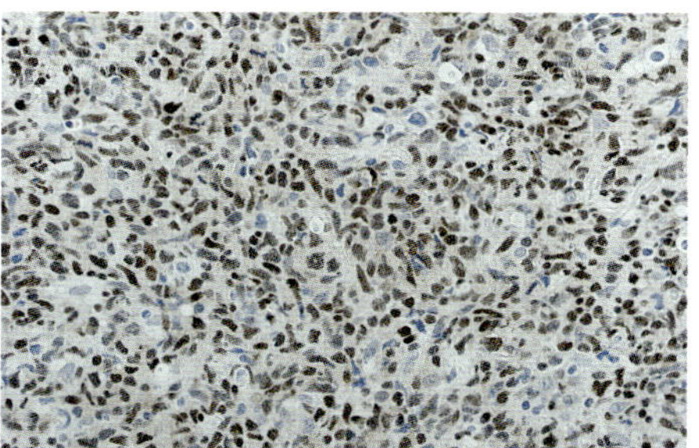

**Fig. 4.105** Blastic plasmacytoid dendritic cell neoplasm. The neoplastic cells show nuclear staining for TCF4 (E2-2).

The epidermis is generally spared, separated from the infiltrate by a grenz zone. Tumour cells express CD4 and CD56, as well as the PDC-associated antigens CD123, CD303 {1220,2063}, TCL1 {1071}, CD2AP, MX1 {2678}, SPIB, and TCF4 (E2-2) {1070,1249,1817,2063}. In about 8% of cases, CD4 or CD56 can be negative, but this does not rule out the diagnosis if other PDC-associated antigens are expressed. CD20, granzyme B, and CD34 are negative. CD79a, CD2, CD7, and KIT (CD117) may occasionally be positive. CD68 is detected in 50–80% of cases, in the form of small cytoplasmic dots. S100 protein is expressed in 25–30% of cases and even more frequently in children {1222}. TdT is positive in about one third of cases, with expression in 10–80% of cells. BCL2 is typically expressed (unlike in normal PDCs) {405,2315}. EBV is negative.

## Differential diagnosis

The main differential diagnosis is skin localization of myeloproliferative or myelodysplastic syndromes (myeloid leukaemia cutis) {206}.

## Histogenesis

The normal counterpart is the precursor of the PDC.

## Genetic profile

BPDCN gene expression analysis reveals a signature related to myeloid resting PDCs. Compared with normal PDCs, BPDCN shows overexpression of genes involved in Notch signalling {630}. There is also overexpression of genes involved in the BCL2 and NF-κB pathways, a finding that suggests various potential therapeutic targets {1816,2315}. Recurrent somatic mutations have been detected, affecting *TET2*, *ASXL1*, the RAS gene family, *IKZF3*, *ATM*, *MET*, *KRAS*, *IDH2*, *KIT*, *APC*, *RB1*, *VHL*, *BRAF*, *MLH1*, *TP53*, and *RET* {49,1216,1737,2506}. Several of these genes are involved in DNA methylation and chromatin remodelling. Conflicting findings concerning *NPM1* mutations have been reported {727,1737,2506}. Recently, a druggable TCF4-dependent and BRD4-dependent transcriptional network was described {405}.

## Prognosis and predictive factors

The median survival is 10.0–19.8 months. Most patients (80–90%) show an initial response to multiagent chemotherapy, but relapse shortly thereafter {1201,1250,1966}. Age has an adverse impact on prognosis {2541}, and long-term survival has been reported in 36% of paediatric patients {1222}. Factors that have been associated with shorter survival include extensive marrow or peripheral blood blastosis, low TdT expression {1220}, positivity for CD303 (also called CLEC4C and BDCA2), a low Ki-67 proliferation index, *CDKN2A*/*CDKN2B* deletions {1597}, and mutations in DNA methylation pathway genes {1737}. In one study, lymphoblastic leukaemia induction treatment seemed to be more effective than acute myeloid leukaemia–oriented therapy in both children and adults {2056}. For patients in their first complete remission, allogeneic haematopoietic stem cell transplantation is the best way to achieve long-term survival {566,2228}.

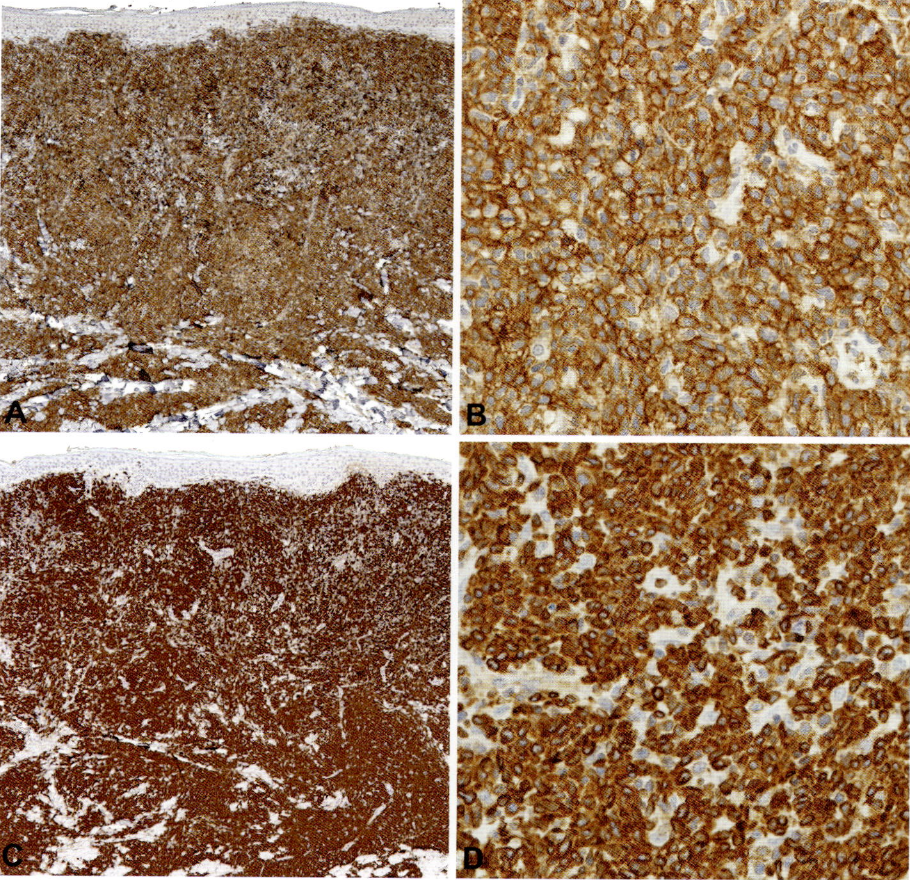


**Fig. 4.106** Blastic plasmacytoid dendritic cell neoplasm. The neoplastic cells show strong immunoreactivity for CD123 (**A**), CD303 (BDCA2) (**B**), TCL1 (**C**), and BCL2 (**D**).

# Cutaneous involvement in myeloid leukaemia

Venkataraman G.
Vardiman J.W.

## Definition

Myeloid leukaemias are clonal neoplastic proliferations of myeloid cells that arise from progenitor cells in the bone marrow. In acute myeloid leukaemia (AML), increased numbers of blasts are found in the bone marrow (and usually in the peripheral blood), and blasts may also infiltrate other tissues such as the skin, either as solid aggregates or as blastic infiltrates of variable density. *BCR-ABL1*+ chronic myeloid leukaemia and chronic myelomonocytic leukaemia are characterized by increased numbers of maturing and mature but abnormal granulocytes and/or monocytes in the marrow and blood; the neoplastic cells may also infiltrate non-haematopoietic tissues such as the skin, most commonly in the blast phase of disease. The finding of a cutaneous infiltrate of blasts in the setting of a previously diagnosed myeloid neoplasm is sufficient evidence for the diagnosis of blast-phase disease.

## ICD-O code 9930/3

## Synonyms

Extramedullary myeloid tumour; granulocytic sarcoma; myeloid sarcoma

## Epidemiology

Cutaneous involvement occurs in 3–10% of AML cases in adults aged > 50 years {25,466,1160}.

## Clinical features

In most cases, cutaneous involvement is concurrent with AML, but it may precede blood or marrow disease and can also be the first manifestation of relapse {1023,1083,1160,1229}. Isolated cutaneous involvement without blood or marrow involvement is rare {14,2877}. Cutaneous involvement is more common in monocytic leukaemias than in other AMLs {1160}, and it tends to be more severe in AML with mutated *NPM1* {1598}.

Skin involvement presents as papules, nodules, or plaques on the torso (in 40% of cases), the extremities (in 41%), or the head and neck region (in 16%). Gingival involvement is characteristic of acute monocytic leukaemia {652}.

## Histopathology

There is diffuse or nodular involvement of the dermis sparing the grenz zone. The blasts are medium-sized monomorphic cells with round, oval, or folded nuclei. They have pale, finely dispersed chromatin and small nucleoli. In chronic myelomonocytic leukaemia, cutaneous involvement often occurs as infiltration by mature plasmacytoid dendritic cells {2739,2747}.

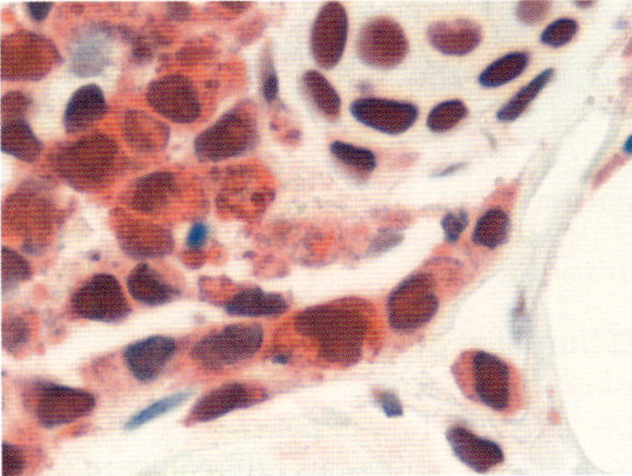

**Fig. 4.108** Cutaneous involvement in myeloid leukaemia. Neoplastic cells with abnormal cytoplasmic NPM1 immunostaining (normal eccrine glands are visible at the right, with a nuclear-restricted pattern); *NPM1*-mutated cases are often negative for CD34.

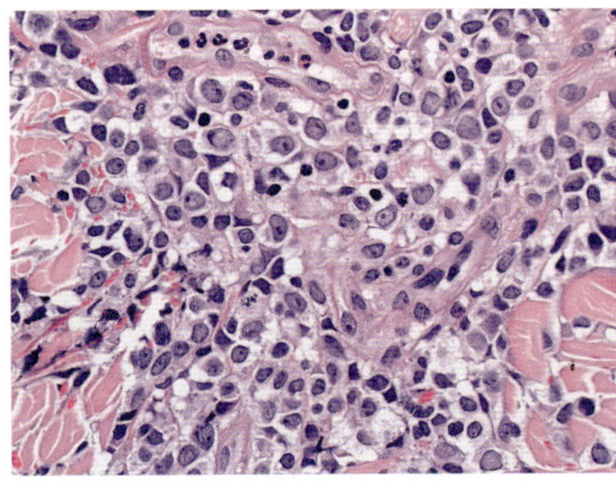

**Fig. 4.109** Acute myeloid leukaemia. Medium-sized blast cells with fine chromatin infiltrate the dermis.

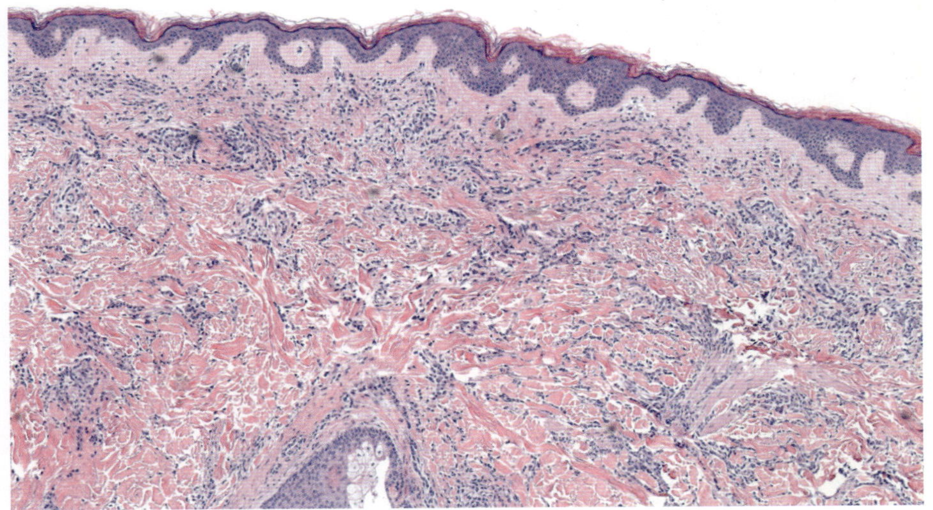

**Fig. 4.107** Cutaneous involvement in myeloid leukaemia. A diffuse blastic infiltrate involving papillary and reticular dermis, separated from the epidermis by a grenz zone.

The neoplastic cells are positive for CD43. CD34 and KIT (CD117) positivity indicates a haematopoietic/precursor phenotype. Expression of lysozyme, CD68, MPO, and/or CD33 confirms a myeloid or monocytic origin {206,1263}. CD14 and KLF4 are both sensitive and specific for monocytic differentiation {1623}. Abnormal cytoplasmic NPM1 immunolocalization is a useful feature because *NPM1*-mutated AMLs are monocytic and often negative for CD34, KIT, and MPO {730}. CD7 and sometimes CD2 are expressed. However, the blasts are typically negative for other B- and T-lineage–associated antigens.

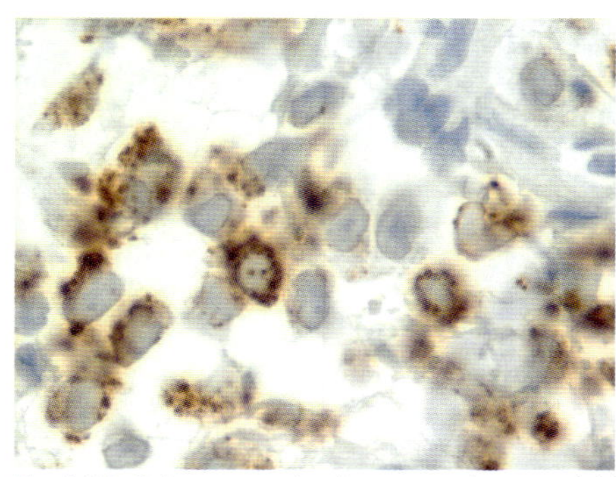

**Fig. 4.110** Cutaneous involvement in myeloid leukaemia. CD68 is expressed in the cytoplasm of leukaemic cells, confirming myeloid/monocytic differentiation.

## Differential diagnosis

Blastic plasmacytoid dendritic cell neoplasm exhibits clinical overlap (leukaemic and cutaneous presentation) and morphological overlap (variable CD4 and CD56 expression) with AML. Expression of CD4, CD56, and CD123 or TCL1 in conjunction with negativity for lysozyme and MPO favours a diagnosis of blastic plasmacytoid dendritic cell neoplasm over a myeloid leukaemia {547,2304}.

## Histogenesis

Myeloid leukaemia arises from myeloid progenitor cells.

## Genetic profile

Few data are available regarding cutaneous-specific cases of myeloid leukaemia. Trisomy 8, del(7q), and 11q23 abnormalities are the most commonly reported chromosomal abnormalities {25,1160}. *NPM1* is the gene most frequently mutated in myeloid leukaemia (followed by *PTPN11*); in AMLs, *NPM1* mutation is associated with the development of cutaneous involvement, with mutation detected in > 50% of leukaemia cases with cutaneous involvement {730,1598}. For cases in which cutaneous involvement precedes evidence of blood and/or bone marrow involvement, every effort should be made to perform cytogenetic or molecular genetic studies on the neoplastic cells from the skin biopsy; the findings of such studies are the most important prognostic indicators and may also provide information regarding targets for therapy.

## Prognosis and predictive factors

Prognosis is largely dependent on the genetics underlying the concurrent AML, and most cutaneous cases follow an aggressive clinical course despite systemic chemotherapy {1160}. In chronic myelomonocytic leukaemia, skin involvement often heralds transformation to AML {1694}.

# Cutaneous mastocytosis

Hartmann K.
Horny H.-P.
Valent P.

## Definition

Mastocytosis is characterized by an abnormal accumulation of clonal tissue mast cells {1128} and can involve various organs, most commonly the skin and bone marrow. The classification of mastocytosis includes cutaneous and systemic categories {1028,2686,2687}. In cutaneous mastocytosis, the skin is the primarily affected site, but cutaneous involvement also occurs in patients with systemic mastocytosis. In adults, cutaneous mastocytosis is diagnosed on the basis of typical skin lesions, absence of bone marrow infiltrates, and absence of other diagnostic criteria for systemic mastocytosis; a bone marrow investigation is therefore required. In children, cutaneous mastocytosis is also diagnosed on the basis of typical cutaneous lesions and symptoms, but because of the well-known rarity of systemic involvement in children, a bone marrow investigation is usually not required. Cutaneous involvement can be categorized into three subforms, based on skin lesion type: maculopapular cutaneous mastocytosis (urticaria pigmentosa), diffuse cutaneous mastocytosis, and cutaneous mastocytoma.

## ICD-O codes

| | |
|---|---|
| Cutaneous mastocytosis | 9740/1 |
| Mast cell sarcoma | 9740/3 |
| Indolent systemic mastocytosis | 9741/1 |
| Aggressive systemic mastocytosis | 9741/3 |
| Systemic mastocytosis with an associated haematological neoplasm | 9741/3 |
| Mast cell leukaemia | 9742/3 |

## Epidemiology

Mastocytosis can occur at any age, but onset in childhood is more common overall. In most paediatric patients, onset occurs during the first 6 months after birth {2820}. Few patients present with congenital disease. Rarely, mastocytosis onset occurs in patients aged 2–15 years. Adult-onset disease typically develops in patients aged < 50 years. Patients with childhood-onset mastocytosis usually have cutaneous mastocytosis, whereas most patients with adulthood-onset disease have systemic mastocytosis. Cutaneous mastocytosis and systemic mastocytosis both affect males and females equally {316,508,2058}. Familial mastocytosis has also been reported, but it is extremely rare {1029,1334}.

**Table 4.05** Classification of mastocytosis

| |
|---|
| **Cutaneous mastocytosis** |
| Maculopapular cutaneous mastocytosis (urticaria pigmentosa) |
| Monomorphic maculopapular cutaneous mastocytosis |
| Polymorphic maculopapular cutaneous mastocytosis |
| Diffuse cutaneous mastocytosis |
| Cutaneous mastocytoma |
| **Systemic mastocytosis** |
| Indolent systemic mastocytosis |
| Smouldering systemic mastocytosis |
| Systemic mastocytosis with an associated haematological neoplasm (systemic mastocytosis with an associated clonal haematological non–mast cell lineage disease) |
| Aggressive systemic mastocytosis |
| Mast cell leukaemia |
| **Mast cell sarcoma** |

## Localization

The localization of skin lesions depends on the subform of cutaneous mastocytosis (Table 4.05) {1028,2820}. Patients with the monomorphic variant of maculopapular cutaneous mastocytosis usually develop lesions on their thighs and trunk. Lesions then slowly spread to the periphery and distal extremities. The face and scalp are only rarely involved. Diffuse

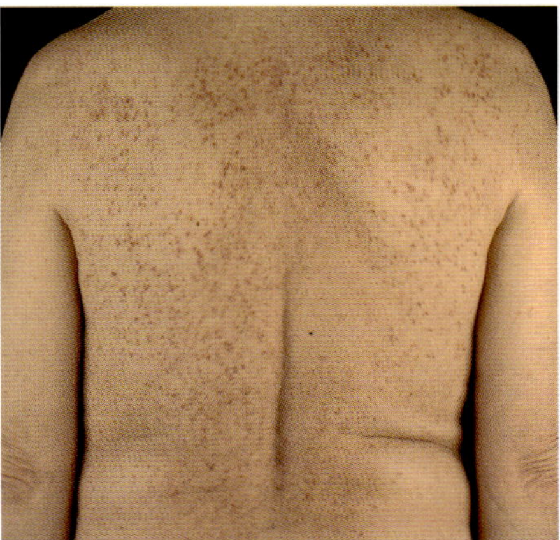

**Fig. 4.111** Maculopapular cutaneous mastocytosis (urticaria pigmentosa), monomorphic variant. This subform is typically characterized by monomorphic, small, symmetrically distributed, brown maculopapular lesions. Usually, the lesions first appear on the thighs and trunk and then spread to the extremities. This variant is mostly observed in adults and is often associated with systemic mastocytosis.

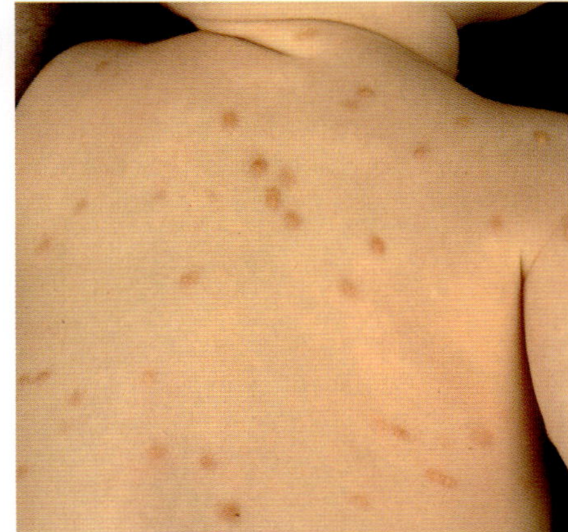

**Fig. 4.112** Maculopapular cutaneous mastocytosis (urticaria pigmentosa), polymorphic variant. This subform presents with polymorphic, large, randomly distributed, brown maculopapular or nodular lesions. All body areas, including the scalp and face, may be involved. This variant only occurs in children; it has a favourable prognosis, with spontaneous resolution after several years.

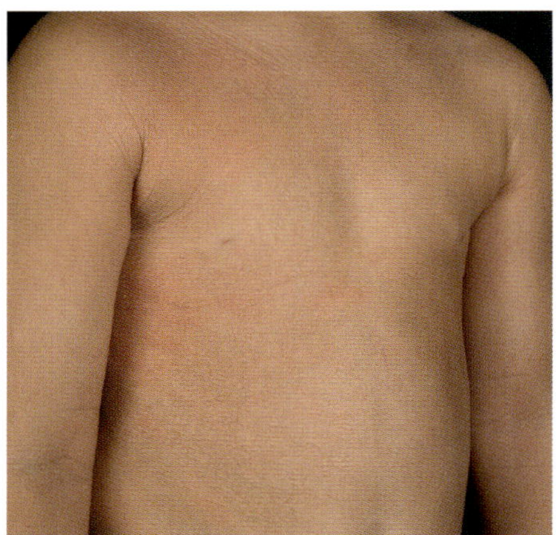

**Fig. 4.113** Diffuse cutaneous mastocytosis. This subform is defined by oedematous erythroderma with a brown or yellow tint; small papules may appear along tension lines; patients show pronounced and persistent dermographism in response to minor mechanical irritation; affected infants frequently develop blisters.

**Table 4.06** Diagnostic criteria for mastocytosis

**Cutaneous mastocytosis**

Major criterion:

- Skin lesions typical of mastocytosis, associated with the Darier's sign

Minor criteria:

- Increased numbers of mast cells in biopsy sections of lesional skin
- (Activating) *KIT* mutation in lesional skin tissue

**Systemic mastocytosis**

Major criterion:

- Multifocal dense infiltrates of mast cells (≥ 15 mast cells in aggregates) in sections of bone marrow and/or other extracutaneous organ(s)

Minor criteria:

- In biopsy sections of bone marrow or other extracutaneous organs, > 25% of mast cells in the infiltrate are spindle-shaped or have atypical morphology, or > 25% of all mast cells in bone marrow aspirate smears are immature or atypical
- An activating point mutation at codon 816 of *KIT* in the bone marrow, blood, or another extracutaneous organ
- Mast cells in bone marrow, blood, or another extracutaneous organ express CD25 (with or without CD2) in addition to normal mast cell markers
- Serum total tryptase is persistently > 20 ng/mL, unless there is an associated myeloid neoplasm, in which case this parameter is not valid

cutaneous mastocytosis usually involves the skin of the whole body. Cutaneous mastocytomas occur at all body sites, with a slight predilection for the trunk and scalp.

## Clinical features

Cutaneous involvement is observed in 100% of patients with cutaneous mastocytosis (by definition), about 80% of patients with indolent systemic mastocytosis, and 30% of patients with advanced systemic mastocytosis {1028}. In all categories of mastocytosis with skin involvement, cutaneous symptoms such as swelling, reddening, pruritus, or (in infants only) blistering can occur, as a result of local mast cell activation. The Darier's sign, which is the classic diagnostic hallmark of cutaneous mastocytosis (and cutaneous involvement in systemic mastocytosis), is defined by swelling and reddening of lesional skin upon stroking. Two clinical variants of cutaneous mastocytosis occur in children {1028}. The polymorphic variant, which is more common, is characterized by brown or red lesions of various sizes. The rarer monomorphic variant is characterized by small round lesions resembling those seen in adults.

Patients with cutaneous mastocytosis or systemic mastocytosis often experience systemic symptoms caused by mast cell–derived mediators; such symptoms include headache, peptic ulcerative disease, diarrhoea, and hypotension. Severe mediator-related symptoms are especially common in patients with a concomitant IgE-dependent allergy {314,2058}. Insect venom allergies are identified in a substantial proportion of patients with cutaneous mastocytosis or indolent systemic mastocytosis {266,1905,2255}, and these patients may develop life-threatening anaphylaxis. Systemic mastocytosis is also associated with a higher risk of osteopenia, osteoporosis, and pathological fractures {316,2121,2240,2241}.

The serum level of tryptase, an enzyme almost exclusively produced by mast cells, serves as a biomarker of mastocytosis (Table 4.06) {1697,2356,2495}. Patients with cutaneous mastocytosis usually have tryptase levels < 20 ng/L, whereas patients with systemic mastocytosis usually have tryptase levels

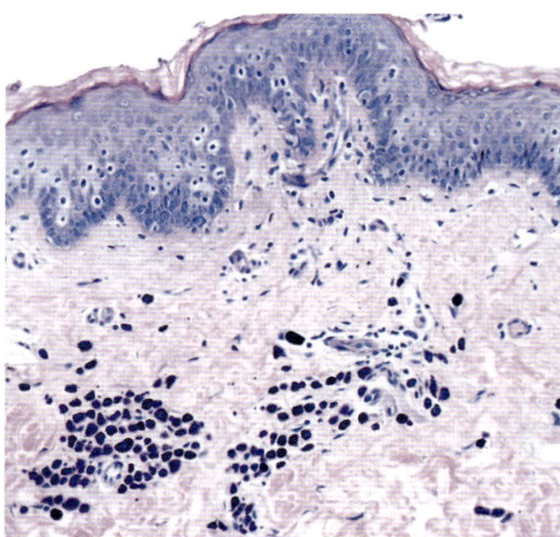

**Fig. 4.116** Maculopapular cutaneous mastocytosis (urticaria pigmentosa) in an adult patient. The typical histological findings in maculopapular cutaneous mastocytosis are loosely scattered or grouped mast cells in the dermis. In this example, the mast cells are exclusively round, with a hypergranular appearance. Phenotypically, these findings can be interpreted as well-differentiated mastocytosis; accordingly, this case showed no bone marrow involvement (Giemsa stain).

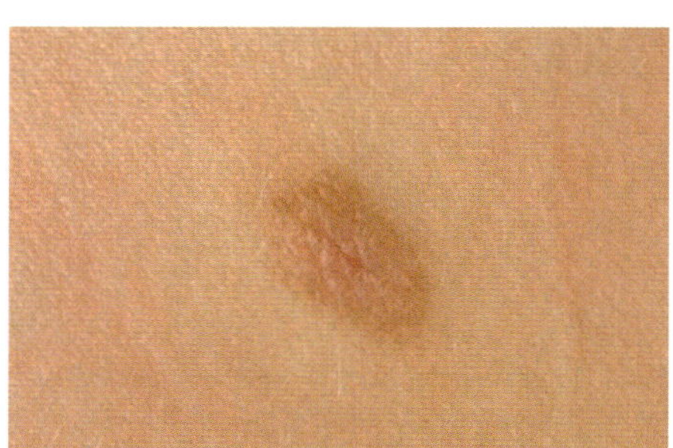

**Fig. 4.114** Cutaneous mastocytoma. This subform is characterized by a brown nodular lesion, often associated with blisters; it usually develops during the first 6 months of life and spontaneously resolves after several years.

**4.115** The Darier's sign. Mechanical irritation of mastocytosis lesions induces swelling, reddening, and itching. This phenomenon is pathognomonic for mastocytosis, and therefore serves as an important diagnostic sign.

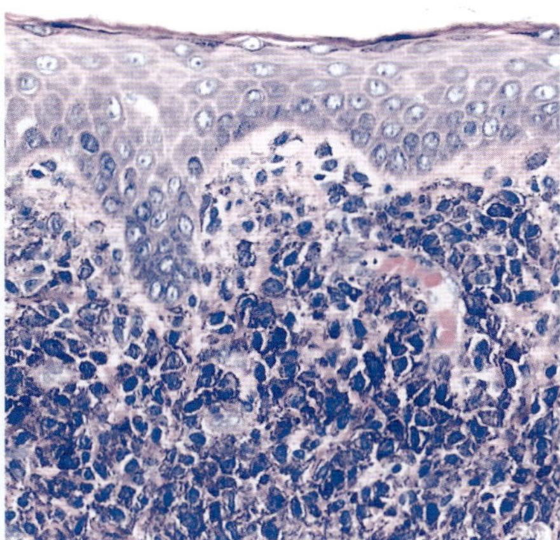

**Fig. 4.117** Indolent systemic mastocytosis with cutaneous involvement. In this adult patient, the upper dermis exhibits packed infiltrates of round mast cells with various degrees of granulation. This patient also showed minor and multifocal mast cell infiltrates in the bone marrow, as well as a *KIT* c.2447A>T (p.D816V) mutation, thus qualifying as systemic mastocytosis (Giemsa stain).

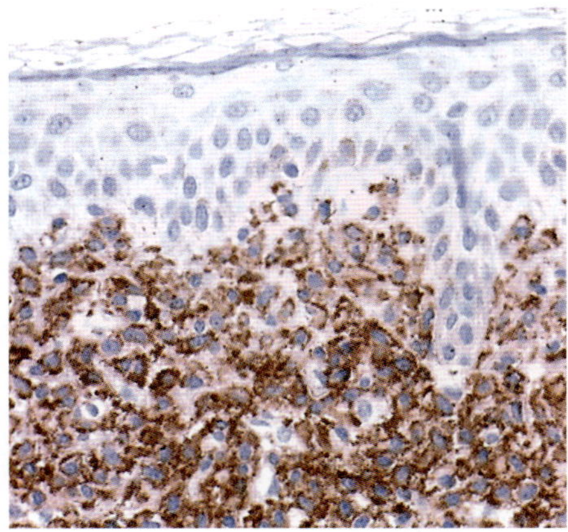

**Fig. 4.118** Indolent systemic mastocytosis with cutaneous involvement. Immunohistochemistry shows expression of tryptase by mast cells; note the typical granular-cytoplasmic staining pattern; there are no mast cells in the epidermis, because of the lack of epidermotropism (ABC staining method).

**Fig. 4.119** Maculopapular cutaneous mastocytosis. Immunohistochemistry shows strong expression of KIT (CD117) by mast cells in this juvenile patient; note the annular (membrane-associated) staining in contrast to the staining with tryptase antibody; weak expression of KIT by adnexal structures (at bottom left) is also observed (ABC staining method).

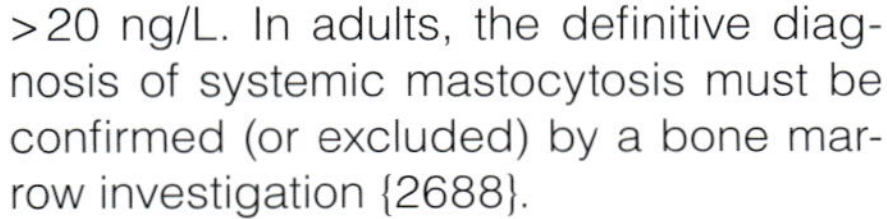

> 20 ng/L. In adults, the definitive diagnosis of systemic mastocytosis must be confirmed (or excluded) by a bone marrow investigation {2688}.

## Histopathology

Cutaneous involvement is characterized by increased numbers of mast cells in the affected dermis (Table 4.06) {350,858,1028,2847}; the numbers of mast cells are usually 4–8 times the numbers seen in the skin of healthy individuals (~40 mast cells/mm$^2$). However, there is considerable variation in mast cell numbers. In typical cases, mast cells are loosely scattered throughout the dermis, with a predilection for the upper dermal layers. Often, mast cells form groups or small clusters in perivascular and periadnexal spaces, but larger compact infiltrates can rarely also occur. Mast cells are particularly numerous in diffuse cutaneous mastocytosis and mastocytomas, often forming band-like aggregates. Involvement of the skin in advanced systemic mastocytosis is uncommon. In rare cases, intradermal mast cell infiltrates as well as leukaemic skin infiltrates are detected (e.g. in patients with chronic myelomonocytic leukaemia). In such cases, it may be difficult to determine the correct diagnosis.

The mast cells in lesional skin may be round or spindle-shaped {1028,2847}. For detection and enumeration of mast cells in lesional skin, immunohistochemistry with antibodies against tryptase and KIT (CD117) is recommended. Similar to bone marrow infiltrates, cutaneous mast cells in mastocytosis may aberrantly express CD25 and/or CD30 {255,706,1107,1490,1830,2484}. This aberrant mast cell phenotype confirms the clonal origin of mast cells, supporting the diagnosis of mastocytosis. However, expression of these markers on skin mast cells is not specific to systemic mastocytosis or to any individual subform of cutaneous mastocytosis. In a few cases, the mast cells are exclusively round and well-granulated and lack CD25 expression, but express CD30. These cases do not carry a *KIT* c.2447A>T (p.D816V) mutation, and they are referred to as well-differentiated mastocytosis; this is a morphological subform that can be seen in almost any mastocytosis category (rather than being considered a separate category unto itself) {1129,2718}. Nevertheless, the well-differentiated morphology of mast cells has prognostic and therapeutic implications; for example, patients with well-differentiated mastocytosis often respond to imatinib {1143,2717}.

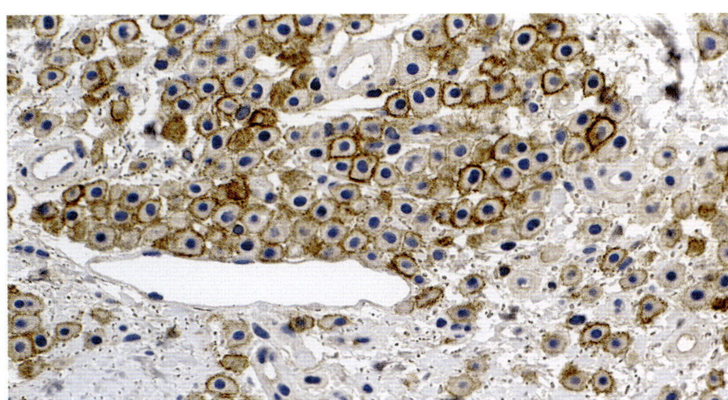

**Fig. 4.120** Maculopapular cutaneous mastocytosis; mast cells show strong staining for CD30.

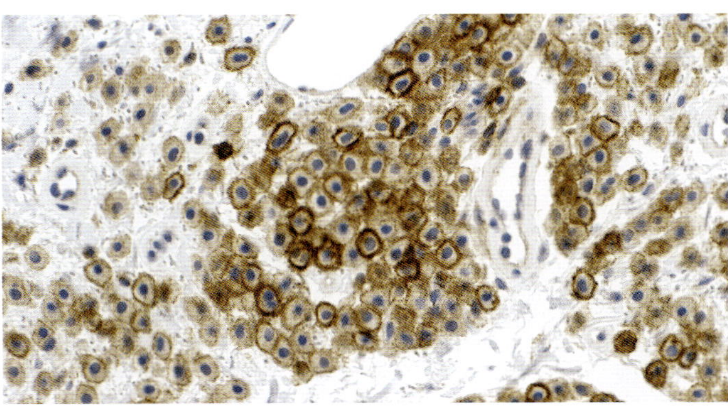

**Fig. 4.121** Maculopapular cutaneous mastocytosis; mast cells show strong staining for CD25.

### Histogenesis

Cutaneous mastocytosis results from a pathological accumulation of clonal mast cells in the skin.

### Genetic profile

The neoplastic mast cells in systemic mastocytosis often exhibit somatic *KIT* mutations {100,1217,1864}, most frequently *KIT* c.2447A>T (p.D816V); this mutation is also detected in about 40% of paediatric patients with cutaneous mastocytosis {263,2820}. However, unlike patients with systemic mastocytosis, children with cutaneous mastocytosis often present with other *KIT* mutations, including mutations in exons 8, 9, and 11.

### Genetic susceptibility

Mastocytosis is usually a sporadic disease associated with somatic *KIT* mutations. Rarely, familial mastocytosis with autosomal dominant inheritance occurs {1029,1334,2076}; in these cases, germline *KIT* mutations may be detected, affecting exons 8, 9, 10, 11, 13, or 17. In patients with sporadic mastocytosis, a higher frequency of certain gene polymorphisms has been reported {564,815,1489,1888}; affected genes include *IL4R*, *IL6*, *IL13*, *IL31*, and *KIT*.

### Prognosis and predictive factors

In adult patients with cutaneous mastocytosis or systemic mastocytosis, cutaneous lesions usually persist, regardless of the subform {1028,2820}. In children, cutaneous lesions often resolve during or shortly after puberty. The polymorphic variant of maculopapular cutaneous mastocytosis is often associated with spontaneous resolution after several years, whereas the monomorphic variant frequently results in chronic disease or even progression to systemic mastocytosis. With regard to overall and progression-free survival, adult-onset cutaneous mastocytosis has a better prognosis than does systemic mastocytosis. Of the systemic mastocytosis variants, indolent systemic mastocytosis has the best prognosis {1561}; advanced systemic mastocytosis is associated with a poor prognosis and short survival times {868}.

# Introduction to histiocytic and dendritic cell neoplasms

Facchetti F.
Berti E.
Jaffe E.S.
Zelger B.

Histiocytes/macrophages and dendritic cells make up the heterogeneous cell population of the mononuclear phagocytic system. The components of this system share histogenetic and differentiation pathways, and the nomenclature for these cells is still evolving {698}. The term "histiocyte" has been used in several very different ways (as has the adjective "histiocytic"); broadly defined, the term encompasses all cells of epithelioid appearance, i.e. cells with prominent cytoplasm such as those seen in dermatofibroma (fibrous histiocytoma), histiocytic (epithelioid) haemangioma, malignant fibrous histiocytoma, and many other entities. In a more restricted sense, the term has been used for the cells of the mononuclear phagocytic system. Even more narrowly, the term can refer specifically to tissue-resident macrophages, which have been shown to derive from embryonal (yolk-sac) or fetal liver cell precursors; they are self-renewing and localized in various tissues, where they are sometimes referred to by more-specific names, such as Langerhans cells, microglia, and Kupffer cells {514,614,1003}. After birth, some subsets of tissue-resident macrophages (notably Langerhans cells) can be replenished by transformation of bone marrow–derived precursors (e.g. monocytes or classic dendritic cell precursors). This replenishment occurs subsequent to cell damage or inflammation, which, in the case of Langerhans cells, is characterized by increased turnover and trafficking to lymph nodes {514,516}. Transformation of circulating monocytes into macrophages typically occurs in inflammatory processes (resulting in so-called inflammatory macrophages), in tissue repair, and in immune responses to tumours {614,1003}.

Non-Langerhans human dendritic cells are classified into two main groups: classic (or myeloid) dendritic cells and plasmacytoid dendritic cells (PDCs). On the basis of antigen expression, classic dendritic cells can be further subdivided into two subsets: DC1 cells express CD141, and DC2 cells express CD1c. Cells with dendritic cell functions can also originate from monocytes during inflammation; such cells are called monocyte-derived inflammatory dendritic cells. Classic dendritic cells, PDCs, Langerhans cells, and monocyte-derived inflammatory dendritic cells all have distinct cell distributions, migratory pathways, functions, and immunophenotypes {514,1003}.

Because of the common origin of the mononuclear phagocytic system components, macrophages and the various dendritic cell populations have some functional overlap, but phagocytosis is typical of macrophages and antigen presentation is maximally developed in dendritic cells. Similarly, several cell markers are shared by macrophages and dendritic cells, but differences do exist and can be useful for tissue recognition, as well as for differential diagnosis with pathological processes involving these cells {728}.

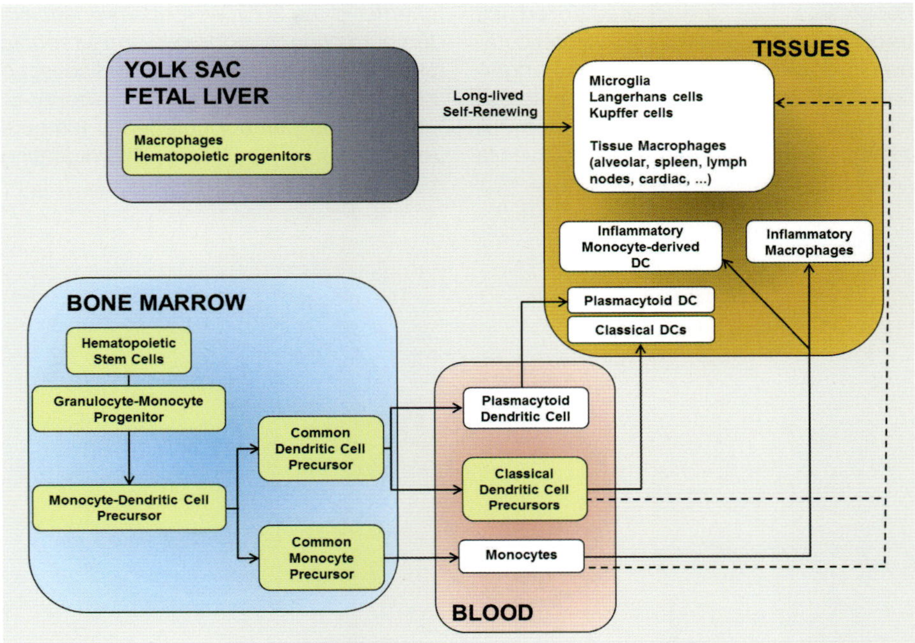


**Fig. 4.122** Organization of the human mononuclear phagocytic system. Tissue-resident macrophages and Langerhans cells are largely derived from embryonal (yolk-sac) or fetal liver cell precursors, and they are maintained in the tissues after birth via long life and self-renewal. Replenishment occurs upon inflammation (dotted-line), from bone marrow–derived precursors. Circulating monocytes typically transform into inflammatory macrophages and a subset of dendritic cells; most dendritic cells (classic and plasmacytoid dendritic cells) derive from a distinct pathway of differentiation.

Neoplasms derived from macrophages and dendritic cells are a heterogeneous group of diseases that can behave in very different ways, ranging from localized clinically indolent conditions to disseminated and aggressive processes. This variability can even be observed among different cases of the same entity, underscoring the importance of comprehensive evaluation of clinical, pathological, imaging, and molecular findings.

A classification of the histiocytoses and neoplasms of the macrophage–dendritic cell lineages was published in 1987 by the Histiocyte Society {1089} and revised in 2016 {686}. The revised classification defines five distinct groups of diseases on the basis of histology, phenotype, molecular alterations, clinical features, and imaging: (1) Langerhans-related histiocytoses, (2) cutaneous and mucocutaneous histiocytoses, (3) malignant histiocytoses, (4) Rosai–Dorfman disease, and (5) haemophagocytic lymphohistiocytosis and macrophage activation syndrome.

The following sections specifically discuss the histiocytic and dendritic cell neoplasms that are characterized by frequent (and sometimes prevalent) cutaneous manifestations, including Langerhans cell histiocytosis, indeterminate cell histiocytosis/indeterminate dendritic cell tumour, Rosai–Dorfman disease, juvenile xanthogranuloma, and reticulohistiocytosis. Also discussed is Erdheim–Chester disease, which is now recognized as a distinct entity, separate from the other members of the juvenile xanthogranuloma family.

Some of the entities included in the *Histiocytic and dendritic cell neoplasms* chapter of the 2017 *WHO classification of tumours of haematopoietic and lymphoid tissues* volume {2545} are not discussed here, because of their extreme rarity or absence as primary cutaneous tumours (e.g. histiocytic sarcoma, interdigitating dendritic cell sarcoma, follicular dendritic cell sarcoma, fibroblastic reticular cell tumour, and disseminated juvenile xanthogranuloma). Like in the 2017 haematolymphoid volume, blastic PDC neoplasm (a highly aggressive and frequently skin-involving tumour derived from PDCs) is discussed separately (see *Blastic plasmacytoid dendritic cell neoplasm*, p. 271), along with other neoplasms derived from precursor cells.

# Langerhans cell histiocytosis

Facchetti F.
Berti E.

## Definition

Langerhans cell histiocytosis (LCH) is a clonal neoplastic proliferation of Langerhans cells expressing CD1a, langerin (CD207), and S100 protein and showing Birbeck granules on electron microscopy.

## ICD-O code 9751/1

## Synonyms

Langerhans cell granulomatosis; Hand–Schüller–Christian disease; Letterer–Siwe disease; Hashimoto–Pritzker disease

## Epidemiology

The overall incidence is about 5 cases per 1 million person-years. Most cases occur in childhood, and the male-to-female ratio is 3.7:1 {2062}. LCH is more common in White individuals of northern European descent and is rare in Black populations. There may be an association with Hodgkin and non-Hodgkin lymphomas, myeloid leukaemia, malignant epithelial neoplasms, and Erdheim–Chester disease (ECD) {207,476,663,667,686,745, 746,1075,1628,1894,2208,2809}.

## Etiology

The etiology is unknown. Previously thought to be a reactive condition, LCH is now considered to be an inflammatory myeloid neoplasm, possibly with a mixed inflammatory/neoplastic etiopathogenesis similar to that of ECD {222,1022}. Smoking may have a role in lung-restricted cases of LCH occurring in adults {2722}.

## Localization

LCH can involve any organ, in a wide variety of combinations. The most commonly affected site is bone (involved in > 80% of cases), followed by skin (in one third of cases) {1560,1785,2516,2618}.

## Clinical features

LCH is classified according to the number of organs affected and the extent of involvement. In single-system LCH, only one organ is affected, by either a single lesion (unifocal disease) or multiple lesions (multifocal disease). In multisystem LCH, two or more organs are affected {1045}. The disease has a variable clinical course, ranging from self-limiting to rapidly progressive and lethal {2187}. Single-system cutaneous LCH accounts for as many as 10% of all cases. The skin can also be involved in multisystem cases; low-risk multisystem LCH (formerly called Hand–Schüller–Christian disease) is characterized by bone and pituitary lesions, exophthalmos, and diabetes insipidus, and skin lesions are seen in about 30% of cases. The more aggressive form, high-risk multisystem LCH (formerly called Letterer–Siwe disease), also commonly involves the skin {2187}. Skin lesions in LCH can occur at any site and appear as papules, nodules, erythematous plaques, ulcerative lesions, crusts, and bullae. They may resemble seborrhoeic dermatitis and may be superinfected by *Pseudomonas*. Self-healing single-system cutaneous LCH (formerly called Hashimoto–Pritzker disease) occurs in newborns, manifesting as solitary, localized, or generalized lesions that involute spontaneously within weeks to months of onset {176,220,2497}.

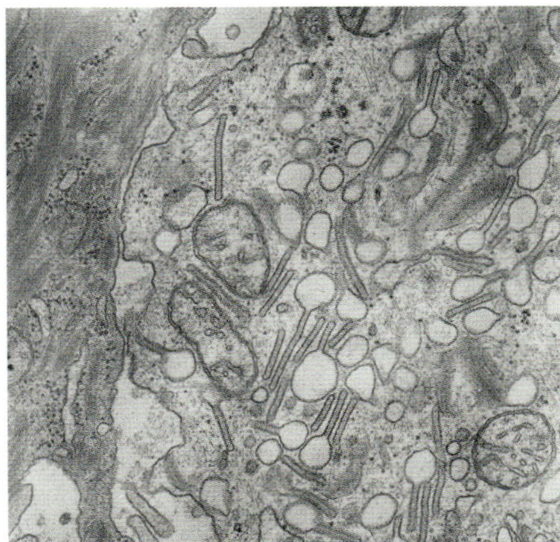

**Fig. 4.125** Langerhans cell histiocytosis. Electron microscopy showing Birbeck granules.

## Histopathology

Skin papules and plaques are composed of a dense infiltrate of LCH cells, with epidermotropism and intraepidermal aggregates. The tumour cells may extend to the dermis and subcutis. LCH cells are round/ovoid medium-sized cells with indented, lobulated, or coffee-bean nuclei; dispersed chromatin; inconspicuous nucleoli; and a thin nuclear membrane. The cytoplasm is moderately abundant and eosinophilic. Atypia is absent or minimal, but mitotic activity can be exuberant, regardless of atypia. Eosinophils, dispersed or clustered into microabscesses, and neutrophils are often present. Over time, the lesions become enriched in

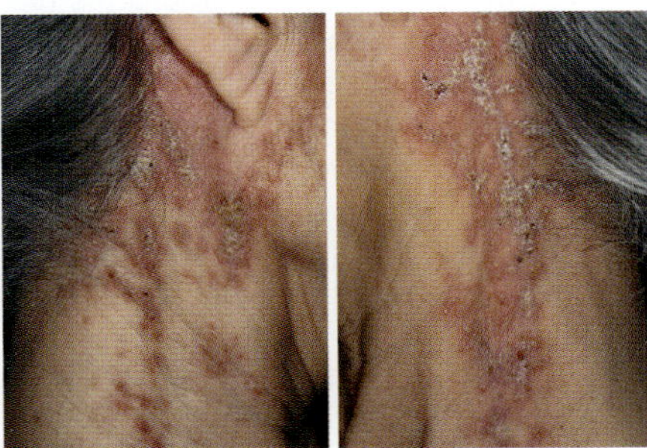

**Fig. 4.123** Low-risk multisystem Langerhans cell histiocytosis. Bilateral erythematous erosive plaques.

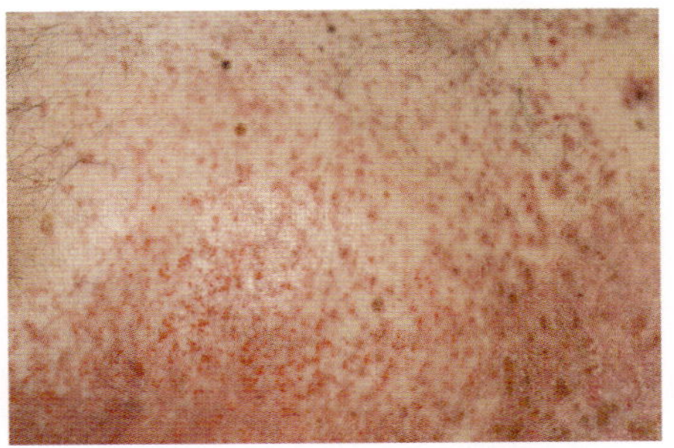

**Fig. 4.124** High-risk multisystem Langerhans cell histiocytosis. Disseminated purpuric papules.

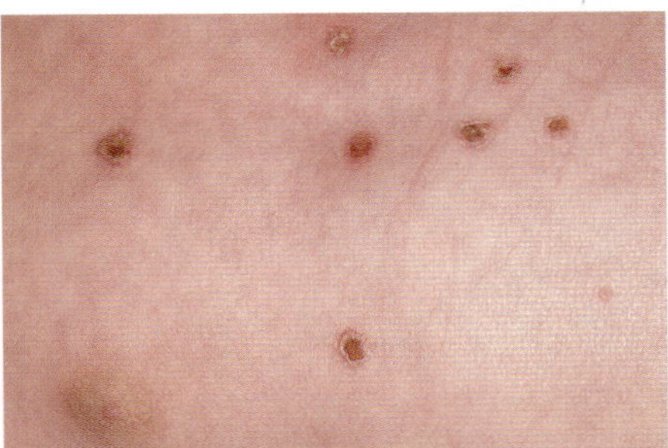

**Fig. 4.126** Self-healing single-system cutaneous Langerhans cell histiocytosis. Multiple papules and nodules.

epithelioid macrophages, foamy cells, multinucleated giant cells, and fibrosis, while the number of LCH cells decreases. Tumour cells consistently express CD1a, langerin (CD207), and S100 protein {458,1446}. Expression of CD68, CD163, and lysozyme is low or absent, but may increase in late-stage lesions. B-cell and T-cell markers (except CD4 and CD56) are absent. Ki-67 expression is highly variable {2062}. BRAF p.V600E can be detected immunohistochemically using the VE1 antibody {48,2193,2207}. Birbeck granules, the ultrastructural hallmark of LCH, are cytoplasmic corpuscles measuring 200–400 nm long and 33 nm wide, with a tennis-racket shape and zipper-like striations.

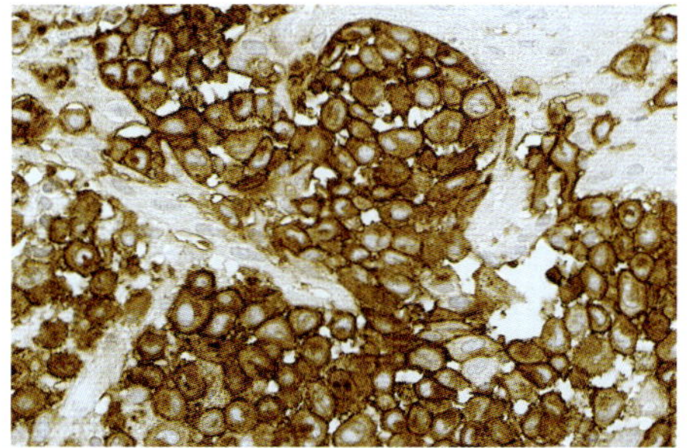

**Fig. 4.127** Langerhans cell histiocytosis (LCH). Dermal infiltrate with epidermotropic, CD1a+ LCH cells.

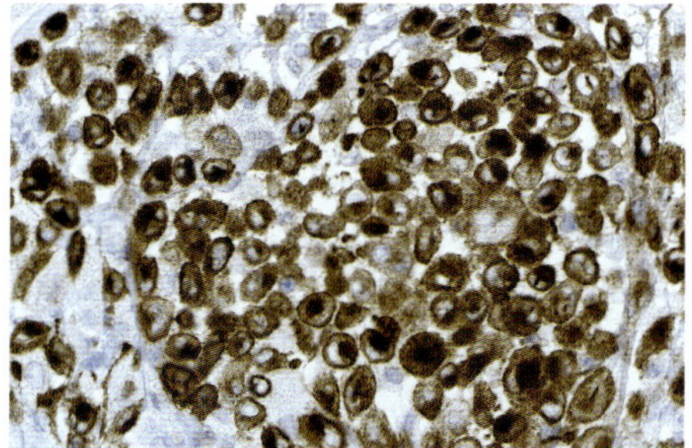

**Fig. 4.128** Langerhans cell histiocytosis (LCH). LCH cells showing langerin (CD207) positivity.

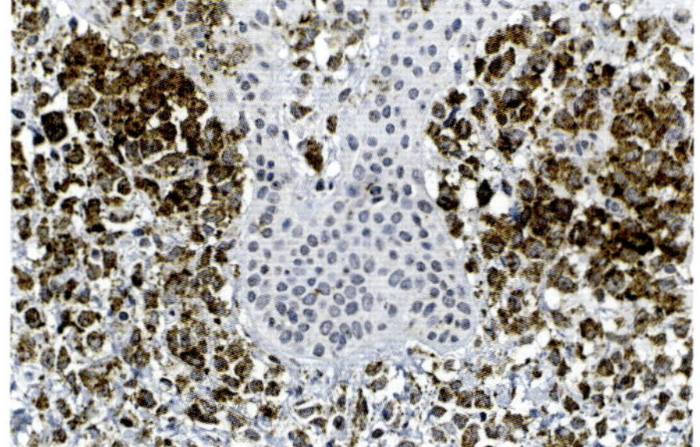

**Fig. 4.129** Langerhans cell histiocytosis (LCH). There is strong immunopositivity for BRAF p.V600E (as detected by the mutation-specific VE1 monoclonal antibody) in LCH cells.

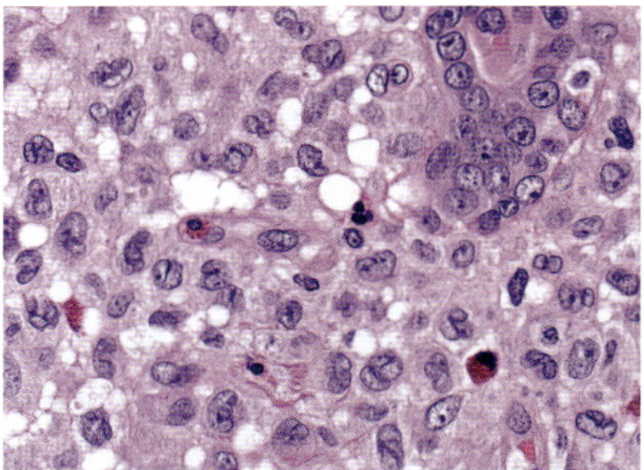

**Fig. 4.130** Langerhans cell histiocytosis (LCH). Typical appearance of LCH cells, with indented, lobulated, or coffee-bean nuclei and eosinophilic cytoplasm.

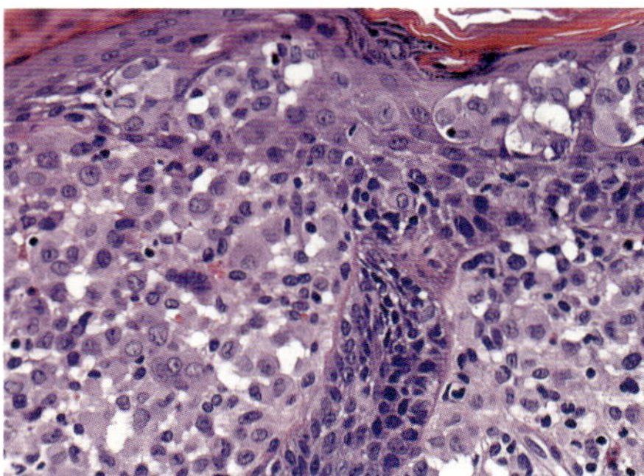

**Fig. 4.131** Langerhans cell histiocytosis. A dermal papule with epidermotropism.

## Differential diagnosis

Indeterminate cell histiocytosis/indeterminate dendritic cell tumour has similar histological features, but is negative for langerin (CD207) and lacks Birbeck granules. Other non-Langerhans cutaneous histiocytoses (particularly juvenile xanthogranuloma) may express S100 protein in some cells, but consistently show a full-blown histiocytic (CD68+, CD163+) phenotype and are negative for CD1a and langerin (CD207). Highly atypical and mitotically active large cell proliferations that variably express all LCH markers are defined as Langerhans cell sarcoma {1528}; this aggressive neoplasm can arise de novo or in association with LCH, indicating tumour progression. Marked dermal Langerhans cell reactions occur in inflammatory and neoplastic skin diseases {2007}, and small intraepithelial aggregates of Langerhans cells are found especially frequently in spongiotic dermatitis {365}.

## Histogenesis

The postulated normal counterparts of LCH are epidermal Langerhans cells {1897}, although they differ in protein and gene expression profiles {55,187}. Molecular data indicate that precursors may include CD34+ haematopoietic stem cells, circulating CD1c+ myeloid dendritic cells, circulating CD14+ monocytes, and/or differentiated tissue-resident Langerhans cells {223,1782}.

## Genetic profile

Recurrent mutations of MAPK pathway components in LCH include mutations in *BRAF* (p.V600E), found in about 50% of cases {126,223,1019,2278}; *MAP2K1*, found in 19% of *BRAF*-wildtype cases {320,423,1890}; and more rarely *ARAF* and *MAP3K1* {1890,1891}. Mutations in *PIK3CA*, *PICK1*, and *PIK3R2* have also been reported {423,1069}. Because of the low allelic frequency of these mutations, the use of highly sensitive detection techniques is recommended {686,687, 710}.

The molecular landscape of LCH is also found in ECD, a tumoural proliferation of differentiated histiocytes {687,710}), whose relationship with LCH is further supported by an association between the two conditions in some cases {686,1075,1239}. ECD shows distinctive clinical and radiological manifestations {710,1781}; cutaneous lesions typically consist of periorbital xanthelasma {686,710}.

LCH and lymphomas may occur synchronously or metachronously {207,476, 663,667,745,746,1628,1894,2208,2809} and often show a clonal relationship, indicating either derivation from a common precursor or so-called transdifferentiation {745,1628,2208}.

## Genetic susceptibility

Familial clustering of LCH has been reported {13,93,2389,2894}, but data on genetic predisposition are lacking.

## Prognosis and predictive factors

Age < 1 year, male sex, advanced stage, involvement of so-called risk organs (i.e. bone marrow, spleen, and/or liver), and unresponsiveness to treatment negatively influence prognosis. BRAF p.V600E mutation correlates with high-risk disease and increased resistance to standard first-line treatment {1067}; its presence in precursor cells or in plasma cell–free DNA is a marker of active and high-risk LCH {223,515,1068,1400,1782}. LCH with BRAF p.V600E mutation has shown sensitivity to BRAF inhibitors in phase II clinical trials {625A,1021}.

# Indeterminate cell histiocytosis/ indeterminate dendritic cell tumour

Facchetti F.
Berti E.
Zelger B.

## Definition

Indeterminate cell histiocytosis/indeterminate dendritic cell tumour is an enigmatic entity thought to derive from indeterminate cells (presumably precursors of Langerhans cells), but these cells have never been reliably and unequivocally identified {2858}. The neoplastic cells express markers of both Langerhans cells (CD1a and S100 protein) and macrophages.

## ICD-O code 9757/3

## Synonym

Indeterminate dendritic cell histiocytosis

## Epidemiology

This is a rare disease; the largest reported series consists of 18 cases affecting adults {2138}, but teenagers {1787,2281} and children {1551,1669} are also occasionally affected.

## Clinical features

Patients present with solitary or multiple papules and nodules, which tend to coalesce {2138}. The lesions are soft and reddish in early stages; in later stages they are firm and dark red to brownish, occasionally eroded {227,1937}. Multiple lesions may be generalized or agminated. Extracutaneous manifestations (in the conjunctiva or bone) are infrequent. Occasionally, lymph nodes may be involved {1414,2138,2730}. As many as 20% of cases have been associated with a non-Hodgkin lymphoma {234,2178}, chronic myelomonocytic leukaemia, acute myeloblastic leukaemia {1119,2730}, or hepatocellular carcinoma {1969}.

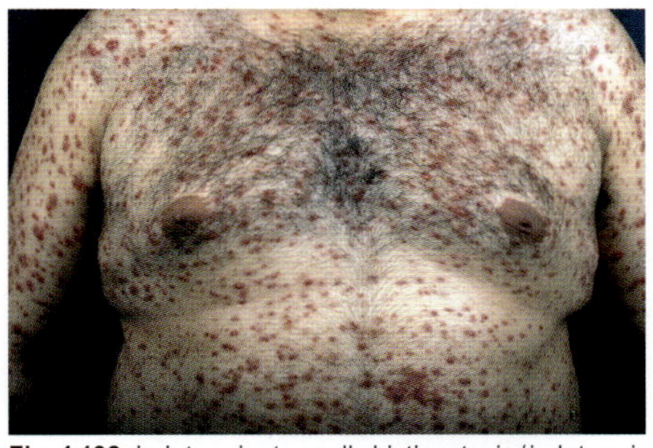

**Fig. 4.132** Indeterminate cell histiocytosis/indeterminate dendritic cell tumour. Multiple firm papules on the trunk and arms, ranging in size from a few millimetres to 1 cm and varying in colour from dark red to brownish.

## Histopathology

The lesions contain sheets of cells resembling Langerhans cells, with kidney-shaped nuclei. Epidermal involvement is typically absent {1119}. A spindle cell variant has been described {2233}. Eosinophils and lymphocytes may be prominent. The immunoprofile is characterized by the expression of CD1a and S100 protein, lacking langerin (CD207); ultrastructurally, no Birbeck granules are recognizable {610,2178}.

## Differential diagnosis

Langerhans cell histiocytosis expresses langerin (CD207) and shows Birbeck granules ultrastructurally {453}. Some indeterminate cell histiocytosis/indeterminate dendritic cell tumour cases may show overlapping features with either xanthogranuloma or Langerhans cell histiocytosis {2138}.

## Histogenesis

The cells of origin are so-called immature Langerhans cells, lacking langerin (CD207) expression and Birbeck granules {2178}.

## Genetic profile

*ETV3-NCOA2* gene fusion has been detected in 4 cases {321,2115}. A clonal relationship with associated B-cell lymphomas has been reported in a few cases {234,2178}. BRAF p.V600E mutation has been found in one case associated with angioimmunoblastic T-cell lymphoma {1932}.

## Prognosis and predictive factors

Most cases show spontaneous regression, without recurrence. Disease progression and malignant behaviour have been reported in cases with atypical cytological features {268,1669} or association with other haematological neoplasms {268,2178}.

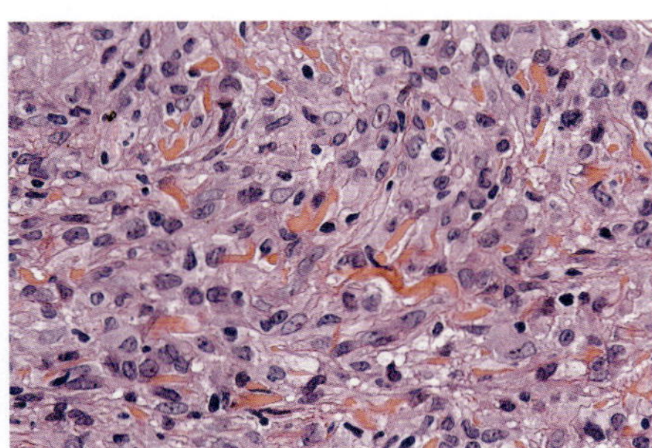

**Fig. 4.133** Indeterminate cell histiocytosis/indeterminate dendritic cell tumour. Diffuse infiltrate of medium-sized cells, with round to oval or indented nuclei and moderately abundant eosinophilic cytoplasm.

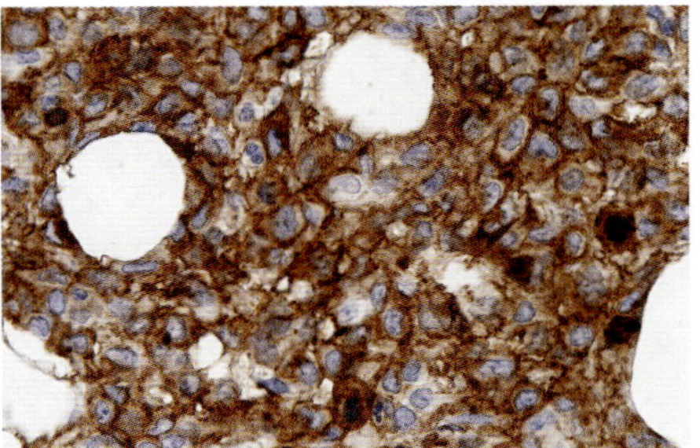

**Fig. 4.134** Indeterminate cell histiocytosis/indeterminate dendritic cell tumour. Tumour cells are positive for CD1a.

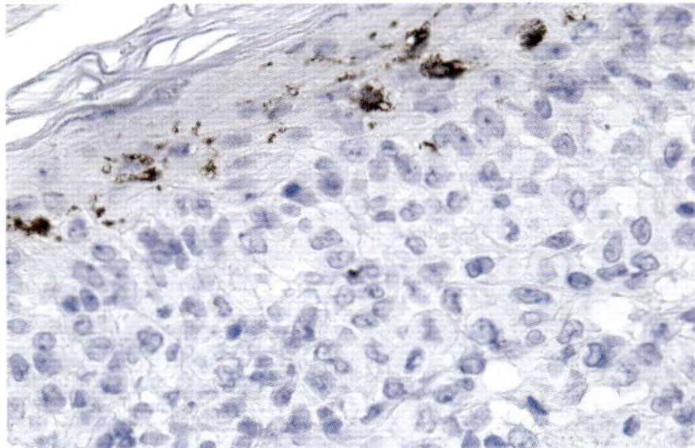

**Fig. 4.135** Indeterminate histiocytosis/indeterminate dendritic cell tumour. Tumour cells are negative for langerin (CD207), which is expressed by epidermal Langerhans cells.

# Rosai–Dorfman disease

Facchetti F.
Zelger B.

## Definition
Rosai–Dorfman disease (RDD) is a reactive proliferation of macrophages expressing S100 protein and showing emperipolesis.

## Synonyms
Sinus histiocytosis with massive lymphadenopathy; Destombes–Rosai–Dorfman disease

## Epidemiology
RDD typically presents with lymphadenopathy, mainly in children and young adults. Extranodal disease is most common in the skin, but involvement restricted exclusively to the skin (cutaneous RDD) is rare {304}. Patients are generally older. Females are affected more frequently, and the incidence is higher among Asians {565,1416}.

## Etiology
The etiology is unknown, but a role of cytokine dysregulation has been proposed {1770}.

## Localization
Cervical lymph node involvement is most characteristic. Cutaneous lesions most commonly involve the trunk, followed by the head and neck {822}.

## Clinical features
Patients present with multiple reddish-brown papules, nodules, or plaques (as large as 30 cm) {565,1416}. In cutaneous RDD, laboratory values are typically normal and lymphadenopathy absent.

## Histopathology
There are sheets of dermal to subcutaneous large macrophages with pale to variably eosinophilic cytoplasm, admixed with inflammatory cells, including eosinophils and plasma cells. As is the case at other extranodal sites, the macrophages may be spindle-shaped, emperipolesis can be subtle, and fibrosis can be prominent {1416}. The macrophages express S100 protein, CD14, CD11c, CD68, and CD163, whereas CD1a, langerin (CD207), and HLA-DR are negative {2013}.

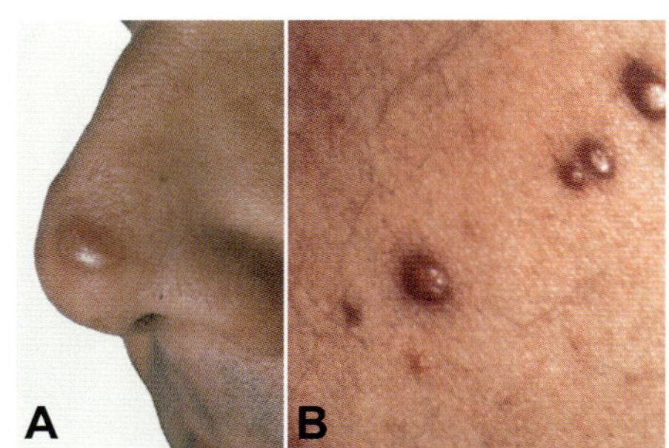

**Fig. 4.136** Rosai–Dorfman disease. **A** Brownish nodule on the nose. **B** Clustered brownish papules on the trunk.

## Differential diagnosis
Juvenile xanthogranuloma may express S100 protein in a variable number of cells, but emperipolesis is absent.

## Histogenesis
RDD is a reactive proliferation of activated macrophages, resulting in S100 protein expression {814,1016,1770}.

## Genetic profile
Mutations involving *KRAS*, *NRAS*, and *MAP2K1* have been reported in about a third of cases, questioning the reactive nature of these cases {625,847,1201A,1701, 2398}.

## Genetic susceptibility
RDD and cutaneous RDD may occur in individuals with germline mutations in *SLC29A3*, i.e. in the setting of histiocytosis–lymphadenopathy plus syndrome (also called Faisalabad histiocytosis, familial RDD, and H syndrome) {1812,1832}. They have also been reported in patients with autoimmune lymphoproliferative syndrome type IA, which is associated with *FAS* (*TNFRSF6*) mutations {1662}.

## Prognosis and predictive factors
RDD is mostly benign, with frequent spontaneous resolution {565}.

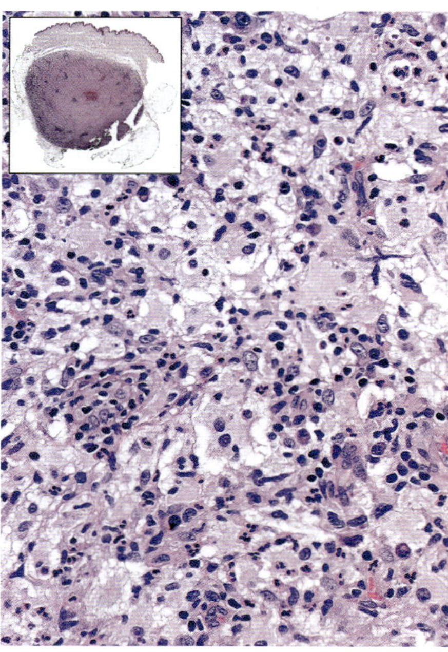

**Fig. 4.137** Rosai–Dorfman disease. A skin nodule largely involving the deep dermis and subcutaneous fat (**inset**), composed of pale large macrophages admixed with heterogeneous inflammatory cells.

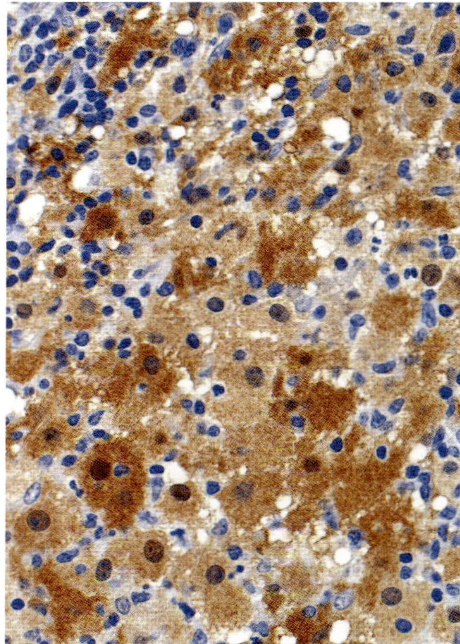

**Fig. 4.138** Rosai–Dorfman disease. Sheets of macrophages positive for S100 protein, occasionally containing lymphocytes in their cytoplasm (i.e. showing emperipolesis).

# Juvenile xanthogranuloma

Facchetti F.
Zelger B.

## Definition

Juvenile xanthogranuloma (JXG) is a benign, self-healing, cutaneous proliferation of macrophages with a variable degree of lipidization, in the absence of a metabolic disorder. The adult form is better termed xanthogranuloma or adult xanthogranuloma.

## Synonyms

Xanthogranuloma; solitary xanthogranuloma; nevoxanthoendothelioma

## Epidemiology

JXG is more common in infancy and childhood, and it may be congenital {601,1215}. Boys are affected more frequently, with a male-to-female ratio of 1.4:1 {1215}. Most cases of the deep, visceral, and disseminated forms occur before the age of 10 years, with onset during the first year of life in 50% of cases {1215}. The rarer adult form shows no sex predilection.

## Localization

JXG can occur at any cutaneous site, with a predilection for the head and neck, upper trunk, and proximal extremities {1215}. Solitary extracutaneous cases, as well as exceptionally rare systemic cases, may involve the mucosal surfaces (most commonly of the upper aerodigestive tract), CNS, pituitary stalk, eye, lung, liver, lymph nodes, and bone marrow {601,1215}.

## Clinical features

The lesions range from small papules, to nodules, to large tumours (as large as 10 cm) {2920}; in the early phase they are reddish-brown, becoming yellowish with maturation. Solitary lesions are most prevalent (seen in 67–81% of cases); when multiple, the lesions are often numerous (as many as 100 in number) {601,2006,2157,2920}. Lichenoid papules {2630}, flat plaques {1837}, and deforming lesions have been reported {373}. JXG develops quickly and typically regresses spontaneously within a year. In adults, xanthogranuloma lesions are usually large, solitary, and persistent, and they are only rarely associated with systemic involvement {2268}.

Extracutaneous involvement occurs in a small proportion of cases. Ocular JXG is almost always unilateral and may lead to permanent blindness due to glaucoma or anterior chamber bleeding {2294}. CNS and pituitary lesions can cause diabetes insipidus, seizures, and hydrocephalus {601,824,1215}. Systemic JXG occurs in 4% of children {601}; patients may present with severe symptoms related to visceral involvement and rarely experience spontaneous resolution {824}. Xanthogranuloma may be associated with café-au-lait spots, neurofibromatosis, and juvenile myelomonocytic leukaemia {335} in children, as well as with other haematological malignancies in adults {2433}.

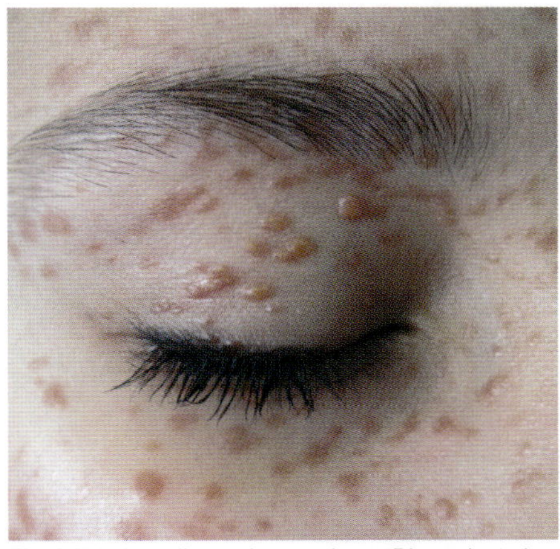

**Fig. 4.139** Juvenile xanthogranuloma. Disseminated brownish papules on the face.

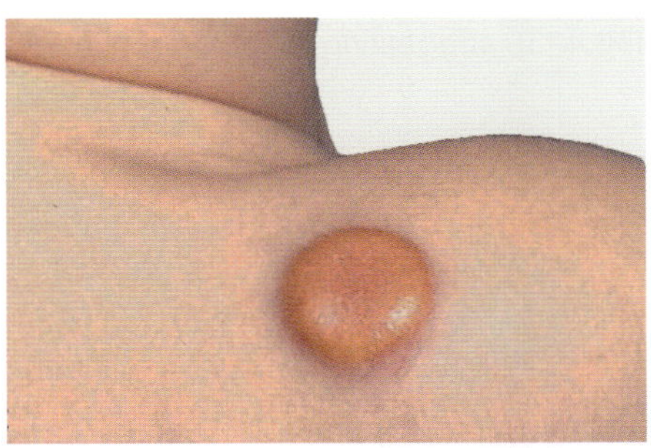

**Fig. 4.140** Juvenile xanthogranuloma, nodular form. A round, high-domed yellowish-brown nodule on the right shoulder.

## Histopathology

JXG generally shows involvement of the superficial and deep dermis by macrophages, which change in appearance over time {1215} from small mononuclear oval to spindled cells with eosinophilic cytoplasm in early lesions, to progressively larger and lipid-laden cells, to frankly foamy macrophages in late lesions. Multinucleated giant cells, including the peculiar Touton-type cells, vary in number and are mainly distributed in the superficial dermis and along the border of the infiltrate. Lymphocytes, eosinophils, neutrophils, and plasma cells are scattered throughout the lesion, and fibrosis increases with time {370,2009}.

JXG cells express CD11c, CD68, CD163, and lysozyme. S100 protein may be positive in rare cases, in as many as 10% of cells {2624}; CD1a and langerin (CD207) are negative {601,1215,2299}.

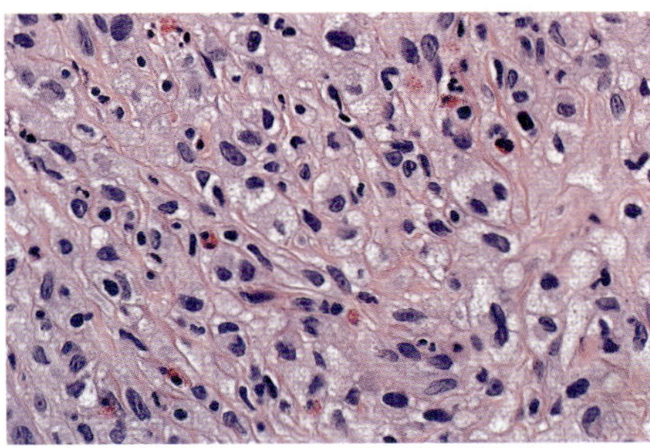

**Fig. 4.141** Juvenile xanthogranuloma. An early lesion showing medium-sized histiocytes (some with incipient cytoplasmic lipidization) and scattered eosinophils.

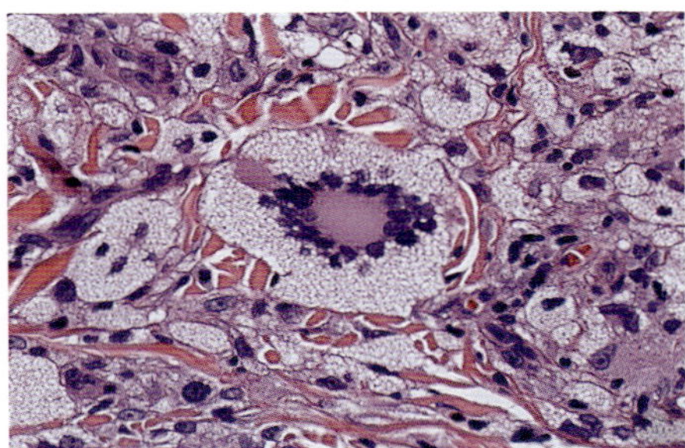

**Fig. 4.142** Juvenile xanthogranuloma. A mature lesion showing numerous xanthomatous cells, including a classic Touton giant cell.

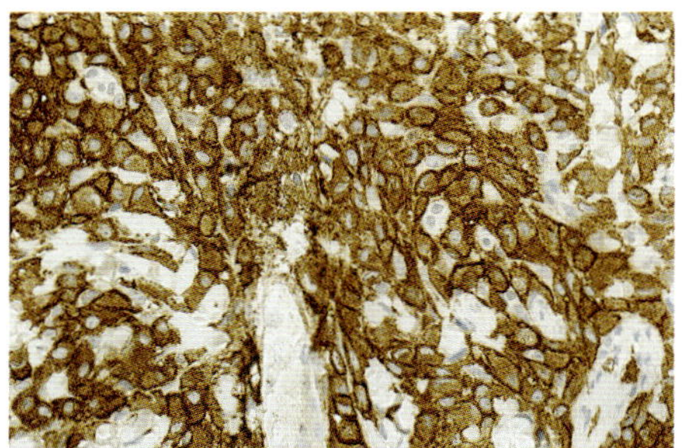

**Fig. 4.143** Juvenile xanthogranuloma. The macrophages are strongly positive for CD163.

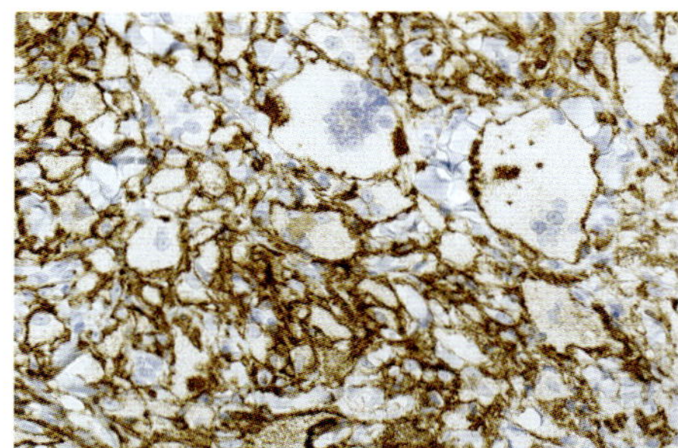

**Fig. 4.144** Juvenile xanthogranuloma. Small and large macrophages (including multinucleated cells) are strongly positive for CD11c.

## Differential diagnosis

Langerhans cell histiocytosis cells express CD1a and langerin (CD207). Reticulohistiocytosis shows cells with ground-glass eosinophilic cytoplasm, a sharply defined nuclear membrane, and a prominent nucleolus, but its distinction from JXG is often subtle {686}. Extracutaneous or disseminated JXG can mimic Erdheim–Chester disease, which should be excluded by careful clinical and/or radiological examination, as well as by molecular analysis for mutations associated with Erdheim–Chester disease {686,1019}.

## Histogenesis

JXG is a benign proliferation of lipid-laden macrophages.

## Genetic profile

Non-recurrent somatic mutations have been reported in 3 cases of JXG, including *PIK3CD* mutations identified in multiple skin specimens in one case {56,423}, suggesting a pathogenetic role of MAPK (ERK) pathway activation {56}. *BRAF* p.V600E mutations have been identified in 2 cases of JXG associated with Langerhans cell histiocytosis, but not in pure JXG {56,423,1019}.

## Genetic susceptibility

Associations with neurofibromatosis types 1 and 2, and juvenile myelomonocytic leukaemia have been documented in approximately 20 cases of JXG {1214}, and the occurrence of JXG in patients with neurofibromatosis has been considered a risk factor for the development of juvenile myelomonocytic leukaemia {2943}. The occurrence of JXG in monozygotic twins indicates the existence of an as-yet undefined genetic susceptibility {438,2570}.

## Prognosis and predictive factors

The prognosis is generally excellent, except for disseminated JXG, which has an overall mortality rate of 5–10% {601,1016}.

# Erdheim–Chester disease

Facchetti F.
Zelger B.
Berti E.
Jaffe E.S.

## Definition

Erdheim–Chester disease (ECD) is a clonal systemic proliferation of macrophages, commonly having a foamy (xanthomatous) component and containing multinucleated (Touton) giant cells. Diagnosis of ECD is based on clinical features, imaging, and histology {624,1018}.

## ICD-O code

9749/3

## Synonym

Polyostotic sclerosing histiocytosis

## Epidemiology

ECD is rare, but recognition of the condition has increased drastically over the past decade {624}. The mean age at diagnosis is 55–60 years, but rare paediatric occurrences (< 15 cases) have also been reported {891}. The male-to-female ratio is 3:1. As many as 20% of patients with ECD also have Langerhans cell histiocytosis (LCH) {1075}, exceptionally even combined with Rosai–Dorfman disease {1979}; the infiltrations characteristic of ECD and LCH may occur within the same biopsy {1075,1781} or at different sites {442}. It has been reported that about 10% of patients with ECD also have a myeloid neoplasm, most commonly in cases associated with LCH {1979}.

## Etiology

Previously thought to be a reactive condition, ECD (like LCH) is now considered to be an inflammatory myeloid neoplasm {95,222,1022}.

## Localization

Virtually any organ or tissue can be infiltrated by ECD. The vast majority of patients have multiorgan disease at presentation {710}, most frequently involving the bones (in particular the long bones, affected in 95% of cases), the cardiovascular system (in particular the aorta, pericardium, and right atrioventricular groove, affected in 50% of cases), the retroperitoneum (in particular the perirenal space, affected in 30% of cases), the CNS (affected in 20–30% of cases), and the periorbital tissues (affected in 20–30% of cases) {710,2401}. The skin (typically of the eyelids or periorbital area, or more rarely of the trunk, back, or legs) is affected in about 30% of cases {442}.

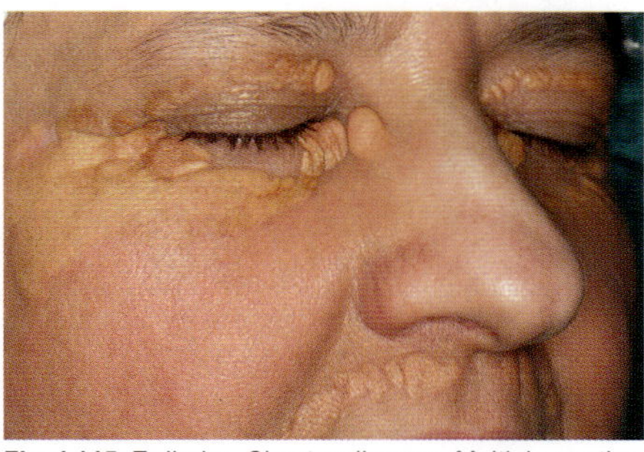

**Fig. 4.145** Erdheim–Chester disease. Multiple xanthomatous plaques involving the periorbital and perioral areas, with extension to the cheek and temple.

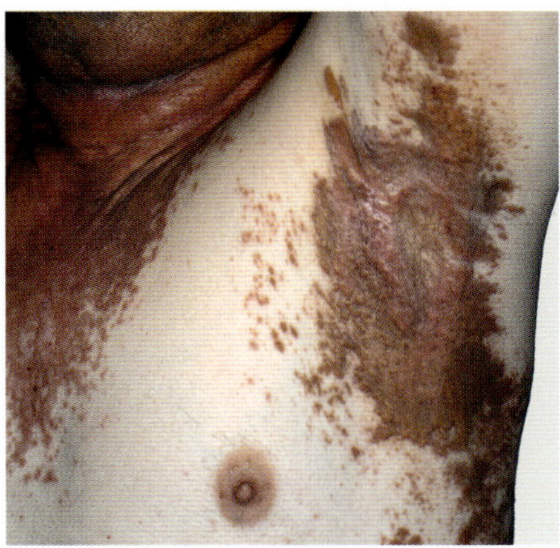

**Fig. 4.146** Erdheim–Chester disease. Multiple red papules that coalesce into extensive plaques involving the neck, upper trunk, and axilla.

## Clinical features

Cutaneous ECD is the first manifestation of disease in 20% of patients {442,710}, sometimes dominating the clinical picture in the so-called asymptomatic or minimally symptomatic clinical variant of ECD {624}. Bilateral xanthelasma of the eyelids or periorbital tissue is the most common cutaneous manifestation. Less frequently, non-xanthelasma lesions occur, consisting of erythematous or brown localized patches, isolated papules, nodules, tumours, or even erythroderma {442}.

The clinical presentation of ECD is extraordinarily protean, and diagnosis is often delayed. ECD can be asymptomatic, and tissue/organ involvement can be detected incidentally by imaging. However, most patients experience several signs and symptoms, most commonly diabetes insipidus and bone pain {710}. CNS symptoms are variable, and severe neurological complications of neurodegenerative cerebellar disease occur in 15–20% of cases {710}. Pericardial involvement can cause pericarditis, effusion, or even tamponade; renovascular hypertension due to renal artery narrowing rarely occurs. Orbital infiltration (often bilateral) produces exophthalmos, pain, oculomotor nerve palsies, or blindness.

Imaging plays a fundamental role in the diagnosis of ECD. Characteristic findings of bone involvement (in particular involvement of the diaphysis and metaphysis of long bones) can be imaged using radiography, 99Tc scintigraphy, and PET {97,1017}. Other typical features are circumferential sheathing of the thoracic or abdominal aorta (so-called coated aorta) {1836,2383}, prominent involvement of the renal capsule (so-called hairy kidney) and ureters {653,1836}, infiltration of right atrium or auriculoventricular sulcus {1020}, and diffuse pleural thickening {98}.

## Histopathology

Skin biopsies show infiltration by macrophages, generally with single small nuclei and foamy (xanthomatous) cytoplasm. Multinucleated cells, including Touton giant cells, are frequently observed. Other macrophages with dense eosinophilic cytoplasm may also be present, as may small lymphocytes, plasma cells, and neutrophils. Fibrosis occurs in most cases and is sometimes abundant. The infiltrate may easily be misdiagnosed as xanthelasma, juvenile xanthogranuloma {442,624}, or even a nonspecific inflammatory process {1781}.

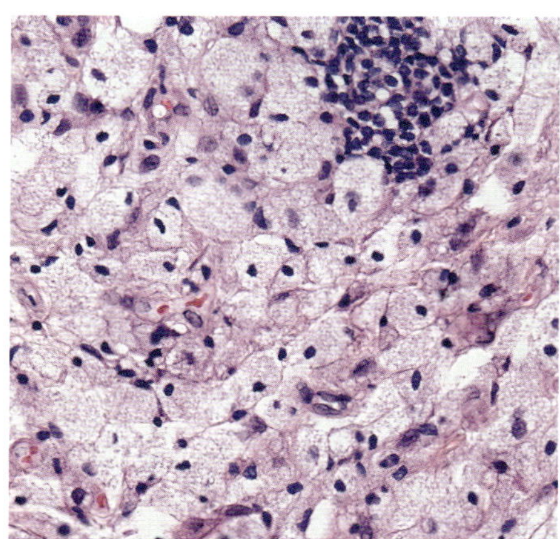

**Fig. 4.147** Erdheim–Chester disease. A subcutaneous infiltrate showing extensive infiltration by foamy macrophages.

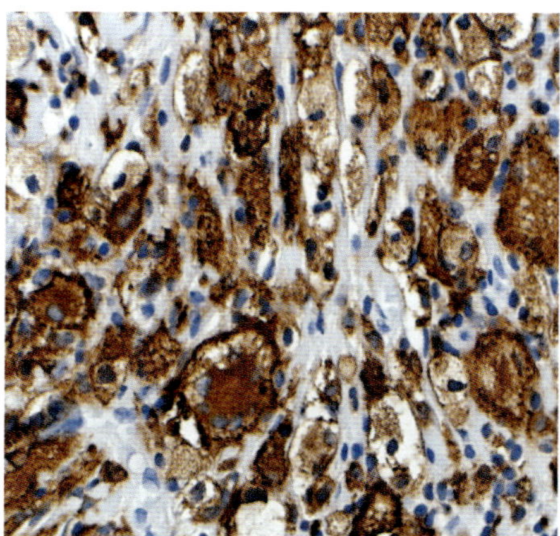

**Fig. 4.148** Erdheim–Chester disease. The foamy, multinucleated cells strongly express CD163.

ECD histiocytes express CD11c, CD14, CD68, and CD163, as well as factor XIIIa and fascin {442,624,710}. Cases focally positive for S100 protein have been reported {686}, but CD1a and langerin are negative. The characteristic immunophenotype is shared by all members of the xanthogranuloma family. Immunohistochemically, ECD cases with mutated *BRAF* stain positively with the monoclonal anti–BRAF p.V600E antibody VE1 {442}.

## Histogenesis

ECD is a benign proliferation of lipid-laden macrophages.

## Genetic profile

In several cases, clonality has been proven by classic cytogenetics and other techniques {626,2729}. Activating mutations in MAPK pathway genes, most notably *BRAF* p.V600E mutations (reported in as many as 66% of cases) {503}, as well as *MAP2K1*, *NRAS*, *KRAS*, and *ARAF* point mutations and *ALK* translocations can be detected in ECD {56,710,1019}. Recurrent mutations in the PI3K pathway gene *PIK3CA* have also been described {56}. Molecular analysis is diagnostically helpful in suspected cases; the presence of characteristic genetic aberrations favour a diagnosis of ECD.

## Prognosis and predictive factors

ECD is a chronic disease; its clinical course depends on the extent and distribution of involvement. Some cases, with lesions limited to the bone, are asymptomatic; others, with systemic disease, may follow an aggressive, rapid clinical course {624,1016}. CNS involvement is a major negative prognostic factor in ECD {96}. The prognosis of ECD was originally reported as poor, with 43% of patients alive after an average follow-up time of 32 months {2741}. For patients treated with interferon alfa, the reported overall 5-year survival rate is 68% {96}. Vemurafenib and cobimetinib (inhibitors of BRAF and MEK, respectively) have recently been used with promising results {362,503,1016,1021}.

# Reticulohistiocytosis

Berti E.
Facchetti F.
Zelger B.

## Definition

The term "reticulohistiocytosis" encompasses a heterogeneous group of monocyte/macrophage proliferative disorders that share the typical histological finding of giant cells with ground-glass cytoplasm. Solitary cutaneous reticulohistiocytosis (SCR) and generalized cutaneous reticulohistiocytosis (GCR) usually lack systemic involvement, whereas multicentric reticulohistiocytosis is invariably associated with erosive polyarthritis and is often multisystemic.

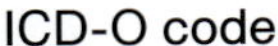

## ICD-O code 8831/0

## Synonym

Reticulohistiocytoma (obsolete)

## Epidemiology

SCR and GCR occur in adults (mean patient age: 35 years) and occasionally in children, with a male-to-female ratio of 1.4:1 {1773,2724}. Multicentric reticulohistiocytosis occurs primarily in adults (mean patient age: 40 years) and more commonly in women, with a female-to-male ratio of 3:1 {2581}.

## Etiology

The etiology is unclear. SCR is probably a reactive condition, occurring in response to a local trauma, insect bite, or infection {372}. GCR may be clonally linked to an underlying leukaemia {840}. Similarly, multicentric reticulohistiocytosis might eventually be shown to occur as the result of a systemic immune derangement, linked to an autoimmune or neoplastic disorder {2378}.

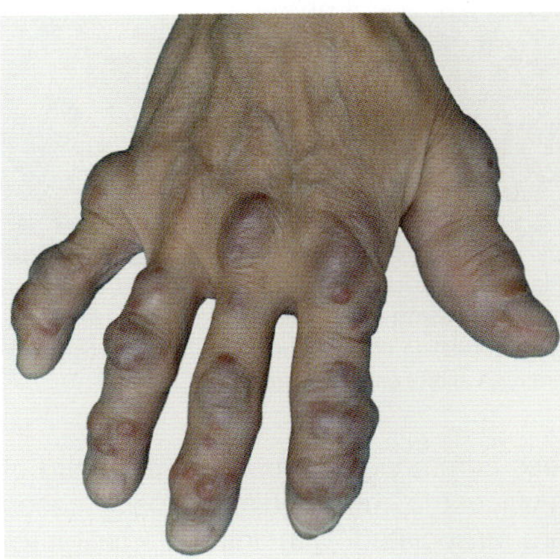

**Fig. 4.149** Multicentric reticulohistiocytosis. Papulonodular lesions preferentially localized on juxta-articular and paronychial areas are typical clinical features.

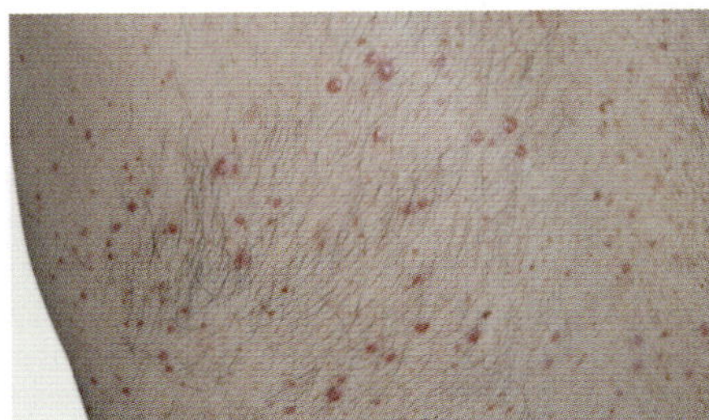

**Fig. 4.150** Generalized cutaneous reticulohistiocytosis. Multiple papular lesions spread over the skin.

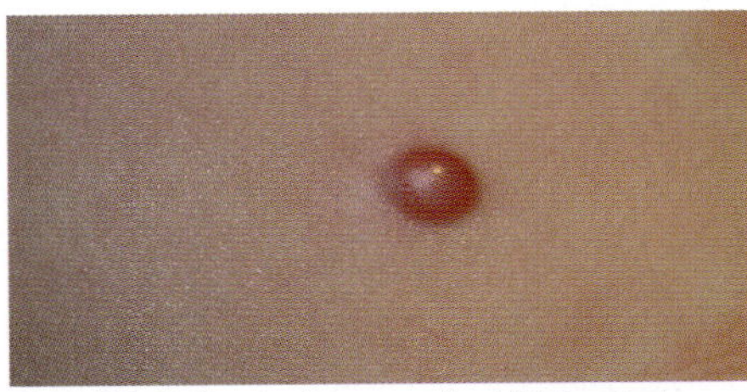

**Fig. 4.151** Solitary cutaneous reticulohistiocytosis. A solitary papular lesion on the back.

## Localization

SCR and GCR occur most commonly on the limbs, trunk, and head and neck region {1773}. GCR may also involve the bone marrow {840}. Multicentric reticulohistiocytosis most frequently involves the acral regions, in particular the head (including mucosae), hands (with the so-called coral-bead sign), and juxta-articular regions of the limbs. The joints are frequently involved, in particular the joints of the hand, as well as the knee and wrist joints {2558}.

## Clinical features

SCR presents with a single, asymptomatic, cutaneous or mucosal, firm xanthomatous to dark-red papule or nodule. It may grow rapidly (but almost never

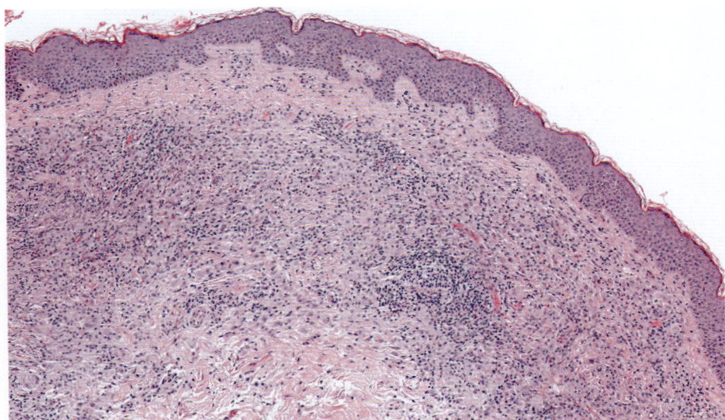

**Fig. 4.152** Generalized cutaneous reticulohistiocytosis. A typical mixed inflammatory infiltrate in the mid-dermis, with several large mononuclear to multinucleated giant cells.

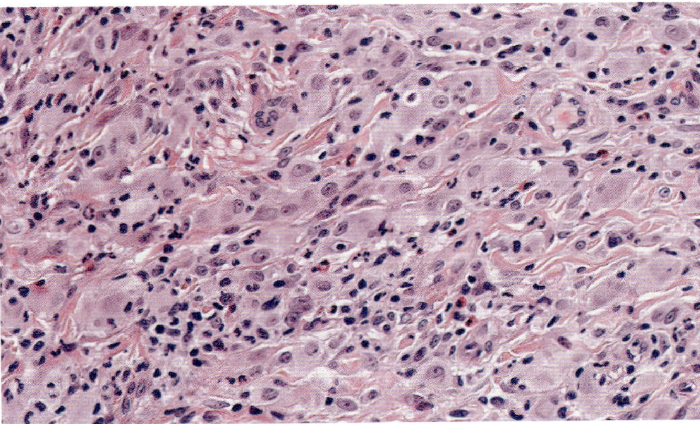

**Fig. 4.153** Generalized cutaneous reticulohistiocytosis. Giant cells with abundant eosinophilic ground-glass cytoplasm, intermingled with small lymphocytes and granulocytes.

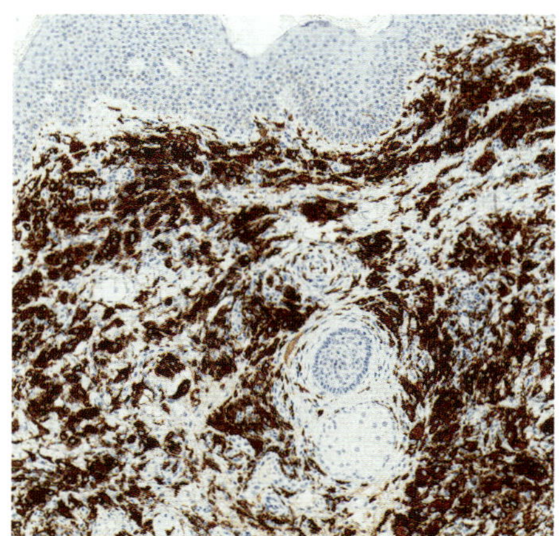

**Fig. 4.154** Generalized cutaneous reticulohistiocytosis. A skin section showing both macrophages and giant cells stained positively for CD163.

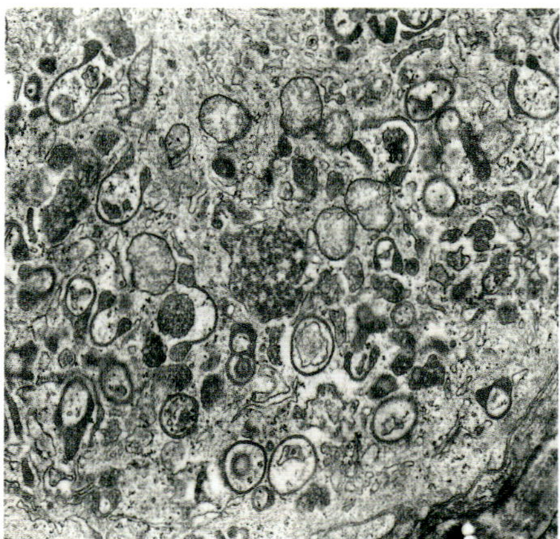

**Fig. 4.155** Multicentric reticulohistiocytosis. Pleomorphic cytoplasmic inclusions are highly complex structures consisting of membranes limiting electron-dense granules and/or containing vesicles.

exceeding 1 cm) and may involute spontaneously {372}. GCR is similar clinically to SCR, but with multiple papulonodular lesions {2724}. GCR diagnoses include pure cutaneous forms and a (less common) cutaneous proliferative disorder of macrophages, concurrent with acute myeloid leukaemia {840,898,2617}. Multicentric reticulohistiocytosis invariably presents with the association of skin lesions and arthritis, often along with fever, weight loss, and weakness. The skin lesions consist of slowly appearing, brownish-red to flesh-coloured papules that are sometimes itchy. The lesions are generally < 1 cm in size but occasionally coalesce into plaques, resulting in a cobblestone appearance. Osteoarticular involvement, the initial symptom in 40% of cases typically manifests as an aggressive erosive peripheral symmetrical polyarthritis. Other organs (e.g. the heart, lungs, and liver) are affected less commonly. As many as one third of multicentric reticulohistiocytosis cases are associated with internal malignancies (e.g. of the lung, bronchus, or ovary) and/or autoimmune disorders (e.g. primary biliary cirrhosis, systemic sclerosis, systemic lupus erythematosus, Sjögren syndrome, and dermatomyositis) {1600,2378,2636}.

## Histopathology

The histology is identical in all variants and tissues. There are large mononuclear (epithelioid), binucleated, or multinucleated giant cells with randomly oriented nuclei and finely granular ground-glass cytoplasm. Early-stage lesions show a mixed infiltrate of lymphocytes, plasma cells, eosinophils, and macrophages, with few multinucleated giant cells. Late-stage lesions show a typical diffuse infiltrate with numerous giant cells. The giant cells sometimes show emperipolesis of neutrophils or lymphocytes {1601,1773}. Immunohistochemically, the macrophages are positive for CD14, CD68 (KP1), CD68 (PGM1), CD163, vimentin, lysozyme, and fascin. They are variably positive for factor XIIIa, and generally negative for CD1a, S100 protein, and langerin (CD207). Giant cells give a positive periodic acid–Schiff (PAS) reaction and stain with Sudan Black B. Electron microscopy reveals peripheral villi on the surface of the giant cells and polylobated nuclei. The cytoplasm is rich in Golgi bodies, mitochondria, activated lysosomes, and myelin figures. Multicentric reticulohistiocytosis shows pleomorphic cytoplasmic inclusions and collagen phagocytosis in 50% of cases {371,1599,1601,1773}.

## Histogenesis

Reticulohistiocytosis is a reactive process of macrophages associated with local trauma or (when systemic) with neoplasms or autoimmune disorders. It is closely related to the xanthogranuloma family of diseases {2804,2921}.

## Prognosis and predictive factors

SCR is cured by excision. GCR can be disfiguring, but it is a benign and sometimes self-healing disorder {1773,2724}. In men, GCR may be associated with acute myeloid leukaemia (upon which the prognosis is dependent) {840,898,2617}. In multicentric reticulohistiocytosis, cutaneous lesions may regress; the prognosis is linked to joint destruction by arthritis and associated neoplasms or autoimmune disorders {2378,2636}.

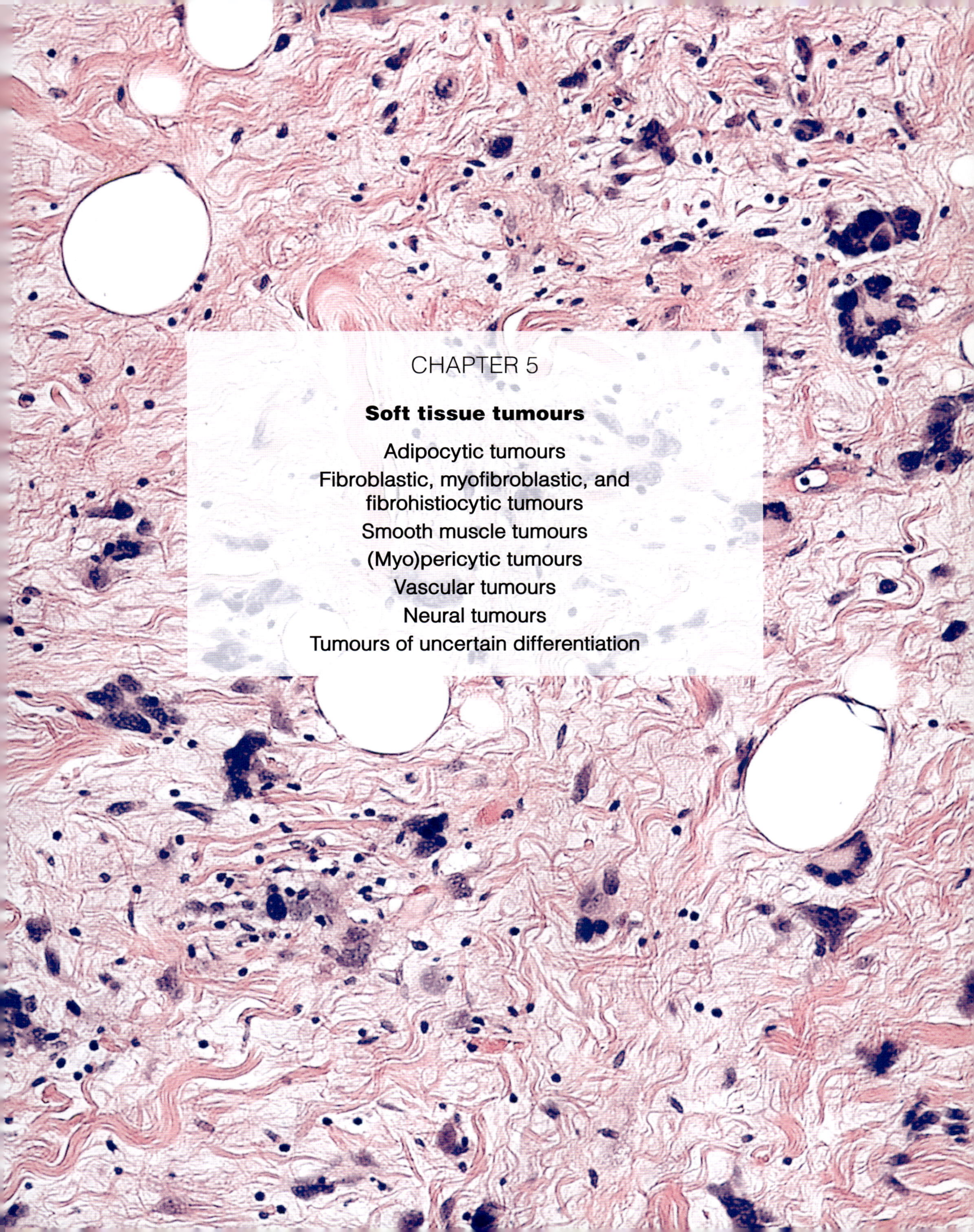

CHAPTER 5

# Soft tissue tumours

# Soft tissue tumours: Introduction

Lazar A.J.
Billings S.D.
Calonje E.
Elder D.E.
Hornick J.L.
Massi D.
Requena L.
Scolyer R.A.

Although this chapter on soft tissue and neural tumours includes only entities that are limited to (or have characteristic expressions in) the skin, a general introduction to soft tissue pathology is provided here for context.

Age-standardized incidence rates of soft tissue sarcomas are fairly constant where adequately tracked, at 30–50 cases per 1 million person-years {861,973,1690,1996}. Benign soft tissue neoplasms as a group are roughly a hundred times as common, with an incidence rate of about 3000 cases per 1 million person-years; the individual entities range from common (e.g. lipoma) to rare (e.g. primitive non-neural granular cell tumour) {1859}. Cutaneous sarcomas are a relatively rare subset of skin tumours, far outnumbered by carcinomas and benign mesenchymal skin neoplasms {2247}. The most common benign mesenchymal tumours are lipomas, dermatofibromas (fibrous histiocytomas), vascular or smooth muscle lesions, and nerve sheath tumours; the vast majority of these tumours are superficial and < 5 cm. Deep soft tissue tumours are covered in the *WHO classification of tumours of soft tissue and bone* volume of this series {792}. Numerically greater and more diverse sarcomas are seen in adults than in children, but sarcomas constitute only 1% of major malignancies in adults {2442}. They arise mainly in the extremities (in particular the thighs), trunk, head and neck, and retroperitoneum. Sarcomas account for about 10–15% of paediatric malignancies, but their overall incidence rate in children is much lower than in adults {979,2836}.

## Etiology

Most soft tissue sarcomas arise spontaneously, with an unknown etiology, but soft tissue tumours (both benign and malignant) are also seen in several inherited syndromes, including Maffucci syndrome (associated with chondroid and vascular tumours) and Cowden syndrome (associated with lipomas and haemangiomas). These syndromes are discussed in more detail in the *WHO classification of tumours of soft tissue and bone* volume {792}. Somatic genetic factors such as recurrent chromosomal translocations drive the pathogenesis of some sarcomas, but how and in what cell these somatic genetic factors arise remains unknown. Viruses associated with soft tissue tumours include EBV (associated with some smooth muscle tumours in immunosuppressed patients) {615} and HHV8 (associated with Kaposi sarcoma) {416}. Angiosarcoma can complicate longstanding lymphoedema, in particular following radical mastectomy (as seen in Stewart–Treves syndrome). Sarcomas can also arise in fields of prior therapeutic irradiation. This is a dose- and time-dependent phenomenon, resulting mostly in subfascial, high-grade pleomorphic sarcomas arising after an average latency period of about 5 years, but cutaneous angiosarcomas can occur as early as 1 year after irradiation for breast carcinoma {1985}.

## Clinical features

Benign and malignant soft tissue and neural tumours typically present as painless masses, and their growth rates vary. Cutaneous lesions form a plaque or elevated nodule, which can ulcerate when malignant. Large (> 5 cm) superficial lesions and all subfascial or deep-seated tumours should be referred to a specialist multidisciplinary centre before biopsy or surgery {573}.

## Histopathology

Malignant soft tissue neoplasms are generally characterized by nuclear pleomorphism, mitotic activity, and necrosis. Some benign tumours can also show one or more of these features; for example, nuclear atypia can be seen in cutaneous pleomorphic fibroma and atypical fibrous histiocytoma (which can also show necrosis), and frequent mitoses can be seen in nodular fasciitis.

## Genetics

Benign soft tissue and neural tumours feature simple genetic properties. In malignancy, two genetic classes exist: simple-karyotype sarcomas associated with a recurrent mutation or translocation (e.g. dermatofibrosarcoma protuberans) and complex-karyotype sarcomas with numerous chromosomal aberrations, including copy-number alterations, but lacking recurrent mutations (e.g. undifferentiated pleomorphic sarcoma) {272}.

## Diagnostic procedures

Investigation includes clinical assessment of the size and depth of the tumour, the use of imaging modalities (CT and MRI), and biopsy. Imaging can be used to assess the extent of a primary tumour, to determine its relationship to normal structures, and to identify metastases.

Superficial lesions < 2–5 cm in diameter can be completely excised. Larger lesions (and all deeper-seated tumours) necessitate diagnostic sampling. Core needle biopsy (often image-guided and preferably using a larger-bore needle) can provide diagnostic information on malignancy, subtype, and grade, with high sensitivity and specificity in experienced hands {1077,2672}. Open biopsy and cytology are less commonly used.

## Tumour behaviour

The *WHO classification of tumours of soft tissue and bone* {792} recognizes four tumour behaviour categories: benign, locally aggressive intermediate, rarely metastasizing intermediate, and malignant. Benign tumours are usually cured by local excision and rarely recur locally (and any recurrences are non-destructive). Intermediate tumours can be either locally aggressive (e.g. fibromatosis, which locally infiltrates surrounding tissues) or rarely metastasizing (generally dermal or subcutaneous tumours with a very low [< 2%] but definite risk of metastasis; e.g. plexiform fibrohistiocytic tumour). Malignant tumours infiltrate and recur locally and commonly metastasize (i.e. in > 20% of cases).

## Grading

Grading, which is an attempt to predict clinical behaviour on the basis of histological variables, can only be performed using material from primary untreated neoplasms. It is not applicable to all sarcomas; for example, angiosarcomas, clear cell sarcomas, and epithelioid sarcomas are always considered to be high-grade. The most widely used system for grading soft tissue sarcomas is the three-tiered system developed by the French Fédération Nationale des Centres de Lutte Contre le Cancer (FNCLCC) {510,1895}. It uses a combination of tumour differentiation, mitotic rate, and necrosis to categorize tumours as being of low, intermediate, or high grade. However, this system is rarely applicable to cutaneous sarcomas. More-broadly applicable molecular approaches are currently in development, but further refinement is needed {457,1548}.

## Staging

The American Joint Committee on Cancer (AJCC)/Union for International Cancer Control (UICC) staging system (the TNM staging system) is widely used {68}. Unlike the staging of many other tumours, sarcoma staging incorporates histological grading and site of involvement along with histological type, tumour size, extent of lymph node involvement, and presence or absence of metastasis. Alternative staging approaches incorporating non-anatomical variables are also under consideration {308,2139}.

## Prognosis and predictive factors

Complete excision is the most important factor in preventing local recurrence {2654,2903}. Some sarcomas (notably epithelioid sarcoma) are relentlessly recurrent, often with late metastases {2284,2496}. Factors generally associated with a greater risk of metastasis are larger tumour size, greater depth of involvement, and higher grade. Accordingly, cutaneous sarcomas have a lower risk of metastasis than do their deeper-seated counterparts {2267}; for example, histologically malignant leiomyosarcomas confined to the dermis are essentially non-metastasizing tumours {1441,1680}. In some instances, histological subtype alone is predictive, but one of the principal factors in assessing prognosis and determining management is histological grade. Site is also important, because low-grade sarcomas in sites where complete surgical excision is difficult (e.g. the retroperitoneum or head and neck) generally have a worse outcome than do similarly staged tumours in the extremities {945}.

# Adipocytic tumours

## Atypical lipomatous tumour

Folpe A.
Kutzner H.
Lazar A.J.

### Definition
Atypical lipomatous tumour is a mesenchymal tumour of borderline malignancy showing adipocytic differentiation. This tumour can recur locally but does not metastasize. The synonym "well-differentiated liposarcoma", historically used for cutaneous and superficial tumours on the extremities, should be avoided for tumours in superficial locations.

### ICD-O codes
| | |
|---|---|
| Atypical lipomatous tumour | 8850/1 |
| Dedifferentiated liposarcoma | 8858/3 |

### Synonym
Well-differentiated liposarcoma (obsolete in dermis and subcutis)

### Epidemiology
Primary cutaneous or dermal atypical lipomatous tumour is exceptionally rare {603,853,1693,1983}; dermal involvement much more commonly constitutes extension from an underlying subcutaneous (or rarely intramuscular) tumour. Exceptionally, dedifferentiation may occur {59,2896}.

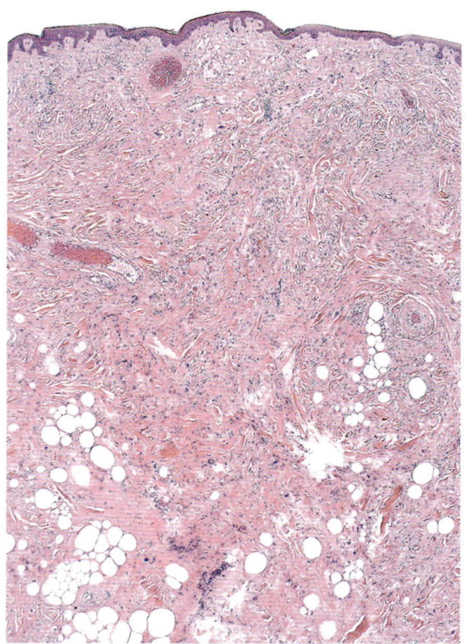

**Fig. 5.01** Primary dermal atypical lipomatous tumour presenting as a dome-shaped mass composed of mature fat and fibrous septa containing hyperchromatic stromal cells. FISH analysis showed that this case harboured a *MDM2* amplification.

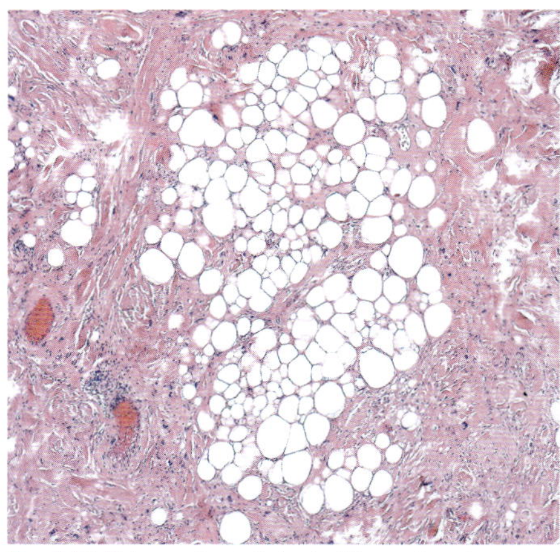

**Fig. 5.02** Primary dermal atypical lipomatous tumour. Medium-power view; note the scattered atypical stromal cells.

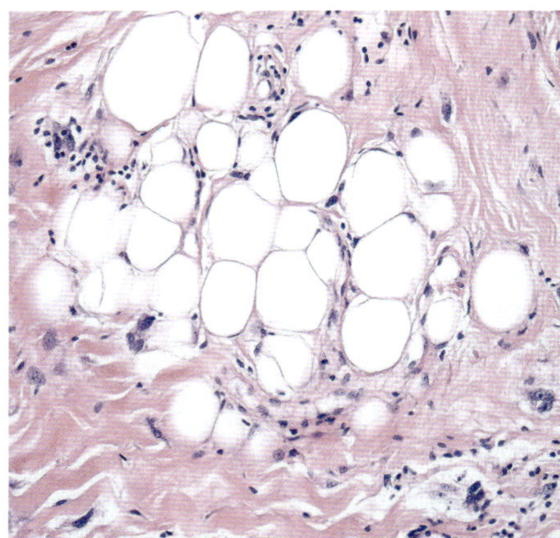

**Fig. 5.03** Primary dermal atypical lipomatous tumour. High-power view of hyperchromatic stromal cells.

### Clinical features
Atypical lipomatous tumour presents as a nonspecific nodule or mass in the dermis or subcutis. Occasional exophytic tumours can mimic an acrochordon (skin tag).

### Histopathology
Atypical lipomatous tumour is composed of a variable proportion of mature adipose tissue, irregular fibrous septa containing hyperchromatic stromal cells, and rare lipoblasts. The atypia can range from subtle to overtly pleomorphic. Dedifferentiated liposarcoma arises in association with a pre-existing atypical lipomatous tumour and most often consists of an undifferentiated pleomorphic sarcoma {717,720,1065}.

### Differential diagnosis
Dermal spindle cell/pleomorphic lipoma may closely simulate dermal atypical lipomatous tumour, but lacks MDM2 overexpression/amplification and shows loss of RB1 expression {446}. Pleomorphic liposarcoma shows greater cellularity, atypia, and mitotic activity, and it frequently consists largely of undifferentiated pleomorphic sarcoma with only scattered lipoblasts {29,44,45}.

### Genetic profile
Atypical lipomatous tumours and dedifferentiated liposarcomas contain giant ring chromosomes containing amplified sequences from the 12q13-15 region {787,1654}. These sequences contain the genes *MDM2*, *CDK4*, *TSPAN31* (*SAS*), *HMGA2* (*HMGIC*), and *CPM*, among others {702,1615,1756,2025,2027}.

### Prognosis and predictive factors
Local recurrence is rare in dermal or subcutaneous atypical lipomatous tumour, and dedifferentiation is extremely rare. Dedifferentiation in cutaneous tumours carries a theoretic risk of metastasis.

# Pleomorphic liposarcoma

Lazar A.J.
Folpe A.
Kutzner H.

## Definition

Pleomorphic liposarcoma is a pleomorphic, high-grade sarcoma containing a variable number of pleomorphic lipoblasts. No areas of well-differentiated liposarcoma or other lines of differentiation are present.

## ICD-O code

8854/3

## Epidemiology

Pleomorphic liposarcomas of the skin and subcutis are extremely rare, with < 75 cases reported (and < 15 of these being dermal) {853,864,1120,2838}. Cases typically occur in older adults {853,864,1120,2838}.

## Localization

These tumours most commonly involve the extremities, followed by the trunk and the head and neck region {853,864,1120,2838}.

## Clinical features

Patients present with a nonspecific or occasionally fatty-looking mass of the skin or subcutis.

## Histopathology

The tumours contain a variable number of pleomorphic lipoblasts in a background of undifferentiated-looking, high-grade, pleomorphic spindle cell sarcoma. Lipoblasts are required for diagnosis, but may be very few in number. Rare cases consist of sheets of pleomorphic lipoblasts, sometimes showing epithelioid or small cell morphology. Myxofibrosarcoma-like histology may be seen {864}.

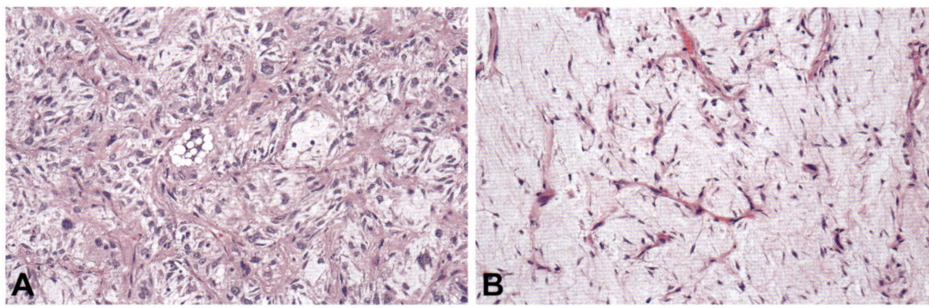


**Fig. 5.05** Pleomorphic liposarcoma. **A** An example consisting chiefly of undifferentiated spindle cell sarcoma, with only very rare pleomorphic lipoblasts. **B** This tumour also shows large areas resembling myxofibrosarcoma, a relatively common finding in subcutaneous pleomorphic liposarcomas.

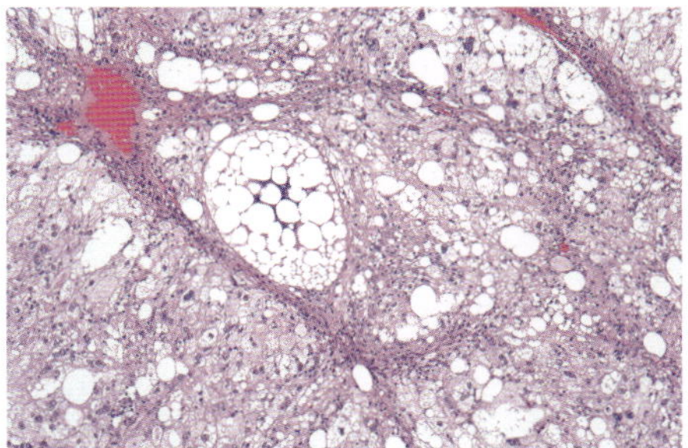

**Fig. 5.06** Pleomorphic liposarcoma. An example composed of sheets of markedly pleomorphic lipoblasts.

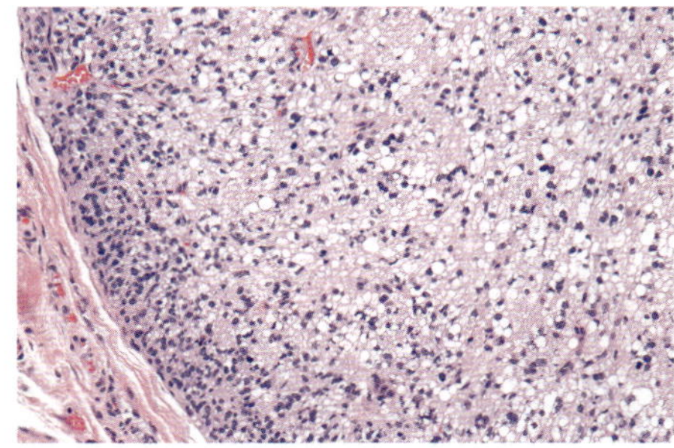

**Fig. 5.07** Pleomorphic liposarcoma. An example with small cell and epithelioid features. Such cases are easily confused with other round cell sarcomas and with lipid-rich carcinomas such as renal cell carcinoma.

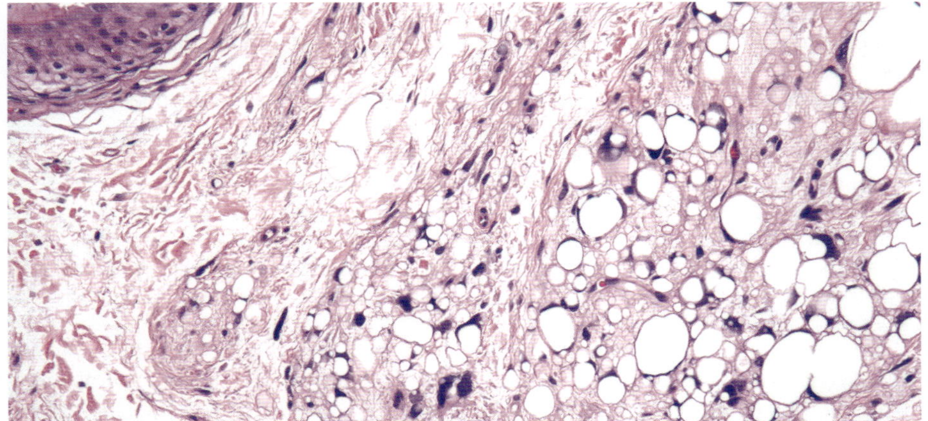

**Fig. 5.04** Primary dermal pleomorphic liposarcoma consisting of a nodule of pleomorphic lipoblasts.

## Differential diagnosis

The differential diagnosis includes other adipocytic neoplasms such as atypical lipomatous tumour, dedifferentiated lipoma, myxoid liposarcoma, and pleomorphic lipoma.

## Genetic profile

Cytogenetic and molecular genetic studies have consistently identified multiple chromosomal copy-number and structural abnormalities (along with *TP53* mutations in deep-seated tumours), similar to the findings in other high-grade pleomorphic sarcomas {879,1756}.

## Prognosis and predictive factors

The prognosis of dermal and subcuticular pleomorphic liposarcoma is very favourable (unlike that of their more common deeply situated counterparts), with only rare reports of metastatic disease {853,864,1120,2838}.

# Lipoma

Low I.
Calonje E.
Ivan D.

## Definition
Lipoma is a benign mesenchymal tumour composed of mature adipocytes.

## ICD-O code 8850/0

## Epidemiology
Lipomas are the most common mesenchymal neoplasms in adults, typically presenting in the fifth or sixth decade of life. They are uncommon in children, unless associated with clinical syndromes. Lipomas are more frequently seen in obese individuals. Some hereditary syndromes are associated with lipomatosis.

## Etiology
The majority of conventional lipomas are idiopathic.

## Localization
The majority of superficial lipomas occur in the subcutaneous tissue of the neck, upper trunk, and proximal limbs; these tumours seldom occur in the face, except in a subfascial location on the forehead. Other than sclerotic (fibroma-like) lipoma, which shows a predilection for acral sites, lipomas rarely involve the distal extremities. Pure cutaneous lipomas are rare {1740}.

## Clinical features
Superficial lipoma typically presents as either solitary or multiple slow-growing, mobile, and painless masses. Multiple lipomas have been reported following total body irradiation therapy. Multiple symmetrical lipomatosis (also called Madelung disease) is characterized by symmetrical lipomatous deposits in the subcutaneous tissue of the neck, back, and upper trunk, usually in middle-aged men. Diffuse lipomatosis typically presents before the age of 2 years, and manifests as infiltrative masses of adipose tissue involving part of a limb or the trunk. There is an association with tuberous sclerosis {1388}. In familial multiple lipomatosis, encapsulated subcutaneous lipomas develop (usually in the third decade of life) on the forearms, trunk, and thighs {1540}. Other hereditary syndromes associated with lipomatosis include Proteus syndrome (characterized by the presence of connective tissue and epidermal naevi, disproportionate overgrowth of body parts, and vascular malformations), Cowden syndrome, and Bannayan–Zonana syndrome (characterized by macrocephaly, subcutaneous and visceral lipomas, and haemangiomas).

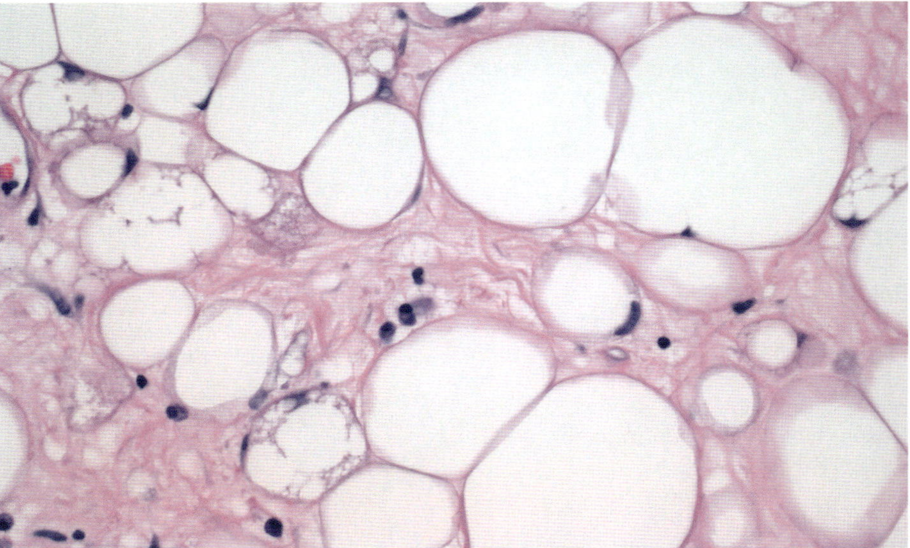

**Fig. 5.08** Fat necrosis. Adipocytes in fat necrosis often show a multivacuolated cytoplasm and substantial variation in cell size and shape; however, the nuclei remain small and normochromatic.

## Histopathology
Conventional lipomas are typically thinly encapsulated masses composed of lobules of mature adipocytes, dissected by thin, incomplete fibrous septa. The histological appearances of lipomas associated with various syndromes are similar, except for the absence of encapsulation in syndromic cases and the more-diffuse infiltrative pattern of the fat in diffuse lipomatosis. Metaplastic bone (osteolipoma) and/or cartilage (chondrolipoma) may occasionally be present in otherwise conventional lipomas, usually in longstanding tumours {2486}. Some lipomas contain a prominent fibrous component (fibrolipomas) or myxoid component (myxolipomas). Myxolipomas that are richly vascular are called angiomyxolipomas {1525}. Sclerotic (fibroma-like) lipoma is an uncommon variant, characterized by sclerotic or myxocollagenous stroma containing sparsely distributed, bland spindle to stellate cells and scattered adipocytes {1494}. Chondroid lipoma is a rare, morphologically distinct lipoma variant that consists of cords and nests of small round vacuolated cells embedded within a myxoid to hyaline chondroid matrix, with interspersed mature adipocytes {2612}. Chondroid lipomas are richly vascular, and secondary changes such as haemorrhage, sclerosis, and calcifications are common. In addition to diffusely expressing S100 protein, the vacuolated cells may occasionally express keratins {1372}.

## Differential diagnosis
Benign lipomas are usually easy to distinguish from atypical lipomatous tumours by the absence of atypical stromal cells and lipoblasts {1983}. Benign adipocytes may display vacuolated nuclei called Lochkern, which should not be confused with lipoblasts. Traumatized lipomas may show marked degenerative changes, such as fibrosis, fat necrosis, and myxoid

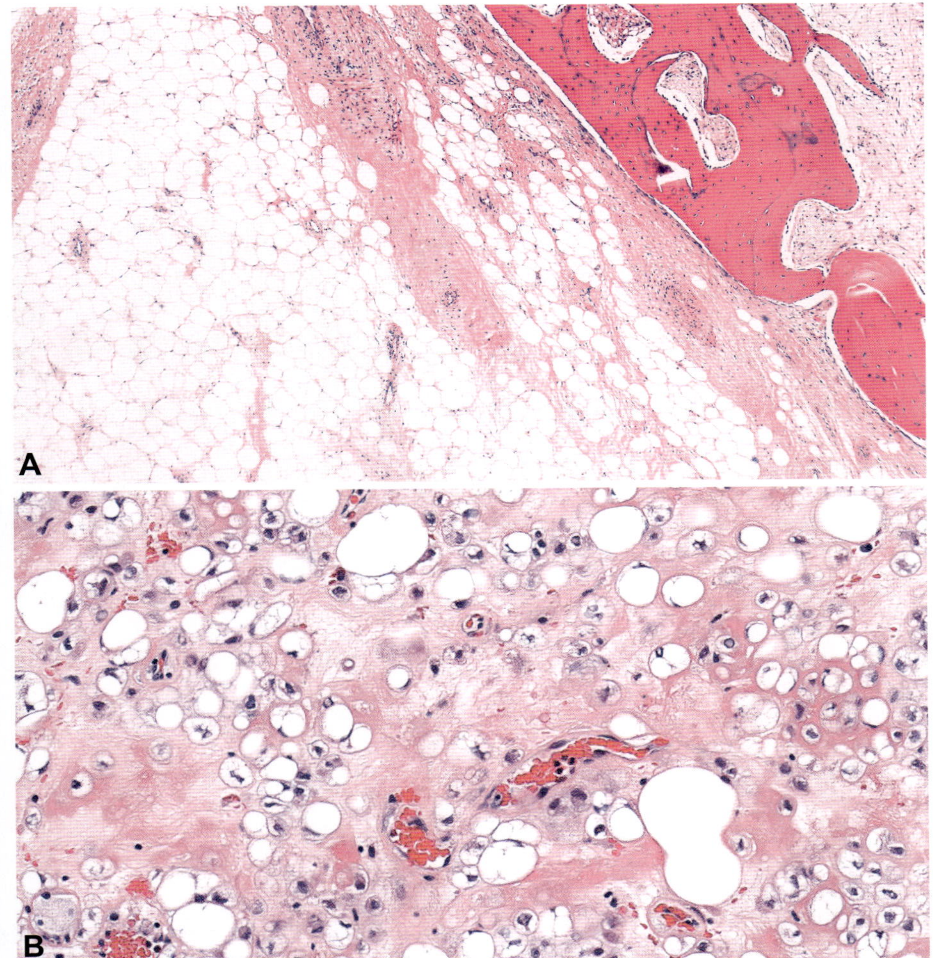

**Fig. 5.09 A** Osteolipoma. Metaplastic bone and/or cartilage may be present in otherwise conventional lipomas, usually in longstanding tumours. **B** Chondroid lipoma. Adipocytes of variable size are present in a chondromyxoid matrix. Small adipocytes have multivacuolated cytoplasm.

change, but they do not show the hyperchromasia of atypical stromal cells seen in atypical lipomatous tumour. Some cases of myxolipoma can be difficult to distinguish from spindle cell lipoma with marked myxoid change, which shows spindle-shaped cells and ropy collagen. Chondroid lipoma should be distinguished from extraskeletal myxoid chondrosarcoma, which is very uncommon in superficial locations, is usually sizeable at presentation, and lacks interspersed adipocytes.

## Histogenesis

Structural aberrations resulting in deregulation of the *HMGA2* gene play an important pathogenic role in a substantial proportion of conventional lipomas. The protein encoded by *HMGA2* contains structural DNA-binding domains that likely act as a transcriptional regulating factor in adipogenesis {2865}.

## Genetic profile

Clonal karyotypic abnormalities are seen in >50% of conventional lipomas. The most common rearrangements are translocations involving 12q13-15, which affect the high-mobility group (HMG) proteins {165,742}. Rearrangements involving 6p21-23 and interstitial deletions of 13q have also been reported. A recurrent t(11;16) chromosomal translocation has been identified in chondroid lipoma {1140}.

## Genetic susceptibility

In familial multiple lipomatosis, the pattern of inheritance is usually autosomal dominant, and the involved gene has been mapped to 12q14.3. Germline mutations in the *PTEN* tumour suppressor gene (located at 10q23.31) are common in patients with Proteus syndrome and Bannayan–Zonana syndrome.

## Prognosis and predictive factors

Lipomas (both conventional types and less common variants) are completely benign, but they rarely (i.e. in < 5% of cases) recur locally.

# Spindle cell/pleomorphic lipoma

Billings S.D.
Patel R.M.
Wong D.D.

## Definition

Spindle cell/pleomorphic lipoma (SCL/PL) is a single entity of which spindle cell lipoma and pleomorphic lipoma are two morphological expressions. Spindle cell lipoma is a benign adipocytic tumour composed of mature fat, bland spindle cells, and ropy collagen {696}. Pleomorphic lipoma additionally features pleomorphic cells and multinucleated floret-like giant cells {2428}.

## ICD-O code 8857/0

## Synonyms

Spindle cell lipoma; pleomorphic lipoma; dendritic fibromyxolipoma

## Epidemiology

SCL/PL is most frequent among men aged 45–60 years; < 10% of cases occur in women {74,696,791,2428}.

## Localization

These tumours most commonly affect the subcutis of the posterior neck, back, and shoulders {696,2428}; about 20% of cases involve other sites, including the face, scalp, oral cavity, upper and lower limbs, chest, and trunk {74,791,2428,2673}. Dermal-based and intramuscular lesions are rarely encountered {823,2673}. In women, the extremities are the most common site {1398}.

## Clinical features

SCL/PL is a painless, mobile, firm, subcutaneous mass measuring 3–5 cm, which develops slowly (over the course of years). A familial predisposition, with multiple lesions, has been described {734,1032}.

## Histopathology

Spindle cell lipomas are well-circumscribed lesions composed of a combination of mature adipocytes, bland spindle cells, and eosinophilic ropy collagen bundles occurring in variable proportions, often in a fibromyxoid stroma {74,696,791}. Mast cells are a consistent finding. The adipocytes vary in size compared with conventional lipomas, and lipoblasts are seen in as many as 50% of cases {1766}. Spindle cells are randomly arranged in short, parallel bundles. Nuclei are bland, elongated, and uniform in size and shape, and they may palisade. Pleomorphic lipomas additionally show pleomorphic spindle cells and multinucleated floret-like giant cells with radially located, hyperchromatic nuclei {124,2428}. Variants include fat-poor lesions, in which spindle cells predominate over the lipomatous component {246,2269}; myxoid variants {2854}; a (pseudo)angiomatous variant with slit-like spaces and pseudopapillary projections {1046,2909}; and lesions with plexiform growth patterns {2922}, extramedullary haematopoiesis {2363}, and focal cartilaginous and osseous metaplasia {791}. SCL/PLs characteristically stain strongly and diffusely for CD34 {2535,2592} and show loss of nuclear RB1 expression {446}.

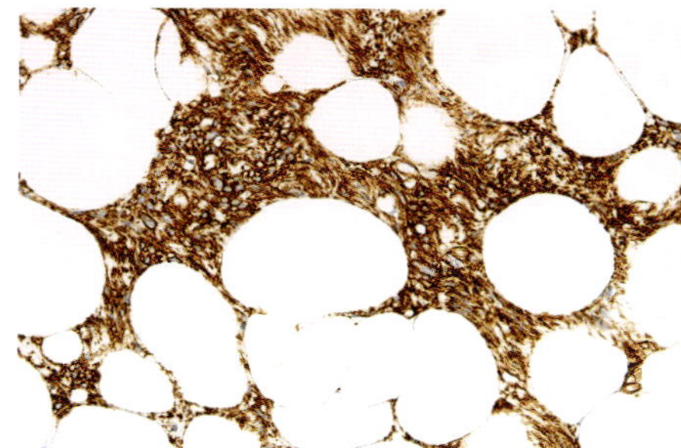

**Fig. 5.12** Spindle cell lipoma. All components are immunoreactive for CD34.

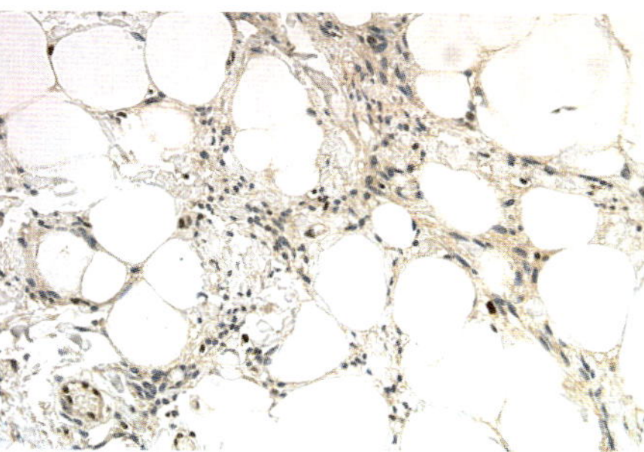

**Fig. 5.13** Spindle cell lipoma. Loss of nuclear RB1 immunoreactivity within constituent cells; note the intact nuclear RB1 expression in endothelial cells (an internal positive control).

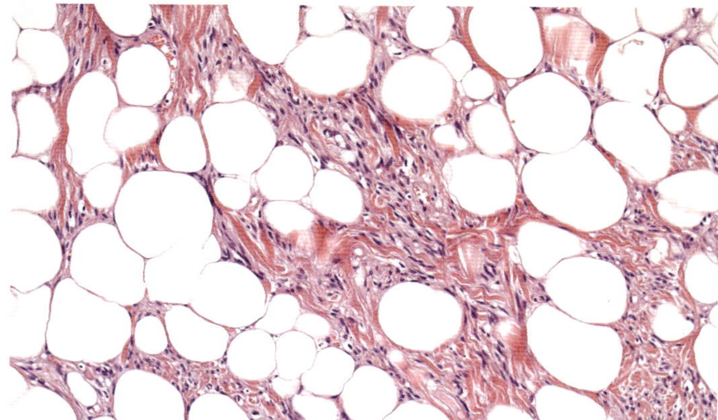

**Fig. 5.10** Spindle cell lipoma. A variable combination of mature fat, bland spindle cells, and ropy collagen.

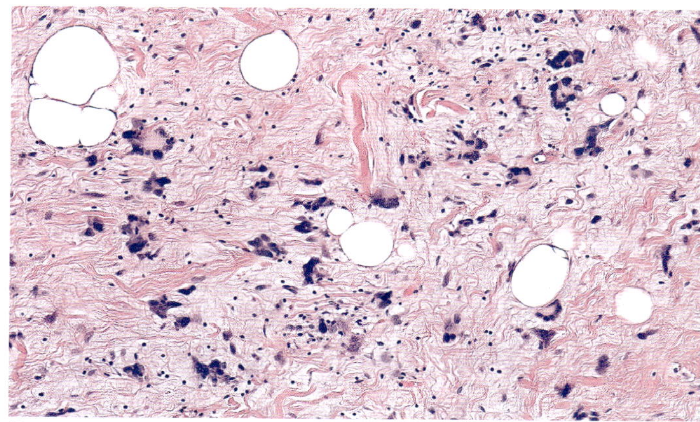

**Fig. 5.11** Pleomorphic lipoma. Features of spindle cell lipoma with the addition of pleomorphic cells and multinucleated floret-like giant cells.

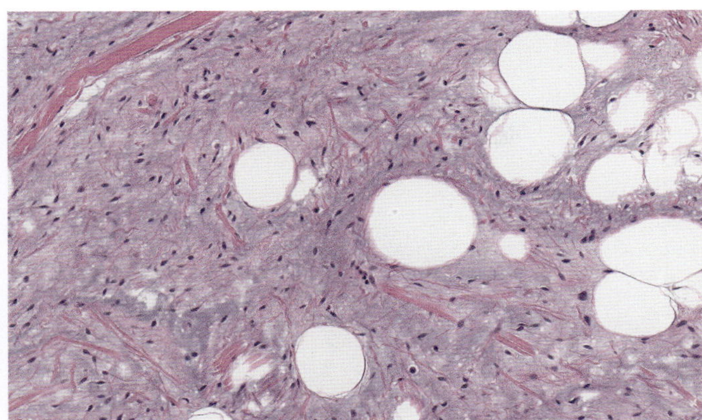

**Fig. 5.14** Myxoid spindle cell lipoma. Bland spindle cells, ropy collagen, and mature adipocytes in an extensively myxoid stroma.

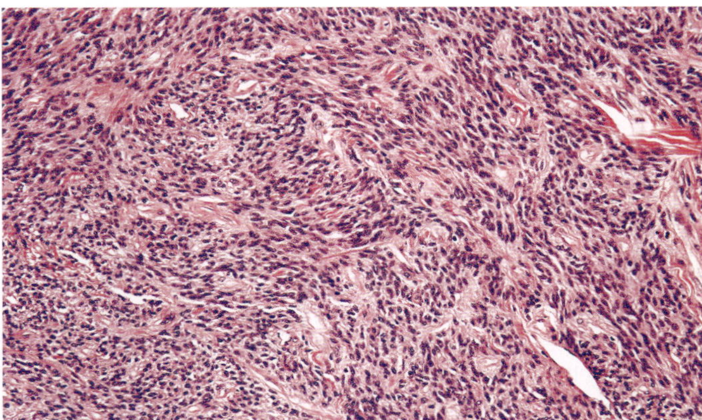

**Fig. 5.15** Fat-free spindle cell lipoma. Intersecting fascicles of bland spindle cells and ropy collagen in the absence of a significant adipocytic component.

## Differential diagnosis

SCL/PLs (particularly fat-poor lesions) must be distinguished from other CD34-positive superficial spindle cell lesions, including myxofibrosarcoma, dermatofibrosarcoma protuberans, solitary fibrous tumour, and neurofibroma {2471}. Pleomorphic lipoma may mimic atypical lipomatous tumour/well-differentiated liposarcoma and pleomorphic liposarcoma {853}. Cellular angiofibroma and mammary-type myofibroblastoma have features overlapping with those of SCL/PL and are related entities {1633,1634,1721,2536}.

## Histogenesis

The histogenesis is likely related to *RB1* loss.

## Genetic profile

Recurrent cytogenetic abnormalities involving deletions of 13q and 16q are characteristic of SCL/PL {560,563,787}. FISH studies indicate that breakpoints in 13q deletions cluster around the region 13q14, where *RB1* resides {560}. Monoallelic and biallelic deletions of *RB1* are found in most cases {164,560}. The same findings are seen in mammary-type myofibroblastoma and cellular angiofibroma, supporting their relation to SCL/PL {796,1626,1721}.

## Prognosis and predictive factors

SCL/PLs are benign tumours {74,696,2428}.

# Angiolipoma

Billings S.D.
Requena L.

## Definition
Angiolipoma is a subcutaneous tumour composed of mature fat cells and clusters of thin-walled capillaries, often with fibrin thrombi.

## ICD-O code 8861/0

## Epidemiology
Angiolipomas are common tumours. They usually present in teenagers and young adults, and are more common in males than in females. Rare cases are familial {6}.

## Etiology
Most cases occur secondary to mutations in *PRKD2* {1104}.

## Localization
Angiolipomas most commonly involve the extremities, followed by the trunk, but a wide variety of sites (including the breast, head and neck, deep soft tissue, and organs) can be involved {88,1104,1449}.

## Clinical features
Angiolipomas usually present as multiple, small, painful subcutaneous nodules.

## Histopathology
Angiolipomas have varying proportions of mature adipocytes admixed with clusters of capillaries embedded in hyalinized stroma with spindled cells. Intravascular fibrin thrombi are common. Rare cases with few fat cells are termed cellular angiolipoma {2405}.

## Differential diagnosis
Spindle cell lipoma lacks clusters of capillaries and has ropy collagen bundles. Kaposi sarcoma is composed of spindled cells with slit-like vascular spaces and is immunoreactive for HHV8. The vessels of angiosarcoma have complex architecture, and the tumour cells have nuclear atypia. Intramuscular haemangiomas have more-variable vessels rather than only clusters of capillaries.

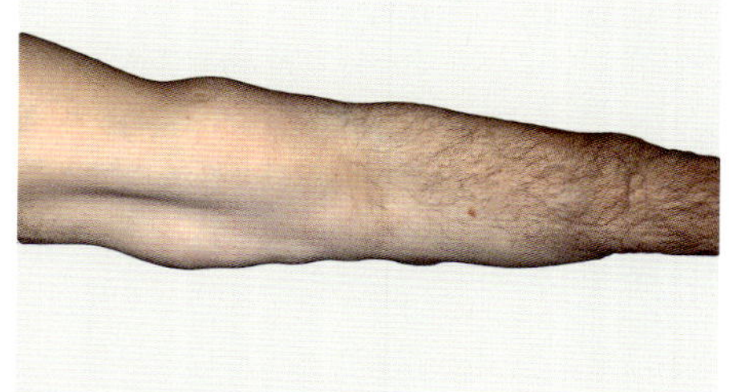

**Fig. 5.16** Multiple angiolipomas.

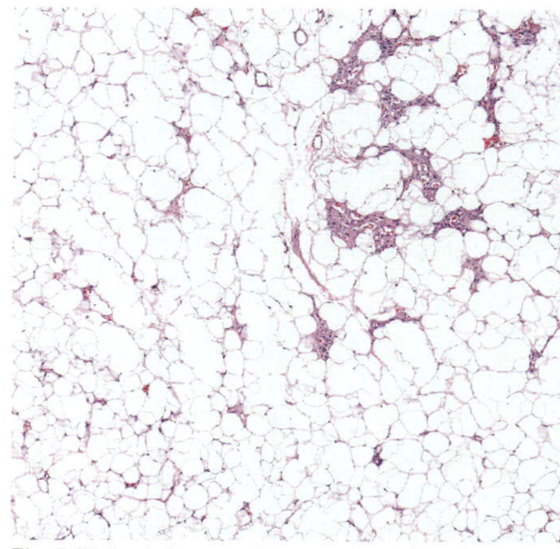

**Fig. 5.17** Angiolipoma. An example with clusters of capillaries and mature adipose tissue.

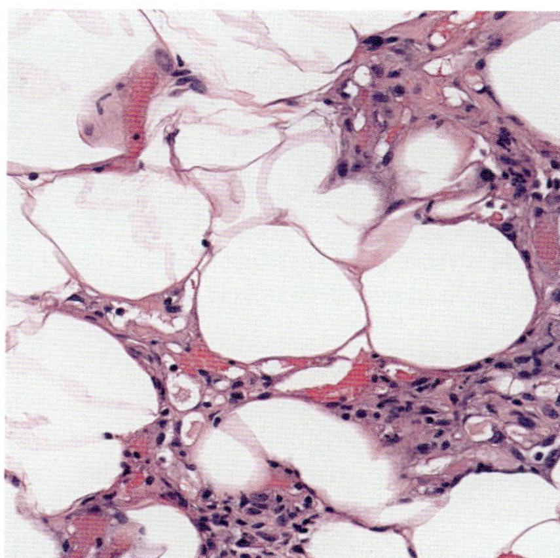

**Fig. 5.18** Angiolipoma. Fibrin thrombi are often seen in the vessels of angiolipoma.

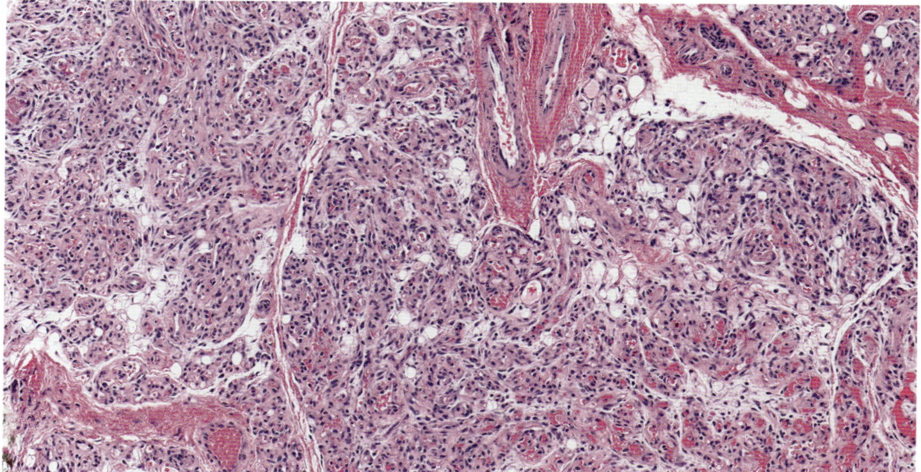

**Fig. 5.19** Angiolipoma. Rare cases, termed cellular angiolipoma, consist almost entirely of the vascular component, with little mature adipose tissue.

## Histogenesis
Mutations in *PRKD2*, found predominantly in the adipocytes, promote angiogenesis {1104}.

## Genetic profile
About 80% of angiolipomas have low-level mutations in *PRKD2* {1104}. The adipocytes have the highest levels of mutation.

## Genetic susceptibility
As many as 5% of cases are familial, with an autosomal dominant pattern of inheritance {854}.

## Prognosis and predictive factors
Angiolipomas are benign, with no risk of malignant progression.

# Naevus lipomatosus superficialis

Requena L.
Cheah A.L.
Patel R.M.

## Definition
Naevus lipomatosus superficialis (NLS) is a developmental anomaly characterized by ectopic adipose tissue within the upper half of the dermis. There are two subtypes: the rare classic form, consisting of multiple lesions in a zonal distribution, and the more common solitary form.

## Synonym
Naevus lipomatosus cutaneous superficialis (of Hoffmann–Zurhelle)

## Epidemiology
NLS is rare. In the classic form, lesions are either present at birth or develop within the first two decades of life {1245}. The solitary form has been reported in a wider age group, ranging from birth to 88 years {974,1043}. There is no sex predilection {1245}.

## Etiology
The etiology is unknown. NLS is a malformation.

## Localization
NLS is typically seen in the gluteal region and neighbouring skin, including the lower back and upper thigh {12,781,2110,2176}. There may be a linear or zosteriform distribution, and the lesions typically do not cross the midline {1245,1732}. The solitary form has additionally been reported to occur at locations outside of the pelvic girdle, including the head and neck {1990,2273,2329,2805}, upper extremities {1245,2423}, distal lower extremities {12,1245,2713}, and clitoris {1043}.

## Clinical features
NLS typically presents as painless, slow-growing, soft, skin-coloured to yellow, dome-shaped papules and nodules with wrinkling of the overlying skin. The papules may coalesce into plaques with a cerebriform surface. Occasional cases may show surface comedones {1245,1732}. The reported sizes range from 0.3 cm to 20 cm {12,1732}. There are usually no associated clinical abnormalities {12}. An extremely rare association with generalized folded skin (Michelin tire baby syndrome) has been reported {852,2246}. Although clinically benign, rare cases may recur locally following excision {12}.

## Histopathology
NLS is composed of groups of mature adipocytes at the level of the papillary dermis, typically around subpapillary blood vessels {12,1732}. The amount of ectopic fat is variable. Accompanying connective tissue changes in the dermis include an increase in the density of small blood vessels, irregularly distributed and sometimes thickened collagen, and increased numbers of fibroblasts {12,1181}. The elastic tissue is decreased in lesional skin. There is an inverse relationship between the vascularity of the lesion and the proportion of fat present {12}. One electron microscopic study suggested that the lesional adipocytes arise from precursor cells lying close to the blood vessels, comparable to the sequence of events seen in fetal adipogenesis {2176}. The epidermis may show irregular acanthosis, follicular plugging {12,781,1732}, and (rarely) abnormalities of folliculosebaceous units {1179,2560,2900}.

## Differential diagnosis
NLS must be differentiated from lipoma and soft tissue fibroma with lipomatous stroma. Lipoma is typically a well-circumscribed subcutaneous nodular lesion composed mostly of mature adipocytes. Although thin connective tissue septa may separate lobules of adipocytes in lipomas, there is no normal dermis between the adipocytes like in NLS. Soft tissue fibroma contains groups of mature adipocytes in the stroma, but the lesion has a pedunculated silhouette. Soft tissue fibromas with fatty metaplasia are considered by some to be a solitary form of NLS.

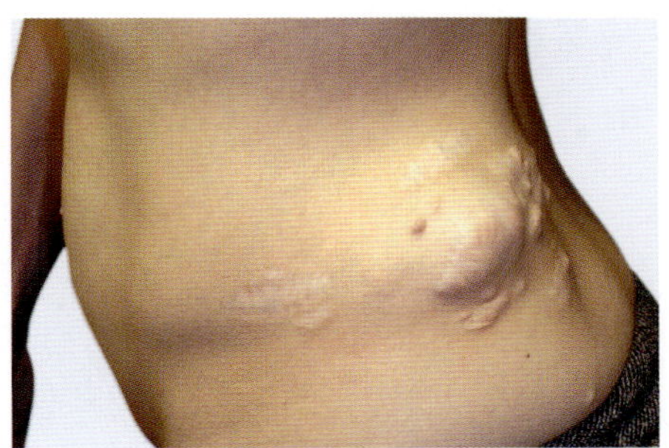

**Fig. 5.20** Naevus lipomatosus superficialis. Soft nodules with a zosteriform distribution on the lateral trunk and lower back.

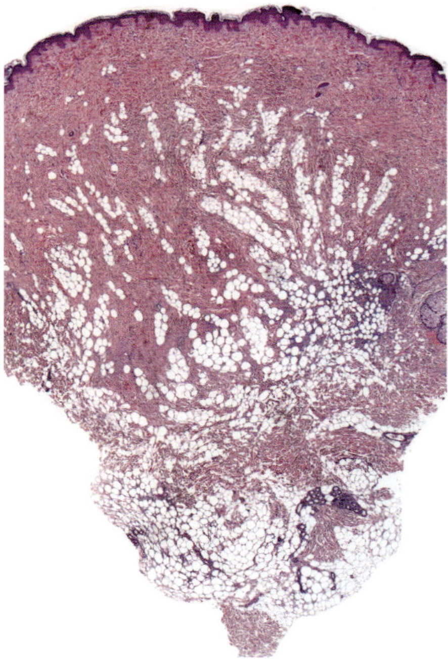

**Fig. 5.21** Naevus lipomatosus superficialis. A scanning view showing groups of mature adipocytes abnormally located in the upper dermis.

## Genetic profile
The single case of NLS that has been analysed cytogenetically showed deletion of 2p24 {377}.

## Genetic susceptibility
No associated hereditary syndromes or susceptibility genes have been reported.

## Prognosis and predictive factors
NLS is a benign lesion. Simple excision is curative.

# Myxoinflammatory fibroblastic sarcoma

Hornick J.L.
Laskin W.B.

## Definition

Myxoinflammatory fibroblastic sarcoma (MIFS) is a low-grade fibroblastic neoplasm with a predilection for acral soft tissue, characterized by prominent inflammation and bizarre ganglion-like and vacuolated, mucin-filled (pseudolipoblast-like) cells.

## ICD-O code 8811/1

## Synonyms

Acral MIFS {1735}; inflammatory myxoid tumour of the soft parts with bizarre giant cells {1763}; inflammatory myxohyaline tumour of the distal extremities with virocyte/Reed–Sternberg–like cells {1820}

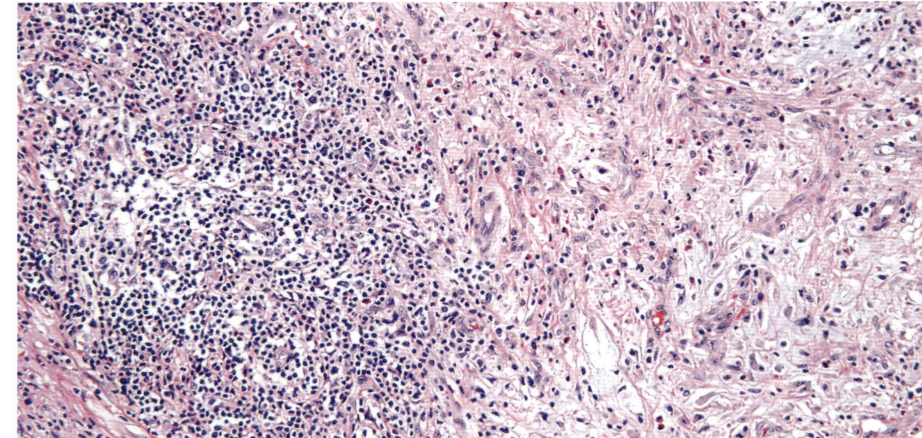

**Fig. 5.22** Myxoinflammatory fibroblastic sarcoma showing an admixture of fibroinflammatory and myxoid areas; note the dense chronic inflammatory infiltrate.

## Epidemiology

MIFS is most common among individuals in the fourth to sixth decades of life; it is rare in children and adolescents {1496,1735,1820}. This entity affects the sexes equally {1496,1735,1820}.

## Etiology

MIFS is sporadic.

## Localization

These tumours occur primarily in the fingers and hands (affected in > 50% of cases), the dorsum of the feet (in > 20%), and the wrists/ankles (in ~15%); rare cases occur in more-proximal and non-appendicular sites {1455,1496,1589}.

## Clinical features

Most patients present with a painless mass clinically resembling a benign process {1496,1735,1820}. As can be seen radiologically and at surgery, MIFS is centred within superficial soft tissue and often spreads along fascia and tendon sheaths to involve the joint space, muscle, and (rarely) bone {1455,1820,2583}.

## Histopathology

The tumour is composed of collagenous and myxohyaline zones, hypovascular pools of mucin, and a variably dense mixed inflammatory infiltrate. The neoplastic elements are mild to moderately atypical plump spindled and epithelioid cells, a lesser number of ganglion-like cells with irregularly contoured nuclei and viral inclusion–like nucleoli (Reed–Sternberg–like cells), and pleomorphic pseudolipoblasts {1496,1735,1820}. Mitoses are usually scarce to absent,

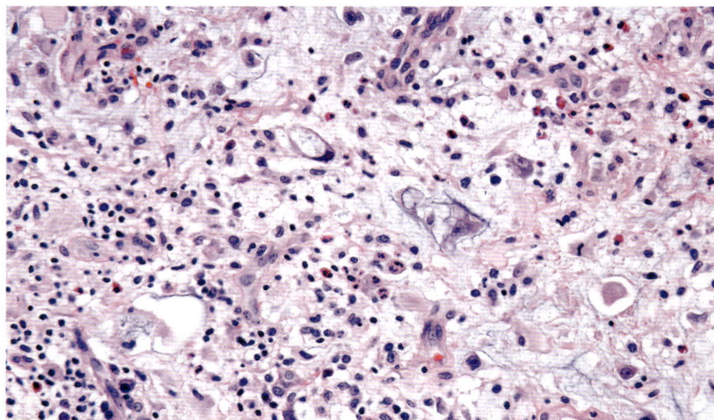

**Fig. 5.23** Myxoinflammatory fibroblastic sarcoma. In the myxoid regions, pseudolipoblasts are usually seen; the inflammatory infiltrate is often polymorphous.

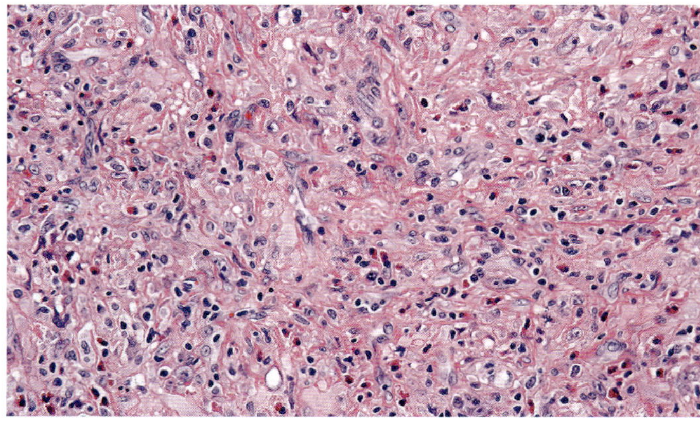

**Fig. 5.24** Myxoinflammatory fibroblastic sarcoma. The variably spindled to epithelioid cells admixed with inflammatory cells are embedded in a hyalinized stroma.

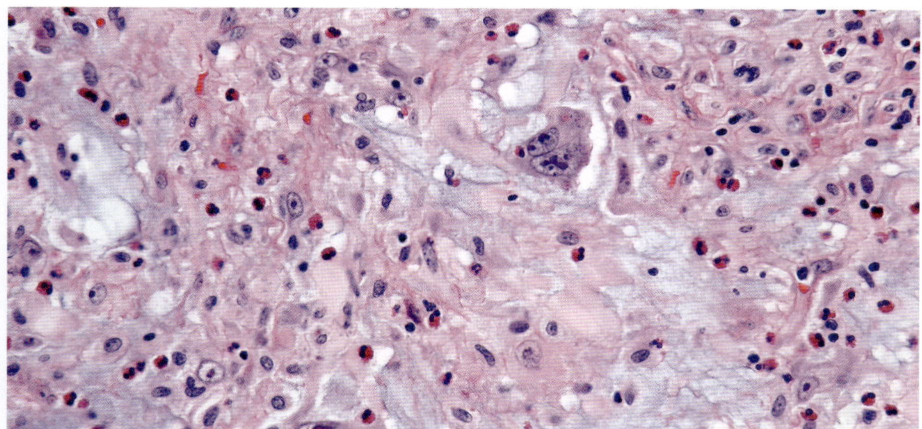

**Fig. 5.25** Myxoinflammatory fibroblastic sarcoma. Occasional pleomorphic cells with inclusion-like macronucleoli are a characteristic finding.

and atypical forms are not seen. The tumour cells demonstrate diffuse vimentin; variable CD34 and podoplanin (recognized by D2-40); and focal keratin, KIT (CD117), CD68, and actin expression {1438,1496,1735}.

## Differential diagnosis

Superficially located haemosiderotic fibrolipomatous tumour {1666}, pleomorphic hyalinizing angiectatic tumour {2468}, and low-grade myxofibrosarcoma {1744,2801} lack Reed–Sternberg-like cells and prominent inflammation. Superficial CD34-positive fibroblastic tumour {393} lacks mucin and exhibits more cytological atypia and diffuse CD34 expression.

## Histogenesis

The tumour cells show fibroblastic differentiation {1735}.

## Genetic profile

Some cases harbour an unbalanced or balanced t(1;10)(p22;q24), involving *TGFBR3* in 1p22 and *MGEA5* in 10q24, along with amplification of 3p11-12 (including *VGLL3*) in the form of supernumerary ring chromosomes {82,994,1485,1658}. The same genetic findings have been reported in haemosiderotic fibrolipomatous tumour and tumours with hybrid features of MIFS and haemosiderotic fibrolipomatous tumour {82,675}. The translocation may be more common in hybrid tumours than in pure MIFS {2941}.

## Prognosis and predictive factors

The recurrence rate averages about 30% for reported cases {1455,1496,1589} and roughly correlates with the completeness of surgical excision {1496}. Approximately 3% of cases metastasize, mainly to regional lymph nodes and less often to the lung {1455,1496,1589}. No particular histological features are predictive of aggressive behaviour.

# Dermatofibrosarcoma protuberans and variants

Lazar A.J.
Mahar A.

## Definition

Dermatofibrosarcoma protuberans (DFSP) is a superficial fibroblastic neoplasm with storiform architecture, harbouring the characteristic translocation t(17;22)(q21.3;q13.1) resulting in *COL1A1-PDGFB* fusion.

## ICD-O codes

| | |
|---|---|
| Dermatofibrosarcoma protuberans | 8832/1 |
| Giant cell fibroblastoma | 8834/1 |
| Bednar tumour | 8833/1 |
| Fibrosarcomatous dermatofibrosarcoma protuberans | 8832/3 |

## Epidemiology

Most cases are sporadic.

## Etiology

*COL1A1-PDGFB* fusions drive tumorigenesis.

## Localization

DFSP is most common on the trunk, followed by the proximal extremities and the head and neck region {285,2615}.

## Clinical features

These neoplasms usually present as a painless, firm, slow-growing plaque or nodule. Discolouration may be seen (brown, reddish-blue, or violaceous). Longstanding lesions may develop a multinodular or so-called protuberant appearance. Rapid growth in a longstanding lesion may herald fibrosarcomatous transformation.

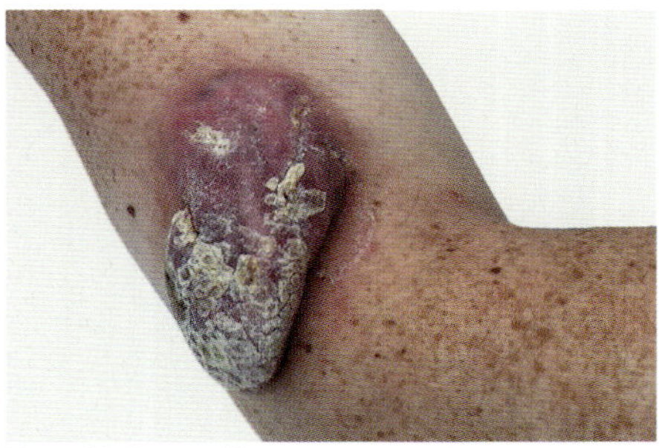

**Fig. 5.26** Dermatofibrosarcoma protuberans on the arm.

## Histopathology

*Classic DFSP*

The classic form is characterized by a proliferation of uniform, medium-sized spindle cells with a storiform or cartwheel pattern of growth centred in the dermis. It is separated from the epidermis by a grenz zone and infiltrates the subcutaneous adipose tissue in a lace-like or honeycomb pattern. It lacks the overlying epidermal hyperplasia of a dermatofibroma. The periphery is poorly defined and the tumour can show subtle tentacle-like extension along tissue planes and around lobules of subcutaneous adipose tissue. Less commonly, it can be centred in the subcutis, with minimal or no dermal involvement. Mitotic figures are infrequent. There is minimal atypia. Intense staining for CD34 is characteristic.

*Giant cell fibroblastoma*

This variant is most commonly seen in childhood (and is considered a paediatric variant of DFSP). Compared with the classic form, giant cell fibroblastoma has a similar location and storiform spindle cell morphology but shows additional features, including numerous multinucleated giant cells with wreath-like arrangement of nuclei around pseudovascular spaces, as well as prominent myxoid change {1227,2598}.

*Myxoid DFSP*

This uncommon subtype is defined as DFSP with >50% myxoid change. The tumours show multinodular growth with abundant pale myxoid stroma, frequently branching small thin-walled vessels, and scattered mast cells {1751,2150}. This variant is diagnostically challenging, because the storiform pattern can be obscured by myxoid stroma.

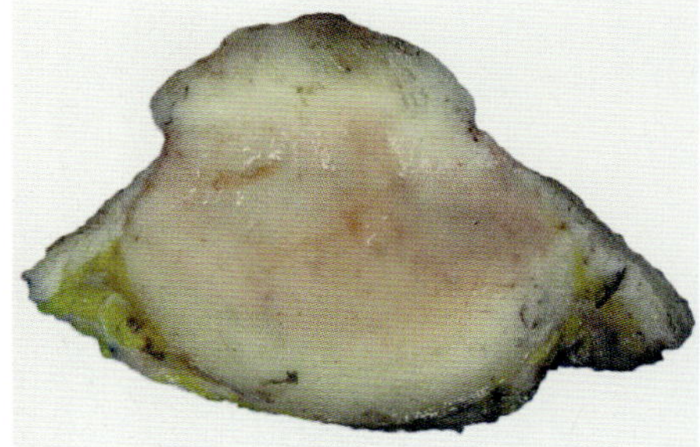

**Fig. 5.27** Dermatofibrosarcoma protuberans. Cut section showing a firm, fibrous tumour.

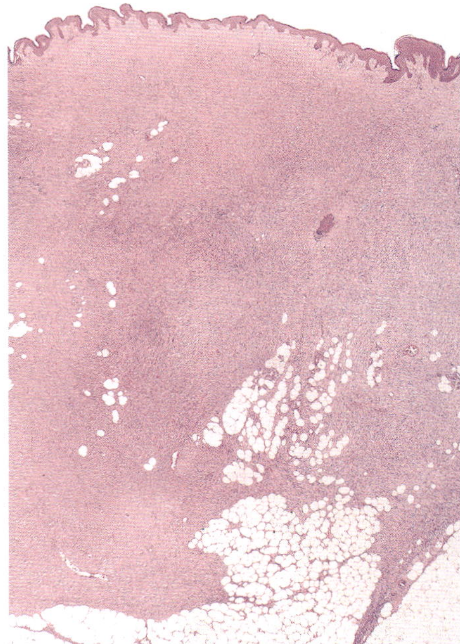

**Fig. 5.28** Dermatofibrosarcoma protuberans. Tumour fills the dermis and extends into the subcutis.

*Pigmented DFSP (Bednar tumour)*

This variant contains numerous dendritic cells containing melanin pigment. The pigmented cells can show positive staining for S100 protein.

*Myoid DFSP*

This variant is characterized by pale nodules of spindle-shaped cells with eosinophilic cytoplasm. It has well-defined margins and is often centred on a blood vessel and associated with stromal hyalinization. The nodules are positive for SMA and negative for CD34 and desmin {2831}.

*Other morphological variants*

Granular cell, sclerosing, and atrophic variants have also been described; hybrids of these and all of the above-mentioned forms can also be encountered.

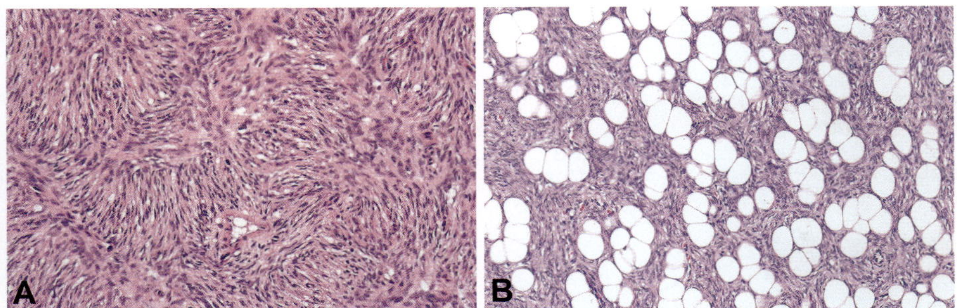


**Fig. 5.29** Dermatofibrosarcoma protuberans. **A** The classic storiform pattern. **B** Infiltration through fat cells.

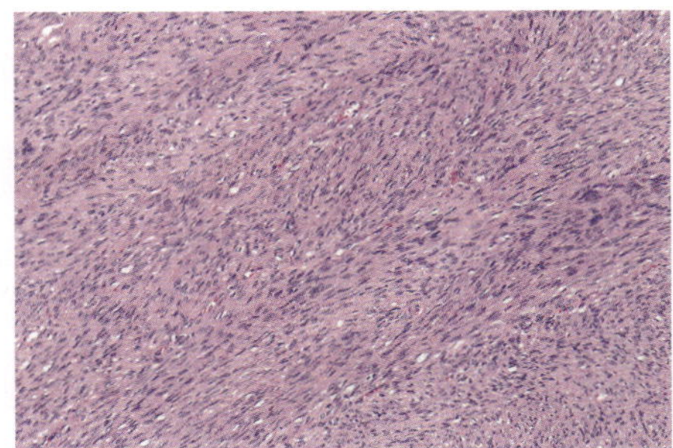

**Fig. 5.30** Fibrosarcomatous dermatofibrosarcoma protuberans. This variant shows a herringbone (rather than storiform) pattern.

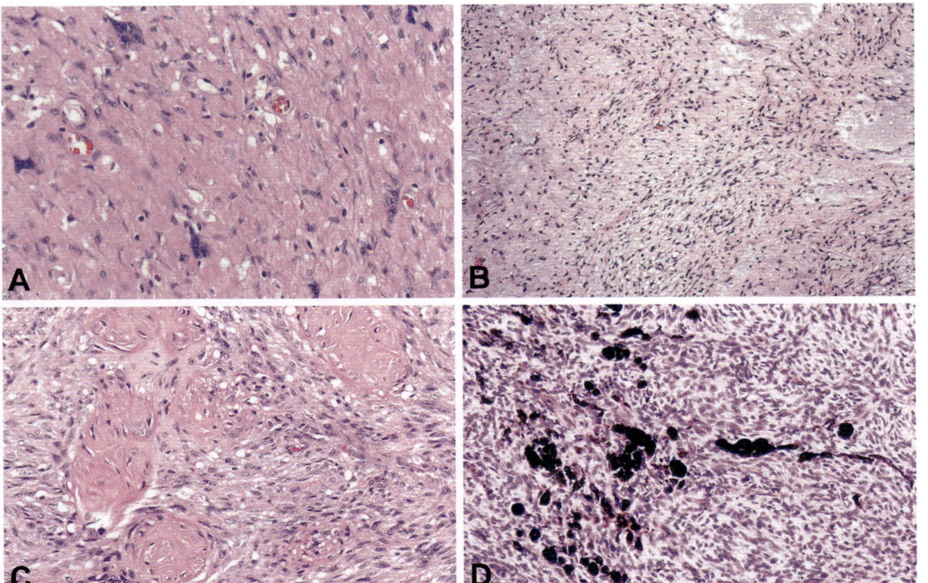


**Fig. 5.31** Dermatofibrosarcoma protuberans. **A** Giant cell fibroblastoma. **B** The myxoid subtype lacks storiform architecture. **C** Myoid nodules are rarely encountered. **D** The pigmented subtype (Bednar tumour) shows melanin pigmentation.

*Fibrosarcomatous DFSP*
Fibrosarcomatous transformation, which is seen in approximately 10% of DFSP cases, is characterized by transition (often abrupt) to a herringbone or fascicular growth pattern with increased cellularity, increased atypia, and increased mitotic activity. This variant may form a discrete nodule in a background of DFSP and often shows diminished or lost CD34 expression. Fibrosarcomatous transformation can occur de novo or in recurrent tumour {1742}.

DFSP shows strong diffuse staining for CD34 in most cases (80–90%). CD34 positivity can be lost in fibrosarcomatous areas.

## Differential diagnosis
Distinction from dermatofibroma can be difficult on a small or superficial biopsy. Dermatofibroma has less-uniform cytology, with variability of the spindle cell morphology and admixture with other cell types, including macrophages, lymphocytes, and multinucleated giant cells. Dermatofibroma is usually associated with overlying epidermal hyperplasia. Entrapment of collagen is seen peripherally; it is usually CD34 negative.

Tumours in the differential diagnosis of DFSP lack rearrangement of *PDGFB* (for which both FISH and PCR tests are available), but morphology and immunohistochemistry are most often sufficient {1999,2287}.

## Histogenesis
The tumour is considered to be fibroblastic in type.

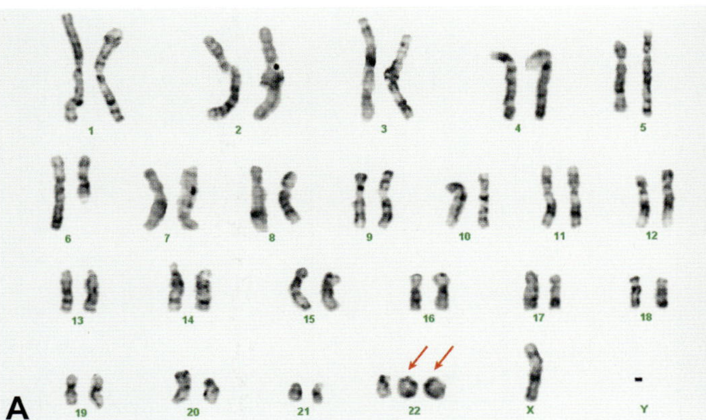


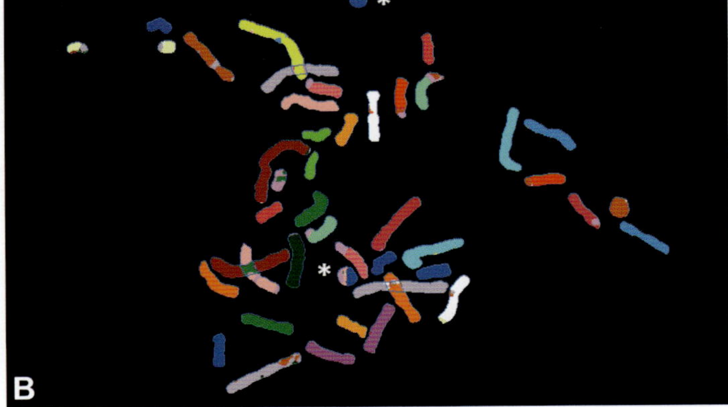


**Fig. 5.32** Dermatofibrosarcoma protuberans. **A** The classic G-banded karyotype shows two supernumerary chromosomes (arrows). **B** Multiplexed spectral in situ hybridization of a chromosomal spread shows supernumerary chromosomes pseudocoloured to demonstrate material from both 22 and 17, in pink and blue, respectively (asterisks).

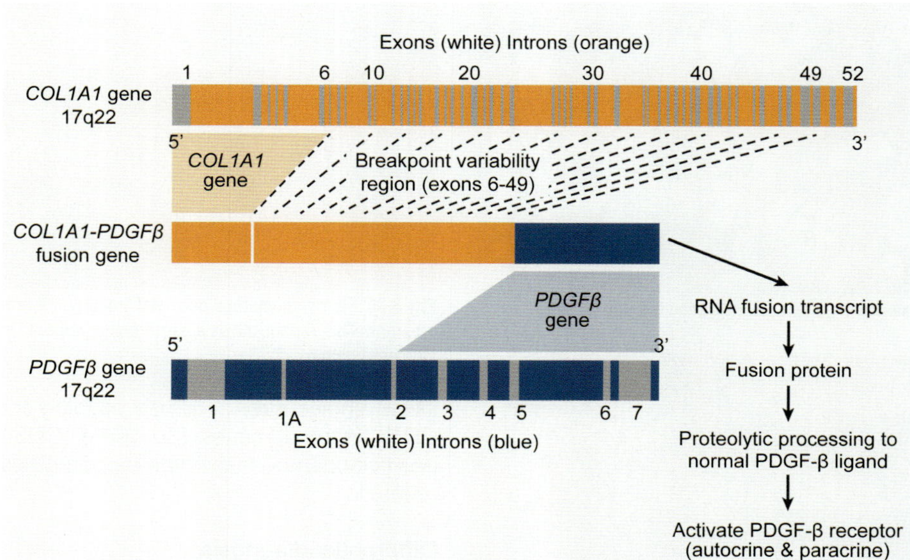


**Fig. 5.33** Dermatofibrosarcoma protuberans. Both t(17;22) and supernumerary r(22) with material from chromosome 17 result in a gene fusion whereby *PDGFB* is brought under the control of the strong, constitutive *COL1A1* promoter. The resulting fusion protein is proteolytically processed to normal PDGFB ligand, which drives oncogenesis.

## Genetic profile

Supernumerary ring chromosomes containing centromere from 22 and material from both 22 and 17 are the characteristic cytogenetic finding {1653,2024,2026}. Another alteration, unbalanced t(17;22)(q21.3;q13.1), is more common in paediatric cases. Both aberrations bring the *PDGFB* gene under the control of the *COL1A1* promoter {2447}. There are numerous breakpoints in the *COL1A1* gene (which consists of 52 exons), whereas the *PDGFB* breakpoint is restricted and always allows expression of *PDGFB* exon 2 {1928,1999}. After proteolytic processing that removes the COL1A1 protein leader sequence, there is massive overexpression of normal PDGFB ligand to ignite downstream pathways, likely in an autocrine fashion. Gains in genomic copies of *COL1A1-PDGFB* can be seen in fibrosarcomatous transformation {8}.

## Genetic susceptibility

Rarely, multicentric atrophic DFSP is seen in association with adenosine deaminase–deficient severe combined immunodeficiency {539,1351}.

## Prognosis and predictive factors

DFSP has a substantial risk of local recurrence (which occurs in 20–50% of cases), in particular when incompletely excised {2615}. Fibrosarcomatous DFSP has an increased risk of local recurrence and additionally has metastatic potential; metastasis occurs in 10–15% of cases, usually after multiple local recurrences, most commonly to lung {10,285,1102,2615}.

Because the forced overexpression of *PDGFB* leads to activation of the PDGF receptors, tyrosine kinase inhibitors can be used to interfere with the phosphorylation and activation of PDGFB when clinically appropriate {1646,1705,2262}.

# Plexiform fibrohistiocytic tumour

Kutzner H.
Fanburg-Smith J.C.
Luzar B.

## Definition

Plexiform fibrohistiocytic tumour (PFHT) is a dermal/subcutaneous tumour of intermediate malignant potential, with frequent recurrences and rare metastases {697,1611,2152,2290}. It is composed of plexiform myofibroblastic fascicles and multinodular histiocytoid clusters.

## ICD-O code 8835/1

## Epidemiology

PFHT occurs predominantly in children and young adults, with a wide age range (1–77 years, median: 20 years {1824}) and a balanced sex distribution {1109,1517}.

## Localization

PFHT most commonly involves the upper extremities, followed by the lower limbs, trunk, and head and neck region {1824}.

## Clinical features

PFHT presents as a slow-growing, poorly circumscribed, small (< 3 cm) plaque-like lesion, extending from the mid-dermis into the subcutaneous fat.

## Histopathology

PFHT is a predominantly dermal/subcutaneous tumour with a plexiform architecture composed of myofibroblastic fascicles in conjunction with whorling histiocyte-rich nodules in a cannonball-like pattern. Three histological subtypes have been defined on the basis of the predominant cell type: myofibroblastic, histiocytoid, and mixed {1824}.

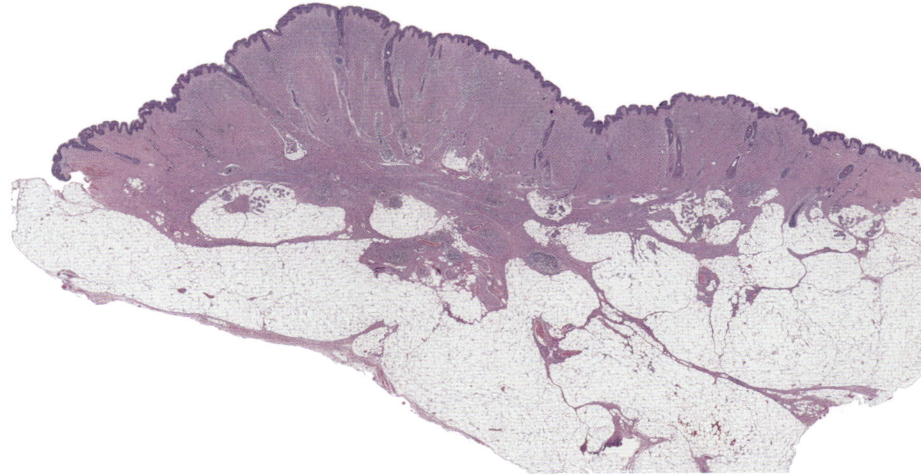

**Fig. 5.34** Plexiform fibrohistiocytic tumour composed of intermingling fascicles and histiocytoid nodules extending into the subcutaneous fat.

The small cellular nodules are composed of densely packed histiocytoid cells and large multinucleated osteoclast-like giant cells, most of which express CD68. There may be accompanying metaplastic alterations, haemorrhage, and inflammation, resulting in a pseudogranulomatous pattern. The intermingling short plexiform fascicles show spindled SMA-positive myofibroblasts. Mitotic activity is low; cytological atypia and atypical mitoses are exceedingly rare {697,1109,1824,2557}.

## Differential diagnosis

Because of its pseudogranulomatous pattern, PFHT can easily be confused with a reactive process. Depending on the PFHT subtype, the differential diagnosis can include fibromatosis, lipofibromatosis, myofibromatosis, fibrous hamartoma of infancy, nodular fasciitis, giant cell tumour of soft parts, and cellular neurothekeoma {54,1126,1207,1824,2786}.

## Genetic profile

To date, no recurring cytogenetic or molecular genetic abnormalities have been reported {1518}.

## Prognosis and predictive factors

Wide local excision is the preferred treatment {2123}. PFHT generally follows a favourable clinical course {697,1824,2152}.

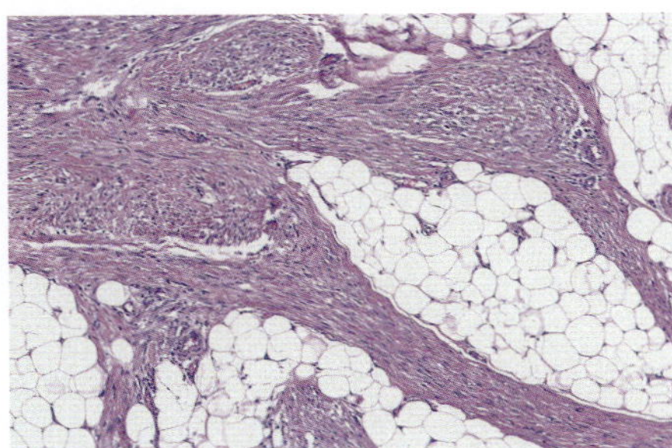

**Fig. 5.35** Plexiform fibrohistiocytic tumour. Intermingling myofibroblastic fascicles.

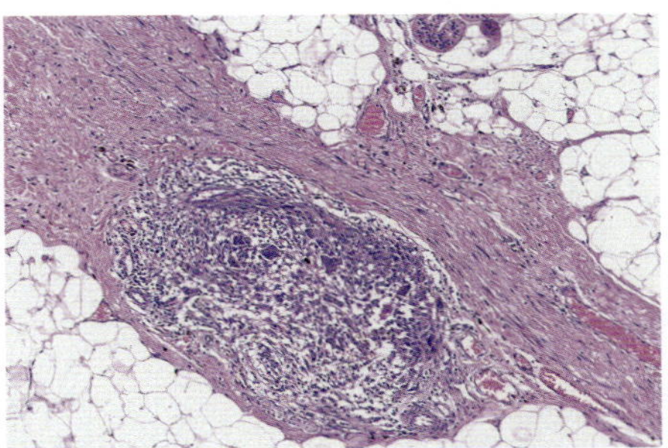

**Fig. 5.36** Plexiform fibrohistiocytic tumour. Histiocytoid nodule with siderophages and characteristic multinucleated osteoclast-like cells.

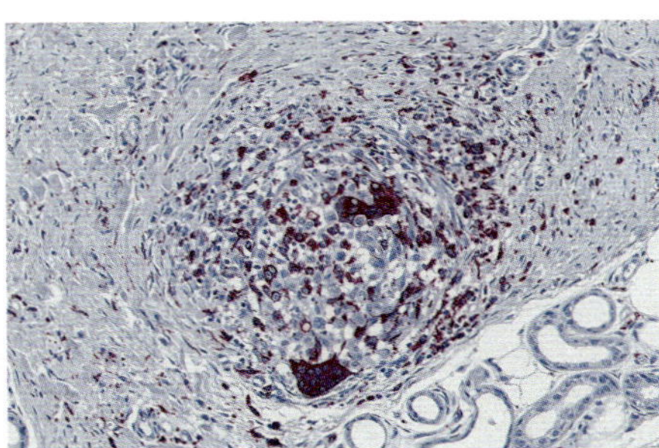

**Fig. 5.37** Plexiform fibrohistiocytic tumour. CD68 (PGM1) expression in the osteoclast-like cells and some of the histiocytoid cells.

# Superficial fibromatosis

Prieto V.G.
Andea A.A.

## Definition

Superficial fibromatosis is a fibroblastic proliferation derived from fascia or aponeurosis, with infiltrative growth and frequent recurrence.

## ICD-O code 8813/1

## Synonyms

Dupuytren disease;
Dupuytren contracture (palmar);
Ledderhose disease (plantar);
Peyronie disease (penile)

## Epidemiology

The prevalence of palmar fibromatosis ranges from 0.6% (in dark-skinned populations) to 30% (in people of northern European descent aged >60 years). The male-to-female ratio of between 3:1 and 9:1 decreases with age, reaching 1:1 by the ninth decade of life. Plantar fibromatosis is less common, is slightly more frequent in males, and tends to occur at a younger age (with a female predominance in children) than palmar lesions. Some patients present with concurrent forms of superficial fibromatosis {312,771,1080,1491,1926}.

## Etiology

There is an autosomal dominant inheritance pattern with incomplete penetrance, as well as multiple predisposing factors, such as smoking, alcohol consumption, trauma, diabetes, epilepsy, use of anticonvulsant drugs, treatment with BRAF inhibitors, and exposure to vibration {337,1080}. Other etiological factors include immune-mediated microvasculature damage, aberrations in the WNT signalling pathway, and abnormal secretion of TGF-β {1704,2595,2650}.

## Localization

Palmar fibromatosis occurs on the volar aspect of the hand (either the ulnar half of the palm or the proximal phalanx); 25–50% of cases are bilateral. Plantar fibromatosis affects the medial half of the sole (the medial plantar arch in children). The tunica albuginea is affected in penile fibromatosis {312,599,771,2679}.

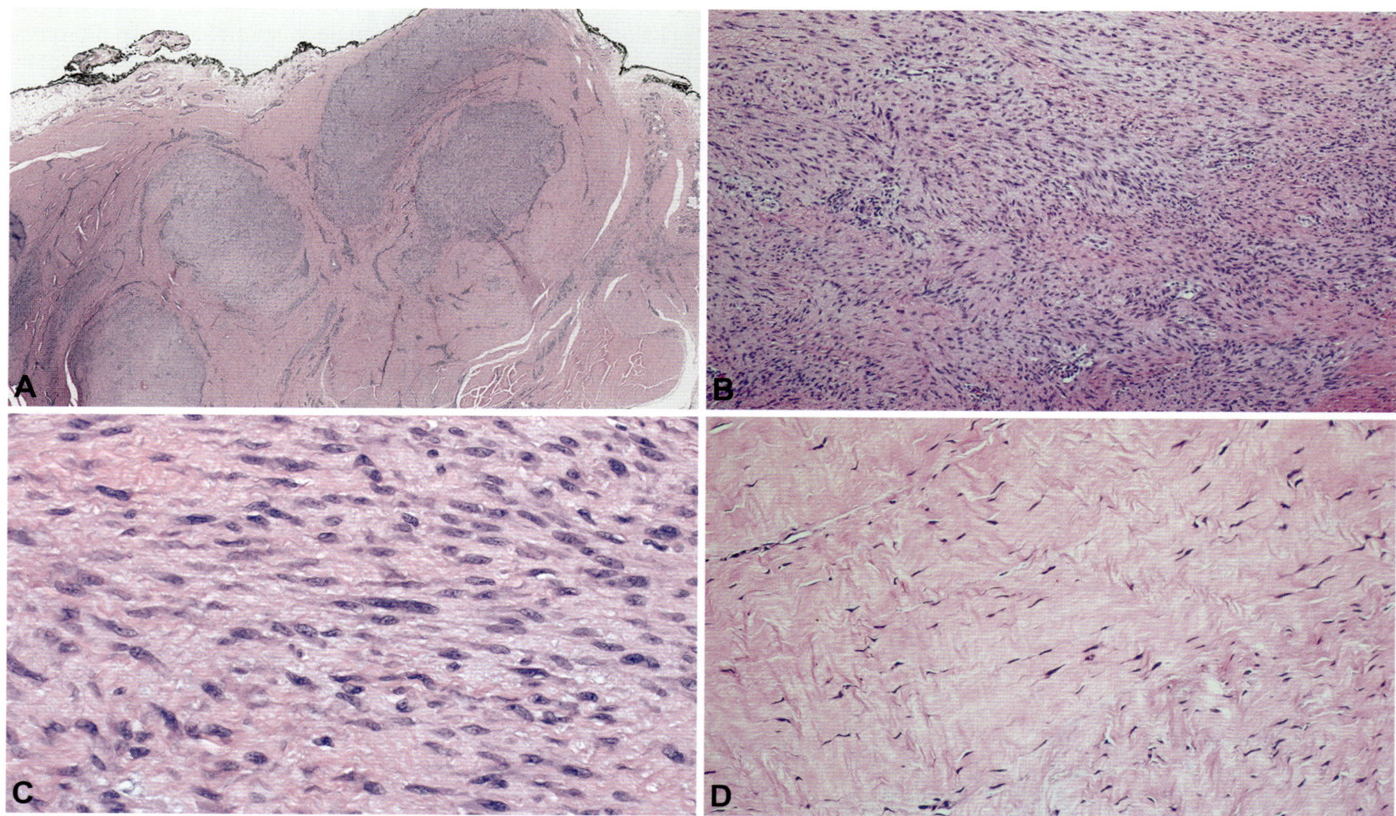

**Fig. 5.38** Superficial fibromatosis. **A** Low-power view showing a characteristic multinodular growth pattern. **B** Tumour cells are arranged in parallel fascicles separated by a collagenous stroma. **C** The tumour is composed of spindle cells with bland ovoid nuclei with open chromatin and small nucleoli. **D** Late-stage lesions are hypocellular and consist mostly of densely hyalinized fibrous tissue.

## Clinical features

This entity typically has three phases: proliferative, involutive, and residual. Initial solitary or multiple nodules evolve to show cord-like indurations or bands between nodules in the residual phase. With the exception of plantar lesions, superficial fibromatosis lesions usually develop contractures {312,2679}.

## Histopathology

Grossly, superficial fibromatosis manifests as multiple rubbery to firm nodules with a white to grey surface. There is a multinodular growth pattern with fascicles of uniform spindle cells (fibroblasts or myofibroblasts) containing oval nuclei with open or finely granular chromatin, small nucleoli, and eosinophilic to amphophilic cytoplasm, together with long curvilinear blood vessels. Occasional cases, more commonly in the paediatric population, may show more-pronounced atypia or focal mitotic figures of normal shape. Hypocellular older lesions show densely hyalinized stroma. Plantar lesions tend to form distinctive, hypercellular nodules with a paucicellular centre and occasional multinucleated giant cells {719,771,2679}. There is variable expression of actins. Focal nuclear expression of β-catenin is seen in about 50% of cases, in the absence of *CTNNB1* mutation {1819}.

## Differential diagnosis

The main differential diagnosis is scarring, which can be histologically indistinguishable; therefore, clinical information regarding prior trauma to the area (including surgical trauma) is required.

## Genetic profile

Gains of whole chromosomes 7 and 8 in palmar fibromatosis and 8 and 14 in plantar fibromatosis have been reported. Palmar fibromatosis also shows copy-number alterations involving 14q11.2 and 7p14.1 {599,2412}.

## Genetic susceptibility

See *Etiology*.

## Prognosis and predictive factors

Local recurrence is more common in patients with multiple nodules, bilateral lesions, coexisting palmoplantar disease, early disease onset, and a family history of the disease {771}.

# Dermatofibroma (fibrous histiocytoma) and variants

Glusac E.J.
Kutzner H.
Luzar B.
O'Brien B.H.

## Definition
Dermatofibroma (fibrous histiocytoma) is a common benign papular or nodular skin lesion composed of variable combinations of fibroblastic cells, macrophages, and coarse collagen.

## ICD-O code
| | |
|---|---|
| Dermatofibroma (fibrous histiocytoma) | 8832/0 |

## Synonyms
Benign fibrous histiocytoma; histiocytoma (cutis); fibroma durum; subepidermal nodular fibrosis or sclerosis; sclerosing haemangioma {946}

## Epidemiology
Dermatofibroma can arise at any age, but is most common in the third and fourth decades of life. The classic type is more common in younger females, particularly on the legs. Other variants have a more equal sex distribution.

## Etiology
It has been debated whether dermatofibroma is inflammatory or neoplastic. Some lesions have shown clonality and recurrent translocations {449,2712,2769}, suggesting neoplasia. This entity has also been reported to arise after trauma, insect bites, or folliculitis, suggesting an inflammatory origin {2917}. More recently, gene fusions involving *PRKCB* and *PRKCD* (encoding protein kinase C isoforms) have been noted in a subset of cases, confirming a neoplastic nature {2769}.

## Localization
The lesions are most commonly seen on the legs, followed by the arms and trunk. Occasional lesions are seen on the hands, feet, and head and neck {894,1193,1244,1748}. The cellular variant is the subtype most commonly involving the head and neck.

## Clinical features
Most dermatofibromas are isolated asymptomatic papules that evolve rapidly and then stabilize. Early-stage lesions are typically erythematous, but older ones are brown or skin-toned, often with a peripheral brown rim. The lesions are typically ≤ 1 cm in diameter but are occasionally ≥ 5–10 cm. They are typically firm, well circumscribed, and symmetrical. Most lesions are raised and dome-shaped and show a central dimple when squeezed. They may be cystic, eroded, or crusted. Occasionally several lesions are present, and rarely there can be dozens, either widely distributed or agminated. Multiple lesions may have no clinical significance, but they have been reported in conditions associated with immunosuppression and in association with immunosuppressive drugs.

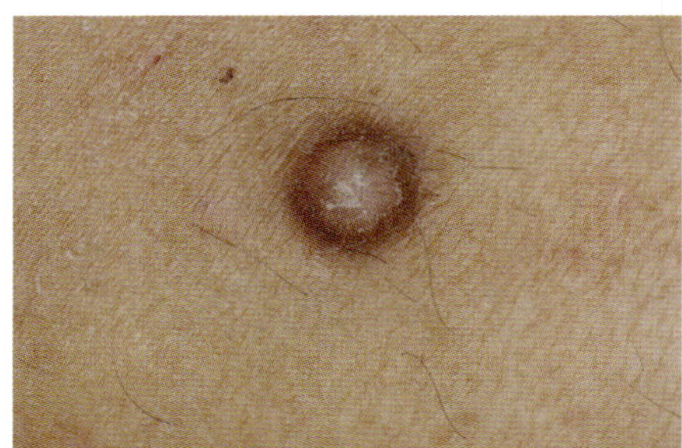

**Fig. 5.39** Dermatofibroma. Symmetrical, firm papulonodule with a peripheral brown rim.

## Histopathology
The lesions are typically centred in the mid-reticular dermis, with a rounded to slightly wedge-shaped outline. Early-stage lesions typically show abundant plump spindled to rounded cells dispersed among coarse collagen bundles. The nuclei are rounded to elongated, and may be triangular. At the periphery, collagen is typically trapped, forming collagen balls. Older lesions typically show more-abundant collagen and fewer macrophages. A storiform pattern may be seen. Lesions commonly involve the upper subcutis and occasionally deeper aspects. In such cases, the septa are typically expanded, resulting in a starfish or spoke-like configuration {1271}. The epidermis overlying dermatofibroma typically exhibits elongated hyperpigmented rete ridges and may exhibit induction of rudimentary hair follicles and/or

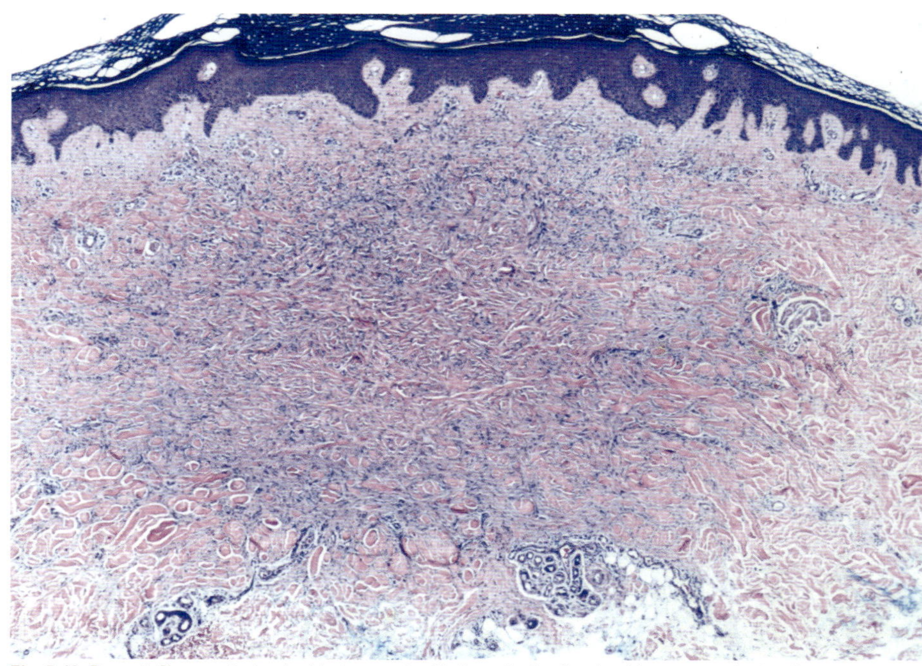

**Fig. 5.40** Dermatofibroma. A standard lesion, centred in the reticular dermis with a symmetrical outline.

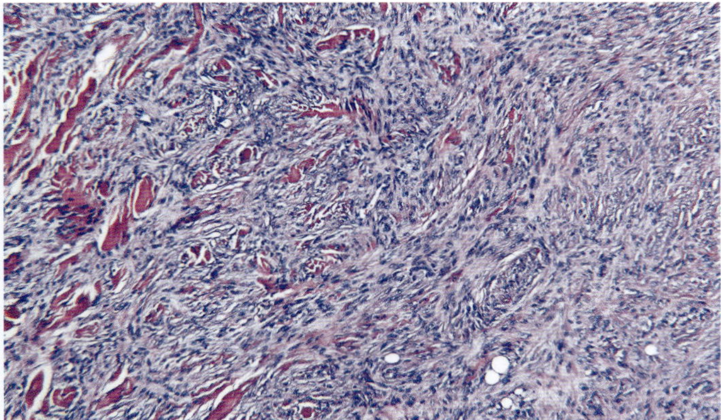
**Fig. 5.41** Cellular dermatofibroma with densely packed spindled cells.

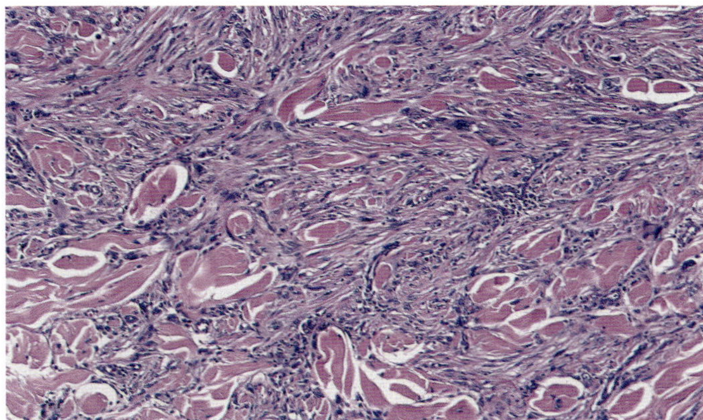
**Fig. 5.42** Atypical dermatofibroma with pleomorphic and spindled cells.

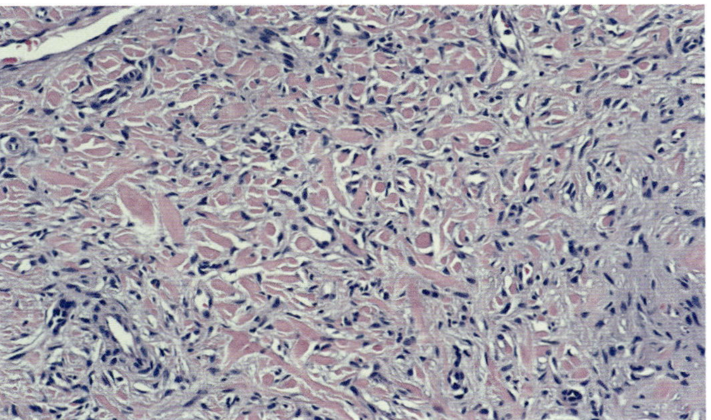
**Fig. 5.43** Dermatofibroma. An older lesion, with spindled and triangular cells with coarse collagen.

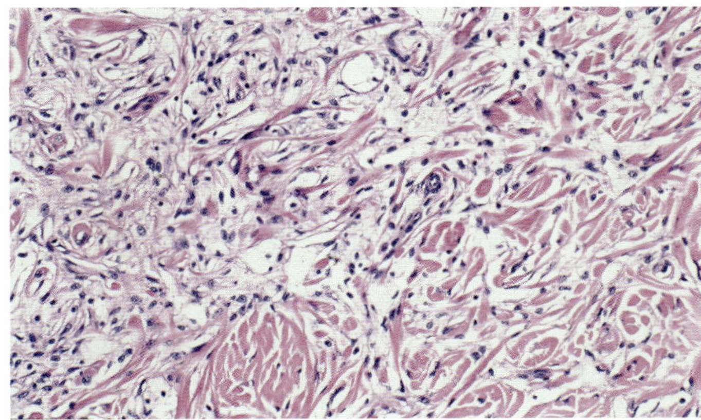
**Fig. 5.44** Dermatofibroma with foamy macrophages.

sebaceous glands. Junctional melanocytic hyperplasia may be present. Older lesions may be hypocellular, with marked fibrosis.

Dermatofibroma shows a large number of histological variants, and lesions with combined features also occur {2918}. Cellular lesions are densely cellular with a fascicular growth pattern and less abundant stroma {357}. Deep variants are centred in the deep dermis or subcutis {2915}; such lesions are generally larger, more cellular, and less fibrous. Both the cellular and deep variants tend to be more circumscribed. Angiomatous variants have abundant small blood vessels and numerous siderophages {946,2924}. The aneurysmal variant is distinctive, with large blood-filled spaces occupying much of the lesion. In lipidized variants (or lipidized components), the histiocytoid cells and giant cells typically contain abundant, clear, vacuolated cytoplasm. Dermatofibromas can show ossification, myofibroblastic features {2923}, keloidal collagen {1463}, and/or myxoid change {2918}. Rarely, there is clear-cell/balloon-cell change {2002,2644,2771} and granular cytoplasm {2685}. Some lesions may show marked pleomorphism, necrosis, and atypical mitotic figures (atypical fibrous histiocytoma/dermatofibroma with monster cells) {2565}. These lesions typically contain scattered pleomorphic cells (often binucleated or multinucleated) in a background of more-conventional dermatofibroma.

Epithelioid fibrous histiocytoma (also called epithelioid cell histiocytoma) has *ALK* rearrangement and overexpression, and may be a distinct entity unrelated to conventional dermatofibroma (see *Epithelioid fibrous histiocytoma*, p. 313) {649}.

Immunohistochemistry does not play a prominent role in the diagnosis of dermatofibroma. This entity is typically positive for nonspecific markers such as CD68 and factor XIIIa, but the labelling is variable and can also be seen in a variety of other lesions. Early proliferative lesions and cellular dermatofibroma may be positive for SMA {2923}. Peripheral and variable CD34 positivity may sometimes be seen, in contrast to the diffuse immunoreactivity seen in dermatofibrosarcoma protuberans.

## Differential diagnosis

Dermatofibroma is more polymorphous and lacks the infiltrative pattern and diffuse CD34 positivity of dermatofibrosarcoma protuberans. Atypical fibrous histiocytoma has a different clinical presentation than atypical fibroxanthoma. Despite the overlapping nomenclature, aneurysmal fibrous histiocytoma should not be confused with angiomatoid fibrous histiocytoma. Sclerosing perineurioma has more-uniform epithelioid cells and EMA (epithelial membrane antigen) positivity. Bland forms of spindle cell melanoma, spindle cell carcinoma, or superficial leiomyosarcoma may be excluded by immunostains in more cellular variants of benign fibrous histiocytoma (dermatofibroma).

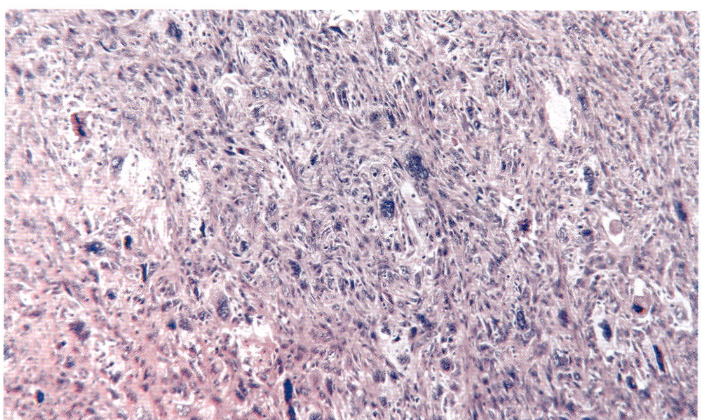

**Fig. 5.45** Atypical dermatofibroma with pleomorphic giant cells.

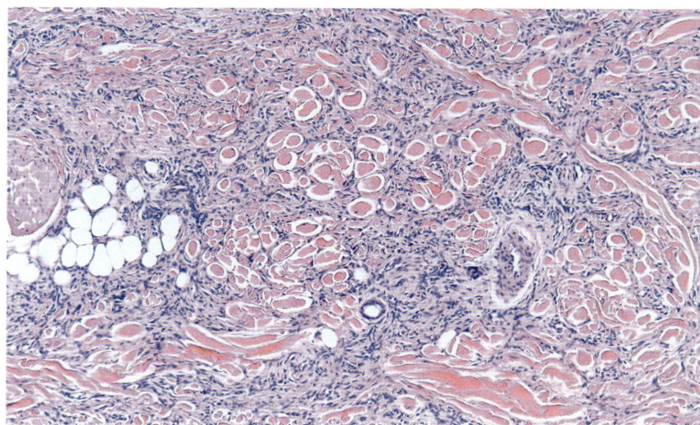

**Fig. 5.46** Dermatofibroma with spindled cells and macrophages, coarse collagen, and collagen balls.

## Histogenesis

There is evidence of fibroblastic, myofibroblastic, and/or macrophage differentiation {2097}.

## Prognosis and predictive factors

Dermatofibroma is a benign lesion. Incomplete excision may result in local non-destructive recurrence. There is conflicting evidence as to whether dermatofibroma of the face behaves more aggressively than dermatofibroma at other anatomical sites {709,1748}. The risk of local recurrence is higher with the cellular, atypical, and aneurysmal subtypes {357}. Extraordinarily rare lesions have metastasized to lymph nodes and/or lung; most have been of the cellular, atypical, or aneurysmal subtype {21,647,887,1261,1753}. There is some evidence suggesting that metastasizing tumours have more chromosomal aberrations than are typical of standard indolent dermatofibroma {1753}.

# Epithelioid fibrous histiocytoma

Requena L.
Hornick J.L.

## Definition

Epithelioid fibrous histiocytoma is a distinctive, usually exophytic and well-circumscribed benign cutaneous neoplasm composed of epithelioid cells, including binucleated forms. *ALK* rearrangement is present in the vast majority of cases.

## ICD-O code 8830/0

## Synonym

Epithelioid cell histiocytoma

## Epidemiology

Epithelioid fibrous histiocytoma typically arises in young to middle-aged adults (median patient age: 40 years), with a female predominance {893,1244,2451}.

## Etiology

Epithelioid fibrous histiocytoma is sporadic.

## Localization

Epithelioid fibrous histiocytoma most commonly affects the lower extremities, followed by the upper extremities. The trunk and the head and neck region are uncommon sites {893,894,1244,2451}.

## Clinical features

Epithelioid fibrous histiocytoma presents as an exophytic nodule, often with a vascular appearance {1244}.

## Histopathology

Epithelioid fibrous histiocytoma is usually well circumscribed; exophytic examples often have an epidermal collarette. The tumour is composed of uniform plump epithelioid cells with vesicular nuclei, small nucleoli, and abundant pale eosinophilic or amphophilic cytoplasm, often including binucleated forms. Small, thin-walled blood vessels may be prominent, sometimes with perivascular accentuation of tumour cells. ALK is overexpressed in about 90% of cases {649}, and EMA (epithelial membrane antigen) is positive in 65% {646}. CD30 expression may be seen {649,2552}. SMA and desmin are usually negative {646}.

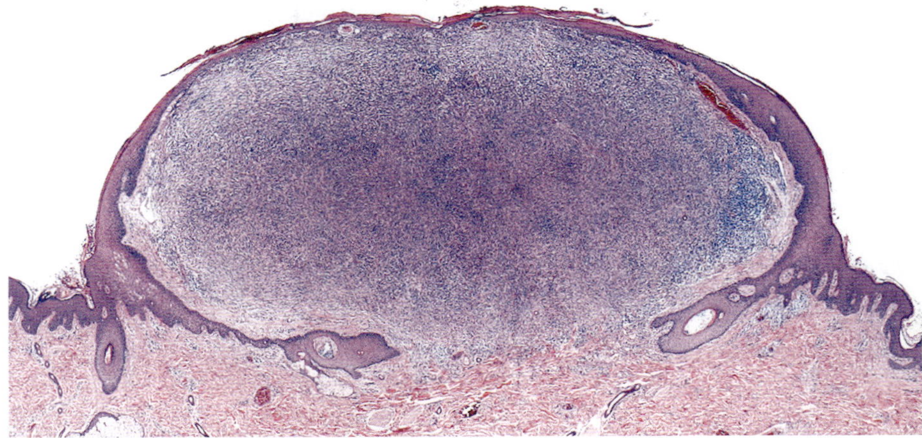

**Fig. 5.47** Epithelioid fibrous histiocytoma. An exophytic, well-circumscribed tumour with an epidermal collarette.

## Differential diagnosis

The differential diagnosis includes Spitz naevus, cutaneous syncytial myoepithelioma, epithelioid sarcoma, and cellular neurothekeoma.

## Histogenesis

Although the histogenesis is unknown, epithelioid fibrous histiocytoma is likely biologically distinct from dermatofibroma (conventional fibrous histiocytoma) and variants {534,649}.

## Genetic profile

About 90% of epithelioid fibrous histiocytomas harbour *ALK* rearrangements {649,2552}; *VCL-ALK* and *SQSTM1-ALK* fusions have been reported {1221}.

## Prognosis and predictive factors

Epithelioid fibrous histiocytoma is benign and rarely recurs locally {1244,2451}.

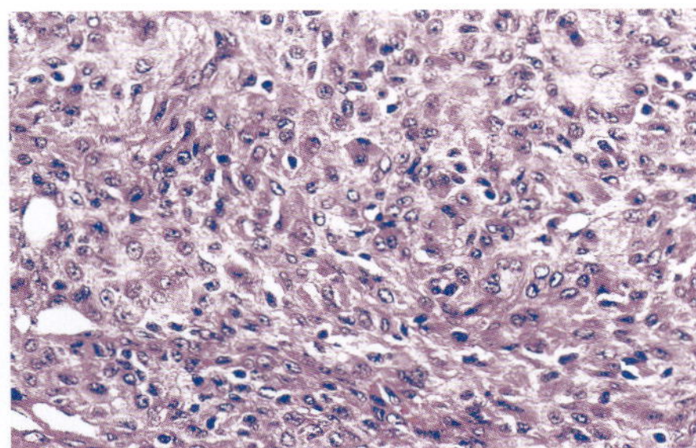

**Fig. 5.48** Epithelioid fibrous histiocytoma. The epithelioid tumour cells may contain eosinophilic cytoplasm; note the thin-walled blood vessels and occasional binucleated forms.

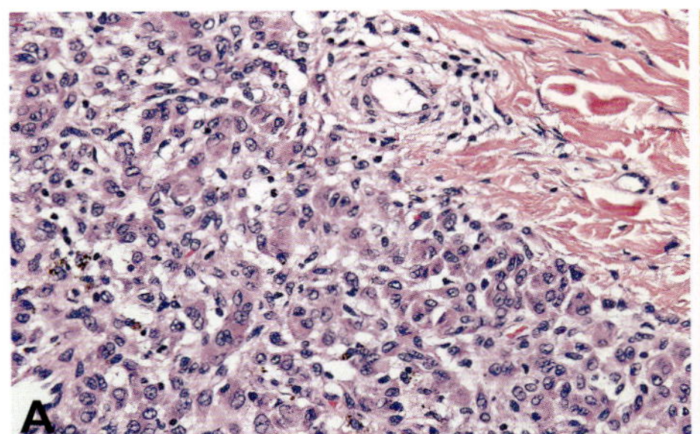


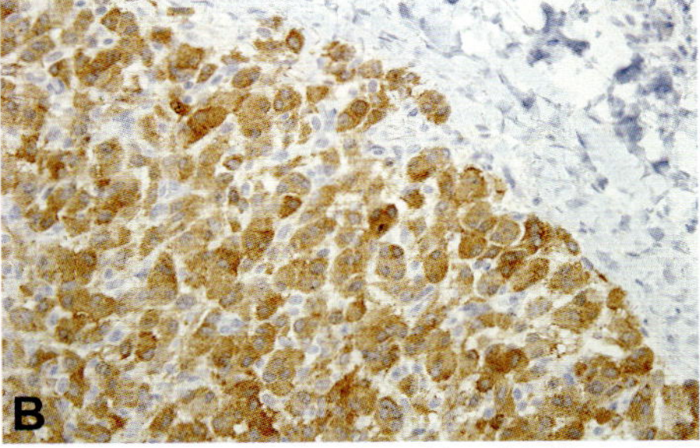


**Fig. 5.49** Epithelioid fibrous histiocytoma. **A** The epithelioid tumour cells contain round to ovoid nuclei with vesicular chromatin, small nucleoli, and amphophilic cytoplasm; note the sharply circumscribed margin. **B** Tumour cells show strong cytoplasmic immunostaining for ALK, reflecting the presence of *ALK* rearrangement.

# Fibromas

Kutzner H.
Lazar A.J.
Patel R.M.
Wang W.-L.

## Fibroma of tendon sheath

### Definition
Fibroma of tendon sheath is a rare benign tumour, presumably of (myo)fibroblastic origin, that arises in the tenosynovial soft tissue and occurs predominantly in the upper extremities.

### ICD-O code 8813/0

### Epidemiology
These fibromas are rare. They occur most frequently in middle-aged men {42,392,480}.

### Localization
The most common sites are the tendons of the fingers, hand, and wrist. Less common sites include the forearm, foot, and knee {392,480}.

### Clinical features
Most tumours present as an asymptomatic to mildly painful, small (< 2 cm), slow-growing, and solitary mass, although multiple nodules have also been reported {42,480,1994}.

### Histopathology
The tumours are well circumscribed and composed of small to medium-sized stellate spindle cells arranged in fascicles or a storiform pattern set within a dense hyalinized matrix with slit-like spaces and dilated vascular channels. Some myxoid change, extravasated red blood cells, mononuclear inflammatory cells, and (rarely) giant cells can be seen. Cellular areas may also be present {480}.

### Differential diagnosis
Cellular variants can show overlap with nodular fasciitis and benign fibrous histiocytoma.

### Genetic profile
Traditional karyotyping reveals translocations including t(2;11)(q31-32;q12) and t(9;11)(p24;q13-14), although this may not be a consistent finding {1908}. A subset of these tumours (6 of 9 cases in one series) have been found to have *USP6* rearrangements, although a partner was not identified. This finding has led researchers to speculate that a subset may in fact be tenosynovial nodular fasciitis {392}.

### Prognosis and predictive factors
Fibroma of tendon sheath is benign, but recurs locally in about 25% of cases {480}.

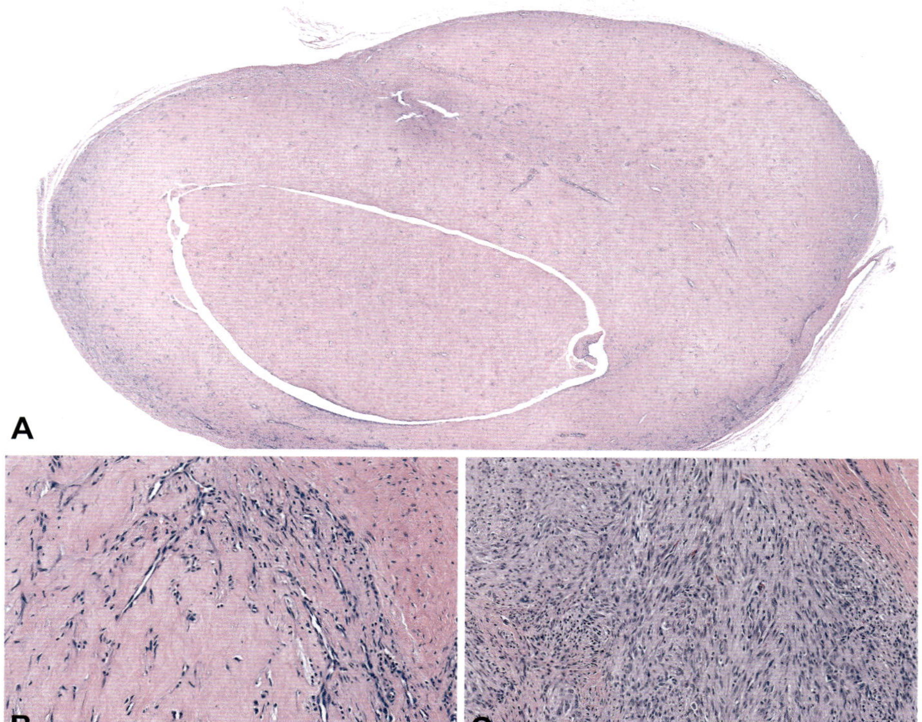


**Fig. 5.50** Fibroma of tendon sheath. **A** Sharply circumscribed hypocellular tumour with a hyalinized matrix containing slit-like spaces and blood vessels. **B** Bland fibroblasts and slit-like capillary vessels within a hyalinized matrix. **C** Example showing foci of increased cellularity, with constituent spindle cells arrayed in a fascicular to storiform growth pattern resembling nodular fasciitis.

## Calcifying aponeurotic fibroma

### Definition
Calcifying aponeurotic fibroma is a benign, locally infiltrative fibroblastic tumour with chondro-osseous foci, predominantly occurring in the distal extremities of children.

### ICD-O code 8816/0

### Synonym
Juvenile aponeurotic fibroma

### Epidemiology
Calcifying aponeurotic fibroma is rare; it predominantly occurs in children (typically boys). Adults are rarely affected {775}.

### Localization
Calcifying aponeurotic fibromas most commonly involve aponeurotic soft tissue of the palms and feet. Other sites include the thigh, arm, elbow, and knee {775}.

### Clinical features
These fibromas typically present as a solitary painless mass, but they can be multiple {775}.

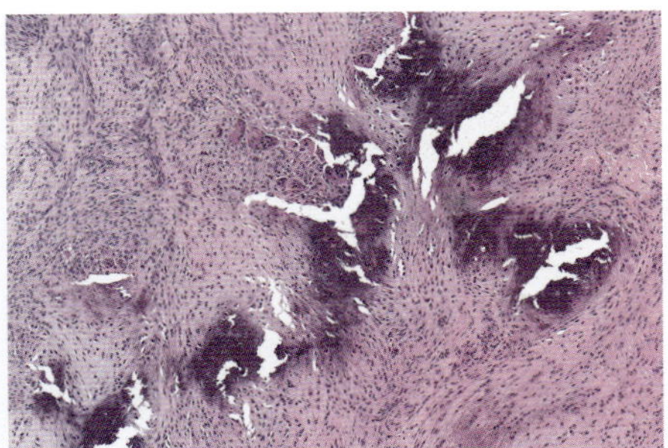

**Fig. 5.51** Calcifying aponeurotic fibroma. Spindle cells arranged in fascicles surrounding areas of calcification containing epithelioid and chondroid cells and occasional multinucleated osteoclast-like giant cells.

### Histopathology
The tumour is composed of spindled cells arranged in parallel fascicles. Epithelioid/chondroid cells can be seen, with or without calcification {775,1335}. There is variable expression of MSA, SMA, CD99, S100 protein, and CD68. Rare cases also label for CD34, CD57, progesterone receptor, and EMA (epithelial membrane antigen). β-catenin is negative {2613}.

### Differential diagnosis
The differential diagnosis includes infantile fibromatosis (inclusion body fibromatosis) and superficial fibromatosis.

### Genetic profile
Calcifying aponeurotic fibromas have recently been reported to have a recurrent translocation involving the promoter region of *FN1* (exon 23, 27, or 42) on 2q35 and *EGF* (exon 17 or 19) on 4q25, resulting in the aberrant overexpression of EGF, which can be detected immunohistochemically {2108}.

### Genetic susceptibility
Calcifying aponeurotic–like lesions have been reported in a family with Albright hereditary osteodystrophy {1257}.

### Prognosis and predictive factors
These fibromas are benign, but the rate of local recurrence may be as high as 50% {775}. Rare cases of metastasis and malignant (fibrosarcomatous) transformation have been reported {65,612,1479}.

## Sclerotic fibroma

### Definition
Sclerotic fibroma is a benign cutaneous fibrous tumour with a prominent storiform pattern and clefting. The tumours can be sporadic or associated with Cowden syndrome.

### ICD-O code 8823/0

### Synonym
Storiform collagenoma

### Epidemiology
There is a predilection for middle-aged adults. Cases associated with Cowden syndrome have a male predominance {1759}, and sporadic cases have a female predominance {2136}.

### Localization
Sclerotic fibroma is most common on the head and neck region and arms {1759}.

### Clinical features
The tumours are solitary or multiple, slow-growing, painless, white to skin-coloured papules to nodules of long duration {1759,2136}.

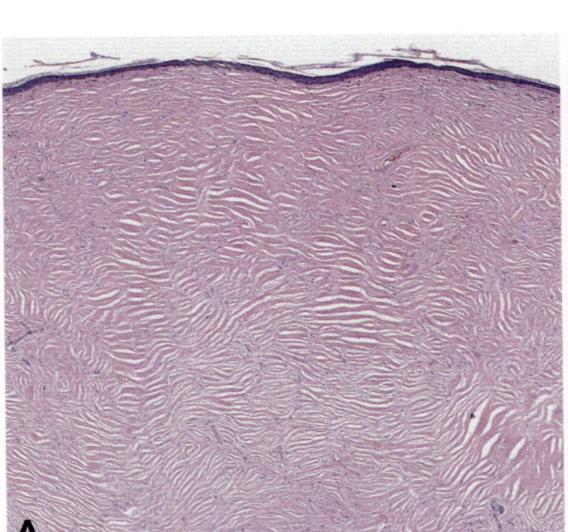

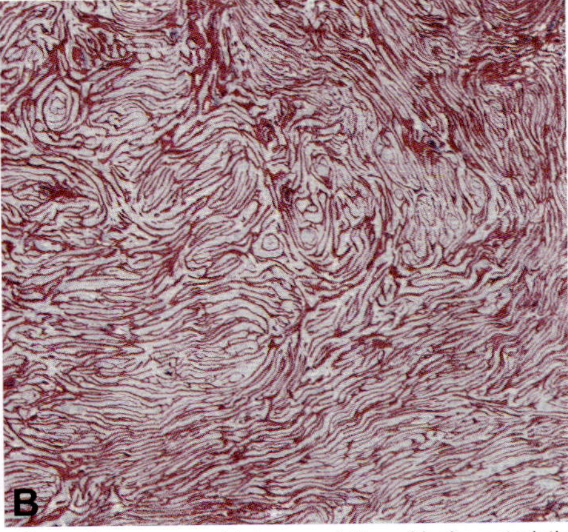

**Fig. 5.52** Sclerotic fibroma. **A** Hypocellular fibrotic tumour with a collagenous matrix in association with characteristic plywood-like clefting. **B** Characteristic CD34-positive fingerprint pattern.

### Histopathology
Sclerotic fibromas are polypoid well-circumscribed hypocellular lesions with abundant collagen (with plywood-like clefting) admixed with banal small spindle cells arranged in a storiform pattern. Myxoid change can be seen {1759,2136}. The tumours express CD34 {1002}.

### Differential diagnosis
These tumours must be distinguished from dermatofibroma.

### Genetic profile
Tumours that arise in association with Cowden syndrome have loss of *PTEN* (10q23.3), resulting in loss of its expression.

### Genetic susceptibility
Sclerotic fibroma (in particular when multiple) has been associated with Cowden syndrome {1759,2155}.

### Prognosis and predictive factors
Sclerotic fibroma is benign.

## Nuchal-type fibroma

### Definition
Nuchal-type fibroma is a benign fibroblastic tumour characterized by abundant thick collagen bundles, most commonly arising in the posterior neck.

### ICD-O code 8810/0

### Epidemiology
This fibroma most commonly occurs in middle-aged adults, with a male predominance {134,1765}.

### Localization
The most common site is the posterior neck {1765}, but other sites can also be involved. Nuchal-type fibroma most often involves the subcutaneous soft tissue, and there is occasionally dermal and skeletal muscle involvement.

### Clinical features
Patients typically present with a long history of solitary superficial to deep, painless swelling. These fibromas are rarely multiple {134,1512,1765}.

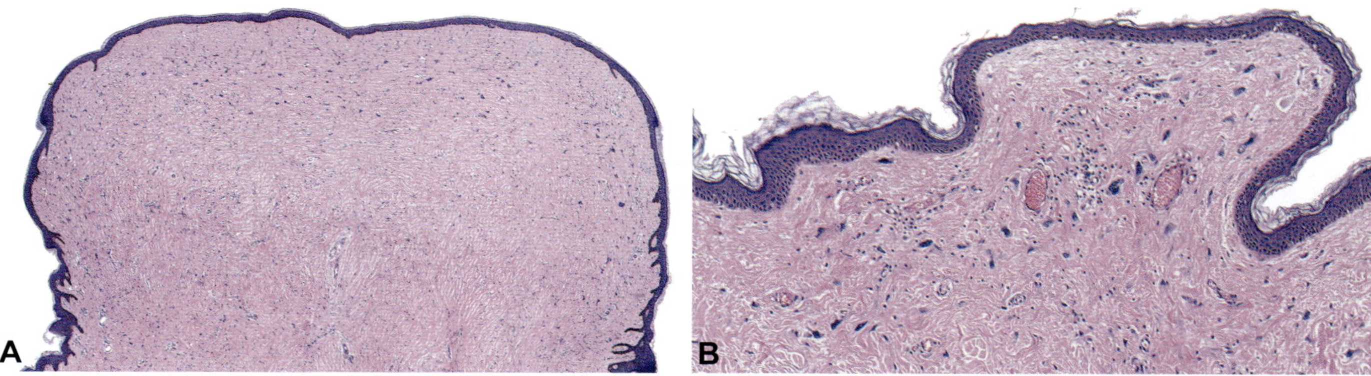


**Fig. 5.53** Pleomorphic fibroma. **A** A dome-shaped papule with stellate hyperchromatic fibroblasts. **B** Collagen bundles admixed with atypical fibroblasts demonstrating degenerative nuclear pleomorphism and hyperchromasia.

### Histopathology
The tumours are poorly circumscribed masses, 1–8 cm in size. They are hypocellular and characterized by thick collagen fibres and small fibroblasts. Entrapped islands of fat and nerves with traumatic neuroma–like changes can be seen. Immunohistochemistry is not specific; the tumours are negative for desmin, actin, S100 protein, and EMA (epithelial membrane antigen) {134,1765}. There may be nuclear expression of β-catenin.

### Differential diagnosis
The differential diagnosis includes desmoid-type fibromatosis and Gardner fibroma.

### Genetic profile
A few tested cases have been found to harbour *APC* mutations. One case harboured a mutation in *MUTYH*, which encodes a base excision repair protein; *MUTYH* mutations have also been implicated in familial adenomatous polyposis and attenuated familial adenomatous polyposis {1570}.

### Genetic susceptibility
There is an association with diabetes; in one series, 11 of 25 patients with nuchal-type fibroma (44%) also had diabetes {1765}. Some tumours are associated with Gardner syndrome {1765}.

### Prognosis and predictive factors
These tumours have an excellent prognosis. Rare local recurrence has been reported. Local excision is curative {134,1765}.

## Gardner fibroma

### Definition
Gardner fibroma is a benign fibroblastic tumour usually occurring in children with familial adenomatous polyposis.

### ICD-O code 8810/0

### Epidemiology
Most cases occur in children (in particular boys); Gardner fibroma is uncommon in adults {502}.

### Localization
The strongest predilection is for the back and the head and heck region, followed by the extremities and chest wall.

### Clinical features
These fibromas are typically solitary or (rarely) multiple. They are sometimes associated with desmoid-type fibromatosis {2795}.

### Histopathology
These are poorly defined tumours with a plaque-like growth pattern and a wide range of sizes (examples as large as 12 cm have been reported). The tumours are composed of dense collagen with clefts and cracks and bland spindle cells. Entrapped fat and mast cells can be seen. β-catenin is positive {502}.

### Differential diagnosis
The differential diagnosis includes nuchal-type fibroma and desmoid-type fibromatosis. Some authors have proposed that a subset of nuchal-type fibromas are in fact Gardner fibromas {2795}.

### Genetic profile
These tumours have mutations in *APC* {2795}.

### Genetic susceptibility
There is an association with Gardner syndrome {2795}.

### Prognosis and predictive factors
Gardner fibroma is a benign tumour with a rate of recurrence as high as 50%. Some patients develop desmoid-type fibromatosis {612,1479}.

## Pleomorphic fibroma

### Definition
Pleomorphic fibroma is a benign, often polypoid, fibroblastic neoplasm characterized by bizarre pleomorphic cells.

### ICD-O code 8832/0

### Epidemiology
This fibroma occurs in middle-aged adults, with a slight female predominance {45,1272}.

### Localization
Pleomorphic fibroma affects the extremities, trunk, and (less commonly) head and neck {45,1272}.

### Clinical features
The tumours are painless, single, slow-growing, fleshy polyps to papules {45,1272}.

### Histopathology
Pleomorphic fibromas are small, often polypoid, and relatively well circumscribed. They are mildly to moderately cellular, composed of haphazardly

arranged collagen bundles admixed with large pleomorphic cells with hyperchromatic multilobulated nuclei with smudgy chromatin {45,1272}. They are positive for CD34 and show loss of RB1 {1081}.

### Differential diagnosis
The differential diagnosis includes superficial atypical lipomatous tumour, pleomorphic lipoma, and atypical fibroxanthoma.

### Genetic profile
These tumours have *RB1* deletion and are negative for *MDM2* amplification {1081,1272}.

### Prognosis and predictive factors
These are benign tumours, with rare recurrence {45,1272}.

## Elastofibroma

### Definition
Elastofibroma is a benign soft tissue tumour characterized by abnormal elastic fibres, bland fibroblasts, and myxoid stroma.

### ICD-O code
8820/0

### Epidemiology
Elastofibroma most commonly affects elderly adults, with a female predominance.

### Localization
Elastofibroma is subscapular but can also involve the chest wall.

### Clinical features
These fibromas present as slow-growing, predominantly solitary tumours and can occasionally cause symptoms such as swelling, discomfort, stiffness, and pain {1862,1997}.

### Histopathology
Elastofibromas are large and have poorly defined borders. They are hypocellular, with fragmented and thickened to globular elastic fibres, which can be highlighted with Verhoeff elastic staining. Scattered small bland spindle cells are seen {1862}.

### Genetic profile
Elastofibromas have a variety of chromosomal abnormalities. Copy gains (including gains of Xq) {1910}, alterations to chromosome 1 and t(8;12)(q22;q24.3) {1709A}, and/or t(2;19) and (X;1) rearrangements {174} have been found in some of the cases.

### Genetic susceptibility
Some cases run in families {2342}; in one series, one third of the patients reported a familial history {1862}.

### Prognosis and predictive factors
Elastofibroma has an excellent prognosis {1862,1997}.

## Collagenous fibroma

### Definition
Collagenous fibroma (desmoplastic fibroblastoma) is a benign soft tissue tumour characterized by stellate fibroblasts in a fibromyxoid background.

### ICD-O code
8810/0

### Synonym
Desmoplastic fibroblastoma

### Epidemiology
These rare tumours predominantly affect middle-aged adults, with a male predominance {718,1038,1772,1906}.

### Localization
The tumours occur in wide variety of locations and are predominantly subcutaneous {718,1772,1906}.

### Clinical features
Collagenous fibroma presents as a painless, solitary, slow-growing mass {1772}.

### Histopathology
The tumours are circumscribed and can be as large as 20 cm. They are hypocellular lesions characterized by spindled to stellate-shaped fibroblasts set within a fibromyxoid to delicate collagenous background {718,1772,1906}. Immunohistochemistry is nonspecific; desmin, keratin, and CD34 are negative {1906}.

### Differential diagnosis
The differential diagnosis includes desmoid-type fibromatosis.

### Genetic profile
Collagenous fibromas have been reported to have translocations involving 11q12, including t(2;11)(q31;q12) and t(11;17)(q12;p11.2) {216,1627}. The *FOSL1* gene is located nearby (at 11q13.1), and the FOSL1 protein is overexpressed in these tumours {1289,1616}.

### Prognosis and predictive factors
Collagenous fibromas are benign, with no local recurrence after excision {718,1772,1906}.

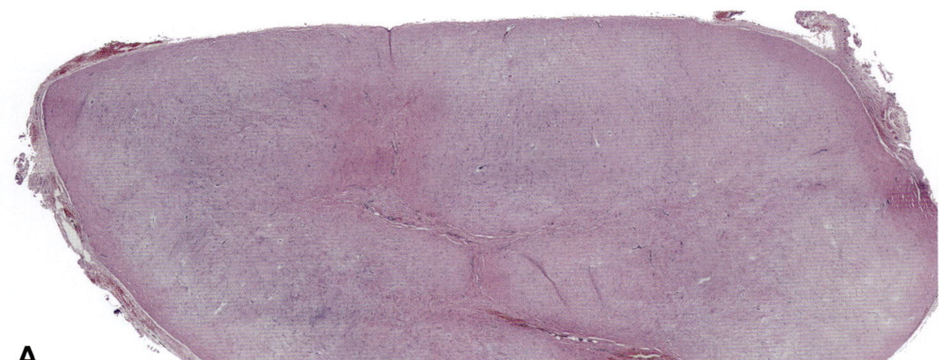


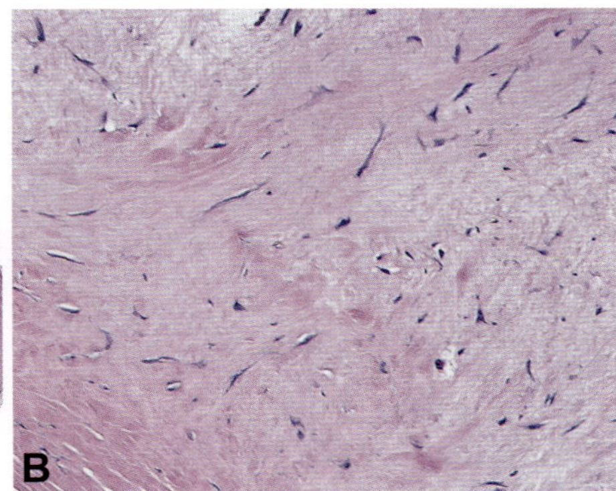


**Fig. 5.54** Collagenous fibroma (desmoplastic fibroblastoma). **A** Hypocellular proliferation of distinctive, widely spaced, spindled to stellate fibroblasts in a fibromyxoid stroma. **B** Hypocellular area with bland stellate fibroblasts.

# Superficial acral fibromyxoma

Billings S.D.
Fetsch J.F.
Kutzner H.

## Definition
Superficial acral fibromyxoma is a benign fibroblastic tumour typically restricted to acral sites, with a predilection for the periungual region of the digits.

## ICD-O code 8811/0

## Synonyms
Digital fibromyxoma; cellular digital fibroma

## Epidemiology
Most cases present in the fifth decade of life, but people of any age can be affected {769,1106}. There is a male predominance, with a male-to-female ratio of 2:1 {23,41,553,769,2094}.

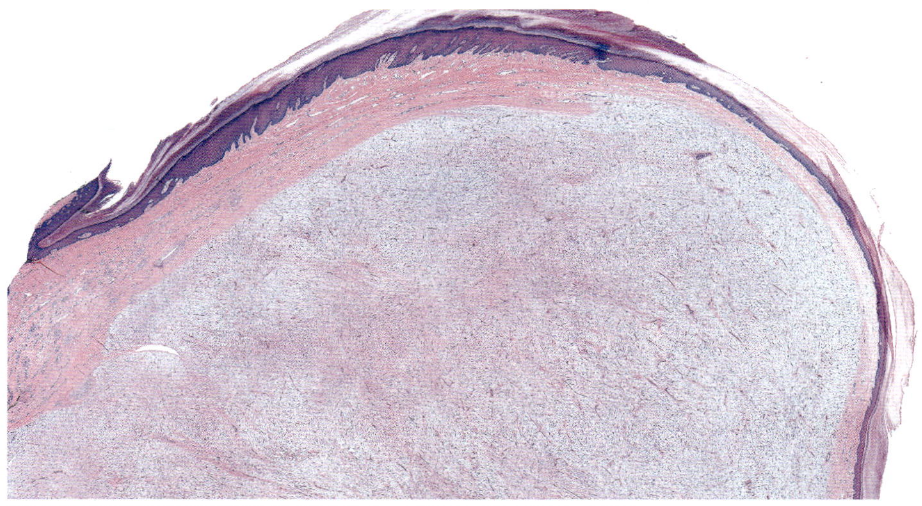
**Fig. 5.55** Superficial acral fibromyxoma. Low-power image of a periungual case.

## Localization
Superficial acral fibromyxomas typically present as 0.5–5 cm (median: 1.5 cm) masses in periungual locations on the fingers and toes. Less commonly, the palm or sole, leg, or ankle is involved {41,769,1106,2094}.

## Clinical features
Most cases present as solitary, slow-growing, sometimes painful masses of the digits. Nail deformities are common, and scalloping/invasion of underlying bone can be seen in a minority of cases {769,1106,2719}.

## Histopathology
Superficial acral fibromyxoma has a lobular to infiltrative low-power appearance and is composed of bland spindled to stellate cells in a storiform to loose fascicular pattern, with a variably prominent vasculature embedded in a myxoid to fibromyxoid to collagenous stroma {41,769,2094}. The mitotic rate is low. Atypical mitotic figures are not seen. Multinucleated cells are seen in about half of all cases. Rare cases show focal pleomorphism. The rare cellular variant (cellular digital fibroma) has increased cellularity with little intervening stroma {964,1725}. The tumours are CD34-positive (in 70–90% of cases) and CD99-positive, and show loss of RB1 expression {23,41,769,1602,2094}. The reported prevalence of EMA (epithelial membrane antigen) expression varies from < 10% to > 70% {769,1106}; when present, expression is focal {41}. Occasional cases are

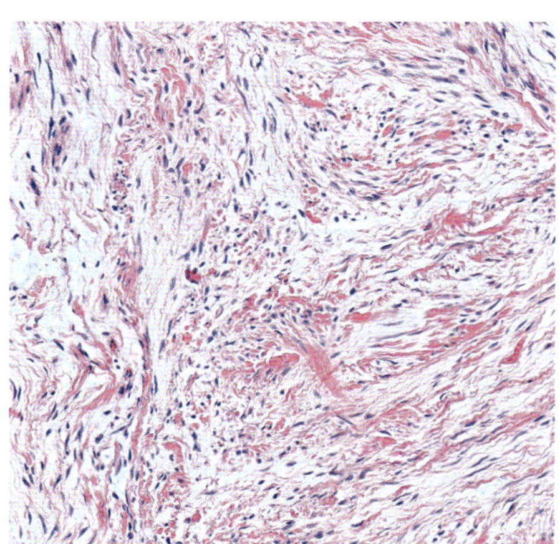
**Fig. 5.56** Superficial acral fibromyxoma. Bland spindled cells arranged in irregular fascicles in a myxoid to collagenous stroma.

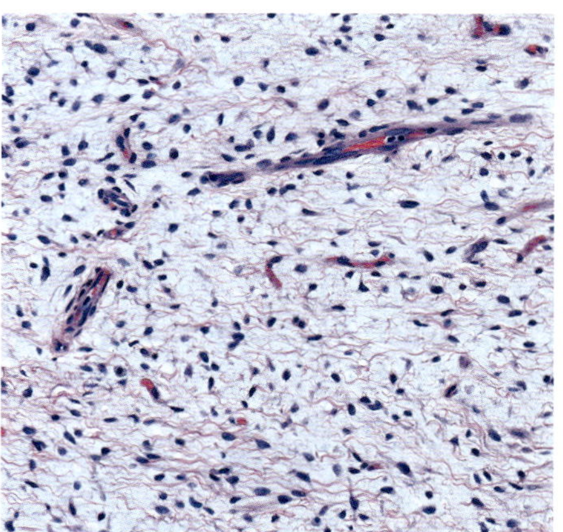
**Fig. 5.57** Superficial acral fibromyxoma. A case with predominantly myxoid stroma and prominent vasculature.

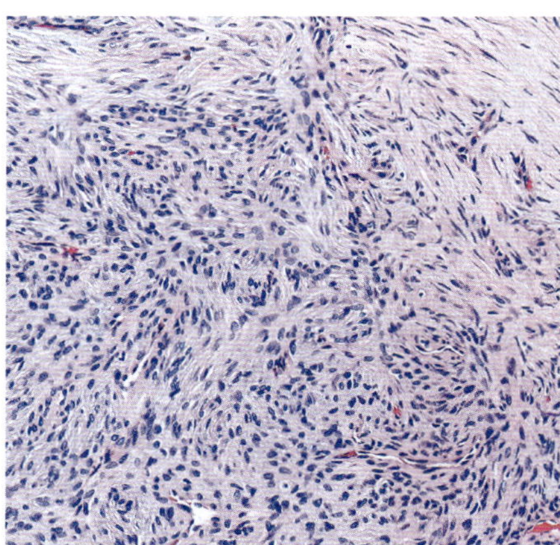
**Fig. 5.58** Cellular superficial acral fibromyxoma (cellular digital fibroma). Cellular cases show a fascicular to storiform arrangement of bland spindled cells in a fibrous to somewhat myxoid stroma.

positive for SMA {1106}. One small series showed consistent immunoreactivity for nestin {553}. The tumours are negative for MUC4, BCL2, keratin, S100 protein, STAT6, and GFAP {1106}.

### Differential diagnosis
Benign fibrous histiocytoma rarely involves acral sites, and has characteristic peripheral collagen trapping. Superficial angiomyxoma has a purely myxoid stroma, which often contains scattered neutrophils. Sclerosing perineurioma occurs in acral locations, but has an epithelioid morphology and purely collagenous stroma {818}. More-cellular superficial acral fibromyxomas can be confused with dermatofibrosarcoma protuberans, but dermatofibrosarcoma protuberans rarely involves acral sites, and it harbours rearrangements of *PDGFB* {1582}. Low-grade fibromyxoid sarcoma rarely involves acral sites, is positive for MUC4, and has *FUS* rearrangement {650}. Acquired digital fibrokeratoma is less cellular, with vertically oriented collagen bundles {769}.

### Histogenesis
The histogenesis is unknown, but may be related to loss of *RB1* {23}.

### Genetic profile
Loss of *RB1* is seen in 90% of cases {23}.

### Prognosis and predictive factors
All reported cases with follow-up have behaved in a benign manner, but local recurrence is relatively common following incomplete removal; the rate may exceed 20% {41,769,1106}.

# Cutaneous myxoma

Requena L.

Cutaneous myxoma is a benign multilobular lesion composed mostly of myxoid material; it shows sparse cellularity and abundant vascularization.

### ICD-O code
8840/0

### Synonyms
Angiomyxoma;
superficial angiomyxoma

### Epidemiology
Cutaneous myxoma is an uncommon neoplasm occurring mostly in adults. The sex distribution is equal. Most cases are sporadic, but multiple lesions can arise in the setting of Carney complex (see *Carney complex*, p. 391).

### Etiology
The etiology is unknown. Multiple cutaneous myxomas may be a marker of Carney complex; most patients with such cases have a mutation in the *PRKAR1A* gene, which encodes one of the four subunits of protein kinase A {2740}.

### Localization
Solitary lesions, which are not associated with Carney complex, are usually located on distal areas of the limbs or the head {57,2830}. Multiple cutaneous myxomas in patients with Carney complex are particularly frequent in the external auditory canal and on the eyelids {761}.

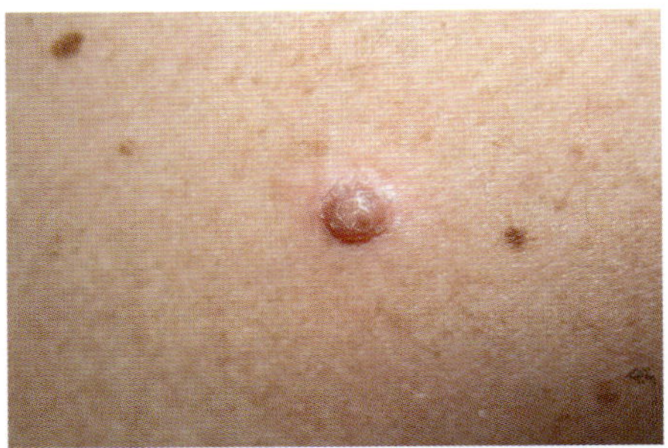

**Fig. 5.59** Cutaneous myxoma. A translucent papule on the anterior aspect of the leg.

### Clinical features
Cutaneous myxomas present as slow-growing nodules that have usually been present for many years before they are surgically removed. In patients with multiple lesions, the possibility of Carney complex should be investigated. The syndrome is inherited as an autosomal dominant trait and consists of the association of endocrine hyperactivity (Cushing syndrome, testicular tumours, and acromegaly); spotty skin pigmentation; psammomatous melanotic schwannoma; and multiple cutaneous, cardiac, and mammary myxomas {383,385,665,1001,1133}. Multiple cutaneous myxomas in the absence of any other anomalies associated with Carney complex have also been described {217,1853}.

### Histopathology
Cutaneous myxoma presents as a well-circumscribed multilobular lesion with an abundant vascular component. When the vascular component is predominant the lesion is called angiomyxoma. Collagenous septa compartmentalize the lesion, and the vascular component is more prominent at the periphery {356}. Each lobule is composed of abundant myxoid material, with sparse cellularity. The stromal cells have fusiform or stellate morphology. Adnexal induction (of various degrees) in the epidermis covering the lesion is frequently seen in the myxomas of patients with Carney complex. Scattered neutrophils in the stroma are

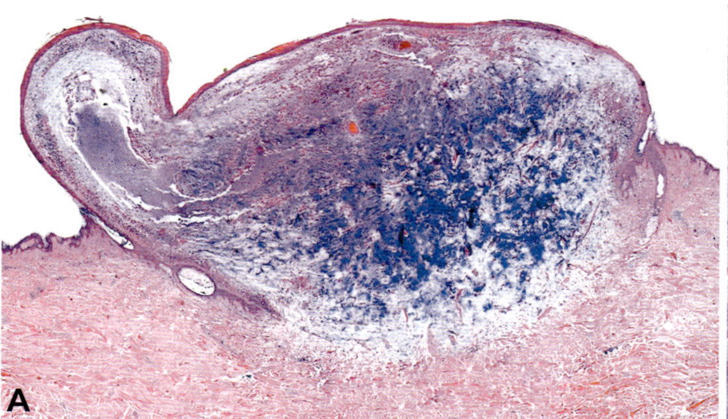
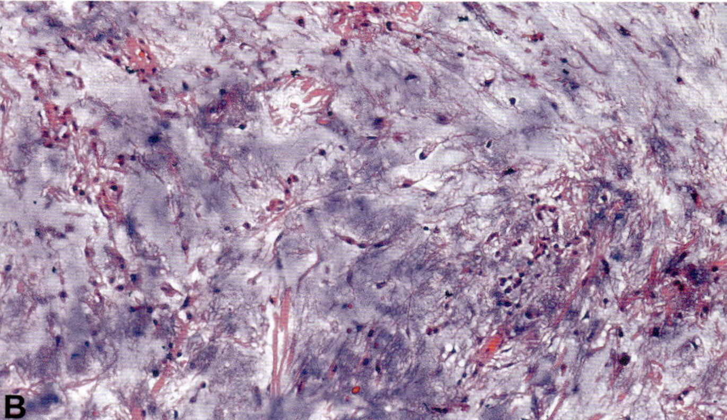

**Fig. 5.60** Cutaneous myxoma. **A** Scanning view showing a well-circumscribed mucinous nodule involving the upper half of the dermis. **B** Higher magnification showing fusiform and stellate cells, as well as numerous thin-walled blood vessels, embedded in a mucinous stroma.

also characteristic of cutaneous myxoma {356}.
Immunohistochemistry shows positivity for vimentin and α-SMA. The lesions are negative for CD34, S100 protein, factor XIIIa, CD57 (LEU7), CD68 (as recognized by KP1), S100A9 (as recognized by MAC387), and desmin {356,2830}.

## Differential diagnosis

Focal mucinosis lacks the cellular and vascular components seen in cutaneous myxoma. Cutaneous myxomas may involve the genital area {772}; therefore, the histopathological differential diagnosis must be established with aggressive angiomyxoma. Aggressive angiomyxoma is a larger lesion that extends deeply to subcutaneous structures and displays a vascular component characterized by variably sized vessels, from small thin-walled capillary vessels to large thick-walled vessels with perivascular hyalinization.

## Genetic susceptibility

Multiple lesions may be seen in patients with Carney complex, and most of these patients have a mutation in the *PRKAR1A* gene, which encodes one of the four subunits of protein kinase A {2740}.

## Prognosis and predictive factors

Cutaneous myxomas are benign neoplasms. Simple excision is curative, although persistence has been reported in as many as 38% of the cases after incomplete surgical resection {356,385}.

# Dermatomyofibroma

Kutzner H.
Rongioletti F.

## Definition
Dermatomyofibroma is a rare benign cutaneous mesenchymal neoplasm of fibroblastic/myofibroblastic differentiation {1146,1273}.

## ICD-O code
8824/0

## Synonym
Plaque-like dermal fibromatosis (obsolete)

## Epidemiology
Dermatomyofibroma most frequently occurs in young females {1146,1747}; it is rare in young children {1613,2578}.

## Localization
The sites of strongest predilection are the upper trunk, upper arm, shoulder, axillary folds, and neck, followed by the abdominal wall and thigh {1146,1273,1747}.

## Clinical features
Dermatomyofibroma presents as an asymptomatic, small, circumscribed, coin-sized, longstanding or slow-growing, flat or plaque-like, moderately indurated and slightly erythematous/pigmented lesion {1146,1273,1747}. The lesions only rarely are multicentric or reach a considerable size {1450}.

## Histopathology
Throughout the dermis, there is a horizontally oriented arrangement of densely packed slender bundles and long fascicles of cytologically bland fusiform spindle cells showing fibroblastic and myofibroblastic differentiation. The epidermis is bland; adnexal structures are spared. Elastic fibres are preserved or even slightly increased, which may be a helpful differential diagnostic clue. Dermatomyofibroma extension into the superficial subcutis is rare. Early and active lesions may express α-SMA. Mature lesions (which constitute the majority) are negative for SMA, desmin, h-caldesmon, CD34, and S100 protein {1747}.

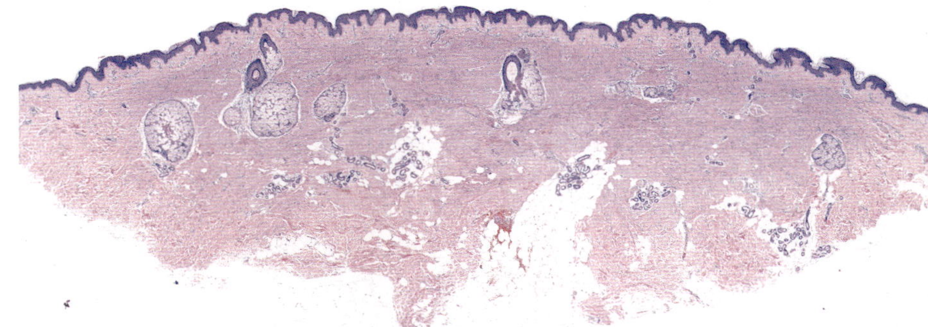

**Fig. 5.62** Dermatomyofibroma. Horizontally oriented strands and fascicles of closely packed myofibroblasts throughout the dermis; adnexal structures are preserved.

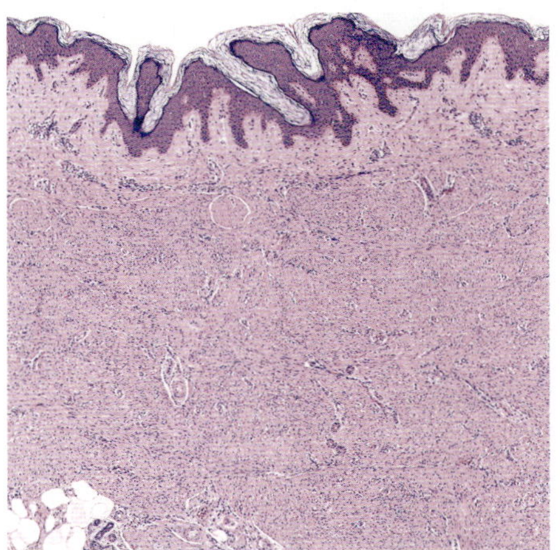

**Fig. 5.63** Dermatomyofibroma. Densely packed myofibroblasts in horizontal array.

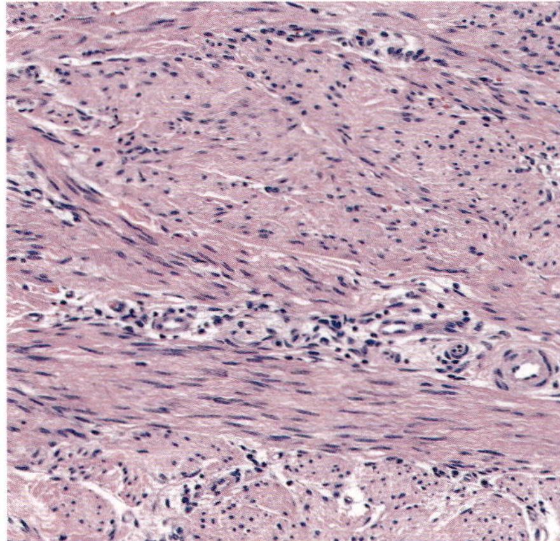

**Fig. 5.64** Dermatomyofibroma. Typical myofibroblasts/fibroblasts with elongated nuclei and fusiform cytoplasm; there is no mitotic activity or pleomorphism.

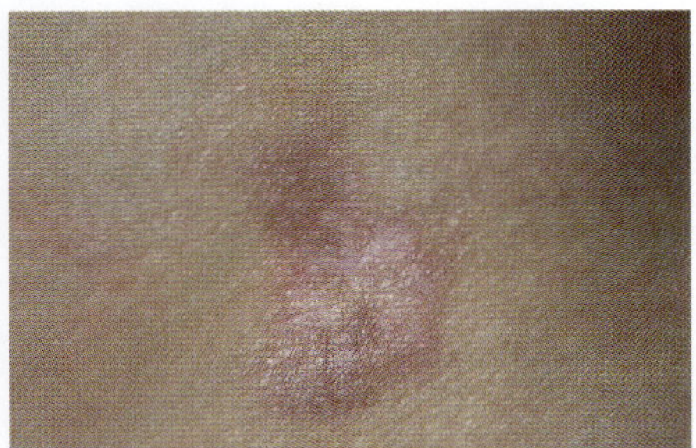

**Fig. 5.61** Dermatomyofibroma. A flat, plaque-like, and slightly indurated lesion.

## Differential diagnosis
The differential diagnosis includes dermatofibrosarcoma protuberans, dermatofibroma, myofibroma, smooth muscle tumours and smooth muscle hamartoma, fibroblastic connective tissue naevus, fibrous hamartoma of infancy, and desmoid-type fibromatosis.

## Histogenesis
Dermatomyofibroma is a myofibroblastic tumour {1273,1898}.

## Prognosis and predictive factors
Dermatomyofibroma is benign; no instances of recurrence have been reported, even in the setting of incomplete excision {1747}.

# Myofibroma and myofibromatosis

Agaimy A.
Michal M.
Wick M.R.

## Definition

Myofibroma and myofibromatosis are benign neoplasms of presumed myofibroblastic histogenesis and phenotype.

## ICD-O codes

| | |
|---|---|
| Myofibroma | 8824/0 |
| Myofibromatosis | 8824/1 |

## Synonyms

Infantile myofibroma;
infantile myofibromatosis; congenital generalized fibromatosis (obsolete); solitary myofibroma; adult myofibroma

## Epidemiology

Myofibroma accounts for 12% of paediatric soft tissue lesions. The age range varies from newborn (including for congenital lesions) to 70 years. Overall, 90% of cases are paediatric and 65% occur during the first 2 years of life {1964}. Multicentric lesions exclusively affect children (more commonly girls).

## Etiology

Other than inherited germline mutations in the familial form, no predisposing or etiological factors are known.

## Localization

Solitary myofibroma typically presents as a dermal or subcutaneous nodule in the skin of the head and neck, upper extremities, or trunk, in addition to other soft tissue sites, including muscle and (less commonly) bone. Multicentric disease has a similar site distribution and other features similar to those of solitary myofibroma. The generalized form additionally shows visceral involvement {1964}.

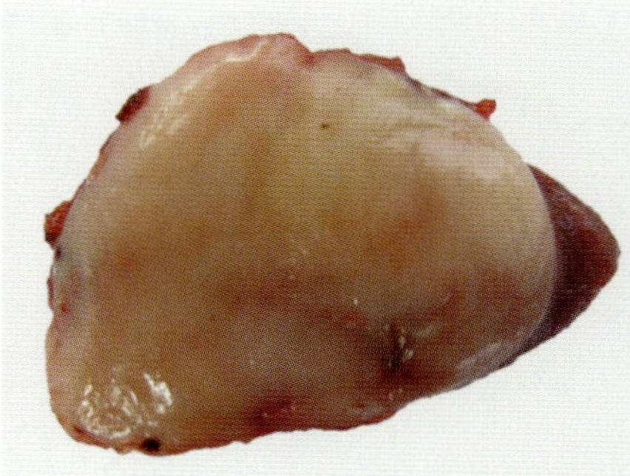

**Fig. 5.65** Cellular infantile myofibroma. Example with a fleshy tan-yellow bulging cut surface. Reprinted with permission from: Agaimy A et al. (2017) Am J Surg Pathol. 41:195-203.

## Clinical features

Myofibroma presents as a well-circumscribed, unencapsulated violaceous dermal or subcutaneous nodule measuring a few millimetres to several centimetres, with a firm, fibrous consistency. On the basis of clinical evaluation, myofibromas can be categorized into three clinicopathological forms: solitary, multicentric, and generalized {1964}. The solitary form has a predilection for males, whereas the multicentric form is more common in females.

## Histopathology

Myofibroma is characterized by biphasic growth of darker-staining rounded or plump spindled cells associated with numerous thin-walled haemangiopericytoma-like vessels and mature eosinophilic spindled myoid cells with frequent myointimal nodules (vascular balls). The stroma is characteristically myxohyaline. Foci of calcification may be present. Mitotic activity is variable. Atypical mitoses are absent. Foci of ischaemic-type necrosis can be seen. A subset of lesions show atypical features such as diffuse cellularity, increased mitotic activity, nerve entrapment, and infiltrative growth. These features are not associated with aggressive behaviour and should not be mistaken for evidence of sarcoma {1568}. The cells of myofibroma stain diffusely for SMA, but h-caldesmon is absent or only focally positive. Myofibroma is usually desmin-negative.

## Differential diagnosis

The differential diagnosis of myofibroma is defined by this entity's varied histological appearance and includes myopericytoma, angioleiomyoma, glomus tumour,

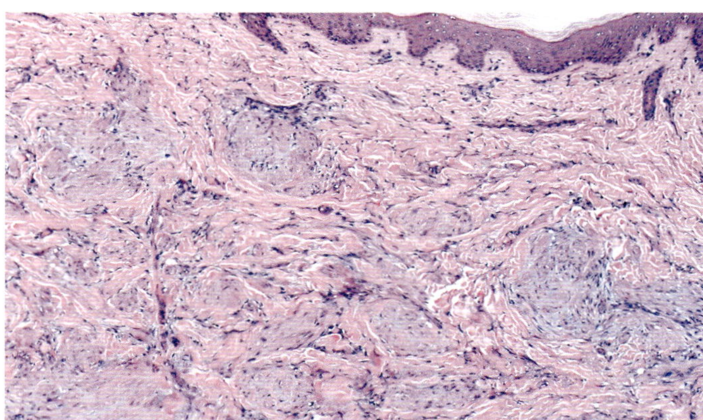

**Fig. 5.66** Cutaneous infantile myofibroma. An example showing irregular myxohyaline nodules and bundles dissecting between dermal collagen. Reprinted with permission from: Agaimy A et al. (2017) Am J Surg Pathol. 41:195-203.

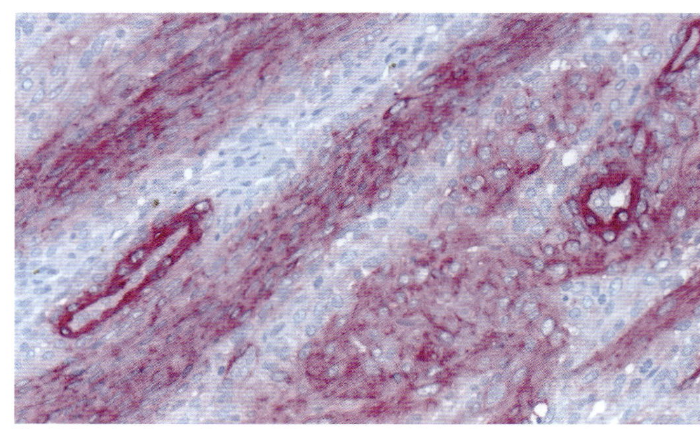

**Fig. 5.67** Infantile myofibroma. SMA staining highlights the myoid cell bundles.

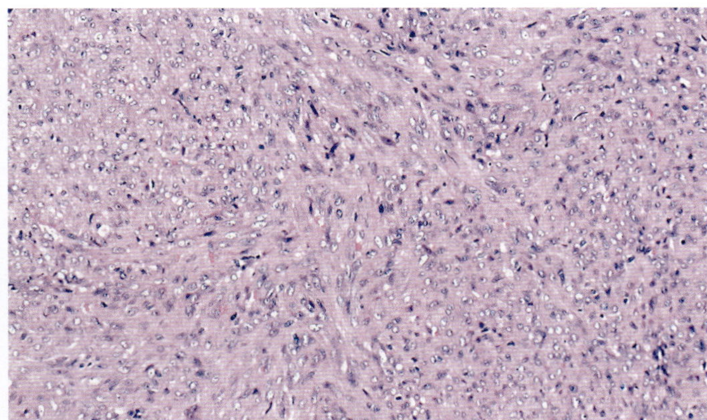

**Fig. 5.68** Atypical infantile myofibroma. Because of its diffuse cellular growth pattern, this variant can be mistaken for infantile fibrosarcoma.

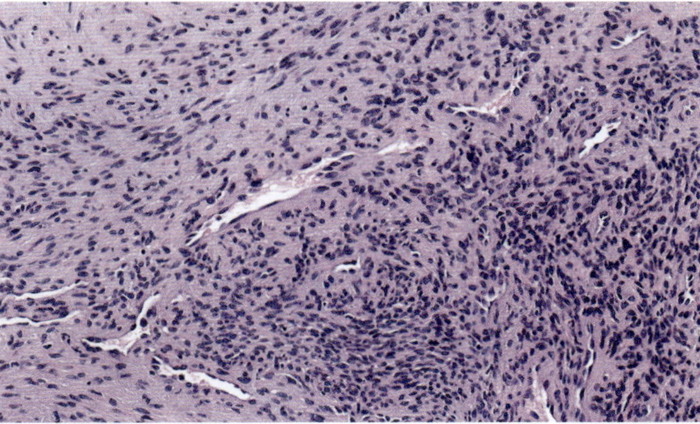

**Fig. 5.69** Myofibroma. At the periphery there are spindled myoid cells and centrally there are uniform round cells associated with a prominent vasculature.

leiomyoma, solitary fibrous tumour, infantile fibrosarcoma, synovial sarcoma with prominent haemangiopericytoma-like features, leiomyosarcoma, and paediatric and adult low-grade and high-grade sarcomas with myopericytic features.

## Histogenesis

Although myofibroma is presumed to be of myofibroblastic origin {1743}, it also shows features of modified myopericytes – a characteristic it shares with other lesions categorized as perivascular myoid cell neoplasms {1745}.

## Genetic profile

Germline and somatic *PDGFRB* mutations are seen in the familial and sporadic forms {22,455,1668}. Mutation types differ between familial and non-familial (sporadic) myofibromatosis.

Other reported cytogenetic aberrations include unbalanced whole-arm translocation between chromosomes 9 and 16 {2456}. Infantile myofibromatosis lacks the *ETV6-NTRK3* and *LMNA-NTRK1* gene fusions that are seen in infantile fibrosarcoma {281} and a subset of paediatric myopericytic sarcomas {990}.

## Genetic susceptibility

Activating germline mutations in *PDGFRB* (identified in 89% of studied families) and *NOTCH3* (in 11%) are associated with familial infantile myofibromatosis {1668}.

## Prognosis and predictive factors

Myofibroma is benign and does not recur after local excision. Fatality associated with the generalized form is due to extensive visceral involvement with limited options for surgical intervention. Atypical histological features do not correlate with adverse outcome {1568}.

# Plaque-like CD34+ dermal fibroma

Kutzner H.
Patterson J.W.

## Definition

Plaque-like CD34+ dermal fibroma is a congenital or acquired dermal spindle cell neoplasm with histopathological features mimicking those of superficial dermal dermatofibrosarcoma protuberans.

## ICD-O code 8810/0

## Synonym

Medallion-like dermal dendrocyte hamartoma {1413,2212}

## Epidemiology

This congenital or acquired neoplasm affects all ages, with a slight female predominance {1857}.

## Localization

There is no specific site predilection {1857}.

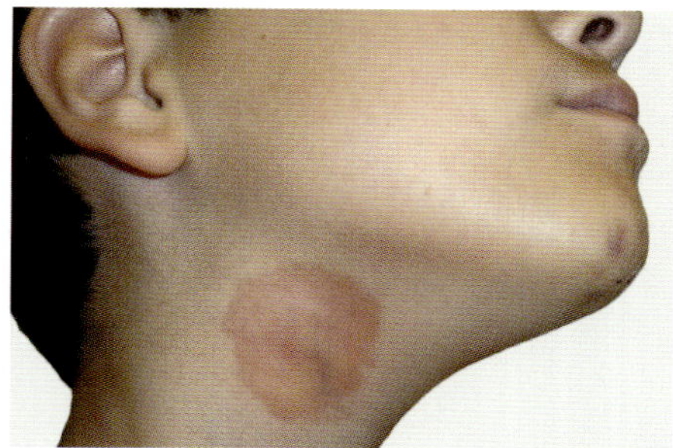

**Fig. 5.70** Plaque-like CD34+ dermal fibroma. A flat, slightly indurated circumscribed tumour on the anterior aspect of the neck of a young boy.

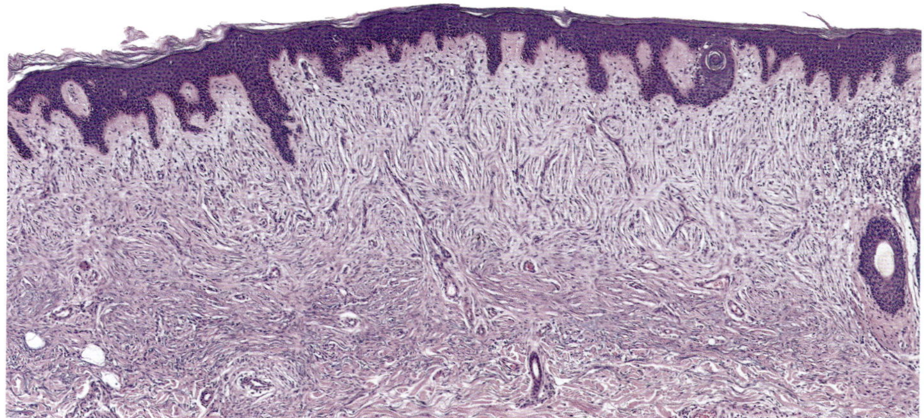

**Fig. 5.71** Plaque-like CD34+ dermal fibroma. Characteristic zonation of tumour cells, with perpendicular arrangement in the upper portion and horizontal arrangement in the deeper part.

## Clinical features

Plaque-like CD34+ dermal fibroma presents as a congenital or slowly enlarging, flat, well-demarcated, plaque-like, moderately indurated, erythematous to slightly brownish lesion ranging from coin-sized to several centimetres in diameter. The tumour surfaces may appear atrophic, depressed, or wrinkled. Nodular variants are rare {1857,2523}.

## Histopathology

There is a band-like proliferation of small cytologically bland spindled fibroblasts in the upper and mid-dermis, with a marked subepidermal grenz zone. Tumour extension into the deep dermis (and in particular into the subcutaneous fat) is rare. Most cases show a richly vascularized, vaguely storiform pattern. There may be slight zonation, with cells of the superficial tumour portion being oriented perpendicular to the epidermis and cells of the deeper portion proliferating in a storiform pattern. A concentric array of tumour cells around small vessels and peripheral nerves may be seen. There is no fat entrapment as is seen in dermatofibrosarcoma protuberans. Cytologically, the tumour cells are bland and have inconspicuous nucleoli. Mitoses are scarce. Immunohistochemically, the tumour cells are strongly positive for CD34, fascin, and vimentin, whereas fac-

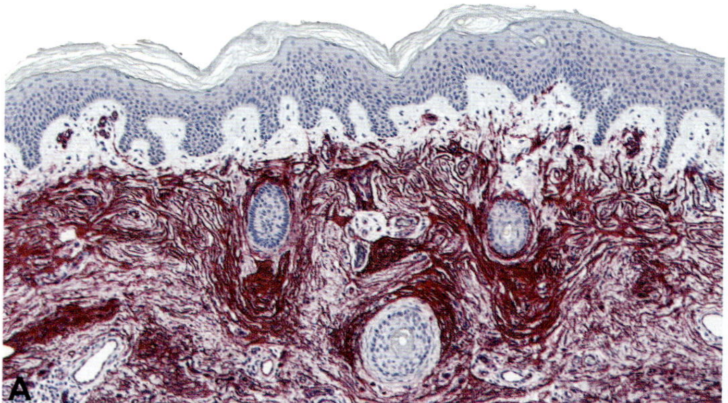

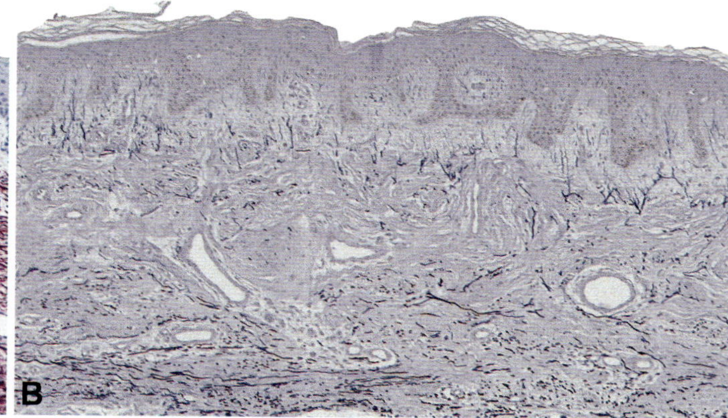

**Fig. 5.72** Plaque-like CD34+ dermal fibroma. **A** CD34 staining reveals the characteristic fingerprint pattern of a fibroblastic tumour. **B** Verhoeff elastic staining reveals a marked reduction of elastic fibres.

tor XIIIa expression is inconsistent. SMA is not significantly expressed {1471,2523}.

### Differential diagnosis

The differential diagnosis includes fibroblastic connective tissue naevus {594,2726} and dermatomyofibroma. The morphological features of plaque-like CD34+ dermal fibroma overlap substantially with those of dermatofibrosarcoma protuberans {450,1665,2577}; the main differentiating feature is the absence of t(17;22)(q22;q13) in plaque-like CD34+ dermal fibroma.

Lesions clinically resembling plaque-like CD34+ dermal fibroma have been described in children with adenosine deaminase–deficient severe combined immunodeficiency. Microscopically, such lesions contain CD34+ dermal cells but are relatively hypocellular. All reported cases have been found to have the *COL1A1-PDGFB* fusion characteristic of dermatofibrosarcoma protuberans {539}.

### Histogenesis

Recent findings suggest that plaque-like CD34+ dermal fibroma is a neoplastic fibroblastic proliferation {1471} rather than a dendrocytoma {1413,2212}.

### Prognosis and predictive factors

Plaque-like CD34+ dermal fibroma is benign, without recurrences {1857}.

# Nodular fasciitis

Lazar A.J.
Karim R.

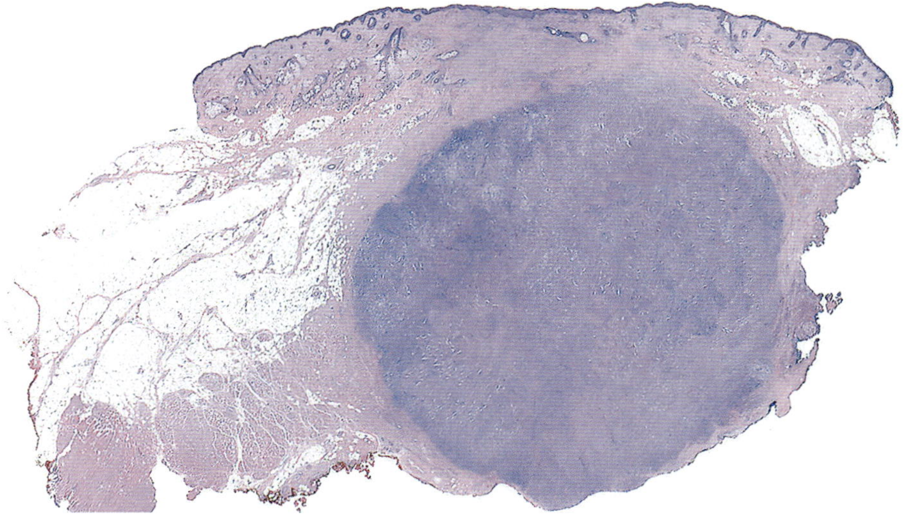

Fig. 5.73 Nodular fasciitis. Low-power view.

## Definition

Nodular fasciitis is a self-limited benign clonal process, classically occurring in the subcutis, composed of fibroblasts/myofibroblasts in a disorganized tissue culture–like array.

## ICD-O code

8828/0

## Synonyms

Pseudosarcomatous fasciitis; nodular pseudosarcomatous fasciitis; subcutaneous pseudosarcomatous fibromatosis

## Epidemiology

Nodular fasciitis can occur at any age, but has a peak incidence in the third and fourth decades, with equal distribution between males and females {1389,2095}.

## Etiology

Nodular fasciitis was previously thought to be a reactive process, and as many as 10% of patients report a prior history of trauma. It is now recognized as a translocation-driven neoplasm that consistently regresses (a so-called transient neoplasia) {701}.

## Localization

Nodular fasciitis can arise from the superficial fascia, from the subcutaneous septa, or (rarely) in the dermis, and it usually bulges into the subcutis. Intramuscular, intra-articular, and visceral lesions are rare {593,1125,1454,2096,2818}. The most common sites are the forearm, thigh, and upper arm, which account for more than half of all cases {2418}; however, nodular fasciitis can involve any part of the body {2799}. Well-described variants include intravascular fasciitis and cranial fasciitis {1500,1998,2316}.

## Clinical features

Nodular fasciitis presents clinically as a relatively rapidly growing subcutaneous mass that enlarges (typically over the course of 3–6 weeks, but in some cases over a period as long as 3 months) and then regresses. It is typically < 2–3 cm in maximal diameter, but rare cases reaching 10 cm have been reported {221}. The mass may be tender or painless {2418}.

## Histopathology

Nodular fasciitis may be circumscribed or infiltrative along subcutaneous septa. It is composed of fibroblasts and/or myofibroblasts without overt cytological atypia. Mitotic activity can be frequent, but the mitoses are not atypical. Cellularity varies between and within lesions. Feathery tissue culture–like areas are typical of the entity, but more-cellular areas can form fascicles. Stroma can be myxoid and/or collagenous, even keloidal. The vasculature is rich and fine, resembling granulation tissue. Extravasated red cells are usually seen, often in the tissue culture–like areas. Osteoclastic giant cells and chronic inflammatory cells can be present. The lesions tend to be partially infiltrative. Strong expression of SMA is characteristic.

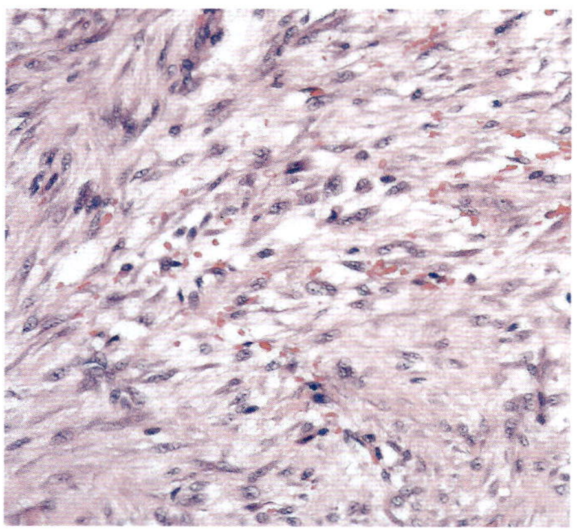

Fig. 5.74 Nodular fasciitis. Disorganized spindle cells and extravasated red blood cells are characteristic.

## Differential diagnosis

The histological differential diagnosis depends on the location, the proportion of collagen and myxoid stroma, and cellularity. Collagenous variants can be mistaken for fibromatosis, collagenous fibroma (desmoplastic fibroblastoma), or granulation tissue. Neural tumours, nerve sheath tumours, myositis ossificans, proliferative fasciitis, proliferative myositis, dermatofibrosarcoma protuberans, and inflammatory myofibroblastic tumours can also be differential diagnoses. Large and/or mitotically active nodular fasciitis can be mistaken for sarcoma {86}.

## Histogenesis

Nodular fasciitis is postulated to originate from fibroblastic/myofibroblastic cells; however, given the wide histological spectrum, it may have a heterogeneous origin.

## Genetic profile

Nodular fasciitis has been shown to harbour a translocation between

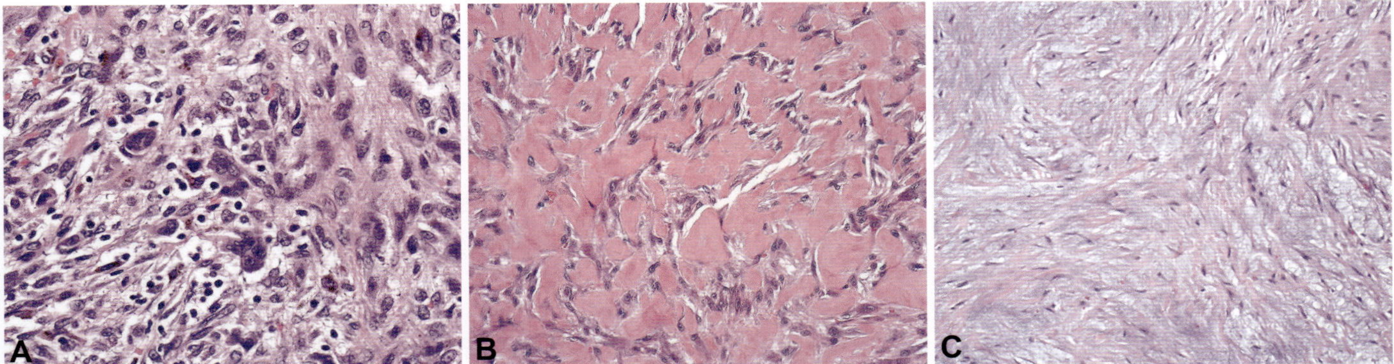

**Fig. 5.75** Nodular fasciitis. The recognition of this entity can be complicated by features such as inflammatory and multinucleated giant cells (**A**), keloidal collagen deposition (**B**), and extensive myxoid change (**C**).

chromosomes 17 and 22, t(17;22)(p13;q13), which results in *MYH9-USP6* gene fusion and subsequent overexpression of USP6 {701}. This translocation is also seen in aneurysmal bone cyst {1944,1945}. USP6 is a deubiquitinating enzyme with roles in cell trafficking, cell signalling, protein breakdown, and inflammation. *MYH9* encodes a non-muscle myosin heavy chain that has roles in cell motility, shape, adhesion, and differentiation. Other gene promoters can also be substituted for *MYH9* in this characteristic gene fusion; *PPP6R3-USP6* fusion was reported in a case of nodular fasciitis that recurred (with metastasis) several times over a period of 10 years {967}.

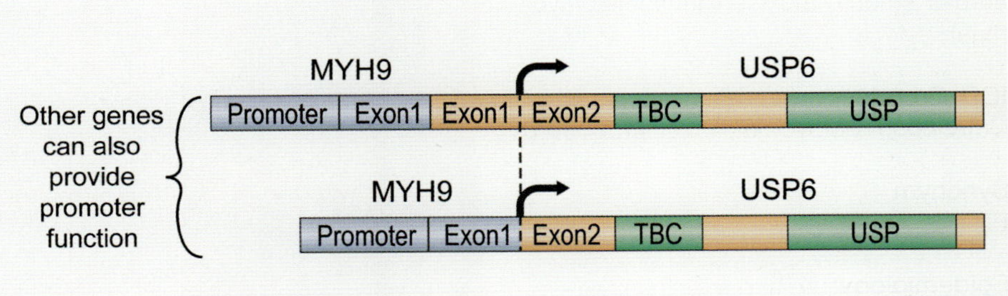


**Fig. 5.76** Nodular fasciitis. Schematic representation of the characteristic *MYH9-USP6* gene fusion.

## Prognosis and predictive factors

Nodular fasciitis can very rarely recur following incomplete excision, most commonly when surgical margins are positive.

# Smooth muscle tumours

## Cutaneous leiomyomas and variants

Folpe A.
Fullen D.R.

### Definition
Cutaneous leiomyomas are benign dermal smooth muscle tumours derived from intrinsic dermal arrector pili smooth muscle (pilar leiomyomas) or dartoic/vulvar/areolar smooth muscle (genital leiomyomas).

### ICD-O code
Cutaneous leiomyoma 8890/0

### Synonym
Piloleiomyoma

### Epidemiology
Pilar leiomyomas are rare. Cases involving multiple tumours typically have an earlier onset than do solitary leiomyomas {1648}. Solitary tumours are more common in females than in males.

### Etiology
Multiple pilar leiomyomas are commonly inherited in an autosomal dominant pattern, with variable penetrance.

### Localization
The extensor surfaces of the extremities are most commonly affected, followed by the trunk and the head and neck region {1111}. Genital leiomyomas can involve the scrotum, vulva, nipple, or areola.

### Clinical features
Cutaneous leiomyomas are flesh-coloured to reddish-brown, firm, dome-shaped papules or nodules. Multiple leiomyomas are more often painful and may be distributed in linear, segmental, or zosteriform patterns {1362}. Solitary leiomyomas are usually no larger than 2 cm {1648}. Genital leiomyomas are usually solitary raised to pedunculated papules or nodules, usually < 2 cm but occasionally larger, and asymptomatic. Vulvar tumours may enlarge during pregnancy {1648}.

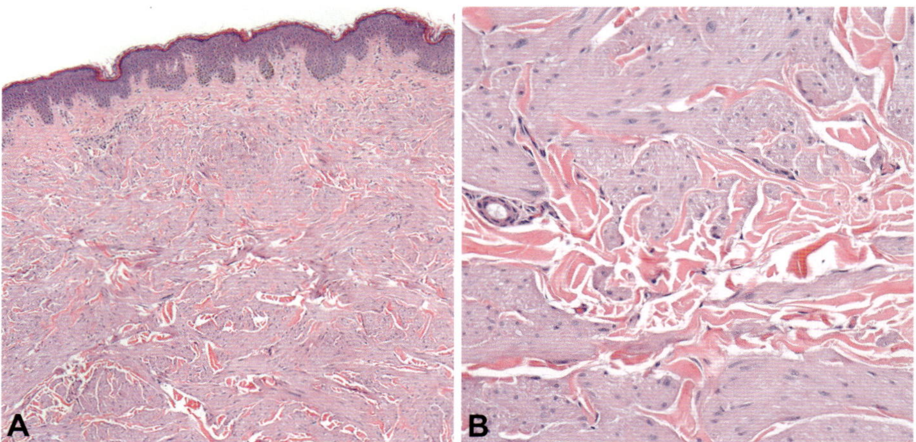


**Fig. 5.77** Pilar leiomyoma. **A** Low-power view of a haphazard, poorly circumscribed proliferation of well-differentiated smooth muscle. **B** Higher-power view showing well-differentiated smooth muscle cells with no nuclear atypia or mitotic activity.

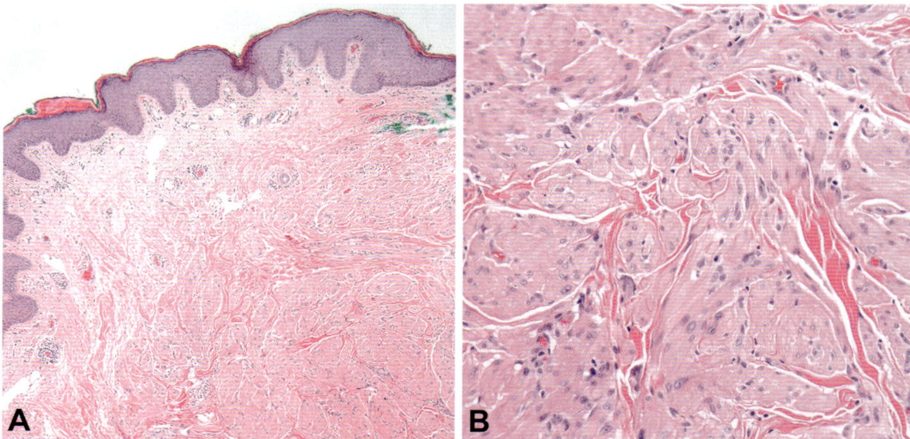


**Fig. 5.78** Dartoic leiomyoma. **A** A tumour of scrotal dartoic muscle, consisting of a hypocellular proliferation of well-differentiated smooth muscle arranged in intersecting bundles. **B** Higher-power view of well-differentiated, benign-looking smooth muscle.

### Histopathology
Pilar leiomyomas are poorly circumscribed dermal nodules of intersecting, well-differentiated smooth muscle bundles composed of spindle cells with elongated, blunt-ended nuclei, perinuclear vacuoles, and eosinophilic cytoplasm {1111,1647,1648}. Rare mitotic figures may be seen {2125}. Enlarged, hyperchromatic cells similar to those seen in symplastic uterine leiomyomas may be encountered {521,1637,1757}. SMA, desmin, and caldesmon are typically expressed. Demonstration of loss of fumarate hydratase expression is useful in identifying possible cases of hereditary leiomyomatosis and renal cell cancer syndrome {329,389,1579,1580}.

### Differential diagnosis
Smooth muscle hamartoma is an uncommon, usually congenital hyperplasia of

dermal smooth muscle bundles, thought to result from abnormal migration and proliferation of arrector pili muscle during fetal development; it is distinguished from pilar leiomyoma by its congenital or earlier onset, patch or plaque appearance, lack of associated tenderness, and more-haphazardly arranged and discrete smooth muscle bundles. Cutaneous leiomyosarcoma (atypical smooth muscle tumour) shows cytological atypia, increased cellularity, mitotic activity, and infiltrative growth. Cutaneous metastases from deep soft tissue leiomyosarcomas typically show marked pleomorphism, very brisk mitotic activity, and necrosis.

## Genetic susceptibility

Heterozygous germline loss-of-function mutations in *FH*, located at 1q43, predisposes individuals to hereditary leiomyomatosis and renal cell cancer syndrome, which manifests as cutaneous and uterine leiomyomas and renal cell carcinoma {182,851,1543,2749} and is very rare {1648}.

## Prognosis and predictive factors

Pilar leiomyomas are benign. Multiple leiomyomas may be associated with aggressive type 2 papillary renal cell carcinoma in hereditary leiomyomatosis and renal cell cancer syndrome, influencing patient management and prognosis.

# Cutaneous leiomyosarcoma (atypical smooth muscle tumour)

Folpe A.
Elston D.
Kutzner H.

## Definition

Cutaneous leiomyosarcoma (atypical smooth muscle tumour) is a primary dermal neoplasm composed of generally well-differentiated spindled cells closely resembling (and likely derived from) normal arrector pili smooth muscle, but showing nuclear enlargement, hyperchromatism, and mitotic activity.

## ICD-O code 8897/1

## Synonyms

Atypical intradermal smooth muscle neoplasm; piloleiomyosarcoma

## Epidemiology

Cutaneous leiomyosarcomas are rare. They most often occur in older adult men, with a mean patient age of 56 years and a male-to-female ratio of 3:1 to 4:1 {1441,1680}.

## Etiology

Rare cases have been described in association with Li–Fraumeni syndrome {1441}. EBV-associated leiomyosarcomas may occur in immunosuppressed patients.

## Localization

The tumours most commonly involve the trunk and lower extremities {1441,1680}.

## Clinical features

The tumours typically present as small (0.5–3 cm), solitary, and occasionally painful nodules.

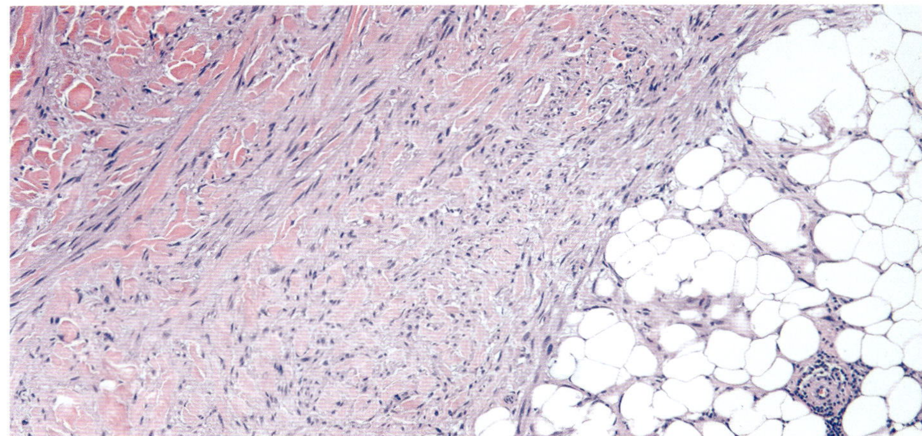

**Fig. 5.79** Cutaneous leiomyosarcoma (atypical smooth muscle tumour). Cases in which the tumour extends into the subcutaneous adipose tissue probably have a higher risk for metastasis than do cases confined to the dermis, but data are limited.

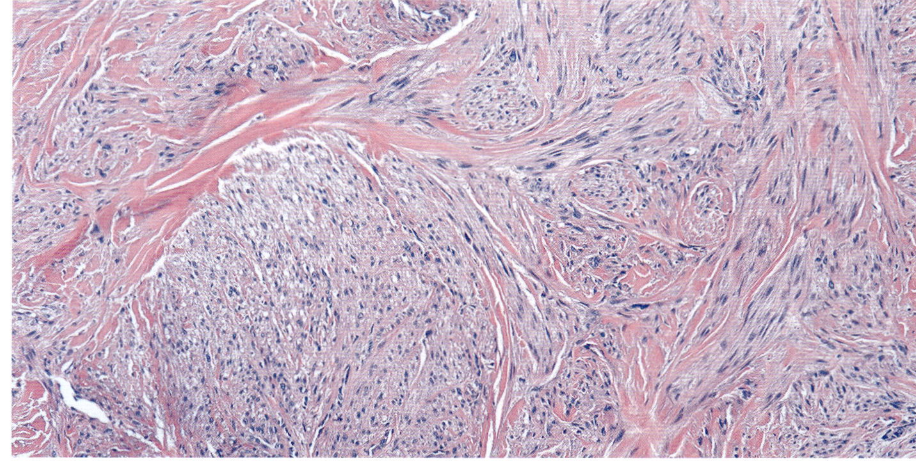

**Fig. 5.80** Cutaneous leiomyosarcoma (atypical smooth muscle tumour). An example with hyalinized collagen; such lesions can be mistaken for cellular fibrous histiocytoma, but demonstration of SMA, desmin, and h-caldesmon expression establishes the diagnosis of a true smooth muscle tumour.

## Histopathology

Cutaneous leiomyosarcomas are typically well differentiated, consisting of fascicles of relatively uniform, eosinophilic spindled cells with perinuclear vacuoles and cigar-shaped nuclei. Compared with normal pilar smooth muscle, leiomyosarcomas show greater cellularity, nuclear enlargement, and hyperchromatism, and they show mitotic activity. Marked nuclear pleomorphism and necrosis are rare; the presence of such features should raise concern for metastasis from a deeply situated leiomyosarcoma {2779}. Cutaneous leiomyosarcomas typically grow in an infiltrative fashion into the surrounding dermis, and they may show limited involvement of the subcutaneous fat. Immunohistochemically, these tumours are essentially always positive for SMA and desmin, and almost always positive for caldesmon {1441,1680}. Expression of keratins may be seen in as many as 45% of cases {1441}.

## Genetic profile

The genetic events underlying the development of cutaneous leiomyosarcoma are unknown. There does not seem to be an increased incidence among patients with germline *FH* mutation {2463}.

## Prognosis and predictive factors

The prognosis of these tumours is superb, with no metastases noted in the largest series to date (84 cases) of tumours confined to the dermis {1441}. Data are limited, but dermal leiomyosarcomas showing subcutaneous involvement may have a low risk of metastasis. Grading is not of prognostic value.

# (Myo)pericytic tumours

## Glomus tumour and variants

Patterson J.W.
Folpe A.
Jackett L.

### Definition
Glomus tumours are mesenchymal neoplasms composed of cells resembling the modified smooth muscle cells of the normal glomus body.

### ICD-O codes

| | |
|---|---|
| Glomus tumour | 8711/0 |
| Glomuvenous malformation (glomangiomyoma) | 8713/0 |
| Glomus tumour of uncertain malignant potential | 8711/1 |
| Malignant glomus tumour | 8711/3 |

### Synonyms
Glomangioma; glomangiosarcoma

### Epidemiology
Glomus tumours of the skin are more common than their soft tissue counterparts {1841,2234}. Digital and subungual lesions have a slight female predominance. Glomus tumours are most common in the fourth to sixth decades of life {1839}. Paediatric malignant glomus tumours are extremely rare {2848}.

### Localization
The tumours are most frequently located in the distal extremities, in particular in the subungual region, digits, hand, wrist, and foot {807,2437,2511}. Glomuvenous malformation is more common on the trunk. Rare malignant glomus tumours of the skin occur in various locations {485,807}.

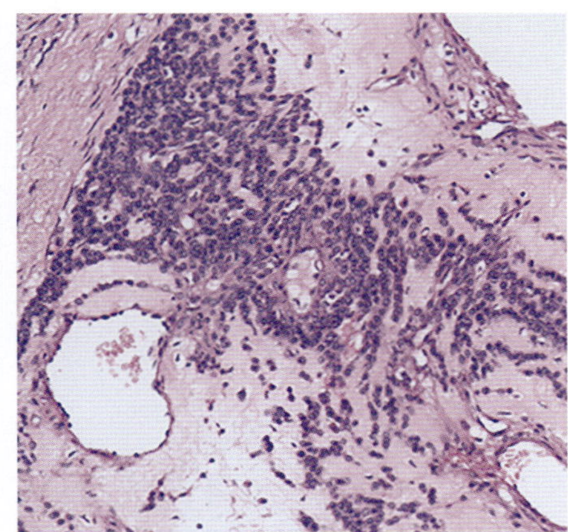
**Fig. 5.81** Glomuvenous malformation. There are ectatic vascular channels and clustered glomus cells.

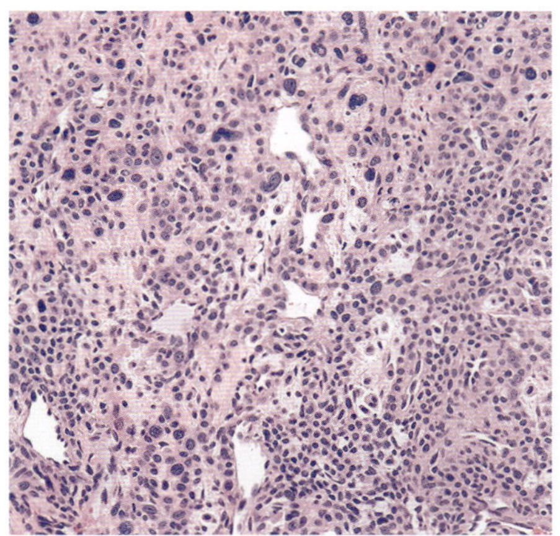
**Fig. 5.82** Symplastic glomus tumour. There is striking nuclear atypia in the absence of mitoses and other atypical features.

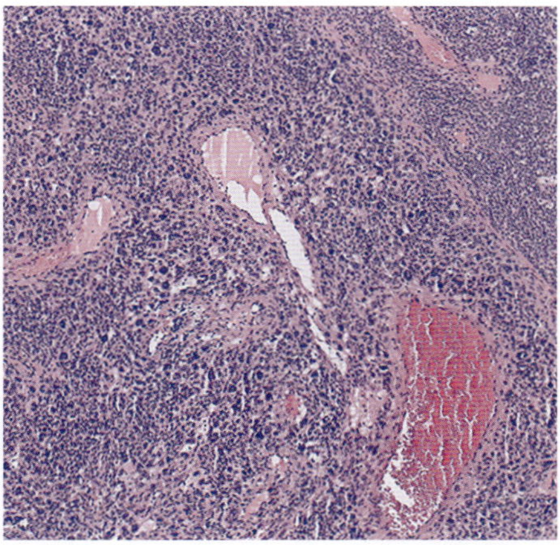
**Fig. 5.83** Glomus tumour of uncertain malignant potential with coexisting typical and atypical components. The atypical component shows a moderate nuclear grade but insufficient mitotic activity for a diagnosis of malignancy.

### Clinical features
Most cutaneous glomus tumours present as solitary, small (< 1 cm), painful nodules or plaques, with a pink to blue hue {1226}. Pain in response to temperature change or light touch is characteristic {1973,2450}. Glomuvenous malformations, which may be large, are most common in patients with multiple or familial lesions.

### Histopathology
Glomus cells are small, uniform, and round, with a central round nucleus, amphophilic to lightly eosinophilic cytoplasm, and a sharp cellular outline with peripheral basal lamina. Oncocytic, epithelioid, myxoid, and hyalinized variants are recognized {2105,2462}. Solid glomus tumours, which account for approximately 75% of all cases, are composed of nests of glomus cells surrounding capillary sized vessels. Small cuffs of glomus cells are often seen around small vessels located outside the main mass. Glomuvenous malformations, which account for 20% of cases, feature dilated vascular channels with intervening small clusters of glomus cells. Glomus tumours may also contain spindled cells resembling smooth muscle (glomangiomyoma) or a branching, haemangiopericytoma-like vasculature (glomangiopericytoma) {927}. Glomangiomatosis is an extremely rare variant of glomus tumour with an overall architectural resemblance to diffuse angiomatosis {807,1988,2934}, but containing nests of glomus cells within vessel walls. Symplastic tumours show striking nuclear atypia in the absence of other worrisome features {807,1270,2302}.

Histologically and/or clinically malignant glomus tumours are extremely rare {807,1486,2892}. The diagnosis of malignant glomus tumour should be reserved only for tumours showing marked nuclear atypia (with any level of mitotic activity) and/or atypical mitotic figures. A component of pre-existing benign-looking

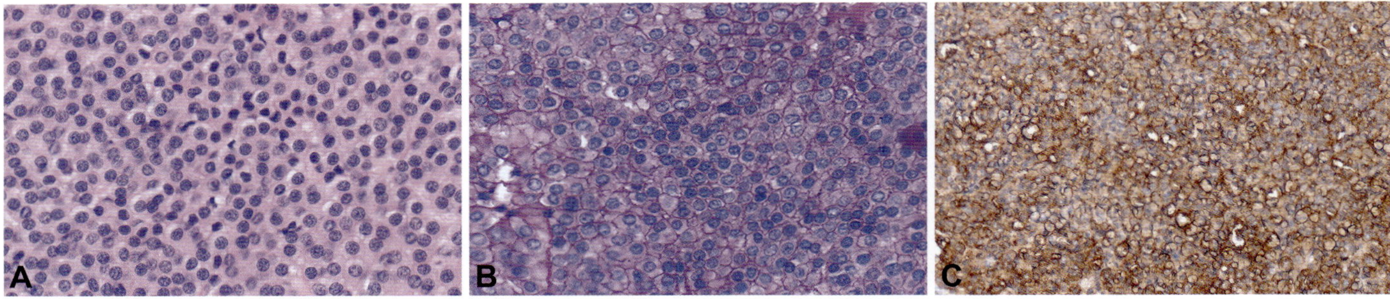


**Fig. 5.84** Typical glomus tumour. **A** Glomus cells have a central round nucleus, eosinophilic cytoplasm, and a well-defined cytoplasmic membrane. **B** Periodic acid–Schiff (PAS) staining highlights pericellular basal lamina. **C** Glomus cells show uniform strong immunostaining for SMA.

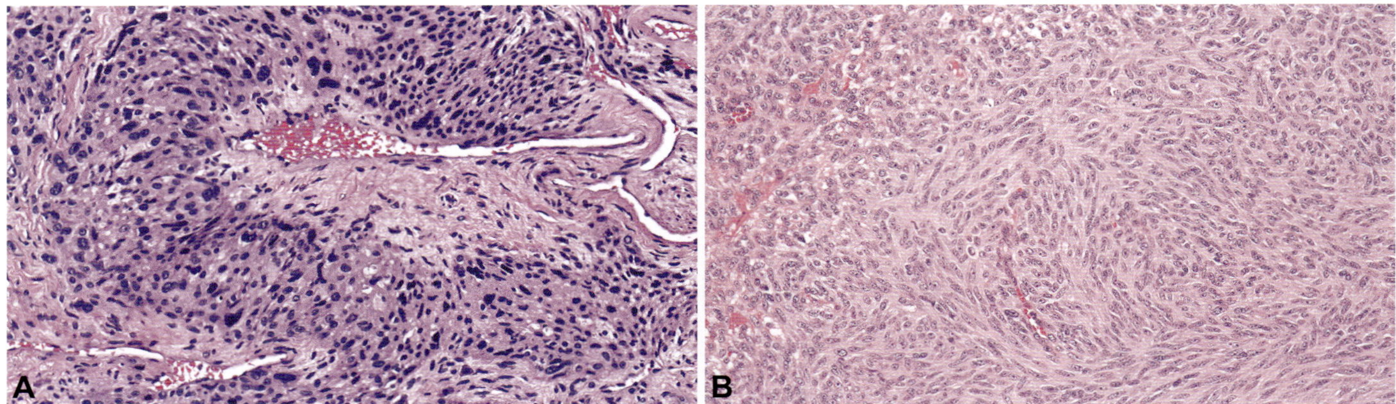


**Fig. 5.85** Malignant glomus tumour. **A** Marked atypia and mitotic activity are clues to malignancy. **B** A spindle cell–type example with mitotic activity.

glomus tumour is often present. Malignant glomus tumours may retain an overall architectural resemblance to normal glomus tumour (but with malignant-looking round cells), or they may consist of a spindled component resembling leiomyosarcoma or fibrosarcoma. Immunohistochemical demonstration of SMA and pericellular collagen IV is required for diagnosis of round cell forms of malignant glomus tumour, in the absence of a clear-cut benign precursor. Glomus tumours not fulfilling the criteria for malignancy but having at least one atypical feature other than nuclear pleomorphism should be diagnosed as glomus tumours of uncertain malignant potential.

Glomus tumours of all types typically express SMA and caldesmon. Pericellular collagen IV can be demonstrated. Other markers are usually negative {807}.

## Genetic profile

Multiple familial glomus tumours appear to have an autosomal dominant pattern of inheritance {260,2642}. They are caused by inactivating mutations in *GLMN* (1p22.1), which encodes the glomulin protein (normally expressed in vascular smooth muscle cells) {807}. A somatic mutation on the second allele has been identified in glomangioma tissue. An association between digital glomus tumours and neurofibromatosis type 1, with biallelic *NF1* inactivation, has been reported, with frequent involvement of multiple digits {302,1025,1026}. Mitotic recombination of chromosome 17q has been identified as another somatic inactivation mechanism in glomus tumours associated with neurofibromatosis type 1 {2510}. There is no evidence of *NF1* inactivation or overactivation of the RAS/MAPK pathway in sporadic glomus tumours {301}. In general, glomus tumours associated with neurofibromatosis type 1 are benign {2437}.

Fusions involving the microRNA gene *MIR143* and NOTCH genes, as well as NOTCH gene rearrangements alone, have been found in both benign and malignant glomus tumours {1835}.

## Prognosis and predictive factors

Malignant glomus tumours are highly aggressive, with metastasis occurring in approximately 40% of cases, resulting in the death of the patient {807,1486}. It is uncertain whether cutaneous malignant glomus tumours harbour the same risk of metastasis.

# Myopericytoma and variants

Agaimy A.
Luzar B.
Michal M.
Patterson J.W.

## Definition

Myopericytoma is a benign neoplasm with perivascular myoid cell differentiation.

## ICD-O code

Myopericytoma 8824/0

## Epidemiology

Myopericytoma occurs preferentially in adults but can occur at any age from birth to old age, with a predilection for males.

## Etiology

There are no known etiological or predisposing factors. Rare lesions have occurred in association with EBV in people with AIDS; such cases tend to be multifocal and originate at unusual visceral or intracranial sites {1499}.

## Localization

Myopericytoma is dermal-based or subcutaneous {1745}. The most commonly affected sites are the distal extremities, followed by the proximal extremities, head and neck (including the oral cavity), and trunk. Deep-seated, visceral, and intracranial lesions are rare. Myopericytoma and myointimoma of the glans penis may constitute the same entity {2210}.

## Clinical features

Myopericytoma presents as a solitary painless dermal or subcutaneous nodule. Multifocal lesions are uncommon {1745}. Intravascular lesions may be painful {1399}.

## Histopathology

Myopericytoma forms a morphological spectrum with perivascular myoid cell neoplasms, ranging from glomus tumour to glomangiomyoma to myofibroma. Myopericytomas are well-circumscribed unencapsulated nodules measuring < 2 cm. They are composed of bland oval or spindled cells with eosinophilic cytoplasm, round to ovoid nuclei, and frequent concentric perivascular growth. The cellularity and vasculature vary greatly. Cellular solid lesions resemble myofibroma.

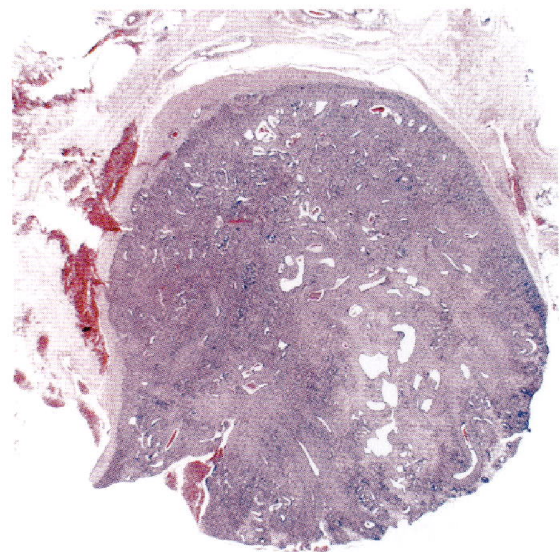

**Fig. 5.86** Myopericytoma presenting as a small, well-circumscribed subcutaneous nodule.

Some lesions contain thin-walled communicating vascular channels, whereas others display angioleiomyoma-like muscular vessels. Other histological variants include hypocellular fibroma–like myopericytoma, haemangiopericytoma-like myopericytoma {1745}, and myopericytoma with glomoid features (termed glomangiopericytoma). Anastomosing multinodular growth, which is rare {1180}, has been referred to as myopericytomatosis {1154}. Less common variants include intramural and intravascular lesions. Secondary changes (e.g. hyalinization, metaplastic ossification, ischaemic-type necrosis, and degenerative atypia) are uncommon.

Myopericytoma cells stain diffusely and strongly for SMA and h-caldesmon. Positive staining for MSA has also been reported {115}. Desmin is usually absent or only focally positive {1745}.

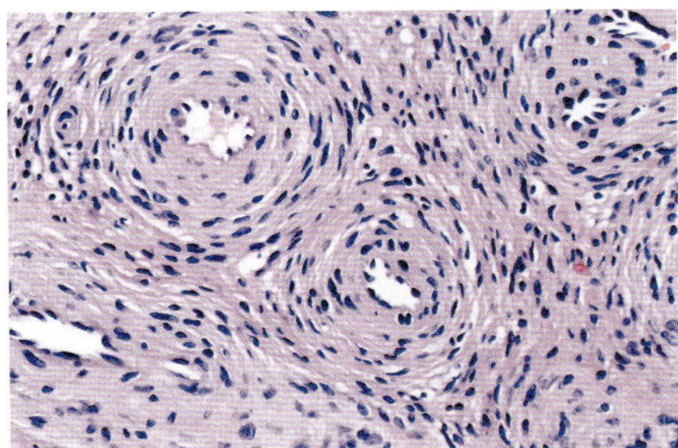

**Fig. 5.87** Myopericytoma. Uniform ovoid cells with concentric (onion skin–like) perivascular growth.

## Differential diagnosis

The differential diagnosis of myopericytoma includes the morphological spectrum of myofibroma, angioleiomyoma, and glomus tumour. Solitary fibrous tumour and EBV-associated smooth muscle tumours are also considerations.

## Histogenesis

Myopericytoma differentiates towards the myopericyte {1745}. Myointimal cells possibly contribute to the tumorigenesis of myopericytoma {122}.

## Genetic profile

Genetic alterations detected in subsets of myopericytoma include t(7;12)(p21-22;q13-15) resulting in *ACTB-GLI1* gene fusion {561}, *BRAF* mutations (found in 15% of cases) {22,2272}, *SRF-RELA* gene fusion in cellular myopericytoma {81}, and *PDGFRB* mutations in so-called myopericytomatosis. The few classic cases examined in one study lacked *PDGFRB* mutations {22}.

## Prognosis and predictive factors

Myopericytoma is benign and does not usually recur, even after marginal or incomplete excision. Malignant transformation has not been conclusively documented. Myopericytoma is likely unrelated to paediatric or adult sarcomas with myopericytic features {990,1722}.

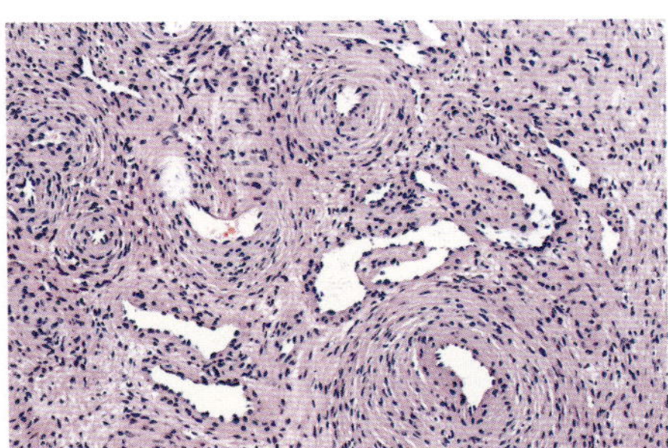

**Fig. 5.88** Myopericytoma. Some cases show an admixture of haemangiopericytoma-like and onion skin–like vasculature.

# Angioleiomyoma

Patel R.M.
Requena L.

## Definition
Angioleiomyoma is a common, benign, often painful, mesenchymal tumour composed of thick-walled blood vessels surrounded by dense, reduplicated smooth muscle cells. It is a member of the so-called perivascular myoid family of tumours, which also includes myopericytoma, myofibroma, and glomus tumour.

## ICD-O code 8894/0

## Synonyms
Vascular leiomyoma; angiomyoma

## Epidemiology
Angioleiomyomas account for about 5% of all benign soft tissue tumours. They are more common in females. These tumours can occur at any age, but they most commonly arise in the fourth to sixth decades of life {977,1699}.

## Etiology
Trauma and venous stasis are potential causal factors {2130}. Lesions in immunosuppressed patients can be associated with EBV {432,615,2038}.

## Localization
Angioleiomyomas can occur anywhere, but they are typically dermal or subcutaneous lesions in the lower extremities, head, or trunk {977,1699}. Intraosseous and subfascial sites have also been reported {1936,2680}.

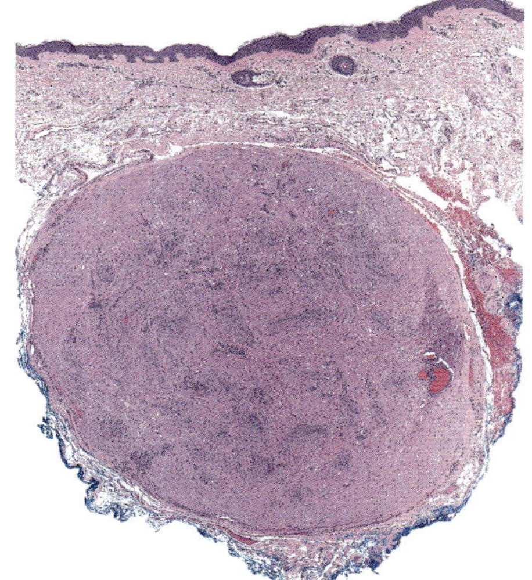

**Fig. 5.89** Angioleiomyoma. Well-circumscribed lesion composed of blood vessels surrounded by bundles of well-developed smooth muscle.

## Clinical features
The tumours are solitary, small, firm, slow-growing, painful nodules {977,1037,1699}.

## Histopathology
Angioleiomyoma is a circumscribed proliferation of bland smooth muscle cells concentrically arrayed around blood vessels. Mitotic activity is inconspicuous. Solid, venous, and cavernous variants have been described {977}. The constituent cells are immunoreactive for SMA, MSA, calponin, and (variably) caldesmon. Desmin is expressed in most cases {1699}. In EBV-associated lesions, in situ hybridization for EBV-encoded small RNA (EBER) is positive {615}.

## Differential diagnosis
The differential diagnosis includes myopericytoma, myofibroma, glomus tumour, and leiomyoma.

## Histogenesis
Lesional spindle cells demonstrate the typical ultrastructural features of smooth muscle cells {123,2373}.

## Genetic profile
Simple karyotypes with varied structural changes have been reported {2806}. As revealed by comparative genomic hybridization, the most common DNA losses involve 22q11.2. The most common gains are at Xq {1909}.

## Prognosis and predictive factors
Angioleiomyomas are benign lesions cured by simple excision. Only rare recurrences have been reported {977,1640}.

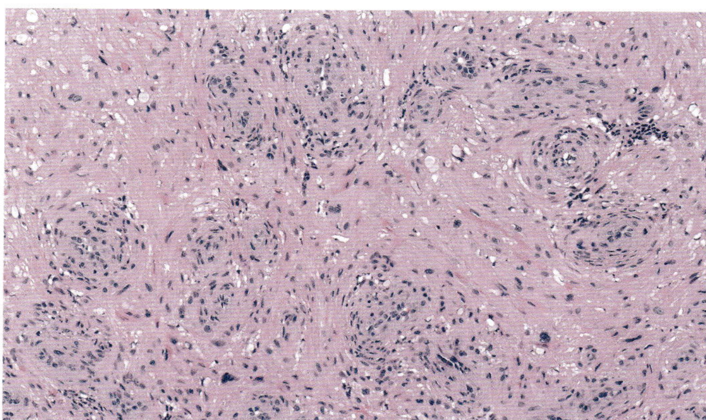

**Fig. 5.90** Angioleiomyoma. Multiple blood vessels surrounded by concentric bland smooth muscle cells.

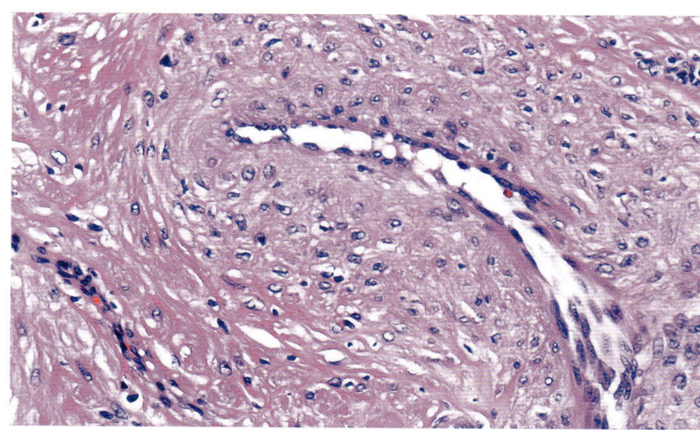

**Fig. 5.91** Angioleiomyoma. Blood vessels surrounded by bundles of bland smooth muscle. Note the lack of cytological atypia and mitoses.

# Vascular tumours
# Cutaneous angiosarcoma

Billings S.D.
Brenn T.
Hornick J.L.

## Definition
Cutaneous angiosarcoma is a highly malignant neoplasm with endothelial differentiation.

## ICD-O code
9120/3

## Synonyms
Lymphangiosarcoma; haemangiosarcoma

## Epidemiology
Cutaneous angiosarcoma most commonly occurs in sun-damaged skin of the head and neck in elderly patients {274,645}. It also occurs secondary to radiation therapy (most commonly in breast cancer patients) or chronic lymphoedema {248,306,552,2030,2429}.

## Etiology
Most primary cutaneous angiosarcomas are likely related to chronic sun damage. In secondary cutaneous angiosarcoma, radiation therapy (most commonly for breast cancer) and chronic lymphoedema related to radical mastectomy are the most common predisposing factors {248,306,552,2030}. Angiosarcoma can also occur secondary to lymphoedema (in particular following mastectomy, as seen in Stewart–Treves syndrome) due to other causes, including obesity {2429}.

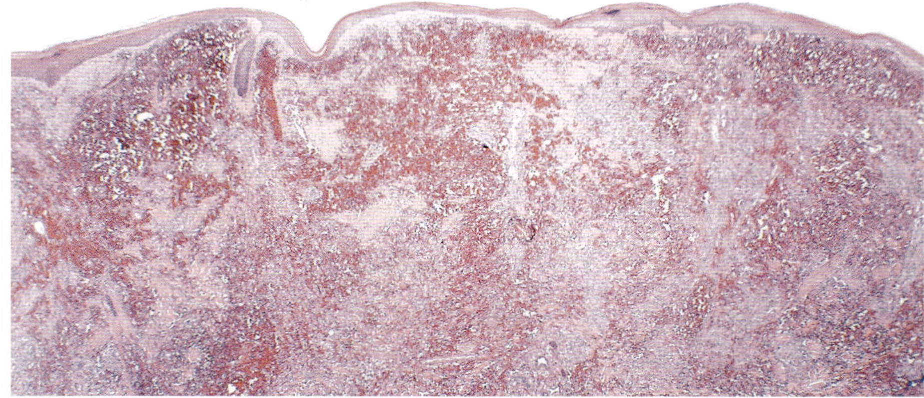

**Fig. 5.92** Angiosarcoma. Low-power image showing multiple erythematous, haemangioma-like areas.

## Localization
Primary cutaneous angiosarcoma typically presents in sun-damaged skin of the head and neck in elderly patients {645}. Radiation-induced angiosarcoma is most commonly seen in the skin of the breast and/or chest wall in breast cancer patients {248,306}. Lymphoedema-associated angiosarcoma is most common in the ipsilateral upper extremity or chest wall of patients treated with radical mastectomy, but it can also arise in other locations in association with longstanding lymphoedema {552,2199,2429,2432}.

## Clinical features
Early-stage lesions can be subtle bruise-like or haemangioma-like areas, which progress to solitary or multifocal erythematous and violaceous plaques and nodules {2017}. Radiation-induced angiosarcomas arise in irradiated skin of the breast, with an average latency period of about 5 years (range: 1 year to > 20 years) {248,306}. Lymphoedema-associated angiosarcomas tend to have a longer latency period, averaging ≥ 10 years {552,2030}.

## Histopathology
Cutaneous angiosarcoma has a wide histopathological range {248,306,616,2857}. Classically, cutaneous angiosarcoma is composed of complex anastomosing vessels lined by hyperchromatic endothelial cells, with multilayering of tumour cells. The tumours can also show a sieve-like pattern of back-to-back neoplastic vessels, a solid spindle cell pattern, prominent epithelioid morphology with

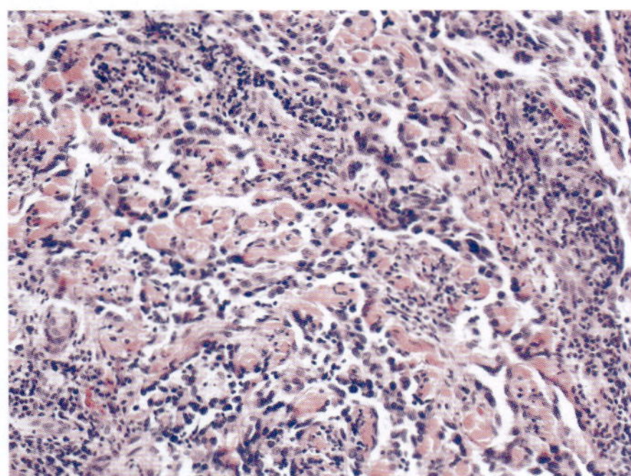

**Fig. 5.93** Angiosarcoma. A medium-power image of neoplastic vessels dissecting dermal collagen.

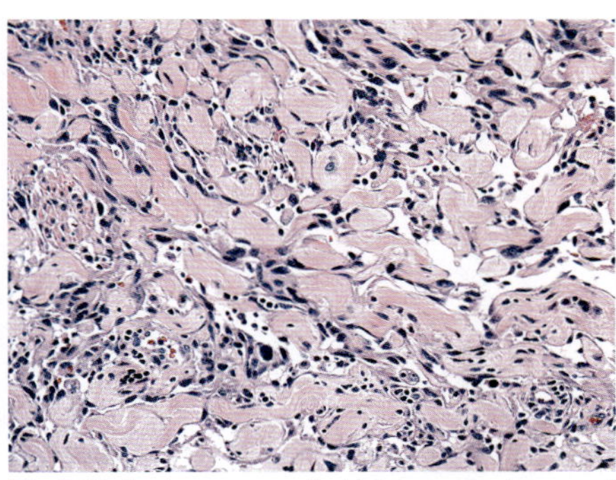

**Fig. 5.94** Angiosarcoma. A higher-power image of neoplastic vessels dissecting dermal collagen bundles.

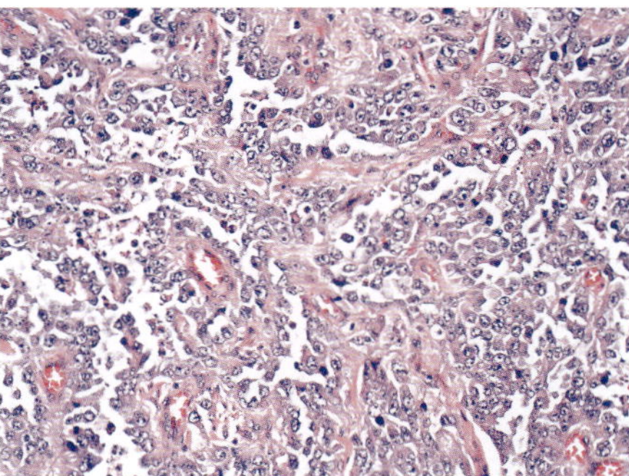

**Fig. 5.95** Epithelioid angiosarcoma. Neoplastic vascular channels lined by epithelioid endothelial cells with abundant eosinophilic cytoplasm.

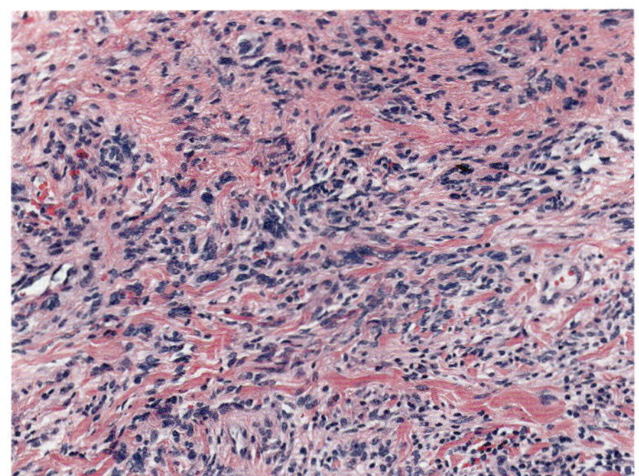

**Fig. 5.96** Angiosarcoma. Occasional cases have a predominantly spindle cell morphology.

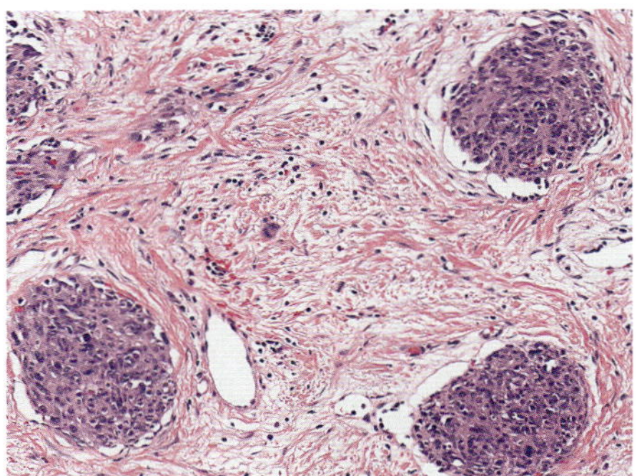

**Fig. 5.97** Radiation-induced angiosarcoma with a characteristic capillary lobule pattern.

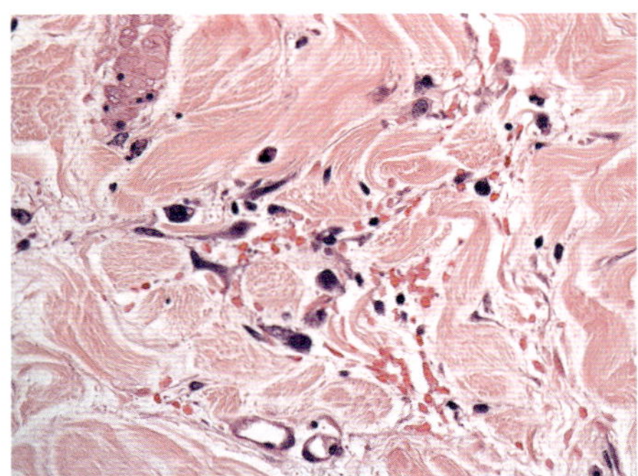

**Fig. 5.98** Radiation-induced angiosarcoma. Rare cases consist of atypical cells forming very subtle vascular channels, which can mimic radiation dermatitis; the presence of haemorrhage is an important clue to the correct diagnosis.

neoplastic vessels lined by epithelioid tumour cells with abundant amphophilic cytoplasm, or solid sheets of epithelioid tumour cells. A given tumour can have a combination of different patterns, ranging from obvious vasoformative areas to more solid areas. In radiation-induced angiosarcoma, a distinctive capillary lobule-like pattern and radiation dermatitis–like pattern have been described {575,622}. Immunohistochemically, the tumours are consistently positive for CD31, CD34, FLI1, and ERG {806,1715}. Epithelioid angiosarcomas may be positive for cytokeratins {788}. Both radiation-induced and lymphoedema-associated angiosarcomas are positive for MYC in nearly 100% of cases, but MYC expression is uncommon in primary cutaneous angiosarcoma {750,1752,2431,2674}.

## Differential diagnosis

Haemangiomas lack atypia and architectural complexity. Epithelioid haemangioendothelioma has a nested to cord-like growth pattern, blander nuclear features, and positivity for CAMTA1 {648}. Angiosarcomas with solid spindled areas can be confused with atypical fibroxanthoma and pleomorphic dermal sarcoma, but these tumours lack expression of CD34 and ERG (although they may express CD31 and FLI1) {2611}. Radiation-induced angiosarcomas must be distinguished from atypical vascular lesions. Atypical vascular lesions lack significant atypia and are negative for MYC expression and *MYC* amplification {750,885,968,1752}. Epithelioid angiosarcoma can be confused with poorly differentiated carcinoma, but poorly differentiated carcinoma is negative for ERG and CD31.

## Genetic profile

No consistent genetic abnormalities have been found in primary cutaneous angiosarcomas, but mutations in *PTPRB* and *PLCG1* have been reported in a subset of cases {192,1144}. *MYC* amplification is seen in > 90% of cases of secondary cutaneous angiosarcoma {750,1144,1752} but is uncommon in primary cutaneous angiosarcoma {2431}. Rare primary cases have rearrangement or mutation of *CIC* {1144}.

## Prognosis and predictive factors

Angiosarcomas are aggressive tumours regardless of grade, with high rates of recurrence and metastasis (most commonly to the lungs but also to lymph nodes). In radiation-induced angiosarcoma, the contralateral breast is a common metastatic site {248}. In one large study, factors associated with an adverse prognosis included patient age > 70 years, necrosis, large tumour size, greater tumour depth, and epithelioid morphology {616}.

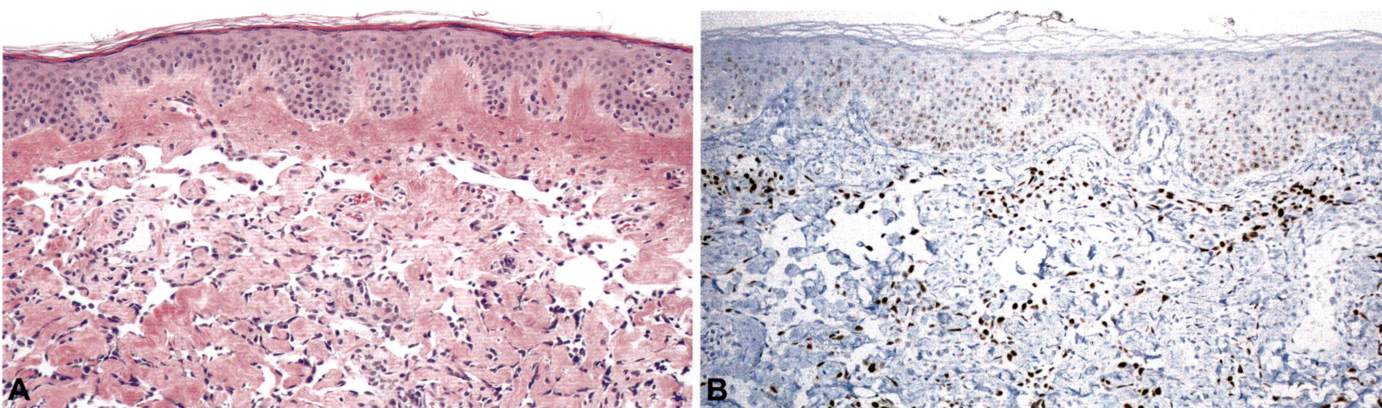



**Fig. 5.99** Radiation-induced angiosarcoma. **A** Within the dermis, there is a proliferation of architecturally complex vessels lined by atypical endothelial cells. **B** Immunostaining for MYC reveals diffuse, strong nuclear positivity.

# Haemangioendotheliomas

Hornick J.L.
Billings S.D.
Requena L.

## Introduction

The term "haemangioendothelioma" encompasses five distinct endothelial neoplasms: four of intermediate biological potential (composite, kaposiform, pseudomyogenic, and retiform haemangioendotheliomas) and one malignant (epithelioid haemangioendothelioma).

## Composite haemangioendothelioma

### Definition

Composite haemangioendothelioma is a locally aggressive, rarely metastasizing endothelial neoplasm composed of an admixture of components, each resembling other vascular lesions.

### ICD-O code 9136/1

### Epidemiology

Composite haemangioendothelioma affects young adults, with a female predominance; infants and children are rarely affected {836,1886,2658}.

### Localization

The distal extremities are affected {1886}.

### Clinical features

The lesions are longstanding reddish-blue nodules or plaques {1886}. Some patients have a history of lymphoedema.

### Histopathology

There is a complex and variable admixture of histological patterns, including retiform, spindle cell, epithelioid, lymphangioma, haemangioma, and well-differentiated angiosarcoma-like components {1886}. Immunohistochemically, the endothelial markers CD31, CD34, FLI1, and ERG are positive.

### Differential diagnosis

The differential diagnosis includes retiform haemangioendothelioma, epithelioid haemangioendothelioma, and angiosarcoma.

### Histogenesis

There is endothelial differentiation.

### Prognosis and predictive factors

Multiple local recurrences over a protracted course are common; lymph node metastasis is rare {836,1886,2159}.

## Kaposiform haemangioendothelioma

### Definition

Kaposiform haemangioendothelioma is a locally aggressive endothelial neoplasm that may mimic Kaposi sarcoma. It is often associated with Kasabach–Merritt syndrome.

### ICD-O code 9130/1

### Epidemiology

There is a marked predilection for infants and young children, with a male predominance {1612,2942}.

### Localization

The kaposiform haemangioendothelioma affects the extremities and may involve the skin and subcutaneous tissue or deep soft tissue {1612}.

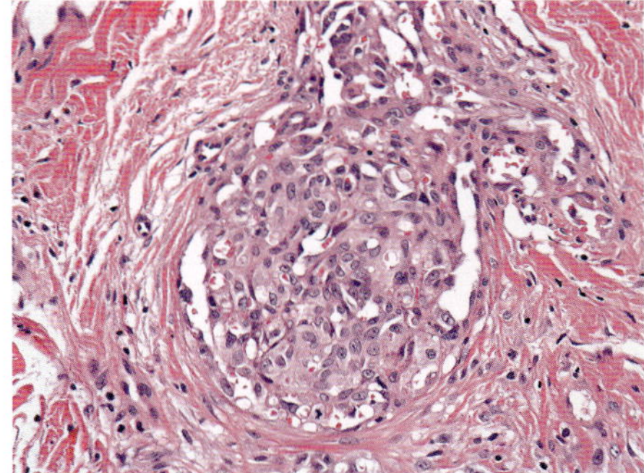

**Fig. 5.101** Kaposiform haemangioendothelioma. Glomeruloid structures are a typical feature.

### Clinical features

The lesion presents as a violaceous mass, sometimes associated with Kasabach–Merritt syndrome (consumptive coagulopathy) {1612}.

### Histopathology

The lesion is a lobular and infiltrative mass composed of capillary haemangioma-like and spindle cell (Kaposi sarcoma-like) areas, including glomeruloid structures {1612}. This tumour type is histologically identical to (and believed to lie on a continuum with) tufted haemangioma {460}. Adjacent lymphangiomatosis is seen in some cases. Immunohistochemically, endothelial markers and lymphatic markers – such as podoplanin (recognized by D2-40) and PROX1 – are positive {1509,1775}. HHV8 and GLUT1 are negative.

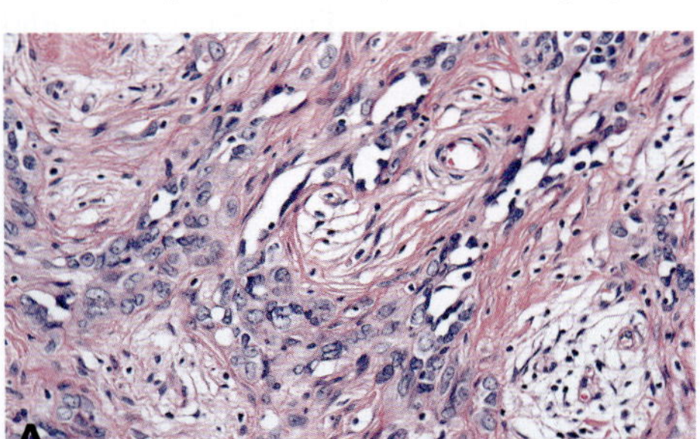


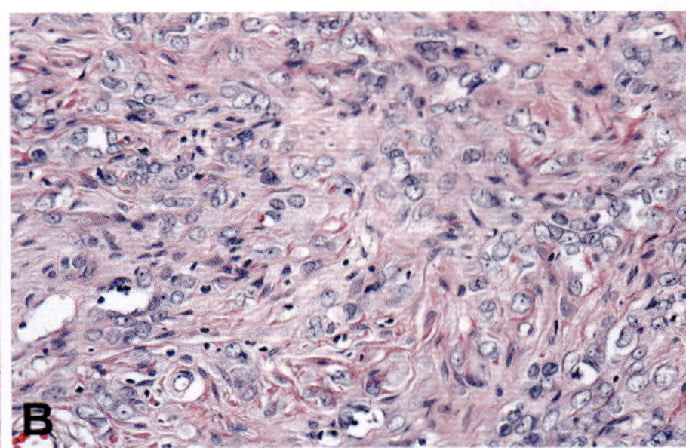


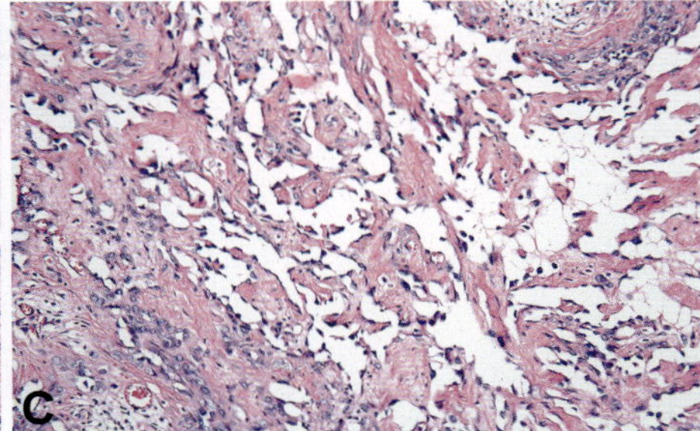


**Fig. 5.100** Composite haemangioendothelioma. This tumour consists of retiform (**A**), epithelioid (**B**), and well-differentiated angiosarcoma-like (**C**) components.

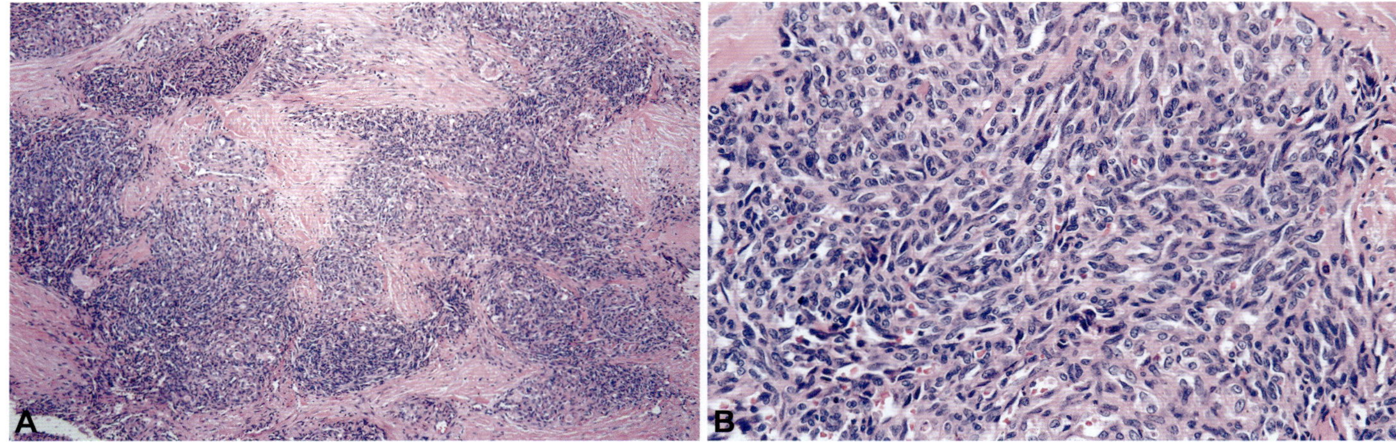


**Fig. 5.102** Kaposiform haemangioendothelioma. The tumour shows a lobular and infiltrative growth pattern (**A**) and consists of bland spindle cells resembling those of Kaposi sarcoma (**B**).

### Differential diagnosis
The differential diagnosis includes Kaposi sarcoma and infantile haemangioma.

### Histogenesis
There is endothelial differentiation.

### Prognosis and predictive factors
The mortality rate is 10–20%, because of complications of Kasabach–Merritt syndrome or extensive local disease {1612,2942}.

## *Pseudomyogenic haemangioendothelioma*

### Definition
Pseudomyogenic haemangioendothelioma is a spindled to epithelioid, rarely metastasizing endothelial neoplasm that often presents as multiple discontiguous nodules in different tissue planes and histologically mimics a myoid tumour or epithelioid sarcoma. *SERPINE1-FOSB* fusion is a consistent feature.

### ICD-O code 9138/1

### Synonym
Epithelioid sarcoma–like haemangioendothelioma

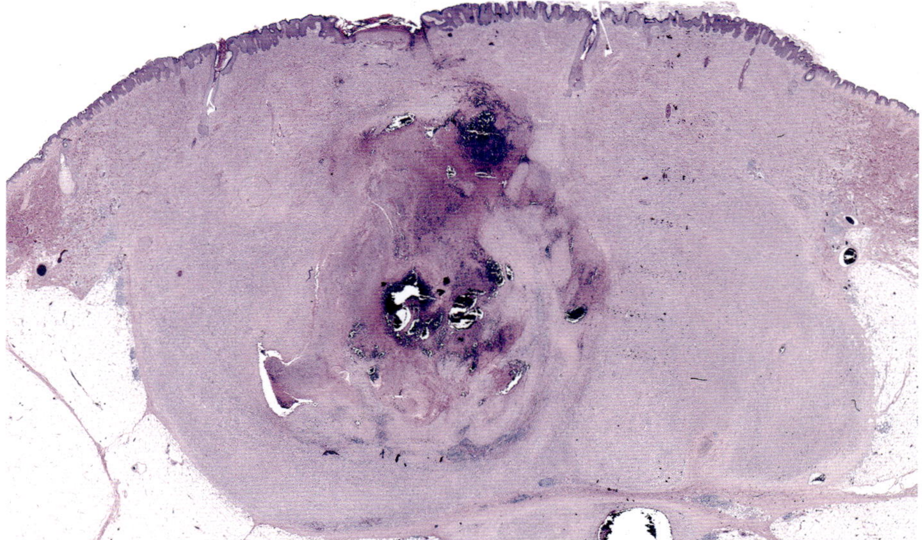

**Fig. 5.103** Pseudomyogenic haemangioendothelioma. This tumour type often involves the dermis and extends into the subcutis; note the overlying epidermal hyperplasia.

### Epidemiology
Pseudomyogenic haemangioendothelioma affects young adults. There is a marked male predominance, with a male-to-female ratio of 5:1 {247,1127}.

### Localization
These lesions affect the lower extremities or (less often) the upper extremities or trunk {1127}.

### Clinical features
Pseudomyogenic haemangioendotheliomas are painless or painful nodules. They are multifocal in two thirds of cases, often involving multiple tissue planes (e.g. skin and subcutis, skeletal muscle, and bone) {247,1127}.

### Histopathology
The lesion is composed of loose fascicles of mildly atypical, plump spindled to epithelioid cells with brightly eosinophilic cytoplasm, a subset of which resemble rhabdomyoblasts; prominent stromal neutrophils are seen in 50% of cases {247,1127}. Immunohistochemically, pseudomyogenic haemangioendothelioma is positive for ERG, FLI1, and cytokeratin AE1/AE3, but negative for cytokeratin MNF116 and CD34; 50% of cases are positive for CD31 {247,1127}. FOSB is consistently positive {1153,2529}.

### Differential diagnosis
The differential diagnosis includes cellular fibrous histiocytoma, spindle cell squamous cell carcinoma, and epithelioid sarcoma.

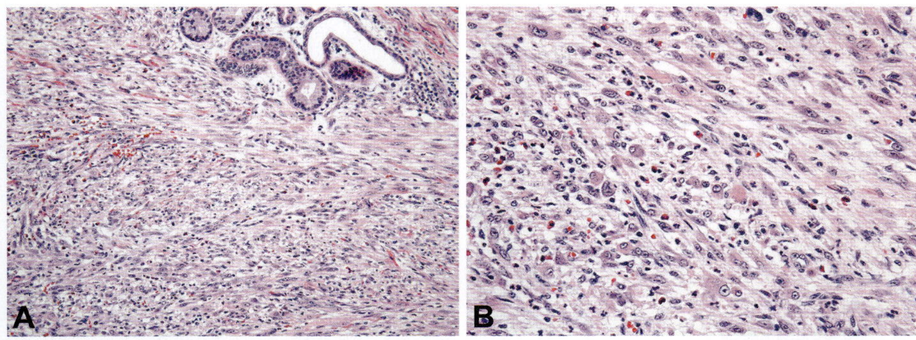

**Fig. 5.104** Pseudomyogenic haemangioendothelioma. **A** The tumour is composed of fascicles of plump spindle cells. **B** Note the occasional cells with brightly eosinophilic cytoplasm (mimicking rhabdomyoblasts) and the scattered neutrophils.

### Histogenesis
There is endothelial differentiation.

### Genetic profile
The lesions show t(7;19) with *SERPINE1-FOSB* {2651,2770}.

### Prognosis and predictive factors
Patients often develop additional lesions in the same anatomical region. Lymph node and distant metastases are uncommon and typically follow a protracted course {1127}.

## Retiform haemangioendothelioma

### Definition
Retiform haemangioendothelioma is a locally aggressive endothelial neoplasm composed of distinctive arborizing blood vessels lined by endothelial cells with hobnail features.

### ICD-O code
9136/1

### Synonym
Hobnail haemangioendothelioma

### Epidemiology
Retiform haemangioendothelioma occurs in children and young adults {355}.

### Localization
The distal extremities are affected, in particular the lower limbs {355}.

### Clinical features
The lesions are reddish-blue nodules or plaques {355}.

### Histopathology
Retiform haemangioendothelioma is composed of hyperchromatic endothelial cells with protuberant (hobnail) nuclei lining narrow, arborizing vascular channels, resembling rete testis, often with focally sheet-like growth. A prominent lymphocytic infiltrate is seen in 50% of cases {355}. Immunohistochemically, CD31, CD34, FLI1, and ERG are positive; expression of lymphatic markers, such as podoplanin (recognized by D2-40) and PROX1, is variable {1775}.

### Differential diagnosis
The differential diagnosis includes papillary intralymphatic angioendothelioma, angiosarcoma, and hobnail haemangioma.

### Histogenesis
There is endothelial differentiation.

### Prognosis and predictive factors
Multiple local recurrences occurring over a protracted course of disease are common; lymph node metastasis is rare {355}.

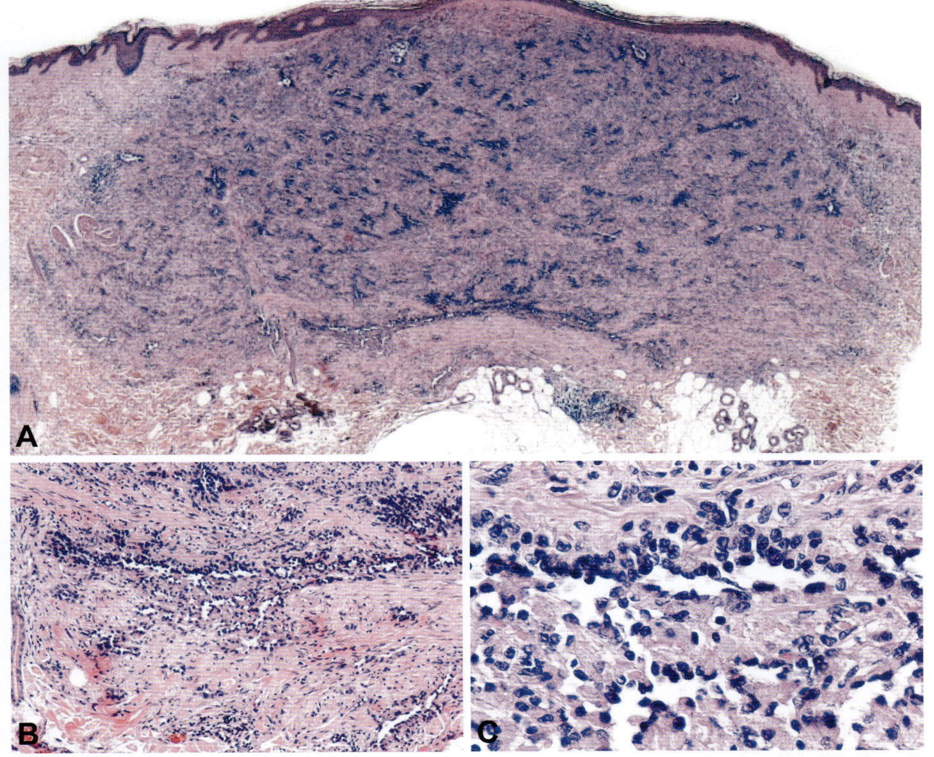

**Fig. 5.105** Retiform haemangioendothelioma. This tumour type often involves the dermis with relatively well-circumscribed margins (**A**) and consists of arborizing, slit-like vascular channels (**B**) lined by endothelial cells with protuberant (hobnail) nuclei and minimal cytoplasm (**C**).

## Epithelioid haemangioendothelioma

### Definition
Epithelioid haemangioendothelioma is a malignant endothelial neoplasm composed of cords of epithelioid cells in a myxohyaline stroma. *WWTR1-CAMTA1* is a consistent gene fusion in this tumour.

### ICD-O code
9133/3

### Epidemiology
This entity most often presents in middle-

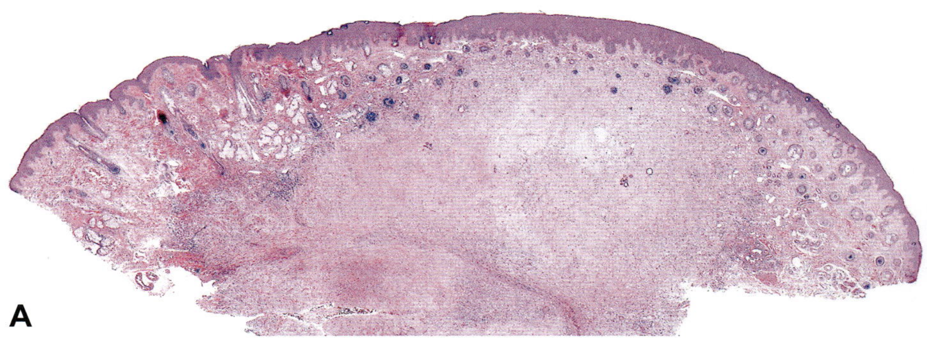


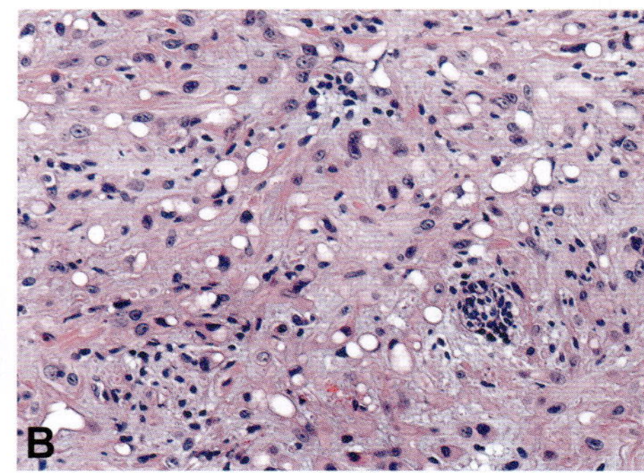


**Fig. 5.106** Epithelioid haemangioendothelioma. **A** Overview showing a well-demarcated neoplasm. **B** The tumour is composed of cords of epithelioid cells with glassy eosinophilic cytoplasm and occasional intracytoplasmic vacuoles in a myxohyaline stroma.

aged adults, with a slight female predominance {387,1741,2113,2270}.

## Localization

The lesion has no site predilection, but only rarely arises in the skin {2113}.

## Clinical features

Most cutaneous examples are nondescript nodules, sometimes with a thickened epidermis {387,2113,2270} and rarely with ulceration {1995}.

## Histopathology

Epithelioid haemangioendothelioma is composed of relatively bland epithelioid cells, often with intracytoplasmic vacuoles, arranged in cords and nests embedded in a variably myxohyaline stroma {2802}. Immunohistochemically, epithelioid haemangioendothelioma is positive for the typical endothelial markers CD31, CD34, FLI1, and ERG, as well as CAMTA1. Keratins are expressed in 20–30% of cases {648,797}.

## Differential diagnosis

The differential diagnosis includes epithelioid haemangioma, cutaneous epithelioid angiomatous nodule, pseudomyogenic haemangioendothelioma, epithelioid angiosarcoma, and carcinomas.

## Histogenesis

There is endothelial differentiation.

## Genetic profile

More than 90% of epithelioid haemangioendotheliomas have t(1;3) with *WWTR1-CAMTA1* fusion {703,2571}; a small subset have *YAP1-TFE3* fusions {79}.

## Prognosis and predictive factors

Metastasis develops in 20–30% of cases. Prognosis has not been specifically studied in cutaneous examples, but in one large series, a higher mitotic rate and size >3 cm were found to be adverse prognostic factors {617}.

# Kaposi sarcoma

Grayson W.
Landman G.

## Definition

Kaposi sarcoma is an HHV8-associated vascular proliferation. Whether it qualifies as a true sarcoma is still a matter of debate {658}. In immunocompromised individuals, HHV8 infection induces vascular proliferation characterized by disorganized endothelial cell growth, resulting in the formation of erythrocyte-containing clefts, organized neovascularization, and an associated inflammatory infiltrate {436}.

## ICD-O code 9140/3

## Synonyms

HHV8-associated vascular proliferation; Kaposi tumour

## Epidemiology

Kaposi sarcoma can affect individuals of any age or sex, but it occurs most commonly in adults and shows a general predilection for men. However, a high proportion of children and women are affected by AIDS-associated Kaposi sarcoma in Africa {1976}. The estimated worldwide crude and age-standardized incidence rates of Kaposi sarcoma are both 0.6 cases per 100 000 person-years, with a male-to-female ratio of 1.9:1. However, there are striking geographical differences, with the highest crude and age-standardized incidence rates (of 8.8 and 11.2 cases per 100 000 person-years, respectively) seen in eastern Africa. The estimated worldwide crude and age-standardized mortality rates are both 0.4 deaths per 100 000 person-years, with the highest crude and age-standardized mortality rates recorded in eastern Africa (6.9 and 9.9 deaths per 100 000 person-years, respectively). The global incidence of Kaposi sarcoma is highest among men who have sex with men, at 5.7 cases per 100 person-years {110}.

## Etiology

The causative agent is HHV8, also known as Kaposi sarcoma–associated herpesvirus. It is a member of

**Table 5.01** Conventional histopathological subtypes and differential diagnoses of cutaneous Kaposi sarcoma (KS)

| Histopathological subtype | Differential diagnoses |
|---|---|
| Patch-stage KS | Early microvenular haemangioma<br>Interstitial (so-called incomplete) granuloma annulare<br>Mild inflammatory dermatosis |
| Plaque-stage KS | Microvenular haemangioma<br>Tufted haemangioma<br>Hobnail haemangioma (targetoid haemosiderotic haemangioma)<br>Acroangiodermatitis (so-called pseudo-KS) |
| Well-developed (nodular) KS | Vascular tumours composed of spindled cells (e.g. spindle cell haemangioma, kaposiform haemangioendothelioma, angiosarcoma)<br>Dermatofibroma variants (e.g. cellular, aneurysmal, haemosiderotic, atypical)<br>Angiomatoid fibrous histiocytoma<br>Spindle cell sarcoma (e.g. dermatofibrosarcoma protuberans, leiomyosarcoma)<br>Spindle cell amelanotic melanoma<br>Dermal fasciitis<br>Bacillary angiomatosis |

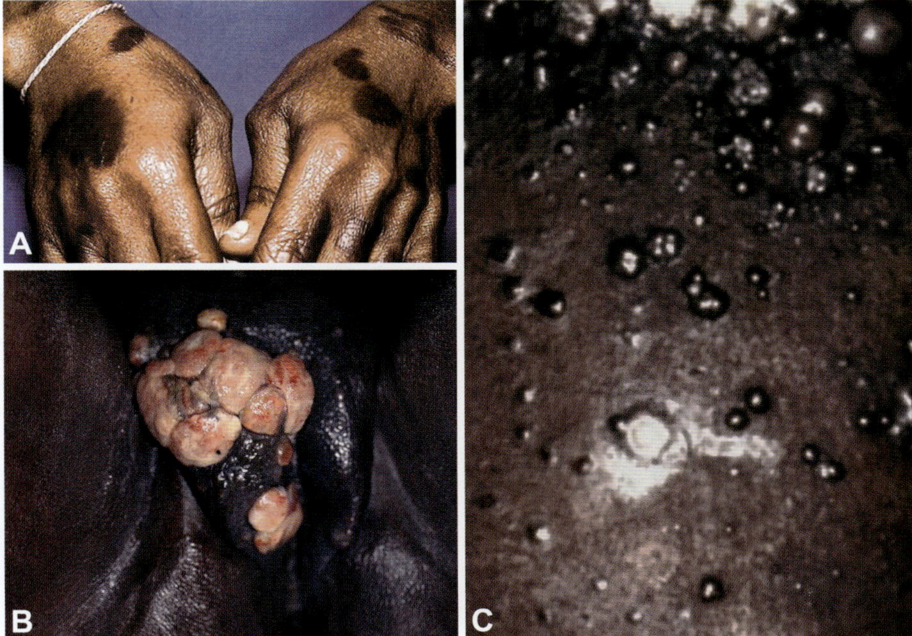


**Fig. 5.107** Kaposi sarcoma. **A** Plaque-stage Kaposi sarcoma; hyperpigmented plaques are present on the hands. **B** Nodular Kaposi sarcoma; a large vulval tumour with ulceration. **C** Verrucous Kaposi sarcoma; numerous hyperkeratotic lesions are present on the lower leg.

the *Gammaherpesvirinae* subfamily of viruses {436}.

## Localization

The skin is the principal site of involvement. Lesions occur most commonly on the lower limbs, followed by the face and genitalia. Mucosal involvement (in particular in the oral cavity) is also common. Classic Kaposi sarcoma tends to affect the lower extremities of elderly non–HIV-infected men. Visceral Kaposi sarcoma in the absence of cutaneous lesions is encountered most frequently in the setting of AIDS {1976}.

## Clinical features

Four clinicopathological subtypes are recognized: iatrogenic (transplant-related), AIDS-associated (epidemic), African (endemic), and classic Kaposi sarcoma. The spectrum of conventional cutaneous lesions encompasses patches, plaques, and nodules. Lower limb involvement may be accompanied by painful lymphoedema. Rarely, verrucous or bullous lesions occur. There is currently no universal staging system applicable to all four clinicopathological subtypes of Kaposi sarcoma. The AIDS Clinical Trial Group (ACTG) staging system was shown to have good correlation with survival in the pre-antiretroviral therapy era, but a more recently proposed prognostic scoring system may have greater relevance today {1976,2504}.

## Histopathology

All four clinicopathological subtypes have a similar histomorphological spectrum. Patch-stage lesions are characterized by abnormal vessels or subtle endothelial cell proliferation with dermal collagen dissection, in particular around the skin adnexa; the promontory sign may also be seen {16}. Plaque-stage Kaposi sarcoma is characterized by abnormal vessels, greater cellularity, and a spindle cell proliferation. Additional features include slit-like spaces containing erythrocytes, surrounding spindled cells, siderophages, and occasional hyaline globules that give a positive periodic acid–Schiff (PAS) reaction; subcutaneous extension can occur. Well-developed (nodular) Kaposi sarcoma lesions show greater cellularity and resultant tumour formation, with haphazardly intersecting fascicles of spindled cells, often accompanied by a plasma cell–predominant inflammatory

**Table 5.02** Less common histopathological variants and differential diagnoses of cutaneous Kaposi sarcoma (KS)

| Histopathological variant | Differential diagnoses |
|---|---|
| Anaplastic (pleomorphic) KS | Spindle cell sarcoma (e.g. leiomyosarcoma, malignant peripheral nerve sheath tumour, spindle cell rhabdomyosarcoma, fibrosarcoma, fibrosarcomatous dermatofibrosarcoma protuberans)<br>Amelanotic spindle cell melanoma<br>Spindle cell carcinoma |
| Lymphangioma-like (lymphangiomatous) KS | Lymphangioma (e.g. acquired progressive lymphangioma, lymphangioma circumscriptum)<br>Postradiation atypical vascular proliferation<br>Angiosarcoma |
| Lymphangiectatic KS[a,b] | Lymphangioma |
| Telangiectatic KS[c] | Intratumoural congestion and ectasia of native (i.e. non-neoplastic) blood vessels<br>Sinusoidal haemangioma |
| Bullous KS[b] | Re-epithelializing subepidermal bulla unrelated to KS |
| Cavernous haemangioma–like KS[c] | Cavernous haemangioma |
| Hyperkeratotic (verrucous) KS[b] | Verruciform epidermal hyperplasia and hyperkeratosis unrelated to underlying KS |
| Keloidal KS | True keloid scar (e.g. arising at a previous punch biopsy site for confirmation of KS) |
| Micronodular KS | Early intradermal spindle cell sarcoma<br>Early cellular dermatofibroma |
| Pyogenic granuloma–like KS | Lobular capillary haemangioma (pyogenic granuloma)<br>Bacillary angiomatosis |
| Ecchymotic KS | Intradermal haemorrhage/ecchymosis due to another cause (e.g. biopsy-related trauma) |
| Intravascular KS | Intravenous pyogenic granuloma<br>Intravascular papillary endothelial hyperplasia<br>Intravascular fasciitis<br>Papillary intralymphatic angioendothelioma<br>Intravascular myopericytoma |
| Glomeruloid KS | Glomeruloid haemangioma<br>Tufted haemangioma |
| KS with myoid nodules[c] | Dermatofibrosarcoma protuberans with myoid nodules |
| Pigmented KS | Intralesional haemosiderin pigment deposition in a neoplasm other than KS<br>Melanocytic proliferation (e.g. spindle cell melanoma, cellular blue naevus)<br>Pigmented dermatofibrosarcoma protuberans (Bednar tumour) |
| Regressing/regressed KS | Inflammatory dermatosis<br>Dermal neovascularization |

[a] Lymphangiectatic KS may be associated with bullous lesions clinically, hence forming part of the clinical spectrum of bullous KS.
[b] Lymphangiectatic, bullous, and hyperkeratotic (verrucous) KSs may be associated with chronic lymphoedema, hence forming part of the clinical spectrum of lymphoedematous KS.
[c] Telangiectatic KS, cavernous haemangioma–like KS, and KS with myoid nodules are usually associated with background features of classic nodular KS.

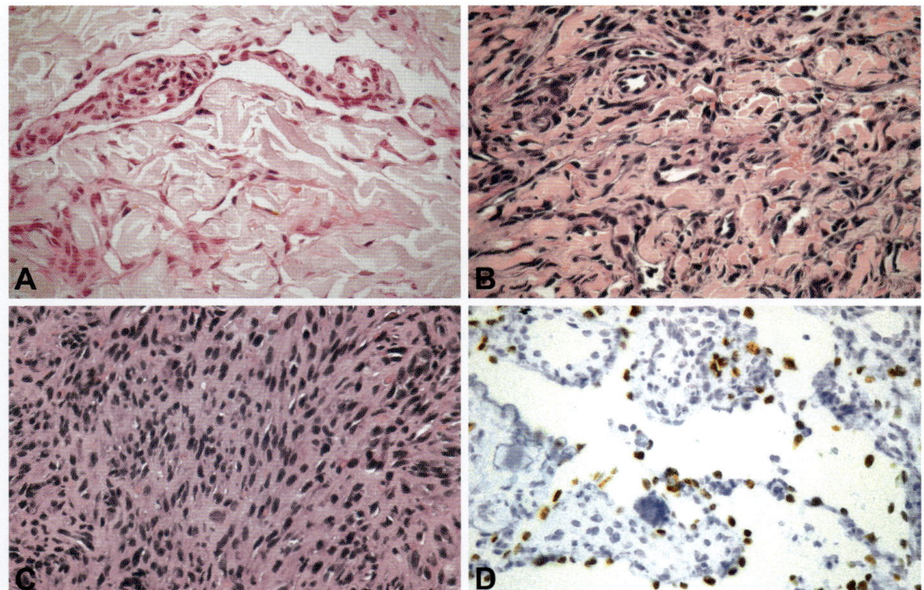

**Fig. 5.108** Kaposi sarcoma. **A** Patch-stage Kaposi sarcoma; there is dissection of dermal collagen by a subtle vasoformative cellular proliferation, and the promontory sign is evident. **B** Plaque-stage Kaposi sarcoma; a more cellular proliferation, erythrocytic extravasation, and a subtle plasma cell infiltrate are seen. **C** Nodular Kaposi sarcoma; there are cellular spindle cell fascicles lining compressed, slit-like spaces containing red blood cells. **D** Lymphangioma-like Kaposi sarcoma; HHV8 immunostaining of the lesional endothelial nuclei.

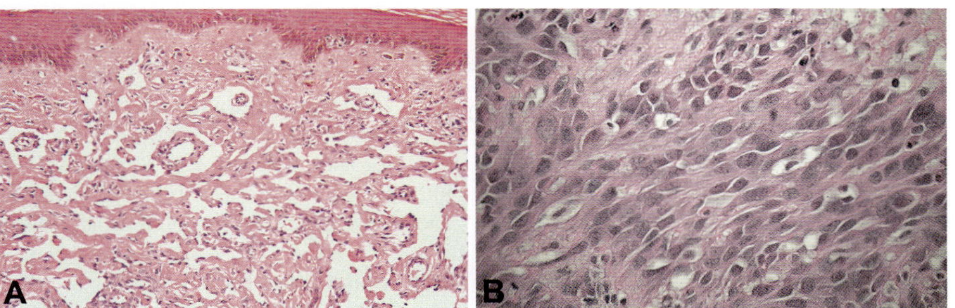

**Fig. 5.109** Kaposi sarcoma. **A** Lymphangioma-like Kaposi sarcoma; the dermis is expanded by interanastomosing and ectatic, lymphangiomatous-looking channels. **B** Anaplastic (pleomorphic) Kaposi sarcoma; there is cellular atypia, mitotic activity, focal necrosis, and an absence of obvious vasoformative features.

infiltrate. Mitoses and mild atypia can be seen.

The lesional cells show immunoreactivity for the HHV8-associated protein LANA-1, as well as CD34, CD31, and podoplanin (recognized by D2-40). Lesions that have regressed following chemotherapy or antiretroviral therapy show increased microvascular density around native dermal vessels {930}. Numerous less common histopathological variants have been described (see Table 5.02), including lymphangioma-like Kaposi sarcoma and anaplastic Kaposi sarcoma {930,931,1930}. Rare AIDS-associated cases can harbour an opportunistic pathogen {929}.

## Differential diagnosis

The differential diagnoses of the more conventional histopathological subtypes of Kaposi sarcoma and the less common histopathological variants are listed in Table 5.01 and Table 5.02, respectively.

## Histogenesis

HHV8 infection alone is insufficient for the development of Kaposi sarcoma; host immune dysfunction, genetic factors, and environmental factors also play a role. Initially, there is infection by HHV8 of resident and circulating endothelial cells and mononuclear inflammatory cells. LANA-1 upregulates viral homologues of FLICE inhibitory protein (vFLIP) and cyclin D (viral cyclin). Viral oncoproteins (e.g. vIL-6) and antiapoptotic proteins (e.g. LANA-1, vIAP, and vBCL2) potentiate the proliferation of infected endothelial cells and immune evasion, while expression of matrix metalloproteinases and proangiogenic molecules leads to migration of infected endothelial cells. An inflammatory phase follows, with secretion of proinflammatory cytokines and chemotaxis of T helper 2 (Th2) inflammatory cells. Subsequent tumorigenesis involves activation of autocrine and paracrine pathways, secretion of stimulatory molecules by inflammatory cells, induction of angiogenesis (e.g. via vGPCR-induced upregulation of VEGF), and spindle cell proliferation. There is reprogramming of blood vessel endothelial cells and a resultant expression profile more akin to that of lymphatic endothelium {1976}. Kaposi sarcoma is a predominantly multifocal disease, with oligoclonality evident in the vast majority of cases and not all lesions arising from a single clone {658,881}.

## Genetic profile

There are seven major HHV8 genotypes, and their relative frequency varies according to geographical region and race {2132,2638}. Genetic variants of HHV8 may be associated with greater susceptibility to the development of classic Kaposi sarcoma {529}.

## Genetic susceptibility

*HLA-DMB* has been identified as a candidate susceptibility gene for AIDS-associated Kaposi sarcoma, and *STAT4* for classic Kaposi sarcoma {2,35}. Familial clustering has been documented {1254}.

## Prognosis and predictive factors

Although advanced cutaneous Kaposi sarcoma often results in substantial morbidity (in particular when associated with lymphoedema), visceral disease may be more invasive, leading to potentially catastrophic organ dysfunction, haemorrhage, and death {881}. Anaplastic Kaposi sarcoma tends towards local aggressiveness and deeper invasion {2634}. The scoring system proposed by Stebbing et al. {2504} may have prognostic and therapeutic relevance in AIDS-associated Kaposi sarcoma.

# Atypical vascular lesion

Requena L.
Calonje E.
Fisher C.
Wick M.R.

### Definition

Atypical vascular lesion is a benign vascular proliferation with histopathological features mimicking those of angiosarcoma, arising in irradiated skin.

### ICD-O code 9126/0

### Synonyms

Post-radiation therapy lymphangiectasia {67}; benign lymphangiomatous papule {121}; post-radiation therapy lymphangioma {1547}; benign vascular lesion in previously irradiated skin {920}

### Epidemiology

Presentation is in adults, predominantly in elderly women following radiotherapy for breast cancer. The latency period varies, but the lesions typically appear 2–3 years after radiotherapy {306}.

### Etiology

These lesions are induced by radiotherapy. Total radiation doses range from 37.5 Gy to 60 Gy (mean total radiation dose: 50 Gy) {306}.

### Localization

Most patients are women with breast cancer who develop lesions on irradiated skin of the anterior chest, but identical lesions can also occur in other areas after irradiation for cervical cancer, endometrial cancer, ovarian cancer, Hodgkin lymphoma, myeloma, melanoma, or vascular malformations {306}.

### Clinical features

The lesions are papules, small vesicles, or erythematous ecchymotic plaques with prominent telangiectases.

### Histopathology

Atypical vascular proliferations usually involve the upper and mid-dermis (sparing the epidermis). They sometimes extend to the deep reticular dermis but (unlike radiation-induced angiosarcoma) not into the subcutis. At scanning magnification, the lesions show V-shaped architecture, with broader extension and larger lumina in superficial than in deeper areas. The lesion is composed of irregular, branched, anastomosing, thin-walled vascular channels lined by a single discontinuous layer of flattened endothelial cells and an empty lumen, resembling lymphatics. In places, the vascular channels are back-to-back, with the lumina separated by a thin layer of endothelial cells. Small intravascular papillations are frequently seen.

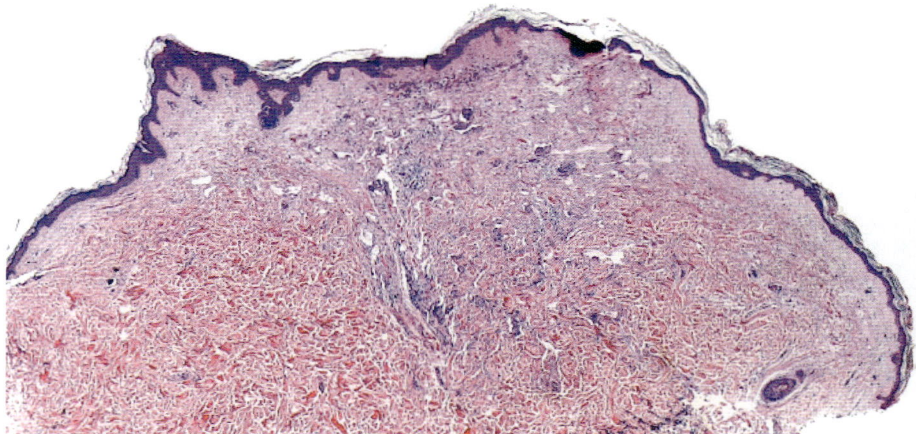

**Fig. 5.110** Atypical vascular lesion. Histopathological features in irradiated skin. Scanning view showing wedge-shaped involvement of the superficial dermis and mid-dermis.

Two histopathological variants of atypical vascular lesions in irradiated skin have been described: the lymphatic type (described above) and the vascular type {2010}. The vascular type resembles hobnail or microvenular haemangioma, with proliferation of small capillary vessels that do not form lobules. Very rare cases of atypical vascular lesion progressing to angiosarcoma have been reported {2010}.

As demonstrated immunohistochemically, the endothelial lining cells express CD31, podoplanin (recognized by D2-40), PROX1, and LYVE1, evidencing a lymphatic endothelial nature. The Ki-67 proliferation index is low {2158}. In lesions of vascular type, the endothelial cells express CD31 and CD34, but not podoplanin. HHV8 is always negative.

Atypical vascular lesions can coexist with radiation-induced angiosarcoma, and superficially sampled radiation-induced angiosarcomas can be indistinguishable from atypical vascular lesions {306,307,2010,2380}. Early-stage radiation-induced angiosarcoma shows endothelial MYC expression and a high Ki-67 proliferation index (> 10%), whereas atypical vascular lesions are MYC-negative and show no substantial proliferation.

### Differential diagnosis

The histopathological differential diagnosis of atypical vascular lesions in irradiated skin includes radiation-induced angiosarcoma. Clinicopathological correlation with immunohistochemical studies and investigation of MYC expression by immunohistochemistry or of *MYC* amplification by FISH is usually sufficient for a confident diagnosis {750,968,1657,1752}. Other differential diagnoses include lymphatic malformations, benign lymphangioendothelioma, and Kaposi sarcoma.

### Histogenesis

Radiation-induced endothelial cell proliferation is considered the main histogenetic factor.

### Prognosis and predictive factors

Atypical vascular lesions are benign, but they can coexist with (and in rare cases progress to) angiosarcoma {306,307,2010,2380}.

# Cutaneous epithelioid angiomatous nodule

Brenn T.
Kutzner H.
Sangüeza O.P.

## Definition

Cutaneous epithelioid angiomatous nodule is a distinctive benign cutaneous vascular proliferation with prominent epithelioid cell morphology.

## ICD-O code 9125/0

## Epidemiology

The age of presentation has a wide range, with peak incidence in young to middle-aged adults (median age: 37 years) {305,2308}. There is no strong sex predilection.

## Etiology

These lesions appear to be reactive.

## Localization

Cutaneous epithelioid angiomatous nodule affects a wide range of anatomical sites, with a predilection for the trunk and extremities. Mucosal surfaces may also be involved {305,2308,2853}.

## Clinical features

The lesions present as solitary papules and nodules with erythematous to bluish discolouration, measuring < 1.5 cm (median: 0.5 cm). Rarely, the tumours are multiple. An eruptive presentation has also been reported {305,2015,2308}.

## Histopathology

The tumours occur as well-circumscribed nodules in the superficial to mid-dermis. They are composed of solid sheets of large polygonal epithelioid cells with abundant cytoplasm containing vesicular nuclei with small eosinophilic nucleoli. Intracytoplasmic vacuoles are frequently observed. Mitotic figures are seen, but atypical mitoses and nuclear pleomorphism are absent. Intralesional vascular channels are a focal feature. The tumours show haemosiderin deposition; an inflammatory cell infiltrate composed of lymphocytes, plasma cells, and eosinophils; and variable perilesional fibrosis. The overlying epidermis may be acanthotic with collarette formation. Rarely, there is involvement of deep dermis and superficial subcutis. Immunohistochemically, the tumour cells express endothelial cell markers (CD31, CD34, and factor VIII), and intralesional SMA-positive pericytes are present.

## Differential diagnosis

Differentiation from epithelioid angiosarcoma is particularly important because of its aggressive behaviour, and both tumours can occur in a similar clinical context. Epithelioid angiosarcoma is larger and involves deeper structures, with infiltrative margins; it is characterized by nuclear pleomorphism with numerous and atypical mitotic figures. Tumour necrosis may also be present. Epithelioid haemangioendothelioma is characterized by epithelioid endothelial cells arranged in cords and strands in a chondromyxoid stroma rather than the solid sheet-like growth seen in epithelioid angiomatous nodule. Epithelioid haemangioma is multinodular and shows more vasoformative elements lined by epithelioid endothelial cells in a fibrous stroma; there is also a variably prominent inflammatory cell infiltrate with eosinophils and lymphoid follicles.

## Histogenesis

The tumours are endothelial cell neoplasms.

## Prognosis and predictive factors

Cutaneous epithelioid angiomatous nodule is entirely benign, and no adverse outcome has been documented in the literature {305,2308}.

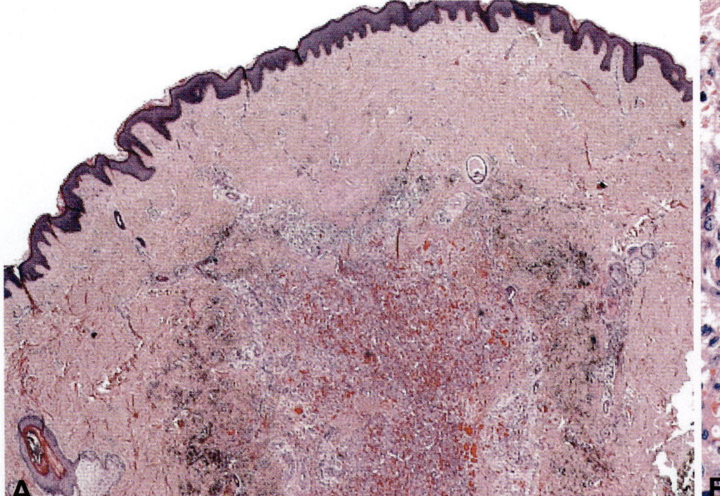


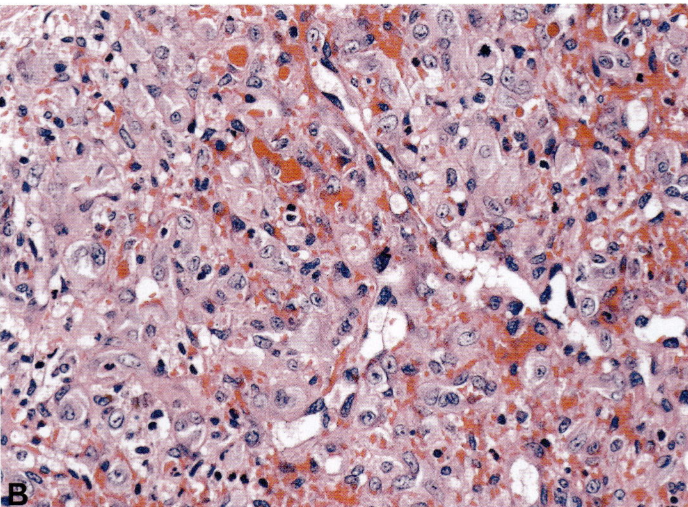


**Fig. 5.111** Cutaneous epithelioid angiomatous nodule. **A** The tumour is nodular and well circumscribed; it is based within the dermis, with surrounding haemosiderin deposition. **B** Epithelioid endothelial cells are arranged in sheets. They have abundant eosinophilic cytoplasm and contain vesicular nuclei with small eosinophilic nucleoli; intracytoplasmic lumina are focally present. A mitotic figure is visible in the upper-right corner; also note the presence of well-formed intralesional vascular channels.

# Haemangiomas

Calonje E.
Glusac E.J.
Mihm M.C. Jr
North P.E.
Piris A.
Requena L.
Sangüeza O.P.
Wick M.R.

## *Cherry haemangioma*

### Definition
Cherry haemangioma, a variant of capillary haemangioma, is a benign superficial dermal capillary proliferation with a lobular architecture.

### ICD-O code 9120/0

### Synonyms
Cherry angioma; senile angioma; Campbell de Morgan spot

### Epidemiology
This haemangioma affects middle-aged to elderly adults, with no sex predilection.

### Localization
The most common location is the trunk, followed by the upper limbs and (less commonly) the lower limbs.

### Clinical features
The lesions are multiple, tiny, bright-red, asymptomatic papules that increase in number with age.

### Histopathology
The papillary dermis is expanded by a slightly polypoid lobular proliferation of small congested and dilated capillaries with surrounding loose stroma, often with an epithelial collarette.

### Genetic profile
*HRAS* and *KRAS* mutations are found in a small proportion of cases {942}.

### Prognosis and predictive factors
Cherry haemangioma is benign.

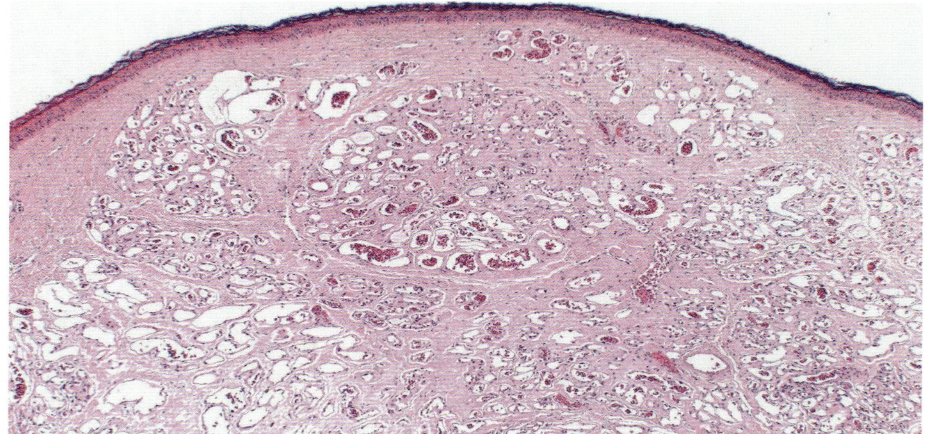

**Fig. 5.112** Cherry haemangioma. Lobules of thin-walled, variably dilated capillaries surrounded by hyalinized stroma.

## *Sinusoidal haemangioma*

### Definition
Sinusoidal haemangioma is a histologically distinctive benign vascular lesion, with features resembling those of anastomosing haemangioma (a lesion seen mainly in the kidney) {354,1235,1818}.

### ICD-O code 9120/0

### Epidemiology
These rare haemangiomas occur mainly in middle-aged adults, with a predilection for women. In men, they frequently develop in the setting of gynaecomastia.

### Etiology
The etiology is unknown, but many consider this lesion to be a histologically distinct form of venous malformation.

### Localization
The most common location is the trunk. Subcutaneous tissue of the breast and extremities can be affected.

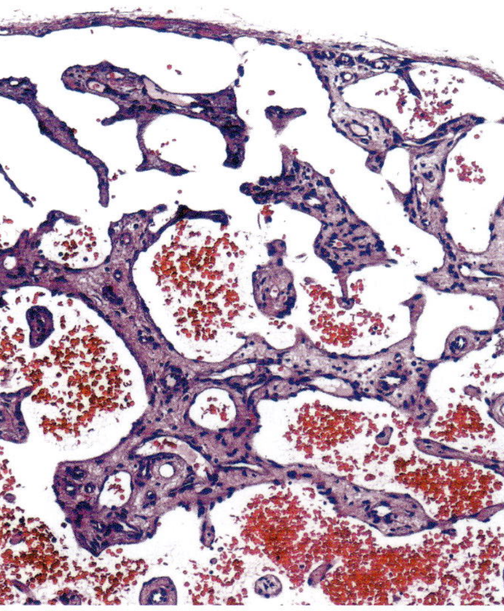

**Fig. 5.113** Sinusoidal haemangioma. Note the distinctive sinusoidal appearance of the vascular channels.

### Clinical features
The lesion is a small, asymptomatic, bluish, dermal or subcutaneous nodule.

### Histopathology
The lesions are lobular and relatively well circumscribed, composed of irregular, dilated, congested, thin-walled vascular channels with scant smooth muscle in a sinusoidal or sieve-like pattern with little intervening stroma. The endothelial cells are uniform. Mitotic activity is absent. Thrombosis and dystrophic calcification are often present. A similar vascular pattern is commonly seen focally in venous malformations.

### Differential diagnosis
In the breast, the differential diagnosis includes well-differentiated angiosarcoma. However, angiosarcoma shows multilayering of endothelial cells, cytological atypia, and mitotic activity.

### Prognosis and predictive factors
Sinusoidal haemangioma is benign.

## Microvenular haemangioma

### Definition

Microvenular haemangioma is a mitotically quiescent vascular lesion – likely a variant of venous malformation {1157,1873}.

### ICD-O code 9120/0

### Epidemiology

This rare haemangioma presents mainly in young adults, with no sex predilection.

### Localization

This lesion affects the extremities and rarely the trunk.

### Clinical features

The lesion is a single small (or occasionally larger), red, asymptomatic, papule or plaque. Exceptional eruptive or multiple lesions have been reported {1569,1873,2870}.

### Histopathology

The lesions are poorly defined, usually involve superficial and deep reticular dermis, and consist of elongated (often irregular) small vascular channels resembling venules. The vessels dissect somewhat hyalinized-looking collagen bundles. Extension of channels into arrector pili muscles is common. A single layer of pericytes, which can be highlighted by SMA staining, is consistently present. The endothelial cells are bland and lack mitotic activity; they are positive for ERG, CD31, and CD34 but negative for podoplanin (recognized by D2-40) {2647}.

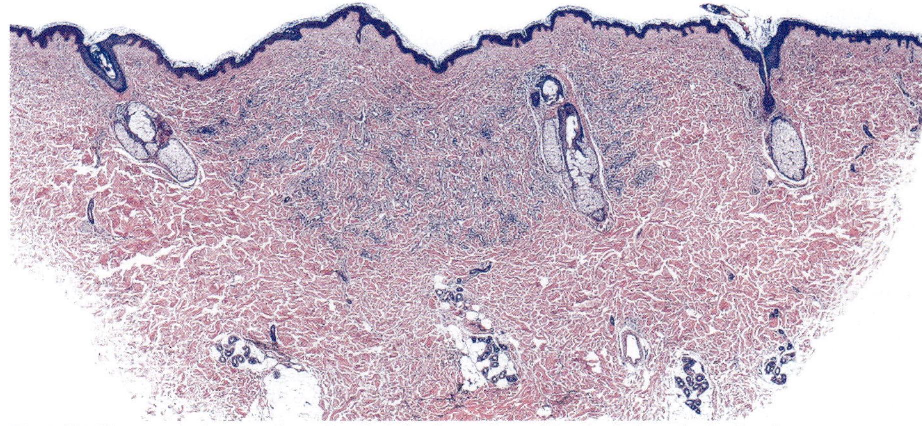

**Fig. 5.115** Microvenular haemangioma. Poorly defined vascular proliferation in the reticular dermis.

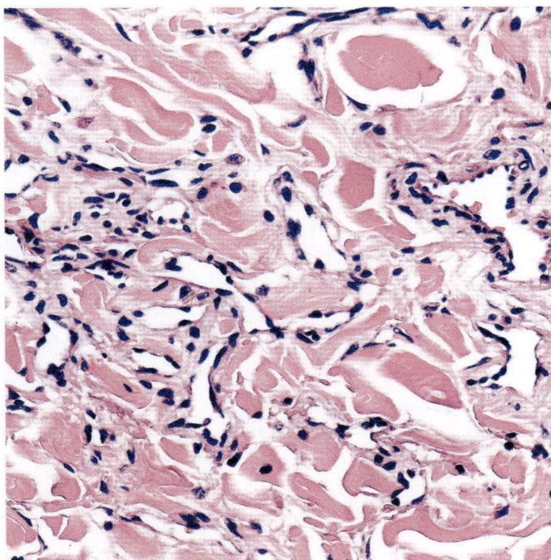

**Fig. 5.114** Microvenular haemangioma. Angulated venule-like channels lined by a single layer of bland endothelial cells.

### Differential diagnosis

The dissection of collagen may prompt consideration of angiosarcoma or Kaposi sarcoma. Microvenular haemangioma lacks atypia and multilayering, has a pericyte layer, and is HHV8-negative.

### Prognosis and predictive factors

Microvenular haemangioma is benign, with only exceptional local recurrence.

## Hobnail haemangioma

### Definition

Hobnail haemangioma is a benign vascular proliferation of lymphatic lineage, with hobnail endothelial cells {821,958,1749}.

### ICD-O code 9120/0

### Synonyms

Targetoid haemosiderotic haemangioma; superficial haemosiderotic lymphovascular malformation {15};
targetoid haemosiderotic lymphatic malformation {821,1248,2648}

### Epidemiology

This relatively rare haemangioma presents mainly in young and middle-aged adults, with a male predilection.

### Etiology

The etiology is unknown. Expression of lymphatic markers and negativity for WT1 and mitotic markers support the conclusion that these are superficial lymphatic malformations {37,2648}.

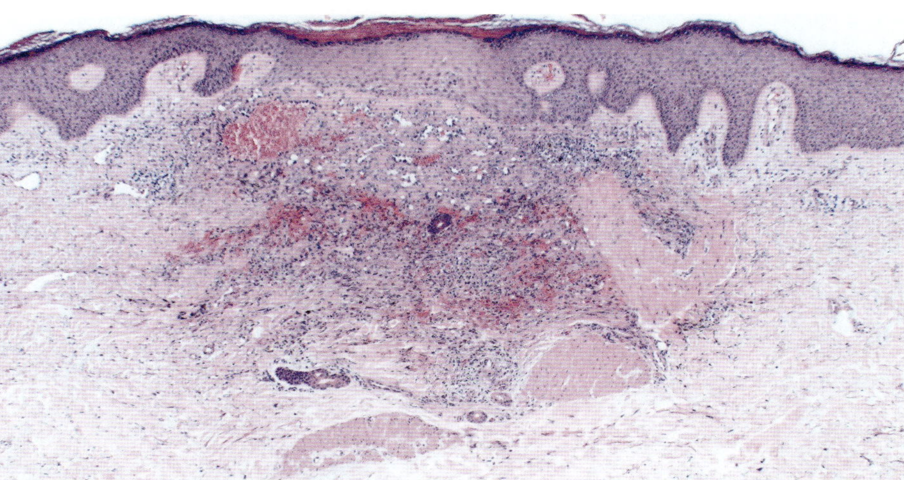

**Fig. 5.116** Hobnail haemangioma presenting as a superficial wedge-shaped vascular proliferation with the base towards the epidermis.

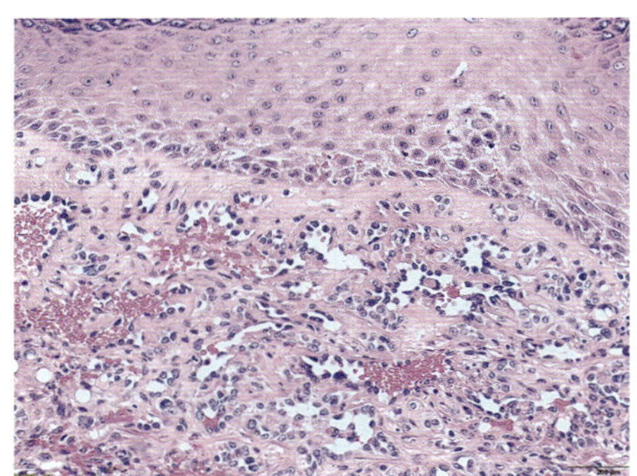

**Fig. 5.117** Hobnail haemangioma. Thin-walled lymphatic-like vascular channels are more prominent in the superficial part of the proliferation and are lined by distinctive hobnail endothelial cells.

### Localization
This lesion affects the trunk and extremities.

### Clinical features
Most hobnail haemangiomas present as a small nondescript erythematous papule. Uncommonly, the lesion is a small reddish-brown or purple papule surrounded by concentric ecchymotic haloes, hence the original name "targetoid haemosiderotic haemangioma".

### Histopathology
The lesions are wedge-shaped and consist of scattered, thin-walled, irregular vascular channels lined by bland endothelial cells with a hobnail appearance and focal intraluminal papillary projections. Vessels deeper in the lesion become smaller, flattened, and inconspicuous, without hobnail endothelial cells. Red blood cell extravasation, haemosiderin deposition, and perivascular lymphocytes are common. The endothelial cells are strongly positive for podoplanin (recognized by D2-40) and usually negative or weakly positive for CD34, suggesting a lymphatic lineage.

### Differential diagnosis
Identical lesions, usually lacking wedge-shaped architecture, may be seen in atypical vascular lesions occurring after radiotherapy. Papillary intralymphatic angioendothelioma (Dabska tumour) and retiform haemangioendothelioma have hobnail endothelial cells but have a distinctive pattern and are larger and more infiltrative.

### Prognosis and predictive factors
Hobnail haemangioma is benign, with no tendency for recurrence.

## *Glomeruloid haemangioma*

### Definition
Glomeruloid haemangioma is a reactive vascular proliferation associated with multicentric Castleman disease and POEMS syndrome (polyneuropathy, organomegaly, endocrinopathy, myeloma protein, and skin changes) {426,483,2224}.

### ICD-O code 9120/0

### Epidemiology
This rare haemangioma shows no sex predilection. Examples occurring outside the setting of multicentric Castleman disease or POEMS syndrome are likely to in fact be papillary haemangioma (see *Differential diagnosis*) {812,912,2537,2538}.

### Etiology
The etiology is unknown. Glomeruloid haemangioma is generally considered to be a reactive process.

### Localization
This lesion affects the trunk and extremities.

### Clinical features
The lesions are multiple erythematous papules.

### Histopathology
There is dermal proliferation of dilated vascular channels containing clusters of capillaries that resemble renal glomeruli. The endothelial cells often contain intracytoplasmic inclusions that give a positive periodic acid–Schiff (PAS) reaction; these inclusions may be immunoglobulins, enlarged lysosomes, or thanatosomes.

### Differential diagnosis
Papillary haemangioma has a predilection for the head and neck and presents as a single lesion consisting of dermal dilated channels lined by endothelial cells with frequent papillary projections and lacking glomeruloid architecture {2537}.

### Prognosis and predictive factors
Glomeruloid haemangioma is benign but tends to persist, paralleling underlying systemic disease.

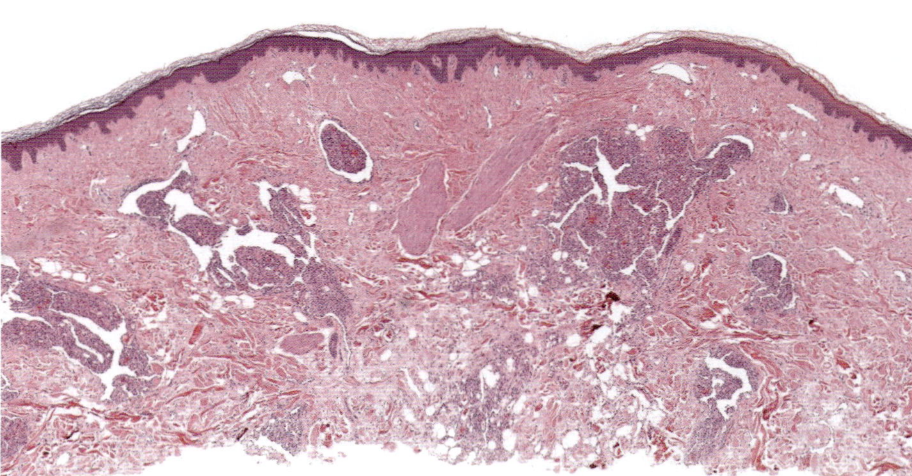

**Fig. 5.118** Glomeruloid haemangioma. Multiple intravascular capillary nodules in the dermis.

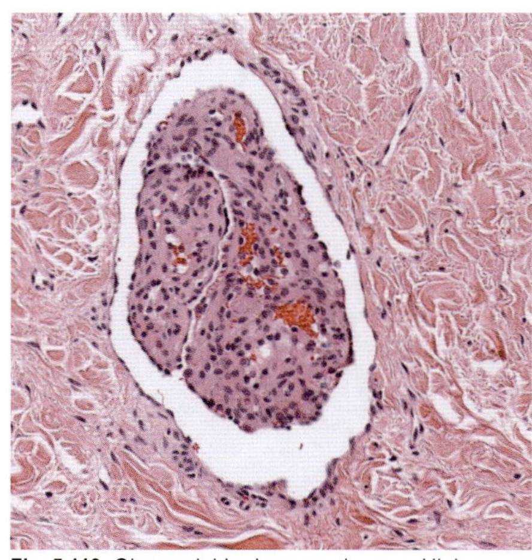

**Fig. 5.119** Glomeruloid haemangioma. High-power image showing an intravascular capillary proliferation resembling a renal glomerulus.

## Spindle cell haemangioma

### Definition
Spindle cell haemangioma is a benign neoplasm composed of spindled cells, ectatic vascular spaces, and vacuolated endothelial cells {789,1464,2032,2803}.

### ICD-O code
9120/0

### Synonym
Spindle cell haemangioendothelioma (obsolete) {2803}

### Epidemiology
This rare haemangioma is more common in the second and third decades of life, with no sex predilection.

### Localization
This lesion affects the distal extremities and occasionally the neck.

### Clinical features
The lesions are multiple asymptomatic bluish nodules developing over many years, with little tendency for regression. There is a strong association with Maffucci syndrome and less common associations with lymphoedema, early-onset varicose veins, and Klippel–Trénaunay syndrome {733,789,1464,2032}.

### Histopathology
The tumours are relatively well circumscribed, often partially intravascular, or sometimes poorly defined. They occupy the dermis, with frequent extension into the subcutis, and they consist of irregular, dilated, thin-walled, congested, cavernous-like vascular channels mixed with solid areas of vacuolated epithelioid endothelial cells scattered among bland spindle-shaped cells with pericytic and fibroblastic features and poorly defined eosinophilic cytoplasm. The cavernous vascular channels are lined by a single layer of bland endothelial cells. Thrombi, with or without dystrophic calcification, are common. Smooth muscle cells may be seen focally. Degenerative cytological atypia is sometimes present. The endothelial cells within the vascular channels and the epithelioid vacuolated cells show positive immunostaining for endothelial markers. Spindle cells may show focal positivity for SMA and/or desmin.

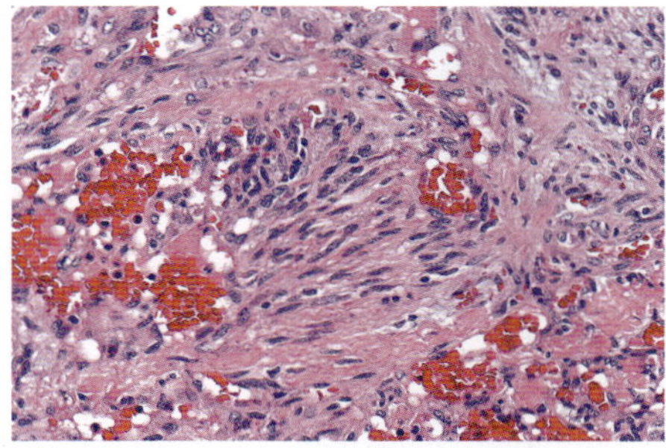

**Fig. 5.120** Spindle cell haemangioma. Dilated and congested thin-walled vascular channels, bland spindle-shaped cells, and vacuolated epithelioid endothelial cells.

### Differential diagnosis
Nodular Kaposi sarcoma lacks cavernous vascular channels and epithelioid vacuolated cells and is positive for HHV8.

**Fig. 5.121** Spindle cell haemangioma. A somewhat circumscribed vascular proliferation with dilated cavernous-like channels intermixed with more-solid cellular areas.

### Genetic profile
Sporadic lesions and lesions associated with Maffucci syndrome are associated with IDH1 p.R132C hotspot mutations {1464,1975,2594}. Frequent somatic alterations in 2p22.3, 2q24.3, and 14q11.2 are also found in spindle cell haemangiomas and enchondromas occurring in patients with Maffucci syndrome {72}.

### Genetic susceptibility
Spindle cell haemangioma is associated with Maffucci syndrome {733,1464}.

### Prognosis and predictive factors
Spindle cell haemangiomas are benign and do not usually recur, but multiple new lesions may develop over time {789}.

## Epithelioid haemangioma

### Definition
Epithelioid haemangioma is a benign vascular proliferation with vessels lined by epithelioid endothelial cells, often with an associated inflammatory component.

### ICD-O code
9125/0

### Synonyms
Angiolymphoid hyperplasia with eosinophilia; histiocytoid haemangioma; pseudopyogenic granuloma {58,2229,2659}

### Epidemiology
This haemangioma is most common in young adults (with a slight predilection for males), but all ages and racial groups are affected {1947}.

### Etiology
The etiology is unknown. Some cases may be reactive, related to trauma, acquired arteriovenous fistulas, or congenital arteriovenous malformations {776}. Epithelioid haemangiomas may be a heterogeneous group of histologically overlapping disorders, some neoplastic and others reactive to shunting.

### Localization
These lesions have a predilection for the head and neck and the trunk {1947}.

### Clinical features
The lesions are single or multiple, persistent, skin-coloured to erythematous papules and nodules. Peripheral eosinophilia is seen in 15% of patients {1947}. Similar

lesions may occur in deeper soft tissue and internal organs, including bone.

### Histopathology

A lobular vascular proliferation of vascular channels is lined by bland epithelioid endothelial cells with abundant eosinophilic or amphophilic cytoplasm and vesicular nuclei that protrude into the lumen, resembling cobblestones. A focal intravascular component may be seen, and rare examples are entirely intravenous. Inflammation is typically prominent, consisting of lymphocytes, histiocytes, plasma cells, and numerous eosinophils. Fibrosis occurs in late-stage lesions, which are also characterized by less inflammation and less-prominent epithelioid endothelial cells. In many cases, mural damage in a medium to large artery is present. Immunohistochemically, the endothelial cells are positive for blood vascular markers, lack lymphatic markers, and are accompanied by an SMA-positive pericyte layer. The epithelioid endothelial cells do not express EMA (epithelial membrane antigen) or keratins.

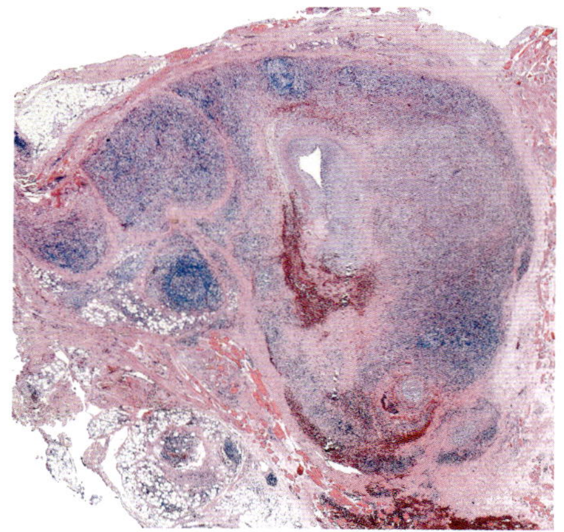

**Fig. 5.122** Epithelioid haemangioma. A lobular, solid proliferation of vascular channels obscured by a prominent inflammatory cell infiltrate.

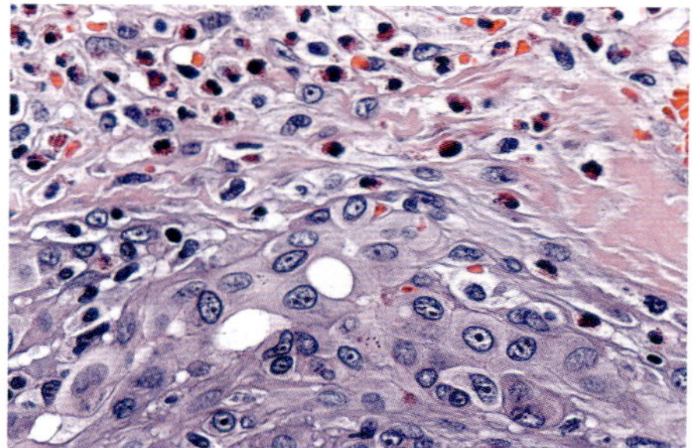

**Fig. 5.123** Epithelioid haemangioma. Vascular channels are typically lined by epithelioid endothelial cells; note the abundant eosinophils in the background.

### Differential diagnosis

Epithelioid haemangioma must be distinguished from Kimura disease, which occurs mainly in Asian males, presents with larger and deeper lesions, and is often associated with systemic symptoms and involvement of lymph nodes. Histologically, although the composition of the inflammatory cell infiltrate of Kimura disease is similar to that of epithelioid haemangioma, the vascular channels are not lined by epithelioid endothelial cells {1459}.

### Genetic profile

*FOS* gene rearrangements have been reported in bone and soft tissue epithelioid haemangiomas, but are rare in cutaneous epithelioid haemangioma and absent in examples with classic histological features (angiolymphoid hyperplasia with eosinophilia) {1145}.

### Prognosis and predictive factors

Epithelioid haemangioma is benign, but recurrences are common.

## *Tufted haemangioma*

### Definition

Tufted haemangioma is a benign cutaneous vascular tumour sometimes associated with Kasabach–Merritt syndrome and likely synonymous biologically with the kaposiform haemangioendothelioma {548,2386}.

### ICD-O code 9161/0

### Synonyms

Acquired tufted angioma; angioblastoma

### Epidemiology

This rare haemangioma has a strong predilection for infants and children, with no sex predilection {1246,1959}.

### Localization

These lesions have a predilection for the neck and upper trunk.

### Clinical features

The tumours present as slow-growing poorly defined macules, papules, nodules, and plaques, with rare focal regression {1074,2239}. Patients with large cutaneous lesions may develop Kasabach–Merritt syndrome {693}. This and other features suggest that tufted haemangioma is likely a smaller, superficial clinical variant of kaposiform haemangioendothelioma.

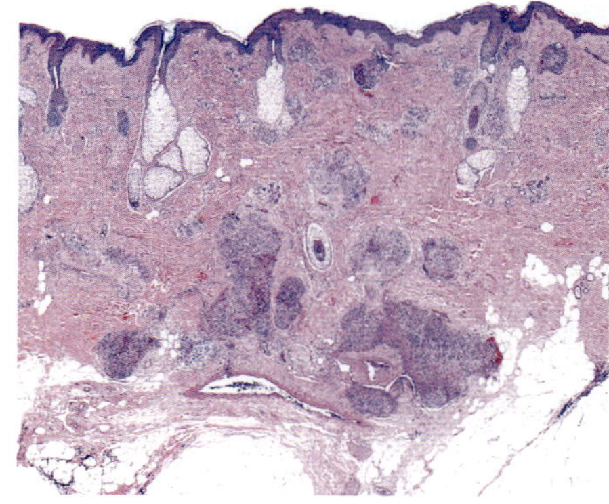

**Fig. 5.124** Tufted haemangioma. Multiple well-defined lobules of vascular channels in a so-called cannonball distribution.

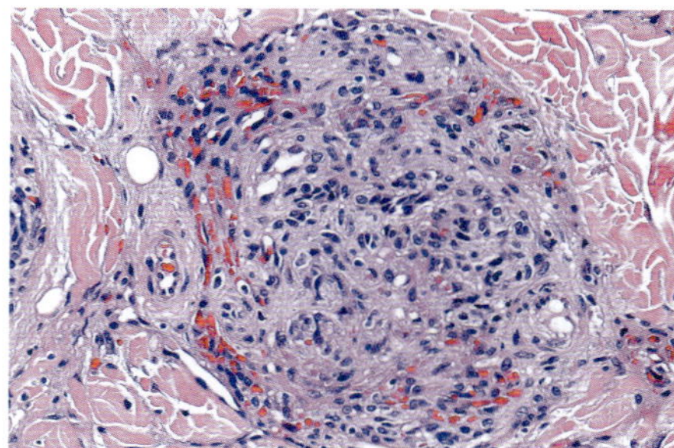

**Fig. 5.125** Tufted haemangioma. A typical tuft composed of small congested vascular channels surrounded by a slightly dilated crescent-like lymphatic channel.

### Histopathology

Multiple, scattered, tightly packed lobules of capillaries are present throughout the dermis and more rarely the subcutis, in a so-called cannonball pattern. The lumen of vascular channels is often difficult to discern, and pericytes are prominent. The endothelial cells are flat and occasionally contain intracytoplasmic hyaline structures. A distinctive feature is the presence of a crescent-like lymphatic channel around each tumour lobule. The stroma between tumour lobules may be desmoplastic and contain lymphatic-like channels. Focal fascicles of spindled endothelial cells, which are positive for podoplanin (recognized by D2-40), CD31, and CD34, may be seen within the capillary lobules.

### Differential diagnosis

Nodular Kaposi sarcoma lacks a cannonball architecture and is positive for HHV8.

## Prognosis and predictive factors

Tufted haemangioma is benign but often progressive. It may wax and wane, but does not completely regress.

# *Angiokeratoma*

## Definition

Angiokeratoma is a superficial vascular ectasia associated with variable overlying epidermal changes {1173}.

## ICD-O code 9141/0

## Epidemiology

Four clinicopathological types of angiokeratomas have been described {1173}. Angiokeratoma corporis diffusum (ACD) is associated with Fabry disease and presents in late childhood. Angiokeratoma of Fordyce (AF) most commonly presents in adult males. Angiokeratoma of Mibelli (AM) most commonly presents in adults, with no sex predilection. Solitary angiokeratoma (SA) or angiokeratoma circumscriptum also presents in adults, with no sex predilection.

## Etiology

The etiology of sporadic angiokeratomas is unknown. In Fabry disease, the lesions seem to develop because of accumulation of globotriaosylceramide in endothelial cells as a result of α-galactosidase deficiency. ACD may also develop as a result of deficiency in other enzymes, including α-L-fucosidase {699}, β-mannosidase {2540}, and α-N-acetylgalactosaminidase {1402}. Rare cases with no enzyme deficiency may be seen {1110}.

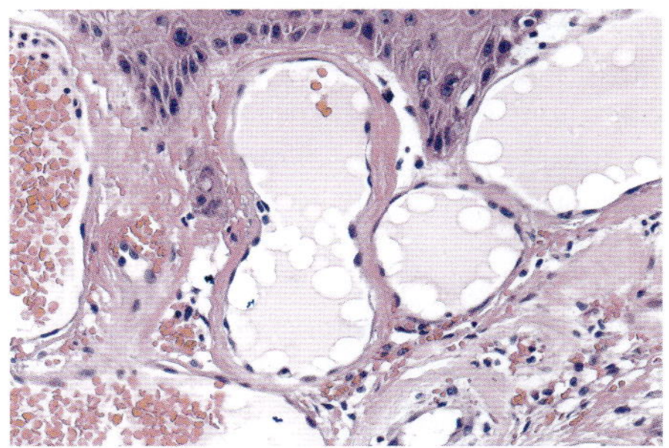

**Fig. 5.126** Angiokeratoma. Congested and dilated vascular channels lined by a single flattened layer of endothelial cells.

## Localization

ACD is characterized by lesions in a bathing-trunk distribution. AF presents on the scrotum and vulva {1171,1172}. AM presents on the dorsum of fingers and toes {2344}. SA presents mainly on the lower limbs {2344}.

## Clinical features

ACD presents with numerous asymptomatic pinpoint papules with minimal epidermal change. AF and AM present with single or multiple small red keratotic papules. SA presents as a single keratotic (often crusted) papule or nodule.

## Histopathology

ACD shows dilated, congested vascular channels in the papillary dermis, with minimal epidermal change. Endothelial cells, pericytes, and fibroblasts show cytoplasmic vacuoles representing lipid. AF, AM, and SA show dilated, thin-walled vascular channels in the papillary dermis associated with overlying epidermal changes consisting of acanthosis and hyperkeratosis.

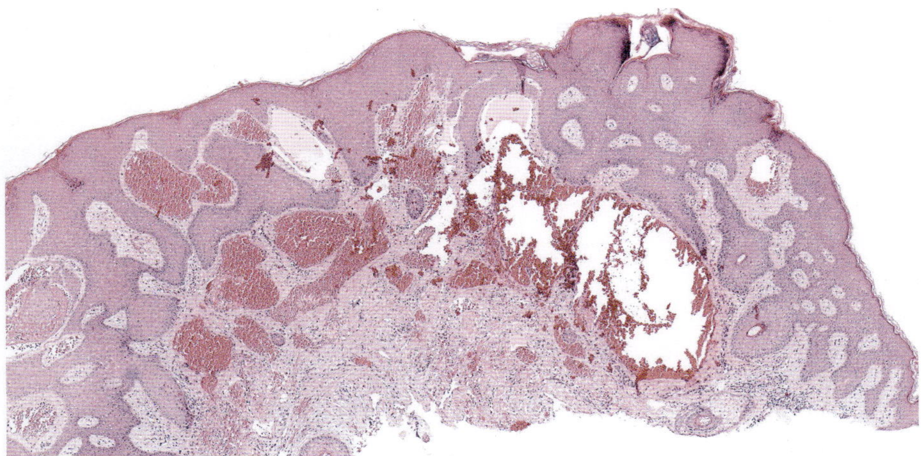

**Fig. 5.127** Angiokeratoma. Low-power image showing large, congested vascular epidermal channels.

## Differential diagnosis

SA must be distinguished from verrucous venous malformation (see below).

## Genetic susceptibility

ACD is associated with Fabry disease, an X-linked genetic disorder of α-galactosidase deficiency.

## Prognosis and predictive factors

In ACD, lesions continue to develop throughout life.

# *Infantile haemangioma*

## Definition

Infantile haemangioma is a benign tumour characterized by a proliferation of lobules of capillaries with a distinctive immunophenotype presenting exclusively in infancy and showing spontaneous slow regression.

## ICD-O code 9131/0

## Synonyms

Infantile haemangioendothelioma; cellular haemangioma of infancy; juvenile haemangioma; strawberry naevus

## Epidemiology

This haemangioma, which occurs in about 3–5% of the population, is the most common tumour of infancy. It shows a female predilection and is more common in White populations {1358,1846}.

## Localization

These lesions are most common on the head and neck and the extremities, but they also occur on the trunk, genitals, and in some viscera (notably, the liver and intestines).

## Clinical features

Nascent tumours may be evident at birth, but typically appear in the first 2–6 weeks of life, as a bright red or blue nodule or plaque, often with a strawberry-like appearance. There is initial rapid growth over a period of months, transitioning to a longer involuting phase of a few years {1358,1846}.

## Histopathology

The histology of infantile haemangioma defines the three stage of the lesion: proliferation, partial regression, and complete regression. Early proliferative

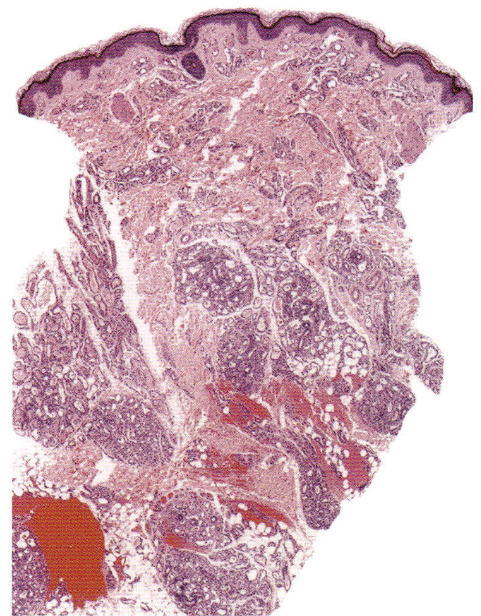

**Fig. 5.128** Infantile haemangioma. Dermal and subcutaneous proliferation of lobules of capillaries.

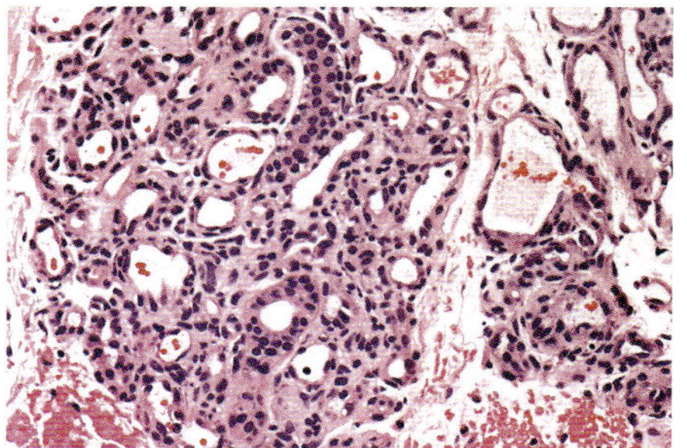

**Fig. 5.129** Infantile haemangioma. Note the uniform dilated capillaries lined by a single layer of bland endothelial cells and surrounded by a layer of pericytes.

lesions consist of cellular dermal and/or subcutaneous masses of tightly packed capillaries with small lumina, lined by plump endothelial cells rimmed by pericytes. The capillaries are interspersed with immature dendritic-type cells and arranged in lobules separated by delicate fibrous septa or normal intervening stroma. Perineural extension is common {358}, and the feeding and draining vessels may be quite large. During active involution, the lesional capillaries become variably dilated and congested, and gradually disappear. The basement membranes thicken and show apoptotic dust, and the pericapillary mast cells increase in number. Nearing end-stage, the tumour lobules are replaced by loose fibrous or fibrofatty stroma containing a few residual ghost capillaries composed of thickened multilayered rinds of basement membrane material with little or no cellular lining. The endothelial cells show a complex immunophenotype shared only by placental capillaries, including positivity for GLUT1, LeY, CD15, CCR6, IDO, and IGF2 {1920}.

### Differential diagnosis

Infantile haemangioma must be distinguished from congenital non-progressive haemangiomas on the basis of careful clinicopathological correlation and GLUT1 immunohistochemistry. All infantile haemangiomas have endothelial GLUT1 positivity, whereas congenital non-progressive haemangioma endothelial cells are negative for this marker {1921}.

### Histogenesis

The fact that infantile haemangioma's immunoreactivity for GLUT1, LeY, and other markers is identical to that of placental microvessels suggests that this tumour results from embolization of placental cells or stem cells differentiating towards placental vascular cells {1922}.

### Genetic profile

Cultured infantile haemangioma endothelial cells are clonal, a finding consistent with a neoplastic process {287}. No underlying genetic abnormalities have been identified.

### Genetic susceptibility

Although racial distributions suggest genetic predilections, there is no evidence to support a primary genetic driver. Rare families show increased incidence.

### Prognosis and predictive factors

These tumours are benign, but treatment is necessary when there is associated morbidity due to location or size. All cases show spontaneous regression, albeit of variable rates and degrees.

## *Congenital non-progressive haemangiomas: rapidly involuting congenital haemangioma and non-involuting congenital haemangioma*

### Definition

Congenital non-progressive haemangiomas are a distinct group of vascular lesions that arise in utero and are fully formed at birth. There are two clinical variants: rapidly involuting congenital haemangioma (RICH) and non-involuting congenital haemangioma (NICH) {270,691,1845}. For cases that regress incompletely, the term "partially involuted congenital haemangioma (PICH)" has been proposed {1881}.

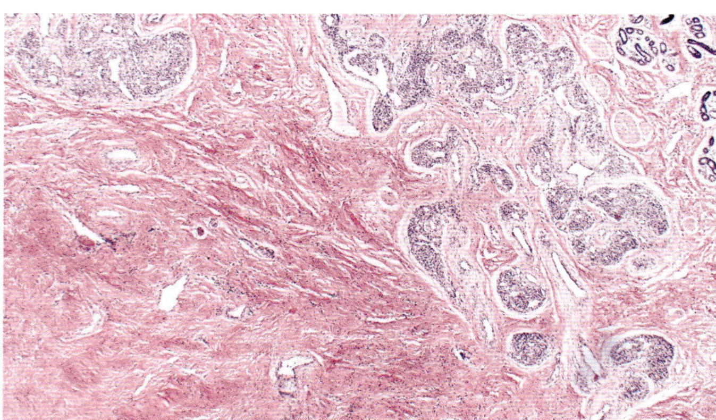

**Fig. 5.130** Rapidly involuting congenital haemangioma. Lobules of capillaries, scattered larger vascular channels, and an area of fibrosis indicative of regression.

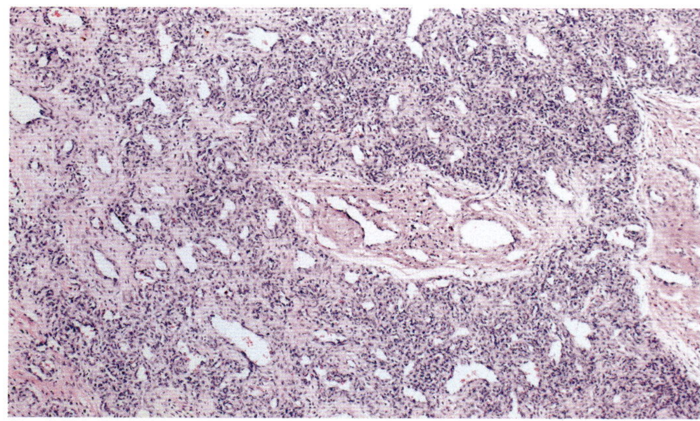

**Fig. 5.131** Rapidly involuting congenital haemangioma. Lobules of capillaries.

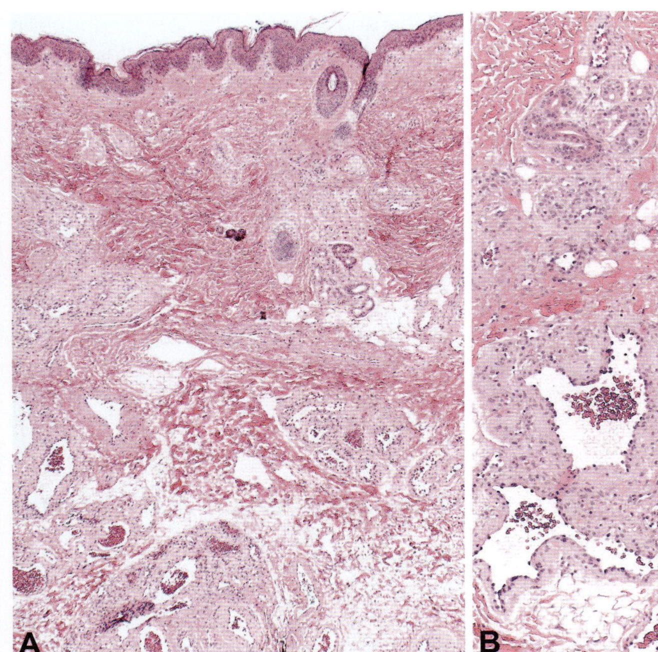

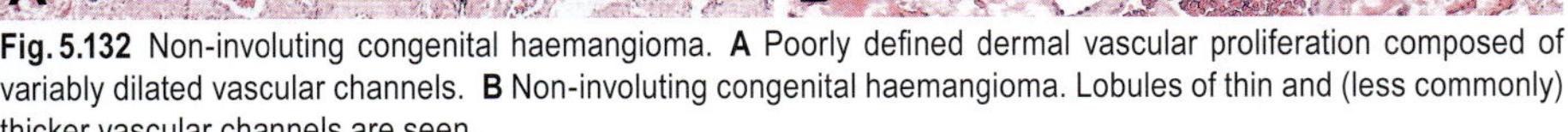

**Fig. 5.132** Non-involuting congenital haemangioma. **A** Poorly defined dermal vascular proliferation composed of variably dilated vascular channels. **B** Non-involuting congenital haemangioma. Lobules of thin and (less commonly) thicker vascular channels are seen.

### ICD-O codes

| | |
|---|---|
| Rapidly involuting congenital haemangioma | 9131/0 |
| Non-involuting congenital haemangioma | 9131/0 |

### Epidemiology

Congenital non-progressive haemangiomas present at birth, with no sex predilection. They are less common than infantile haemangioma.

### Localization

The most common location is the head, followed by the extremities.

### Clinical features

The lesions are usually fully formed at birth, typically following either a persistent clinical course (NICH) or a very rapidly regressive course through infarction (RICH) during the first 6 months of life {212}. Initial lesions vary in size and consist of a vascular red or bluish mass with overlying telangiectasia and occasionally associated with ulceration. Rare tumours regress incompletely (PICH) {1881}. NICH increases in size proportionally as the patient grows, and it does not regress {692}. Exceptional cases show limited postnatal growth.

### Histopathology

RICH, PICH, and NICH vary along a histopathological spectrum, largely dependent on the degree of infarction. All are composed of variably well-circumscribed capillary lobules within dermis and/or subcutis. Interlobular stroma is often fibrotic and may contain arteries, veins, and sometimes lymphatic channels of moderate size. Intralobular capillary endothelial cells and pericytes can be plump, but they lack the increased mitotic activity, GLUT1-positivity, and basement membrane multilamination of infantile haemangioma. Persistent lesions (NICHs and PICHs) are more likely to display arteriovenous shunts, hobnail endothelial cells, and a large vessel in the centre of the vascular lobules {692}. The endothelial cells of all variants are negative for GLUT1 {1845}.

### Differential diagnosis

Distinction from infantile haemangioma is usually straightforward, on the basis of presentation at birth and the lack of endothelial positivity for GLUT1 in congenital non-progressive haemangiomas.

### Genetic profile

Somatic activating mutations in *GNAQ* and *GNA11* at Glu209 have been identified in both NICH and RICH {119}.

### Prognosis and predictive factors

Most RICHs involute spontaneously, and NICHs tend to persist. Persistent congenital non-progressive haemangiomas often require surgical or laser intervention.

## Lobular capillary haemangioma

### Definition

Lobular capillary haemangioma is a common vascular cutaneous and mucosal neoplasm that consists of a proliferation of capillaries with a lobular architecture.

### ICD-O code 9131/0

### Synonym

Pyogenic granuloma

### Epidemiology

This haemangioma (including rare congenital cases) presents over a wide age range, with no sex predilection {239,1024,2003}.

### Etiology

Because of the prominent secondary inflammatory changes present in the tumour and the frequent association with trauma, lobular capillary haemangioma was previously considered to be a reactive inflammatory process. However, the presumption that it is a neoplastic vascular proliferation is now favoured {2675}.

### Localization

These lesions have a predilection for the fingers and the head and neck, in particular the nasal and oral mucosae. Gingival lesions occur in pregnant women (granuloma gravidarum). Involvement of internal organs is rare {2707}.

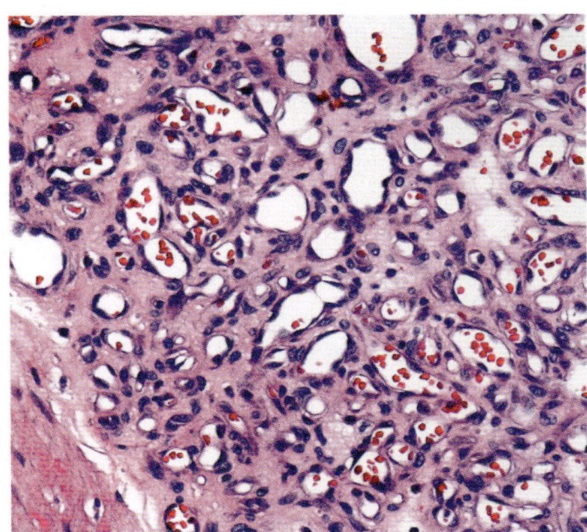

**Fig. 5.133** Lobular capillary haemangioma. The tumour lobules are composed of small capillaries.

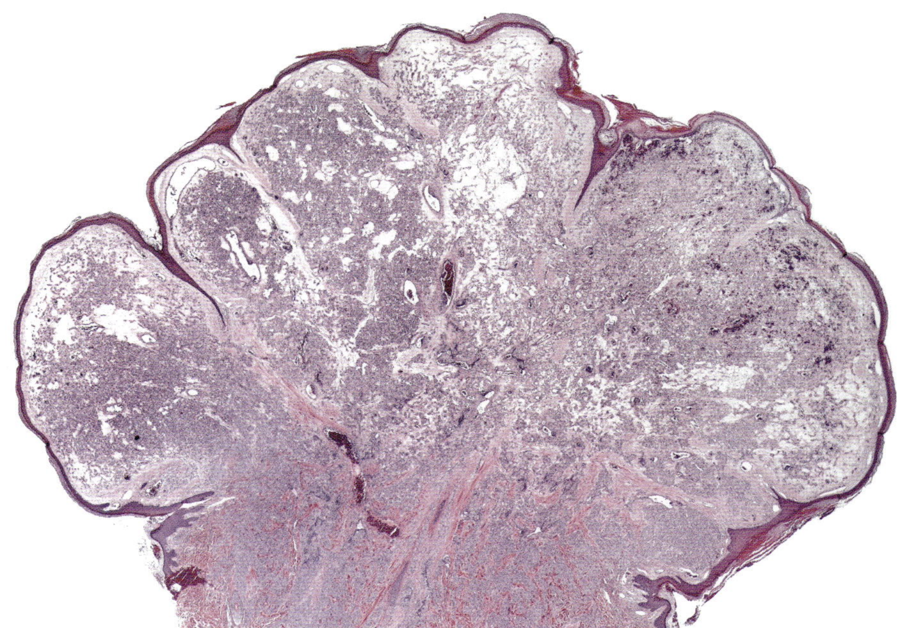

**Fig. 5.134** Lobular capillary haemangioma. A polypoid lobular proliferation of vascular channels with an epidermal collarette.

### Clinical features

The lesion is a rapidly growing, polypoid, haemorrhagic, and frequently ulcerated blue or red nodule. Multiple lesions occasionally develop; in children, recurrences may be associated with multiple satellites {193,1875,2784}. Lesions can occur in association with port wine stain and other vascular malformations. They are also associated with many medications and biological agents, including retinoids and BRAF inhibitors {558,724,1064,1361}. Rare tumours present in deep dermal/ subcutaneous or intravenous locations {526}.

### Histopathology

The tumours are polypoid, with an epidermal collarette and frequent ulceration with prominent inflammation consisting of neutrophils, usually restricted to the superficial aspect of the lesion. Variably dilated capillaries lined by plump endothelial cells rimmed by a pericyte layer are arranged in lobules within oedematous stroma. Mitotic activity is common, and focal cytological atypia may be noted, in particular in mucosal lesions. Older lesions show variable fibrosis. Deep-seated and intravenous lesions are identical but lack inflammation.

### Differential diagnosis

Nodular Kaposi sarcoma shows a similar architecture but consists of bundles of spindle-shaped cells with clefting, intracytoplasmic eosinophilic globules, and HHV8 positivity. Bacillary angiomatosis (an infectious vascular proliferation caused mainly by *Rochalimaea henselae*) is histologically similar, but the vascular channels are lined by pale epithelioid endothelial cells and aggregates of neutrophils, and nuclear dust and

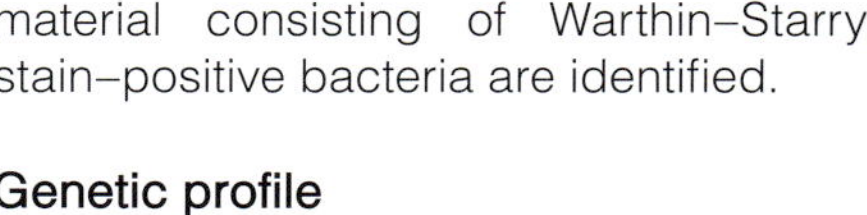

amorphous basophilic or amphophilic material consisting of Warthin–Starry stain–positive bacteria are identified.

### Genetic profile

Sporadic lobular capillary haemangiomas and those occurring within port wine stain may be associated with RAS family and *BRAF* mutations (mainly c.1799T>A) {942}.

### Prognosis and predictive factors

Complete regression is not typical, and local recurrence occurs in approximately 10% of cases.

## Verrucous venous malformation

### Definition

Verrucous venous malformation is a distinctive localized vascular malformation associated with overlying prominent epidermal changes {352,1174,2775}.

### ICD-O code

9142/0

### Synonyms

Verrucous haemangioma;
verrucous venulocapillary malformation

### Epidemiology

This is a rare congenital lesion, with no sex predilection.

### Localization

These lesions have a predilection for the lower extremities, and occasionally occur on the trunk.

### Clinical features

The lesions are slightly raised singular, grouped, or confluent red-to-purple plaques that become more hyperkeratotic and may bleed and slowly enlarge over time.

### Histopathology

An epidermis with prominent acanthosis, papillomatosis, hyperkeratosis, parakeratosis, and crusting overlies an expanded papillary dermis with numerous dilated and congested capillaries and venules, often extending into the investing dermis of skin adnexae. The subcutaneous tissue displays a notably increased density of variably congested capillaries and venules. Mitotic activity is rare to absent. WT1 is negative in the endothelial cells,

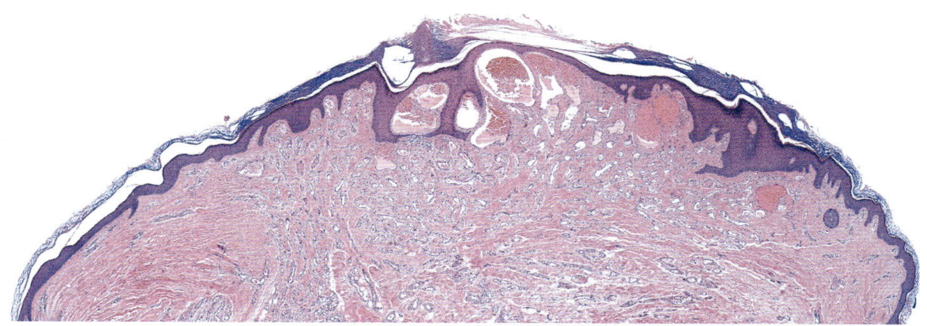

**Fig. 5.135** Verrucous venous malformation. At low power.

supporting the conclusion that these lesions are malformations {2775}.

### Differential diagnosis

The superficial dermal changes closely resemble angiokeratoma. Histological distinction relies on the identification of a deep dermal/subcutaneous component.

### Genetic profile

Verrucous venous malformation is non-familial. A somatic missense mutation in *MAP3K3* has been identified in some cases {538}.

### Prognosis and predictive factors

Verrucous venous malformation shows persistence and slow expansion following incomplete excision.

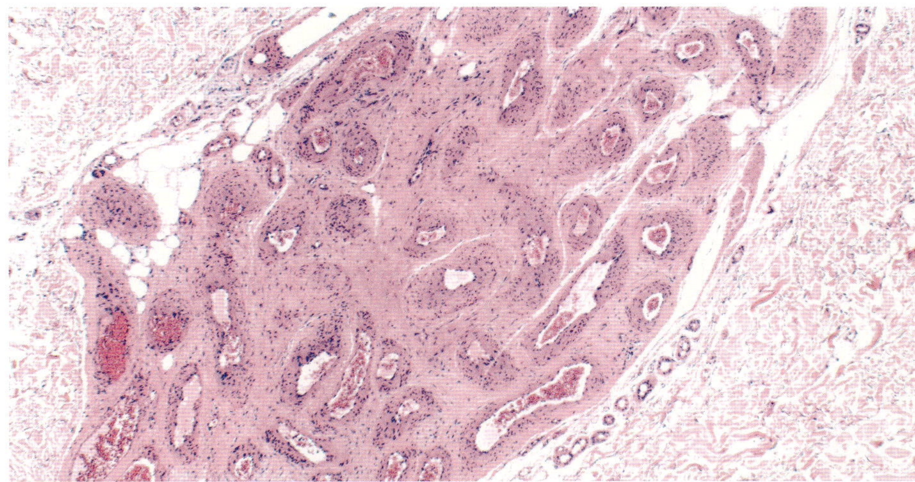

**Fig. 5.136** Arteriovenous malformation. A dermal proliferation of thick-walled and thin-walled vascular channels.

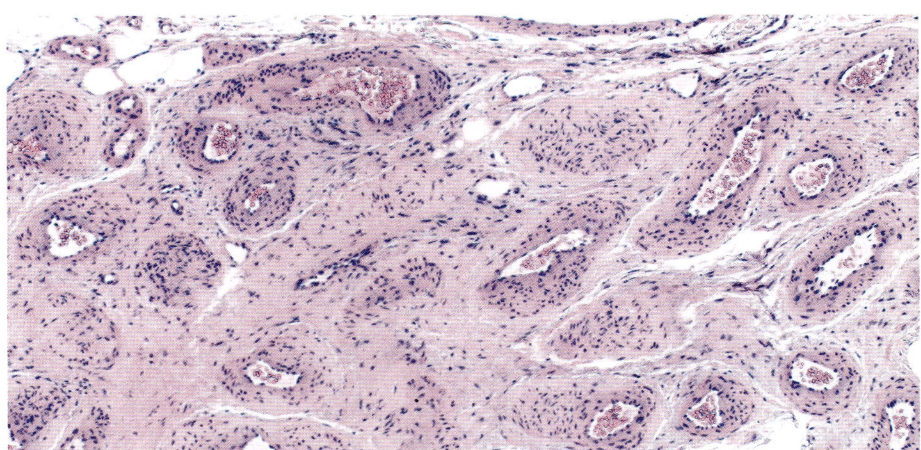

**Fig. 5.137** Arteriovenous malformation. The vascular channels resemble small arteries and veins.

## Arteriovenous malformation

### Definition

Arteriovenous malformation (AVM) is a congenital vascular anomaly characterized by abnormal arteriovenous connections and high-flow arteriovenous shunting. Deep and superficial clinical variants have been described {972,2812}.

### ICD-O code 9123/0

### Synonyms

Arteriovenous haemangioma;
cirsoid aneurysm;
acral arteriovenous tumour

### Epidemiology

AVMs have no sex predilection and are congenital, but may not become clinically evident until later in life. Most are solitary and sporadic.

### Localization

AVM can involve the skin, subcutis, bone, and viscera and has a marked predilection for the head, neck, and limbs. Small, superficial vascular lesions with a predilection for the lips, perioral skin, nose, and eyelids of middle-aged to elderly men, traditionally called acral arteriovenous tumour, may not be true AVMs.

### Clinical features

AVMs involving skin and deep soft tissue are characterized by a poorly defined bluish or red mass that may be pulsatile, with variably severe arteriovenous shunting, sometimes leading to local tissue necrosis, haemorrhage, or high-output heart failure. The superficial variant is typically a small red or blue papule.

### Histopathology

The lesions are histologically heterogeneous, but primarily show beds of arterioles, capillaries, and venules set within a fibromyxomatous background, intermixed with larger-calibre arteries and thick-walled veins. In lesions with high-grade shunting, the arteries are tortuous, with fragmented mural elastic laminae, and the veins show irregular intima and/or mural fibrosis, reflective of elevated venous pressure and turbulence. The overlying skin often contains a small-vessel proliferation similar to that seen in ischaemia and stasis. Superficial scalp AVMs, which are limited in depth by cranial bone, are histologically similar.

### Differential diagnosis

Diagnosis typically requires careful clinicopathological correlation and radiological studies, in particular in small samples. Focal cellular small vessel proliferations in AVM can mimic infantile haemangioma, but are GLUT1 negative {2701}.

### Genetic profile

Most cases are sporadic. Inherited lesions occurring as part of the rare capillary malformation–AVM syndrome are associated with germline *RASA1* mutations, which are probably causative {2605}.

### Prognosis and predictive factors

Incompletely excised lesions recur, often with recruitment of new collateral flow through the residual AVM nidus.

# Lymphangioma (superficial lymphatic malformation)

Requena L.
Kutzner H.
Mihm M.C. Jr

## Definition

The term "lymphangioma" is a misnomer; these lesions are probably superficial lymphatic malformations.

## ICD-O code 9170/0

## Synonyms

Lymphangioma simplex; circumscribed lymphangioma; cystic hygroma

## Epidemiology

Superficial lymphatic malformations are present at birth or appear during the first few months of life. There is no sex predilection.

## Etiology

Lymphatic malformations result from embryological development anomalies of the lymphatic system. Superficial lymphatic malformations result from defects in the connection between distal lymphatic vessels and deeper lymphatic channels. Therefore, these superficial lymphatic malformations are not connected to the general lymphatic circulation.

## Localization

These lymphatic malformations may be found in any area of the body surface, but they have a preference for the axillary folds, shoulders, neck, proximal part of the limbs, genital region, and tongue {784,2022,2810}.

## Clinical features

Superficial lymphatic malformations appear as multiple small translucent or yellowish vesicles grouped in a plaque (with a so-called frogspawn appearance). Frequently, the lesions have a wart-like surface. Purpuric areas are sometimes seen inside the lesion, due to the presence of a blood vessel component either as part of the malformation or as part of a fistula attached to the malformed lymphatic vessels. Most superficial lymphatic malformations are accompanied by deeper malformed lymphatic vessels in the subcutis {1971}, and rare cases are associated with visceral involvement {1185,1827}. They are also among the vascular anomalies associated with Maffucci syndrome {2533} and Cobb syndrome {2413}.

Cystic hygroma is a variant of subcutaneous macrocystic lymphatic malformation located in areas of loose connective tissue such as the neck, armpits, and groin folds {244}. Lesions involving the posterior triangle of the neck may be associated with hydrops fetalis, Turner syndrome (45,X0 karyotype), diverse congenital malformations, several chromosomal aneuploidies, and fetal death {451}.

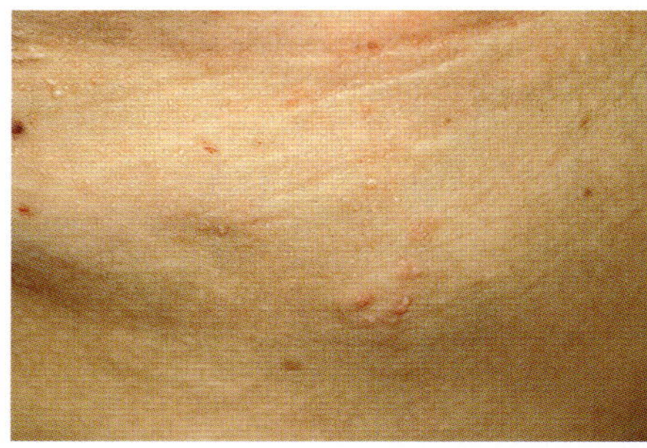

**Fig. 5.139** Lymphangioma (superficial lymphatic malformation) presenting as multiple small translucent papules scattered on the lateral aspect of the chest.

Lymphangiomatosis is a rare disorder characterized by the presence of abnormal lymphatic vessels diffusely distributed within an anatomical region. Cases of lymphangiomatosis with bone and visceral involvement have poor prognosis and high mortality {2129}, whereas lesions involving only soft tissues and bone have an indolent course {2022}.

A recently described lymphatic disorder is multifocal lymphangioendotheliomatosis with thrombocytopenia. The disorder consists of the association of congenital cutaneous and gastrointestinal lymphatic

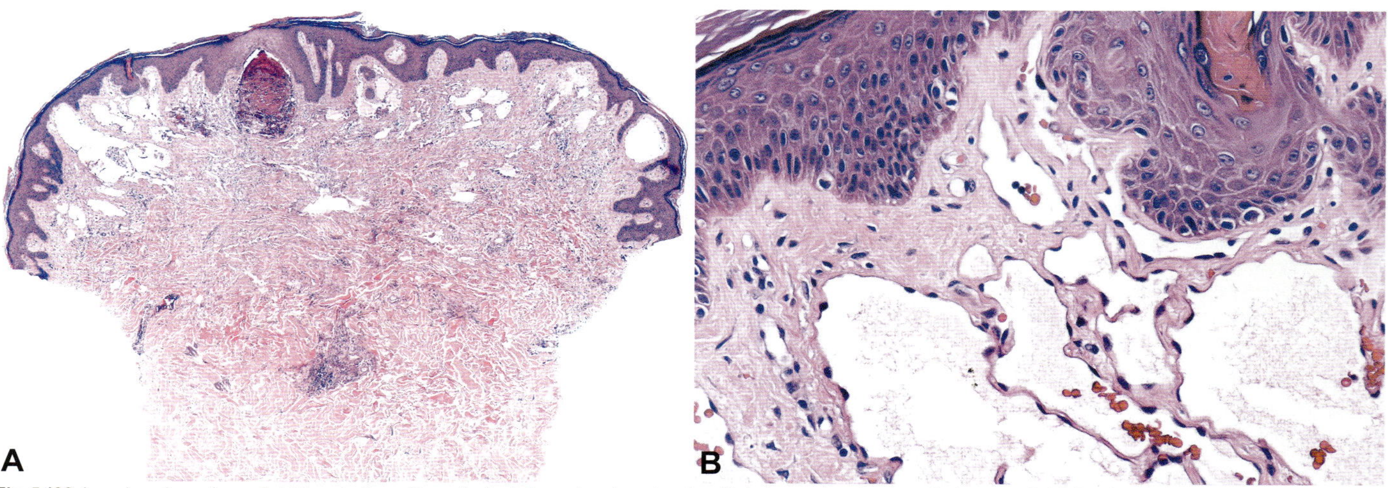


**Fig. 5.138** Lymphangioma (superficial lymphatic malformation). **A** Scanning view showing dilated vascular structures in the superficial dermis. **B** Higher magnification reveals that these vessels are lined by a discontinuous layer of flattened endothelial cells.

malformations and coagulopathy, which in severe cases may evolve to massive consumptive coagulopathy, as seen in Kasabach–Merritt syndrome {1919}.

## Histopathology

Superficial lymphatic malformations involve the papillary dermis, although they sometimes extend to the reticular dermis and even the subcutaneous tissue. The lesions consist of dilated thin-walled vascular structures lined by a single discontinuous layer of flattened endothelial cells, many arranged in papillae {178,784}. The lumina of these dilated lymphatic vessels look empty, but are filled with eosinophilic homogeneous lymphatic fluid and sometimes erythrocytes. Small delicate valves are a clue to diagnosis. Foamy macrophages and multinucleated giant cells are sometimes also present, and a discrete lymphocytic inflammatory infiltrate is frequently seen in the underlying dermis. Macrocystic and deeper lymphatic malformations appear as interconnected, irregular, dilated vessels in the subcutaneous fat and adjacent tissues, some with a muscular layer in their vessel walls {2261}. Immunohistochemically, the endothelial cells lining the lymphatic malformations express podoplanin (recognized by D2-40), LYVE1, and PROX1 {794,1113,2334}.

## Differential diagnosis

Superficial lymphatic malformations may be difficult to distinguish from angiokeratomas, in particular when blood is also present in the lumina. In such cases, immunomarkers specific for lymphatic endothelium, such as podoplanin (recognized by D2-40), LYVE1, and PROX1, may be helpful. However, many classic circumscribed angiokeratomas are lined by cells that also have a lymphatic endothelial cell immunophenotype, and these two lesions are probably more closely related than was previously thought {2649,2778}.

## Histogenesis

VEGFR3 and its ligands VEGF-C and VEGF-D seem to be involved in the lymphangiogenesis. It has been shown that transgenic mice with VEGF-C hyperexpression develop lymphatic hyperplasia {1223}.

## Genetic profile

Families with Milroy disease, which is a congenital inherited lymphatic disorder transmitted in an autosomal dominant fashion, show mutations in *FLT4* (*VEGFR3*) on chromosome 5q {762,763}. It seems that mutations in *PROX1* {2829} and *FOXC2* {737} are also involved in the development of lymphatic malformations.

## Prognosis and predictive factors

The prognosis of superficial lymphatic malformations is good when they are not associated with deeper or visceral involvement.

# Neural tumours

## Neurofibroma and variants

Shea C.
Tetzlaff M.

### Definition

Cutaneous neurofibroma is a benign tumour of axons, Schwann cells, fibroblasts, and perineurial cells, within a collagenous to variably myxoid stroma with mast cells {1238,1562,1729,2183}.

### ICD-O code

Neurofibroma 9540/0

### Epidemiology

Cutaneous neurofibroma occurs equally in both sexes, with peak incidence in the third decade of life {80}.

### Etiology

The etiological factors for sporadic neurofibroma have not been identified. For those associated with neurofibromatosis, see *Genetic profile*.

### Localization

Sporadic neurofibromas arise anywhere on the skin or mucosa, slightly more commonly on the trunk. Diffuse neurofibromas most commonly arise on the head and neck {2143,2341}. Plexiform neurofibromas most commonly involve deep soft tissue of the trunk.

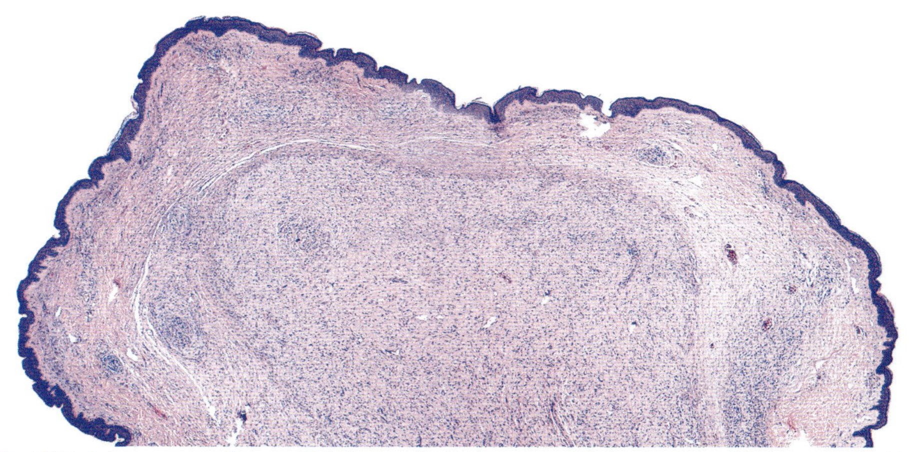

**Fig. 5.140** Cutaneous neurofibroma. Well-circumscribed but unencapsulated, pale eosinophilic tumour centred in the dermis.

### Clinical features

Sporadic (solitary) neurofibromas typically arise as slow-growing, painless, soft, skin-coloured papules to nodules. Diffuse neurofibromas present as large plaques, and plexiform neurofibromas present as large multinodular masses. Diffuse and plexiform neurofibromas more commonly affect children and young adults {1253,2143,2702}. Multiple neurofibromas or plexiform and diffuse variants are clues to an association with neurofibromatosis type 1 (NF1), a spectrum of disorders producing cutaneous, neural, and skeletal lesions. The clinical diagnosis of NF1 requires two or more of the following criteria: ≥ 6 café-au-lait macules, ≥ 2 neurofibromas of any type or 1 plexiform neurofibroma, axillary and/or inguinal freckles, optic glioma, ≥ 2 Lisch nodules (pigmented hamartomas of the iris), characteristic bone lesions (sphenoid dysplasia and/or tibial pseudoarthrosis), and a first-degree relative with NF1 {487,659,825,1542,2181,2182,2183}.

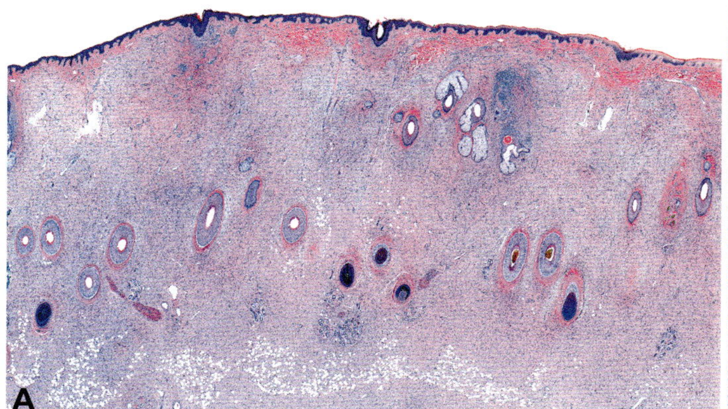

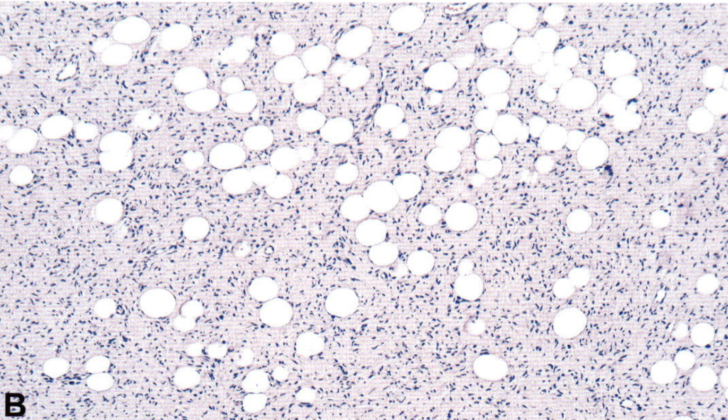

**Fig. 5.141** Diffuse neurofibroma. **A** Pale eosinophilic tumour infiltrating the dermis (without effacing endogenous structures) and extending into the subcutis. **B** High-magnification view of tumour cells insinuating within subcutaneous adipose tissue.

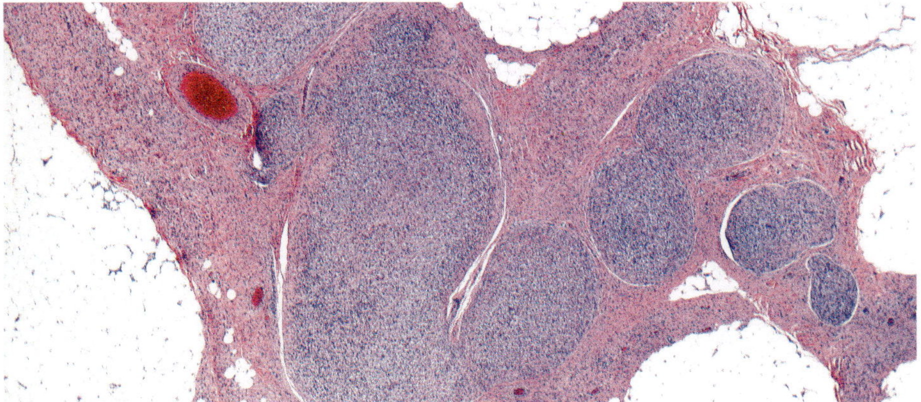
**Fig. 5.142** Plexiform neurofibroma. Serpiginous, expanded nerve bundles infiltrated by tumour.

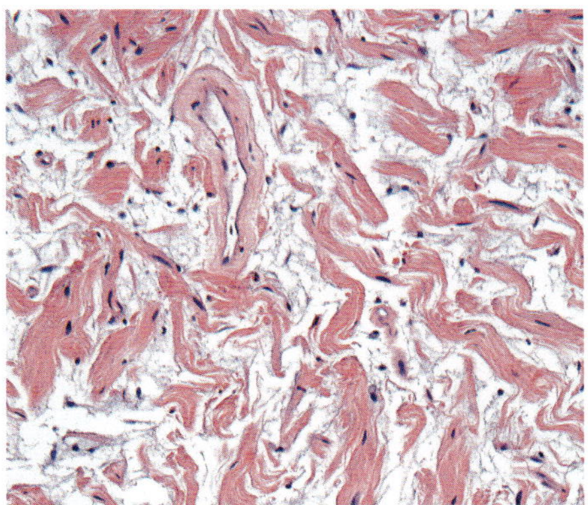
**Fig. 5.143** Cutaneous neurofibroma. Spindle cells in a matrix composed of strands of collagen.

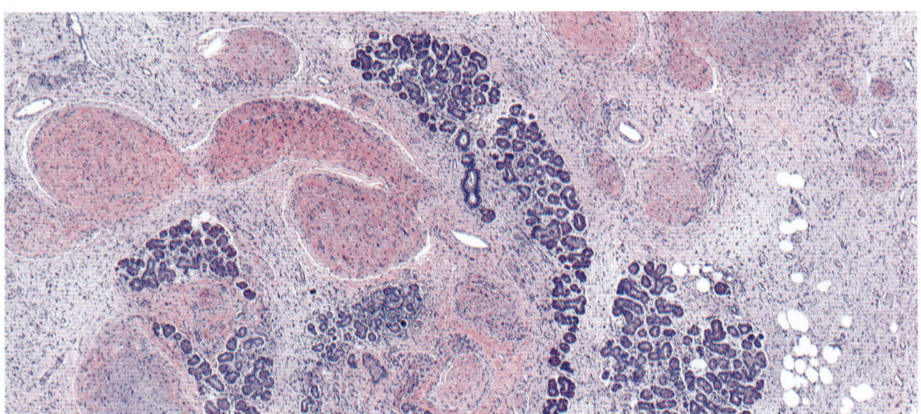
**Fig. 5.144** Mixed-pattern (plexiform and diffuse) neurofibroma. Tortuous nerve bundles expanded by tumour with spillage into the surrounding tissue, without effacement of architecture; note the preservation of glandular structures.

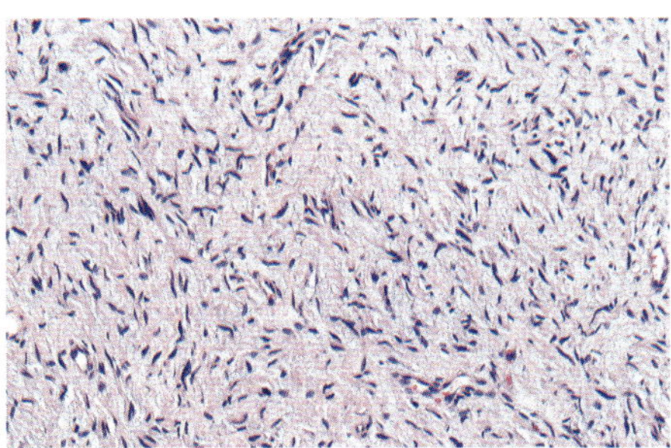
**Fig. 5.145** Cutaneous neurofibroma. Spindle cells with thin, wavy, hyperchromatic nuclei and delicate, pale eosinophilic cytoplasmic processes; these spindle cells are embedded in a matrix of thin strands of collagen and interstitial mucin, with an associated infiltrate of small mature lymphocytes, histiocytes, and conspicuous mast cells.

## Histopathology

Solitary neurofibroma is usually a relatively circumscribed, unencapsulated, pale eosinophilic dermal tumour composed of spindle cells with thin, wavy nuclei and delicate, pale eosinophilic cytoplasm in a collagenous and variably myxoid stroma admixed with mast cells {1238}. Dermal glands and hair follicles are preserved. In myxoid neurofibroma, myxoid stroma predominates {142,922,1729}. In sclerotic neurofibroma, scant spindle cells are embedded in a sclerotic, collagenous matrix {913,1870}. Lipomatous neurofibroma contains admixed adipocytes {33,2682,2684}. Pigmented neurofibroma contains variable melanin, often towards the periphery {773,1252}.

Diffuse neurofibroma is an infiltrative tumour involving the dermis and subcutis, often entrapping adnexa or adipocytes {1729,2170,2702}. The cellular constituents are similar to those of solitary neurofibroma, with the addition of frequent Meissner bodies.

Plexiform neurofibroma, which is highly specific for NF1, consists of tortuous, swollen nerves expanded by axons, Schwann cells, and fibroblasts, within a myxoid/collagenous matrix {1253}. Plexiform neurofibroma may coexist with diffuse neurofibroma extending into the surrounding tissue. This diagnosis should be reserved for large, deeply situated masses; small, superficial neurofibromas with an incidental plexiform pattern do not qualify.

Immunohistochemical studies of neurofibroma demonstrate expression of S100 protein and SOX10 in some tumour cells {501,2170}. CD34 staining highlights fibroblasts in a characteristic so-called fingerprint pattern {2885}.

## Differential diagnosis

The differential diagnosis includes schwannoma, perineurioma, dermatofibroma, myxoid dermatofibrosarcoma protuberans with diffuse neurofibroma, neurotized naevus, and desmoplastic melanoma.

## Histogenesis

The cell of origin of neurofibroma is the subject of controversy, as is its designation as a neoplasm versus a hamartoma, given its admixed composition of peripheral nerve axons, Schwann cells, fibroblasts, perineurial cells, and associated inflammation {249,1729,2183,2307,2503}

## Genetic profile

NF1 is an autosomal dominant disorder caused by alterations in the *NF1* gene on chromosome 17. Many affected patients lack a family history; their disease is attributed to de novo mutations.

## Prognosis and predictive factors

Solitary sporadic neurofibromas do not usually cause clinical problems, although this depends on the anatomical location. Neurofibromas occurring in the setting of neurofibromatosis can cause considerable patient morbidity, depending on their number and/or location. An additional concern (most commonly in patients with NF1) is transformation to malignant peripheral nerve sheath tumour.

# Solitary circumscribed neuroma

Ferguson P.M.
Scolyer R.A.
Argenyi Z.B.
Hollmann T.

## Definition
Solitary circumscribed neuroma (SCN) is a benign circumscribed tumour composed of nerve fibres, typically occurring as a small papule on the face.

## ICD-O code 9570/0

## Synonym
Palisaded encapsulated neuroma

## Epidemiology
SCN occurs equally in both sexes. It is most common in the fifth to seventh decades of life, but can occur at any age.

## Localization
Although 90% of lesions arise on the face, SCN can be found in skin at any site, preferentially near mucocutaneous junctions {786,1241,2145}. Mucosal involvement is well documented, with the oral cavity being the second most common location {1437}.

## Clinical features
SCN typically presents as an asymptomatic, solitary, small (2–6 mm), firm, and pink to flesh-coloured papule. Rare examples of multiple SCNs have been reported in patients with no evidence of any associated systemic disease {1571}.

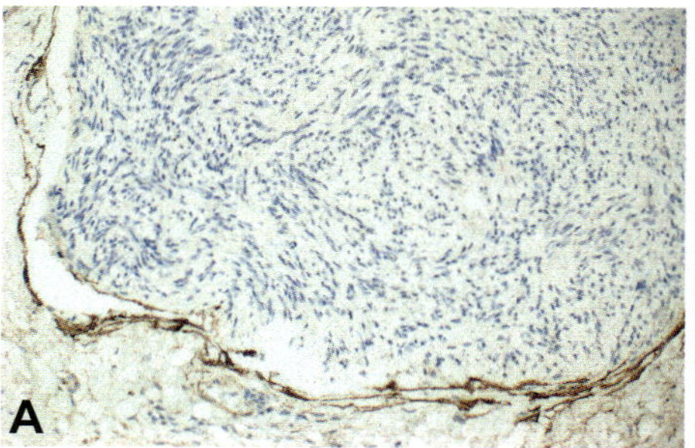
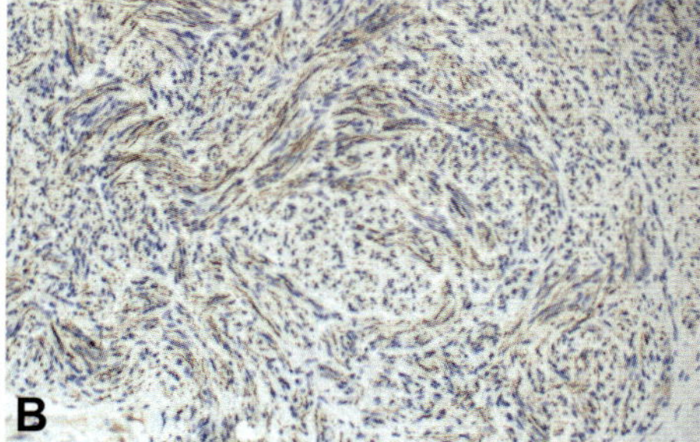

**Fig. 5.146** Solitary circumscribed neuroma. **A** Expression of EMA (epithelial membrane antigen) is limited to the peripheral perineurial component. **B** Axons are present throughout the lesion, as highlighted by staining for NFP.

## Histopathology
SCN forms a well-circumscribed round to oval dermal nodule encased by a delicate fibrous capsule, which is often superficially incomplete. The tumour is composed of bland, elongated spindle cells in broad fascicles that are often separated by artefactual clefts. Occasional non-atypical mitotic figures may be seen. The nuclei of SCN may show a focal parallel, palisaded arrangement, but prominent palisading and Verocay bodies are usually absent. A plexiform or multinodular growth pattern may be present, but the usual internal structure is retained {91}.

The capsular perineurial cells stain for EMA (epithelial membrane antigen); the fascicular spindle cells are positive for S100 protein and negative for GFAP. NFP is present in axons throughout the lesion. SCN is negative for SMA, desmin, and melanocytic markers {90,786}.

## Differential diagnosis
It is important to distinguish SCN from entities associated with systemic diseases, especially in the context of multiple lesions. Neurofibromas are unencapsulated, hypocellular tumours and lack the peripheral EMA staining seen in the perineurium of SCN. Schwannomas are histologically similar but lack the artefactual clefting of SCN.

## Histogenesis
SCN is a benign tumour of nerve fibres, with Schwann cells predominating over axons {786}.

## Prognosis and predictive factors
SCN is benign, and it does not recur after excision.

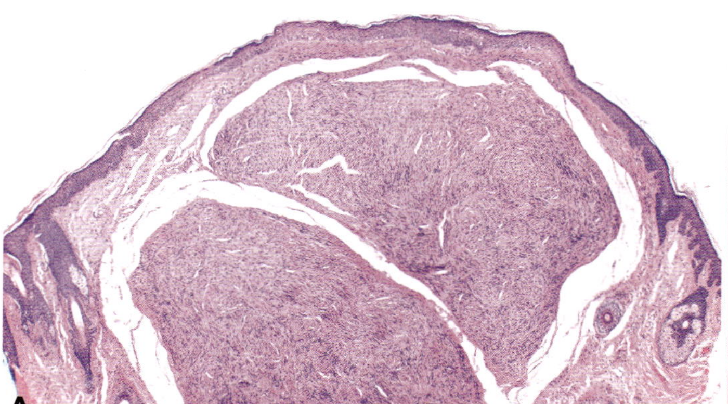
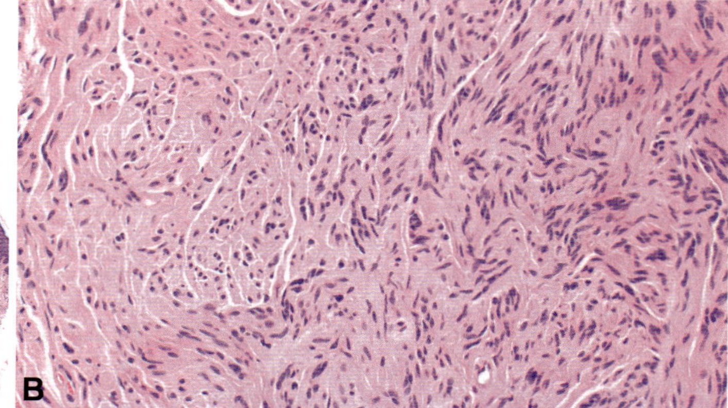

**Fig. 5.147** Solitary circumscribed neuroma. **A** Well-circumscribed dermal tumour shows partial encapsulation. Occasionally, as seen in this case, there is multinodular growth. **B** Bland, elongated spindle cells in fascicles are often separated by artefactual clefts; the nuclei show focal parallel alignment, but prominent palisading is usually absent.

# Dermal nerve sheath myxoma

Kutzner H.

## Definition
Dermal nerve sheath myxoma (NSM) is a benign myxoid cutaneous tumour with nerve sheath differentiation.

## ICD-O code
9562/0

## Synonym
Myxoid neurothekeoma

## Epidemiology
NSM affects all ages (reported range: 8–84 years, median age: 34 years). There is no sex predilection {770}.

## Localization
NSM typically arises in the dermis or subcutis of the limbs, most commonly on the fingers {770}. Involvement of the head and neck region, including the oral cavity, is rare {2250}.

## Clinical features
The tumour presents as a small, painless, slow-growing mass {770}.

## Histopathology
NSM is a characteristically unencapsulated multilobulated tumour composed of highly myxomatous nodules delineated by collagenous septa {1495}. Within the abundant myxoid matrix, there are small spindled to epithelioid Schwann cells in corded, nested, or syncytial-like aggregates; there are also Schwann cells with a ring-like appearance, often with cytoplasmic–nuclear invaginations {770}. Mitoses are uncommon. The tumour cells express S100 protein, GFAP, neuron-specific enolase, p75, and CD57 and are negative for CD63 (NKI/C3) and SMA. There are interspersed CD34-positive stromal fibroblasts and adjacent perineurial fibroblasts positive for EMA (epithelial membrane antigen) {770,1495}.

## Differential diagnosis
Despite its name, so-called cellular neurothekeoma is not a true nerve sheath tumour, as evidenced by its lack of expression of S100 protein and SOX10 {768}. Other differential diagnoses include cutaneous myxoma and myxoid neurofibroma.

## Histogenesis
NSM is of peripheral nerve sheath origin; it is most likely a myxoid variant of schwannoma.

## Genetic profile
There are similarities between the molecular genetic signatures of NSM and dermal schwannoma {2406}, whereas cellular and mixed variants of neurothekeoma closely resemble cellular fibrous histiocytomas, which are composed of myofibroblasts and histiocytes {768}.

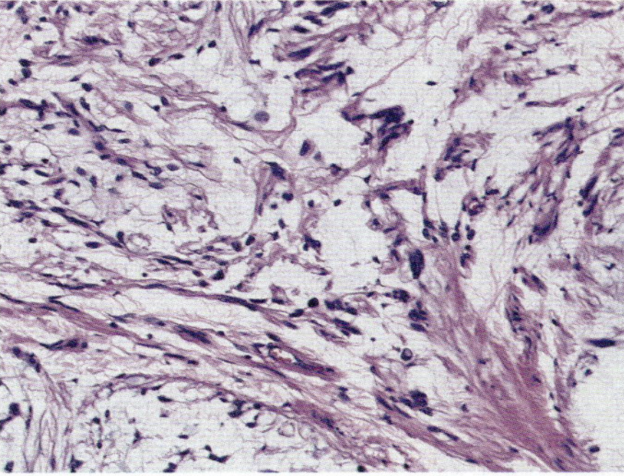

**Fig. 5.150** Dermal nerve sheath myxoma. Slightly pleomorphic tumour cells and delicate collagen fibres in a highly myxoid stroma.

## Prognosis and predictive factors
NSM is a benign tumour, albeit with a high rate of recurrence after incomplete excision {770}.

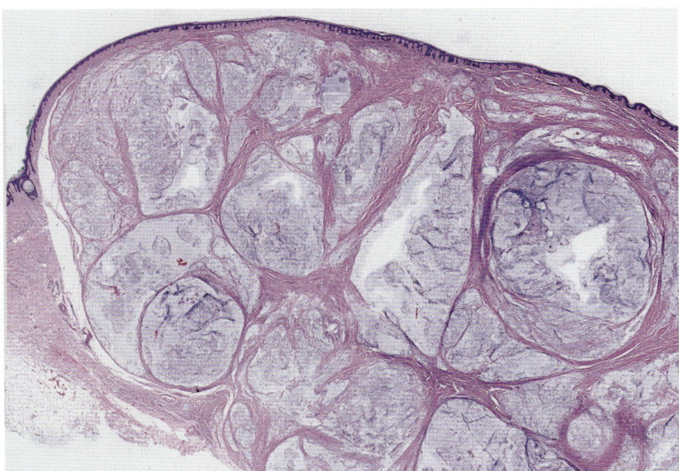

**Fig. 5.148** Dermal nerve sheath myxoma. Multilobulated, unencapsulated dermal tumour.

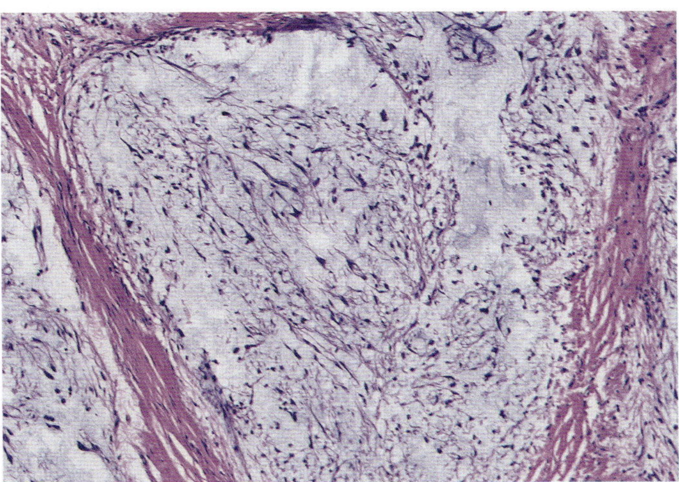

**Fig. 5.149** Dermal nerve sheath myxoma. Stellate and spindled tumour cells within abundant myxoid stroma.

# Perineurioma

Zelger B.
Hornick J.L.

## Definition

Perineurioma is a peripheral nerve sheath tumour with perineurial differentiation arising in the skin, intestinal mucosa {1123}, intraneural tissue {688}, and soft tissue.

## ICD-O codes

| | |
|---|---|
| Perineurioma | 9571/0 |
| Malignant perineurioma | 9571/3 |

## Synonym

Perineurial cell tumour

## Epidemiology

This rare tumour is slightly more common in females. It has a wide age range, with peak incidence among middle-aged adults {1124}. Sclerosing perineuriomas are more common in young adults {774,2872}.

## Localization

Perineurioma has a wide distribution. The most common location is the lower limbs, followed by the upper limbs, trunk, and (rarely) head and neck. Sclerosing perineurioma is more common on the fingers and palms.

## Clinical features

The lesions are well-circumscribed, painless, skin-coloured papules, nodules, or tumours measuring from <5 mm to 20 cm. They occur subcutaneously more often than they involve deep soft tissues; 10% are dermal {1124}. They are rarely multiple {2253}.

## Histopathology

There is a storiform to fascicular growth pattern, with lamellar arrangement, perivascular whorls, and collagenous to myxoid stroma. Rare cases are plexiform {1746,2916} or lipomatous {1614}. Slender spindle cells with wavy, tapering nuclei and delicate bipolar cytoplasmic processes are apparent. Occasionally, degenerative nuclear atypia and/or pleomorphism and multinucleated cells (ancient change) can be seen. Sclerosing perineuriomas show strands of small epithelioid to spindle cells (rarely granular {40}) in dense collagen. Reticular perineuriomas show anastomosing cords of elongated spindle cells with reticular architecture.

Immunohistochemically, EMA (epithelial membrane antigen) is positive, but often only focally. Collagen IV, laminin {364}, claudin-1, and GLUT1 are often positive {805,2872}; about 60% of soft tissue perineuriomas are positive for CD34 {2885}. There is no immunoreactivity for S100 protein or GFAP.

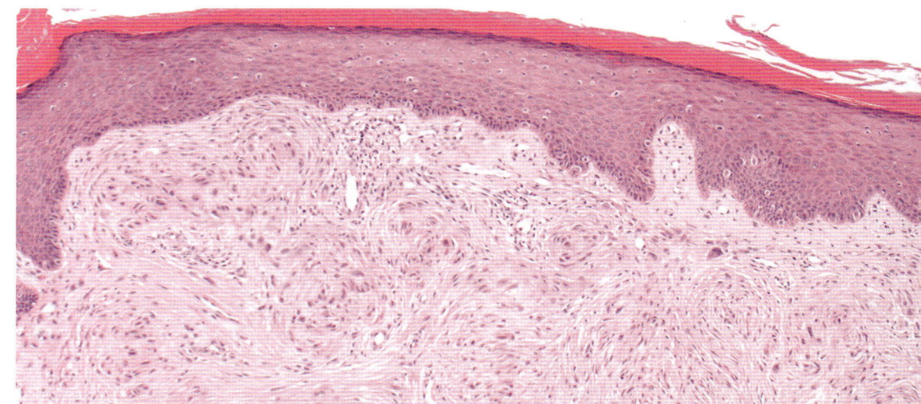

**Fig. 5.151** Cutaneous perineurioma from the hand of a 14-year-old girl. Note the characteristic whorls of short spindled to epithelioid cells.

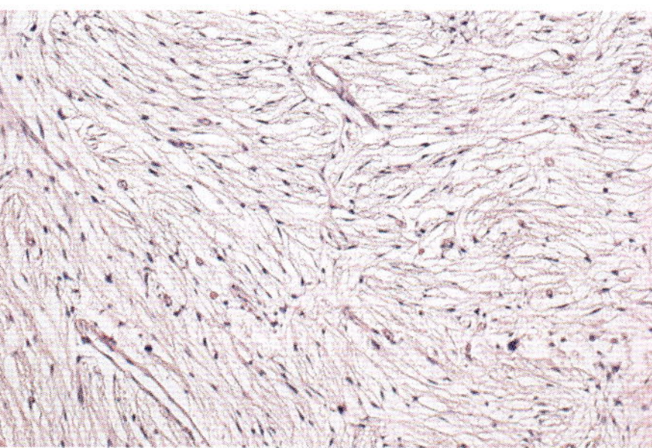

**Fig. 5.152** Reticular perineurioma. Myxoid stroma and reticular arrangement of spindle cells.

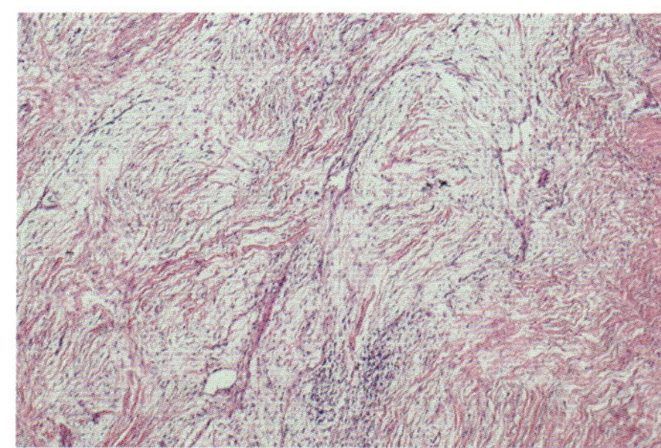

**Fig. 5.153** Soft tissue perineurioma with variably myxoid to collagenous stroma, mimicking low-grade fibromyxoid sarcoma.

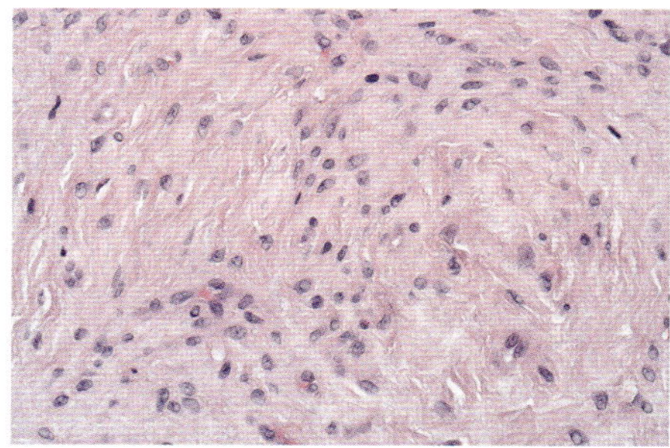

**Fig. 5.154** Sclerosing perineurioma. Epithelioid morphology with sclerotic stroma.

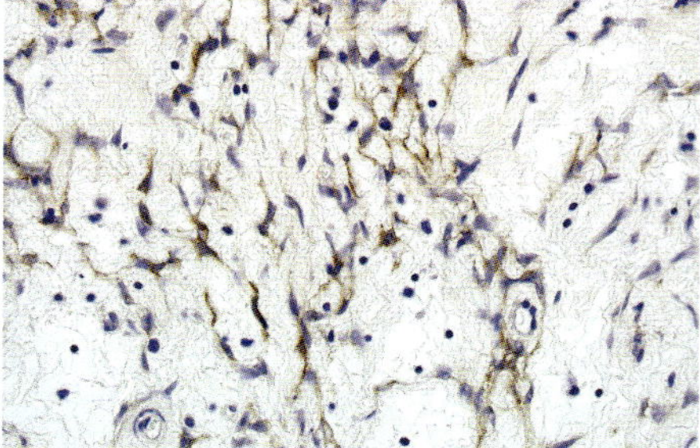

**Fig. 5.155** Perineurioma. EMA (epithelial membrane antigen) marks scattered cells; staining is often patchy and can be faint.

### Differential diagnosis

The differential diagnosis includes epithelioid fibrous histiocytoma, fibroma of tendon sheath, sclerotic fibroma {2206}, extracranial meningioma, and low-grade fibromyxoid sarcoma {774}.

### Histogenesis

Perineurioma shows perineurial differentiation.

### Genetic profile

Chromosome 22 deletions and monosomies are seen, similar to those found in schwannomas {1498,2069}. Chromosome 10q aberrations are found in sclerosing perineuriomas {313,1755}.

### Genetic susceptibility

In rare cases, perineurioma occurs in the setting of neurofibromatosis type 1 or neurofibromatosis type 2 {117,2069}.

### Prognosis and predictive factors

Perineuriomas are benign and rarely recur locally. Exceptionally rare malignant perineuriomas may metastasize, but they are less aggressive than conventional malignant peripheral nerve sheath tumour {1087}.

# Granular cell tumour

Lazar A.J.
Argenyi Z.B.

## Definition

Granular cell tumour is a benign neuroectodermal tumour composed of large, round to oval cells with abundant and distinctly granular cytoplasm.

## ICD-O codes

| | |
|---|---|
| Granular cell tumour | 9580/0 |
| Malignant granular cell tumour | 9580/3 |

## Synonyms

Abrikossoff tumour;
granular cell myoblastoma (obsolete)

## Epidemiology

Granular cell tumour can occur at any age, but most cases arise in the fourth to sixth decades of life. The male-to-female ratio is between 2:1 and 3:1 {1478}.

## Localization

Common sites include the head and neck (in particular the tongue), breast, proximal extremities, gastrointestinal tract, and respiratory tract. Involvement of the skin/subcutis or submucosa is common, but deeper visceral involvement can also occur.

## Clinical features

Lesions in the skin are firm, flesh-coloured to red, and 0.5–3 cm. As many as 10% of cases are multifocal. Exceptionally, granular cell tumours can show malignant change {735}.

## Histopathology

Granular cell tumours most commonly involve the skin/cutis or mucosa. Pseudoepitheliomatous hyperplasia is common {1917}. The tumour borders are poorly defined, and the tumour is composed of packets and trabeculae of large, round to oval cells with distinctly granular and abundant cytoplasm. The cell borders are indistinct and appear syncytial. The centrally located nuclei range from small, uniform, and hyperchromatic to enlarged and vesicular with prominent nucleoli. The finely granular cytoplasm results from massive accumulation of lysosomes, punctuated by larger intracytoplasmic granules surrounded by clear haloes (pustulo-ovoid bodies of Milian). Perineural involvement is frequent. Malignant granular cell tumour (which is exceedingly rare) is recognized by aggressive histological features {735}. The immunohistochemical profile of granular cell tumours includes S100 positivity. CD68, CD63 (NKI/C3), and neuron-specific enolase staining are also positive, but this is likely due to nonspecific reactivity with cytoplasmic lysosomes. Strong nuclear TFE3 and MITF are common, but HMB45 staining is negative, and melan-A is rare and focal {889,2350}. Staining for keratins, GFAP, and NFP is negative.

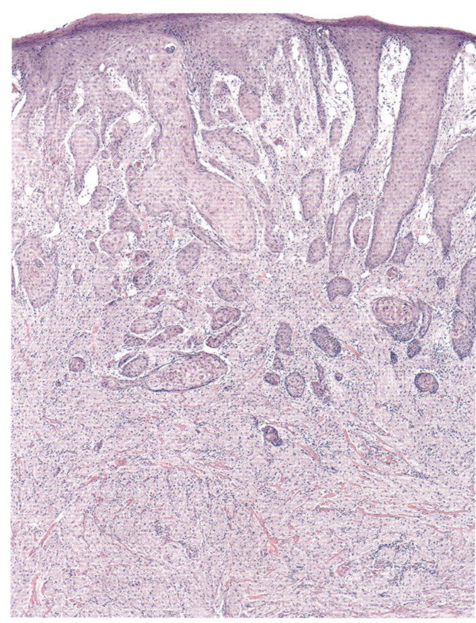

**Fig. 5.156** Granular cell tumour. A dermal example with extensive pseudoepitheliomatous hyperplasia.

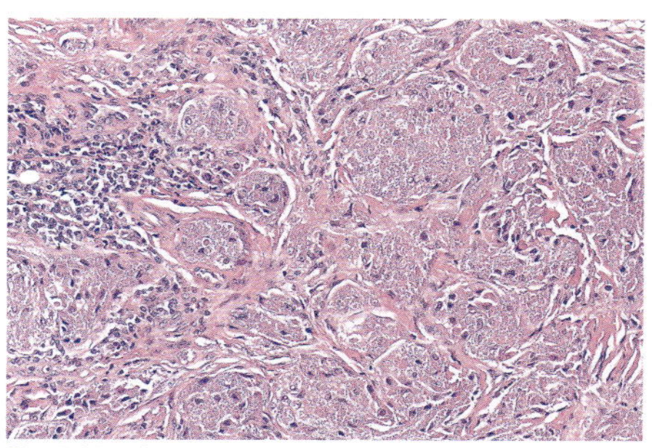

**Fig. 5.157** Granular cell tumour. Packets of granular cells are present in the dermis.

## Differential diagnosis

The differential diagnosis includes primitive non-neural granular cell tumour and rare granular variants of diverse tumours including naevi, melanomas, fibrous histiocytomas, atypical fibroxanthoma, and leiomyosarcoma.

## Histogenesis

Granular cell tumour shows peripheral nerve sheath tumour (Schwannian) differentiation.

## Genetic profile

The genetic profile of granular cell tumour is largely unexplored {378}. In malignant cases analysed as single case reports, no recurrent mutations were found {1880,2796,2869}. These tumours appear to have a low mutation burden.

## Genetic susceptibility

Multiple granular cell tumours have been described in association with Noonan syndrome, LEOPARD syndrome (multiple lentigines, electrocardiographic conduction abnormalities, ocular hypertelorism, pulmonic stenosis, abnormal genitalia, retardation of growth, and sensorineural deafness), and *PTEN* hamartoma tumour syndromes, but most multiple cases are sporadic {830,1587,1660,2352}.

## Prognosis and predictive factors

Granular cell tumour may show local recurrence {1478}. The rare malignant form (accounting for < 1% of all cases) can give rise to metastasis, including distant dissemination.

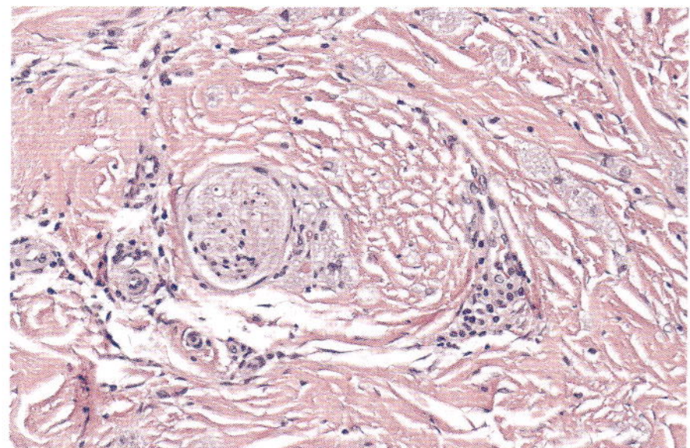

**Fig. 5.158** Granular cell tumour. Perineural infiltration is common.

# Schwannoma

Messina J.
Yeh I.

## Definition
Schwannoma is a benign neoplasm composed of Schwann cells.

## ICD-O code
9560/0

## Synonym
Neurilemmoma

## Epidemiology
Schwannomas typically arise in the fourth to sixth decades of life.

## Etiology
Conventional schwannomas harbour somatic loss-of-function mutations in *NF2* {1203}. Other recurrently mutated tumour suppressors include *ARID1A/B* (mutated in 29% of cases) and *TSC1/2* (in 15%). *SH3PXD2A-HTRA1* fusions (found in 10% of cases) activate the MAPK pathway and are mutually exclusive with mutations in the receptor tyrosine kinase gene *DDR1* (found in 11% of cases) {27}.

## Localization
Schwannomas occur in the soft tissue of the extremities, head and neck, and trunk. Subcutaneous localization is more common than dermal.

## Clinical features
Schwannomas are slow-growing and occasionally painful. They are typically solitary.

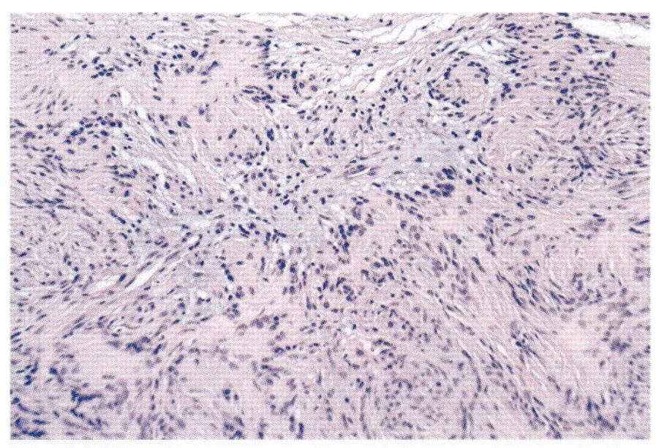
**Fig. 5.159** Schwannoma. Antoni A area demonstrating palisading Verocay bodies.

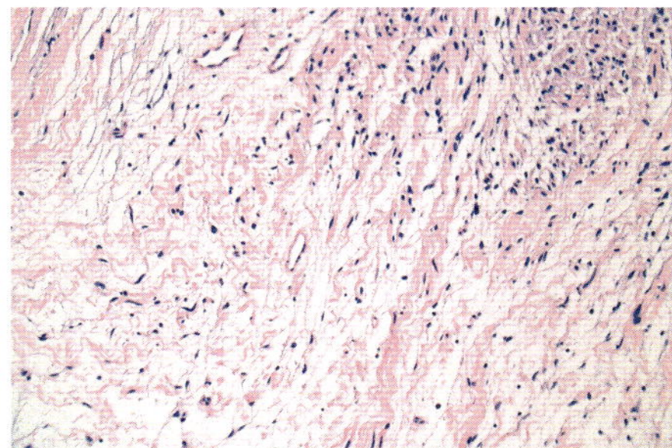
**Fig. 5.160** Schwannoma. Antoni B area demonstrating a hypocellular myxoid region adjacent to Antoni A changes.

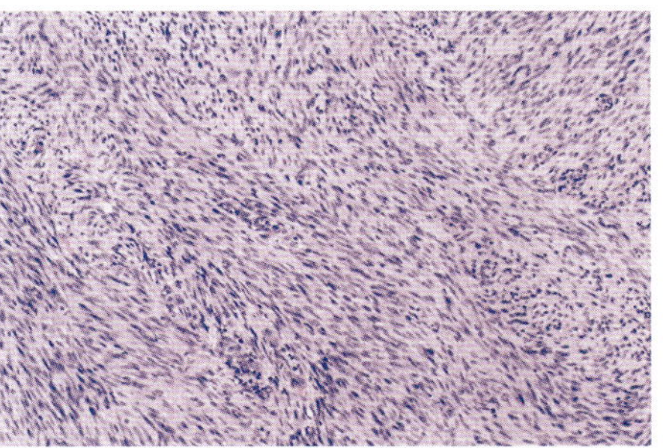
**Fig. 5.161** Cellular schwannoma. Increased cellularity with fascicular architecture.

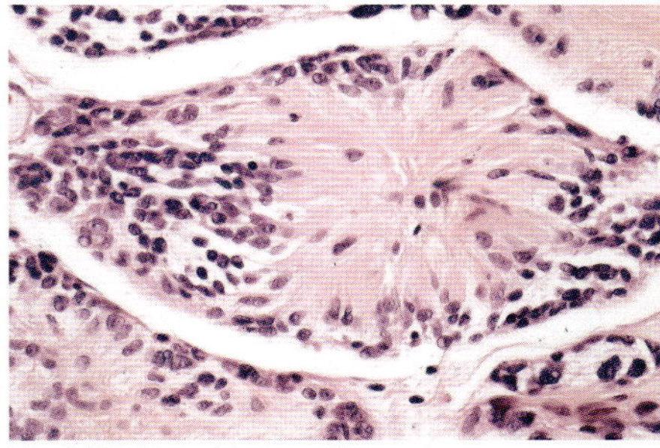
**Fig. 5.162** Neuroblastoma-like schwannoma with a characteristic pseudorosette.

## Histopathology
Antoni A areas containing spindle cells with wavy nuclei alternate with hypocellular Antoni B areas, which contain blood vessels in a myxoid matrix. Within the Antoni A areas, parallel rows of nuclei (Verocay bodies) may be seen. Schwannomas are strongly positive for S100 protein and SOX10, and they have a perineurial capsule that is positive for EMA (epithelial membrane antigen). Mitoses are rare. In so-called ancient schwannoma, there is degenerative nuclear atypia. Rare variants include plexiform, epithelioid, cellular, neuroblastoma-like, and microcystic/reticular schwannoma {790,903,1283,1607,2464}.

## Differential diagnosis
The differential diagnosis includes soli-

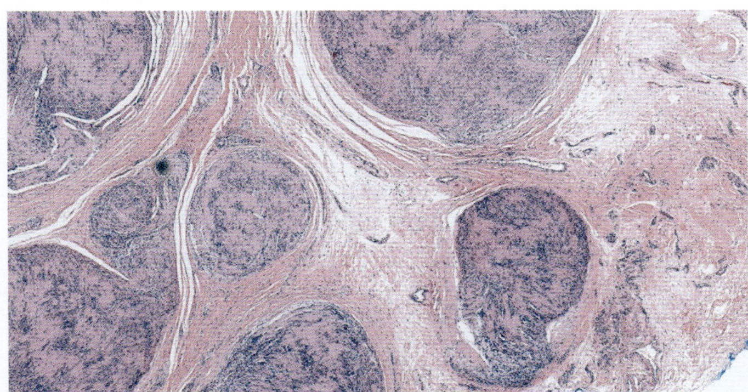
**Fig. 5.163** Plexiform schwannoma. Multiple schwannoma nodules in the dermis.

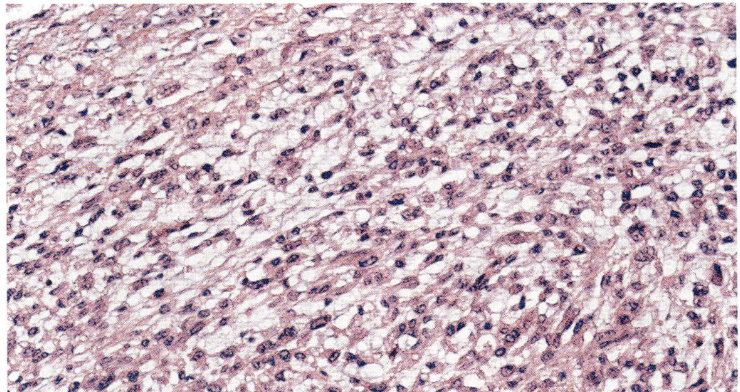
**Fig. 5.164** Epithelioid schwannoma. Epithelioid tumour cells.

tary circumscribed neuroma. For epithelioid schwannoma, it also includes myoepithelioma and ossifying fibromyxoid tumour.

## Histogenesis

Schwannomas arise from the nerve sheath of cranial, spinal, and peripheral nerves.

## Genetic susceptibility

Germline loss-of-function mutations in the tumour suppressors *NF2*, *LZTR1*, and *SMARCB1* are associated with schwannoma susceptibility. Vestibular schwannomas are the hallmark of neurofibromatosis type 2. Schwannomatosis 1 and schwannomatosis 2 are due to germline mutations of *SMARCB1* (which encodes SMARCB1 [INI1]) and *LZTR1*, respectively {1148,2065}; patients with these disorders typically show loss of two tumour suppressors (*NF2* and either *SMARCB1* or *LZTR1*) {1337}. Cutaneous plexiform schwannoma can be seen in the spectrum of neurofibromatosis type 2 {2683}.

## Prognosis and predictive factors

Schwannoma recurs infrequently; malignant transformation is extraordinarily rare.

# Malignant peripheral nerve sheath tumour

Kutzner H.

## Definition

Malignant peripheral nerve sheath tumour (MPNST) is a tumour arising from a peripheral nerve, from a neurofibroma, or in conjunction with neurofibromatosis type 1 {1604,1606,2607}.

## ICD-O codes

| | |
|---|---|
| Malignant peripheral nerve sheath tumour | 9540/3 |
| Epithelioid malignant peripheral nerve sheath tumour | 9542/3 |
| Malignant triton tumour | 9561/3 |

## Synonym

Malignant schwannoma

## Epidemiology

Sporadic cases typically arise in the fourth or fifth decade of life. Cases associated with neurofibromatosis type 1 occur in younger patients. Cutaneous MPNSTs account for 2–5% of all cases {2607,2816}.

## Localization

MPNST affects the lower extremities and trunk {1604}; epithelioid cases can also affect the head and neck {1606}.

## Clinical features

There is a characteristic prolonged period of slow growth, followed by rapid proliferation {2607}.

## Histopathology

Conventional (spindle cell) MPNST shows pleomorphism and varying cellularity (a marbled growth pattern), often with heterologous components. There is often an associated (precursor) neurofibroma. S100 protein is negative to focally positive, and there is frequent loss of H3K27me3 {1604,2099,2335}.

Epithelioid MPNST shows strands and cords of polygonal epithelioid tumour cells (> 50%) surrounded by hyalinized or myxoid stroma, often with divergent heterologous differentiation {1231,1497,1604,1606,2607}. S100 protein is strongly positive, and there is loss of SMARCB1 (INI1) in 50% of cases {391,1231}.

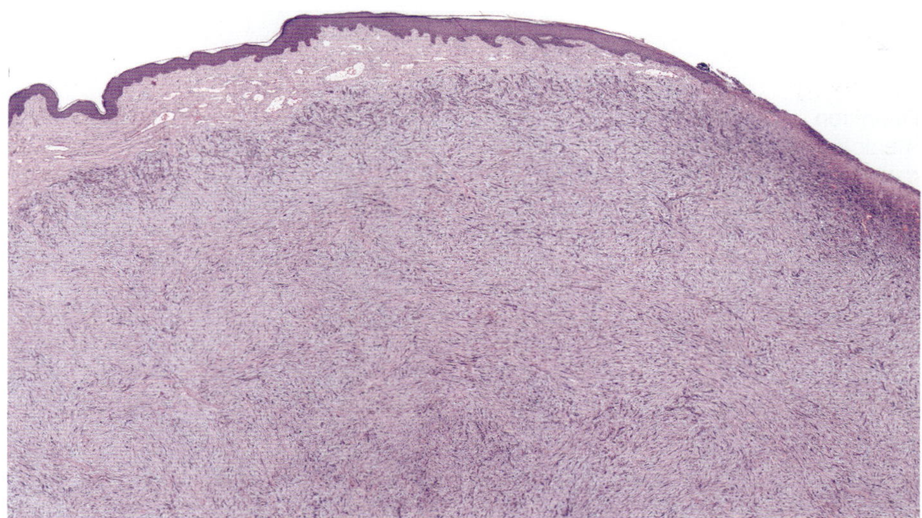

**Fig. 5.165** Malignant peripheral nerve sheath tumour. Sarcomatous tumour with a subepidermal grenz zone and sheets of pleomorphic spindle cells.

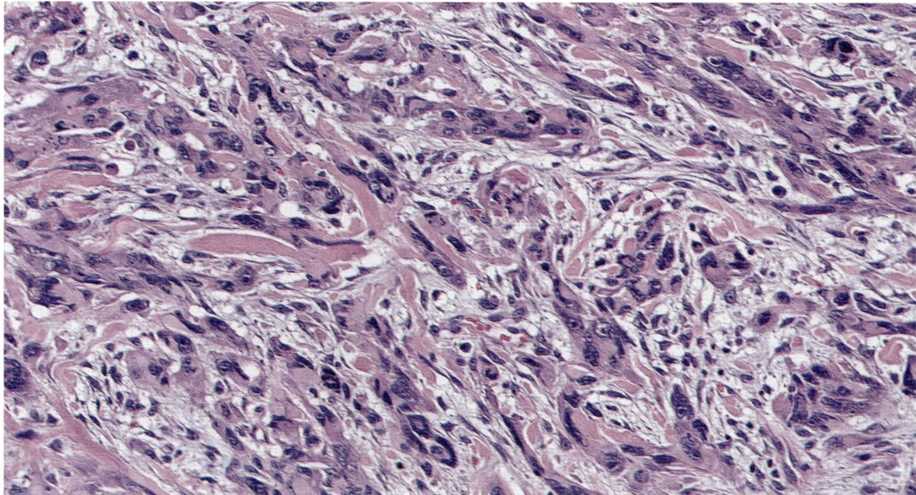

**Fig. 5.166** Malignant peripheral nerve sheath tumour. Marked pleomorphism and a slightly myxoid stroma.

## Differential diagnosis

The differential diagnosis includes spindle cell melanoma, fibrosarcomatous dermatofibrosarcoma protuberans, melanoma, and (myoepithelial) carcinoma.

## Histogenesis

MPNST is of neuroectodermal origin.

## Genetic profile

MPNSTs show complex clonal abnormalities {190,747,1534,2335}.

## Genetic susceptibility

The association of cutaneous MPNST with neurofibromatosis type 1 is somewhat weaker than that of deep-seated MPNST {747,1604}.

## Prognosis and predictive factors

The available data are limited, but cutaneous MPNST may have an aggressive course {60,747,1231,1606}.

# Tumours of uncertain differentiation

## Atypical fibroxanthoma and variants

Beer T.W.
Calonje E.
Wick M.R.

### Definition

Atypical fibroxanthoma (AFX) is a dermally based neoplasm of uncertain histogenesis. Tumours that meet the strict diagnostic criteria generally behave in a low-grade fashion. Most cases arise on sun-damaged sites in elderly individuals. The diagnosis requires evaluation of multiple immunostains.

### ICD-O code

Atypical fibroxanthoma 8830/1

### Synonyms

Superficial malignant fibrous histiocytoma (obsolete); dermal undifferentiated pleomorphic sarcoma

### Epidemiology

These rare tumours occur most commonly in sun-damaged skin of elderly White individuals, in particular those living in areas with high solar radiation {189,1182,1603}. Males are affected more often than females. AFXs have also been reported in young patients with Li–Fraumeni syndrome (i.e. with germline mutation of *TP53* {1533}) and xeroderma pigmentosum {2399,2485}.

### Etiology

Evidence of an association with ultraviolet (UV) radiation exposure includes clinical factors, the association with Li–Fraumeni syndrome and xeroderma pigmentosum, and the finding of UV radiation signature mutations in *TP53* {602,2282,2399,2485}. Some cases have occurred in fields of radiotherapy {1182,1590}, as well as in the contexts of immunosuppression and organ transplantation {1710}.

### Localization

The tumours usually develop at sun-exposed sites, especially on the head and neck. The ear is a particularly common location. Purported examples developing on the limbs of young people are likely to in fact be other entities, such as atypical fibrous histiocytoma.

### Clinical features

AFX often presents as a solitary, localized nodule as large as 2 cm in diameter, occurring on sun-damaged skin {189,1603,1788,2938}. Ulceration is common, often with a short history of rapid growth. Although there are no specific clinical features, the diagnosis can sometimes be suspected given the context and lack of pigmentation or features pointing to a diagnosis of basal cell carcinoma or squamous cell carcinoma (SCC).

### Histopathology

A frequently circumscribed dermal tumour is present, with no involvement of the subcutis. The lesions are typically highly cellular, with striking nuclear enlargement, pleomorphism, and atypia.

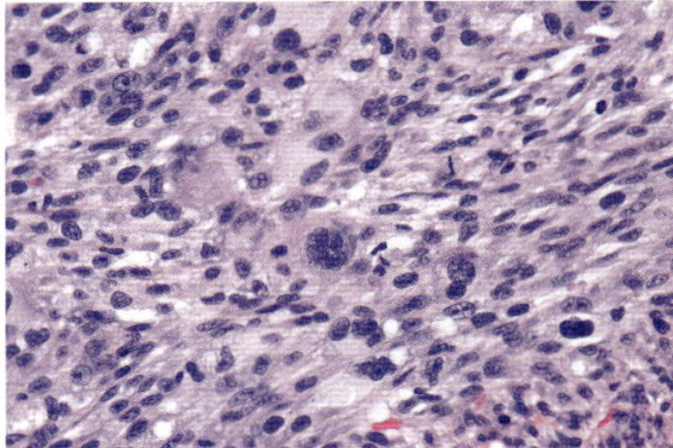

**Fig. 5.167** Atypical fibroxanthoma. Multinucleated tumour cells and mitoses are frequently identifiable.

Mitoses (including atypical forms) are frequent. Enlarged spindle or epithelioid cells are seen, some with a histiocyte-like appearance. Irregular fascicles may be present, with scattered inflammatory cells and occasionally with areas of haemorrhage. Ulceration is common, sometimes with an epidermal collarette or atrophy. Necrosis is not a feature in most cases; when present, it is of very limited extent microscopically. Plaque-like growth is occasionally seen, with a band of cells parallel to the epidermis; these lesions may be less well circumscribed {189}.

Spindle cell AFX shows exclusively spindle-shaped cells in fascicles with eosinophilic cytoplasm, vesicular nuclei, and prominent nucleoli {1010}. Sometimes the cytological features of this variant are relatively bland. Clear cell AFX exhibits cells with clear to foamy cytoplasm and hyperchromatic, pleomorphic nuclei

**Table 5.03** Selected immunostaining results for the differential diagnosis of atypical fibroxanthoma (AFX)

| Marker(s) | AFX | Cellular and atypical dermatofibroma (fibrous histiocytoma) | Poorly differentiated SCC (primary or secondary) | Melanoma | Leiomyosarcoma |
|---|---|---|---|---|---|
| S100 protein and SOX10 | – | – | – | + | – |
| Desmin and h-caldesmon | – | – | – | – | + |
| Cytokeratins | – | – | + | – | Rarely + |
| EMA (epithelial membrane antigen) | Rarely + | – | Variable | – | – |
| SMA | Often + | Variable | Rarely + | Variable | + |
| +/– (if not otherwise qualified), positive/negative staining is typical; SCC, squamous cell carcinoma. | | | | | |

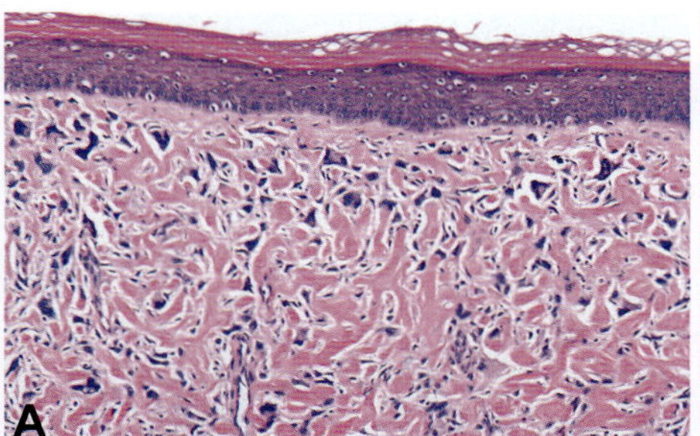
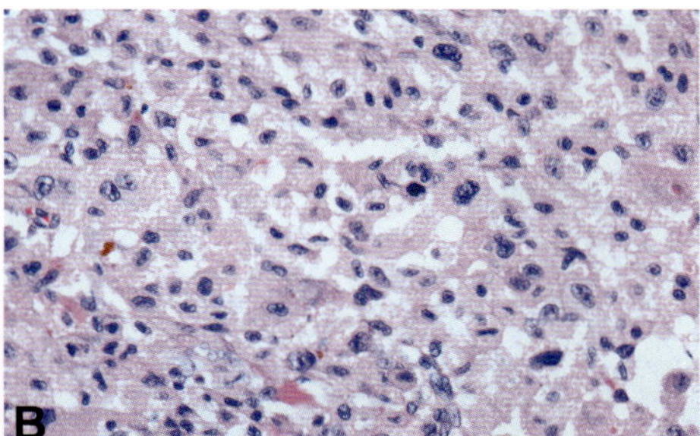
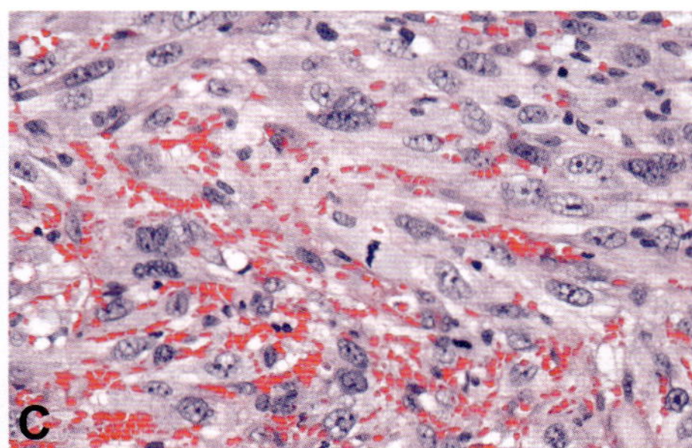

**Fig. 5.168** Atypical fibroxanthoma (AFX) variants. **A** This tumour shows keloidal change; in other zones, the lesion was almost entirely composed of eosinophilic collagen fibres, with only very sparse remaining malignant cells. **B** This example of AFX exhibits granular cells with haemorrhage and pigmentation due to haemosiderin deposition. **C** Extensive haemorrhage in AFX sometimes raises the differential diagnosis of angiosarcoma.

{2579}. Glycogen is of limited extent or absent. Other variants include granular cell, keloidal, myxoid, and sclerotic forms. Regression (which can be extensive) is sometimes seen, making diagnosis on a partial biopsy challenging. Pigmented AFXs show haemosiderin deposition and haemorrhage {120}. By definition, AFX is a diagnosis of exclusion; markers of specific differentiation must be negative (see below).

## Differential diagnosis

Lesions that resemble AFX but are large or show substantial invasion of the subcutis or beyond, perineural invasion, lymphovascular invasion, or necrosis should instead be classified as pleomorphic dermal sarcoma (PDS) {1778}. The diagnosis of AFX should be rendered with caution on partial biopsies if the depth of permeation and extent of the lesion cannot be ascertained, since the lesion could be PDS. Because primary or secondary melanoma and SCC can mimic AFX, evidence of junctional activity, melanin, or keratinization should be sought. Leiomyosarcoma and angiosarcoma are also considerations. Atypical fibrous histiocytoma (dermatofibroma with monster cells) generally occurs in younger patients, with an absence of severe solar elastosis and sometimes with surrounding changes of more-typical dermatofibroma {1261}.

Immunohistochemistry is vital for excluding other malignancies, in particular melanoma, leiomyosarcoma, and poorly differentiated SCC (see Table 5.03). A broad panel of immunostains is essential. In particular, melanocyte markers (e.g. SOX10, melan-A, and S100 protein) and keratinocyte markers (e.g. MNF116, AE1/AE3, 34βE12, p63, and p40) are negative in AFX {189,886,1061,1603}. Included S100-positive Langerhans cells, which can be numerous, can be confirmed with staining for langerin or CD1a. Many AFXs are MITF-positive {2564}. In some studies, most tumours stained for SMA, but strong desmin or h-caldesmon staining could suggest leiomyosarcoma {1010}. CD10 is frequently strongly expressed in AFX (and may be the only positive stain), but it is nonspecific and can also be seen in melanoma and SCC. CD68 and CD163, although often positive, are of limited diagnostic value and also stain included macrophages. Multinucleated tumour giant cells may show nonspecific staining for HMB45 antigen and calponin. In vascular-looking AFX, negative staining for CD34 and ERG may be required to exclude angiosarcoma. Some AFXs express CD31 and EMA (epithelial membrane antigen) without evidence of other epithelial marker positivity.

## Genetic susceptibility

Comparative genomic hybridization has revealed various genomic changes, with most tumours found to have 9p and 13q deletions {1776}. Activating mutations have been identified in the promoter region of the *TERT* gene {938}. AFXs have occurred in the setting of Li–Fraumeni syndrome (with germline *TP53* mutation) {1533} and xeroderma pigmentosum {439,2008,2399}. One patient with AFX and xeroderma pigmentosum was found to harbour both *TP53* mutation and germline mutation of the *CDKN2A* (*INK4a-ARF*) gene {2485}.

## Prognosis and predictive factors

Most AFXs behave in a benign fashion, provided that stringent criteria are used for diagnosis. As many as 5% of cases recur, usually due to incomplete excision. Metastases have been reported rarely {523,1060,2781}. Some of the reported cases may in fact be other entities (including PDS), because some reports predate immunohistochemistry, or only limited immunostains were documented, or there was no clear distinction between AFX and PDS.

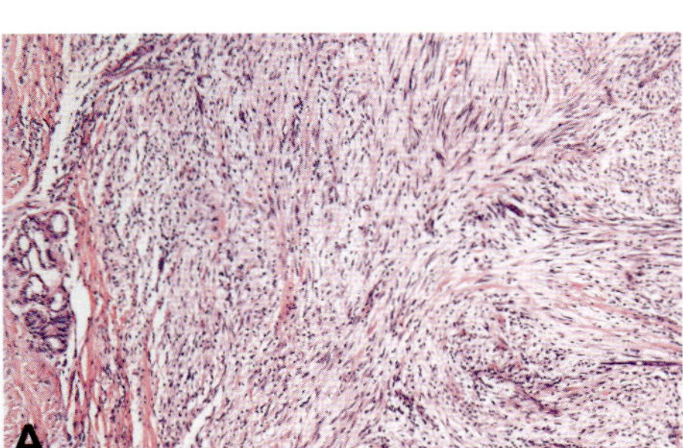
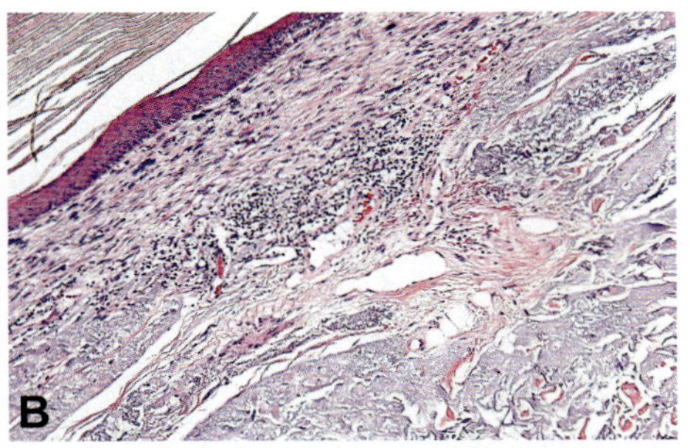

**Fig. 5.169** Atypical fibroxanthoma. **A** Myxoid variant. **B** Plaque-like variant, with cells lying parallel to the epidermis. Centrally, this tumour showed features more typical of atypical fibroxanthoma, with a nodule invading deep into the dermis.

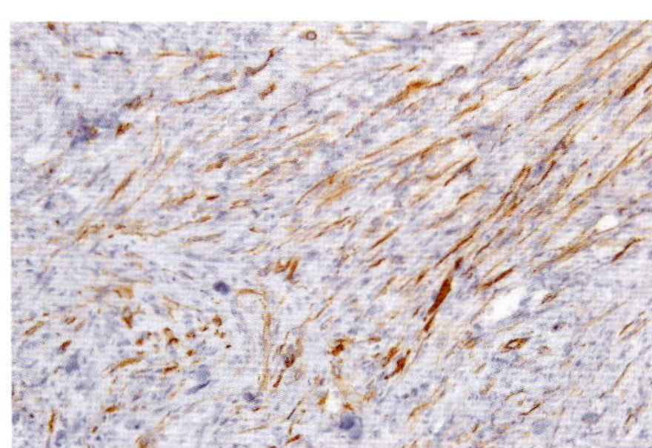

**Fig. 5.170** Atypical fibroxanthoma. SMA positivity is frequent.

# Pleomorphic dermal sarcoma

Brenn T.
Wick M.R.

## Definition

Pleomorphic dermal sarcoma (PDS) is an undifferentiated pleomorphic tumour possibly related to (and with clinical, histological, and immunohistochemical features similar to those of) atypical fibroxanthoma. The additional presence of subcutaneous tissue invasion, tumour necrosis, and perineurial or lymphovascular invasion confers risk for more-aggressive behaviour.

## ICD-O code 8802/3

## Synonyms

Undifferentiated pleomorphic sarcoma of the skin; superficial malignant fibrous histiocytoma (obsolete)

## Epidemiology

PDS exclusively presents on sun-damaged skin of elderly patients (median patient age: 81 years) {1778,2580}. White populations are affected more commonly, with a male predominance {1778}.

## Etiology

Ultraviolet (UV) radiation–induced damage and immunosuppression are etiological factors {938,1778,2580}.

## Localization

These tumours typically affect the head, with a predilection for the scalp {1778,2580}.

## Clinical features

The tumours are rapidly growing large nodules or plaques, measuring several centimetres (median size: 2.5 cm). Ulceration is common.

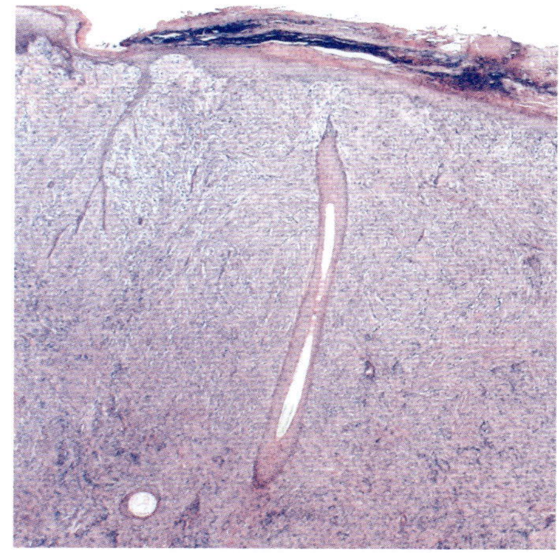

**Fig. 5.171** Pleomorphic dermal sarcoma. This large and cellular tumour is based within the dermis and extends to the overlying epidermis.

## Histopathology

The tumours are centred within the dermis, with an expansile nodular or plaque-like growth pattern. They are poorly demarcated, with irregular edges and diffuse infiltration of subcutaneous adipose tissue, skeletal muscle, or fascia. Ulceration of the overlying epidermis is common. PDS is composed of sheets of pleomorphic tumour cells containing an admixture of epithelioid, spindle, and multinucleated giant cells. The tumour cells vary in size but are typically large, with abundant and variably frothy cytoplasm containing hyperchromatic or vesicular nuclei with prominent and often multiple eosinophilic nucleoli. Nuclear pleomorphism is a striking feature and mitotic activity (including atypical mitoses) is brisk. Tumour necrosis is identified in 50% of cases, and perineural infiltration and lymphovascular invasion in approximately 30%. A subset of cases are composed mainly of atypical spindle cells in a fascicular arrangement. Additional findings include myxoid, desmoplastic, or keloidal stromal change; pseudoangiomatous features; a storiform growth pattern; and admixed osteoclast-like multinucleated giant cells.

Immunohistochemically, the tumour cells are consistently negative for S100 protein, HMB45 antigen, cytokeratins, CD34, ERG, and desmin {1778,2580,2611}. CD10 staining is strong and diffuse. SMA is expressed in 70% of cases, CD31 in 30%, EMA (epithelial membrane antigen) in 16%, and melan-A in 6% {1778,2580,2610,2611}.

## Differential diagnosis

The main differential diagnoses are atypical fibroxanthoma, melanoma, poorly differentiated carcinoma, leiomyosarcoma, and angiosarcoma. PDS can be distinguished from atypical fibroxanthoma by the demonstration of subcutaneous tissue invasion, tumour necrosis, or lymphovascular or perineurial invasion. Melanoma and carcinoma are excluded by negative staining for S100 protein and cytokeratins, respectively.

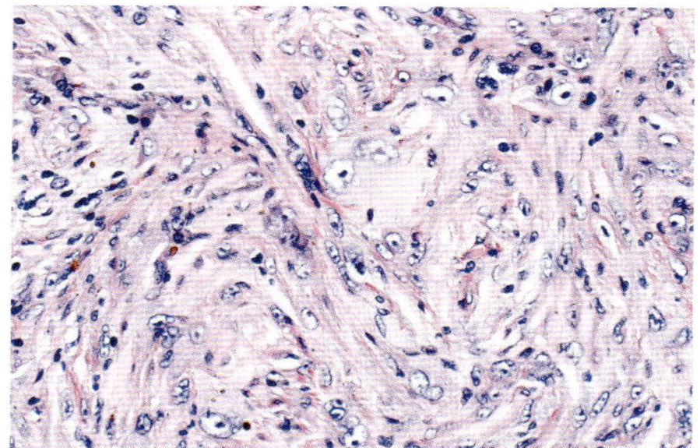

**Fig. 5.172** Pleomorphic dermal sarcoma. Tumour cells are epithelioid and spindled, showing marked nuclear atypia; multinucleated tumour giant cells are admixed.

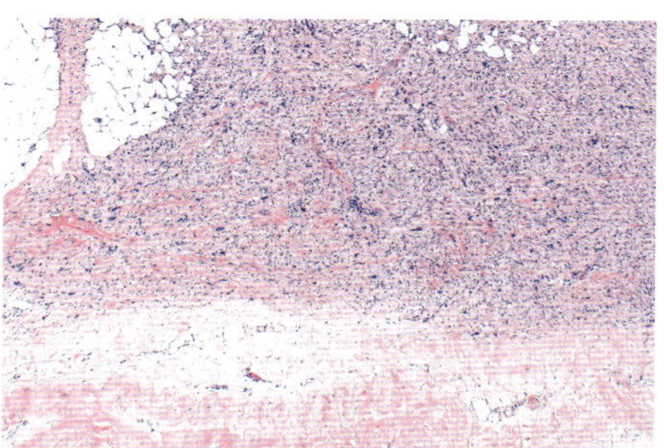

**Fig. 5.173** Pleomorphic dermal sarcoma. This tumour is characterized by infiltrative growth, with invasion of subcutaneous adipose tissue and the underlying galea.

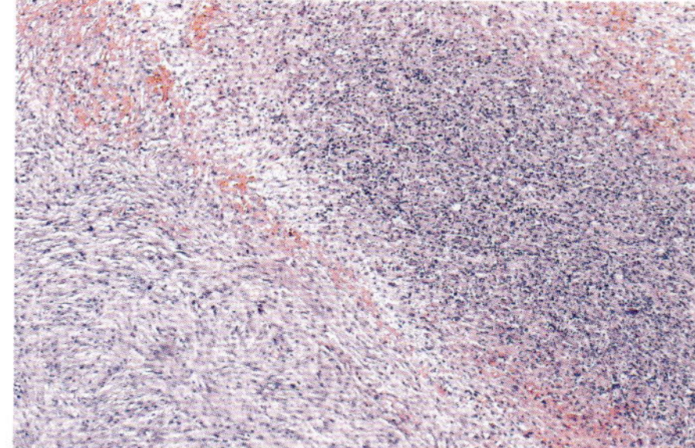

**Fig. 5.174** Pleomorphic dermal sarcoma with focal necrosis on the right.

Leiomyosarcoma is characterized by a more brightly eosinophilic cytoplasm and by desmin expression. Poorly differentiated angiosarcoma and PDS may show overlapping clinical and histological features, and they share immunoexpression of CD31 and FLI1. ERG immunohistochemistry is a reliable differentiating tool in difficult cases: cutaneous angiosarcoma consistently expresses ERG, whereas there is no expression in PDS.

### Histogenesis

PDS is an undifferentiated tumour of uncertain histogenesis, closely related to atypical fibroxanthoma.

### Genetic profile

PDS is associated with sun damage, and the tumours carry the *TP53* UV radiation signature mutation as well as mutations in the *TERT* promoter {938,1058,2282}. Other reported genetic alterations include activating mutations in *HRAS* and *PIK3CA*.

### Prognosis and predictive factors

PDS has a 20–30% risk for local recurrence and metastasis to skin, lymph nodes, and lung {1778,2580}. The presence of metastatic disease is associated with high mortality rates {2580,2781}.

# Myxofibrosarcoma

Billings S.D.
Lazar A.J.

### Definition

Myxofibrosarcoma is a variably cellular, lobular, and infiltrative spindle cell sarcoma with myxoid stroma and often curvilinear vasculature.

### ICD-O code 8811/3

### Synonym

Myxoid malignant fibrous histiocytoma (historical, now obsolete)

### Epidemiology

Myxofibrosarcoma is one of the most common sarcomas in elderly individuals. Most patients are in their sixth to eighth decades of life, with a slight male predominance; occurrence before the age of 30 years is exceptional.

### Localization

These tumours most commonly involve the extremities, with the lower limbs (in particular the thigh) involved more commonly than the upper limbs. Approximately half of all cases occur in the dermis and subcutis; the rest involve deeper compartments {1519,1744,2303,2801}.

### Clinical features

A painless, slow-growing mass is the usual presentation. Repeated local recurrence is common, often with histological progression over time. Intermediate-grade and high-grade myxofibrosarcomas have an increased risk of metastasis, typically to the lung.

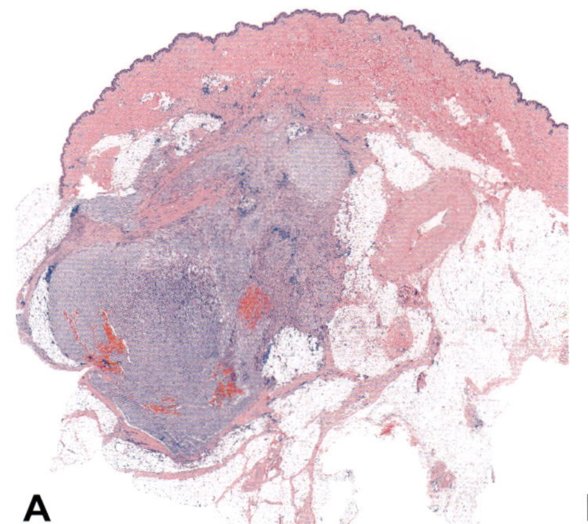


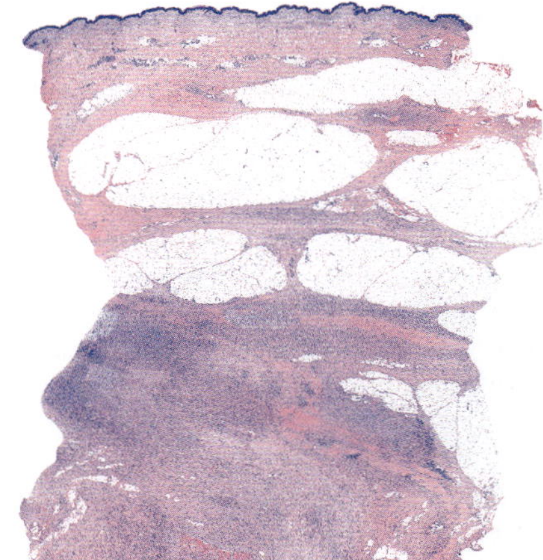


**Fig. 5.175** Myxofibrosarcoma. These tumours are usually multinodular (**A**), and they can be very infiltrative along fibrous septa (**B**).

### Histopathology

Myxofibrosarcoma has a spectrum of appearances, ranging from a hypocellular and extensively myxoid low-grade form to a more cellular spindle cell form in which the myxoid component is less prominent. Low-grade myxofibrosarcoma is a multinodular, infiltrative tumour that extends along fibrous septa of the subcutis, composed variably of spindle cells lacking overt atypia admixed with more-pleomorphic forms {736,2219}. Curvilinear vessels are frequently conspicuous, and tumour cells often cluster around the vessels. Pseudolipoblasts with multivacuolated cytoplasm due to mucinous content are common. Mitoses are sparse in low-grade myxofibrosarcoma. Higher-grade lesions, which show increased mitoses, cellularity, and sometimes necrosis, can become indistinguishable from undifferentiated pleomorphic sarcoma. A transition from low-grade to higher-grade areas is often present. Rare epithelioid variants exist {1877}. Consistent with the presumed fibroblastic/myofibroblastic differentiation, patchy SMA expression is common, but most other immunostains are negative. CD34 expression may be seen {2471}.

## Differential diagnosis

The differential diagnosis includes cutaneous myxoma, myxoid dermatofibrosarcoma protuberans, low-grade fibromyxoid sarcoma, myxoid spindle cell lipoma, and other higher-grade sarcomas that can show myxoid features.

## Histogenesis

Myxofibrosarcoma is believed to show fibroblastic differentiation.

## Genetic profile

Myxofibrosarcoma is a complex-karyotype sarcoma, with chromosomal structure rearrangements, copy-number alterations, and aneuploidy seen even in low-grade cases. Recurrence with histological progression is associated with increasing genomic complexity.

## Prognosis and predictive factors

The 5-year overall survival rate is about 77% {2303}. The prognosis for low-grade myxofibrosarcoma is good, despite local recurrence rates being 18–54%, independent of grade {1744,2303}. Lower extremity cases can have lower rates of local recurrence than other sites {1519}. The rates of local recurrence are similar in superficial and deep cases, but survival is inferior in deep cases (as they tend to be larger and of higher grade), but this has not been found to be an independent risk factor in multivariate analyses {1519,1744,2303}. Intermediate-grade and high-grade myxofibrosarcomas appear to be less aggressive (with metastasis rates of 15–23%) than undifferentiated pleomorphic sarcoma or other higher-grade sarcomas in the extremities {944,1858,2801}. Higher myxoid content is associated with better outcome; a recognizable myxoid component of even 5% confers superior outcome {1519,2801}. Compared with conventional cases, myxofibrosarcomas with epithelioid features are more aggressive, and they have a substantial risk of lymph node metastasis {1877}.

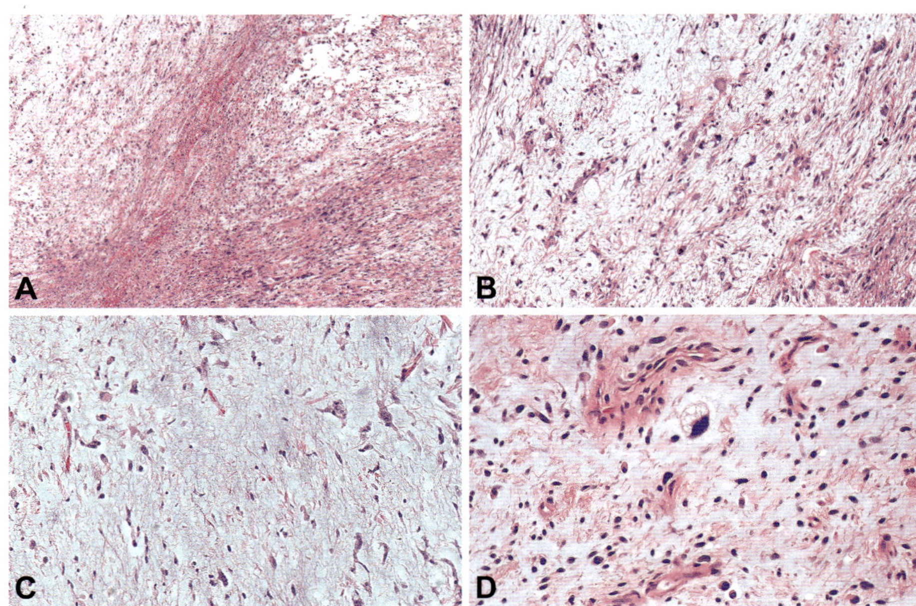

**Fig. 5.176** Myxofibrosarcoma. **A** Nodules are separated by fibrous septa. **B** Atypical and pleomorphic cells surround curvilinear vessels. **C** The myxoid component can be extensive, with only rare atypical cells. **D** Pseudolipoblasts can be seen.

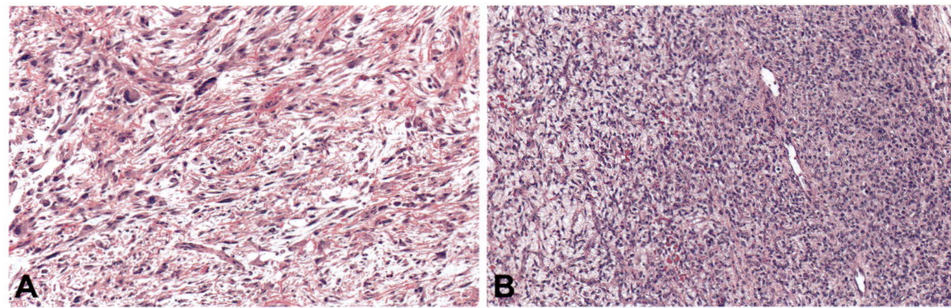

**Fig. 5.177** Myxofibrosarcoma. The higher-grade forms show variable cellularity, from intermediate (**A**) to high (**B**). The proportion of the myxoid component and the tumour cell morphology can also vary.

# Epithelioid sarcoma

Hornick J.L.
Patel R.M.

## Definition

Epithelioid sarcoma is a rare soft tissue sarcoma composed of epithelioid cells with an epithelial phenotype. Classic (distal) and proximal types have been described. Classic epithelioid sarcoma often involves the skin.

## ICD-O code 8804/3

## Epidemiology

Epithelioid sarcoma accounts for 0.6–1% of all sarcomas and 4–8% of childhood sarcomas {395,1575,2236}. It is most common among individuals aged 10–35 years (median age: 25 years) and shows a male predominance {275,441,860,993}.

## Etiology

Epithelioid sarcoma is sporadic.

## Localization

Epithelioid sarcoma arises most commonly in the hands, fingers, and forearms, followed by the feet, toes, and ankles {275,695,993}.

## Clinical features

Epithelioid sarcoma presents as single or multiple painless, slow-growing, ulcerated nodules, which are often mistaken for a reactive or infectious process. A low level of clinical suspicion for malignancy may lead to a delay in diagnosis. Epithelioid sarcoma can also present as a larger, deep-seated, infiltrative mass. Unlike other sarcomas, epithelioid sarcoma often metastasizes to lymph nodes, as well as more distant sites.

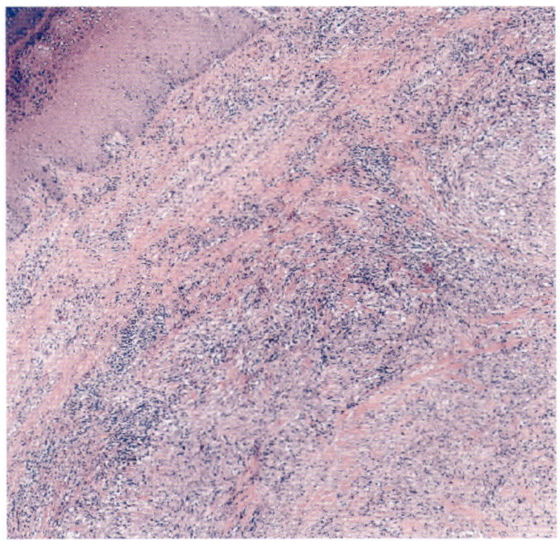

**Fig. 5.178** Epithelioid sarcoma. Nodular growth pattern within the dermis; note the areas of necrosis resembling a necrotizing granulomatous process.

## Histopathology

Epithelioid sarcoma is composed of infiltrative, cellular nodules of epithelioid cells with eosinophilic cytoplasm and uniform, vesicular nuclei. Central necrosis of tumour nodules can mimic the appearance of a necrobiotic granuloma {695,1056}. Spindle cells sometimes predominate. Pseudoglandular and pseudovascular architecture, myxoid change, calcification, and bone formation may be seen {441,1430,1771,2750}. Proximal-type epithelioid sarcoma, which has more nuclear atypia, prominent nucleoli, eccentric nuclei, and eosinophilic cytoplasm, resembles extrarenal rhabdoid tumour {959}.

Epithelioid sarcoma expresses low-molecular-weight and high-molecular-weight cytokeratins, EMA (epithelial membrane antigen), and CD34 (in 50% of cases) {1563,1771}. More than 90% of cases show loss of SMARCB1 (INI1) {1108,1121,1953,2284,2614}. Epithelioid sarcoma may express ERG and FLI1 {1774,2515}.

## Differential diagnosis

The differential diagnosis includes granulomatous processes, carcinomas, and epithelioid vascular tumours.

## Genetic profile

Monoallelic or biallelic *SMARCB1* deletion is a consistent finding in epithelioid sarcoma {1511,1809,2531} and is often accompanied by overexpression of particular microRNAs, implicating both genetic and epigenetic silencing {1411,1980,2314}. Epithelioid sarcoma has a high mutation rate and a complex genome {1213}.

## Prognosis and predictive factors

Epithelioid sarcoma recurs in >70% of cases, and about 50% of patients develop metastases, often following a protracted course {144,445,2496}. The 5-year and 10-year survival rates for all types of epithelioid sarcoma combined are 60–80% and 42–62%, respectively {144,353,860}. Adverse prognostic factors include male sex, older age, multifocality, high mitotic rate, nodal involvement, proximal location, size >5 cm, deep location, and extensive necrosis {144,445,1200}.

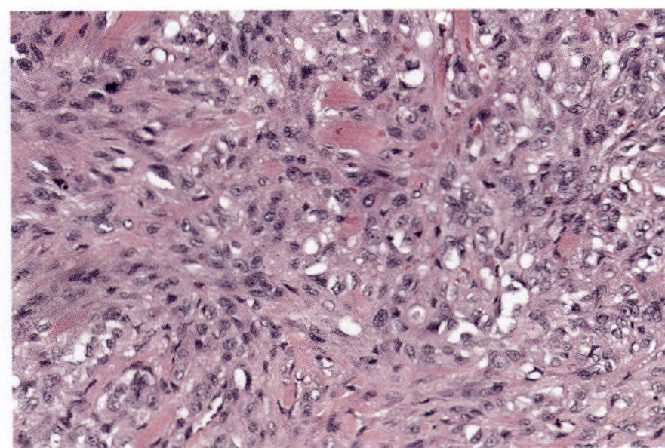

**Fig. 5.179** Epithelioid sarcoma. Epithelioid cells with vesicular chromatin and abundant eosinophilic cytoplasm.

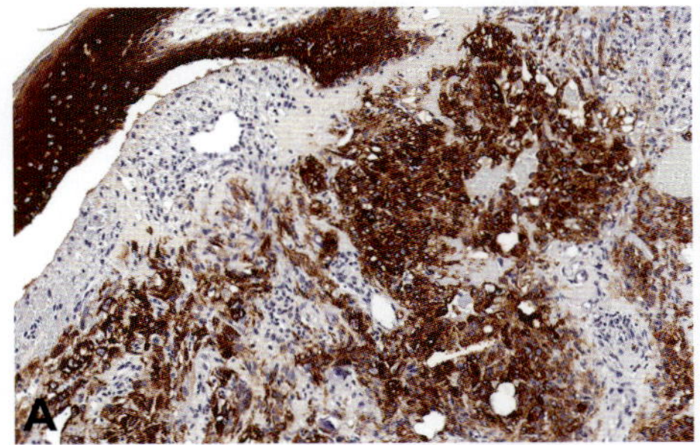


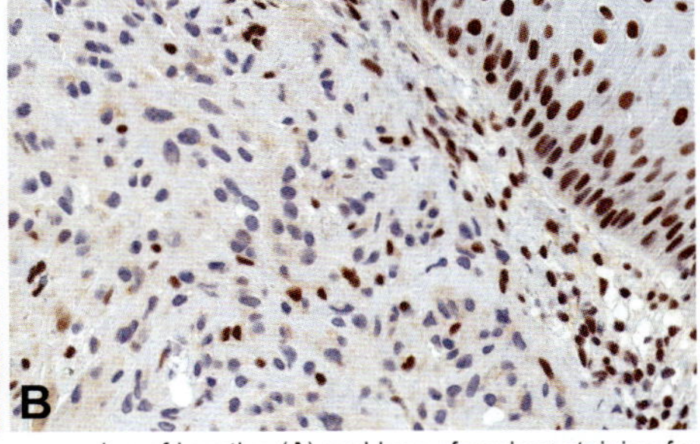


**Fig. 5.180** Epithelioid sarcoma. This entity shows diffuse expression of keratins (**A**) and loss of nuclear staining for SMARCB1 (INI1) (**B**).

# Dermal clear cell sarcoma

Busam K.J.
Kutzner H.

## Definition

Dermal clear cell sarcoma is a malignant neoplasm of uncertain histogenesis showing melanocytic differentiation.

## ICD-O code 9044/3

## Synonym

Melanoma of soft parts {481}

## Epidemiology

This tumour tends to affect young adults, most commonly arising during the third to fourth decades of life {481,694,1005}.

## Localization

The tumour predominantly affects the distal extremities {1005,1382,2440}.

## Clinical features

The tumours present as amelanotic nodules {2440}.

## Histopathology

Dermal clear cell sarcoma is characterized by fascicles and nests of usually amelanotic spindled and epithelioid cells. Their cytoplasm may display clear cell features. Multinucleated wreath-type giant cells and collagenous septa may be seen. The nuclear features and number of mitoses are variable. A grenz zone is present in most tumours {1005}. Rare cases may show junctional nests or solitary tumour cells in the epidermis (compound clear cell sarcoma) {1382}. Immunohistochemically, the tumour cells express S100 protein and SOX10, as well as melanocyte differentiation antigens such as HMB45 antigen, melan-A, and MITF {2440}.

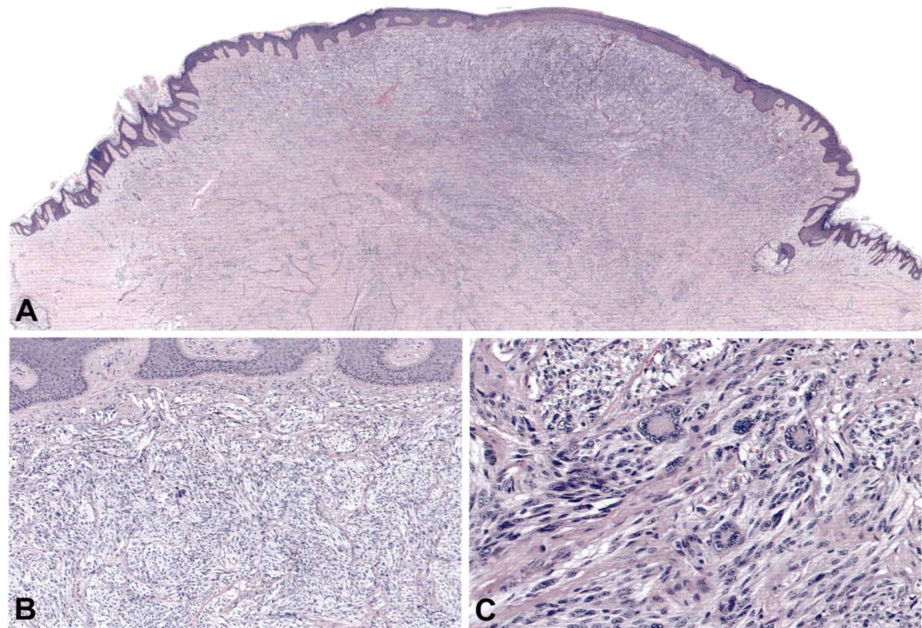


**Fig. 5.181** Dermal clear cell sarcoma. **A** Amelanotic dermal tumour extending into the superficial subcutis. A grenz zone separates the epidermis from the dermal neoplasm. **B** Compact fascicles of spindle and epithelioid cells are present in the dermis, separated by thin strands of collagen. Some tumour cells display clear cell features. **C** Multinucleated wreath-like giant cells are present.

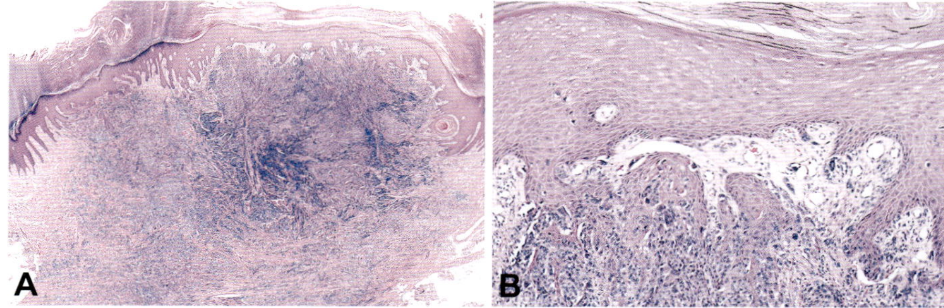


**Fig. 5.182** Compound clear cell sarcoma. **A** Amelanotic infiltrative tumour in the dermis and superficial subcutis associated with epidermal hyperplasia and hyperkeratosis. **B** Tumour cells are present not only in the dermis, but also in the epidermis, appearing as solitary units and junctional nests. Cytogenetic analysis confirmed the presence of a t(12;22) translocation.

## Differential diagnosis

Dermal clear cell sarcoma may be confused with spitzoid melanocytic tumours, cellular blue naevus, primary nodular or metastatic melanoma, epithelioid sarcoma, or other sarcomas.

## Histogenesis

The cell of origin is unknown. Gene expression and immunohistochemical studies confirm melanocytic differentiation {1088,2372}.

## Genetic profile

It has been reported that >90% of cases of clear cell sarcoma harbour the translocation t(12;22)(q13;q12), which fuses the *EWSR1* gene and the *ATF1* gene. A rare variant translocation, t(2;22)(q34;q12), which fuses *EWSR1* and *CREB1*, has also been identified {631,2780}.

## Prognosis and predictive factors

Dermal clear cell sarcoma is clinically characterized by a propensity for local recurrences with late metastases. The survival rate of patients with metastasis is approximately 50% at 5 years and 33% at 10 years {481,694}. There are no known clinical or pathological features that correlate with outcome.

# Ewing sarcoma

Patel R.M.
Scolyer R.A.

## Definition

Ewing sarcoma is a prototypical small round blue cell sarcoma. About 10–20% of all cases are extraskeletal, and primary cutaneous and superficial cases are rare.

## ICD-O code 9364/3

## Synonyms

Ewing family tumour; primitive neuroectodermal tumour

## Epidemiology

Cutaneous Ewing sarcoma typically arises in children and young adults, but has also been reported in older individuals (median age: 17 years, range: 2–77 years). There is a female predilection {139,1036,2424,2597}.

## Etiology

The pathogenesis of Ewing sarcoma is driven by transcription factors encoded by chimeric FET-ETS family gene fusions, most commonly *EWSR1-FLI1* {469,1036,1523,1619}.

## Localization

Ewing sarcoma most commonly involves the lower limbs (affected in 38% of cases), followed by the upper limbs (in 26%), head (in 20%), and trunk (in 16%) {139,1619,2424,2597}.

## Clinical features

The lesions consist of dermal or subcutaneous nodules that may be painful, polypoid, or ulcerated {139,1036,2424,2597}.

## Histopathology

The tumour nodules are composed of sheets of mitotically active, uniform, small round cells with indistinct cell borders and round nuclei with fine chromatin and inconspicuous nucleoli. The constituent cells have a high N:C ratio and only a scant amount of lightly eosinophilic to clear glycogenated cytoplasm that gives a positive periodic acid–Schiff (PAS) reaction {139,1036,1583}. Homer Wright rosettes are rarely present in cases with neuroectodermal differentiation {1620}. Membranous CD99 immunoreactivity is a highly sensitive but nonspecific finding in nearly all cases. Neural markers (e.g. neuron-specific enolase, S100 protein, synaptophysin, PGP9.5, and CD57) {394} and epithelial markers (AE1/AE3 and CAM5.2) may also occasionally be expressed, but desmin positivity is rare and typically very focal {517,808,953,1583}. Nonspecific immunoreactivity for FLI1 is present in 94% of cases with the *EWSR1-FLI1* fusion {808,809,1583,2238}. Staining for ERG is positive in cases with *ERG* rearrangements, and it may also be positive in cases with *FLI1* rearrangements {2625}. Recently described immunostaining for NKX2-2 is sensitive but imperfectly specific {1152,2895}.

## Differential diagnosis

The differential diagnosis of cutaneous and superficial Ewing sarcomas depends on the age of the patient and includes a wide variety of primary and metastatic malignant neoplasms with small round blue cell morphology, such as Merkel cell carcinoma, malignant glomus tumour, lymphoma, and melanoma {469,1620,2424}.

## Histogenesis

A possible neural crest {1139,2751} or mesenchymal stem cell origin has been proposed for Ewing sarcoma by some experts {2188,2189,2616,2626}.

## Genetic profile

The *EWSR1-FLI1* fusion is seen in >95% of cutaneous and superficial Ewing sarcomas {607,1036,1277,2035}. Rarely, an *EWSR1-ERG* fusion is present {1224,1813,2483,2597}.

## Prognosis and predictive factors

Cutaneous and superficial Ewing sarcomas have a better outcome than their counterparts in deep soft tissue and bone {606,844,2091}. Long-term survival has been reported both with and without adjuvant therapy {396,475,619,2586}. The overall survival rate is 93%, and the 10-year probability of survival is estimated at approximately 90% {606,859}.

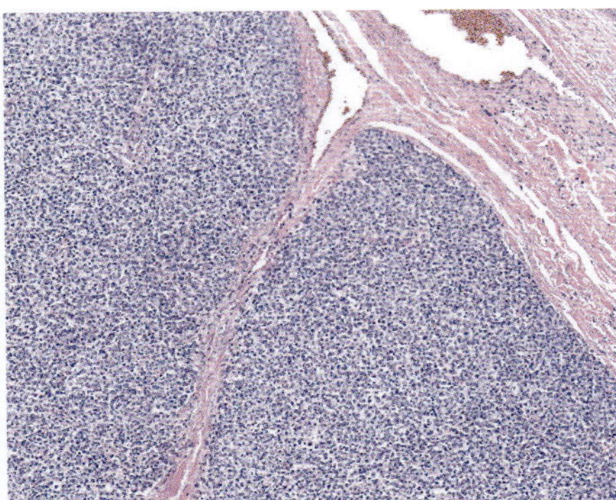

**Fig. 5.183** Primary cutaneous Ewing sarcoma. Small round blue cell tumour within the dermis.

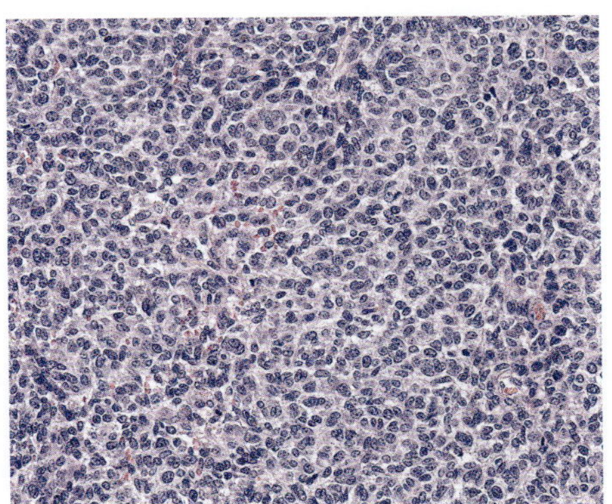

**Fig. 5.184** Primary cutaneous Ewing sarcoma composed of regular small round blue cells.

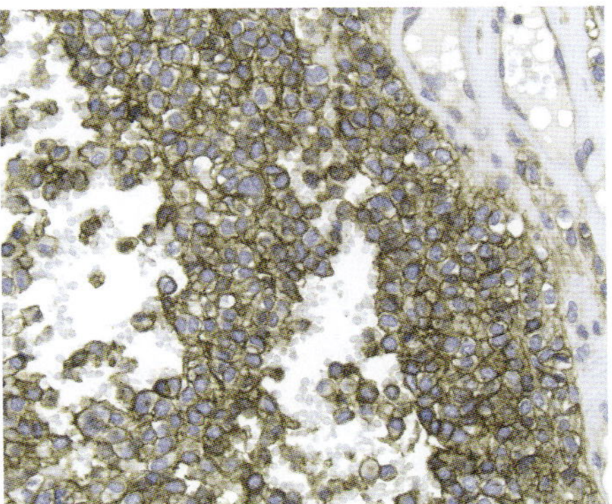

**Fig. 5.185** Ewing sarcoma. Membranous CD99 immunoreactivity.

# Primitive non-neural granular cell tumour

LeBoit P.E.
Lazar A.J.

## Definition

Primitive non-neural granular cell tumour (PNNGCT) is a rare, low-grade neoplasm of mesenchymal cells of unknown lineage with prominent cytoplasmic granularity.

## ICD-O code 8990/1

## Synonyms

Primitive polypoid granular cell tumour; non-neural granular cell tumour; dermal non-neural granular cell tumour

## Epidemiology

The majority of reported cases have presented in children or young adults {756,1514}. Some reported cases in elderly patients may in fact be granular cell variants of atypical fibroxanthoma {189,1603,2192}.

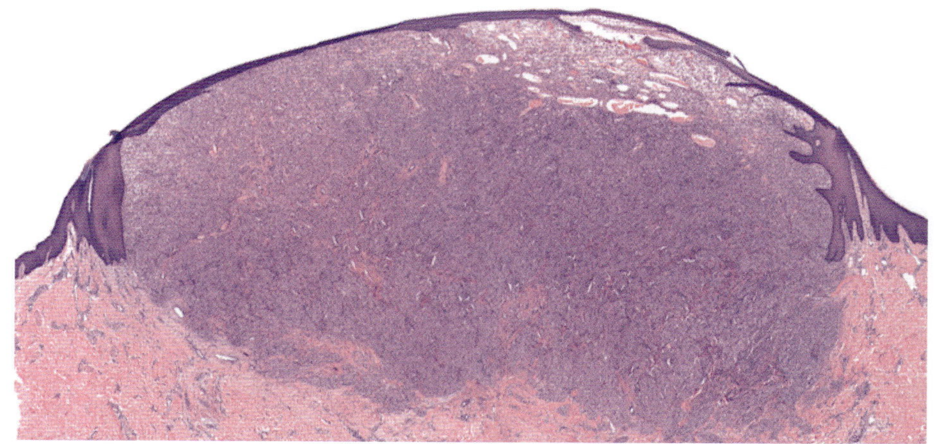

**Fig. 5.186** Primitive non-neural granular cell tumour. The lesions are often polypoid, with an epithelial collarette.

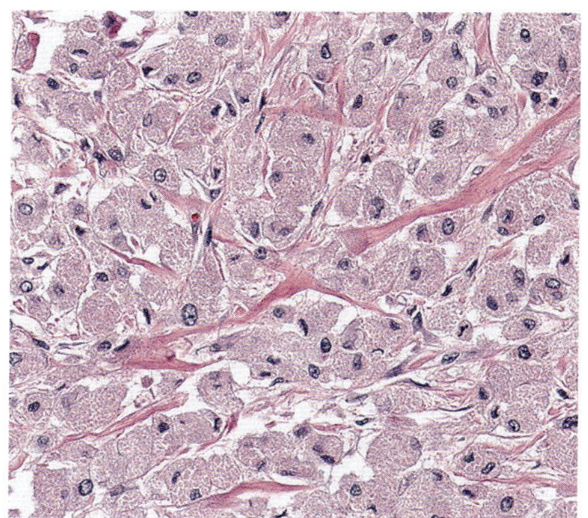

**Fig. 5.187** Primitive non-neural granular cell tumour. Note the large oval cells with abundant cytoplasmic eosinophilic granules.

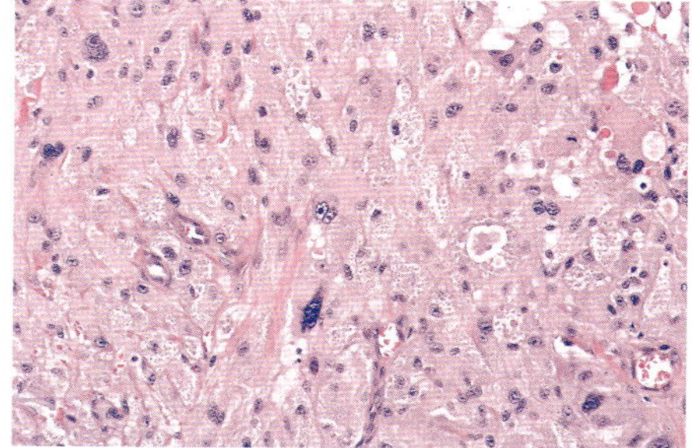

**Fig. 5.188** Primitive non-neural granular cell tumour. Cytological atypia and pleomorphism may be encountered, but do not correlate with a more aggressive course; note the pustulo-ovoid bodies of Milian in the right side of the field.

## Localization

The back was the preferred site in one series; in another, the lesions were widely distributed on the torso, limbs, and face {444,1504}.

## Clinical features

The lesions are most commonly non-ulcerated papules or nodules.

## Histopathology

PNNGCTs can be polypoid. Some lesions are gently domed. The lesional cells often extend to the base of the dermis or into the subcutis. The overlying epidermis is usually thin, with epithelial collarettes defining the lateral edges. The granular cells form sheets and are large and oval, with coarse eosinophilic granules. The cellular granularity is due to the accumulation of lysosomes in the cytoplasm of the affected cells. The largest granules are surrounded by clear haloes (pustulo-ovoid bodies of Milian). The nuclei can vary from moderately sized and monomorphous to large, pleomorphic, and heterochromatic. Mitoses can range from few to many, and atypical mitoses can occur. A few cases have shown lymphatic invasion. The cells of PNNGCTs fail to stain for S100 protein or SOX10. They usually stain positively for CD68 and CD63 (NKI/C3), likely because of reactivity with lysosomes in the cytoplasm, but such positivity is not lineage-specific; it can also be seen in the cells of many other neoplasms.

## Differential diagnosis

Conventional granular cell tumour of Schwannian origin is the most important differential diagnosis. Polypoid configuration, epithelial collarettes, nuclear pleomorphism, and easily detectable mitoses favour PNNGCT over granular cell tumour. Unlike PNNGCTs, conventional granular cell tumours are positive for S100 protein and SOX10. Unlike granular cell atypical fibroxanthoma, PNNGCT occurs in younger patients and most often not on the face or scalp. Granular cell fibrous papules are usually found on the nose, are smaller dome-surfaced lesions, and have nearly clear cytoplasm with paler granules. Granular cell variants of basal cell carcinoma, dermatofibroma, and dermatofibrosarcoma protuberans have areas in which the conventional aspects of these neoplasms are apparent.

## Prognosis and predictive factors

Most cases are indolent, despite worrisome histopathological features. Few cases with regional lymph node metastasis have been reported {38,1504}.

# Cellular neurothekeoma

Requena L.
Hornick J.L.

## Definition

Cellular neurothekeoma is a benign cutaneous neoplasm of uncertain histogenesis. Although this entity was originally considered to be related to dermal nerve sheath myxoma, there is no compelling evidence that cellular neurothekeoma shows nerve sheath differentiation.

## ICD-O code

9562/0

## Synonym

Neurothekeoma

## Epidemiology

Cellular neurothekeoma is most common in children and young adults, with a female predominance {770,842,1126,2230}.

## Localization

Cellular neurothekeoma has a predilection for the face (in particular the nasomalar and nasolabial areas), shoulders, and upper limbs {770,842,1126,2230}. It is usually solitary, although rare examples of multiple neurothekeomas have been reported {768,1636}.

## Clinical features

Cellular neurothekeoma presents as a solitary firm papule or nodule with no distinctive clinical features.

## Histopathology

Cellular neurothekeoma is a lobulated or micronodular neoplasm composed of nests of usually epithelioid but occasionally spindled cells with a vesicular nucleus, small nucleolus, and palely eosinophilic cytoplasm, often separated by dense collagenous stroma {1126}. Some tumours contain prominent myxoid stroma. Occasional neoplastic cells may be multinucleated or may show hyperchromatic nuclei, and mitotic figures are common {154,158,2518}. In rare cases, areas of calcification {897}, ossification {2227}, perineural invasion {2518}, and a plexiform pattern with hybrid features of both cellular neurothekeoma and perineurioma can be seen {2172}.

Immunohistochemically, the most consistent markers expressed in cellular neurothekeoma are CD63 (NKI/C3) {149}, neuron-specific enolase {92}, PGP9.5 {2772}, and S100A6 {837}, whereas expression of MITF, SMA, and podoplanin (recognized by D2-40) is more variable {1260,1967,2518}. Cellular neurothekeoma does not express S100 protein, GFAP, CD57, or EMA (epithelial membrane antigen) {154,158,770,2230}.

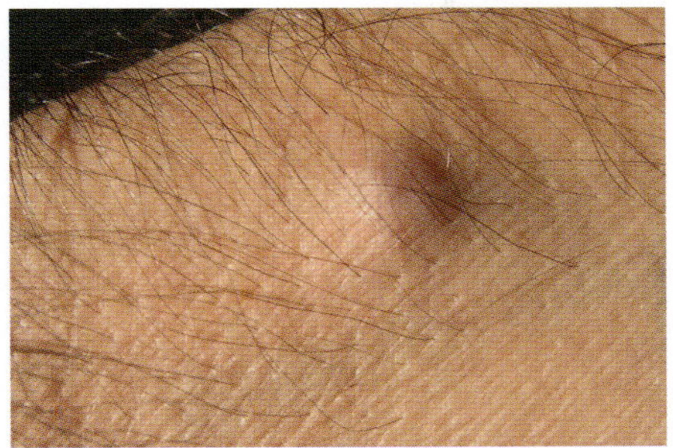

**Fig. 5.189** Cellular neurothekeoma. A nodular lesion on the forearm of a young male patient.

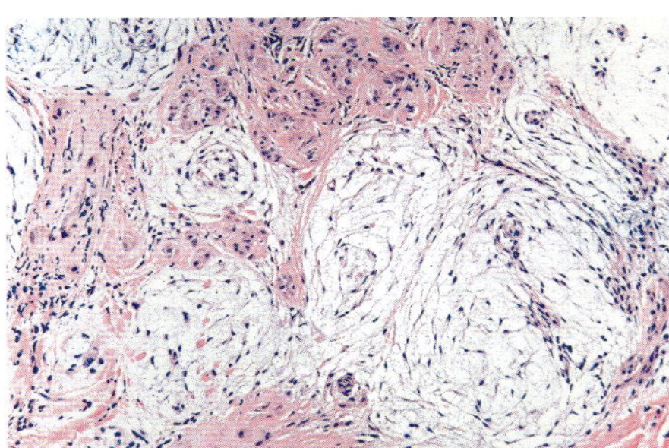

**Fig. 5.190** Cellular neurothekeoma. Some tumours show prominent myxoid stromal change and can mimic dermal nerve sheath myxoma.

## Differential diagnosis

The differential diagnosis includes dermal nerve sheath myxoma, Spitz naevus, and plexiform fibrohistiocytic tumour. Dermal nerve sheath myxomas and Spitz naevi are positive for S100 protein. Cutaneous leiomyoma has an intersecting fascicular pattern and is desmin-positive. Plexiform fibrohistiocytic tumour has a biphasic appearance and a plexiform growth pattern.

## Histogenesis

The histogenesis is uncertain, but the gene expression profile is similar to that of cellular fibrous histiocytoma, suggesting myofibroblastic differentiation {2406}.

## Prognosis and predictive factors

Cellular neurothekeoma is benign, and complete surgical removal is curative.

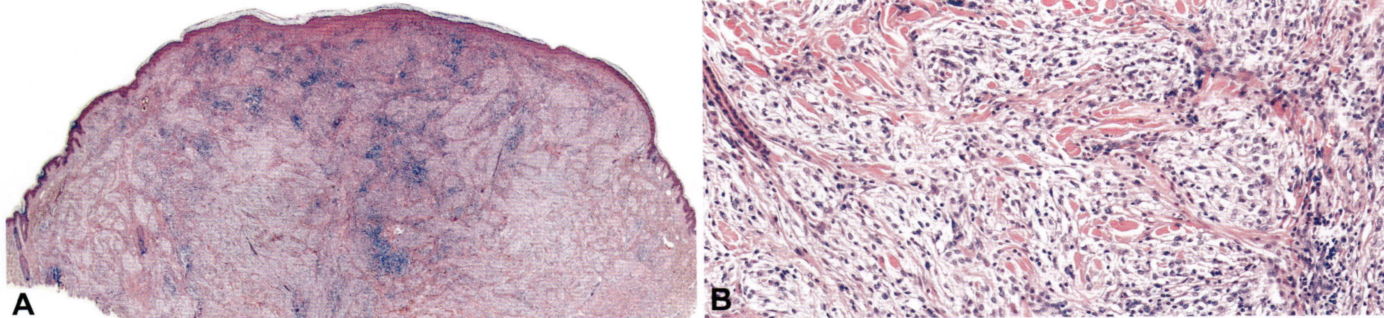


**Fig. 5.191** Cellular neurothekeoma. **A** Scanning magnification reveals a nested growth pattern. **B** The tumour is composed of nests of epithelioid to spindled cells in a collagenous stroma.

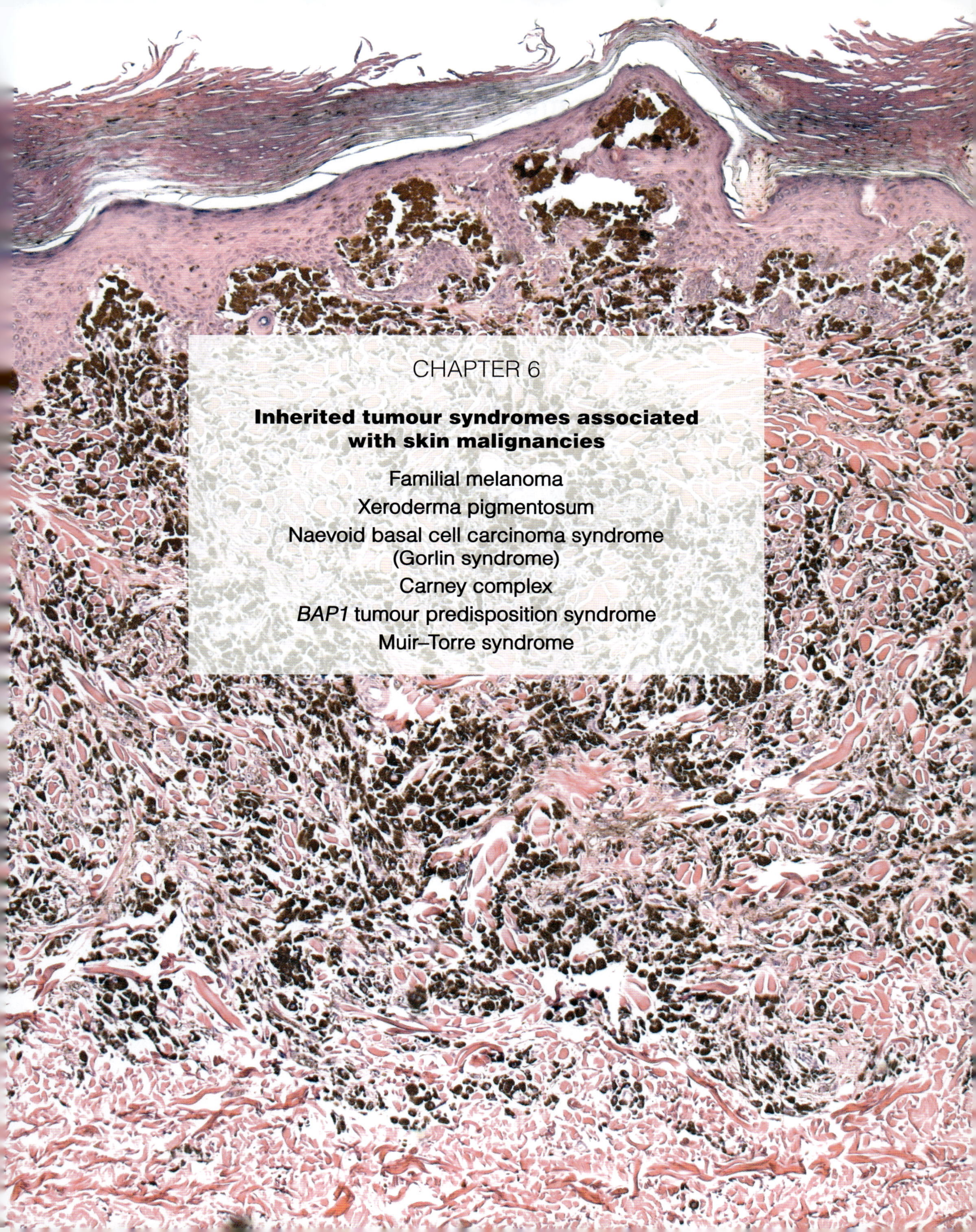

CHAPTER 6

# Inherited tumour syndromes associated with skin malignancies

# Inherited tumour syndromes associated with skin malignancies: Introduction

Scolyer R.A.
Cree I.A.
Elder D.E.
Lazar A.J.
Massi D.

Cancer is a disease of the genome characterized by a series of DNA perturbations selected for as a result of malignant properties such as uncontrolled cell division, resistance to apoptosis, and the ability to migrate beyond the site of initiation and survive and proliferate at metastatic sites. The study of familial cancer syndromes with simple Mendelian inheritance patterns led to the discovery of key genes that are important not only for the roles they play in genetic susceptibility to cancer, but also for the insight they provide into the molecular pathogenesis of many sporadic cancers and their classification. For example, in the recently described *BAP1* tumour predisposition syndrome, germline *BAP1* mutations are associated with an increased risk of developing a variety of tumour types, including characteristic cutaneous melanocytic naevi/tumours as well as uveal and cutaneous melanomas, mesothelioma, and renal cell carcinoma. This discovery has also improved our understanding of the molecular basis of some cutaneous melanocytic tumours, which has led to a more rational taxonomy (as detailed in the *Melanocytic tumours* chapter of this volume).

Contemporary genomic sequencing techniques, greatly bolstered by large international consortium initiatives such

**Table 6.01** Inherited disorders associated with skin tumours

| Disease/phenotype | MIM number | Inheritance | Tumour type | Locus | Gene | Protein | Normal protein function [notes] |
|---|---|---|---|---|---|---|---|
| Familial melanoma[a] (CMM2) | 155601 | AD | M | 9p21.3 | *CDKN2A* | p16, p14ARF | Cell-cycle control; inhibits cyclin-dependent kinase phosphorylation of RB1<br>Promotes apoptosis; stabilizes p53 by inhibiting MDM2 |
| Familial melanoma[a] (CMM3) | 609048 | AD | M | 12q14.1 | *CDK4* | CDK4 | Drives cell cycle; phosphorylates RB1 |
| Familial atypical mole–malignant melanoma syndrome[a] (CMM1) | 155600 | AD | M | 1p36 | Unknown | Unknown | [*CDKN2A* and *CDK4* mutations excluded] |
| Xeroderma pigmentosum (XP) | | | | | | | |
| XPA | 278700 | AR | BCC, SCC, M | 9q22.3 | *XPA* | XPA | Helps repair damaged DNA via binding interactions with TFIIH, XPF, and XPG |
| XPB | 610651 | | | 2q14.3 | *ERCC3* | XPB | A 3' to 5' helicase; part of the TFIIH transcription factor complex |
| XPC | 278720 | | | 3p25.1 | *XPC* | XPC | Global genomic nucleotide excision repair; binds to damaged DNA |
| XPD | 278730 | | | 19q13.3 | *ERCC2* | XPD | A 5' to 3' helicase; part of the TFIIH transcription factor complex |
| XPE | 278740 | | | 11p11.2 | *DDB2* | XPE (p48) | Global genomic nucleotide excision repair; binds to damaged DNA |
| XPF | 278760 | | | 16p13.1 | *ERCC4* | XPF | A 5' endonuclease; forms a heterodimer with ERCC1 |
| XPG | 278780 | | | 13q33.1 | *ERCC5* | XPG | A 3' endonuclease; stabilizes open complex |
| XPV | 278750 | | | 6p21.1 | *POLH* | POLH | A translesion DNA polymerase |
| Naevoid basal cell carcinoma syndrome | 109400 | AD | BCC | 9q22.3 | *PTCH1* | PTCH1 | Plays a role in embryonic development; regulates hedgehog signalling |
| | | | | 10q24.3 | *SUFU* | SUFU | Inhibits hedgehog signalling |
| Carney complex | 160980 | AD | PEM | 17q24.2 | *PRKAR1A* | PRKAR1A | A regulatory subunit; *PRKAR1A* mutation results in overactive protein kinase A |
| *BAP1* tumour predisposition syndrome | 614327 | AD | M | 3p21.1 | *BAP1* | BAP1 | A ubiquitin C-terminal hydrolase; a tumour suppressor |

| Disease/phenotype | MIM number | Inheritance | Tumour type | Locus | Gene | Protein | Normal protein function [notes] |
|---|---|---|---|---|---|---|---|
| Cowden syndrome (a *PTEN* hamartoma tumour syndrome) | 158350 | AD | TL, MH | 10q23.3 | *PTEN* | PTEN | A lipid phosphatase; downregulates the PI3K/AKT pathway |
| MTS (a variant of Lynch syndrome) | 158320 | AD | CSN | 2p21-p16.3 | *MSH2* | MSH2 | DNA mismatch repair [*MSH2* mutation is the most common cause of MTS] |
| | | | | 3p22.2 | *MLH1* | MLH1 | DNA mismatch repair |
| | | | | 2p16.3 | *MSH6* | MSH6 | DNA mismatch repair |
| | | | | 7p22.1 | *PMS2* | PMS2 | DNA mismatch repair [to date, *PMS2* mutation is known to cause Lynch syndrome, but not the MTS variant] |
| *MUTYH*-associated polyposis (a rare cause of the MTS phenotype) | 608456 | AR | CSN | 1p34.1 | *MUTYH* | MUTYH | A DNA glycosylase; repairs oxidative DNA damage |
| Gardner syndrome | 175100 | AD | EC | 5q22.2 | *APC* | APC | Negatively regulates β-catenin and WNT signalling |
| Multiple endocrine neoplasia type 1 | 131100 | AD | MFA | 11q13 | *MEN1* | Menin | Inhibits JUND-activated transcription |
| Multiple endocrine neoplasia type 2A | 171400 | AD | CLA | 10q11.2 | *RET* | RET | A receptor tyrosine kinase |
| Tuberous sclerosis type 1 | 191100 | AD | MSL | 9q34 | *TSC1* | Hamartin | Interacts with tuberin; inhibits growth |
| Tuberous sclerosis type 2 | 613254 | AD | MSL | 16p13.3 | *TSC2* | Tuberin | Interacts with hamartin; inhibits growth |
| Neurofibromatosis type 1 (von Recklinghausen disease) | 162200 | AD | FTK | 17q11.2 | *NF1* | Neurofibromin (NF1) | Interacts with hamartin; inhibits growth |
| Neurofibromatosis type 2 | 101000 | AD | ST | 22q12.2 | *NF2* | Merlin (NF2) | Integrates cytoskeletal signalling |
| Peutz–Jeghers syndrome | 175200 | AD | MML | 19p13.3 | *STK11* | STK11 | A serine/threonine kinase; a tumour suppressor |
| Bloom syndrome | 210900 | AR | ST | 15q26.1 | *BLM* | BLM | A DNA helicase; unwinds blocked replication forks |
| Rothmund–Thomson syndrome | 268400 | AR | D | 8q24.3 | *RECQL4* | RECQL4 | A DNA helicase; unwinds blocked replication forks |
| Werner syndrome | 277700 | AR | SSL | 8p12 | *WRN* | WRN | A DNA helicase; unwinds blocked replication forks |
| Birt–Hogg–Dubé syndrome | 135150 | AD | HFH | 17p11.2 | *FLCN* | Folliculin | A tumour suppressor [precise mechanism unknown] |
| *CYLD*-related syndrome family | | | | | | | |
| Brooke–Spiegler syndrome | 605041 | AD | C, TE, SPA | 16q12.1 | *CYLD* | CYLD | Negatively regulates NF-κB activation |
| Familial cylindromatosis | 132700 | | C | | | | |
| Multiple familial trichoepithelioma 1 | 601606 | | TE | | | | |
| Hereditary leiomyomatosis and renal cell cancer | 150800 | AD | CLM | 1q43 | *FH* | Fumarase | Involved in the Krebs cycle |

**AD**, autosomal dominant; **AR**, autosomal recessive; **BCC**, basal cell carcinoma; **C**, cylindroma; **CLA**, cutaneous lichen amyloidosis; **CLM**, cutaneous leiomyoma; **CMM1–3**, cutaneous malignant melanoma 1–3; **CSN**, cutaneous sebaceous neoplasia; **D**, dermatosis; **EC**, epidermoid cyst; **FTK**, fibromatous tumours of the skin; **HFH**, hair follicle hamartomas; **M**, melanoma; **MFA**, multiple facial angiofibromas; **MH**, multiple hamartomas; **MML**, melanocytic macules of the lip; **MSL**, multiple skin lesions; **MTS**, Muir–Torre syndrome; **PEM**, pigmented epithelioid melanocytoma (also called epithelioid blue naevus); **SCC**, squamous cell carcinoma; **SPA**, eccrine spiradenoma; **SSL**, scleroderma-like skin changes; **ST**, skin tumours; **TE**, trichoepithelioma; **TL**, trichilemmoma; **XPA–XPG**, xeroderma pigmentosum complementation groups A–G; **XPV**, xeroderma pigmentosum variant.

[a] Germline mutations in multiple genes are associated with genetic susceptibility to melanoma (discussed in greater detail in Chapter 2: *Melanocytic tumours*); only the three most common phenotypes are listed here.

as the International Cancer Genome Consortium (ICGC) and The Cancer Genome Atlas (TCGA), are now important sources of cancer gene discovery. However, cancer syndromes continue to provide critical insights into the important interaction of the genome with the environment, as mediated by genetic susceptibility and dramatically demonstrated by the extreme sensitivity to ultraviolet (UV) radiation seen in xeroderma pigmentosum. We have also learned how the tissue context (i.e. epigenetically determined cellular differentiation) influences genetic susceptibility; although all cells harbour a given germline mutation, only certain malignancies are regularly encountered. For example, in Muir–Torre syndrome (a variant of Lynch syndrome), colon and endometrial cancers are common, but melanoma and sarcoma are very uncommon, suggesting that certain tissues are more permissive to microsatellite instability–mediated oncogenic transformation. Inherited cancer syndromes also provide new insights into cancer precursor lesions and how neoplasia evolves over time. Examples of these principles are included in the following sections.

Many inherited tumour syndromes have cutaneous manifestations. This chapter contains detailed descriptions of clinical, pathological, and genetic information about selected major and well-characterized inherited syndromes specifically associated with malignant tumours of the skin. Associations of specific benign cutaneous tumours with other inherited tumour syndromes (including syndromes associated with internal malignancies), such as hereditary leiomyomatosis and renal cell cancer, Brooke–Spiegler syndrome, Birt–Hogg–Dubé syndrome, and Cowden syndrome (part of the *PTEN* hamartoma tumour syndrome spectrum), are briefly highlighted in the sections describing those tumours elsewhere in this volume. A summary of the genetic basis, inheritance patterns, and tumour types associated with the syndromes detailed in this chapter, as well as many others described elsewhere in this volume, is presented in Table 6.01 (p. 380).

# Familial melanoma

Tsao H.
Berwick M.
Demenais F.
Elder D.E.
Mann G.J.
Newton-Bishop J.
Tucker M.

## Definition

Familial melanoma is generally defined as melanoma occurring in two or more first-degree relatives. The term "familial melanoma" excludes conditions such as xeroderma pigmentosum and albinism with extreme sensitivity to ultraviolet (UV) radiation.

## MIM numbers

See Table 6.02.

## Synonyms

Familial dysplastic naevi/melanoma; familial atypical mole–malignant melanoma syndrome

## Epidemiology

In the time since familial melanoma was first described by Norton (in 1820) and later by Cawley (in 1952) {400}, a family history of melanoma has been recognized as an important melanoma risk factor. A meta-analysis of 60 observational studies found the relative risk conferred by a family history of melanoma (defined as > 1 first-degree relative with the disease) to be 1.74 (95% CI: 1.41–2.14) {846}. Generally, countries with higher levels of UV radiation exposure have a greater proportion of melanoma cases associated with a family history (Australia: 10.8% {2790}, USA: 8.1% {2266}, Denmark: 3% {1960}). In a pooled dataset from 15 case–control studies, 6.3% of cases were associated with a family history of melanoma, with a very similar relative risk of melanoma of 1.74 (95% CI: 1.21–2.46) {581}. Many families with familial melanoma also have dysplastic (atypical) naevi, identifying individuals at an increased risk of developing melanoma. In about half of all families with familial melanoma, heritability is due to high-risk susceptibility genes (see *Genetics*). In a substantial proportion of the other half, heritability is probably due to intermediate/lower-penetrance susceptibility genes, likely related to pigmentation and naevi {2140}.

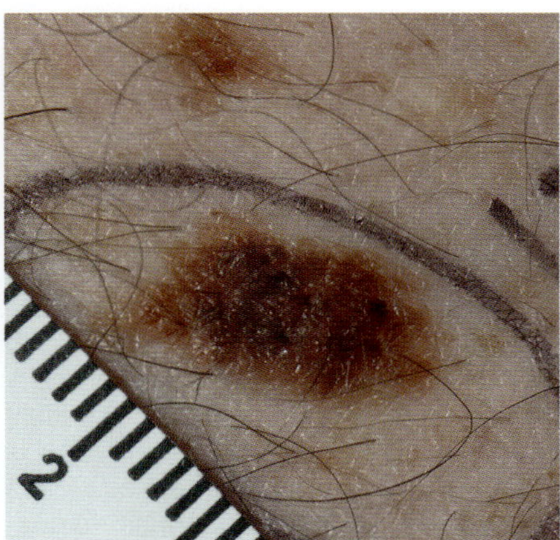

**Fig. 6.01** Atypical naevi. An atypical (dysplastic) naevus showing clinical atypia.

**Table 6.02** Genetic susceptibility to melanoma

| Susceptibility phenotype | MIM number | Locus | Gene | Gene/locus MIM no. | Inheritance |
|---|---|---|---|---|---|
| CMM1 | 155600 | 1p36 | Unknown | n/a | AD |
| CMM2 | 155601 | 9p21.3 | *CDKN2A* | 600160 | AD |
| Melanoma–pancreatic cancer syndrome | 606719 | | | | |
| Melanoma–astrocytoma syndrome | 155755 | | | | |
| CMM3 | 609048 | 12q14.1 | *CDK4* | 123829 | AD |
| CMM4 | 608035 | 1p22 | Unknown | n/a | Unknown |
| CMM5 | 613099 | 16q24.3 | *MC1R* | 155555 | Additive |
| CMM6 | 613972 | 14q32.3 | *XRCC3* | 600675 | Unknown |
| CMM7 | 612263 | 20q11.2 | Unknown | n/a | Unknown |
| CMM8 | 614456 | 3p13 | *MITF* | 156845 | Probably AD |
| CMM9 | 615134 | 5p15.3 | *TERT* | 187270 | AD |
| CMM10 | 615848 | 7q31.3 | *POT1* | 606478 | AD |
| *BAP1* tumour predisposition syndrome (CMM11) | 614327 | 3p21.1 | *BAP1* | 603089 | AD |

AD, autosomal dominant; CMM1–11, cutaneous malignant melanoma 1–11; n/a, not applicable.

## Clinical features

In the past, attempts to identify highly penetrant melanoma susceptibility genes selected families for inclusion on the basis of melanoma clustering alone. The most common germline mutation established as causal for familial clustering of melanoma is in *CDKN2A*. However, an increased frequency of germline *CDKN2A* mutations is also associated with an increased risk of pancreatic cancer; this association is particularly strong in families living in North America and mainland Europe, and weaker in the United Kingdom and Australia {907}. The apparent variation in susceptibility to pancreatic cancer may reflect genetic diversity (given that the melanoma-susceptible populations in the United Kingdom and Australia are genetically similar), but this has not yet been confirmed. More recently, smoking-related cancers have also been shown to be more common in families with *CDKN2A* founder mutations (in the Netherlands {592} and in Sweden {1059}), so environmental factors may also explain some of the variation in susceptibility to cancers other than cutaneous melanoma. *CDKN2A* encodes p16 (p16INK4a), which binds to CDK4, and germline *CDK4* mutations also lead to an increased melanoma risk. Families with *CDKN2A* mutations are very phenotypically similar to those with *CDK4* mutations {2109}; both groups tend to have a relatively early onset of melanoma (~10 years earlier than in the general population), multiple primaries, and a variable association with clinically atypical naevi.

The identification of germline susceptibility genes (e.g. *POT1*) in families at risk of mixed cancer types has resulted in the recognition of different phenotypes. Some families with germline *POT1* mutations may have susceptibility to cutaneous melanoma {2200,2407}, but other families studied for different cancers have shown different susceptibilities, such as to angiosarcoma {359} or glioma {128}. The true risk of various cancers in these rare families with *POT1* mutations remains to be determined. Families with inactivating germline mutations in the *BAP1* gene have a distinctive phenotype described in a separate section (see *BAP1 tumour predisposition syndrome*, p. 393).

In a study of sporadic melanomas and familial melanomas from families with and without *CDKN2A* germline mutations, the tumours in mutation carriers tended to have histological features of superficial spreading melanoma, including higher levels of pigmentation and increased pagetoid scatter. The presence of spindle cell morphology in the vertical growth phase was a strong negative predictor of a mutated genotype; of the 15 cases with this phenotype, none harboured a *CDKN2A* mutation {2317}. To date, no large series of melanomas in the setting of familial melanoma with histopathological and outcome data have been reported.

**Table 6.03** Low/medium-risk melanoma susceptibility loci identified by genome-wide association studies

| Chromosomal region | Peak SNP in the region | Nearby gene(s) | Odds ratio[a] | Pigmentation-related? | Naevus gene(s)? | Reference |
|---|---|---|---|---|---|---|
| 1q21.3 | rs7412746 | *ARNT, SETDB1* | 0.87 | | | {1617} |
| 1q42.12 | rs3219090 | *PARP1* | 0.87 | | | {1617} |
| 2p22.2 | rs6750047 | *RMDN2, CYP1B1* | 1.10 | | | {1503} |
| 2q33.1 | rs13016963 | *CASP8* | 1.14 | | | {162} |
| 5p15.33 | rs401681 | *TERT, CLPTM1L* | 1.15 | | Yes | {443} |
| 5p13.3-13.2 | rs16891982 | *SLC45A2* | 0.40 | Yes | | {162} |
| 6p22.3 | rs6914598 | *CDKAL1* | 1.11 | | | {1503} |
| 7p21.1 | rs1636744 | *AGR3* | 1.10 | | | {1503} |
| 9p21.3 | rs7023329 | *MTAP, CDKN2A* | 0.85 | | Yes | {252} |
| 9p31.2 | rs10739221 | *TMEM38B, RAD23B* | 1.13 | | | {1503} |
| 10q24.33 | rs2995264 | *STN1 (OBFC1)* | 1.17 | | | {1503} |
| 11q13.3 | rs498136 | *CCND1* | 1.13 | | Yes | {1503} |
| 11q14.3 | rs1393350 | *TYR* | 1.29 | Yes | | {252} |
| 11q22.3 | rs1801516 | *ATM* | 0.84 | | | {162} |
| 15q12-13.1 | rs4778138 | *OCA2, HERC2* | 0.84 | Yes | | {71,1503} |
| 16q12.2 | rs16953002 | *FTO* | 1.16 | | | {1168} |
| 16q24.3 | rs258322 | *MC1R* | 1.69 | Yes | | {252} |
| 20q11.22 | rs910873 | *PIGU, ASIP* | 1.72 | Yes | | {319} |
| 21q22.3 | rs45430 | *MX2* | 0.88 | | | {162} |
| 22q13.1 | rs2284063 | *PLA2G6* | 0.83 | | Yes | {252,729} |

[a] Each odds ratio estimate listed is from the first genome-wide association study reporting the locus as having genome-wide significance.

## Genetics

Intermittent exposure to intense sunlight is an important environmental risk factor for melanoma {437}, but inherited genetic variation is key. Melanoma is largely a disease of pale-skinned people, in whom the two well-established high-penetrance genes are *CDKN2A* and *CDK4*. Mutations of these genes are identified in 30–40% of families with ≥ 3 melanoma cases. Five other genes (*BAP1*, *POT1* {2200,2407}, *ACD*, *TERF2IP* {83}, and *TERT* {1011,1117}) have recently been identified as very rare high-penetrance melanoma susceptibility genes (with mutations of each currently found in < 1% of families with familial melanoma).

Genetic susceptibility to melanoma can also be due to the combined effect of multiple inherited medium- to low-penetrance genes. To date, three medium-penetrance genes (*MC1R*, *MITF*, and *SLC45A2*) have been identified {2140}, all of which are involved in pigmentation. To date, genome-wide association studies have revealed 20 low/medium-risk loci, including *MC1R* and *SLC45A2* (Table 6.03). Nine of these loci are associated with pigmentation or number of naevi; others are involved in telomere biology, DNA repair, or regulation of the cell cycle. For some of the loci, the biological role in melanoma susceptibility is still unknown. Gene–gene interactions may also contribute to the polygenic inheritance of melanoma {318}. Interactions between melanoma susceptibility genes and environmental factors (e.g. UV radiation exposure and tobacco smoke) are also likely to exist, further study is needed.

The Cancer Genome Atlas (TCGA) melanoma initiative has provided the most comprehensive view of somatic changes in melanoma tumours. Overall, 91% of melanoma tumours exhibit evidence of RAS pathway activation; 51%, 28%, and 14% contain mutations in *BRAF*, *NRAS*, and *NF1*, respectively {867}, suggesting that constitutive RAS circuit stimulation is a core driver of melanoma growth. The RB1 and MDM2/p53 tumour-suppressive pathways are also crippled in 69% and 19% of tumours, respectively. Non-coding *TERT* promoter mutations are present in 65% of specimens, and *TERT* itself is amplified in about 10% of cases. There are no known unique somatic signatures associated with any of the familial melanoma syndromes, but certain *MC1R* variants are associated with an increased somatic-mutation burden; some (called R alleles {2201}) show a strong association with red hair, and others (r alleles {1233}) show only a weak association.

### Prognosis and predictive factors

The mutation penetrance of the most common high-penetrance susceptibility gene (*CDKN2A*) has been reported {251}. The overall penetrance was estimated to be 0.30 (95% CI: 0.12–0.62) by the age of 50 years and 0.67 (95% CI: 0.31–0.96) by the age of 80 years. There was a statistically significant effect of residing in a geographical area with a high population incidence rate of melanoma ($P = 0.003$). *CDKN2A* mutation penetrance by the age of 50 years was found to be 0.13 in Europe, 0.50 in the USA, and 0.32 in Australia; by the age of 80 years it was 0.58 in Europe, 0.76 in the USA, and 0.91 in Australia. The penetrance of rarer gene mutations (e.g. *POT1* and *BAP1* mutations) in melanoma and other cancers has not yet been established. The penetrance of all genes may be modulated by other factors; this has been observed for atypical (dysplastic) naevi and *MC1R* variants, which increase melanoma risk in *CDKN2A* mutation carriers {608}.

# Xeroderma pigmentosum

Kraemer K.H.
Sarasin A.

## Definition

Xeroderma pigmentosum (XP) is an autosomal recessive disease characterized by sensitivity to sunlight, photophobia, and early-onset freckling followed by neoplastic changes in sun-exposed sites {627,1439}. There is cellular hypersensitivity to ultraviolet (UV) radiation due to deficient nucleotide excision repair (NER) of DNA damage. There are seven complementation groups of XP (XPA–XPG), each caused by mutations in one of seven NER genes. There is also a variant form of XP (XPV), in which NER is normal but there is a defect in a translesion DNA polymerase {1951}.

## MIM numbers

| | | | |
|---|---|---|---|
| XPA | 278700 | XPE | 278740 |
| XPB | 610651 | XPF | 278760 |
| XPC | 278720 | XPG | 278780 |
| XPD | 278730 | XPV | 278750 |

## Synonym

De Sanctis–Cacchione syndrome

## Epidemiology

The incidence of XP is about 1 case per 1 million live births in Europe {1387} and the USA, 1 per 22 000 in Japan {1084}, and 1 per 5000 in the Comorian archipelago {388}. Patients (of all races) have been reported worldwide.

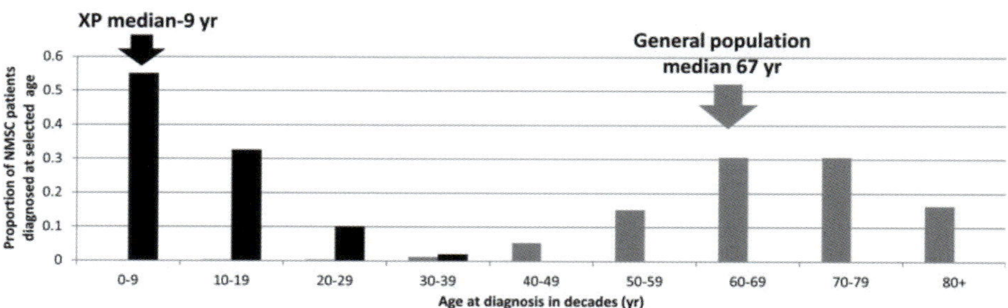


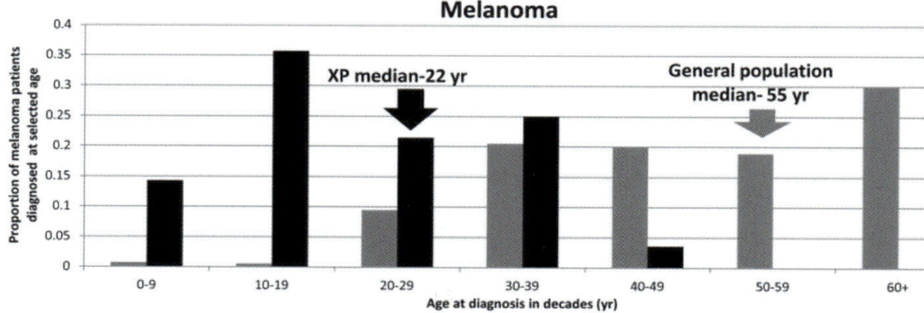


**Fig. 6.03** Skin cancer in the setting of xeroderma pigmentosum (XP). These graphs show the proportions of non-melanoma skin cancer cases (upper panel) and melanoma cases (lower panel) first diagnosed within each of the age groups indicated, among patients with XP (black bars) and in the general population of the USA (grey bars); individuals with both non-melanoma skin cancer and melanoma are included in both graphs. The median age at first diagnosis of non-melanoma skin cancer was 9 years among the patients with XP versus 67 years in the general population. The median age at first diagnosis of melanoma was 22 years among the patients with XP versus 55 years in the general population.

## Diagnostic criteria

Diagnosis is based on clinical features and confirmed by DNA sequencing and by tests of cellular hypersensitivity to (and DNA repair after) UV radiation–induced damage {1439}.

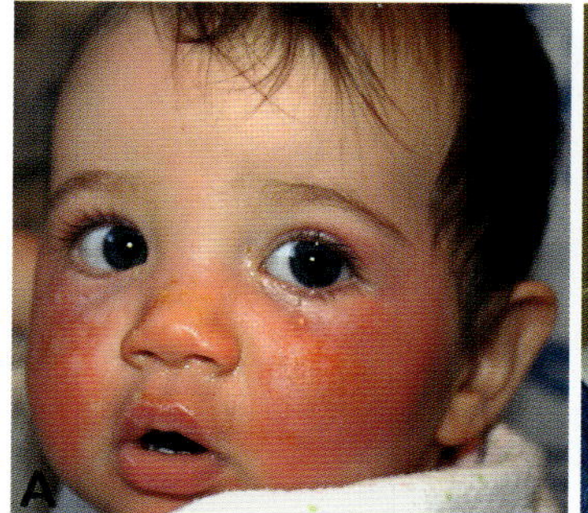

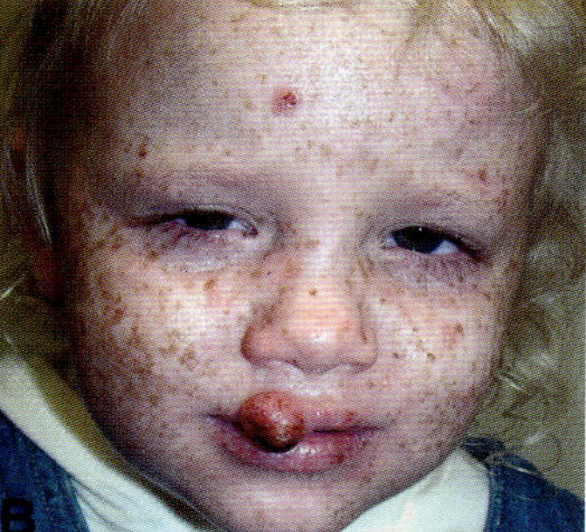

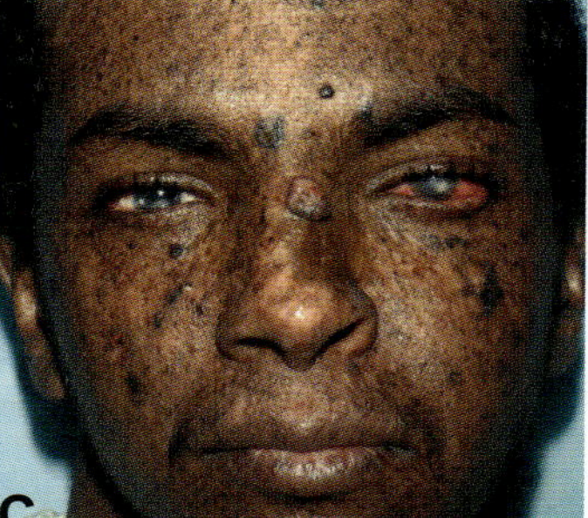

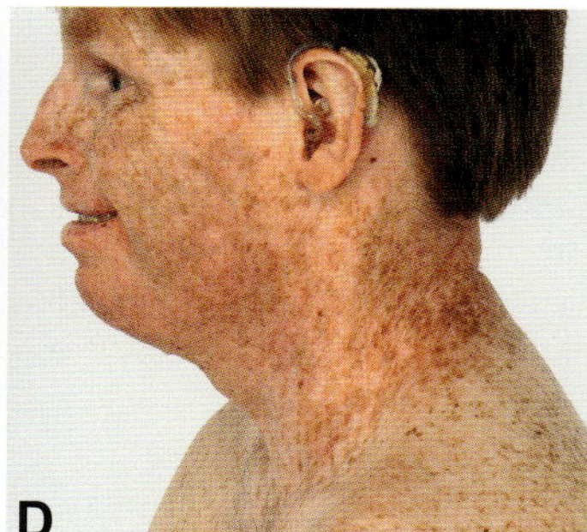


**Fig. 6.02** Xeroderma pigmentosum (XP). **A** A 9-month-old girl with XP complementation group D (XPD) with severe blistering erythema of the cheeks following minimal sun exposure. Note the sparing of her forehead and eyes, which were protected by a hat. **B** A 2-year-old girl with XP complementation group C (XPC) who did not sunburn easily but developed multiple hyperpigmented macules on her face. A rapidly growing keratoacanthoma or other squamous cell carcinoma grew on her upper lip and a precancerous lesion appeared on her forehead. **C** A 23-year-old northern African man with XPC with numerous hyperpigmented macules on his face. A nodular basal cell carcinoma is present on his left nasal root and a pigmented basal cell carcinoma on his left cheek. His eyes show corneal scarring from unprotected sun exposure. **D** A 35-year-old man with XP complementation group A (XPA) with neurological degeneration. He has numerous hyperpigmented macules on the sun-exposed areas of his face and neck. Progressive sensorineural deafness necessitates the use of a hearing aid.

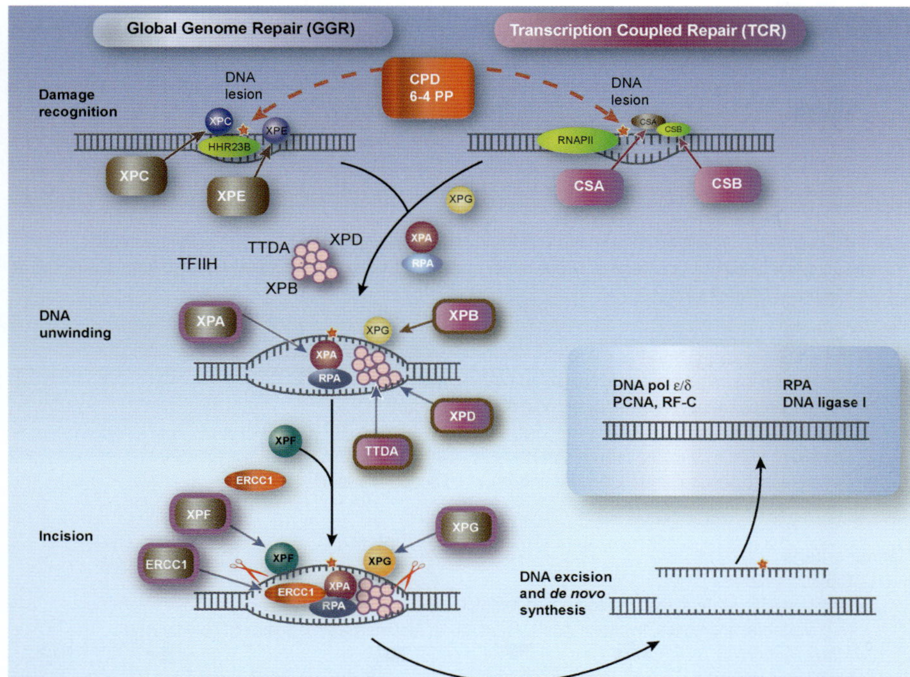


**Fig. 6.04** The nucleotide excision repair pathway. Transcription-coupled repair removes damage from actively transcribed genes, and global genome repair removes damage from the remainder of the genome. In global genome repair, DNA damage such as ultraviolet (UV) radiation–induced cyclobutane pyrimidine dimers (CPDs) and 6-4 photoproducts (6-4 PPs) is recognized by proteins including the *DDB2* (*XPE*) and *XPC* gene products. In transcription-coupled repair, the lesion appears to block the progress of RNA polymerase II (RNAPII) in a process involving the *ERCC8* (*CSA*) and *ERCC6* (*CSB*) gene products. Following initial damage recognition, the two pathways converge. The XPB (ERCC3) and XPD (ERCC2) helicases unwind the DNA region surrounding the lesion, along with the *XPA* and *ERCC5* (*XPG*) gene products and replication protein A (RPA). The XPF and XPG (ERCC5) endonucleases perform incisions to excise the lesion in a fragment of B30 nucleotides. The resulting gap is filled in via de novo DNA synthesis. If any individual part of this highly coordinated system is mutated, the entire pathway fails to function normally. Mutations in the genes shown in rounded rectangles have been associated with clinical disease. DNA pol ε/δ, DNA polymerase ε/δ; PCNA, proliferating cell nuclear antigen; RF-C, replication factor C.

## Clinical features

### *Skin*

Approximately half of the patients with XP have a history of acute sunburn following minimal sun exposure {290}. The other half have a history of almost-normal tanning. However, in all patients, numerous freckle-like hyperpigmented macules appear on sun-exposed skin, usually before the age of 2 years. Eyelid papillomas may be present. Basal cell carcinoma and squamous cell carcinoma are common, as is melanoma in the UV radiation–exposed portions of the eye {317}.

### *Eyes*

Ocular findings are limited to the anterior (UV radiation–exposed) structures. Photophobia may be associated with prominent conjunctival redness. UV irradiation of the eye may result in severe keratitis, leading to corneal opacification and vascularization. Patients may have loss of eyelashes, ectropion, entropion, or complete loss of the lids. Benign conjunctival inflammatory masses have been reported.

### *Nervous system*

Neurological abnormalities have been reported in approximately 25% of cases {290}. Onset may occur early in infancy (de Sanctis–Cacchione syndrome) or may be delayed until the second decade of life. The neurological abnormalities may initially be mild (e.g. isolated hyporeflexia), but often lead to progressive sensorineural deafness (beginning with high-frequency hearing loss) {2633}, mental retardation, microcephaly, spasticity, and/or seizures. In one study, the predominant neuropathological abnormality found at autopsy was loss of neurons, particularly in the cerebrum and cerebellum {1482}.

### *Cancer*

Among XP patients aged < 20 years, the risk of skin cancer (basal cell carcinoma, squamous cell carcinoma, and melanoma) in sun-exposed sites, including the anterior eye and the tip of the tongue, is more than 10 000 times the risk in the general population {290,388}. Multiple primary skin cancers are common. The reported median age of onset of non-melanoma skin cancer in the USA is 9 years – 50 years earlier than in the general population. Tumours of the brain (glioma and medulloblastoma) {290,1440}, CNS (astrocytoma of the spinal cord) {628}, lung, uterus {1482}, breast, pancreas, stomach, kidney, and testicle {1440}, as well as leukaemia {1440}, have also been reported in small numbers of patients. These reports suggest an overall risk of internal neoplasms about 10–20 times that in the general population {290,1482}.

## Genetics

XP has been associated with mutations in seven NER genes: *XPA*, *ERCC3 (XPB)*, *XPC*, *ERCC2 (XPD)*, *DDB2 (XPE)*, *ERCC4 (XPF)*, and *ERCC5 (XPG)* {627,1149}. *XPC* and *DDB2 (XPE)* code for proteins that recognize bulky DNA lesions produced by UV radiation and some other DNA-damaging agents. *ERCC3 (XPB)* and *ERCC2 (XPD)* are helicases necessary to open the double helix at the site of the lesion. *ERCC4 (XPF)* and *ERCC5 (XPG)* are endonucleases that cut the damaged strand at the 5' and 3' sites, respectively. There is marked clinical and molecular heterogeneity in XP. Patients with XPC, XPE, or XPV do not have neurological involvement, whereas patients with XPA, XPB, XPD, and XPG may have neurological abnormalities in addition to skin involvement. Patients with XPD may have one of at least five known clinical phenotypes: XP with skin disease, XP with neurological disease, XP–Cockayne syndrome complex, trichothiodystrophy (a disorder characterized by sulfur-deficient brittle hair), and XP–trichothiodystrophy complex {627}.

## Prognosis and predictive factors

Management of patients with XP is based on early diagnosis, lifelong protection from UV radiation exposure, and early detection and treatment of neoplasms {2566}. Gene therapy using corrected XP skin cells is being investigated {660,661,2785}.

# Naevoid basal cell carcinoma syndrome (Gorlin syndrome)

Granter S.
Evans D.G.
Sekulic A.

## Definition

Naevoid basal cell carcinoma syndrome (NBCCS), also known as Gorlin syndrome, is a complex syndrome involving multiple organ systems, caused by germline mutations in genes involved in the hedgehog signalling pathway (most commonly *PTCH1*).

## MIM number 109400

## Synonyms

Basal cell naevus syndrome; Gorlin syndrome; Gorlin–Goltz syndrome

## Epidemiology

Estimates of the prevalence of NBCCS have ranged from 1 case per 164 000 population to 1 case per 30 827 population {715,2397}, with an incidence of 1 case per 15 000 births {715}.

## Diagnostic criteria

Diagnosis is relatively straightforward in most patients, but in others it can be challenging because of the variable expressivity of the syndrome, in particular in dark-skinned patients, who may not develop basal cell carcinomas (BCCs). The diagnosis of NBCCS requires confirmation either of two major criteria or of one major criterion plus two minor criteria, as summarized in Table 6.04 {297}.

**Table 6.04** Diagnostic criteria for naevoid basal cell carcinoma syndrome (NBCCS). The diagnosis requires confirmation either of two major criteria or of one major criterion plus two minor criteria. Adapted from: Evans DG et al. J Med Genet. 30:460–4 {716}

**Major criteria**
- Basal cell carcinoma onset at < 20 years of age, or an excessive number of basal cell carcinomas (out of proportion to prior sun exposure and skin type)
- Odontogenic keratocyst (keratocystic odontogenic tumour)
- Palmar or plantar pitting
- Lamellar calcification of the falx cerebri
- Desmoplastic or nodular medulloblastoma in a child aged < 4 years[a]
- A first-degree relative with NBCCS

**Minor criteria**
- Rib abnormalities
- Other specific skeletal malformations and radiological changes (e.g. vertebral anomalies, kyphoscoliosis, short fourth metacarpals, or postaxial polydactyly)
- Macrocephaly
- Cleft lip or palate
- Ovarian or cardiac fibroma
- Lymphomesenteric cysts
- Ocular abnormalities (e.g. strabismus, hypertelorism, congenital cataracts, glaucoma, or coloboma)

[a] The diagnostic criteria have been adapted to include early-onset childhood medulloblastoma as a major criterion; however, in order to protect specificity (i.e. to prevent cases from spuriously meeting the criteria on the basis of radiation-induced basal cell carcinomas from non-NBCCS medulloblastoma), only the medulloblastoma histologies specifically associated with NBCCS (desmoplastic and nodular) are included, and only when occurring in a child aged < 4 years.

## Clinical features

Numerous clinical abnormalities are associated with NBCCS. Here we focus on the most common abnormalities, which constitute major and minor diagnostic criteria.

BCCs typically appear in childhood or early adulthood, with a mean age at presentation of 21.4 years {1370}. The tumours vary in number from one to more than a thousand, and tend to occur on sun-damaged skin of the face, elsewhere in the head and neck region, the trunk, and limbs {1370}. It is important to note that although 97% of White patients with NBCCS aged > 40 years were found to have developed BCCs, only about 40% of Black patients were found to have developed BCCs by the age of 35 years {1370}. The tumour behaviour is variable, ranging from indolent to locally aggressive {1370}. The development of BCCs at sites of radiation therapy

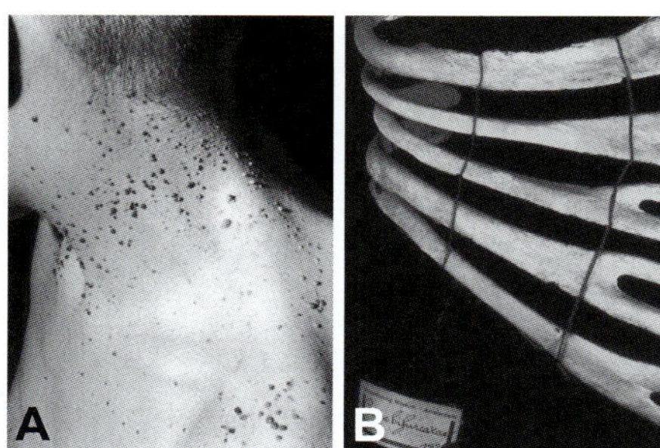


**Fig. 6.05** Naevoid basal cell carcinoma syndrome (Gorlin syndrome). **A** Numerous basal cell carcinomas in the head and neck area and upper trunk. **B** Multiple bifid ribs.

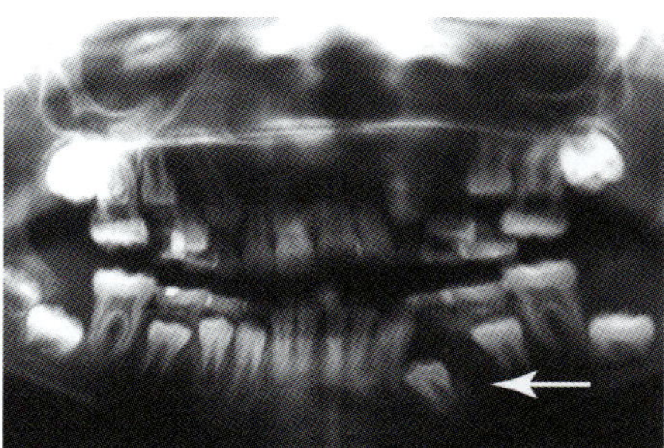

**Fig. 6.06** Naevoid basal cell carcinoma syndrome (Gorlin syndrome). Multiple odontogenic keratocysts (keratocystic odontogenic tumours) are highlighted by the presence of displaced teeth (arrow).

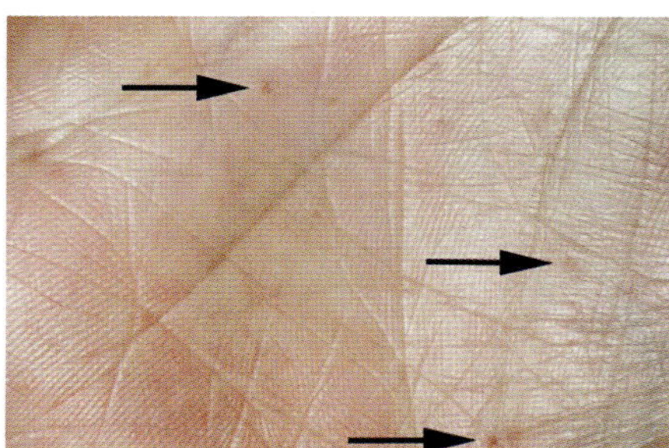

**Fig. 6.07** Naevoid basal cell carcinoma syndrome (Gorlin syndrome). Palmar pitting (arrows) can be extremely subtle; it is easier to detect in less-clean hands, because dirt tends to become trapped in the pits.

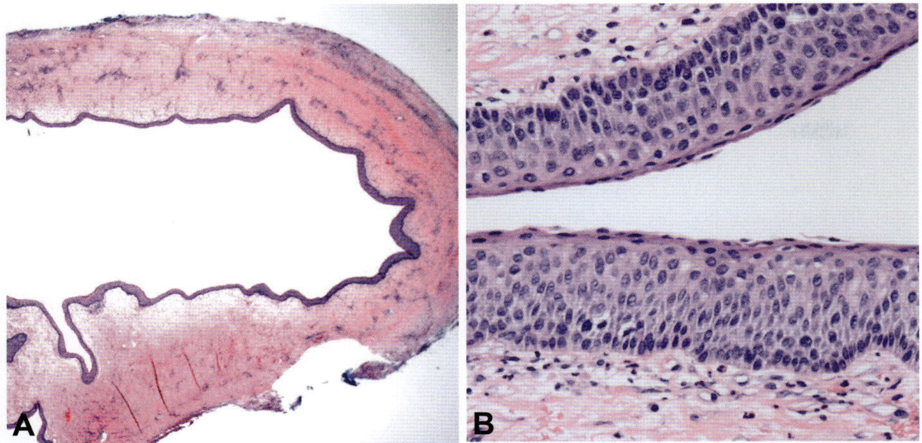

**Fig. 6.08** Naevoid basal cell carcinoma syndrome (Gorlin syndrome): odontogenic keratocyst (keratocystic odontogenic tumour). **A** Scanning magnification shows a squamous lined cyst. **B** Higher magnification shows expansion of the basal and parabasal layers and parakeratosis.

is a well-documented complication of NBCCS {1370}. Odontogenic keratocysts (keratocystic odontogenic tumours) of the jaw are seen in 75% of patients, with a mean age at presentation of 15.5 years in one large study and 17.7 years in another {1370,2397}. Three quarters of patients develop cysts by the age of 20 years {1370}. The cysts are most commonly located in the mandible. Multiple cysts are typical; in one study, they numbered up to 28 (mean: 5.1) {1370}. The cysts are usually symptomatic (causing swelling, jaw pain, etc.) but about one third are asymptomatic, detected by radiological exam {2397}. The cysts have a marked tendency to recur, often requiring multiple surgeries; in one series, the recurrence rate was 60% {1727}.

Palmar or plantar pitting is seen in as many as 87% of patients, with the palms being slightly more commonly affected than the soles (in 86% and 81% of cases, respectively) {716,1370}. Pitting can develop in patients as young as 5 months.

Lamellar calcification of the falx cerebri is seen in as many as 92% of patients {716,2397}. Less commonly, calcification of the diaphragma sellae, tentorium cerebelli, and petroclinoid ligaments may be seen.

Medulloblastoma, most often the desmoplastic variant, is seen in 5% of patients and is often diagnosed in the first few years of life {297}. Desmoplastic medulloblastoma in the setting of NBCCS has a more favourable prognosis compared with classic medulloblastoma in the absence of NBCCS. Recently, another variant of medulloblastoma (medulloblastoma with extensive nodularity) has been shown to also be associated with NBCCS {856}. Patients with NBCCS and medulloblastoma should be considered for *SUFU* testing {2469}.

Rib abnormalities, most commonly fusion, splaying, bifurcation, or hypoplasia, are seen in approximately half of patients and most commonly affect the third, fourth, and fifth ribs {1370}.

Other skeletal malformations and radiological changes are also common, including vertebral anomalies, kyphoscoliosis, short fourth metacarpals, postaxial polydactyly, pectus deformities, Sprengel deformity, and syndactyly.

Macrocephaly is seen in 80% of patients {716,2397}. Hypertelorism is also a common finding, seen in as many as 42% of patients {1370}.

Cleft lip or palate is seen in approximately 6% of patients {716}. However, high-arched palate or prominent palatine ridges were seen in nearly half of the patients in one study {1370}, and high-arched palate was seen in 63% of patients in another {2397}.

Ovarian fibromas, which are usually bilateral and calcified, are found in as many as 24% of patients {716}.

Cardiac fibromas are uncommon, seen in 3% of patients {716}; although often asymptomatic and discovered during screening imaging studies, some cases may be associated with life-threatening arrhythmias {277}. Ovarian fibroma is also a minor diagnostic criterion for NBCCS.

Lymphomesenteric cysts (cystic lymphangiomas) are present in as many as 8%

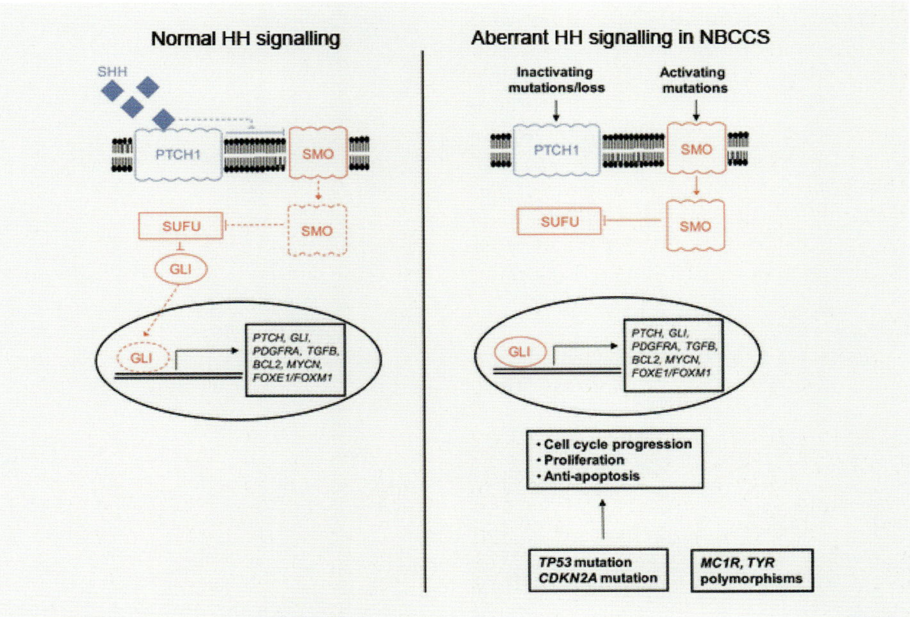


**Fig. 6.09** The hedgehog (HH) signalling pathway: normal HH signalling and aberrant HH signalling in naevoid basal cell carcinoma syndrome (NBCCS). In the normal HH signalling pathway (left panel), in the presence of the sonic hedgehog signalling protein (SHH), PTCH1 suppresses smoothened (SMO), which in turn allows SUFU to inhibit GLI transcription factors; in the absence of SHH, SMO is released from inhibition by PTCH1 and translocates to the cytosol, where it inhibits SUFU, thereby relieving inhibition of GLI transcription factors (normal signalling, left panel). In NBCCS (right panel), *PTCH1* mutations lead to constitutive activation of GLI transcription factors; in rare NBCCS cases, *SMO* mutations (which are common in sporadic basal cell carcinoma) or *SUFU* mutations may lead to the same result.

of patients and tend to be asymptomatic {2488}.

Ocular abnormalities, including strabismus, nystagmus, congenital cataracts, glaucoma, coloboma, and microphthalmia, are seen in as many as 26% of patients {716}.

## Genetics

NBCCS is caused by mutations in the hedgehog signalling pathway, most commonly (in ~70% of patients) loss-of-function mutations in the *PTCH1* gene located at 9q22.3 {986}. In the absence of its ligand – the sonic hedgehog (SHH) protein – the membrane-bound protein PTCH1 maintains smoothened (SMO) in its inactive state, and SMO is incapable of activating GLI transcription factors (see Fig. 6.09, p. 389). SUFU (encoded by the *SUFU* gene) also negatively regulates GLI transcription factors. Mutations in *PTCH1*, or (much less commonly) *SMO* or *SUFU*, result in constitutive activation of the hedgehog signalling pathway. A phase II clinical trial has shown that treatment with vismodegib, an SMO antagonist, reduces the development of surgically eligible BCCs in patients with NBCCS {2573}. Vismodegib treatment has also been shown to decrease the size of odontogenic keratocysts (keratocystic odontogenic tumours) {62}.

Much of what is known about the molecular pathogenesis of sporadic BCCs comes from research on NBCCS. Approximately 90% of sporadic BCCs harbour two somatic mutations in *PTCH1*, and approximately 10% of sporadic BCCs have activating mutations in *SMO* {2866}.

# Carney complex

Zembowicz A.
Stratakis C.A.

## Definition

Carney complex is characterized by skin pigmentation abnormalities, myxomas, endocrine tumours or overactivity, and psammomatous melanotic schwannomas {530,2517}.

## MIM number

160980

## Synonyms

LAMB syndrome (lentigines, atrial myxomas, and blue naevi); NAME syndrome (naevi, atrial myxomas, myxoid neurofibromas, and ephelides)

Carney complex was first described by Dr J. Aidan Carney, as "the complex of myxomas, spotting pigmentation and endocrine over-reactivity" {530}.

## Epidemiology

Carney complex is very rare, with up to 800 reported cases. The majority of cases are familial, but 25–40% of patients have no family history.

**Table 6.05** Diagnostic criteria for Carney complex; the diagnosis requires confirmation of at least two major criteria

**Major criteria**

- Spotty skin pigmentation with typical distribution (i.e. lips, conjunctiva, inner or outer canthi, and vaginal or penile mucosa)
- Myxoma[a] (cutaneous and mucosal)
- Cardiac myxoma[a]
- Breast myxomatosis[a], or fat-suppressed MRI findings suggestive of this diagnosis
- Primary pigmented nodular adrenocortical diseasea, or paradoxical positive response of urinary glucocorticosteroid excretion to dexamethasone administration during the high-dose dexamethasone suppression test (the Liddle test)
- Acromegaly as a result of growth hormone–producing adenoma[a]
- Large cell calcifying Sertoli cell tumour[a], or characteristic calcification seen on testicular ultrasound
- Thyroid carcinoma[a], or multiple hypoechoic nodules seen on thyroid ultrasound in a child aged < 18 years
- Psammomatous melanotic schwannomas[a]
- Pigmented epithelioid melanocytoma (epithelioid blue naevus)[a]
- Breast ductal adenoma[a]
- Osteochondromyxoma[a]

**Supplementary criteria**

- A first-degree relative with Carney complex
- Inactivating pathogenic variants of *PRKAR1A*

[a] These criteria require histological confirmation.

## Diagnostic criteria

The diagnostic criteria for Carney complex are listed in Table 6.05.

## Clinical features

Manifestations of Carney complex typically develop by early in the third decade of life {530,2517}. Pale-brown to black lentigines involving the lips, conjunctiva, inner or outer corners of the eyes (the canthi), and the genital areas are the most common presenting feature of Carney complex; these lentigines typically increase in number at puberty. Some patients develop larger pigmented papules or nodules, which correspond to pigmented epithelioid melanocytomas (also called epithelioid blue naevi) {384}. Cardiac myxomas can occur in any (or all) cardiac chambers and can lead to intracardiac obstruction of blood flow, embolic phenomena, and/or heart failure. Myxomas can also involve the skin, breast, oropharynx, and female genital tract. Cushing syndrome associated with primary pigmented nodular adrenocortical disease is the most frequent endocrine manifestation. Although people with Carney complex have an increased risk of cancer, most of the tumours associated with Carney complex are benign; large cell calcifying Sertoli cell tumour affects one third of boys within the first decade and almost all adult men. As many as 75% of individuals with Carney complex have multiple thyroid nodules, most of which are thyroid follicular adenomas. Although > 75% of patients have abnormal growth hormone secretion, clinically evident acromegaly as a result of a growth hormone–producing pituitary adenoma is evident in only 10–15%; a

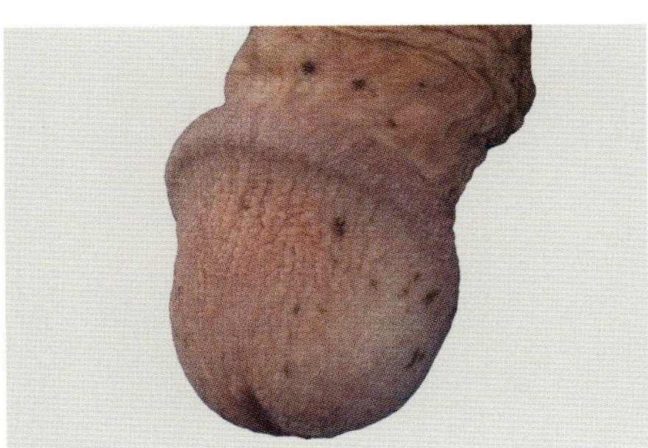

**Fig. 6.10** Carney complex. Mucosal lentiginosis.

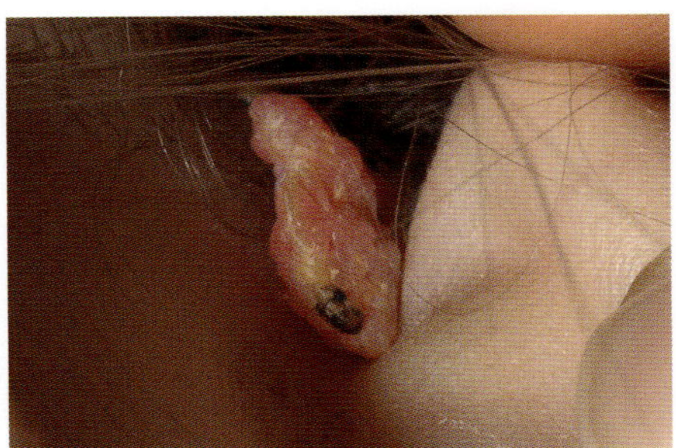

**Fig. 6.11** Carney complex. Superficial angiomyxoma.

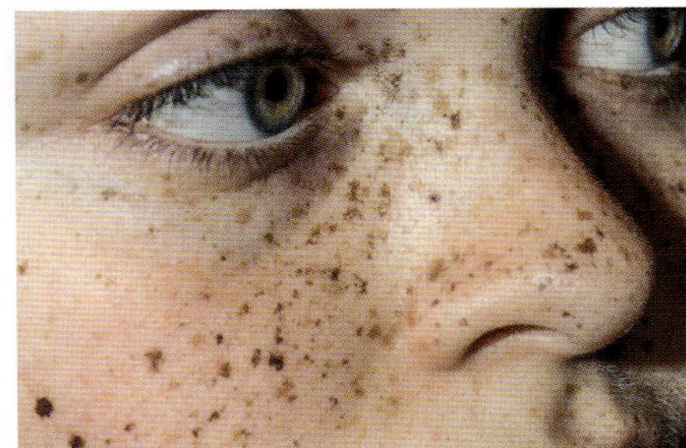

**Fig. 6.12** Carney complex. Cutaneous lentiginosis.

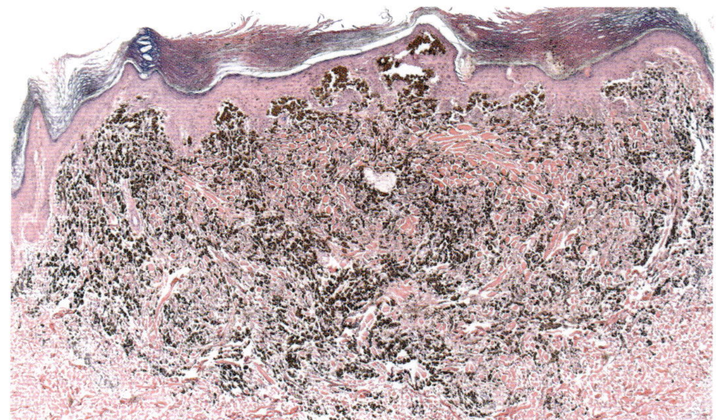

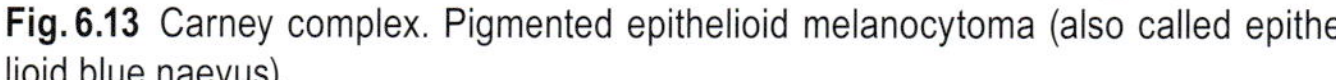

**Fig. 6.13** Carney complex. Pigmented epithelioid melanocytoma (also called epithelioid blue naevus).

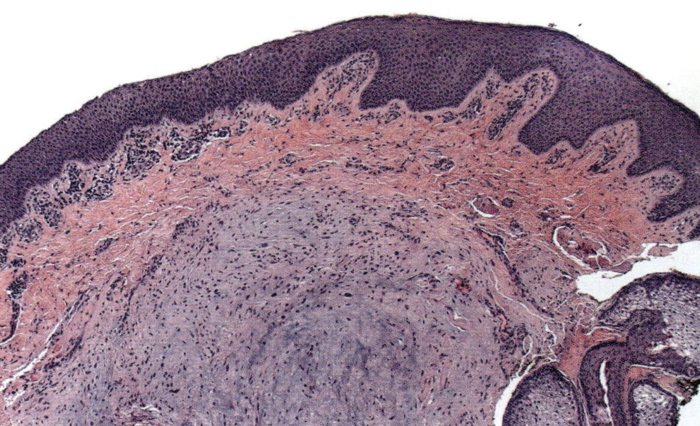

**Fig. 6.14** Carney complex. Superficial angiomyxoma.

few individuals present with gigantism in adolescence. Psammomatous melanotic schwannoma, a rare nerve sheath tumour (which can be aggressive), occurs in an estimated 10% of affected individuals. The median age at diagnosis is 20 years.

## Genetics

About 62% of the families with Carney complex have pathogenic mutations in *PRKAR1A* (located on chromosome 17q24.2), the gene that encodes the regulatory subunit 1α of the cAMP-dependent protein kinase A {224,1130,1380}; the frequency is even higher (80%) among individuals presenting with Cushing syndrome caused by primary pigmented nodular adrenocortical disease. Approximately 20% of individuals with Carney complex who are negative for *PRKAR1A* single-nucleotide variants carry *PRKAR1A* deletions resulting in *PRKAR1A* haploinsufficiency {1131,2291}. In another 20% of families affected by Carney complex, the condition has been linked to a locus on chromosome 2p16 {1381}, but no gene has been found to be mutated in these cases.

Pathogenic germline duplications of *PRKACA*, the gene that encodes the catalytic subunit Cα of protein kinase A, have been detected in patients with adrenal tumours and Cushing syndrome who do not have other manifestations of Carney complex {235,1584}. It is unclear whether these patients in fact have Carney complex or not. *PRKACB* gene amplification has been identified in one patient with Carney complex {811}. *PRKACB* encodes the catalytic subunit Cβ of protein kinase A. Both the *PRKACA* and *PRKACB* defects are gain-of-function mutations, and the effects are thus similar in many ways to those of the inactivating *PRKAR1A* defects; all of these defects lead to protein kinase A activation.

The overall penetrance of Carney complex among individuals with a pathogenic *PRKAR1A* variant is > 95% by the age of 50 years {530,2517}. To date, only two *PRKAR1A* mutations are known to result in incomplete penetrance of Carney complex {224,950,1130}. When expressed, these two pathogenic variants lead to a relatively mild version of Carney complex, manifesting mostly as primary pigmented nodular adrenocortical disease, which can be accompanied by lentigines.

## Prognosis and predictive factors

Most patients with Carney complex do well if they are enrolled in a clinical surveillance programme. It is appropriate to evaluate relatives at risk in order to identify as early as possible those who would benefit from initiation of treatment and preventive measures.

# *BAP1* tumour predisposition syndrome

Bastian B.C.
de la Fouchardière A.
Hayward N.
Murali R.
Scolyer R.A.
Wiesner T.

## Definition

*BAP1* tumour predisposition syndrome (*BAP1*-TPDS) is caused by germline mutations in the *BAP1* gene and is inherited in an autosomal dominant pattern. Individuals carrying heterozygous *BAP1* mutations have an increased risk of developing various tumour types, most commonly *BAP1*-inactivated naevi/melanocytomas of the skin, uveal and cutaneous melanomas, peritoneal and pleural mesotheliomas, clear cell renal cell carcinoma, and basal cell carcinoma.

## MIM number

614327

## Synonyms

Tumour predisposition syndrome; *BAP1* loss familial cancer syndrome; *BAP1* hereditary cancer syndrome; COMMON syndrome (cutaneous/ocular melanoma, atypical melanocytic proliferations, and other internal neoplasms)

## Epidemiology

The prevalence is unknown, but *BAP1*-TPDS is likely a rare hereditary cancer syndrome; approximately 100 affected families have been reported in the literature to date.

## Diagnostic criteria

Affected individuals are often first clinically suspected of having *BAP1*-TPDS when they manifest tumours associated with the syndrome, particularly when the tumours develop at a young age. The diagnosis of *BAP1*-TPDS should be confirmed by the detection of loss-of-function *BAP1* mutations in the germline DNA {1850,2828}.

## Clinical features

The most common manifestations of *BAP1*-TPDS are multiple *BAP1*-inactivated naevi/melanocytomas of the skin. Beginning in the second decade of life, affected patients usually develop multiple inconspicuous, skin-coloured to reddish-brown, dome-shaped to pedunculated, well-circumscribed papules, predominantly on sun-exposed skin. Some of these *BAP1*-inactivated melanocytic tumours display small areas of brown colour at their periphery, likely because they evolve from common acquired naevi. The number of lesions varies, typically ranging from a few to > 50 {2828}.

Histologically, *BAP1*-inactivated naevi/melanocytomas of the skin are predominantly composed of intradermal melanocytes with varying degrees of atypia, ranging from clearly benign lesions with naevoid cells and minimal atypia (*BAP1*-inactivated naevi) to highly atypical tumours with large epithelioid cells with well-defined cytoplasmic borders, abundant amphophilic cytoplasm, pleomorphic vesicular nuclei, and prominent nucleoli (*BAP1*-inactivated melanocytomas). Tumour-infiltrating lymphocytes are often seen. Many of these skin lesions appear as combined melanocytic naevi with areas of small, oval melanocytes (a common naevus component) adjacent to the larger, epithelioid melanocytes. In

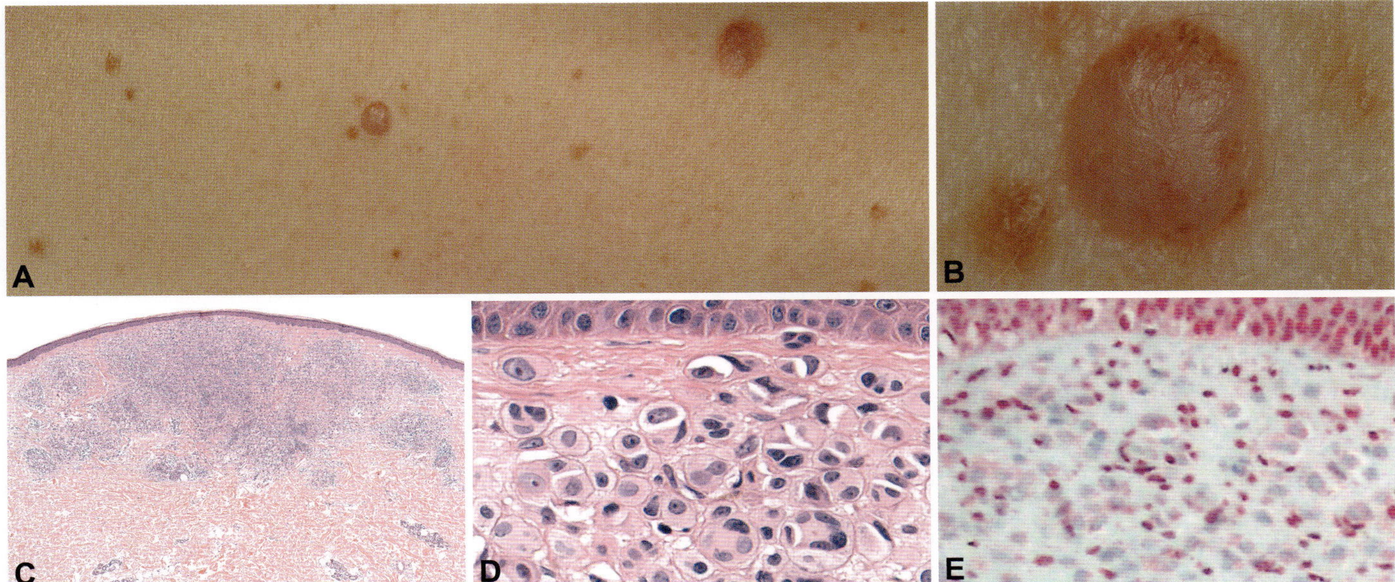

**Fig. 6.15** *BAP1*-inactivated naevi (skin lesions typical of *BAP1* tumour predisposition syndrome). **A** Multiple skin-coloured to slightly reddish dome-shaped papules on the right upper arm, together with common acquired naevi. **B** One *BAP1*-inactivated naevus is shown in detail. **C** Symmetrical, predominantly intradermal tumour. **D** Higher magnification shows enlarged, epithelioid melanocytes with distinct cell borders, abundant cytoplasm, large nuclei with vesicular chromatin, and conspicuous nucleoli. **E** Immunohistochemistry shows loss of nuclear BAP1 expression in the large, epithelioid melanocytes, but not in the keratinocytes or the tumour-infiltrating lymphocytes.

most lesions, the wildtype *BAP1* allele is inactivated (by various somatic alterations), resulting in a lack of nuclear BAP1 expression on immunohistochemistry. Most lesions also harbour BRAF p.V600E mutations {1578,2827}.

In addition to *BAP1*-inactivated naevi/melanocytomas of the skin, individuals with germline *BAP1* mutations have an increased risk of developing uveal and cutaneous melanomas {1009,2828}; peritoneal and pleural mesotheliomas {2601,2823}; clear cell renal cell carcinoma {2088}; basal cell carcinoma {589,2760}; and probably other cancer types, including cholangiocarcinoma {1228,2060}, meningioma {183,454}, lung adenocarcinoma {84,183}, thyroid cancer {1711,2088}, leptomeningeal melanoma {588}, and paraganglioma {2759}.

## Genetics

*BAP1*-TPDS is caused by germline mutations in the *BAP1* tumour suppressor gene, which is located on the short arm of chromosome 3 (at 3p21.1) and encodes a ubiquitin carboxy-terminal hydrolase. The BAP1 protein, which is part of the polycomb repressive deubiquitinase complex, deubiquitinates histone H2A and is involved in chromatin modification and transcriptional regulation. Inactivation of BAP1 may occur as a result of chromosomal deletions involving the *BAP1* locus or because of loss-of-function mutations altering the *BAP1* nucleotide sequence. The mutations are most commonly deleterious nonsense, frameshift, or splice-site mutations that result in a truncated and non-functional protein, or deleterious missense mutations that interfere with the ubiquitin hydrolase function of BAP1 {1850}.

## Prognosis and predictive factors

Penetrance is incomplete, but the precise risk of an individual patient with *BAP1*-TPDS developing one or more of the associated tumours has not yet been determined. Additional environmental factors may increase the risk; for example, ultraviolet (UV) radiation and asbestos exposure may increase the risk of melanoma and mesothelioma, respectively. Prognosis depends on the tumour type and stage of the malignancies. *BAP1*-inactivated naevi/melanocytomas of the skin have a good prognosis and rarely metastasize {1850}.

# Muir–Torre syndrome

Lazar A.J.
Calonje E.
Wood B.A.

## Definition

Muir–Torre syndrome (MTS) is a hereditary condition characterized by the development of cutaneous sebaceous neoplasia and visceral malignancies. MTS is considered a variant of Lynch syndrome (MIM number 120435). The phenotype of sebaceous neoplasia and visceral malignancy can also be seen in patients with abnormalities of *MUTYH* (familial adenomatous polyposis 2, MIM number 608456).

## MIM number 158320

## Epidemiology

The population incidence of MTS has not yet been determined, but the syndrome has been identified in approximately 9% of individuals from families with Lynch syndrome {2080,2487}.

## Diagnostic criteria

MTS is characterized by synchronous or metachronous development of cutaneous sebaceous neoplasia and visceral malignancy. The presence of multiple keratoacanthomas and visceral malignancy in a patient with a family history of MTS may also be diagnostic {2360}. Molecular confirmation by germline assessment of DNA mismatch repair genes such as *MSH2*, *MLH1*, and *MSH6* can play an important role in diagnostic confirmation and in the screening of individuals with a definite risk due to family history.

## Clinical features

The cutaneous lesions seen in MTS include sebaceous adenoma, sebaceoma, and sebaceous carcinoma {334,1234,2263}. The strongest association is with sebaceous adenoma; the association with sebaceous carcinoma (in particular periocular sebaceous carcinoma) is weaker {2082}. Sebaceous tumours with cystic changes can be seen, but are not pathognomonic {9,104,2263}. Sebaceous neoplasms outside the head and neck region are characteristic; conversely, periocular sebaceous lesions are only occasionally associated with MTS. Multiple sebaceous neoplasms are a very strong indicator. There is no association with sebaceous hyperplasia. Keratoacanthomas, sometimes showing sebaceous differentiation, in particular multiple lesions in younger patients at sites without chronic sun exposure, can be a feature, but these are less frequently reported in the recent literature.

Gastrointestinal malignancies, in particular carcinomas involving the right side of the colon, occur in about 50% of patients. Adenocarcinoma of the small bowel and gastric carcinoma are also seen {2596,2789}. Colon polyps are found in about one quarter of patients. Urothelial carcinoma, in particular involving the renal pelvis and ureter, occurs in approximately 20–25% of patients {582}, and 15% of female patients develop endometrial carcinoma {505}. Other reported malignancies include ovarian carcinoma, gliomas, breast carcinoma, prostate carcinoma, sarcoma, and tumours of the lung and haematolymphoid system.

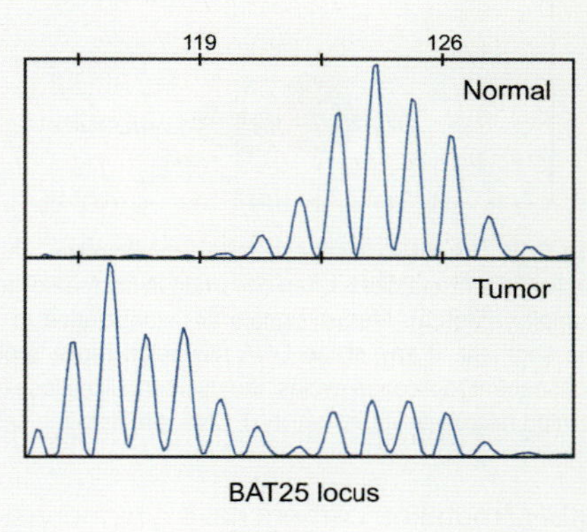


**Fig. 6.17** Microsatellite instability. The BAT25 microsatellite shows instability in the tumour compared with normal tissue, indicating DNA mismatch repair deficiency, as is seen in most cases of Lynch syndrome and Muir–Torre syndrome.

## Genetics

About 70% of cases of MTS are associated with inherited germline abnormalities of DNA mismatch repair protein genes. Loss of the remaining wildtype allele leads to microsatellite instability in the associated tumours. Abnormalities of *MSH2* are strongly associated with the MTS phenotype, with *MSH2* mutations present in 90% of cases. Most of the remaining cases harbour *MLH1* abnormalities. This strongly contrasts with Lynch syndrome, where germline deficits of *MLH1* and *MSH2* have roughly equal incidence. Compared with *MLH1* mutation carriers,

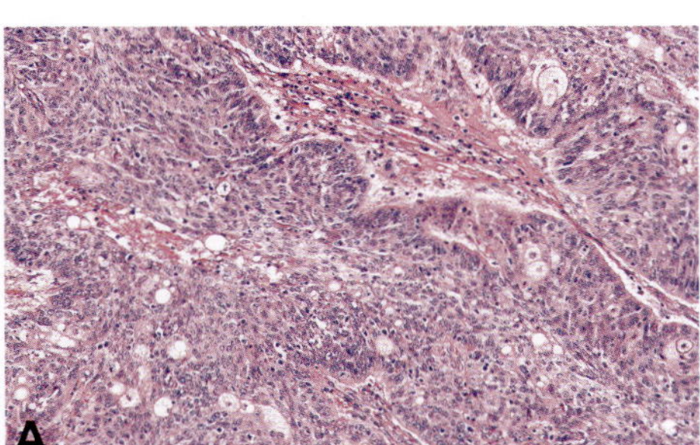

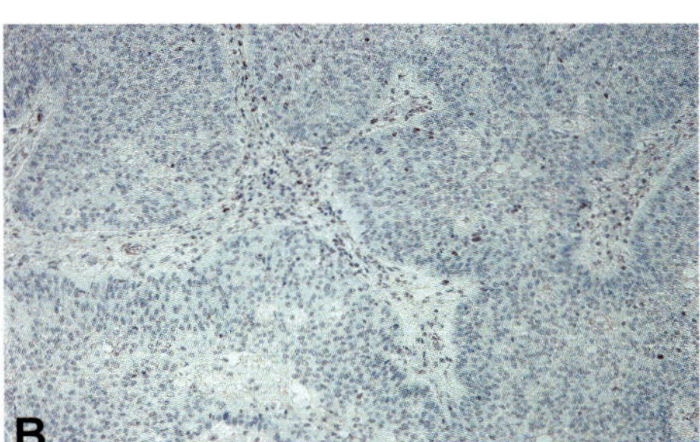

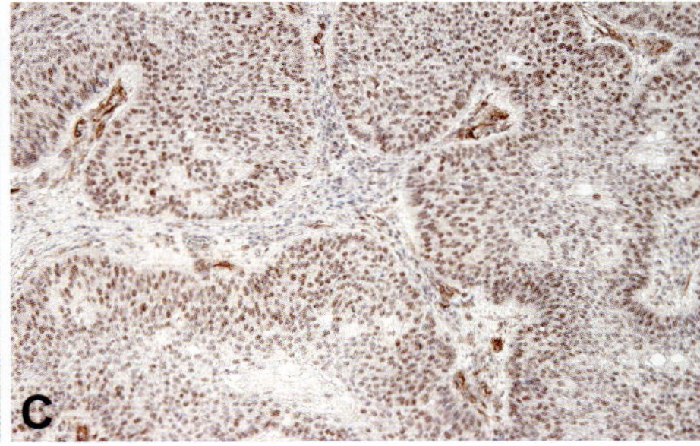


**Fig. 6.16** Sebaceous carcinoma. **A** Sebaceous carcinoma of the trunk. **B** Loss of nuclear MSH2 is seen in this case associated with Muir–Torre syndrome. **C** Nuclear MLH1 is retained.

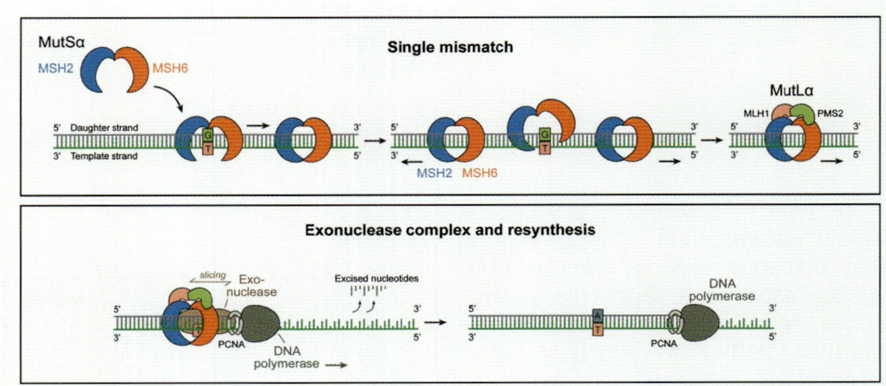


**Fig. 6.18** The DNA mismatch repair mechanism. The MSH2–MSH6 complex (MutSα) detects single base-pair replication mismatches, often occurring in microsatellites (areas of repetitive DNA sequence). With the MLH1–PMS2 complex (MutLα), MutSα signals an exonuclease to excise the mismatch. DNA polymerase then resynthesizes the segment. If any of the DNA mismatch repair proteins are not functional, then mismatches accumulate; with subsequent replication cycles, the microsatellites lose (or sometimes gain) base pairs, resulting in changes in length, termed microsatellite instability. PCNA, proliferating cell nuclear antigen.

*MSH2* mutation carriers have a higher risk of urothelial, ovarian, and CNS tumours {895,2789}. Abnormalities of *MSH6* are an uncommon cause of MTS and may be associated with a somewhat distinct presentation, including relatively higher risks of colorectal and endometrial cancers, but lower risks of gastric and small bowel carcinomas {367,1635,2596}. *PMS2* mutations have been reported only anecdotally.

Immunohistochemically, approximately one half to two thirds of unselected sebaceous neoplasms are deficient in DNA mismatch repair proteins (MSH2, MLH1, and MSH6) {723,1225,2453}. The rates of loss vary; in the head and neck region, adenomas show 30–40% loss, whereas loss in carcinomas is rare. Outside the head and neck region, both adenomas and carcinomas commonly show loss (in > 80% of cases). DNA-based testing to directly demonstrate microsatellite instability strongly correlates with immunohistochemistry {1448,1695}. These rates of loss are much higher than the incidence of MTS. Immunohistochemistry on all patients may not be effective as a screening tool; genetic testing and careful correlation with clinical history are often needed {2196}. Somatic mutation of either *MSH2* or *MLH1* has been seen in sebaceous tumours, explaining the lack of germline concordance {1242,2602}. Published positive predictive values for immunohistochemistry in the detection of germline DNA mismatch repair defects range from 22% to 37%, although negative predictive values were as high as 95% {723,2197}.

As many as one third of MTS cases display a microsatellite-stable phenotype. Some cases are associated with *MSH6* mutation, and a proportion show biallelic inactivation of the base excision repair gene *MUTYH* and an autosomal recessive inheritance pattern {1234}.

## Prognosis and predictive factors

The visceral malignancies of MTS and Lynch syndrome are generally found to have less-aggressive behaviour than their sporadic counterparts {2360}.

# Contributors

* Indicates participation in the Working Group Meeting on the WHO Classification of Skin Tumours that was held in Lyon, France, 24–26 September 2017

\# Indicates disclosure of interests


**Dr Abbas AGAIMY**
Institute of Pathology
University of Erlangen
Krankenhausstraße 8-10
91054 Erlangen
GERMANY
Tel. +49 9131 85 22288
Fax +49 9131 85 24745
abbas.agaimy@uk-erlangen.de

**Dr Aleodor A. ANDEA**
Department of Pathology
Michigan Medicine, University of Michigan
University Hospital, Floor 2,
1500 East Medical Center Drive, SPC 5054
Ann Arbor MI 48109
USA
Tel. +1 734 764 4460
Fax +1 734 764 4690
andeaa@med.umich.edu

**Dr Zsolt B. ARGENYI**
Department of Dermatopathology
University of Washington Medical Center
1959 Northeast Pacific Street
Seattle WA 98195-6100
USA
Tel. +1 206 598 4615
zsolt@uw.edu

**Dr Bruce ARMSTRONG**
48 Austin Street, Unit 14
Shenton Park WA 6008
AUSTRALIA
Tel. +61 403 496 404
bruce.armstrong@uwa.edu.au

**Dr Armita BAHRAMI**
Department of Pathology
St. Jude Children's Research Hospital
262 Danny Thomas Place
Memphis TN 38105
USA
Tel. +1 901 595 7116
Fax +1 901 595 3100
armita.bahrami@stjude.org

**Dr Raymond L. BARNHILL** *#
Department of Pathology
Institut Curie, Faculty of Medicine
University of Paris Descartes
26 Rue d'Ulm
75005 Paris
FRANCE
Tel. +33 6 21 04 86 74
Fax +33 1 53 10 40 10
raymond.barnhill@gmail.com

**Dr Boris C. BASTIAN** *
Department of Dermatology
University of California San Francisco
555 Mission Bay Boulevard South
Room 252K, Box 3118
San Francisco CA 94143-3118
USA
Tel. +1 415 502 0267
boris.bastian@ucsf.ed

**Dr Maxime BATTISTELLA**
Pathology Department
Hôpital Saint Louis, AP-HP
Université Paris 7
1 Avenue Claude Vellefaux
75010 Paris
FRANCE
Tel. +33 1 42 49 45 61
Fax +33 1 42 49 99 54
maxime.battistella@aphp.fr

**Dr Trevor W. BEER**
Department of Anatomical Pathology
Clinipath Pathology
310 Selby Street North
Osborne Park WA 6017
AUSTRALIA
Tel. +61 8 9371 4507
Fax +61 8 9382 9446
trevorbeer@gmail.com

**Dr Emilio BERTI** *
Department of Dermatology
Fondazione IRCCS Cà Granda
Ospedale Maggiore Policlinico
Via Pace 9
20122 Milano
ITALY
Tel. +39 2 5503 5107
Fax +39 2 5032 0779
emilio.berti@unimi.it

**Dr Marianne BERWICK**
Department of Dermatology and
Internal Medicine
University of New Mexico
2703 Frontier Avenue Northeast
Albuquerque NM 87131-0001
USA
Tel. +1 505 272 4369
Fax +1 505 272 2570
mberwick@salud.unm.edu

**Dr Steven D. BILLINGS** *
Anatomic Pathology Department
Cleveland Clinic Main Campus
Mail Code L25
9500 Euclid Avenue
Cleveland OH 44195
USA
Tel. +1 216 444 2826
billins@ccf.org

**Dr Thomas BRENN** *
Depts. of Pathology & Laboratory Medicine
University of Calgary
Diagnostic & Scientific Centre
9–3535 Research Road NW
Calgary AB
CANADA T2L 2K8
Tel. +1 403 770 3201
Fax +1 403 770 3295
thomas.brenn@ucalgary.ca

**Dr Klaus J. BUSAM**
Department of Pathology
Memorial Sloan Kettering Cancer Center
1275 York Avenue
New York NY 10065
USA
Tel. +1 212 639 5905
Fax +1 323 321 5015
busamk@mskcc.org

**Dr Eduardo CALONJE** *
Dermatopathology Laboratory
St John's Institute of Dermatology
St Thomas' Hospital
Westminster Bridge Road
London SE1 7EH
UNITED KINGDOM
Tel. +44 20 7188 6408
Fax +44 20 7188 6382
jaime.calonje@kcl.ac.uk

**Dr Elias CAMPO**
Hematopathology Unit
Hospital Clinic
University of Barcelona
Carrer de Villarroel 170
08036 Barcelona
SPAIN
Tel. +34 93 227 5450
Fax +34 93 227 5717
ecampo@clinic.ub.es

**Dr David S. CASSARINO**
Southern California Permanente
Department of Pathology
Sunset Medical Center
4867 Sunset Boulevard, 2nd Floor
Los Angeles CA 90027
USA
Tel. +1 323 783 3595
Fax +1 323 783 7825
dsc9w@yahoo.com

**Dr Rino CERIO** #
Department of Morbid Anatomy
Institute of Pathology
Royal London Hospital
Whitechapel Road
London E1 1BB
UNITED KINGDOM
Tel. +44 20 324 60215
Fax +44 20 324 60216
r.cerio@qmul.ac.uk

**Dr Lorenzo CERRONI**
Department of Dermatology
Medical University of Graz
Auenbruggerplatz 8
8036 Graz
AUSTRIA
Tel. +43 316 385 80316
Fax +43 316 385 12466
lorenzo.cerroni@medunigraz.at

**Dr John K.C. CHAN**
Department of Pathology
Queen Elizabeth Hospital
Gascoigne Road, Kowloon
Hong Kong SAR
CHINA
Tel. +852 3506 6830
Fax +832 2385 2455
jkcchan@ha.org.hk

**Dr Alison L. CHEAH**
Histopathology
Douglass Hanly Moir Pathology
14 Giffnock Avenue
Macquarie Park NSW 2113
c/o Locked Bag 145
North Ryde NSW 2113
AUSTRALIA
Tel. +61 2 9855 5150
acheah@dhm.com.au

**Dr Emily CHU**
Department of Dermatology
Hospital of the University of Pennsylvania
3400 Spruce Street
Philadelphia PA 19104
USA
Tel. +1 215 662 2737
emily.chu@uphs.upenn.edu

**Dr Alistair J. COCHRAN** *
Departments of Pathology and
Laboratory Medicine and Surgery
David Geffen School of Medicine at UCLA
54-140 CHS, 10833 Le Conte Avenue
Los Angeles CA 90095
USA
Tel. +1 310 825 2743
Fax +1 310 267 2058
acochran@mednet.ucla.edu

**Dr Martin G. COOK** *
Histopathology
Royal Surrey County Hospital
Egerton Road
Guildford GU2 7XX
UNITED KINGDOM
Tel. +44 1483 464 065
Fax +44 1483 452 718
m.cook@nhs.net

**Dr Sarah COUPLAND**
Molecular and Clinical Cancer Medicine
Institute of Translational Medicine
University of Liverpool
William Henry Duncan Building, 3rd Floor
Liverpool L7 8TX
UNITED KINGDOM
Tel. +44 151 706 5885
Fax +44 151 706 5859
s.e.coupland@liverpool.ac.uk

**Dr Ian A. CREE** *
WHO Classification of Tumours Group
International Agency for Research on Cancer
150 Cours Albert Thomas
69372 Lyon
FRANCE
Tel. +33 4 72 73 85 34
Fax +33 4 72 73 86 98
creei@iarc.fr

**Dr A. Neil CROWSON** #
Pathology Laboratory Associates
St. John Medical Center
4142 South Mingo Road
Tulsa OK 74123
USA
ncrowson@sjmc.org

**Dr Diona DAMIAN**
Dermatology
GH3, Royal Prince Alfred Hospital
Missenden Road
Camperdown NSW 2050
AUSTRALIA
Tel. +61 2 9515 8295
Fax +61 2 9565 1048
diona.damian@sydney.edu.au

**Dr Arnaud DE LA FOUCHARDIÈRE** *#
Département de Biopathologie
Centre Léon Bérard
28 Rue Laennec
69008 Lyon
FRANCE
Tel. +33 4 78 78 28 20
Fax +33 4 78 78 27 13
arnaud.delafouchardiere@lyon.unicancer.fr

**Dr Louis P. DEHNER**
Department of Pathology and Immunology
Washington University School of Medicine
Peters Building, 3rd Floor
Campus Box 8118
660 South Euclid Avenue
St. Louis MO 63110
USA
Tel. +1 314 362 0150
dehner@wustl.edu

**Dr Florence DEMENAIS**
Genetic Variation and Human Diseases Unit
INSERM, Université Paris Diderot
UMR-946 Bâtiment IGM
27 Rue Juliette Dodu
75010 Paris
FRANCE
Tel. +33 1 53 72 50 05
Fax +33 1 53 72 50 49
florence.demenais@inserm.fr

**Dr Stefan DOJCINOV**
Department of Cellular Pathology
University Hospital of Wales
Heath Park
Cardiff CF14 4XW
UNITED KINGDOM
Tel. +44 29 20 746436
dojcinov@cf.ac.uk

**Dr Lyn M. DUNCAN**
Department of Pathology
Massachusetts General Hospital
55 Fruit Street, Warren 825
Boston MA 02114
USA
Tel. +1 617 726 8890
Fax +1 617 726 8711
duncan@helix.mgh.harvard.edu

**Dr David E. ELDER *#**
Division of Anatomic Pathology
Hospital of the University of Pennsylvania
3400 Spruce Street
Philadelphia PA 19104
USA
Tel. +1 215 662 6503
Fax +1 215 349 8088
elder@pennmedicine.upenn.edu

**Dr Rosalie ELENITSAS *#**
Department of Dermatology
University of Pennsylvania
3600 Spruce Street
2 Maloney Building
Philadelphia PA 19104
USA
Tel. +1 215 662 4497
Fax +1 215 349 5615
rosalie.elenitsas@uphs.upenn.edu

**Dr George W. ELGART**
Department of Dermatology and
Cutaneous Surgery
University of Miami School of Medicine
1444 Northwest 9th Avenue, 3rd Floor
Miami FL 33136
USA
Tel. +1 305 243 6272
Fax +1 305 243 5810
gelgart@med.miami.edu

**Dr Dirk ELSTON**
Medical University of South Carolina
135 Rutledge Avenue, Rutledge Tower
Charleston SC 29425
USA
Tel. +1 843 792 3021
elstond@musc.edu

**Dr Ervin H. EPSTEIN Jr**
Department of Dermatology
University of California
San Francisco CA 94143-1214
USA
Tel. +1 415 647 3992
Fax +1 415 647 3996
eepstein@chori.org

**Dr D. Gareth EVANS**
Department of Medical Genetics and
Cancer Epidemiology
University of Manchester
Oxford Road
Manchester M13 9PL
UNITED KINGDOM
Tel. +44 161 701 5104
gareth.d.evans@manchester.ac.uk

**Dr Fabio FACCHETTI ***
Department of Pathology
University of Brescia
Spedali Civili di Brescia
25123 Brescia
ITALY
Tel. +39 303995 426
Fax +39 303995 377
fabio.facchetti@unibs.it

**Dr Julie C. FANBURG-SMITH**
Pathology and Orthopedic Surgery
Penn State Health Milton S. Hershey
Medical Center
Hershey PA 17033
USA
Tel. +1 703 623 7013
jcfsmd@gmail.com

**Dr Andrew FELDMAN**
Department of Laboratory Medicine and
Pathology
Mayo Clinic
200 First Street Southwest
Rochester MN
USA
Tel. +1 507 284 4939
Fax +1 507 284 5115
feldman.andrew@mayo.edu

**Dr Peter M. FERGUSON**
Royal Prince Alfred Hospital
Melanoma Institute Australia
University of Sydney
Missenden Road, Building 94
Camperdown NSW 2050
AUSTRALIA
Tel. +61 2 9515 8339
Fax +61 2 9515 8405
peter.ferguson@melanoma.org.au

**Dr Judith A. FERRY**
Department of Pathology
Massachusetts General Hospital
55 Fruit Street, Warren 2
Boston MA 02114
USA
Tel. +1 617 726 4826
Fax +1 617 726 7474
jferry@partners.org

**Dr John F. FETSCH**
Soft Tissue Pathology
Joint Pathology Center
606 Stephen Sitter Avenue
Silver Spring MD 20910
USA
Tel. +1 301 295 7275
Fax +1 301 295 7184
john.f.fetsch.civ@mail.mil

**Dr Cyril FISHER**
Department of Histopathology
Royal Marsden NHS Foundation Trust
203 Fulham Road
London SW3 6JJ
UNITED KINGDOM
Tel. +44 207 808 2630
Fax +44 207 808 2578
cyril.fisher@rmh.nhs.uk

**Dr Robert FOLBERG**
William Beaumont School of Medicine
Oakland University
O'Dowd Hall, Room 428
586 Pioneer Drive
Rochester MI 48309-4482
USA
Tel. +1 248 370 2452
Fax +1 248 370 3638
rfolberg@oakland.edu

**Dr Andrew FOLPE**
Division of Anatomic Pathology
Mayo Clinic
200 First Street Southwest
Rochester MN 55905
USA
Tel. +1 507 284 2511
folpe.andrew@mayo.edu

**Dr Douglas R. FULLEN**
Departments of Pathology and Dermatology
University of Michigan
Medical Science I, Suite 3261
1301 Catherine Street
Ann Arbor MI 48109
USA
Tel. +1 734 764 4460
Fax +1 734 764 4690
dfullen@umich.edu

**Dr Philippe GAULARD**
Department of Pathology
Henri Mondor University Hospital, AP-HP
INSERM U955
51 Av. du Maréchal de Lattre de Tassigny
94010 Créteil
FRANCE
Tel. +33 1 49 81 27 43
Fax +33 1 49 81 27 33
philippe.gaulard@aphp.fr

**Dr Pedram GERAMI**
Department of Dermatology
Feinberg School of Medicine
Northwestern University
NMH/Arkes Family Pavilion, Suite 1600
676 North Saint Clair Street
Chicago IL 60611
USA
Tel. +1 312 695 1413
pgerami1@nm.org

**Dr Earl J. GLUSAC**
Department of Pathology and Dermatology
Yale School of Medicine
LMP 5031
15 York Street, Box 208059
New Haven CT 06520-8059
USA
Tel. +1 203 785 4094
Fax +1 203 785 6869
earl.glusac@yale.edu

**Dr Scott GRANTER**
Department of Pathology
Brigham and Women's Hospital
75 Francis Street, Amory 3
Boston MA 02115
USA
Tel. +1 617 732 5628
sgranter@partners.org

**Dr Wayne GRAYSON** *
Ampath National Laboratories
University of the Witwatersrand
63 Cedar Avenue West, Fourways
2055 Johannesburg
SOUTH AFRICA
Tel. +27 11 709 1244
Fax +27 12 682 2464
wayne.grayson@live.com

**Dr Joan GUITART** #
Departments of Dermatology and Pathology
Feinberg School of Medicine
Northwestern University
NMH/Arkes Family Pavilion, Suite 1600
676 North Saint Clair Street
Chicago IL 60611
USA
Tel. +1 312 695 1413
j-guitart@northwestern.edu

**Dr Eckart HANEKE**
Department of Dermatology
University of Bern
*Private address:*
Schlippehof 5
79110 Freiburg im Breisgau
GERMANY
Tel. +49 761 8978368
Fax +49 761 3837401
haneke@gmx.net

**Dr Karin HARTMANN** #
Department of Dermatology
University of Lübeck
Ratzeburger Allee 160
23562 Lübeck
GERMANY
Tel. +49 451 500 41520
Fax +49 451 500 41644
karin.hartmann@uksh.de

**Dr Nick HAYWARD**
Oncogenomics Department
QIMR Berghofer
Medical Research Institute
300 Herston Road
Herston QLD 4006
AUSTRALIA
Tel. +61 7 3362 0306
nick.hayward@qimrberghofer.edu.au

**Dr Peter J. HEENAN**
Department of Pathology
University of Western Australia
35 Stirling Highway
Crawley WA 6009
AUSTRALIA
Tel. +61 8 9389 6834
peter.heenan37@gmail.com

**Dr Klaus F. HELM** #
Department of Dermatology and Pathology
Penn State Health
Milton S. Hershey Medical Center
500 University Drive, Room C7714C
Hershey PA 17033
USA
Tel. +1 717 531 1677
Fax +1 717 531 4278
khelm@psu.edu

**Dr Emmilia HODAK**
Department of Dermatology
Rabin Medical Center
Beilinson Hospital
Tel Aviv University
Ze'ev Jabotinsky Road 39
49100 Petah Tikva
ISRAEL
Tel. +972 544 895189
Fax +972 3 9223353

**Dr Travis HOLLMANN**
Department of Pathology
Memorial Sloan Kettering Cancer Center
1275 York Avenue
New York NY 10065
USA
Tel. +1 212 639 8134
Fax +1 212 717 3203
hollmant@mskcc.org

**Dr Jason L. HORNICK**
Department of Pathology
Brigham and Women's Hospital
75 Francis Street
Boston MA 02115
USA
Tel. +1 617 525 7257
Fax +1 617 566 3897
jhornick@partners.org

**Dr Hans-Peter HORNY**
Institute of Pathology
Ludwig Maximilian University
Thalkirchner Straße 36
80337 München
GERMANY
Tel. +49 89 2180 73698
Fax +49 1 2180 73604
hans-peter.horny@med.uni-muenchen.de

**Dr Vicki HOWARD**
Douglass Hanly Moir Pathology
14 Giffnock Avenue
Macquarie Park NSW 2113
AUSTRALIA
Tel. +61 2 9855 5101
Fax +61 2 9878 5077
vhoward@dhm.com.au

**Dr Doina IVAN**
Departments of Pathology and Dermatology
University of Texas MD Anderson Cancer
1515 Holcombe Boulevard, Unit 85
Houston TX 77030
USA
Tel. +1 713 563 1844
Fax +1 713 792 3696
dsivan@mdanderson.org

**Dr Keiji IWATSUKI** #
Department of Dermatology
Graduate School of Medicine,
Dentistry and Pharmaceutical Sciences
Okayama University
2-5-1 Shikata-cho, Okayama City
Okayama 700-8558
JAPAN
keijiiwa@cc.okayama-u.ac.jp

**Dr Louise JACKETT**
Tissue Pathology and Diagnostic Oncology
Royal Prince Alfred Hospital
Missenden Road
Camperdown NSW 2050
AUSTRALIA
Tel. +61 2 9515 7533
Fax +61 2 9515 8405
louise.jackett@health.nsw.gov.au

**Dr Elaine S. JAFFE** *
Laboratory of Pathology
Center for Cancer Research, NCI, NIH
Building 10, Room 3S-235
10 Center Drive, MSC-1500
Bethesda MD 20892-1500
USA
Tel. +1 301 480 8461
Fax +1 301 480 8089
ejaffe@mail.nih.gov

**Dr Craig JAMES**
Clinpath Laboratories
19 Fullarton Road
Kent Town SA 5067
AUSTRALIA
Tel. +61 8 8366 2000
cjames@senet.com.au

**Dr Patty M. JANSEN**
Department of Pathology
Leiden University Medical Center
Room L2-69
Albinusdreef 2
2333 ZA Leiden
THE NETHERLANDS
p.m.jansen@lumc.nl

**Dr Denisa KACEROVSKA**
Sikl Department of Pathology
Faculty of Medicine Hospital
Charles University
Alej Svobody 80
304 60 Pilsen
CZECH REPUBLIC
Tel. +420 737 22 0482
kacerovska@biopticka.cz

**Dr Steven KADDU**
Department of Dermatology
Medical University of Graz
Auenbruggerplatz 8
8036 Graz
AUSTRIA
Tel. +43 385 3012/80494
steven.kaddu@medunigraz.at

**Dr Marshall E. KADIN** #
Department of Dermatology and Skin Surgery
Roger Williams Medical Center
Boston University School of Medicine
50 Maude Street
Providence RI 02908
USA
Tel. +1 401 456 2521
Fax +1 401 456 6449
mkadin@rwmc.org

**Dr Jean KANITAKIS**
Department of Dermatology
Edouard Herriot Hospital Group (Pav. R)
5 Place d'Arsonval
69437 Lyon Cedex 03
FRANCE
Tel. +33 4 72 11 03 01
Fax +33 4 72 11 03 23
jean.kanitakis@univ-lyon1.fr

**Dr Grace F. KAO**
Department of Dermatology
George Washington University School of Medicine, Suite 2B-430
2150 Pennsylvania Avenue Northwest
Washington DC 20037
USA
Tel. +1 410 964 0281
Fax +1 410 730 2812
graycekao@gmail.com

**Dr Rooshdiya KARIM**
Tissue Pathology and Diagnostic Oncology
Royal Prince Alfred Hospital
Building 94
Missenden Road
Camperdown NSW 2050
AUSTRALIA
rooshdiya.karim@health.nsw.gov.au

**Dr Dmitry V. KAZAKOV** *
Sikl Department of Pathology
Medical Faculty in Pilsen
Charles University
Alej Svobody 80
304 60 Pilsen
CZECH REPUBLIC
Tel. +420 737 220405
kazakov@medima.cz

**Dr Werner KEMPF** *
Kempf und Pfaltz Histologische Diagnostik and Department of Dermatology,
University Hospital Zurich
Affolternstrasse 56
8050 Zurich
SWITZERLAND
Tel. +41 44 233 3377
Fax +41 44 233 3378
werner.kempf@uzh.ch

**Dr Jinah KIM** #
Department of Pathology
Stanford University
300 Pasteur Drive, Room L235, MC 5324
Stanford CA 94305
USA
Tel. +1 650 736 1068
Fax +1 650 725 7409
jinahkim@stanford.edu

**Dr Tero KIVELÄ**
Ophthalmic Pathology Laboratory
Helsinki University Central Hospital
Haartmaninkatu 4 C PL220
00029 Helsinki
FINLAND

**Dr Young-Hyeh KO**
Samsung Medical Center
Department of Pathology
Sungkyunkwan University
School of Medicine
Seoul
REPUBLIC OF KOREA
yhko310@skku.edu

**Dr Anastasia M. KONSTANTINOVA**
Department of Pathology
Clinical Research and Practical Center for Specialized Oncological Care
4 Linea VO 39-9
Saint Petersburg 199004
RUSSIAN FEDERATION
Tel. +7 921 3117415
anastasia.konstantynova@gmail.com

**Dr Steven KOSSARD**
Kossard Dermatopathologists
Laverty Pathology, Level 2
60 Waterloo Road
Macquarie Park NSW 2118
AUSTRALIA
Tel. +61 2 9005 7441
Fax +61 2 8353 3040
steven.kossard@kossard.com.au

**Dr Kenneth H. KRAEMER**
Basic Research Laboratory
National Cancer Institute
Building 37, Room 4002
Bethesda MD 20892
USA
Tel. +1 301 496 9033
Fax +1 301 594 3409
kraemerk@nih.gov

**Dr Heinz KUTZNER**
Dermatopathology Friedrichshafen
Siemensstraße 6/1
88048 Friedrichshafen
GERMANY
Tel. +49 7541 6044 0
Fax +49 7541 6044 23
kutzner@dermpath.de

**Dr Gilles LANDMAN**
Department of Pathology
Escola Paulista de Medicina
Universidade Federal de São Paulo
Rua Botucatu 740, Edificio Lemos Torres
São Paulo 04023-900
BRAZIL
Tel. +55 11 5576 4996
Fax +55 11 3289 3227
glandman@unifesp.br

**Dr William B. LASKIN**
Department of Pathology
Yale School of Medicine
Box 208023
New Haven CT 06520-8023
USA
Tel. +1 203 384 3591
Fax +1 203 384 3237
william.laskin@yale.edu

**Dr Alexander J. LAZAR** *
Departments of Pathology,
Genomic Medicine and Dermatology
University of Texas MD Anderson Cancer
1515 Holcombe Boulevard, Unit 85
Houston TX 77030
USA
Tel. +1 713 563 1843
Fax +1 713 563 1849
alazar@mdanderson.org

**Dr Rossitza LAZOVA**
Department of Pathology
California Skin Institute
2420 Samaritan Drive
San Jose CA 95124
USA
Tel. +1 408 369 5600, ext. 246
Fax +1 408 558 7949
drlazova@caskin.com

**Dr Philip E. LeBOIT**
Dermatopathology Section
University of California San Francisco
1701 Divisadero Street, Suite 280
San Francisco CA 94115
USA
Tel. +1 415 353 7550
Fax +1 415 353 7553
philip.leboit@ucsf.edu

**Dr Irene LOW**
Department of Histopathology
Middlemore Hospital
Bray Building, Level 1
100 Hospital Road
Otahuhu, Auckland 2104
NEW ZEALAND
Tel. +64 9 276 0154
Fax +64 9 270 4753
irene.low@middlemore.co.nz

**Dr Lori LOWE**
Departments of Pathology and Dermatology
Michigan Medicine, University of Michigan
Medical Science I, Suite 3261
1300 Catherine Street
Ann Arbor MI 48109
USA
Tel. +1 734 764 4460
Fax +1 734 615 2964
lorilowe@med.umich.edu

**Dr Boštjan LUZAR**
Institute of Pathology
Faculty of Medicine
University of Ljubljana
Korytkova 2
1000 Ljubljana
SLOVENIA
Tel. +386 1 543 7130
bostjan.luzar@mf.uni-lj.si

**Dr Cynthia MAGRO**
Dermatopathology
Weill Cornell Medicine
1300 York Avenue, Room F-309
Box 58
New York NY 10065
USA
Tel. +1 212 746 6434
Fax +1 212 746 8570
cym2003@med.cornell.edu

**Dr Annabelle MAHAR**
Tissue Pathology and Diagnostic Oncology
Royal Prince Alfred Hospital
Missenden Road, Building 94
Camperdown NSW 2050
AUSTRALIA
Tel. +61 02 9515 6870
Fax +61 02 9515 8405
annabelle.mahar@health.nsw.gov.au

**Dr Graham J. MANN**
Centre for Cancer Research
Westmead Institute for Medical Research
University of Sydney
176 Hawkesbury Road
Westmead NSW 2145
AUSTRALIA
Tel. +61 2 8627 3777
graham.mann@sydney.edu.au

**Dr Magdalena MARTINKA**
Vancouver General Hospital
University of British Columbia
855 West 12th Avenue
Vancouver BC V5Z 1M9
CANADA
Tel. +1 604 875 5555
Fax +1 604 875 5707
magda.martinka@vch.ca

**Dr Daniela MASSI** *
Division of Pathological Anatomy,
Department of Surgery and Translational
Medicine, University of Florence
Largo Brambilla 3
50134 Firenze
ITALY
Tel. +39 055 4478 137
Fax +39 055 275 1716
daniela.massi@unifi.it

**Dr Guido MASSI**
Department of Pathology
Catholic University Medical School
Largo F. Vito 1
00168 Roma
ITALY
Tel. +39 069521 9335
gmassi@rm.unicatt.it

**Dr Stanley W. McCARTHY**
Royal Prince Alfred Hospital
Melanoma Institute Australia
University of Sydney
Missenden Road, Building 94
Camperdown NSW 2050
AUSTRALIA
Tel. +61 2 9515 8339
Fax +61 2 9515 8405
stan.mccarthy@health.nsw.gov.au

**Dr Catriona McKENZIE**
Tissue Pathology and Diagnostic Oncology
Royal Prince Alfred Hospital
Missenden Road, Building 94
Camperdown NSW 2050
AUSTRALIA
Tel. +61 2 9515 8076
Fax +61 2 9515 8405
catriona.mckenzie@health.nsw.gov.au

**Dr Darius R. MEHREGAN**
Wayne State University School of Medicine
and Pinkus Dermatopathology Laboratory
1314 North Macomb Street
Monroe MI 48162
USA
Tel. +1 734 242 6870
Fax +1 734 242 4962
darmehregan@pinkuslab.com

**Dr David A. MEHREGAN**
Pinkus Dermatopathology Laboratory
1314 North Macomb Street
Monroe MI 48162
USA
Tel. +1 734 344 4971
davmehregan@pinkuslab.com

**Dr Jane MESSINA***
Departments of Anatomic Pathology and
Cutaneous Oncology
Moffitt Cancer Center and Research Institute
12902 USF Magnolia Drive
Tampa FL 33612
USA
Tel. +1 813 745 3910
Fax +1 813 745 1708
jane.messina@moffitt.org

**Dr Michal MICHAL**
Sikl Department of Pathology
Faculty of Medicine Hospital
Charles University
Alej Svobody 80
304 60 Pilsen
CZECH REPUBLIC
michal@medima.cz

**Dr Daniela MIHIC-PROBST**
Department of Pathology and
Molecular Pathology
University Hospital Zurich
Schmelzbergstrasse 12
8091 Zurich
SWITZERLAND
Tel. +41 44 255 25 95
Fax +41 44 255 44 16
daniela.mihic@usz.ch

**Dr Martin C. MIHM Jr** *#
Department of Dermatology
Brigham and Women's Hospital
41 Avenue Louis Pasteur, Room 317
Boston MA 02115
USA
Tel. +1 617 264 5910
Fax +1 617 264 3013
martin.mihm@bwh.harvard.edu

**Dr Rajmohan MURALI**
Department of Pathology
Memorial Sloan Kettering Cancer Center
1275 York Avenue
New York NY 10065
USA
Tel. +1 212 639 5905
muralir@mskcc.org

**Dr George F. MURPHY**
Program in Dermatopathology
Brigham and Women's Hospital
221 Longwood Avenue, EBRC4
Boston MA 02115
USA
Tel. +1 617 525 7485
gmurphy@bwh.harvard.edu

**Dr Eduardo NAGORE**
Department of Dermatology
Instituto Valenciano de Oncología
Carrer del Professor Beltrán Báguena 8
46009 Valencia
SPAIN
Tel. +34 96111 4015
Fax +34 96111 4341
eduyame@ono.com

**Dr Shigeo NAKAMURA**
Department of Pathology and
Laboratory Medicine
Nagoya University Hospital
65 Tsurumai-cho, Showa-ku
Nagoya 466-8560
JAPAN
Tel. +81 52 744 2896
Fax +81 52 744 2897
snakamur@med.nagoya-u.ac.jp

**Dr Julia NEWTON-BISHOP**
Faculty of Medicine and
Health Institute of Cancer and Pathology
Cancer Genetics Building
St James's University Hospital
Beckett Street
Leeds LS9 7TF
UNITED KINGDOM
Tel. +44 113 206 4919
j.a.newton-bishop@leeds.ac.uk

**Dr Paula E. NORTH**
Department of Pathology
Children's Hospital of Wisconsin
Milwaukee Campus
8915 West Connell Court
Milwaukee WI 53226
USA
Tel. +1 414 266 2526
Fax +1 414 266 2779
pnorth@mew.edu

**Dr Blake Hugh O'BRIEN**
Sullivan Nicolaides Pathology
24 Hurworth Street
Bowen Hills QLD 4006
AUSTRALIA
Tel. +61 7 3377 8666
Fax +61 7 3377 8722
blake_o'brien@snp.com.au

**Dr Hiroko OHGAKI** *
Institute of Neuropathology
Charité University Hospital
Charitéplatz 1
10117 Berlin
GERMANY
Tel. +49 30 450 564 678
hiroko.ohgaki@charite.de

**Dr Nicolas ORTONNE**
Department of Pathology
Henri Mondor University Hospital, AP-HP
INSERM U955
51 Av. du Maréchal de Lattre de Tassigny
94000 Créteil
FRANCE
Tel. +33 1 49 81 27 38
nicolas.ortonne@hmn.aphp.fr

**Dr Rajiv M. PATEL**
Departments of Pathology and Dermatology
Michigan Medicine, University of Michigan
Medical Science I, Suite 3261
1301 Catherine Street
Ann Arbor MI 48109
USA
Tel. +1 734 764 4460
Fax +1 734 764 4690
rajivpat@med.umich.edu

**Dr James W. PATTERSON**
Department of Pathology
University of Virginia Health System
Box 800214
Charlottesville VA 22908
USA
Tel. +1 434 982 4402
Fax +1 343 243 6757
jwp9e@virginia.edu

**Dr Marco PAULLI**
Pathology, Department of Molecular Medicine
Fondazione IRCCS Policlinico San Matteo
University of Pavia
Via Forlanini 14
27100 Pavia
ITALY
Tel. +39 38 250 1241
Fax +39 38 252 5866
m.paulli@smatteo.pv.it

**Dr Tony PETRELLA**
Department of Pathology
Maisonneuve-Rosemont Hospital
5415 Boulevard de l'Assomption
Montreal QC H1T 2M4
CANADA
Tel. +1 514 377 4412
tony.petrella@umontreal.ca

**Dr John D. PFEIFER**
Department of Pathology and Immunology
Washington University School of Medicine
Campus Box 8118
660 South Euclid Avenue
St. Louis MO 63110
USA
Tel. +1 314 747 0276
Fax +1 314 362 4096
pfeifer@path.wustl.edu

**Dr Michael PIEPKORN** #
Division of Dermatology
University of Washington School of Medicine
Dermatopathology NW
2330 130th Avenue Northeast, #201
Bellevue WA 98005
USA
Tel. +1 425 455 9945
Fax +1 425 455 9947
mpiepkor@uw.edu

**Dr Stefano A. PILERI** #
Unit of Haematopathology
European Institute of Oncology
Via Ripamonti 435
20141 Milano
ITALY
Tel. +39 2 57489521
stefano.pileri@ieo.it

**Dr Laura B. PINCUS**
Departments of Dermatology and Pathology
Section of Dermatopathology
University of California
1701 Divisadero Street, Suite 280
San Francisco CA 94115
USA
Tel. +1 415 353 7553
Fax +1 415 353 7593
laura.pincus@ucsf.edu

**Dr Adriano PIRIS**
Mihm Cutaneous Pathology
Brigham and Women's Hospital
Harvard Medical School
41 Avenue Louis Pasteur, Suite 317
Boston MA 02115
USA
Tel. +1 617 264 3030
Fax +1 617 264 3013
apiris@bwh.harvard.edu

**Dr Stefania PITTALUGA**
Laboratory of Pathology
Center for Cancer Research
National Cancer Institute
Building 10, Room 2S235A
Bethesda MD 20892-1500
USA
Tel. +1 301 480 8465
Fax +1 301 480 8089
stefpitt@mail.nih.gov

**Dr Maurilio PONZONI**
Unit of Lymphoid Malignancies
San Raffaele Scientific Institute
Ateneo Vita-Salute University
Via Olgettina 60
20132 Milano
ITALY
Tel. +39 2 2643 2544
Fax +39 2 2643 2409
ponzoni.maurilio@hsr.it

**Dr Victor G. PRIETO** *
Department of Pathology
University of Texas MD Anderson Cancer
1515 Holcombe Boulevard, Unit 85
Houston TX 77030
USA
Tel. +1 713 792 3187
Fax +1 713 745 3674
vprieto@mdanderson.org

**Dr Melissa P. PULITZER**
Memorial Sloan Kettering Cancer Center
1275 York Avenue, C528
New York NY 10065
USA
Tel. +1 212 639 2038
pulitzem@mskcc.org

**Dr Leticia QUINTANILLA-MARTINEZ**
Institute of Pathology
University Hospital Tübingen
Eberhard Karls University of Tübingen
Liebermeisterstraße 8
72076 Tübingen
GERMANY
Tel. +49 707 1298 2266
Fax +49 707 1292 258
leticia.quintanilla-fend@med.uni-tuebingen.de

**Dr Michael RABKIN**
Rabkin Dermatopathology Laboratory, P.C.
419 East Second Avenue
Tarentum PA 15084
USA
Tel. +1 412 968 9266
Fax +1 412 968 5673
msrabkin@gmail.com

**Dr Luis REQUENA**
Department of Dermatology
Fundación Jiménez Díaz
Universidad Autónoma de Madrid
Avenida Reyes Católicos 2
28040 Madrid
SPAIN
Tel. +34 91 550 4800
Fax +39 91 544 2636
irequena@fjd.es

**Dr Alistair ROBSON**
Departamento de Diagnóstico Laboratorial
IPOLFG – Serviço de Anatomia Patológica
Rua Prof. Lima Basto
1099-023 Lisboa
PORTUGAL
Tel. +351 910 729 277
a.robson@ldpath.com

**Dr Franco RONGIOLETTI** *
Unit of Dermatology
University of Cagliari
Via dell'Ospedale 54
09124 Cagliari
ITALY
Tel. +39 335 6917222
Fax +39 070 6092580
rongioletti@unica.it

**Dr Brian ROUS** *
National Cancer Registration Service
Victoria House, Capital Park
Fulbourn CB21 5XA
UNITED KINGDOM
Tel. +44 1223 213 625
Fax +44 1223 213 571
brian.rous@phe.gov.uk

**Dr Christian A. SANDER**
Department of Dermatology
Asklepios Klinik St. Georg
Lohmühlenstraße 5
20099 Hamburg
GERMANY
Tel. +49 40 18 18 85 2220
Fax +49 40 18 18 85 2462
c.sander@asklepios.com

**Dr Omar P. SANGÜEZA**
Department of Pathology and Dermatology
Wake Forest School of Medicine
Medical Center Boulevard
Winston-Salem NC 27157-1072
USA
Tel. +1 336 716 4096
Fax +1 336 716 6359
osanguez@wakehealth.edu

**Dr Daniel J. SANTA CRUZ**
Division of Dermatology
Department of Medicine
Washington University School of Medicine
2199 White Lane Drive
Chesterfield MO 63017
USA
Tel. +1 314 230 5044
Fax +1 314 230 5044
dsantacruz@aol.com

**Dr Marco SANTUCCI**
Division of Pathological Anatomy
Department of Surgery and Translational Medicine, University of Florence
Largo Brambilla 3
50134 Firenze
ITALY
Tel. +39 55 447 8105
Fax +39 55 432 144
marco.santucci@unifi.it

**Dr Alain SARASIN**
Laboratory of Genetic Instability and Oncogenesis, UMR 8200 CNRS
Institut Gustave Roussy
114 Rue Edouard Vaillant
95805 Villejuif Cedex
FRANCE
Tel. +33 1 42 11 63 28
Fax +33 1 42 11 50 08
alain.sarasin@gustaveroussy.fr

**Dr Birgitta SCHMIDT**
Department of Pathology
Boston Children's Hospital and
Harvard Medical School
300 Longwood Avenue
Boston MA 02115
USA
Tel. +1 617 355 8588
Fax +1 617 730 0207
birgitta.schmidt@childrens.harvard.edu

**Dr Tilman SCHULZ**
Institute for Pathology
Klinikum Bayreuth
Preuschwitzer Straße 101
95445 Bayreuth
GERMANY
Tel. +49 921 499 5610
Fax +49 921 400 5609
dr.tilman_schulz@gmx.de

**Dr Richard A. SCOLYER***
Tissue Pathology and Diagnostic Oncology
Royal Prince Alfred Hospital
Missenden Road, Building 94
Camperdown NSW 2050
AUSTRALIA
Tel. +61 2 9515 7011
Fax +61 2 9515 8405
richard.scolyer@health.nsw.gov.au

**Dr Aleksandar SEKULIC**
Department of Dermatology
Mayo Clinic
13400 East Shea Boulevard
Scottsdale AZ 85259
USA
Tel. +1 480 301 8508
sekulic.aleksandar@mayo.edu

**Dr Christopher SHEA**#
Section of Dermatology
University of Chicago Medicine
5841 South Maryland Avenue
Chicago IL 60637
USA
Tel. +1 773 702 6559
Fax +1 773 702 8398
cshea@medicine.bsd.uchicago.edu

**Dr Rajendra (Raj) SINGH***
Dermatopathology Section
Icahn School of Medicine at Mount Sinai
Annenberg Building, Floor 15, Room 05
1468 Madison Avenue
New York NY 10029
USA
rajendra.singh@mountsinai.org

**Dr Bruce R. SMOLLER**
Department of Pathology and Laboratory
Medicine, University of Rochester School of
Medicine and Dentistry
601 Elmwood Avenue, Box 626
Rochester NY 14642
USA
Tel. +1 585 275 3183
Fax +1 585 276 2802
bruce_smoller@urmc.rochester.edu

**Dr H. Peter SOYER**#
Dermatology Research Centre
University of Queensland
Diamantina Institute
37 Kent Street
Woolloongabba QLD 4102
AUSTRALIA
Tel. +61 7 344 38017
Fax +61 7 344 37779
p.soyer@uq.edu.au

**Dr Constantine A. STRATAKIS**#
Eunice Kennedy Shriver National Institute of
Child Health and Human Development
Building 31, Room 2A46, MSC2425
Bethesda MD 20892
USA
Tel. +1 301 594 5984
Fax +1 301 480 6480
stratakc@mail.nih.gov

**Dr Paul E. SWANSON**
Department of Pathology
University of Washington School of Medicine
Box 356100
1959 Northeast Pacific Street
Seattle WA 98195-6100
USA
Tel. +1 206 598 0574
Fax +1 206 598 3803
ps3@uw.edu

**Dr Steven H. SWERDLOW**
Division of Hematopathology
UPMC Presbyterian
Hill Building, Room 359
3477 Euler Way
Pittsburgh PA 15213
USA
Tel. +1 412 647 5191
Fax +1 412 647 4008
swerdlowsh@upmc.edu

**Dr Ben TALLON**
Skin Dermatology Institute
752 Cameron Road
Tauranga, Bay of Plenty 3112
NEW ZEALAND
Tel. +64 7 571 5548
bentallon@gmail.com

**Dr Kong Bing TAN**
Department of Pathology
Yong Loo Lin School of Medicine
National University of Singapore
5 Lower Kent Ridge Road
Singapore 119074
SINGAPORE
Tel. +65 6772 2057
Fax +65 6778 0671
pattankb@nus.edu.sg

**Dr Michael TETZLAFF**
Department of Pathology
University of Texas MD Anderson Cancer
1515 Holcombe Boulevard, Unit 85
Houston TX 77030
USA
Tel. +1 713 792 2585
mtetzlaff@mdanderson.org

**Dr Yoshiki TOKURA**#
Department of Dermatology
Hamamatsu University School of Medicine
1-20-1 Handayama, Higashi-ku
Hamamatsu 431-3192
JAPAN
Tel. +81 53 435 2303
Fax +81 53 435 2368
tokura@hama-med.ac.jp

**Dr Massimo TOMMASINO**
Infections and Cancer Biology Group
International Agency for Research on Cancer
150 Cours Albert Thomas
69372 Lyon
FRANCE
Tel. +33 4 72 73 81 91
Fax +33 4 72 73 85 75
tommasino@iarc.fr

**Dr Carlos A. TORRES-CABALA**
Departments of Pathology and Dermatology
University of Texas MD Anderson Cancer
1515 Holcombe Boulevard, Unit 85
Houston TX 77030
USA
Tel. +1 713 792 3151
Fax +1 713 745 8228
ctcabala@mdanderson.org

**Dr Hensin TSAO**
Wellman Center for Photomedicine and
Department of Dermatology
Massachusetts General Hospital
50 Blossom Street, Edwards 211
Boston MA 02114-2517
USA
Tel. +1 617 726 2914
Fax +1 617 726 7768
htsao@mgh.harvard.edu

**Dr Margaret TUCKER**
Human Genetics Program
National Institutes of Health
Room SG/7E542
9609 Medical Center Drive
Rockville MD 20850-9779
USA
Tel. +1 240 276 7396
tuckerp@mail.nih.gov

**Dr Hisashi UHARA** #
Department of Dermatology
Sapporo Medical University
School of Medicine
South 1, West 16, Chuo-ku
Sapporo 060-8543
JAPAN
uharah@sapmed.ac.jp

**Dr Carmelo URSO**
Dermatopathology Study Center of Florence
Via Della Cernaia 88
50129 Firenze
ITALY
Tel. +39 55 417 375
cylaur@libero.it

**Dr Peter VALENT**
Department of Internal Medicine I
Division of Hematology and Hemostaseology
Medical University of Vienna
1090 Vienna
AUSTRIA
Tel. +43 1 40400 60850
Fax +43 1 40400 40300
peter.valent@meduniwien.ac.at

**Dr Joost VAN DEN OORD**
Translational Cell and Tissue Research
Department of Imaging and Pathology
KU Leuven, O&N IV
Herestraat 49, Box 7003 24
3000 Leuven
BELGIUM
Tel. +32 16 336591
Fax +32 16 336548
joost.vandenoord@kuleuven.be

**Dr James W. VARDIMAN**
Department of Pathology
University of Chicago
TW-055, MC 008
5841 South Maryland Avenue
Chicago IL 60637
USA
Tel. +1 773 702 6196
Fax +1 773 702 9207
james.vardiman@uchospitals.edu

**Dr Camilla VASSALLO**
Department of Dermatology
Fondazione IRCCS Policlinico San Matteo
University of Pavia
Viale Camillo Golgi 19
27100 Pavia
ITALY
Tel. +39 0382 503492
Fax +39 0382 526379
c.vassallo@smatteo.pv.it

**Dr Girish VENKATARAMAN**
Department of Pathology
University of Chicago
MC 0008, Room TW-055B
5841 South Maryland Avenue
Chicago IL 60637
USA
Tel. +1 773 702 5273
Fax +1 773 702 9207
girish.venkataraman@uchospitals.edu

**Dr Beatrice VERGIER**
Service de Pathologie (Sud)
Hôpital Haut-Lévêque
CHU de Bordeaux
Avenue de Magellan
33604 Pessac
FRANCE
Tel. +33 5 57 65 60 26
Fax +33 5 57 65 63 72
beatrice.vergier@chu-bordeaux.fr

**Dr Maarten H. VERMEER** #
Department of Dermatology
Leiden University Medical Center
Room B1-Q-93
Albinusdreef 2
2333 ZA Leiden
THE NETHERLANDS
Tel. +31 71 526 1952
m.h.vermeer@lumc.nl

**Dr Noreen WALSH**
Division of Anatomical Pathology
Nova Scotia Health Authority, QEII Site
MacKenzie Building, Suite 721
5788 University Avenue
Halifax NS B3H 1V8
CANADA
Tel. +1 902 473 6897
Fax +1 902 473 7978
noreen.walsh@nshealth.ca

**Dr Wei-Lien (Billy) WANG**
Department of Pathology
University of Texas MD Anderson Cancer
Unit 85
1515 Holcombe Boulevard
Houston TX 77030
USA
Tel. +1 713 792 4240
Fax +1 713 745 8228
wlwang@mdanderson.org

**Dr Sean J. WHITTAKER** #
Division of Genetics and Molecular Medicine
KCL, St John's Institute of Dermatology
Tower Wing, 9th Floor
Guy's Hospital, Great Maze Pond
London SE1 9RT
UNITED KINGDOM
Tel. +44 207 188 8076
Fax +44 207 188 8050
sean.whittaker@kcl.ac.uk

**Dr Mark R. WICK**
Division of Surgical Pathology and
Cytopathology, University Hospital
University of Virginia Health System
1215 Lee Street, Room 3020
Charlottesville VA 22908-2014
USA
Tel. +1 434 243 4818
Fax +1 434 924 9617
mrw9c@hscmail.mcc.virginia.edu

**Dr Thomas WIESNER** #
Department of Dermatology
Medical University of Vienna
Währinger Gürtel 18-20
1090 Vienna
AUSTRIA
Tel. +43 1 404 007 7060
Fax +43 1 404 007 5740
thomas.wiesner@meduniwien.ac.at

**Dr Rein WILLEMZE** *
Leiden University Medical Center
Building 1
Albinusdreef 2, Box 9600
2333 ZA Leiden
THE NETHERLANDS
Tel. +31 71 526 2421
willemze.dermatology@lumc.nl

**Dr Christian WITTEKIND**
Leipzig University Hospital
Pathology Institute
Liebigstr. 26
04103 Leipzig
GERMANY
Tel. +49 341 971 5000
Fax +49 341 971 5009
christian.wittekind@medizin.uni-leipzig.de

**Dr Daniel D. WONG**
PathWest Laboratory Medicine
School of Pathology and Laboratory
Medicine, University of Western Australia
QEII Medical Centre, J Block, Level 1
Nedlands WA 6009
AUSTRALIA
Tel. +61 8 6457 2727
Fax +61 8 6457 3009
daniel.wong@health.wa.gov.au

**Dr Benjamin A. WOOD**
PathWest Laboratory Medicine
School of Pathology and Laboratory Medicine, University of Western Australia
QEII Medical Centre, J Block, Ground Floor
Nedlands WA 6009
AUSTRALIA
Tel. +61 8 6457 1862
Fax +61 8 6457 4122
benjamin.wood@health.wa.gov.au

**Dr Xiaowei XU**
Department of Pathology and Laboratory Medicine
Hospital of the University of Pennsylvania
6 Founders Pavilion
Philadelphia PA 19104-4283
USA
Tel. +1 215 662 6503
Fax +1 215 349 5910
xug@pennmedicine.upenn.edu

**Dr Iwei YEH**
Dermatopathology Section
University of California San Francisco
1701 Divisadero Street, Suite 336
San Francisco CA 94115-1790
USA
Tel. +1 415 353 7536
Fax +1 415 353 7546
iwei.yeh@ucsf.edu

**Dr Sook Jung YUN** *
Department of Dermatology
Chonnam National University Medical School
160 Baekseo-ro, Dong-gu
Gwangju 61469
REPUBLIC OF KOREA
Tel. +82 61 379 7698
Fax +82 62 222 4058
sjyun@chonnam.ac.kr

**Dr Iris ZALAUDEK**
Department of Dermatology
Medical University of Graz
Auenbruggerplatz 8
8036 Graz
AUSTRIA
Tel. +43 316 385 2423
Fax +43 316 385 2466
iris.zalaudek@medunigraz.at

**Dr Bernhard ZELGER** *
Dermatohistopathological Laboratory
Department of Dermatology and Venereology
Innsbruck Medical University
Anichstraße 35
6020 Innsbruck
AUSTRIA
Tel. +43 664 228 1209
Fax +43 512 504 22990
bernhard.zelger@i-med.ac.at

**Dr Artur ZEMBOWICZ** *
Dermatopathology Consultations, LLC
152 Second Avenue
Needham Heights, MA 02494
USA
Tel. +1 617 549 1168
dr.z@dermatopathologyconsultations.com

# Declaration of interests

**Dr Barnhill** reports having received personal consultancy fees from Myriad Genetics.

**Dr Elder** reports having received personal consultancy fees from Myriad Genetics and from SciBase.

**Dr Cerio** reports benefiting from honoraria from Leo Pharma, Almirall, Janssen Pharmaceutica, and Meda Pharmaceuticals, and that his unit at Queen Mary University of London has received research funding from Terumo BCT.

**Dr Crowson** reports owning stocks in Pathology Laboratory Associates, Inc., in his capacity as president of the company.

**Dr de la Fouchardière** reports having received personal consultancy fees from Roche and Bristol-Myers Squibb.

**Dr Elenitsas** reports having received personal consultancy fees from Myriad Genetics.

**Dr Guitart** reports having received personal consultancy fees from Actelion and Leo Pharma. He also reports that the Department of Dermatology at the Feinberg School of Medicine, Northwestern University, receives research funding from Actelion, Soligenix, Medivir, and Mallinckrodt, and has received research funding from Celgene.

**Dr Hartmann** reports having received personal consultancy fees from Novartis, Deciphera, and ALK, and honoraria from Novartis and AbbVie.

**Dr Helm** reports having received personal consultancy fees from Myriad Genetics.

**Dr Iwatsuki** reports having received honoraria from Minophagen Pharmaceutical, and that the Department of Dermatology, Okayama University Graduate School of Medicine, Dentistry and Pharmaceutical Sciences, has received research funding from Minophagen Pharmaceutical.

**Dr Kadin** reports having received research support from the Drs Martin & Dorothy Spatz Charitable Foundation.

**Dr Kim** reports having provided expert testimony on behalf of Neal H. Howard & Associates.

**Dr Mihm** reports having received personal consultancy fees from Novartis and Alnylam, and providing unpaid consulting for Mela Sciences. He also reports serving on the advisory boards of Caliber I.D. and Biocoz Global.

**Dr Piepkorn** reports owning and having financial interests in Dermatopathology Northwest.

**Dr Pileri** reports having received personal consultancy fees from Takeda.

**Dr Shea** reports having received personal consultancy fees from Myriad Genetics.

**Dr Soyer** reports having received personal consultancy fees from Pierre Fabre, and that the University of Queensland receives research funding from Leo Pharma.

**Dr Stratakis** reports that his laboratory at the Eunice Kennedy Shriver National Institute of Child Health and Human Development holds patents on *PRKAR1A* and *PDE11A* genes.

**Dr Tokura** reports having received personal consultancy fees from Kyowa Kirin Pharmaceutical Development and Minophagen Pharmaceutical, and that the Department of Dermatology, Hamamatsu University School of Medicine, has received research funding from Novartis.

**Dr Uhara** reports having received personal consultancy fees and having benefited from research funding from Chugai, Ono, Bristol-Myers Squibb, and MSD.

**Dr Vermeer** reports that the Department of Dermatology, Leiden University Medical Center, receives consultancy fees for his work with Innate Pharma.

**Dr Whittaker** reports that the Division of Genetics and Molecular Medicine, St John's Institute of Dermatology, receives research funding from Galderma, and that the Institute receives consultancy fees for his work with Takeda and Actelion.

**Dr Wiesner** reports that the Memorial Sloan Kettering Cancer Center and the Medical University of Graz have applied for a patent on *BAP1* detection.

## IARC/WHO Committee for the International Classification of Diseases for Oncology (ICD-O)

**Dr Ian A. CREE**
WHO Classification of Tumours Group
International Agency for Research on Cancer
150 Cours Albert Thomas
69372 Lyon
FRANCE
Tel. +33 4 72 73 85 34
Fax +33 4 72 73 86 98
creei@iarc.fr

**Dr Robert JAKOB**
Data Standards and Informatics
World Health Organization (WHO)
20 Avenue Appia
1211 Geneva 27
SWITZERLAND
Tel. +41 22 791 58 77
Fax +41 22 791 48 94
jakobr@who.int

**Dr Brian ROUS**
National Cancer Registration Service
Victoria House, Capital Park
Fulbourn CB21 5XA
UNITED KINGDOM
Tel. +44 1223 213 625
Fax +44 1223 213 571
brian.rous@phe.gov.uk

**Dr Ariana ZNAOR**
Section of Cancer Surveillance
International Agency for Research on Cancer
150 Cours Albert Thomas
69372 Lyon
FRANCE
Tel. +33 4 72 73 83 52
Fax +33 4 72 73 86 96
znaora@iarc.fr

# Sources of figures and tables

## Sources of figures

| Figure | Source |
|---|---|
| 1.01–1.05 | Messina J. |
| 1.06 | Scolyer R.A. |
| 1.07–1.08 | Messina J. |
| 1.09 | Scolyer R.A. |
| 1.10 | Messina J. |
| 1.11 | Singh R. |
| 1.12 | Patterson J.W. |
| 1.13 | Messina J. |
| 1.14 | Scolyer R.A. |
| 1.15–1.16 | Messina J. |
| 1.17–1.18 | Patterson J.W. |
| 1.19–1.20 | Singh R. |
| 1.21–1.23 | Patel R.M. |
| 1.24 | Messina J. |
| 1.25 | Reproduced with permission from: Murphy G.F., Herzberg A.J. (1996) Atlas of Dermatopathology. WB Saunders, Philadelphia |
| 1.26 –1.27 | Murphy G.F. |
| 1.28 | Gaspari A.A.<br>University of Maryland Medical Center<br>Baltimore MD, USA |
| 1.29 | Singh R. |
| 1.30 | Kao G.F. |
| 1.31–1.32 | Singh R. |
| 1.33 A,B | Murphy G.F. |
| 1.34–1.35 | Singh R. |
| 1.36 | Myskowski P.L.<br>Department of Medicine/ Dermatology Service<br>Memorial Sloan Kettering Cancer Center<br>New York NY, USA |
| 1.37–1.38 | Pulitzer M.P. |
| 1.39–1.41 | Cerio R. |
| 1.42–1.43 | Yu L.L.<br>Reproduced from: Pathology and Genetics of Skin Tumours, IARC Press, Lyon: 2006 |
| 1.44–1.45 | Beer T.W. |
| 1.46–1.48 | Murphy G.F. |
| 1.49 | Kao G.F.<br>Reproduced from: Pathology and Genetics of Skin Tumours, IARC Press, Lyon: 2006 |
| 1.50 A,B | Scolyer R.A. |
| 1.51 | Singh R. |
| 1.52–1.57 | Busam K.J. |
| 1.58 | Sanchez-Carpintero I.<br>Clinica Dermatologica Internacional<br>Madrid, Spain |
| 1.59 | Soyer H.P. |
| 1.60 A,B | Craig J. |
| 1.61–1.62 | Massi D. |
| 1.63 | Cerroni L. |
| 1.64–1.65 | Martinka M. |
| 1.66 | Tan K.-B. |
| 1.67 | Grayson W. |
| 1.68 | Weedon D.<br>Reproduced from: Pathology and Genetics of Skin Tumours, IARC Press, Lyon: 2006 |
| 1.69–1.72 | Tan K.-B. |
| 1.73 | Wee J.<br>Department of Medicine<br>Jurong Health<br>Ng Teng Fong General Hospital<br>National University Health System<br>Singapore, Singapore |
| 1.74 | Tan K.-B. |
| 1.75–1.88 | Brenn T. |
| 1.89 A,B | Piris A. |
| 2.01–2.02 | Elder D. |
| 2.03 | Reprinted with permission from: Landi MT, Bauer J, Pfeiffer RM, Elder DE, Hulley B, Minghetti P, et al. (2006) MC1R germline variants confer risk for BRAF-mutant melanoma. Science; 313:521–2 |
| 2.04 | Bastian B.C. |
| 2.05 | Duncan L.M. |
| 2.06 | de la Fourchardiere A. |
| 2.07 | Duncan L.M. |
| 2.08 | Bastian B.C. |
| 2.09–2.10 | Elder D. |
| 2.11 | Cerroni L. |
| 2.12 | Elder D. |
| 2.13–2.15 | Elder D. |
| 2.16 | Lazova R. |
| 2.17–2.18 | Bastian B.C. |
| 2.19–2.20 | Lazova R. |
| 2.21–2.26 | Rongioletti F. |
| 2.27 | Cerroni L. |
| 2.28–2.29 | Chu E. |
| 2.30 | Weedon D.<br>Reproduced from: Pathology and Genetics of Skin Tumours, IARC Press, Lyon: 2006 |
| 2.31–2.32 | Messina J. |
| 2.33 | Courtesy of Dr C. Chung<br>Department of Dermatology and Pathology<br>The Ohio State University Wexner Medical Center<br>Gahanna OH, USA |
| 2.34 | Helm K.F. |
| 2.35 | Cerroni L. |
| 2.36–2.37 | Barnhill R.L. |
| 2.38 A–E | Zembowicz A. |
| 2.39 | Valencia A.<br>Department of Pediatrics<br>Hospital Angeles Pedregal<br>Mexico, D.F. La Magdalena Contreras, Mexico |
| 2.40–2.41 | Zembowicz A. |
| 2.42 | Tsao H. |
| 2.43 | Scolyer R.A. |
| 2.44 | Reprinted by permission from Macmillan Publishers Ltd: Nat Genet. Wiesner T, Obenauf AC, Murali R, Fried I, Griewank KG, Ulz P, et al. Germline mutations in BAP1 predispose to melanocytic tumors. 43:1018-21. Copyright 2011. |
| 2.45–2.46 | Scolyer R.A. |
| 2.47 | Bastian B.C. |
| 2.48–2.49 | Elder D. |
| 2.50 | Cerroni L. |
| 2.51–2.55 | Scolyer R.A |
| 2.56 A–D | Bahrami A. |
| 2.57 | Cerroni L. |
| 2.58–2.59 | Barnhill R.L. |
| 2.60 | Cerroni L. |
| 2.61–2.62 | Barnhill R.L. |
| 2.63–2.64 | Yun S.J. |
| 2.65 | Uhara H. |
| 2.66 | Yun S.J. |
| 2.67 | Uhara H. |
| 2.68–2.70 | Yun S.J. |
| 2.71 A–C | Uhara H. |
| 2.72–2.73 | Yun S.J. |
| 2.74–2.76 | Singh R. |
| 2.77 A,B | Prieto V.G. |
| 2.78 | Kerl H.<br>Reproduced from: Pathology and Genetics of Skin Tumours, IARC Press, Lyon: 2006 |
| 2.79–2.82 | de la Fouchardière A. |
| 2.83 A,B | Cerroni L. |
| 2.84–2.87 | de la Fouchardière A. |
| 2.88–2.90 | Yun S.J. |
| 2.91–2.92 A | Uhara H. |
| 2.92 B | Yun S.J. |
| 2.93 | Uhara H. |
| 2.94 | Mihm M.C. Jr<br>Reproduced from: Pathology and Genetics of Skin Tumours, IARC Press, Lyon: 2006 |
| 2.95–2.96 | Prieto V.G. |
| 2.97–2.98 | Cerroni L. |
| 2.99 | Massi G. |
| 2.100 | Elder D. |
| 2.101–2.102 | Massi G. |
| 2.103 | Cerroni L. |
| 2.104 A–C | Massi G. |
| 2.105 | Cree I.A. |
| 2.106–2.107 | Coupland S. |
| 2.108–2.115 | Zembowicz A. |
| 2.116 A,B | Puig S.<br>Melanoma: Imaging, genetics and immunology – IDIBAPS Melanoma Unit, Dermatology Department – Hospital Clinic, University of Barcelona<br>Barcelona, Spain |
| 2.117 A–D | Elder D. |

| | |
|---|---|
| 2.118–2.126 | Cook M.G.<br>Reprinted with permission from: Cook MG, Massi D, Blokx WAM, et al. New insights into naevoid melanomas: a clinicopathological reassessment. Histopathology. 2017; 71(6):943–50 |
| 2.127 A,B | Elder D. |
| 2.128–2.129 | Messina J. |

| | |
|---|---|
| 3.01 A–C | Prieto V.G. |
| 3.02–3.07 | Kazakov D.V. |
| 3.08 A,B | Brenn T. |
| 3.09–3.13 | Kazakov D.V. |
| 3.14–3.16 | Zembowicz A. |
| 3.17 A,B | Kazakov D.V. |
| 3.18 | Murdoch M.<br>Wits Donald Gordon Medical Centre<br>Parktown, Johannesburg, South Africa |
| 3.19–3.25 | Kazakov D.V. |
| 3.26 A–D | Brenn T. |
| 3.27–3.28 | Kazakov D.V. |
| 3.29 | Requena L. |
| 3.30 | Kazakov D.V. |
| 3.31–3.41 | Sangüeza O.P. |
| 3.42 | Hornick J.L. |
| 3.43 | Fisher C. |
| 3.44 A,B | Hornick J.L. |
| 3.45–3.48 | Requena L. |
| 3.49–3.51 | Kazakov D.V. |
| 3.52–3.53 | Prieto V.G. |
| 3.54 | Kutzner H. |
| 3.55 | Requena L. |
| 3.56–3.57 | Kutzner H. |
| 3.58 | Singh R. |
| 3.59 A,B | Requena L. |
| 3.60–3.62 | Schulz T. |
| 3.63–3.64 | Requena L. |
| 3.65–3.67 | Kutzner H. |
| 3.68 A,B | Requena L. |
| 3.69–3.70 | Kutzner H. |
| 3.71–3.72 | Singh R. |
| 3.73–3.74 | Prieto V.G. |
| 3.75–3.77 | Singh R. |
| 3.78–3.79 | Kacerovska D. |
| 3.80 | Singh R. |
| 3.81 | Kacerovska D. |
| 3.82 A,B | Sangüeza O.P. |
| 3.83–3.84 | Kazakov D.V. |

| | |
|---|---|
| 4.01–4.15 | Cerroni L. |
| 4.16 | Willemze R. |
| 4.17 | Cerroni L. |
| 4.18–4.19 | Willemze R. |
| 4.20 | Cerroni L. |
| 4.21–4.25 | Willemze R. |
| 4.26 | Berti E. |
| 4.27 A–D | Kempf W. |
| 4.28–4.29 | Facchetti F. |
| 4.30–4.33 | Willemze R. |
| 4.34 A–C | Ohshima K.<br>Reprinted from: WHO Classification of Tumours of Haematopoietic and Lymphoid Tissues, IARC Press, Lyon: 2017 |
| 4.35 | Jaffe E.S. |
| 4.36 | Tokura Y.<br>Reprinted from: WHO Classification of Tumours of Haematopoietic and Lymphoid Tissues, IARC Press, Lyon: 2017 |
| 4.37–4.38 | Facchetti F. |
| 4.39–4.41 | Willemze R. |
| 4.42 A | Ko Y.-H. |
| 4.42 B | Harada R. |
| 4.43–4.45 | Quintanilla-Martinez L. |
| 4.46 A,C | Modified with permission from: Quintanilla-Martinez L, Ridaura C, Nagl F, Sáez-de-Ocariz M, Durán-McKinster C, Ruiz-Maldonado R, Alderete G, Grube P, Lome-Maldonado C, Bonzheim I, Fend F (2013) Hydroa vacciniforme-like lymphoma: a chronic EBV+ lymphoproliferative disorder with risk to develop a systemic lymphoma. Blood;122:3101-10. |
| 4.46 B,D | Quintanilla-Martinez L. |
| 4.47 A,B | Ko Y.-H. |
| 4.48–4.50 | Chan J.K.C. |
| 4.51–4.58 | Berti E. |
| 4.59 | Dalac S.<br>Department of Dermatology<br>CHU Dijon<br>Dijon, France |
| 4.60 | Kempf W. |
| 4.61–4.65 | Petrella T. |
| 4.66–4.68 | Willemze R. |
| 4.69 | Feldman A. |
| 4.70–4.71 | Facchetti F. |
| 4.72 A,B | Feldman A. |
| 4.73–4.75 | Kempf W. |
| 4.76 | Willemze R.<br>Reproduced from: WHO Classification of Tumours of Haematopoietic and Lymphoid Tissues, IARC Press, Lyon: 2017 |
| 4.77–4.78 | Willemze R. |
| 4.79 A–C | Willemze R.<br>Reproduced from: WHO Classification of Tumours of Haematopoietic and Lymphoid Tissues, IARC Press, Lyon: 2017 |
| 4.80–4.81 | Willemze R. |
| 4.82 | Tokura Y. |
| 4.83 | Murase T.<br>Liaison Medical Marunouchi<br>Nagoya, Japan |
| 4.84 A,B | Matsue K.<br>Division of Hematology/ Oncology<br>Department of Medicine<br>Kameda Medical Center<br>Kamogawa, Japan |
| 4.85 | Dojcinov S. |
| 4.86–4.87 | Jaffe E.S.4.88– 4.89<br>Adapted with permission from: Beaty MW, Toro J, Sorbara L, Stern JB, Pittaluga S, Raffeld M, Wilson WH, Jaffe ES (2001) Cutaneous lymphomatoid granulomatosis: correlation of clinical and biologic features. Am J Surg Pathol. 25:1111-20. Wolters Kluwer. https://journals.lww.com/ajsp/pages/default.aspx |
| 4.90 | Jaffe E.S. |
| 4.91–4.92 | Ferry J.A. |
| 4.93 A,B | Willemze R. |
| 4.94–4.98 | Ferry J.A. |
| 4.99–4.100 | Berti E. |
| 4.101–4.103 | Petrella T. |
| 4.104–4.106 | Facchetti F. |
| 4.107–4.108 | Venkataraman G. |
| 4.109 | Facchetti F. |
| 4.110 | Venkataraman G. |
| 4.111–4.115 | Hartmann K. |
| 4.116–4.119 | Horny H.-P. |
| 4.120–4.122 | Facchetti F. |
| 4.123–4.124 | Berti E. |
| 4.125 | Reprinted with permission from: Romani N, Clausen BE, Stoitzner P (2010) Langerhans cells and more: langerin-expressing dendritic cell subsets in the skin.<br>Immunol Rev; 234:120-41. |
| 4.126 | Berti E. |
| 4.127–4.131 | Facchetti F. |
| 4.132 | Caputo R. (deceased)<br>Reproduced from: Pathology and Genetics of Skin Tumours, IARC Press, Lyon: 2006 |
| 4.133–4.135 | Facchetti F. |
| 4.136 | Caputo R. (deceased)<br>Reproduced from: Pathology and Genetics of Skin Tumours, IARC Press, Lyon: 2006 |
| 4.137–4.138 | Facchetti F. |
| 4.139 | Calzavara P.<br>Division of Dermatology<br>University of Brescia<br>Brescia, Italy |
| 4.140 | Caputo R. (deceased)<br>Reproduced from: World Health Organization Classification of Tumours. Pathology and Genetics of Skin Tumours, IARC Press, Lyon: 2006 |
| 4.141–4.144 | Facchetti F. |
| 4.145–4.146 | Berti E. |
| 4.147–4.148 | Facchetti F. |
| 4.149–4.155 | Berti E. |

| | |
|---|---|
| 5.01–5.03 | Lazar A.J. |
| 5.04–5.07 | Folpe A. |
| 5.08–5.09 A | Low I. |
| 5.09 B | Billings S. |
| 5.10–5.13 | Wong D. |
| 5.14 | Patel R.M. |
| 5.15 | Billings S. |
| 5.16 | Requena L. |
| 5.17–5.19 | Billings S. |
| 5.20–5.21 | Requena L. |
| 5.22–5.25 | Hornick J.L. |
| 5.26–5.28 | Mahar A. |
| 5.29A | Lazar A.J. |
| 5.29B–5.31A | Mahar A. |
| 5.31B | Lazar A.J. |
| 5.31C | Mahar A. |
| 5.31D | Lazar A.J. |
| 5.32–5.33 | Lazar A.J. |
| 5.34–5.37 | Kutzner H. |
| 5.38A–D | Andea A. |
| 5.39–5.41 | Glusac E.J. |
| 5.42 | Kutzner H. |
| 5.43–5.45 | Glusac E.J. |
| 5.46 | O'Brien B.H. |

| | |
|---|---|
| 5.47–5.48 | Requena L. |
| 5.49 A,B | Hornick J.L. |
| 5.50 A | Kutzner H. |
| 5.50 B,C | Patel R.M. |
| 5.51 | Patel R.M. |
| 5.52–5.54 | Kutzner H. |
| 5.55–5.58 | Billings S. |
| 5.59–5.60 | Requena L. |
| 5.61–5.64 | Kutzner H. |
| 5.65–5.66 | Reprinted with permission from: Agaimy A, Bieg M, Michal M, et al. (2017) Recurrent Somatic PDGFRB Mutations in Sporadic Infantile/ Solitary Adult Myofibromas But Not in Angioleiomyomas and Myopericytomas. Am J Surg Pathol;41:195-203. Wolters Kluwer. https://journals.lww.com/ajsp/pages/default.aspx |
| 5.67–5.68 | Agaimy A. |
| 5.69 | Singh R. |
| 5.70 | Requena L. |
| 5.71–5.72 | Kutzner H. |
| 5.73–5.76 | Lazar A. |
| 5.77–5.80 | Folpe A. |
| 5.81 | Jackett L. |
| 5.82 | Folpe A. |
| 5.83–5.84 | Jackett L. |
| 5.85 A | Schowalter M.<br>Department of Dermatology<br>Cleveland Clinic<br>Cleveland OH, USA |
| 5.85 B | Folpe A. |
| 5.86–5.88 | Agaimy A. |
| 5.89–5.90 | Patel R.M. |
| 5.91 | Requena L. |
| 5.92–5.98 | Billings S. |
| 5.99–5.104 | Hornick J.L. |
| 5.105–5.106 | Requena L. |
| 5.107–5.109 | Grayson W. |
| 5.110 | Requena L. |
| 5.111 A,B | Brenn T. |
| 5.112–5.117 | Calonje E. |
| 5.118–5.119 | Singh R. |
| 5.120–5.126 | Calonje E. |
| 5.127 | Singh R. |
| 5.128–5.134 | Calonje E. |
| 5.135 | Singh R. |
| 5.136–5.137 | Calonje E. |
| 5.138–5.139 | Requena L. |
| 5.140–5.145 | Tetzlaff M. |
| 5.146–5.147 | Ferguson P.M. |
| 5.148–5.150 | Kutzner H. |
| 5.151–5.153 | Zelger B. |
| 5.154–5.155 | Calonje E. |
| 5.156–5.158 | Lazar A.J. |
| 5.159–5.160 | Messina J. |
| 5.161 | Lazar A.J. |
| 5.162 | Calonje E. |
| 5.163–5.164 | Singh R. |
| 5.165–5.166 | Kutzner H. |
| 5.167–5.170 | Beer T.W. |
| 5.171–5.174 | Brenn T. |
| 5.175 A,B | Lazar A.J. |
| 5.176 A,B | Billings S. |
| 5.176 C,D | Lazar A.J. |
| 5.177 A | Billings S. |
| 5.177 B | Lazar A.J. |
| 5.178–5.180 | Patel R.M. |
| 5.181 A–C | Kutzner H. |
| 5.182 A,B | Busam K.J. |
| 5.183–5.185 | Patel R.M. |
| 5.186–5.188 | Lazar A.J. |
| 5.189 | Requena L. |
| 5.190 | Hornick J.L. |
| 5.191 A,B | Requena L. |

| | |
|---|---|
| 6.01 | Tucker M. |
| 6.02–6.03 | Bradford PT, Goldstein AM, Tamura D, Khan SG, Ueda T, Boyle J, et al. (2011) Cancer and neurologic degeneration in xeroderma pigmentosum: long term follow-up characterises the role of DNA repair. J Med Genet.48:168-76. Adapted by permission from: BMJ Publishing Group Limited and<br>DiGiovanna JJ, Kraemer KH (2012). Shining a light on xeroderma pigmentosum. J Invest Dermatol. 132(3 Pt 2):785–96. Copyright 2012, adapted with permission from Elsevier. |
| 6.04 | Adapted from: J Invest Dermatol. Shining a light on xeroderma pigmentosum. DiGiovanna JJ, Kraemer KH. 132(3 Pt 2):785-96. Copyright 2012; and Neuroscience. Xeroderma pigmentosum, trichothiodystrophy and Cockayne syndrome: a complex genotype-phenotype relationship. Kraemer KH, Patronas NJ, Schiffmann R, Brooks BP, Tamura D, DiGiovanna JJ. 145(4):1388-96. Copyright 2007; and Mol Med Today. van Steeg H, Kraemer KH. Xeroderma pigmentosum and the role of UV-induced DNA damage in skin cancer. 5(2):86-94. Copyright 1999. All with permission from Elsevier. |
| 6.05 A,B | Sarasin A.<br>Reproduced from: Pathology and Genetics of Skin Tumours, IARC Press, Lyon: 2006 |
| 6.06 | Padwa B.<br>Department of Plastic and Oral Surgery<br>Boston Children's Hospital<br>Boston MA, USA |
| 6.07 | Reproduced from: Bresler SC, Padwa BL, Granter SR (2016) Nevoid Basal Cell Carcinoma Syndrome (Gorlin Syndrome). Head Neck Pathol. 10:119-24. With permission of Springer. |
| 6.08 A,B | Woo S.B.<br>Division of Oral Medicine and Dentistry<br>Brigham and Women's Hospital<br>Boston MA, USA<br>Reproduced from: Bresler SC, Padwa BL, Granter SR (2016). Nevoid Basal Cell Carcinoma Syndrome (Gorlin Syndrome). Head Neck Pathol. 10(2):119-24. With permission of Springer. |
| 6.09 | Adapted from: Kraft S, Granter SR. Molecular pathology of skin neoplasms of the head and neck. Arch Pathol Lab Med. 2014 Jun;138(6):759-87. With permission from: Archives of Pathology & Laboratory Medicine. Copyright 2014 College of American Pathologists. |
| 6.10–6.12 | Stratakis C.A. |
| 6.13–6.14 | Zembowicz A. |
| 6.15 A–E | Wiesner T. |
| 6.16–6.17 | Lazar A.J. |
| 6.18 | Adapted from: Boland CR, Goel A (2010) Microsatellite instability in colorectal cancer: Gastroenterology. 138(6): 2073–2087.e3. Copyright 2010, with permission from Elsevier. |

## Sources of tables

| | |
|---|---|
| 1.01 | Messina J. |
| 1.02 | Mihm M.C. Jr |

| | |
|---|---|
| 2.01 | Elder D. |
| 2.02 | Elder D. |
| 2.03 | Adapted from: Piepkorn MW, Barnhill RL, Elder DE, Knezevich SR, Carney PA, Reisch LM, et al. (2014) The MPATH-Dx reporting schema for melanocytic proliferations and melanoma. J Am Acad Dermatol. 70(1):131–41. Copyright 2014, with permission from Elsevier |
| 2.04–2.05 | Bastian B.C. |
| 2.06 | Elder D. |
| 2.07–2.12 | Adapted from: Shors AR, Kim S, White E, Argenyi Z, Barnhill RL, Duray P, et al. (2006) Dysplastic naevi with moderate to severe histological dysplasia: a risk factor for melanoma. Br J Dermatol. 155(5):988–93; and adapted from: Xiong MY, Rabkin MS, Piepkorn MW, Barnhill RL, Argenyi Z, Erickson L, et al. (2014) Diameter of dysplastic nevi is a more robust biomarker of increased melanoma risk than degree of histologic dysplasia: a case-control study. J Am Acad Dermatol. 71:1257–1258 e4. |
| 2.13 | Elder D. |
| 2.14–2.15 | Barnhill R.L. |

| | |
|---|---|
| 4.01 | Willemze R. |
| 4.02 | Reprinted with permission from: Olsen E, Vonderheid E, Pimpinelli N, Willemze R, Kim Y, Knobler R, et al. (2007) Revisions to the staging and classification of mycosis fungoides and Sezary syndrome: a proposal of the International Society for Cutaneous Lymphomas (ISCL) and the cutaneous lymphoma task force of the European Organization of Research and Treatment of Cancer (EORTC). Blood. 110(6):1713–22. |
| 4.03 | Adapted from: Swerdlow SH, Campo E, Harris NL, Jaffe ES, Pileri S, Stein H, Thiele J. (Eds): WHO Classification of Tumours of Haematopoietic and Lymphoid Tissues (Revised 4th edition), IARC Press, Lyon: 2017 |
| 4.04 | Jaffe ES, Arber DA, Campo E, Harris NL, Quintanilla-Fend L. Primary cutaneous B-cell lymphomas. Hematopathology. 2nd Edition. Elsevier: 2017 |
| 4.05 | Adapted from: Swerdlow SH, Campo E, Harris NL, Jaffe ES, Pileri S, Stein H, Thiele J. (Eds): WHO Classification of Tumours of Haematopoietic and Lymphoid Tissues (Revised 4th edition), IARC Press, Lyon: 2017 |
| 4.06 | Hartmann K. |
| 5.01–5.02 | Grayson W. |
| 5.03 | Beer T.W. |
| 6.01 | Modified by Lazar A.J., Scolyer R.A., with permission, from: LeBoit PE, Burg G, Weedon D, Sarasain A (Eds): World Health Organization Classification of Tumours. Pathology and Genetics of Skin Tumours, IARC Press, Lyon: 2006 |
| 6.03 | Newton-Bishop J. |
| 6.04 | Adapted from: Evans DG, Ladusans EJ, Rimmer S, Burnell LD, Thakker N, Farndon PA. Complications of the naevoid basal cell carcinoma syndrome: results of a population based study. J Med Genet. 1993 Jun; 30(6):460-4. With permission from BMJ Publishing Group Ltd. |
| 6.05 | Stratakis C.A. |

**Sources of figures on front cover**

| | |
|---|---|
| Top left | Stratakis C.A. (Fig. 6.12) |
| Top centre | Bastian B.C. (Fig. 2.04) |
| Top right | Weedon D. (Fig. 1.68) |
| Middle left | Messina J. (Fig. 2.32) |
| Middle centre | Facchetti F. (Fig. 4.142) |
| Middle right | Willemze R. (Fig. 4.78 B) |
| Bottom left | Lazar A.J. (Fig. 5.33) |
| Bottom centre | Lazar A.J. (Fig. 5.32 B) |
| Bottom right | DiGiovanna JJ, Kraemer KH and Kraemer KH, et al. Adapted from: J Invest Dermatol. Shining a light on xeroderma pigmentosum. DiGiovanna JJ, Kraemer KH. 132(3 Pt 2):785-96. Copyright 2012; and Neuroscience. Xeroderma pigmentosum, trichothiodystrophy and Cockayne syndrome: a complex genotype-phenotype relationship. Kraemer KH, Patronas NJ, Schiffmann R, Brooks BP, Tamura D, DiGiovanna JJ. 145(4):1388-96. Copyright 2007; and Mol Med Today. van Steeg H, Kraemer KH. Xeroderma pigmentosum and the role of UV-induced DNA damage in skin cancer. 5(2):86-94. Copyright 1999. All with permission from Elsevier. |

# References


**1.** Aarts WM, Willemze R, Bende RJ, Meijer CJ, Pals ST, van Noesel CJ (1998). VH gene analysis of primary cutaneous B-cell lymphomas: evidence for ongoing somatic hypermutation and isotype switching. Blood. 92(10):3857–64. PMID:9808579

**2.** Aavikko M, Kaasinen E, Nieminen JK, Byun M, Donner I, Mancuso R, et al. (2015). Whole-genome sequencing identifies STAT4 as a putative susceptibility gene in classic Kaposi sarcoma. J Infect Dis. 211(11):1842–51. PMID:25492914

**3.** Abbas O, Mahalingam M (2009). Cutaneous sebaceous neoplasms as markers of Muir-Torre syndrome: a diagnostic algorithm. J Cutan Pathol. 36(6):613–9. PMID:19515040

**4.** Abbas O, Mahalingam M (2009). Tumor of the follicular infundibulum: an epidermal reaction pattern? Am J Dermatopathol. 31(7):626–33. PMID:19633534

**5.** Abbas O, Richards JE, Mahalingam M (2010). Fibroblast-activation protein: a single marker that confidently differentiates morpheaform/infiltrative basal cell carcinoma from desmoplastic trichoepithelioma. Mod Pathol. 23(11):1535–43. PMID:20711172

**6.** Abbasi NR, Brownell I, Fangman W (2007). Familial multiple angiolipomatosis. Dermatol Online J. 13(1):3. PMID:17511936

**7.** Abbott JJ, Ahmed I (2006). Adenocarcinoma of mammary-like glands of the vulva: report of a case and review of the literature. Am J Dermatopathol. 28(2):127–33. PMID:16625074

**8.** Abbott JJ, Erickson-Johnson M, Wang X, Nascimento AG, Oliveira AM (2006). Gains of COL1A1-PDGFB genomic copies occur in fibrosarcomatous transformation of dermatofibrosarcoma protuberans. Mod Pathol. 19(11):1512–8. PMID:16980946

**9.** Abbott JJ, Hernandez-Rios P, Amirkhan RH, Hoang MP (2003). Cystic sebaceous neoplasms in Muir-Torre syndrome. Arch Pathol Lab Med. 127(5):614–7. PMID:12708909

**10.** Abbott JJ, Oliveira AM, Nascimento AG (2006). The prognostic significance of fibrosarcomatous transformation in dermatofibrosarcoma protuberans. Am J Surg Pathol. 30(4):436–43. PMID:16625088

**11.** Abdulkader M, Kuhar M, Hattab E, Linos K (2016). GATA3 positivity in endocrine mucin-producing sweat gland carcinoma and invasive mucinous carcinoma of the eyelid: report of 2 cases. Am J Dermatopathol. 38(10):789–91. PMID:27533071

**12.** Abel R, Dougherty JW (1962). Nevus lipomatosus cutaneus superficialis (Hoffman-Zurhelle); report of two cases. Arch Dermatol. 85(4):524–6. PMID:13858911

**13.** Aboud MJ, Kadhim MM (2015). Langerhans-cell histiocytosis (LCH) a presentation of two siblings with two different entities. Springerplus. 4:351. PMID:26191478

**14.** Aboutalebi A, Korman JB, Sohani AR, Hasserjian RP, Louissaint A Jr, Le L, et al. (2013). Aleukemic cutaneous myeloid sarcoma. J Cutan Pathol. 40(12):996–1005. PMID:24274424

**15.** AbuHilal M, Breslavet M, Ho N, Taylor G, Pope E (2016). Hobnail hemangioma (superficial hemosiderotic lymphovascular malformation) in children: a series of 6 pediatric cases and review of the literature. J Cutan Med Surg. 20(3):216–20. PMID:26475078

**16.** Ackerman AB (1979). Subtle clues to diagnosis by conventional microscopy. The patch stage of Kaposi's sarcoma. Am J Dermatopathol. 1(2):165–72. PMID:549492

**17.** Ackerman AB, Wade TR (1980). Tricholemmoma. Am J Dermatopathol. 2(3):207–24. PMID:7258553

**18.** Ackerman BA, Reddy VB, Soyer HP, editors (2001). Neoplasms with follicular differentiation. 2nd ed. New York: Ardor Scribendi.

**19.** Acs G, Simpson JF, Bleiweiss IJ, Hugh J, Reynolds C, Olson S, et al. (2003). Microglandular adenosis with transition into adenoid cystic carcinoma of the breast. Am J Surg Pathol. 27(8):1052–60. PMID:12883237

**20.** Adachi Y, Kosami K, Mizuta N, Ito M, Matsuoka Y, Kanata M, et al. (2014). Benefits of skin biopsy of senile hemangioma in intravascular large B-cell lymphoma: a case report and review of the literature. Oncol Lett. 7(6):2003–6. PMID:24932279

**21.** Adamski H, Le Gall F, Coindre JM, Kerbrat P, Chevrant-Breton J (1998). Recurring atypical ("pseudosarcomatous") cutaneous fibrous histiocytoma. Eur J Dermatol. 8(2):122–4. PMID:9649666

**22.** Agaimy A, Bieg M, Michal M, Geddert H, Märkl B, Seitz J, et al. (2017). Recurrent somatic PDGFRB mutations in sporadic infantile/solitary adult myofibromas but not in angioleiomyomas and myopericytomas. Am J Surg Pathol. 41(2):195–203. PMID:27776010

**23.** Agaimy A, Michal M, Giedl J, Hadravsky L, Michal M (2017). Superficial acral fibromyxoma: clinicopathological, immunohistochemical, and molecular study of 11 cases highlighting frequent Rb1 loss/deletions. Hum Pathol. 60:192–8. PMID:27825811

**24.** Agar NS, Wedgeworth E, Crichton S, Mitchell TJ, Cox M, Ferreira S, et al. (2010). Survival outcomes and prognostic factors in mycosis fungoides/Sézary syndrome: validation of the revised International Society for Cutaneous Lymphomas/European Organisation for Research and Treatment of Cancer staging proposal. J Clin Oncol. 28(31):4730–9. PMID:20855822

**25.** Agis H, Weltermann A, Fonatsch C, Haas O, Mitterbauer G, Müllauer L, et al. (2002). A comparative study on demographic, hematological, and cytogenetic findings and prognosis in acute myeloid leukemia with and without leukemia cutis. Ann Hematol. 81(2):90–5. PMID:11907789

**26.** Agnarsson BA, Vonderheid EC, Kadin ME (1990). Cutaneous T cell lymphoma with suppressor/cytotoxic (CD8) phenotype: identification of rapidly progressive and chronic subtypes. J Am Acad Dermatol. 22(4):569–77. PMID:2138636

**27.** Agnihotri S, Jalali S, Wilson MR, Danesh A, Li M, Klironomos G, et al. (2016). The genomic landscape of schwannoma. Nat Genet. 48(11):1339–48. PMID:27723760

**28.** Agoston AT, Liang CW, Richkind KE, Fletcher JA, Vargas SO (2010). Trisomy 18 is a consistent cytogenetic feature in pilomatricoma. Mod Pathol. 23(8):1147–50. PMID:20495544

**29.** Aguilar C, Rosai J (2011). Pleomorphic fibroma of the skin, atypical lipomatous tumor, or both? Int J Surg Pathol. 19(1):63. PMID:21123246

**30.** Aguilera NS, Tomaszewski MM, Moad JC, Bauer FA, Taubenberger JK, Abbondanzo SL (2001). Cutaneous follicle center lymphoma: a clinicopathologic study of 19 cases. Mod Pathol. 14(9):828–35. PMID:11557777

**31.** Ahn CS, Guerra A, Sangüeza OP (2016). Melanocytic nevi of special sites. Am J Dermatopathol. 38(12):867–81. PMID:27870726

**32.** Ahn HK, Suh C, Chuang SS, Suzumiya J, Ko YH, Kim SJ, et al. (2012). Extranodal natural killer/T-cell lymphoma from skin or soft tissue: suggestion of treatment from multinational retrospective analysis. Ann Oncol. 23(10):2703–7. PMID:22547542

**33.** Ahn SK, Ahn HJ, Kim TH, Hwang SM, Choi EH, Lee SH (2002). Intratumoral fat in neurofibroma. Am J Dermatopathol. 24(4):326–9. PMID:12142613

**34.** Aird I, Johnson HD, Lennox B, Stansfeld AG (1954). Epithelioma cuniculatum: a variety of squamous carcinoma peculiar to the foot. Br J Surg. 42(173):245–50. PMID:13219306

**35.** Aissani B, Boehme AK, Wiener HW, Shrestha S, Jacobson LP, Kaslow RA (2014). SNP screening of central MHC-identified HLA-DMB as a candidate susceptibility gene for HIV-related Kaposi's sarcoma. Genes Immun. 15(6):424–9. PMID:25008864

**36.** Akay BN, Saral S, Heper AO, Erdem C, Rosendahl C (2017). Basosquamous carcinoma: dermoscopic clues to diagnosis. J Dermatol. 44(2):127–34. PMID:27570202

**37.** Al Dhaybi R, Lam C, Hatami A, Powell J, McCuaig C, Kokta V (2012). Targetoid hemosiderotic hemangiomas (hobnail hemangiomas) are vascular lymphatic malformations: a study of 12 pediatric cases. J Am Acad Dermatol. 66(1):116–20. PMID:21798621

**38.** Al Habeeb A, Weinreb I, Ghazarian D (2009). Primitive non-neural granular cell tumour with lymph node metastasis. J Clin Pathol. 62(9):847–9. PMID:19734486

**39.** Al-Arashi MY, Byers HR (2007). Cutaneous clear cell squamous cell carcinoma in situ: clinical, histological and immunohistochemical characterization. J Cutan Pathol. 34(3):226–33. PMID:17302606

**40.** Al-Daraji WI (2008). Granular perineurioma: the first report of a rare distinctive subtype of perineurioma. Am J Dermatopathol. 30(2):163–8. PMID:18360122

**41.** Al-Daraji WI, Miettinen M (2008). Superficial acral fibromyxoma: a clinicopathological analysis of 32 tumors including 4 in the heel. J Cutan Pathol. 35(11):1020–6. PMID:18537858

**42.** Al-Qattan MM (2014). Fibroma of tendon sheath of the hand: a series of 20 patients with 23 tumours. J Hand Surg Eur Vol. 39(3):300–5. PMID:23212985

**43.** Al-Zaid T, Ditelberg JS, Prieto VG, Lev D, Luthra R, Davies MA, et al. (2012). Trichilemmomas show loss of PTEN in Cowden syndrome but only rarely in sporadic tumors. J Cutan Pathol. 39(5):493–9. PMID:22486434

**44.** Al-Zaid T, Frieling G, Rosenthal S (2013). Dermal pleomorphic liposarcoma resembling pleomorphic fibroma: report of a case and review of the literature. J Cutan Pathol. 40(8):734–9. PMID:23651098

**45.** Al-Zaid T, Wang WL, Lopez-Terrada D, Lev D, Hornick JL, Hafeez Diwan A, et al. (2013). Pleomorphic fibroma and dermal atypical lipomatous tumor: are they related? J Cutan Pathol. 40(4):379–84. PMID:23506010

**46.** Alain G, Tousignant J, Rozenfarb E (1993). Chronic arsenic toxicity. Int J Dermatol. 32(12):899–901. PMID:8125698

**47.** Alam M, Desai S, Nodzenski M, Dubina M, Kim N, Martini M, et al. (2015). Active ascertainment of recurrence rate after treatment of primary basal cell carcinoma (BCC). J Am Acad Dermatol. 73(2):323–5. PMID:26183979

**48.** Alayed K, Medeiros LJ, Patel KP, Zuo Z, Li S, Verma S, et al. (2016). BRAF and MAP2K1 mutations in Langerhans cell histiocytosis: a study of 50 cases. Hum Pathol. 52:61–7. PMID:26980021

**49.** Alayed K, Patel KP, Konoplev S, Singh RR, Routbort MJ, Reddy N, et al. (2013). TET2 mutations, myelodysplastic features, and a distinct immunoprofile characterize blastic plasmacytoid dendritic cell neoplasm in the bone marrow. Am J Hematol. 88(12):1055–61. PMID:23940084

**50.** Albus J, Batanian J, Wenig BM, Vidal CI (2015). A unique case of a cutaneous lesion resembling mammary analog secretory carcinoma: a case report and review of the literature. Am J Dermatopathol. 37(4):e41–4. PMID:25140660

**51.** Alcaraz I, Cerroni L, Rütten A, Kutzner H, Requena L (2012). Cutaneous metastases from internal malignancies: a clinicopathologic and immunohistochemical review. Am J Dermatopathol. 34(4):347–93. PMID:22617133

**52.** Alikhan A, Ibrahimi OA, Eisen DB (2012). Congenital melanocytic nevi: where are we now? Part I. Clinical presentation, epidemiology, pathogenesis, histology, malignant transformation, and neurocutaneous melanosis. J Am Acad Dermatol. 67(4):495.e1–17. PMID:22980258

**53.** Alkatan HM, Al-Arfaj KM, Maktabi A (2010). Conjunctival nevi: clinical and histopathologic features in a Saudi population. Ann Saudi Med. 30(4):306–12. PMID:20622349

**54.** Alkhalidi H, Ghazarian D (2007). Cellular neurothekeoma with a plexiform morphology: a case report with a discussion of the plexiform lesions of the skin. J Cutan Pathol. 34(3):264–9. PMID:17302611

**55.** Allen CE, Li L, Peters TL, Leung HC, Yu A, Man TK, et al. (2010). Cell-specific gene expression in Langerhans cell histiocytosis lesions reveals a distinct profile compared with epidermal Langerhans cells. J Immunol. 184(8):4557–67. PMID:20220088

**56.** Allen CE, Parsons DW (2015). Biological and clinical significance of somatic mutations in Langerhans cell histiocytosis and related histiocytic neoplastic disorders. Hematology Am Soc Hematol Educ Program. 2015(1):559–64. PMID:26637772

**57.** Allen PW, Dymock RB, MacCormac LB (1988). Superficial angiomyxomas with and without epithelial components. Report of 30 tumors in 28 patients. Am J Surg Pathol. 12(7):519–30. PMID:3389450

**58.** Allen PW, Ramakrishna B, MacCormac LB (1992). The histiocytoid hemangiomas and other controversies. Pathol Annu. 27(Pt 2):51–87. PMID:1584628

**59.** Allen PW, Strungs I, MacCormac LB (1998). Atypical subcutaneous fatty tumors: a review of 37 referred cases. Pathology. 30(2):123–35. PMID:9643489

**60.** Allison KH, Patel RM, Goldblum JR, Rubin BP (2005). Superficial malignant peripheral nerve sheath tumor: a rare and challenging

diagnosis. Am J Clin Pathol. 124(5):685–92. PMID:16203275
**61.** Allon I, Buchner A (2012). Warty dyskeratoma/focal acantholytic dyskeratosis–an update on a rare oral lesion. J Oral Pathol Med. 41(3):261–7. PMID:21936875
**62.** Ally MS, Tang JY, Joseph T, Thompson B, Lindgren J, Raphael MA, et al. (2014). The use of vismodegib to shrink keratocystic odontogenic tumors in patients with basal cell nevus syndrome. JAMA Dermatol. 150(5):542–5. PMID:24623282
**63.** Aloi F, Tomasini C, Pippione M (1993). Cutaneous lymphadenoma. A basal cell carcinoma with unusual inflammatory reaction pattern? Am J Dermatopathol. 15(4):353–7. PMID:7692756
**64.** Altman DA, Mikhail GR, Johnson TM, Lowe L (1995). Trichoblastic fibroma. A series of 10 cases with report of a new plaque variant. Arch Dermatol. 131(2):198–201. PMID:7857118
**65.** Amaravati R (2002). Rare malignant transformation of a calcifying aponeurotic fibroma. J Bone Joint Surg Am. 84-A(10):1889. PMID:12377925
**66.** Ambrojo P, Aguilar A, Simón P, Requena L, Sánchez Yus E (1992). Basal cell carcinoma with matrical differentiation. Am J Dermatopathol. 14(4):293–7. PMID:1503202
**67.** Ambrojo P, Cogolludo EF, Aguilar A, Sánchez Yus E, Sánchez de Paz F (1990). Cutaneous lymphangiectases after therapy for carcinoma of the cervix–a case with unusual clinical and histological features. Clin Exp Dermatol. 15(1):57–9. PMID:2311281
**68.** Amin MB, Edge S, Greene F, Byrd DR, Brookland RK, Washington MK, et al., editors (2017). AJCC cancer staging manual. 8th ed. New York: Springer.
**69.** Amin SM, Beattie A, Ling X, Jennings LJ, Guitart J (2016). Primary cutaneous mammary analog secretory carcinoma with ETV6-NTRK3 translocation. Am J Dermatopathol. 38(11):842–5. PMID:27763904
**70.** Amin SM, Cooper C, Yélamos O, Lee CY, Sholl LM, de la Fouchardiere A, et al. (2015). Combined cutaneous tumors with a melanoma component: a clinical, histologic, and molecular study. J Am Acad Dermatol. 73(3):451–60. PMID:26209219
**71.** Amos CI, Wang LE, Lee JE, Gershenwald JE, Chen WV, Fang S, et al. (2011). Genome-wide association study identifies novel loci predisposing to cutaneous melanoma. Hum Mol Genet. 20(24):5012–23. PMID:21926416
**72.** Amyere M, Dompmartin A, Wouters V, Enjolras O, Kaitila I, Docquier PL, et al. (2014). Common somatic alterations identified in Maffucci syndrome by molecular karyotyping. Mol Syndromol. 5(6):259–67. PMID:25565925
**73.** Andersen WK, Labadie RR, Bhawan J (1997). Histopathology of solar lentigines of the face: a quantitative study. J Am Acad Dermatol. 36(3 Pt 1):444–7. PMID:9091478
**74.** Angervall L, Dahl I, Kindblom LG, Säve-Söderbergh (1976). Spindle cell lipoma. Acta Pathol Microbiol Scand A. 84(6):477–87. PMID:998247
**75.** Ansai S, Kimura T (2009). Rippled-pattern sebaceoma: a clinicopathological study. Am J Dermatopathol. 31(4):364–6. PMID:19461240
**76.** Ansai S, Mihara I (2000). Sebaceous carcinoma arising on actinic keratosis. Eur J Dermatol. 10(5):385–8. PMID:10882948
**77.** Ansai S, Watanabe S, Aso K (1989). A case of tubular apocrine adenoma with syringocystadenoma papilliferum. J Cutan Pathol. 16(4):230–6. PMID:2551940
**78.** Ansai SI (2017). Topics in histopathology of sweat gland and sebaceous neoplasms. J Dermatol. 44(3):315–26. PMID:28256768
**79.** Antonescu CR, Le Loarer F, Mosquera JM, Sboner A, Zhang L, Chen CL, et al. (2013). Novel YAP1-TFE3 fusion defines a distinct subset of epithelioid hemangioendothelioma. Genes Chromosomes Cancer. 52(8):775–84. PMID:23737213
**80.** Antonescu CR, Scheithauer BW, Woodruff JM (2013). Tumors of the peripheral nervous system. In: AFIP atlas of tumor pathology. Series 4, Fascicle 19. Washington, DC: American Registry of Pathology Press.
**81.** Antonescu CR, Sung YS, Zhang L, Agaram NP, Fletcher CD (2017). Recurrent SRF-RELA fusions define a novel subset of cellular myofibroma/myopericytoma: a potential diagnostic pitfall with sarcomas with myogenic differentiation. Am J Surg Pathol. 41(5):677–84. PMID:28248815
**82.** Antonescu CR, Zhang L, Nielsen GP, Rosenberg AE, Dal Cin P, Fletcher CD (2011). Consistent t(1;10) with rearrangements of TGFBR3 and MGEA5 in both myxoinflammatory fibroblastic sarcoma and hemosiderotic fibrolipomatous tumor. Genes Chromosomes Cancer. 50(10):757–64. PMID:21717526
**83.** Aoude LG, Pritchard AL, Robles-Espinoza CD, Wadt K, Harland M, Choi J, et al. (2014). Nonsense mutations in the shelterin complex genes ACD and TERF2IP in familial melanoma. J Natl Cancer Inst. 107(2):dju408. PMID:25505254
**84.** Aoude LG, Wadt K, Bojesen A, Crüger D, Borg A, Trent JM, et al. (2013). A BAP1 mutation in a Danish family predisposes to uveal melanoma and other cancers. PLoS One. 8(8):e72144. PMID:23977234
**85.** Apisarnthanarax P, Bovenmyer DA, Mehregan AH (1984). Combined adnexal tumor of the skin. Arch Dermatol. 120(2):231–3. PMID:6696477
**86.** Arbiser ZK, Folpe AL, Weiss SW (2001). Consultative (expert) second opinions in soft tissue pathology. Analysis of problem-prone diagnostic situations. Am J Clin Pathol. 116(4):473–6. PMID:11601130
**87.** Ardakani NM, Palmer DL, Wood BA (2016). Malignant melanocytic matricoma: a report of 2 cases and review of the literature. Am J Dermatopathol. 38(1):33–8. PMID:26730694
**88.** Arenaz Búa J, Luáces R, Lorenzo Franco F, García-Rozado A, Crespo Escudero JL, Fonseca Capdevila E, et al. (2010). Angiolipoma in head and neck: report of two cases and review of the literature. Int J Oral Maxillofac Surg. 39(6):610–5. PMID:20197228
**89.** Argatoff LH, Connors JM, Klasa RJ, Horsman DE, Gascoyne RD (1997). Mantle cell lymphoma: a clinicopathologic study of 80 cases. Blood. 89(6):2067–78. PMID:9058729
**90.** Argenyi ZB (1990). Immunohistochemical characterization of palisaded, encapsulated neuroma. J Cutan Pathol. 17(6):329–35. PMID:1705947
**91.** Argenyi ZB, Cooper PH, Santa Cruz D (1993). Plexiform and other unusual variants of palisaded encapsulated neuroma. J Cutan Pathol. 20(1):34–9. PMID:8468415
**92.** Argenyi ZB, LeBoit PE, Santa Cruz D, Swanson PE, Kutzner H (1993). Nerve sheath myxoma (neurothekeoma) of the skin: light microscopic and immunohistochemical reappraisal of the cellular variant. J Cutan Pathol. 20(4):294–303. PMID:7693776
**93.** Aricò M, Nichols K, Whitlock JA, Arceci R, Haupt R, Mittler U, et al. (1999). Familial clustering of Langerhans cell histiocytosis. Br J Haematol. 107(4):883–8. PMID:10606898
**94.** Armstrong BK, Kricker A (2001). The epidemiology of UV induced skin cancer. J Photochem Photobiol B. 63(1–3):8–18. PMID:11684447
**95.** Arnaud L, Gorochov G, Charlotte F, Lvovschi V, Parizot C, Larsen M, et al. (2011). Systemic perturbation of cytokine and chemokine networks in Erdheim-Chester disease: a single-center series of 37 patients. Blood. 117(10):2783–90. PMID:21205927
**96.** Arnaud L, Hervier B, Néel A, Hamidou MA, Kahn JE, Wechsler B, et al. (2011). CNS involvement and treatment with interferon-α are independent prognostic factors in Erdheim-Chester disease: a multicenter survival analysis of 53 patients. Blood. 117(10):2778–82. PMID:21239701
**97.** Arnaud L, Malek Z, Archambaud F, Kas A, Toledano D, Drier A, et al. (2009). 18F-fluorodeoxyglucose-positron emission tomography scanning is more useful in followup than in the initial assessment of patients with Erdheim-Chester disease. Arthritis Rheum. 60(10):3128–38. PMID:19790052
**98.** Arnaud L, Pierre I, Beigelman-Aubry C, Capron F, Brun AL, Rigolet A, et al. (2010). Pulmonary involvement in Erdheim-Chester disease: a single-center study of thirty-four patients and a review of the literature. Arthritis Rheum. 62(11):3504–12. PMID:20662053
**99.** Arnulf B, Copie-Bergman C, Delfau-Larue MH, Lavergne-Slove A, Bosq J, Wechsler J, et al. (1998). Nonhepatosplenic gammadelta T-cell lymphoma: a subset of cytotoxic lymphomas with mucosal or skin localization. Blood. 91(5):1723–31. PMID:9473239
**100.** Arock M, Sotlar K, Akin C, Broesby-Olsen S, Hoermann G, Escribano L, et al. (2015). KIT mutation analysis in mast cell neoplasms: recommendations of the European Competence Network on Mastocytosis. Leukemia. 29(6):1223–32. PMID:25650093
**101.** Arps DP, Chan MP, Patel RM, Andea AA (2015). Primary cutaneous cribriform carcinoma: report of six cases with clinicopathologic data and immunohistochemical profile. J Cutan Pathol. 42(6):379–87. PMID:25732813
**102.** Arrese Estrada J, Piérard-Franchimont C, Piérard GE (1990). Histogenesis of recurrent nevus. Am J Dermatopathol. 12(4):370–2. PMID:2203270
**103.** Arrington JH 3rd, Reed RJ, Ichinose H, Krementz ET (1977). Plantar lentiginous melanoma: a distinctive variant of human cutaneous malignant melanoma. Am J Surg Pathol. 1(2):131–43. PMID:602975
**104.** Arsenovic N, Ramaiya A (2009). Is a cystic sebaceous neoplasm always marker for Muir-Torre syndrome? Dermatol Online J. 15(11):11. PMID:19951647
**105.** Arslan H, Diyarbakrl M, Batur S, Demirkesen C (2013). Syringocystadenocarcinoma papilliferum with squamous cell carcinoma differentiation and with locoregional metastasis. J Craniofac Surg. 24(1):e38–40. PMID:23348331
**106.** Arulogun SO, Prince HM, Ng J, Lade S, Ryan GF, Blewitt O, et al. (2008). Long-term outcomes of patients with advanced-stage cutaneous T-cell lymphoma and large cell transformation. Blood. 112(8):3082–7. PMID:18647960
**107.** Asada N, Odawara J, Kimura S, Aoki T, Yamakura M, Takeuchi M, et al. (2007). Use of random skin biopsy for diagnosis of intravascular large B-cell lymphoma. Mayo Clin Proc. 82(12):1525–7. PMID:18053461
**108.** Asgari MM, Moffet HH, Ray GT, Quesenberry CP (2015). Trends in basal cell carcinoma incidence and identification of high-risk subgroups, 1998-2012. JAMA Dermatol. 151(9):976–81. PMID:26039887
**109.** Assor D, Davis JB (1977). Multiple apocrine fibroadenomas of the anal skin. Am J Clin Pathol. 68(3):397–9. PMID:197847
**110.** Atkinson JO, Biggar RJ, Goedert JJ, Engels EA (2004). The incidence of Kaposi sarcoma among injection drug users with AIDS in the United States. J Acquir Immune Defic Syndr. 37(2):1282–7. PMID:15385736
**111.** Attygalle AD, Cabeçadas J, Gaulard P, Jaffe ES, de Jong D, Ko YH, et al. (2014). Peripheral T-cell and NK-cell lymphomas and their mimics; taking a step forward - report on the lymphoma workshop of the XVIth meeting of the European Association for Haematopathology and the Society for Hematopathology. Histopathology. 64(2):171–99. PMID:24128129
**112.** Au JK, Said JW, Sepahdari AR, St John MA (2016). Head and neck Epstein-Barr virus mucocutaneous ulcer: case report and literature review. Laryngoscope. 126(11):2500–4. PMID:27113560
**113.** Au WY, Weisenburger DD, Intragumtornchai T, Nakamura S, Kim WS, Sng I, et al. (2009). Clinical differences between nasal and extranasal natural killer/T-cell lymphoma: a study of 136 cases from the International Peripheral T-Cell Lymphoma Project. Blood. 113(17):3931–7. PMID:19029440
**114.** Aung PP, Batrani M, Mirzabeigi M, Goldberg LJ (2014). Extraocular sebaceous carcinoma in situ: report of three cases and review of the literature. J Cutan Pathol. 41(7):592–6. PMID:24666211
**115.** Aung PP, Goldberg LJ, Mahalingam M, Bhawan J (2015). Cutaneous myopericytoma: a report of 3 cases and review of the literature. Dermatopathology (Basel). 2(1):9–14. PMID:27047931
**116.** Aung PP, Mutyambizi KK, Danialan R, Ivan D, Prieto VG (2015). Differential diagnosis of heavily pigmented melanocytic lesions: challenges and diagnostic approach. J Clin Pathol. 68(12):963–70. PMID:26602414
**117.** Ausmus GG, Piliang MP, Bergfeld WF, Goldblum JR (2007). Soft-tissue perineurioma in a 20-year-old patient with neurofibromatosis type 1 (NF1): report of a case and review of the literature. J Cutan Pathol. 34(9):726–30. PMID:17696922
**118.** Avraham JB, Villines D, Maker VK, August C, Maker AV (2013). Survival after resection of cutaneous adnexal carcinomas with eccrine differentiation: risk factors and trends in outcomes. J Surg Oncol. 108(1):57–62. PMID:23677677
**119.** Ayturk UM, Couto JA, Hann S, Mulliken JB, Williams KL, Huang AY, et al. (2016). Somatic activating mutations in GNAQ and GNA11 are associated with congenital hemangioma. Am J Hum Genet. 98(4):789–95. PMID:27058448
**120.** Diaz-Cascajo C, Borghi S, Bonczkowitz M (1998). Pigmented atypical fibroxanthoma. Histopathology. 33(6):537–41. PMID:9870148
**121.** Diaz-Cascajo C, Borghi S, Weyers W, Retzlaff H, Requena L, Metze D (1999). Benign lymphangiomatous papules of the skin following radiotherapy: a report of five new cases and review of the literature. Histopathology. 35(4):319–27. PMID:10564386
**122.** Díaz-Flores L, Gutiérrez R, García MP, Alvarez-Argüelles H, Díaz-Flores L Jr, Madrid JF (2011). Myopericytoma and arterial intimal thickening: the relationship between myopericytes and myointimal cells. J Cutan Pathol. 38(11):857–64. PMID:21955312
**123.** Díaz-Flores L, Gutiérrez R, Alvarez-Argüelles H, González-Gómez M, del Pino García M, Díaz-Flores L Jr (2016). Ultrastructure and histogenesis of the acral calcified angioleiomyoma. Ultrastruct Pathol. 40(1):24–32. PMID:26691377
**124.** Azzopardi JG, Iocco J, Salm R (1983). Pleomorphic lipoma: a tumour simulating liposarcoma. Histopathology. 7(4):511–23. PMID:6884998
**125.** Bachmeyer C, Bazarbachi A, Rio B, Delmer A, Hunault M, Zittoun R, et al. (1997). Specific cutaneous involvement indicating relapse of Burkitt's lymphoma. Am J Hematol. 54(2):176. PMID:9034303
**126.** Badalian-Very G, Vergilio JA, Degar BA, MacConaill LE, Brandner B, Calicchio ML, et al.

(2010). Recurrent BRAF mutations in Langerhans cell histiocytosis. Blood. 116(11):1919–23. PMID:20519626
**127.** Bae SH, Seon HJ, Choi YD, Shim HJ, Lee JB, Yun SJ (2016). Other primary systemic cancers in patients with melanoma: analysis of balanced acral and nonacral melanomas. J Am Acad Dermatol. 74(2):333–40. PMID:26584878
**128.** Bagcchi S (2015). POT1: a genetic link for familial glioma. Lancet Oncol. 16(1):e12. PMID:25524796
**129.** Baheti AD, Tirumani SH, Sewatkar R, Sachin SS, Shinagare AB, Ramaiya NH (2015). MDCT of extranodal mantle cell lymphoma: a single institute experience. Abdom Imaging. 40(6):1693–9. PMID:25724714
**130.** Bahrami A, Barnhill RL (2018). Pathology and genomics of pediatric melanoma: a critical reexamination and new insights. Pediatr Blood Cancer. 65(2):e26792. PMID:28895292
**131.** Bahrami A, Dalton JD, Krane JF, Fletcher CD (2012). A subset of cutaneous and soft tissue mixed tumors are genetically linked to their salivary gland counterpart. Genes Chromosomes Cancer. 51(2):140–8. PMID:22038920
**132.** Bahrami A, Lee S, Wu G, Kerstetter J, Rahvar M, Li X, et al. (2016). Pigment-synthesizing melanocytic neoplasm with protein kinase C alpha (PRKCA) fusion. JAMA Dermatol. 152(3):318–22. PMID:26676968
**133.** Bahrami S, Malone JC, Lear S, Martin AW (2006). CD10 expression in cutaneous adnexal neoplasms and a potential role for differentiating cutaneous metastatic renal cell carcinoma. Arch Pathol Lab Med. 130(9):1315–9. PMID:16948517
**134.** Balachandran K, Allen PW, MacCormac LB (1995). Nuchal fibroma. A clinicopathological study of nine cases. Am J Surg Pathol. 19(3):313–7. PMID:7872429
**135.** Balch CM, Gershenwald JE, Soong SJ, Thompson JF, Atkins MB, Byrd DR, et al. (2009). Final version of 2009 AJCC melanoma staging and classification. J Clin Oncol. 27(36):6199–206. PMID:19917835
**136.** Baldassano MF, Bailey EM, Ferry JA, Harris NL, Duncan LM (1999). Cutaneous lymphoid hyperplasia and cutaneous marginal zone lymphoma: comparison of morphologic and immunophenotypic features. Am J Surg Pathol. 23(1):88–96. PMID:9888708
**137.** Ban M, Sugie S, Kamiya H, Kitajima Y (2003). Microcystic adnexal carcinoma with lymph node metastasis. Dermatology. 207(4):395–7. PMID:14657634
**138.** Banerjee M, Sarma N, Biswas R, Roy J, Mukherjee A, Giri AK (2008). DNA repair deficiency leads to susceptibility to develop arsenic-induced premalignant skin lesions. Int J Cancer. 123(2):283–7. PMID:18386817
**139.** Banerjee SS, Agbamu DA, Eyden BP, Harris M (1997). Clinicopathological characteristics of peripheral primitive neuroectodermal tumour of skin and subcutaneous tissue. Histopathology. 31(4):355–66. PMID:9363452
**140.** Banks ER, Cooper PH (1991). Adenosquamous carcinoma of the skin: a report of 10 cases. J Cutan Pathol. 18(4):227–34. PMID:1719048
**141.** Baran JL, Duncan LM (2011). Combined melanocytic nevi: histologic variants and melanoma mimics. Am J Surg Pathol. 35(10):1540–8. PMID:21881487
**142.** Baran R, Haneke E (2001). Subungual myxoid neurofibroma on the thumb. Acta Derm Venereol. 81(3):210–1. PMID:11558882
**143.** Baranda L, Torres-Alvarez B, Moncada B, Portales-Pérez D, de la Fuente H, Layseca E, et al. (1999). Presence of activated lymphocytes in the peripheral blood of patients with halo nevi. J Am Acad Dermatol. 41(4):567–72. PMID:10495377
**144.** Baratti D, Pennacchioli E, Casali PG, Bertulli R, Lozza L, Olmi P, et al. (2007). Epithelioid sarcoma: prognostic factors and survival in a series of patients treated at a single institution. Ann Surg Oncol. 14(12):3542–51. PMID:17909905
**145.** Bardach H (1978). Hidroacanthoma simplex with in situ porocarcinoma. A case suggesting malignant transformation. J Cutan Pathol. 5(5):236–48. PMID:730865
**146.** Barnes M, Hestley A, Murray DR, Carlson GW, Parker D, Delman KA (2014). The risk of lymph node involvement in malignant cutaneous adnexal tumors. Am Surg. 80(3):270–4. PMID:24666868
**147.** Barnhill RL, Piepkorn M, Busam KJ, editors (2004). Pathology of melanocytic nevi and malignant melanoma. New York: Springer-Verlag New York.
**148.** Barnhill R, Dy K, Lugassy C (2002). Angiotropism in cutaneous melanoma: a prognostic factor strongly predicting risk for metastasis. J Invest Dermatol. 119(3):705–6. PMID:12230518
**149.** Barnhill RL (1994). Nerve sheath myxoma (neurothekeoma). J Cutan Pathol. 21(1):91–3. PMID:8188941
**150.** Barnhill RL (2006). The Spitzoid lesion: rethinking Spitz tumors, atypical variants, 'Spitzoid melanoma' and risk assessment. Mod Pathol. 19 Suppl 2:S21–33. PMID:16446713
**151.** Barnhill RL, Argenyi ZB, From L, Glass LF, Maize JC, Mihm MC Jr, et al. (1999). Atypical Spitz nevi/tumors: lack of consensus for diagnosis, discrimination from melanoma, and prediction of outcome. Hum Pathol. 30(5):513–20. PMID:10333219
**152.** Barnhill RL, Barnhill MA, Berwick M, Mihm MC Jr (1991). The histologic spectrum of pigmented spindle cell nevus: a review of 120 cases with emphasis on atypical variants. Hum Pathol. 22(1):52–8. PMID:1985078
**153.** Barnhill RL, Cerroni L, Cook M, Elder DE, Kerl H, LeBoit PE, et al. (2010). State of the art, nomenclature, and points of consensus and controversy concerning benign melanocytic lesions: outcome of an international workshop. Adv Anat Pathol. 17(2):73–90. PMID:20179431
**154.** Barnhill RL, Dickersin GR, Nickeleit V, Bhan AK, Muhlbauer JE, Phillips ME, et al. (1991). Studies on the cellular origin of neurothekeoma: clinical, light microscopic, immunohistochemical, and ultrastructural observations. J Am Acad Dermatol. 25(1 Pt 1):80–8. PMID:1880258
**155.** Barnhill RL, Flotte TJ, Fleischli M, Perez-Atayde A (1995). Cutaneous melanoma and atypical Spitz tumors in childhood. Cancer. 76(10):1833–45. PMID:8625056
**156.** Barnhill RL, Kiryu H, Sober AJ, Mihm MC Jr (1990). Frequency of dysplastic nevi among nevomelanocytic lesions submitted for histopathologic examination. Time trends over a 37-year period. Arch Dermatol. 126(4):463–5. PMID:2321991
**157.** Barnhill RL, Kutzner H, Schmidt B, Ali L, Bagot M, Janin A, et al. (2011). Atypical spitzoid melanocytic neoplasms with angiotropism: a potential mechanism of locoregional involvement. Am J Dermatopathol. 33(3):236–43. PMID:21389834
**158.** Barnhill RL, Mihm MC Jr (1990). Cellular neurothekeoma. A distinctive variant of neurothekeoma mimicking nevomelanocytic tumors. Am J Surg Pathol. 14(2):113–20. PMID:2154139
**159.** Barnhill RL, Mihm MC Jr, Magro CM (1991). Plexiform spindle cell naevus: a distinctive variant of plexiform melanocytic naevus. Histopathology. 18(3):243–7. PMID:2045075
**160.** Barón AE, Asdigian NL, Gonzalez V, Aalborg J, Terzian T, Stiegmann RA, et al. (2014). Interactions between ultraviolet light and MC1R and OCA2 variants are determinants of childhood nevus and freckle phenotypes. Cancer Epidemiol Biomarkers Prev. 23(12):2829–39. PMID:25410285
**161.** Barrado-Solis N, Moles-Poveda P, Roca-Estelles MJ, Quecedo-Estebanez E, Gimeno-Carpio E (2016). Melanocytic matricoma with melanocytic atypia: report of a new case. J Eur Acad Dermatol Venereol. 30(5):859–60. PMID:25678301
**162.** Barrett JH, Iles MM, Harland M, Taylor JC, Aitken JF, Andresen PA, et al. (2011). Genome-wide association study identifies three new melanoma susceptibility loci. Nat Genet. 43(11):1108–13. PMID:21983787
**163.** Barrionuevo C, Anderson VM, Zevallos-Giampietri E, Zaharia M, Misad O, Bravo F, et al. (2002). Hydroa-like cutaneous T-cell lymphoma: a clinicopathologic and molecular genetic study of 16 pediatric cases from Peru. Appl Immunohistochem Mol Morphol. 10(1):7–14. PMID:11893040
**164.** Bartuma H, Nord KH, Macchia G, Isaksson M, Nilsson J, Domanski HA, et al. (2011). Gene expression and single nucleotide polymorphism array analyses of spindle cell lipomas and conventional lipomas with 13q14 deletion. Genes Chromosomes Cancer. 50(8):619–32. PMID:21563233
**165.** Bartuma H, Panagopoulos I, Collin A, Trombetta D, Domanski HA, Mandahl N, et al. (2009). Expression levels of HMGA2 in adipocytic tumors correlate with morphologic and cytogenetic subgroups. Mol Cancer. 8:36. PMID:19508721
**166.** Bastiaens M, Hoefnagel J, Westendorp R, Vermeer BJ, Bouwes Bavinck JN (2004). Solar lentigines are strongly related to sun exposure in contrast to ephelides. Pigment Cell Res. 17(3):225–9. PMID:15140067
**167.** Bastiaens MT, Hoefnagel JJ, Bruijn JA, Westendorp RG, Vermeer BJ, Bouwes Bavinck JN (1998). Differences in age, site distribution, and sex between nodular and superficial basal cell carcinoma indicate different types of tumors. J Invest Dermatol. 110(6):880–4. PMID:9620293
**168.** Bastian BC (2014). The molecular pathology of melanoma: an integrated taxonomy of melanocytic neoplasia. Annu Rev Pathol. 9(1):239–71. PMID:24460190
**169.** Bastian BC, Kashani-Sabet M, Hamm H, Godfrey T, Moore DH 2nd, Bröcker EB, et al. (2000). Gene amplifications characterize acral melanoma and permit the detection of occult tumor cells in the surrounding skin. Cancer Res. 60(7):1968–73. PMID:10766187
**170.** Bastian BC, LeBoit PE, Pinkel D (2000). Mutations and copy number increase of HRAS in Spitz nevi with distinctive histopathological features. Am J Pathol. 157(3):967–72. PMID:10980135
**171.** Bastian BC, Olshen AB, LeBoit PE, Pinkel D (2003). Classifying melanocytic tumors based on DNA copy number changes. Am J Pathol. 163(5):1765–70. PMID:14578177
**172.** Bastian BC, Xiong J, Frieden IJ, Williams ML, Chou P, Busam K, et al. (2002). Genetic changes in neoplasms arising in congenital melanocytic nevi: differences between nodular proliferations and melanomas. Am J Pathol. 161(4):1163–9. PMID:12368190
**173.** Batista DA, Vonderheid EC, Hawkins A, Morsberger L, Long P, Murphy KM, et al. (2006). Multicolor fluorescence in situ hybridization (SKY) in mycosis fungoides and Sézary syndrome: search for recurrent chromosome abnormalities. Genes Chromosomes Cancer. 45(4):383–91. PMID:16382449
**174.** Batstone P, Forsyth L, Goodlad J (2001). Clonal chromosome aberrations secondary to chromosome instability in an elastofibroma. Cancer Genet Cytogenet. 128(1):46–7. PMID:11458949
**175.** Battistella M, Carlson JA, Osio A, Langbein L, Cribier B (2014). Skin tumors with matrical differentiation: lessons from hair keratins, beta-catenin and PHLDA-1 expression. J Cutan Pathol. 41(5):427–36. PMID:24673383
**176.** Battistella M, Fraitag S, Teillac DH, Brousse N, de Prost Y, Bodemer C (2010). Neonatal and early infantile cutaneous Langerhans cell histiocytosis: comparison of self-regressive and non-self-regressive forms. Arch Dermatol. 146(2):149–56. PMID:20157025
**177.** Battistella M, Van Eeckhout P, Cribier B (2011). Symplastic trichodiscoma: a spindle-cell predominant variant of trichodiscoma with pseudosarcomatous/ancient features. Am J Dermatopathol. 33(7):e81–3. PMID:21915028
**178.** Bauer BS, Kernahan DA, Hugo NE (1981). Lymphangioma circumscriptum–a clinicopathological review. Ann Plast Surg. 7(4):318–26. PMID:7316423
**179.** Bauer J, Bastian BC (2006). Distinguishing melanocytic nevi from melanoma by DNA copy number changes: comparative genomic hybridization as a research and diagnostic tool. Dermatol Ther. 19(1):40–9. PMID:16405569
**180.** Bauer J, Curtin JA, Pinkel D, Bastian BC (2007). Congenital melanocytic nevi frequently harbor NRAS mutations but no BRAF mutations. J Invest Dermatol. 127(1):179–82. PMID:16888631
**181.** Bax MJ, Johnson TM, Harms PW, Schwartz JL, Zhao L, Fullen DR, et al. (2016). Detection of occult invasion in melanoma in situ. JAMA Dermatol. 152(11):1201–8. PMID:27533878
**182.** Bayley JP, Launonen V, Tomlinson IP (2008). The FH mutation database: an online database of fumarate hydratase mutations involved in the MCUL (HLRCC) tumor syndrome and congenital fumarase deficiency. BMC Med Genet. 9:20. PMID:18366737
**183.** Abdel-Rahman MH, Pilarski R, Cebulla CM, Massengill JB, Christopher BN, Boru G, et al. (2011). Germline BAP1 mutation predisposes to uveal melanoma, lung adenocarcinoma, meningioma, and other cancers. J Med Genet. 48(12):856–9. PMID:21941004
**184.** Abdul-Wahab A, Tang SY, Robson A, Morris S, Agar N, Wain EM, et al. (2014). Chromosomal anomalies in primary cutaneous follicle center cell lymphoma do not portend a poor prognosis. J Am Acad Dermatol. 70(6):1010–20. PMID:24679486
**185.** Beadling C, Jacobson-Dunlop E, Hodi FS, Le C, Warrick A, Patterson J, et al. (2008). KIT gene mutations and copy number in melanoma subtypes. Clin Cancer Res. 14(21):6821–8. PMID:18980976
**186.** Beaty MW, Toro J, Sorbara L, Stern JB, Pittaluga S, Raffeld M, et al. (2001). Cutaneous lymphomatoid granulomatosis: correlation of clinical and biologic features. Am J Surg Pathol. 25(9):1111–20. PMID:11688570
**187.** Bechan GI, Egeler RM, Arceci RJ (2006). Biology of Langerhans cells and Langerhans cell histiocytosis. Int Rev Cytol. 254:1–43. PMID:17147996
**188.** Beckervordersandforth J, Pujari S, Rennspiess D, Speel EJ, Winnepenninckx V, Diaz C, et al. (2016). Frequent detection of human polyomavirus 6 in keratoacanthomas. Diagn Pathol. 11(1):58. PMID:27388771
**189.** Beer TW, Drury P, Heenan PJ (2010). Atypical fibroxanthoma: a histological and immunohistochemical review of 171 cases. Am J Dermatopathol. 32(6):533–40. PMID:20526171
**190.** Beert E, Brems H, Daniëls B, De Wever I, Van Calenbergh F, Schoenaers J, et al. (2011). Atypical neurofibromas in neurofibromatosis

type 1 are premalignant tumors. Genes Chromosomes Cancer. 50(12):1021–32. PMID:21987445
**191.** Behboudi A, Winnes M, Gorunova L, van den Oord JJ, Mertens F, Enlund F, et al. (2005). Clear cell hidradenoma of the skin-a third tumor type with a t(11;19)–associated TORC1-MAML2 gene fusion. Genes Chromosomes Cancer. 43(2):202–5. PMID:15729701
**192.** Behjati S, Tarpey PS, Sheldon H, Martincorena I, Van Loo P, Gundem G, et al. (2014). Recurrent PTPRB and PLCG1 mutations in angiosarcoma. Nat Genet. 46(4):376–9. PMID:24633157
**193.** Behne K, Robertson I, Weedon D (2002). Disseminated lobular capillary haemangioma. Australas J Dermatol. 43(4):297–300. PMID:12423439
**194.** Bekkenk MW, Geelen FA, van Voorst Vader PC, Heule F, Geerts ML, van Vloten WA, et al. (2000). Primary and secondary cutaneous CD30(+) lymphoproliferative disorders: a report from the Dutch Cutaneous Lymphoma Group on the long-term follow-up data of 219 patients and guidelines for diagnosis and treatment. Blood. 95(12):3653–61. PMID:10845893
**195.** Bekkenk MW, Kluin PM, Jansen PM, Meijer CJ, Willemze R (2001). Lymphomatoid papulosis with a natural killer-cell phenotype. Br J Dermatol. 145(2):318–22. PMID:11531801
**196.** Bekkenk MW, Vermeer MH, Jansen PM, van Marion AM, Canninga-van Dijk MR, Kluin PM, et al. (2003). Peripheral T-cell lymphomas unspecified presenting in the skin: analysis of prognostic factors in a group of 82 patients. Blood. 102(6):2213–9. PMID:12750155
**197.** Beljaards RC, Meijer CJ, Van der Putte SC, Hollema H, Geerts ML, Bezemer PD, et al. (1994). Primary cutaneous T-cell lymphoma: clinicopathological features and prognostic parameters of 35 cases other than mycosis fungoides and CD30-positive large cell lymphoma. J Pathol. 172(1):53–60. PMID:7931828
**198.** Bell D, Aung P, Prieto VG, Ivan D (2015). Next-generation sequencing reveals rare genomic alterations in aggressive digital papillary adenocarcinoma. Ann Diagn Pathol. 19(6):381–4. PMID:26386519
**199.** Belliveau MJ, Coupal DJ, Brownstein S, Jordan DR, Prokopetz R (2010). Infundibulocystic basal cell carcinoma of the eyelid in basal cell nevus syndrome. Ophthalmic Plast Reconstr Surg. 26(3):147–52. PMID:20489535
**200.** Bello DM, Chou JF, Panageas KS, Brady MS, Coit DG, Carvajal RD, et al. (2013). Prognosis of acral melanoma: a series of 281 patients. Ann Surg Oncol. 20(11):3618–25. PMID:23838913
**201.** Belousova IE, Nikonova SM, Sima R, Kazakov DV (2007). Granulomatous slack skin with clonal T-cell receptor-gamma gene rearrangement in skin and lymph node. Br J Dermatol. 157(2):405–7. PMID:17573870
**202.** Beltraminelli H, Leinweber B, Kerl H, Cerroni L (2009). Primary cutaneous CD4+ small-/medium-sized pleomorphic T-cell lymphoma: a cutaneous nodular proliferation of pleomorphic T lymphocytes of undetermined significance? A study of 136 cases. Am J Dermatopathol. 31(4):317–22. PMID:19461234
**203.** Beltraminelli H, Müllegger R, Cerroni L (2010). Indolent CD8+ lymphoid proliferation of the ear: a phenotypic variant of the small-medium pleomorphic cutaneous T-cell lymphoma? J Cutan Pathol. 37(1):81–4. PMID:19602068
**204.** Benati E, Ribero S, Longo C, Piana S, Puig S, Carrera C, et al. (2017). Clinical and dermoscopic clues to differentiate pigmented nail bands: an International Dermoscopy Society study. J Eur Acad Dermatol Venereol. 31(4):732–6. PMID:27696528
**205.** Bender RP, McGinniss MJ, Esmay P, Velazquez EF, Reimann JD (2013). Identification of HRAS mutations and absence of GNAQ or GNA11 mutations in deep penetrating nevi. Mod Pathol. 26(10):1320–8. PMID:23599145
**206.** Bénet C, Gomez A, Aguilar C, Delattre C, Vergier B, Beylot-Barry M, et al. (2011). Histologic and immunohistologic characterization of skin localization of myeloid disorders: a study of 173 cases. Am J Clin Pathol. 135(2):278–90. PMID:21228369
**207.** Benharroch D, Guterman G, Levy I, Shaco-Levy R (2010). High content of Langerhans cells in malignant lymphoma–incidence and significance. Virchows Arch. 457(1):63–7. PMID:20473767
**208.** Benner MF, Jansen PM, Meijer CJ, Willemze R (2009). Diagnostic and prognostic evaluation of phenotypic markers TRAF1, MUM1, BCL2 and CD15 in cutaneous CD30-positive lymphoproliferative disorders. Br J Dermatol. 161(1):121–7. PMID:19416236
**209.** Benner MF, Jansen PM, Vermeer MH, Willemze R (2012). Prognostic factors in transformed mycosis fungoides: a retrospective analysis of 100 cases. Blood. 119(7):1643–9. PMID:22160616
**210.** Benner MF, Willemze R (2009). Applicability and prognostic value of the new TNM classification system in 135 patients with primary cutaneous anaplastic large cell lymphoma. Arch Dermatol. 145(12):1399–404. PMID:20026848
**211.** Bennett AK, Mills SE, Wick MR (2003). Salivary-type neoplasms of the breast and lung. Semin Diagn Pathol. 20(4):279–304. PMID:14694981
**212.** Berenguer B, Mulliken JB, Enjolras O, Boon LM, Wassef M, Josset P, et al. (2003). Rapidly involuting congenital hemangioma: clinical and histopathologic features. Pediatr Dev Pathol. 6(6):495–510. PMID:15018449
**213.** Berhane T, Halliday GM, Cooke B, Barnetson RS (2002). Inflammation is associated with progression of actinic keratoses to squamous cell carcinomas in humans. Br J Dermatol. 146(5):810–5. PMID:12000377
**214.** Berman A (1977). Depigmented haloes associated with the involution of flag warts. Br J Dermatol. 97(3):263–5. PMID:921896
**215.** Berman A, Domnitz JM, Winkelmann RK (1982). Plantar warts recently turned black. Clinical and histopathologic findings. Arch Dermatol. 118(1):47–51. PMID:7059201
**216.** Bernal K, Nelson M, Neff JR, Nielsen SM, Bridge JA (2004). Translocation (2;11)(q31;q12) is recurrent in collagenous fibroma (desmoplastic fibroblastoma). Cancer Genet Cytogenet. 149(2):161–3. PMID:15036892
**217.** Bernardeau K, Serpier H, Salmon-Ehr V, Metz D, Pluot M, Kalis B (1998). Multiple isolated cutaneous myxomas. Ann Dermatol Venereol. 125(1):30–3. [French] PMID:9747204
**218.** Bernárdez C, Macías Del Toro E, Ramírez Bellver JL, Martinez Menchón T, Martinez Barba E, Molina-Ruiz AM, et al. (2016). Primary signet-ring cell/histiocytoid carcinoma of the eyelid: a "binocle" presentation of the "monocle tumor". Am J Dermatopathol. 38(8):623–7. PMID:27391452
**219.** Bernengo MG, Novelli M, Quaglino P, Lisa F, De Matteis A, Savoia P, et al. (2001). The relevance of the CD4+ CD26- subset in the identification of circulating Sézary cells. Br J Dermatol. 144(1):125–35. PMID:11167693
**220.** Bernstein EF, Resnik KS, Loose JH, Halcin C, Kauh YC (1993). Solitary congenital self-healing reticulohistiocytosis. Br J Dermatol. 129(4):449–54. PMID:8217762
**221.** Bernstein KE, Lattes R (1982). Nodular (pseudosarcomatous) fasciitis, a nonrecurrent lesion: clinicopathologic study of 134 cases. Cancer. 49(8):1668–78. PMID:6279273
**222.** Berres ML, Allen CE, Merad M (2013). Pathological consequence of misguided dendritic cell differentiation in histiocytic diseases. Adv Immunol. 120:127–61. PMID:24070383
**223.** Berres ML, Lim KP, Peters T, Price J, Takizawa H, Salmon H, et al. (2014). BRAF-V600E expression in precursor versus differentiated dendritic cells defines clinically distinct LCH risk groups. J Exp Med. 211(4):669–83. PMID:24638167
**224.** Bertherat J, Horvath A, Groussin L, Grabar S, Boikos S, Cazabat L, et al. (2009). Mutations in regulatory subunit type 1A of cyclic adenosine 5'-monophosphate-dependent protein kinase (PRKAR1A): phenotype analysis in 353 patients and 80 different genotypes. J Clin Endocrinol Metab. 94(6):2085–91. PMID:19293268
**225.** Berti E, Alessi E, Caputo R, Gianotti R, Delia D, Vezzoni P (1988). Reticulohistiocytoma of the dorsum. J Am Acad Dermatol. 19(2 Pt 1):259–72. PMID:3049688
**226.** Berti E, Cerri A, Cavicchini S, Delia D, Soligo D, Alessi E, et al. (1991). Primary cutaneous gamma/delta T-cell lymphoma presenting as disseminated pagetoid reticulosis. J Invest Dermatol. 96(5):718–23. PMID:1827136
**227.** Berti E, Gianotti R, Alessi E (1988). Unusual cutaneous histiocytosis expressing an intermediate immunophenotype between Langerhans' cells and dermal macrophages. Arch Dermatol. 124(8):1250–3. PMID:3401031
**228.** Berti E, Tomasini D, Vermeer MH, Meijer CJ, Alessi E, Willemze R (1999). Primary cutaneous CD8-positive epidermotropic cytotoxic T cell lymphomas. A distinct clinicopathological entity with an aggressive clinical behavior. Am J Pathol. 155(2):483–92. PMID:10433941
**229.** Alberti-Violetti S, Fanoni D, Provasi M, Corti L, Venegoni L, Berti E (2017). Primary cutaneous acral CD8 positive T-cell lymphoma with extra-cutaneous involvement: a long-standing case with an unexpected progression. J Cutan Pathol. 44(11):964–8. PMID:28796362
**230.** Alberti-Violetti S, Torres-Cabala CA, Talpur R, Corti L, Fanoni D, Venegoni L, et al. (2016). Clinicopathological and molecular study of primary cutaneous CD4+ small/medium-sized pleomorphic T-cell lymphoma. J Cutan Pathol. 43(12):1121–30. PMID:27550169
**231.** Abesamis-Cubillan E, El-Shabrawi-Caelen L, LeBoit PE (2000). Merkel cells and sclerosing epithelial neoplasms. Am J Dermatopathol. 22(4):311–5. PMID:10949455
**232.** Betti R, Alessi E (1996). Nodular trichoblastoma with adamantinoid features. Am J Dermatopathol. 18(2):192–5. PMID:8739995
**233.** Betti R, Inselvini E, Vergani R, Moneghini L, Crosti C (2001). Sebaceoma arising in association with seborrheic keratosis. Am J Dermatopathol. 23(1):58–61. PMID:11176054
**234.** Bettington A, Lai JK, Kennedy C (2011). Indeterminate dendritic cell tumour presenting in a patient with follicular lymphoma. Pathology. 43(4):372–5. PMID:21566494
**235.** Beuschlein F, Fassnacht M, Assié G, Calebiro D, Stratakis CA, Osswald A, et al. (2014). Constitutive activation of PKA catalytic subunit in adrenal Cushing's syndrome. N Engl J Med. 370(11):1019–28. PMID:24571724
**236.** Beutner KR, Becker TM, Stone KM (1991). Epidemiology of human papillomavirus infections. Dermatol Clin. 9(2):211–8. PMID:1647901
**237.** Bevona C, Goggins W, Quinn T, Fullerton J, Tsao H (2003). Cutaneous melanomas associated with nevi. Arch Dermatol. 139(12):1620–4. PMID:14676081
**238.** Bhaijee F, Brown AS (2014). Muir-Torre syndrome. Arch Pathol Lab Med. 138(12):1685–9. PMID:25427047
**239.** Bhaskar SN, Jacoway JR (1966). Pyogenic granuloma–clinical features, incidence, histology, and result of treatment: report of 242 cases. J Oral Surg. 24(5):391–8. PMID:5220911
**240.** Bhawan J (1979). Pilar sheath acanthoma. A new benign follicular tumor. J Cutan Pathol. 6(5):438–40. PMID:521535
**241.** Bice TC, Tran V, Merkley MA, Newlands SD, van der Sloot PG, Wu S, et al. (2015). Disease-specific survival with spindle cell carcinoma of the head and neck. Otolaryngol Head Neck Surg. 153(6):973–80. PMID:26203085
**242.** Biggs PJ, Wooster R, Ford D, Chapman P, Mangion J, Quirk Y, et al. (1995). Familial cylindromatosis (turban tumour syndrome) gene localised to chromosome 16q12-q13: evidence for its role as a tumour suppressor gene. Nat Genet. 11(4):441–3. PMID:7493027
**243.** Bignell GR, Warren W, Seal S, Takahashi M, Rapley E, Barfoot R, et al. (2000). Identification of the familial cylindromatosis tumour-suppressor gene. Nat Genet. 25(2):160–5. PMID:10835629
**244.** Bill AH Jr, Sumner DS (1965). A unified concept of lymphangioma and cystic hygroma. Surg Gynecol Obstet. 120:79–86. PMID:14259790
**245.** Billano RA, Little WP (1982). Hypertrophic actinic keratosis. J Am Acad Dermatol. 7(4):484–9. PMID:7142459
**246.** Billings SD, Folpe AL (2007). Diagnostically challenging spindle cell lipomas: a report of 34 "low-fat" and "fat-free" variants. Am J Dermatopathol. 29(5):437–42. PMID:17890910
**247.** Billings SD, Folpe AL, Weiss SW (2003). Epithelioid sarcoma-like hemangioendothelioma. Am J Surg Pathol. 27(1):48–57. PMID:12502927
**248.** Billings SD, McKenney JK, Folpe AL, Hardacre MC, Weiss SW (2004). Cutaneous angiosarcoma following breast-conserving surgery and radiation: an analysis of 27 cases. Am J Surg Pathol. 28(6):781–8. PMID:15166670
**249.** Bird CC, Willis RA (1969). The histogenesis of pigmented neurofibromas. J Pathol. 97(4):631–7. PMID:5354040
**250.** Birkby CS, Argenyi ZB, Whitaker DC (1989). Microcystic adnexal carcinoma with mandibular invasion and bone marrow replacement. J Dermatol Surg Oncol. 15(3):308–12. PMID:2466067
**251.** Bishop DT, Demenais F, Goldstein AM, Bergman W, Bishop JN, Bressac-de Paillerets B, et al. (2002). Geographical variation in the penetrance of CDKN2A mutations for melanoma. J Natl Cancer Inst. 94(12):894–903. PMID:12072543
**252.** Bishop DT, Demenais F, Iles MM, Harland M, Taylor JC, Corda E, et al. (2009). Genome-wide association study identifies three loci associated with melanoma risk. Nat Genet. 41(8):920–5. PMID:19578364
**253.** Bishop JA, Taube JM, Su A, Binder SW, Kazakov DV, Michal M, et al. (2017). Secretory carcinoma of the skin harboring ETV6 gene fusions: a cutaneous analogue to secretory carcinomas of the breast and salivary glands. Am J Surg Pathol. 41(1):62–6. PMID:27631515
**254.** Blake PW, Bradford PT, Devesa SS, Toro JR (2010). Cutaneous appendageal carcinoma incidence and survival patterns in the United States: a population-based study. Arch Dermatol. 146(6):625–32. PMID:20566926
**255.** Blatt K, Cerny-Reiterer S, Schwaab J, Sotlar K, Eisenwort G, Stefanzl G, et al. (2015). Identification of the Ki-1 antigen (CD30) as a novel therapeutic target in systemic mastocytosis. Blood. 126(26):2832–41. PMID:26486787
**256.** Blessing K, Evans AT, al-Nafussi A (1993). Verrucous naevoid and keratotic malignant melanoma: a clinico-pathological study of 20 cases. Histopathology. 23(5):453–8. PMID:8314219

**257.** Blessing K, Grant JJ, Sanders DS, Kennedy MM, Husain A, Coburn P (2000). Small cell malignant melanoma: a variant of naevoid melanoma. Clinicopathological features and histological differential diagnosis. J Clin Pathol. 53(8):591–5. PMID:11002761
**258.** Blessing K, McLaren KM, Benton EC, Barr BB, Bunney MH, Smith IW, et al. (1989). Histopathology of skin lesions in renal allograft recipients–an assessment of viral features and dysplasia. Histopathology. 14(2):129–39. PMID:2540085
**259.** Blum A, Hofmann-Wellenhof R, Marghoob AA, Argenziano G, Cabo H, Carrera C, et al. (2014). Recurrent melanocytic nevi and melanomas in dermoscopy: results of a multicenter study of the International Dermoscopy Society. JAMA Dermatol. 150(2):138–45. PMID:24226788
**260.** Blume-Peytavi U, Adler YD, Geilen CC, Ahmad W, Christiano A, Goerdt S, et al. (2000). Multiple familial cutaneous glomangioma: a pedigree of 4 generations and critical analysis of histologic and genetic differences of glomus tumors. J Am Acad Dermatol. 42(4):633–9. PMID:10727310
**261.** Boccara O, Blanche S, de Prost Y, Brousse N, Bodemer C, Fraitag S (2012). Cutaneous hematologic disorders in children. Pediatr Blood Cancer. 58(2):226–32. PMID:21445946
**262.** Boccara O, Laloum-Grynberg E, Jeudy G, Aubriot-Lorton MH, Vabres P, de Prost Y, et al. (2012). Cutaneous B-cell lymphoblastic lymphoma in children: a rare diagnosis. J Am Acad Dermatol. 66(1):51–7. PMID:21745698
**263.** Bodemer C, Hermine O, Palmérini F, Yang Y, Grandpeix-Guyodo C, Leventhal PS, et al. (2010). Pediatric mastocytosis is a clonal disease associated with D816V and other activating c-KIT mutations. J Invest Dermatol. 130(3):804–15. PMID:19865100
**264.** Bogle MA, Cohen PR, Tschen JA (2004). Trichofolliculoma with incidental focal acantholytic dyskeratosis. South Med J. 97(8):773–5. PMID:15352674
**265.** Boldrini P (1978). Is exogenous cholesterol a micro-nutrient? Physiol Chem Phys. 10(6):565–8. PMID:754196
**266.** Bonadonna P, Perbellini O, Passalacqua G, Caruso B, Colarossi S, Dal Fior D, et al. (2009). Clonal mast cell disorders in patients with systemic reactions to Hymenoptera stings and increased serum tryptase levels. J Allergy Clin Immunol. 123(3):680–6. PMID:19135713
**267.** Bondi R, Urso C (1996). Syringocystadenocarcinoma papilliferum. Histopathology. 28(5):475–7. PMID:8735727
**268.** Bonetti F, Knowles DM 2nd, Chilosi M, Pisa R, Fiaccavento S, Rizzuto N, et al. (1985). A distinctive cutaneous malignant neoplasm expressing the Langerhans cell phenotype. Synchronous occurrence with B-chronic lymphocytic leukemia. Cancer. 55(10):2417–25. PMID:3886125
**269.** Bonzheim I, Geissinger E, Roth S, Zettl A, Marx A, Rosenwald A, et al. (2004). Anaplastic large cell lymphomas lack the expression of T-cell receptor molecules or molecules of proximal T-cell receptor signaling. Blood. 104(10):3358–60. PMID:15297316
**270.** Boon LM, Enjolras O, Mulliken JB (1996). Congenital hemangioma: evidence of accelerated involution. J Pediatr. 128(3):329–35. PMID:8774499
**271.** Boonchai W, Walsh M, Cummings M, Chenevix-Trench G (2000). Expression of p53 in arsenic-related and sporadic basal cell carcinoma. Arch Dermatol. 136(2):195–8. PMID:10677095
**272.** Borden EC, Baker LH, Bell RS, Bramwell V, Demetri GD, Eisenberg BL, et al. (2003). Soft tissue sarcomas of adults: state of the translational science. Clin Cancer Res. 9(6):1941–56. PMID:12796356
**273.** Albores-Saavedra J, Batich K, Chable-Montero F, Sagy N, Schwartz AM, Henson DE (2010). Merkel cell carcinoma demographics, morphology, and survival based on 3870 cases: a population based study. J Cutan Pathol. 37(1):20–7. PMID:19638070
**274.** Albores-Saavedra J, Schwartz AM, Henson DE, Kostun L, Hart A, Angeles-Albores D, et al. (2011). Cutaneous angiosarcoma. Analysis of 434 cases from the Surveillance, Epidemiology, and End Results Program, 1973-2007. Ann Diagn Pathol. 15(2):93–7. PMID:21190880
**275.** Bos GD, Pritchard DJ, Reiman HM, Dobyns JH, Ilstrup DM, Landon GC (1988). Epithelioid sarcoma. An analysis of fifty-one cases. J Bone Joint Surg Am. 70(6):862–70. PMID:3392084
**276.** Bosisio F, Boi S, Caputo V, Chiarelli C, Oliver F, Ricci R, et al. (2015). Lobular panniculitic infiltrates with overlapping histopathologic features of lupus panniculitis (lupus profundus) and subcutaneous T-cell lymphoma: a conceptual and practical dilemma. Am J Surg Pathol. 39(2):206–11. PMID:25118815
**277.** Bossert T, Walther T, Vondrys D, Gummert JF, Kostelka M, Mohr FW (2006). Cardiac fibroma as an inherited manifestation of nevoid basal-cell carcinoma syndrome. Tex Heart Inst J. 33(1):88–90. PMID:16572881
**278.** Botros N, Cerroni L, Shawwa A, Green PJ, Greer W, Pasternak S, et al. (2015). Cutaneous manifestations of angioimmunoblastic T-cell lymphoma: clinical and pathological characteristics. Am J Dermatopathol. 37(4):274–83. PMID:25794369
**279.** Botton T, Yeh I, Nelson T, Vemula SS, Sparatta A, Garrido MC, et al. (2013). Recurrent BRAF kinase fusions in melanocytic tumors offer an opportunity for targeted therapy. Pigment Cell Melanoma Res. 26(6):845–51. PMID:23890088
**280.** Boulland ML, Wechsler J, Bagot M, Pulford K, Kanavaros P, Gaulard P (2000). Primary CD30-positive cutaneous T-cell lymphomas and lymphomatoid papulosis frequently express cytotoxic proteins. Histopathology. 36(2):136–44. PMID:10672058
**281.** Bourgeois JM, Knezevich SR, Mathers JA, Sorensen PH (2000). Molecular detection of the ETV6-NTRK3 gene fusion differentiates congenital fibrosarcoma from other childhood spindle cell tumors. Am J Surg Pathol. 24(7):937–46. PMID:10895816
**282.** Bourlond F, Velter C, Cribier B (2016). Clinicopathological study of 47 cases of sebaceoma. Ann Dermatol Venereol. 143(12):814–24. PMID:27836252
**283.** Bowen AR, LeBoit PE (2005). Fibroepithelioma of Pinkus is a fenestrated trichoblastoma. Am J Dermatopathol. 27(2):149–54. PMID:15798442
**284.** Bowen S, Gill M, Lee DA, Fisher G, Geronemus RG, Vazquez ME, et al. (2005). Mutations in the CYLD gene in Brooke-Spiegler syndrome, familial cylindromatosis, and multiple familial trichoepithelioma: lack of genotype-phenotype correlation. J Invest Dermatol. 124(5):919–20. PMID:15854031
**285.** Bowne WB, Antonescu CR, Leung DH, Katz SC, Hawkins WG, Woodruff JM, et al. (2000). Dermatofibrosarcoma protuberans: a clinicopathologic analysis of patients treated and followed at a single institution. Cancer. 88(12):2711–20. PMID:10870053
**286.** Boyd AS, Rapini RP (1994). Acral melanocytic neoplasms: a histologic analysis of 158 lesions. J Am Acad Dermatol. 31(5 Pt 1):740–5. PMID:7929919
**287.** Boye E, Yu Y, Paranya G, Mulliken JB, Olsen BR, Bischoff J (2001). Clonality and altered behavior of endothelial cells from hemangiomas. J Clin Invest. 107(6):745–52. PMID:11254674
**288.** Bozan A, Gode S, Kaya I, Yaman B, Uslu M, Akyildiz S, et al. (2015). Long-term follow-up of positive surgical margins in basal cell carcinoma of the face. Dermatol Surg. 41(7):761–7. PMID:26050215
**289.** Bradford PT, Goldstein AM, McMaster ML, Tucker MA (2009). Acral lentiginous melanoma: incidence and survival patterns in the United States, 1986-2005. Arch Dermatol. 145(4):427–34. PMID:19380664
**290.** Bradford PT, Goldstein AM, Tamura D, Khan SG, Ueda T, Boyle J, et al. (2011). Cancer and neurologic degeneration in xeroderma pigmentosum: long term follow-up characterises the role of DNA repair. J Med Genet. 48(3):168–76. PMID:21097776
**291.** Brandt SM, Swistel AJ, Rosen PP (2009). Secretory carcinoma in the axilla: probable origin from axillary skin appendage glands in a young girl. Am J Surg Pathol. 33(6):950–3. PMID:19342945
**292.** Brankov N, Prodanovic EM, Hurley MY (2016). Pigmented basal cell carcinoma: increased melanin or increased melanocytes? J Cutan Pathol. 43(12):1139–42. PMID:27612950
**293.** Bratthauer GL, Lininger RA, Man YG, Tavassoli FA (2002). Androgen and estrogen receptor mRNA status in apocrine carcinomas. Diagn Mol Pathol. 11(2):113–8. PMID:12045715
**294.** Braun RP, Baran R, Le Gal FA, Dalle S, Ronger S, Pandolfi R, et al. (2007). Diagnosis and management of nail pigmentations. J Am Acad Dermatol. 56(5):835–47. PMID:17320240
**295.** Bravo Puccio F, Chian C (2011). Acral junctional nevus versus acral lentiginous melanoma in situ: a differential diagnosis that should be based on clinicopathologic correlation. Arch Pathol Lab Med. 135(7):847–52. PMID:21732773
**296.** Brazzelli V, Larizza D, Martinetti M, Martinoli S, Calcaterra V, De Silvestri A, et al. (2004). Halo nevus, rather than vitiligo, is a typical dermatologic finding of Turner 's syndrome: clinical, genetic, and immunogenetic study in 72 patients. J Am Acad Dermatol. 51(3):354–8. PMID:15337976
**297.** Bree AF, Shah MR (2011). Consensus statement from the first international colloquium on basal cell nevus syndrome (BCNS). Am J Med Genet A. 155A(9):2091–7. PMID:21834049
**298.** Breiting L, Christensen L, Dahlstrøm K, Breiting V, Winther JF (2008). Primary mucinous carcinoma of the skin: a population-based study. Int J Dermatol. 47(3):242–5. PMID:18289323
**299.** Breiting L, Dahlstrøm K, Christensen L, Winther JF, Breiting V (2007). Primary mucinous carcinoma of the skin. Am J Dermatopathol. 29(6):595–6. PMID:18032965
**300.** Bremnes RM, Kvamme JM, Stalsberg H, Jacobsen EA (1999). Pilomatrix carcinoma with multiple metastases: report of a case and review of the literature. Eur J Cancer. 35(3):433–7. PMID:10448295
**301.** Brems H, Legius E, Stewart DR (2012). Molecular basis of glomus tumours. In: Upadhyaya M, Cooper DN, editors. Neurofibromatosis type 1: molecular and cellular biology. Berlin: Springer-Verlag; pp. 367–79.
**302.** Brems H, Park C, Maertens O, Pemov A, Messiaen L, Upadhyaya M, et al. (2009). Glomus tumors in neurofibromatosis type 1: genetic, functional, and clinical evidence of a novel association. Cancer Res. 69(18):7393–401. PMID:19738042
**303.** Brenn T (2012). Pitfalls in the evaluation of melanocytic lesions. Histopathology. 60(5):690–705. PMID:22176022
**304.** Brenn T, Calonje E, Granter SR, Leonard N, Grayson W, Fletcher CD, et al. (2002). Cutaneous Rosai-Dorfman disease is a distinct clinical entity. Am J Dermatopathol. 24(5):385–91. PMID:12357197
**305.** Brenn T, Fletcher CD (2004). Cutaneous epithelioid angiomatous nodule: a distinct lesion in the morphologic spectrum of epithelioid vascular tumors. Am J Dermatopathol. 26(1):14–21. PMID:14726818
**306.** Brenn T, Fletcher CD (2005). Radiation-associated cutaneous atypical vascular lesions and angiosarcoma: clinicopathologic analysis of 42 cases. Am J Surg Pathol. 29(8):983–96. PMID:16006792
**307.** Brenn T, Fletcher CD (2006). Postradiation vascular proliferations: an increasing problem. Histopathology. 48(1):106–14. PMID:16359542
**308.** Brennan MF, Antonescu CR, Moraco N, Singer S (2014). Lessons learned from the study of 10,000 patients with soft tissue sarcoma. Ann Surg. 260(3):416–2. PMID:25115417
**309.** Brenner I, Roth S, Flossbach L, Wobser M, Rosenwald A, Geissinger E (2015). Lack of myeloid differentiation primary response protein MyD88 L265P mutation in primary cutaneous marginal zone lymphoma. Br J Dermatol. 173(6):1527–8. PMID:26099629
**310.** Brenner I, Roth S, Puppe B, Wobser M, Rosenwald A, Geissinger E (2013). Primary cutaneous marginal zone lymphomas with plasmacytic differentiation show frequent IgG4 expression. Mod Pathol. 26(12):1568–76. PMID:23765244
**311.** Breza TS Jr, Zheng P, Porcu P, Magro CM (2006). Cutaneous marginal zone B-cell lymphoma in the setting of fluoxetine therapy: a hypothesis regarding pathogenesis based on in vitro suppression of T-cell-proliferative response. J Cutan Pathol. 33(7):522–8. PMID:16872479
**311A.** Brierly JD, Gospodarowicz MK, Wittekind C, editors (2017). TNM classification of malignant tumours. 8th ed. Oxford: Wiley Blackwell.
**312.** Briganti A, Salonia A, Deho F, Zanni G, Rokkas K, Rigatti P, et al. (2003). Peyronie's disease: a review. Curr Opin Urol. 13(5):417–22. PMID:12917519
**313.** Brock JE, Perez-Atayde AR, Kozakewich HP, Richkind KE, Fletcher JA, Vargas SO (2005). Cytogenetic aberrations in perineurioma: variation with subtype. Am J Surg Pathol. 29(9):1164–9. PMID:16096405
**314.** Brockow K, Jofer C, Behrendt H, Ring J (2008). Anaphylaxis in patients with mastocytosis: a study on history, clinical features and risk factors in 120 patients. Allergy. 63(2):226–32. PMID:18186813
**315.** Broekaert SM, Flux K, Kyrpychova L, Kacerovska D, Ivan D, Schön MP, et al. (2017). Squared-off nuclei and "appliqué" pattern as a histopathological clue to periocular sebaceous carcinoma: a clinicopathological study of 50 neoplasms from 46 patients. Am J Dermatopathol. 39(4):275–8. PMID:28323778
**316.** Broesby-Olsen S, Farkas DK, Vestergaard H, Hermann AP, Møller MB, Mortz CG, et al. (2016). Risk of solid cancer, cardiovascular disease, anaphylaxis, osteoporosis and fractures in patients with systemic mastocytosis: a nationwide population-based study. Am J Hematol. 91(11):1069–75. PMID:27428296
**317.** Brooks BP, Thompson AH, Bishop RJ, Clayton JA, Chan CC, Tsilou ET, et al. (2013). Ocular manifestations of xeroderma pigmentosum: long-term follow-up highlights the role of DNA repair in protection from sun damage. Ophthalmology. 120(7):1324–36. PMID:23601806
**318.** Brossard M, Fang S, Vaysse A, Wei Q, Chen WV, Mohamdi H, et al. (2015). Integrated

pathway and epistasis analysis reveals interactive effect of genetic variants at TERF1 and AFAP1L2 loci on melanoma risk. Int J Cancer. 137(8):1901–9. PMID:25892537
**319.** Brown KM, Macgregor S, Montgomery GW, Craig DW, Zhao ZZ, Iyadurai K, et al. (2008). Common sequence variants on 20q11.22 confer melanoma susceptibility. Nat Genet. 40(7):838–40. PMID:18488026
**320.** Brown NA, Furtado LV, Betz BL, Kiel MJ, Weigelin HC, Lim MS, et al. (2014). High prevalence of somatic MAP2K1 mutations in BRAF V600E-negative Langerhans cell histiocytosis. Blood. 124(10):1655–8. PMID:24982505
**321.** Brown RA, Kwong BY, McCalmont TH, Ragsdale B, Ma L, Cheung C, et al. (2015). ETV3-NCOA2 in indeterminate cell histiocytosis: clonal translocation supports sui generis. Blood. 126(20):2344–5. PMID:26438513
**322.** Brownstein MH (1988). Acantholytic acanthoma. J Am Acad Dermatol. 19(5 Pt 1):783–6. PMID:2461398
**323.** Brownstein MH, Mehregan AH, Bikowski JB, Lupulescu A, Patterson JC (1979). The dermatopathology of Cowden's syndrome. Br J Dermatol. 100(6):667–73. PMID:465314
**324.** Brownstein MH, Shapiro L (1973). Trichilemmoma. Analysis of 40 new cases. Arch Dermatol. 107(6):866–9. PMID:4711118
**325.** Brownstein MH, Wolf M, Bikowski JB (1978). Cowden's disease: a cutaneous marker of breast cancer. Cancer. 41(6):2393–8. PMID:657103
**326.** Brunet V, Marouan S, Routy JP, Hashem MA, Bernier V, Simard R, et al. (2017). Retrospective study of intravascular large B-cell lymphoma cases diagnosed in Quebec: a retrospective study of 29 case reports. Medicine (Baltimore). 96(5):e5985. PMID:28151891
**327.** Buccheri V, Mihaljević B, Matutes E, Dyer MJ, Mason DY, Catovsky D (1993). mb-1: a new marker for B-lineage lymphoblastic leukemia. Blood. 82(3):853–7. PMID:8338949
**328.** Buell JF, Trofe J, Hanaway MJ, Beebe TM, Gross TG, Alloway RR, et al. (2002). Immunosuppression and Merkel cell cancer. Transplant Proc. 34(5):1780–1. PMID:12176573
**329.** Buelow B, Cohen J, Nagymanyoki Z, Frizzell N, Joseph NM, McCalmont T, et al. (2016). Immunohistochemistry for 2-succinocysteine (2SC) and fumarate hydratase (FH) in cutaneous leiomyomas may aid in identification of patients with HLRCC (hereditary leiomyomatosis and renal cell carcinoma syndrome). Am J Surg Pathol. 40(7):982–8. PMID:26945337
**330.** Bugatti L, Filosa G (2007). Dermoscopy of lichen planus-like keratosis: a model of inflammatory regression. J Eur Acad Dermatol Venereol. 21(10):1392–7. PMID:17958847
**331.** Bunn B, van Heerden W (2015). EBV-positive mucocutaneous ulcer of the oral cavity associated with HIV/AIDS. Oral Surg Oral Med Oral Pathol Oral Radiol. 120(6):725–32. PMID:26254983
**332.** Burg G, Kempf W, Cozzio A, Feit J, Willemze R, S Jaffe E, et al. (2005). WHO/EORTC classification of cutaneous lymphomas 2005: histological and molecular aspects. J Cutan Pathol. 32(10):647–74. PMID:16293178
**333.** Burg G, Kempf W, Kazakov DV, Dummer R, Frosch PJ, Lange-Ionescu S, et al. (2003). Pyogenic lymphoma of the skin: a peculiar variant of primary cutaneous neutrophil-rich CD30+ anaplastic large-cell lymphoma. Clinicopathological study of four cases and review of the literature. Br J Dermatol. 148(3):580–6. PMID:12653754
**334.** Burgdorf WH, Pitha J, Fahmy A (1986). Muir-Torre syndrome. Histologic spectrum of sebaceous proliferations. Am J Dermatopathol. 8(3):202–8. PMID:3728878
**335.** Burgdorf WH, Zelger B (2004). JXG, NF1, and JMML: alphabet soup or a clinical issue? Pediatr Dermatol. 21(2):174–6. PMID:15078363
**336.** Burger RA, Marcuse PM (1954). Fibroadenoma of vulva. Am J Clin Pathol. 24(8):965–80. PMID:13197326
**337.** Burke FD, Proud G, Lawson IJ, McGeoch KL, Miles JN (2007). An assessment of the effects of exposure to vibration, smoking, alcohol and diabetes on the prevalence of Dupuytren's disease in 97,537 miners. J Hand Surg Eur Vol. 32(4):400–6. PMID:17950195
**338.** Burkhardt A (1986). Verrucous carcinoma and carcinoma cuniculatum–forms of squamous cell carcinoma? Hautarzt. 37(7):373–83. [German] PMID:3744823
**339.** Burrows NP, Jones RR, Smith NP (1992). The clinicopathological features of familial cylindromas and trichoepitheliomas (Brooke-Spiegler syndrome): a report of two families. Clin Exp Dermatol. 17(5):332–6. PMID:1333921
**340.** Busam KJ (1999). Metastatic melanoma to the skin simulating blue nevus. Am J Surg Pathol. 23(3):276–82. PMID:10078917
**341.** Busam KJ (2005). Cutaneous desmoplastic melanoma. Adv Anat Pathol. 12(2):92–102. PMID:15731577
**342.** Busam KJ, Barnhill RL (1995). Pagetoid Spitz nevus. Intraepidermal Spitz tumor with prominent pagetoid spread. Am J Surg Pathol. 19(9):1061–7. PMID:7661280
**343.** Busam KJ, Jungbluth AA, Rekthman N, Coit D, Pulitzer M, Bini J, et al. (2009). Merkel cell polyomavirus expression in Merkel cell carcinomas and its absence in combined tumors and pulmonary neuroendocrine carcinomas. Am J Surg Pathol. 33(9):1378–85. PMID:19609205
**344.** Busam KJ, Mujumdar U, Hummer AJ, Nobrega J, Hawkins WG, Coit DG, et al. (2004). Cutaneous desmoplastic melanoma: reappraisal of morphologic heterogeneity and prognostic factors. Am J Surg Pathol. 28(11):1518–25. PMID:15489657
**345.** Busam KJ, Shah KN, Gerami P, Sitzman T, Jungbluth AA, Kinsler V (2017). Reduced H3K27me3 expression is common in nodular melanomas of childhood associated with congenital melanocytic nevi but not in proliferative nodules. Am J Surg Pathol. 41(3):396–404. PMID:27849631
**346.** Busam KJ, Sung J, Wiesner T, von Deimling A, Jungbluth A (2013). Combined BRAF(V600E)-positive melanocytic lesions with large epithelioid cells lacking BAP1 expression and conventional nevomelanocytes. Am J Surg Pathol. 37(2):193–9. PMID:23026932
**347.** Busam KJ, Wanna M, Wiesner T (2013). Multiple epithelioid Spitz nevi or tumors with loss of BAP1 expression: a clue to a hereditary tumor syndrome. JAMA Dermatol. 149(3):335–9. PMID:23552620
**348.** Busco S, Buzzoni C, Mallone S, Trama A, Castaing M, Bella F, et al. (2016). Italian cancer figures–Report 2015: the burden of rare cancers in Italy. Epidemiol Prev. 40(1 Suppl 2):1–120. PMID:26951748
**349.** Butsch F, Kind P, Bräuninger W (2012). Bilateral indolent epidermotropic CD8-positive lymphoid proliferations of the ear. J Dtsch Dermatol Ges. 10(3):195–6. PMID:22142195
**350.** Büttner C, Grabbe J, Haas N, Sepp NT, Kunkel G, Henz BM (1999). Comparison of genetic and immunohistochemical findings in childhood and adult onset urticaria pigmentosa. Int Arch Allergy Immunol. 118(2–4):206–7. PMID:10224380
**351.** Caccetta TP, Dessauvagie B, McCallum D, Kumarasinghe SP (2012). Multiple minute digitate hyperkeratosis: a proposed algorithm for the digitate keratoses. J Am Acad Dermatol. 67(1):e49–55. PMID:21050621
**352.** Calduch L, Ortega C, Navarro V, Martínez E, Molina I, Jordá E (2000). Verrucous hemangioma: report of two cases and review of the literature. Pediatr Dermatol. 17(3):213–7. PMID:10886755
**353.** Callister MD, Ballo MT, Pisters PW, Patel SR, Feig BW, Pollock RE, et al. (2001). Epithelioid sarcoma: results of conservative surgery and radiotherapy. Int J Radiat Oncol Biol Phys. 51(2):384–91. PMID:11567812
**354.** Calonje E, Fletcher CD (1991). Sinusoidal hemangioma. A distinctive benign vascular neoplasm within the group of cavernous hemangiomas. Am J Surg Pathol. 15(12):1130–5. PMID:1746680
**355.** Calonje E, Fletcher CD, Wilson-Jones E, Rosai J (1994). Retiform hemangioendothelioma. A distinctive form of low-grade angiosarcoma delineated in a series of 15 cases. Am J Surg Pathol. 18(2):115–25. PMID:8291650
**356.** Calonje E, Guerin D, McCormick D, Fletcher CD (1999). Superficial angiomyxoma: clinicopathologic analysis of a series of distinctive but poorly recognized cutaneous tumors with tendency for recurrence. Am J Surg Pathol. 23(8):910–7. PMID:10435560
**357.** Calonje E, Mentzel T, Fletcher CD (1994). Cellular benign fibrous histiocytoma. Clinicopathologic analysis of 74 cases of a distinctive variant of cutaneous fibrous histiocytoma with frequent recurrence. Am J Surg Pathol. 18(7):668–76. PMID:8017561
**358.** Calonje E, Mentzel T, Fletcher CD (1995). Pseudomalignant perineurial invasion in cellular ('infantile') capillary haemangiomas. Histopathology. 26(2):159–64. PMID:7737662
**359.** Calvete O, Martinez P, Garcia-Pavia P, Benitez-Buelga C, Paumard-Hernández B, Fernandez V, et al. (2015). A mutation in the POT1 gene is responsible for cardiac angiosarcoma in TP53-negative Li-Fraumeni-like families. Nat Commun. 6:8383. PMID:26403419
**360.** Cameselle-Teijeiro J, Alfonsín-Barreiro N, Allegue F, Caeiro M (1997). Apocrine carcinoma with signet ring cells and histiocytoid features. A potentially confusing axillary tumor. Pathol Res Pract. 193(10):713–22. PMID:9505264
**361.** Campbell JJ, Clark RA, Watanabe R, Kupper TS (2010). Sezary syndrome and mycosis fungoides arise from distinct T-cell subsets: a biologic rationale for their distinct clinical behaviors. Blood. 116(5):767–71. PMID:20484084
**362.** Campochiaro C, Tomelleri A, Cavalli G, Berti A, Dagna L (2015). Erdheim-Chester disease. Eur J Intern Med. 26(4):223–9. PMID:25865950
**363.** Campos-do-Carmo G, Ramos-e-Silva M (2008). Dermoscopy: basic concepts. Int J Dermatol. 47(7):712–9. PMID:18613881
**364.** Canales-Ibarra C, Magariños G, Olsoff-Pagovich P, Ortiz-Hidalgo C (2003). Cutaneous sclerosing perineurioma of the digits: an uncommon soft-tissue neoplasm. Report of two cases with immunohistochemical analysis. J Cutan Pathol. 30(9):577–81. PMID:14507408
**365.** Candiago E, Marocolo D, Manganoni MA, Leali C, Facchetti F (2000). Nonlymphoid intraepidermal mononuclear cell collections (pseudo-Pautrier abscesses): a morphologic and immunophenotypical characterization. Am J Dermatopathol. 22(1):1–6. PMID:10698208
**366.** Cao Q, Li Y, Lin H, Ke Z, Liu Y, Ye Z (2013). Mantle cell lymphoma of blastoid variant with skin lesion and rapid progression: a case report and literature review. Am J Dermatopathol. 35(8):851–5. PMID:23928453
**367.** Capelle LG, Van Grieken NC, Lingsma HF, Steyerberg EW, Klokman WJ, Bruno MJ, et al. (2010). Risk and epidemiological time trends of gastric cancer in Lynch syndrome carriers in the Netherlands. Gastroenterology. 138(2):487–92. PMID:19900449
**368.** Cappellesso R, Bellan A, Saraggi D, Salmaso R, Ventura L, Fassina A (2015). YAP immunoreactivity is directly related to pilomatrixoma size and proliferation rate. Arch Dermatol Res. 307(4):379–83. PMID:25516090
**369.** Caprini E, Cristofoletti C, Arcelli D, Fadda P, Citterich MH, Sampogna F, et al. (2009). Identification of key regions and genes important in the pathogenesis of Sezary syndrome by combining genomic and expression microarrays. Cancer Res. 69(21):8438–46. PMID:19843862
**370.** Caputo R (1998). Juvenile xanthogranuloma. In: A text atlas of histiocytic syndromes: a dermatological perspective. London: CRC Press; pp. 39–58.
**371.** Caputo R, Alessi E, Berti E (1981). Collagen phagocytosis in multicentric reticulohistiocytosis. J Invest Dermatol. 76(5):342–6. PMID:7229425
**372.** Caputo R, Grimalt R (1992). Solitary reticulohistiocytosis (reticulohistiocytoma) of the skin in children: report of two cases. Arch Dermatol. 128(5):698–9. PMID:1575538
**373.** Caputo R, Grimalt R, Gelmetti C, Cottoni F (1993). Unusual aspects of juvenile xanthogranuloma. J Am Acad Dermatol. 29(5 Pt 2):868–70. PMID:8408830
**374.** Carbone M, Ferris LK, Baumann F, Napolitano A, Lum CA, Flores EG, et al. (2012). BAP1 cancer syndrome: malignant mesothelioma, uveal and cutaneous melanoma, and MBAITs. J Transl Med. 10:179. PMID:22935333
**375.** Cardoso JC, Calonje E (2011). Cutaneous manifestations of human papillomaviruses: a review. Acta Dermatovenerol Alp Pannonica Adriat. 20(3):145–54. PMID:22131115
**376.** Cardoso JC, Calonje E (2015). Malignant sweat gland tumours: an update. Histopathology. 67(5):589–606. PMID:26114606
**377.** Cardot-Leccia N, Italiano A, Monteil MC, Basc E, Perrin C, Pedeutour F (2007). Naevus lipomatosus superficialis: a case report with a 2p24 deletion. Br J Dermatol. 156(2):380–1. PMID:17223884
**378.** Carinci F, Piattelli A, Rubini C, Fioroni M, Stabellini G, Palmieri A, et al. (2004). Genetic profiling of granular cell myoblastoma. J Craniofac Surg. 15(5):824–34. PMID:15346026
**379.** Carli P, Massi D, Santucci M, Biggeri A, Giannotti B (1999). Cutaneous melanoma histologically associated with a nevus and melanoma de novo have a different profile of risk: results from a case-control study. J Am Acad Dermatol. 40(4):549–57. PMID:10188672
**380.** Carlson JA, Healy K, Slominski A, Mihm MC Jr (1999). Melanocytic matricoma: a report of two cases of a new entity. Am J Dermatopathol. 21(4):344–9. PMID:10446775
**381.** Carlson JA, Mu XC, Slominski A, Weismann K, Crowson AN, Malfetano J, et al. (2002). Melanocytic proliferations associated with lichen sclerosus. Arch Dermatol. 138(1):77–87. PMID:11790170
**382.** Carlson KC, Gibson LE (1991). Cutaneous signs of lymphomatoid granulomatosis. Arch Dermatol. 127(11):1693–8. PMID:1952975
**383.** Carney JA (1995). Carney complex: the complex of myxomas, spotty pigmentation, endocrine overactivity, and schwannomas. Semin Dermatol. 14(2):90–8. PMID:7640202
**384.** Carney JA, Ferreiro JA (1996). The epithelioid blue nevus. A multicentric familial tumor with important associations, including cardiac myxoma and psammomatous melanotic schwannoma. Am J Surg Pathol. 20(3):259–72. PMID:8772778
**385.** Carney JA, Headington JT, Su WP (1986). Cutaneous myxomas. A major component of the complex of myxomas, spotty pigmentation,

and endocrine overactivity. Arch Dermatol. 122(7):790–8. PMID:3729510
**386.** Carr J, Mackie RM (1994). Point mutations in the N-ras oncogene in malignant melanoma and congenital naevi. Br J Dermatol. 131(1):72–7. PMID:8043423
**387.** Carranza-Romero C, Molina-Ruiz AM, Perna Monroy C, Cuevas Santos J, Requena L (2015). Cutaneous epithelioid hemangioendothelioma on the sole of a child. Pediatr Dermatol. 32(3):e64–9. PMID:25782038
**388.** Cartault F, Nava C, Malbrunot AC, Munier P, Hebert JC, N'guyen P, et al. (2011). A new XPC gene splicing mutation has lead to the highest worldwide prevalence of xeroderma pigmentosum in black Mahori patients. DNA Repair (Amst). 10(6):577–85. PMID:21482201
**389.** Carter CS, Skala SL, Chinnaiyan AM, McHugh JB, Siddiqui J, Cao X, et al. (2017). Immunohistochemical characterization of fumarate hydratase (FH) and succinate dehydrogenase (SDH) in cutaneous leiomyomas for detection of familial cancer syndromes. Am J Surg Pathol. 41(6):801–9. PMID:28288038
**390.** Carter JE, Mizell KN, Tucker JA (2008). Mammary-type fibroepithelial neoplasms of the vulva: a case report and review of the literature. J Cutan Pathol. 35(2):246–9. PMID:18190454
**391.** Carter JM, O'Hara C, Dundas G, Gilchrist D, Collins MS, Eaton K, et al. (2012). Epithelioid malignant peripheral nerve sheath tumor arising in a schwannoma, in a patient with "neuroblastoma-like" schwannomatosis and a novel germline SMARCB1 mutation. Am J Surg Pathol. 36(1):154–60. PMID:22082606
**392.** Carter JM, Wang X, Dong J, Westendorf J, Chou MM, Oliveira AM (2016). USP6 genetic rearrangements in cellular fibroma of tendon sheath. Mod Pathol. 29(8):865–9. PMID:27125357
**393.** Carter JM, Weiss SW, Linos K, DiCaudo DJ, Folpe AL (2014). Superficial CD34-positive fibroblastic tumor: report of 18 cases of a distinctive low-grade mesenchymal neoplasm of intermediate (borderline) malignancy. Mod Pathol. 27(2):294–302. PMID:23887307
**394.** Carter RL, al-Sams SZ, Corbett RP, Clinton S (1990). A comparative study of immunohistochemical staining for neuron-specific enolase, protein gene product 9.5 and S-100 protein in neuroblastoma, Ewing's sarcoma and other round cell tumours in children. Histopathology. 16(5):461–7. PMID:2163356
**395.** Casanova M, Ferrari A, Collini P, Bisogno G, Alaggio R, Cecchetto G, et al. (2006). Epithelioid sarcoma in children and adolescents: a report from the Italian Soft Tissue Sarcoma Committee. Cancer. 106(3):708–17. PMID:16353216
**396.** Cash T, McIlvaine E, Krailo MD, Lessnick SL, Lawlor ER, Laack N, et al. (2016). Comparison of clinical features and outcomes in patients with extraskeletal versus skeletal localized Ewing sarcoma: a report from the Children's Oncology Group. Pediatr Blood Cancer. 63(10):1771–9. PMID:27297500
**397.** Cassarino DS, Cabral ES, Kartha RV, Swetter SM (2008). Primary dermal melanoma: distinct immunohistochemical findings and clinical outcome compared with nodular and metastatic melanoma. Arch Dermatol. 144(1):49–56. PMID:18209168
**398.** Cassarino DS, Derienzo DP, Barr RJ (2006). Cutaneous squamous cell carcinoma: a comprehensive clinicopathologic classification–part two. J Cutan Pathol. 33(4):261–79. PMID:16630176
**399.** Castillo L, Moreno A, Tardío JC (2014). Syringocystadenocarcinoma papilliferum in situ: report of a case with late recurrence. Am J Dermatopathol. 36(4):348–52. PMID:24394301
**400.** Cawley EP, Kruse WT, Pinkus HK (1952). Genetic aspects of malignant melanoma. AMA Arch Derm Syphilol. 65(4):440–50. PMID:14902112
**401.** Cazenave H, Maubec E, Mohamdi H, Grange F, Bressac-de Paillerets B, Demenais F, et al. (2013). Genital and anorectal mucosal melanoma is associated with cutaneous melanoma in patients and in families. Br J Dermatol. 169(3):594–9. PMID:23647170
**402.** Cengiz FP, Emiroglu N (2015). An open, comparative clinical study on the efficacy and safety of 10% trichloroacetic acid, 25% trichloroacetic acid and cryotherapy for verruca plana. Cutan Ocul Toxicol. 34(2):144–8. PMID:24938453
**403.** Cengiz FP, Emiroglu N, Wellenhof RH (2015). Dermoscopic and clinical features of pigmented skin lesions of the genital area. An Bras Dermatol. 90(2):178–83. PMID:25830986
**404.** Centeno JA, Mullick FG, Martinez L, Page NP, Gibb H, Longfellow D, et al. (2002). Pathology related to chronic arsenic exposure. Environ Health Perspect. 110 Suppl 5:883–6. PMID:12426152
**405.** Ceribelli M, Hou ZE, Kelly PN, Huang DW, Wright G, Ganapathi K, et al. (2016). A druggable TCF4- and BRD4-dependent transcriptional network sustains malignancy in blastic plasmacytoid dendritic cell neoplasm. Cancer Cell. 30(5):764–78. PMID:27846392
**406.** Cerroni L, editor (2014). Skin lymphoma: the illustrated guide. 4th ed. Oxford: Wiley-Blackwell.
**407.** Cerroni L (2017). Past, present and future of cutaneous lymphomas. Semin Diagn Pathol. 34(1):3–14. PMID:27979336
**408.** Cerroni L, Arzberger E, Pütz B, Höfler G, Metze D, Sander CA, et al. (2000). Primary cutaneous follicle center cell lymphoma with follicular growth pattern. Blood. 95(12):3922–8. PMID:10845929
**409.** Cerroni L, Barnhill R, Elder D, Gottlieb G, Heenan P, Kutzner H, et al. (2010). Melanocytic tumors of uncertain malignant potential: results of a tutorial held at the XXIX Symposium of the International Society of Dermatopathology in Graz, October 2008. Am J Surg Pathol. 34(3):314–26. PMID:20118771
**410.** Cerroni L, El-Shabrawi-Caelen L, Fink-Puches R, LeBoit PE, Kerl H (2000). Cutaneous spindle-cell B-cell lymphoma: a morphologic variant of cutaneous large B-cell lymphoma. Am J Dermatopathol. 22(4):299–304. PMID:10949453
**411.** Cerroni L, Fink-Puches R, Bäck B, Kerl H (2002). Follicular mucinosis: a critical reappraisal of clinicopathologic features and association with mycosis fungoides and Sézary syndrome. Arch Dermatol. 138(2):182–9. PMID:11843637
**412.** Cerroni L, Massone C, Kutzner H, Mentzel T, Umbert P, Kerl H (2008). Intravascular large T-cell or NK-cell lymphoma: a rare variant of intravascular large cell lymphoma with frequent cytotoxic phenotype and association with Epstein-Barr virus infection. Am J Surg Pathol. 32(6):891–8. PMID:18425045
**413.** Cerroni L, Rieger E, Hödl S, Kerl H (1992). Clinicopathologic and immunologic features associated with transformation of mycosis fungoides to large-cell lymphoma. Am J Surg Pathol. 16(6):543–52. PMID:1599034
**414.** Cerroni L, Zenahlik P, Höfler G, Kaddu S, Smolle J, Kerl H (1996). Specific cutaneous infiltrates of B-cell chronic lymphocytic leukemia: a clinicopathologic and prognostic study of 42 patients. Am J Surg Pathol. 20(8):1000–10. PMID:8712287
**415.** Cerroni L, Zöchling N, Pütz B, Kerl H (1997). Infection by Borrelia burgdorferi and cutaneous B-cell lymphoma. J Cutan Pathol. 24(8):457–61. PMID:9331890
**416.** Cesarman E, Knowles DM (1997). Kaposi's sarcoma-associated herpesvirus: a lymphotropic human herpesvirus associated with Kaposi's sarcoma, primary effusion lymphoma, and multicentric Castleman's disease. Semin Diagn Pathol. 14(1):54–66. PMID:9044510
**417.** Cesinaro AM, Bettelli S, Maccio L, Milani M (2014). Primary cutaneous mantle cell lymphoma of the leg with blastoid morphology and aberrant immunophenotype: a diagnostic challenge. Am J Dermatopathol. 36(2):e16–8. PMID:23612032
**418.** Cetinözman F, Jansen PM, Vermeer MH, Willemze R (2012). Differential expression of programmed death-1 (PD-1) in Sézary syndrome and mycosis fungoides. Arch Dermatol. 148(12):1379–85. PMID:23247480
**419.** Cetinözman F, Jansen PM, Willemze R (2012). Expression of programmed death-1 in primary cutaneous CD4-positive small/medium-sized pleomorphic T-cell lymphoma, cutaneous pseudo-T-cell lymphoma, and other types of cutaneous T-cell lymphoma. Am J Surg Pathol. 36(1):109–16. PMID:21989349
**420.** Chabot-Richards D, Zhang Q-Y, Foucar K (2017). B-cell chronic lymphocytic leukemia/small lymphocytic lymphoma, monoclonal B-cell lymphocytosis, and B-cell prolymphocytic leukemia. In: Jaffe ES, Arber DA, Campo E, Harris NL, Quintanilla-Martinez L, editors. Hematopathology. 2nd ed. Philadelphia: Elsevier; pp. 261–84.
**421.** Chahal HS, Lin Y, Ransohoff KJ, Hinds DA, Wu W, Dai HJ, et al. (2016). Genome-wide association study identifies novel susceptibility loci for cutaneous squamous cell carcinoma. Nat Commun. 7:12048. PMID:27424798
**422.** Chahal HS, Rieger KE, Sarin KY (2017). Incidence ratio of basal cell carcinoma to squamous cell carcinoma equalizes with age. J Am Acad Dermatol. 76(2):353–4. PMID:28089000
**423.** Chakraborty R, Hampton OA, Shen X, Simko SJ, Shih A, Abhyankar H, et al. (2014). Mutually exclusive recurrent somatic mutations in MAP2K1 and BRAF support a central role for ERK activation in LCH pathogenesis. Blood. 124(19):3007–15. PMID:25202140
**424.** Chamberlain RS, Huber K, White JC, Travaglino-Parda R (1999). Apocrine gland carcinoma of the axilla: review of the literature and recommendations for treatment. Am J Clin Oncol. 22(2):131–5. PMID:10199445
**425.** Chan AH, Shulman KJ, Lee BA (2017). Differentiating regressed melanoma from regressed lichenoid keratosis. J Cutan Pathol. 44(4):338–41. PMID:28026045
**426.** Chan JK, Fletcher CD, Hicklin GA, Rosai J (1990). Glomeruloid hemangioma. A distinctive cutaneous lesion of multicentric Castleman's disease associated with POEMS syndrome. Am J Surg Pathol. 14(11):1036–46. PMID:2173428
**427.** Chan JK, Sin VC, Wong KF, Ng CS, Tsang WY, Chan CH, et al. (1997). Nonnasal lymphoma expressing the natural killer cell marker CD56: a clinicopathologic study of 49 cases of an uncommon aggressive neoplasm. Blood. 89(12):4501–13. PMID:9192774
**428.** Chan MP, Andea AA, Harms PW, Durham AB, Patel RM, Wang M, et al. (2016). Genomic copy number analysis of a spectrum of blue nevi identifies recurrent aberrations of entire chromosomal arms in melanoma ex blue nevus. Mod Pathol. 29(3):227–39. PMID:26743478
**429.** Chan SA, Hejmadi R, Webster K, Kaur MR (2016). A unexpected growth arising within nevus sebaceous of Jadassohn. Dermatol Online J. 22(1). PMID:26990478
**430.** Chang AE, Karnell LH, Menck HR (1998). The National Cancer Data Base report on cutaneous and noncutaneous melanoma: a summary of 84,836 cases from the past decade. Cancer. 83(8):1664–78. PMID:9781962
**431.** Chang JW (2013). Acral melanoma: a unique disease in Asia. JAMA Dermatol. 149(11):1272–3. PMID:24068331
**432.** Chang JY, Wang C-S, Hung CC, Tsai TF, Hsiao CH (2002). Multiple Epstein-Barr virus-associated subcutaneous angioleiomyomas in a patient with acquired immunodeficiency syndrome. Br J Dermatol. 147(3):563–7. PMID:12207602
**433.** Chang MD, Arthur AK, García JJ, Sukov WR, Shon W (2016). ETV6 rearrangement in a case of mammary analogue secretory carcinoma of the skin. J Cutan Pathol. 43(11):1045–9. PMID:27506949
**434.** Chang SE, Ahn SJ, Choi JH, Sung KJ, Moon KC, Koh JK (1999). Primary adenoid cystic carcinoma of skin with lung metastasis. J Am Acad Dermatol. 40(4):640–2. PMID:10188691
**435.** Chang SE, Kim KJ, Kim ES, Choi JH, Sung KJ, Moon KC, et al. (2002). Two cases of late onset Ota's naevus. Clin Exp Dermatol. 27(3):202–4. PMID:12072008
**436.** Chang Y, Moore P (2014). Twenty years of KSHV. Viruses. 6(11):4258–64. PMID:25386844
**437.** Chang YM, Barrett JH, Bishop DT, Armstrong BK, Bataille V, Bergman W, et al. (2009). Sun exposure and melanoma risk at different latitudes: a pooled analysis of 5700 cases and 7216 controls. Int J Epidemiol. 38(3):814–30. PMID:19359257
**438.** Chantorn R, Wisuthsarewong W, Aanpreung P, Sanpakit K, Manonukul J (2008). Severe congenital systemic juvenile xanthogranuloma in monozygotic twins. Pediatr Dermatol. 25(4):470–3. PMID:18789091
**439.** Chappell AG, Chase EP, Chang B, Cunningham E, Mihm F, Calame A, et al. (2016). Atypical fibroxanthoma in a 13-year-old Guatemalan girl with xeroderma pigmentosum. Pediatr Dermatol. 33(3):e228–9. PMID:27046537
**440.** Charbel C, Fontaine RH, Malouf GG, Picard A, Kadlub N, El-Murr N, et al. (2014). NRAS mutation is the sole recurrent somatic mutation in large congenital melanocytic nevi. J Invest Dermatol. 134(4):1067–74. PMID:24129063
**441.** Chase DR, Enzinger FM (1985). Epithelioid sarcoma. Diagnosis, prognostic indicators, and treatment. Am J Surg Pathol. 9(4):241–63. PMID:4014539
**442.** Chasset F, Barete S, Charlotte F, Cohen-Aubart F, Arnaud L, Le Pelletier F, et al. (2016). Cutaneous manifestations of Erdheim-Chester disease (ECD): clinical, pathological, and molecular features in a monocentric series of 40 patients. J Am Acad Dermatol. 74(3):513–20. PMID:26785805
**443.** Chatzinasiou F, Lill CM, Kypreou K, Stefanaki I, Nicolaou V, Spyrou G, et al. (2011). Comprehensive field synopsis and systematic meta-analyses of genetic association studies in cutaneous melanoma. J Natl Cancer Inst. 103(16):1227–35. PMID:21693730
**444.** Chaudhry IH, Calonje E (2005). Dermal non-neural granular cell tumour (so-called primitive polypoid granular cell tumour): a distinctive entity further delineated in a clinicopathological study of 11 cases. Histopathology. 47(2):179–85. PMID:16045779
**445.** Chbani L, Guillou L, Terrier P, Decouvelaere AV, Grégoire F, Terrier-Lacombe MJ, et al. (2009). Epithelioid sarcoma: a clinicopathologic and immunohistochemical analysis of 106 cases from the French Sarcoma Group. Am J Clin Pathol. 131(2):222–7. PMID:19141382
**446.** Chen BJ, Mariño-Enríquez A, Fletcher CD, Hornick JL (2012). Loss of retinoblastoma protein expression in spindle cell/pleomorphic lipomas and cytogenetically related tumors: an immunohistochemical study with diagnostic

implications. Am J Surg Pathol. 36(8):1119–28. PMID:22790852
**447.** Chen J, Beg M, Chen S (2016). Syringocystadenocarcinoma papilliferum in situ, a variant of cutaneous adenocarcinoma in situ: a case report with literature review. Am J Dermatopathol. 38(10):762–5. PMID:27533073
**448.** Chen JY, Hruby G, Scolyer RA, Murali R, Hong A, Fitzgerald P, et al. (2008). Desmoplastic neurotropic melanoma: a clinicopathologic analysis of 128 cases. Cancer. 113(10):2770–8. PMID:18823042
**449.** Chen TC, Kuo T, Chan HL (2000). Dermatofibroma is a clonal proliferative disease. J Cutan Pathol. 27(1):36–9. PMID:10660130
**450.** Cheon M, Jung KE, Kim HS, Lee JY, Kim HO, Park CK, et al. (2013). Medallion-like dermal dendrocyte hamartoma: differential diagnosis with congenital atrophic dermatofibrosarcoma protuberans. Ann Dermatol. 25(3):382–4. PMID:24003290
**451.** Chervenak FA, Isaacson G, Blakemore KJ, Breg WR, Hobbins JC, Berkowitz RL, et al. (1983). Fetal cystic hygroma. Cause and natural history. N Engl J Med. 309(14):822–5. PMID:6888468
**452.** Chetty R, Serra S, Hsieh E (2005). Basaloid squamous carcinoma of the anal canal with an adenoid cystic pattern: histologic and immunohistochemical reappraisal of an unusual variant. Am J Surg Pathol. 29(12):1668–72. PMID:16327441
**453.** Cheuk W, Cheung FY, Lee KC, Chan JK (2009). Cutaneous indeterminate dendritic cell tumor with a protracted relapsing clinical course. Am J Surg Pathol. 33(8):1261–3. PMID:19471157
**454.** Cheung M, Kadariya Y, Talarchek J, Pei J, Ohar JA, Kayaleh OR, et al. (2015). Germline BAP1 mutation in a family with high incidence of multiple primary cancers and a potential gene-environment interaction. Cancer Lett. 369(2):261–5. PMID:26409435
**455.** Cheung YH, Gayden T, Campeau PM, LeDuc CA, Russo D, Nguyen VH, et al. (2013). A recurrent PDGFRB mutation causes familial infantile myofibromatosis. Am J Hum Genet. 92(6):996–1000. PMID:23731537
**456.** Chiarugi A, Quaglino P, Crocetti E, Nardini P, De Giorgi V, Borgognoni L, et al. (2015). Melanoma density and relationship with the distribution of melanocytic naevi in an Italian population: a GIPMe study–the Italian multidisciplinary group on melanoma. Melanoma Res. 25(1):80–7. PMID:25171087
**457.** Chibon F, Lagarde P, Salas S, Pérot G, Brouste V, Tirode F, et al. (2010). Validated prediction of clinical outcome in sarcomas and multiple types of cancer on the basis of a gene expression signature related to genome complexity. Nat Med. 16(7):781–7. PMID:20581836
**458.** Chikwava K, Jaffe R (2004). Langerin (CD207) staining in normal pediatric tissues, reactive lymph nodes, and childhood histiocytic disorders. Pediatr Dev Pathol. 7(6):607–14. PMID:15630529
**459.** Child FJ, Russell-Jones R, Woolford AJ, Calonje E, Photiou A, Orchard G, et al. (2001). Absence of the t(14;18) chromosomal translocation in primary cutaneous B-cell lymphoma. Br J Dermatol. 144(4):735–44. PMID:11298531
**460.** PDQ Pediatric Treatment Editorial Board (2002). Childhood vascular tumors treatment (PDQ®): health professional version.
**461.** Chiller K, Passaro D, Scheuller M, Singer M, McCalmont T, Grekin RC (2000). Microcystic adnexal carcinoma: forty-eight cases, their treatment, and their outcome. Arch Dermatol. 136(11):1355–9. PMID:11074698
**462.** Chimenti S, Fink-Puches R, Peris K, Pescarmona E, Pütz B, Kerl H, et al. (1999). Cutaneous involvement in lymphoblastic lymphoma. J Cutan Pathol. 26(8):379–85. PMID:10551409
**463.** Chitsazzadeh V, Coarfa C, Drummond JA, Nguyen T, Joseph A, Chilukuri S, et al. (2016). Cross-species identification of genomic drivers of squamous cell carcinoma development across preneoplastic intermediates. Nat Commun. 7:12601. PMID:27574101
**464.** Cho KH, Kim CW, Heo DS, Lee DS, Choi WW, Rim JH, et al. (2001). Epstein-Barr virus-associated peripheral T-cell lymphoma in adults with hydroa vacciniforme-like lesions. Clin Exp Dermatol. 26(3):242–7. PMID:11422165
**465.** Cho KH, Lee SH, Kim CW, Jeon YK, Kwon IH, Cho YJ, et al. (2004). Epstein-Barr virus-associated lymphoproliferative lesions presenting as a hydroa vacciniforme-like eruption: an analysis of six cases. Br J Dermatol. 151(2):372–80. PMID:15327544
**466.** Cho-Vega JH, Medeiros LJ, Prieto VG, Vega F (2008). Leukemia cutis. Am J Clin Pathol. 129(1):130–42. PMID:18089498
**467.** Choi CM, Lew BL, Sim WY (2013). Multiple trichofolliculomas on unusual sites: a case report and review of the literature. Int J Dermatol. 52(1):87–9. PMID:22640019
**468.** Choi EK, Chévez-Barrios P (2014). Inflamed conjunctival nevi: histopathological criteria. Arch Pathol Lab Med. 138(9):1242–6. PMID:25171709
**469.** Choi EY, Gardner JM, Lucas DR, McHugh JB, Patel RM (2014). Ewing sarcoma. Semin Diagn Pathol. 31(1):39–47. PMID:24680181
**470.** Choi HR, Sturgis EM, Rosenthal DI, Luna MA, Batsakis JG, El-Naggar AK (2003). Sarcomatoid carcinoma of the head and neck: molecular evidence for evolution and progression from conventional squamous cell carcinomas. Am J Surg Pathol. 27(9):1216–20. PMID:12960805
**471.** Choi J, Goh G, Walradt T, Hong BS, Bunick CG, Chen K, et al. (2015). Genomic landscape of cutaneous T cell lymphoma. Nat Genet. 47(9):1011–9. PMID:26192916
**472.** Choi YD, Chun SM, Jin SA, Lee JB, Yun SJ (2013). Amelanotic acral melanomas: clinicopathological, BRAF mutation, and KIT aberration analyses. J Am Acad Dermatol. 69(5):700–7. PMID:23972510
**473.** Choi YS, Park SH, Bang D (1989). Pilar sheath acanthoma–report of a case with review of the literature. Yonsei Med J. 30(4):392–5. PMID:2697113
**474.** Chott A, Vonderheid EC, Olbricht S, Miao NN, Balk SP, Kadin ME (1996). The dominant T cell clone is present in multiple regressing skin lesions and associated T cell lymphomas of patients with lymphomatoid papulosis. J Invest Dermatol. 106(4):696–700. PMID:8618007
**475.** Chow E, Merchant TE, Pappo A, Jenkins JJ, Shah AB, Kun LE (2000). Cutaneous and subcutaneous Ewing's sarcoma: an indolent disease. Int J Radiat Oncol Biol Phys. 46(2):433–8. PMID:10661351
**476.** Christie LJ, Evans AT, Bray SE, Smith ME, Kernohan NM, Levison DA, et al. (2006). Lesions resembling Langerhans cell histiocytosis in association with other lymphoproliferative disorders: a reactive or neoplastic phenomenon? Hum Pathol. 37(1):32–9. PMID:16360413
**477.** Chu MB, Slutsky JB, Dhandha MM, Beal BT, Armbrecht ES, Walker RJ, et al. (2014). Evaluation of the definitions of "high-risk" cutaneous squamous cell carcinoma using the American Joint Committee on Cancer staging criteria and National Comprehensive Cancer Network guidelines. J Skin Cancer. 2014:154340. PMID:25309755
**478.** Chu SW, Biswas A (2015). Basal cell carcinomas showing histological features generally associated with cutaneous adnexal neoplasms. J Cutan Pathol. 42(12):1049–62. PMID:26264868
**479.** Chulia MT, Paya A, Niveiro M, Ceballos S, Aranda FI (2001). Phyllodes tumor in ectopic breast tissue of the vulva. Int J Surg Pathol. 9(1):81–3. PMID:11469353
**480.** Chung EB, Enzinger FM (1979). Fibroma of tendon sheath. Cancer. 44(5):1945–54. PMID:91424
**481.** Chung EB, Enzinger FM (1983). Malignant melanoma of soft parts. A reassessment of clear cell sarcoma. Am J Surg Pathol. 7(5):405–13. PMID:6614306
**482.** Chung HJ, Wolpowitz D, Scott G, Gilmore E, Bhawan J (2016). Squamous cell carcinoma with osteoclast-like giant cells: a morphologically heterologous group including carcinosarcoma and squamous cell carcinoma with stromal changes. J Cutan Pathol. 43(2):148–57. PMID:26272477
**483.** Chung WK, Lee DW, Yang JH, Lee MW, Choi JH, Moon KC (2009). Glomeruloid hemangioma as a very early presenting sign of POEMS syndrome. J Cutan Pathol. 36(10):1126–8. PMID:19614998
**484.** Chung-Park M, Zheng Liu C, Giampoli EJ, Emery JD, Shalodi A (2002). Mucinous adenocarcinoma of ectopic breast tissue of the vulva. Arch Pathol Lab Med. 126(10):1216–8. PMID:12296762
**485.** Cibull TL, Gleason BC, O'Malley DP, Billings SD, Wiersema P, Hiatt KM (2008). Malignant cutaneous glomus tumor presenting as a rapidly growing leg mass in a pregnant woman. J Cutan Pathol. 35(8):765–9. PMID:18422692
**486.** Cicchiello M, Lin MJ, Pan Y, McLean C, Kelly JW (2016). An assessment of clinical pathways and missed opportunities for the diagnosis of nodular melanoma versus superficial spreading melanoma. Australas J Dermatol. 57(2):97–101. PMID:26563931
**487.** Cichowski K, Jacks T (2001). NF1 tumor suppressor gene function: narrowing the GAP. Cell. 104(4):593–604. PMID:11239415
**488.** Ackerman LV (1948). Verrucous carcinoma of the oral cavity. Surgery. 23(4):670–8. PMID:18907508
**489.** Clark WH (1991). Tumour progression and the nature of cancer. Br J Cancer. 64(4):631–44. PMID:1911211
**490.** Clark WH Jr, Elder DE, Guerry D 4th, Braitman LE, Trock BJ, Schultz D, et al. (1989). Model predicting survival in stage I melanoma based on tumor progression. J Natl Cancer Inst. 81(24):1893–904. PMID:2593166
**491.** Clark WH Jr, Elder DE, Guerry D 4th, Epstein MN, Greene MH, Van Horn M (1984). A study of tumor progression: the precursor lesions of superficial spreading and nodular melanoma. Hum Pathol. 15(12):1147–65. PMID:6500548
**492.** Clark WH Jr, Elder DE, Van Horn M (1986). The biologic forms of malignant melanoma. Hum Pathol. 17(5):443–50. PMID:3699806
**493.** Clark WH Jr, From L, Bernardino EA, Mihm MC (1969). The histogenesis and biologic behavior of primary human malignant melanomas of the skin. Cancer Res. 29(3):705–27. PMID:5773814
**494.** Clark WH Jr, Hood AF, Tucker MA, Jampel RM (1998). Atypical melanocytic nevi of the genital type with a discussion of reciprocal parenchymal-stromal interactions in the biology of neoplasia. Hum Pathol. 29(1 Suppl 1):S1–24. PMID:9445124
**495.** Clark WH Jr, Reimer RR, Greene M, Ainsworth AM, Mastrangelo MJ (1978). Origin of familial malignant melanomas from heritable melanocytic lesions. 'The B-K mole syndrome'. Arch Dermatol. 114(5):732–8. PMID:646394
**496.** Claudy AL, Garcier F, Kanitakis J (1984). Eccrine porocarcinoma. Ultrastructural and immunological study. J Dermatol. 11(3):282–6. PMID:6092444
**496A.** Clendenning WE, Rappaport HW (1979). Report of the Committee on Pathology of Cutaneous T Cell Lymphomas. Cancer Treat Rep. 63(4):719–24. PMID:376141
**497.** Clevenger J, Joseph C, Dawlett M, Guo M, Gong Y (2014). Reliability of immunostaining using pan-melanoma cocktail, SOX10, and microphthalmia transcription factor in confirming a diagnosis of melanoma on fine-needle aspiration smears. Cancer Cytopathol. 122(10):779–85. PMID:24954720
**498.** Clinical memoranda (1886). Br Med J. 1(1315):491–3. PMID:20751496
**499.** Cobb MW (1990). Human papillomavirus infection. J Am Acad Dermatol. 22(4):547–66. PMID:2156916
**500.** Cockerell CJ (2000). Histopathology of incipient intraepidermal squamous cell carcinoma ("actinic keratosis"). J Am Acad Dermatol. 42(1 Pt 2):11–7. PMID:10607351
**501.** Coffin CM, Dehner LP (1990). Cellular peripheral neural tumors (neurofibromas) in children and adolescents: a clinicopathological and immunohistochemical study. Pediatr Pathol. 10(3):351–61. PMID:1693425
**502.** Coffin CM, Hornick JL, Zhou H, Fletcher CD (2007). Gardner fibroma: a clinicopathologic and immunohistochemical analysis of 45 patients with 57 fibromas. Am J Surg Pathol. 31(3):410–6. PMID:17325483
**503.** Cohen Aubart F, Emile JF, Carrat F, Charlotte F, Benameur N, Donadieu J, et al. (2017). Targeted therapies in 54 patients with Erdheim-Chester disease, including follow-up after interruption (the LOVE study). Blood. 130(11):1377–80. PMID:28667012
**504.** Cohen JN, Joseph NM, North JP, Onodera C, Zembowicz A, LeBoit PE (2017). Genomic analysis of pigmented epithelioid melanocytomas reveals recurrent alterations in PRKAR1A, and PRKCA genes. Am J Surg Pathol. 41(10):1333–46. PMID:28796000
**505.** Cohen PR, Kohn SR, Kurzrock R (1991). Association of sebaceous gland tumors and internal malignancy: the Muir-Torre syndrome. Am J Med. 90(5):606–13. PMID:2029018
**506.** Cohen PR, Schulze KE, Nelson BR (2006). Basal cell carcinoma with mixed histology: a possible pathogenesis for recurrent skin cancer. Dermatol Surg. 32(4):542–51. PMID:16681663
**507.** Cohen PR, Ulmer R, Theriault A, Leigh IM, Duvic M (1997). Epidermolytic acanthomas: clinical characteristics and immunohistochemical features. Am J Dermatopathol. 19(3):232–41. PMID:9185908
**508.** Cohen SS, Skovbo S, Vestergaard H, Kristensen T, Møller M, Bindslev-Jensen C, et al. (2014). Epidemiology of systemic mastocytosis in Denmark. Br J Haematol. 166(4):521–8. PMID:24761987
**509.** Cohen Y, Rosenbaum E, Begum S, Goldenberg D, Esche C, Lavie O, et al. (2004). Exon 15 BRAF mutations are uncommon in melanomas arising in nonsun-exposed sites. Clin Cancer Res. 10(10):3444–7. PMID:15161700
**510.** Coindre JM (2006). Grading of soft tissue sarcomas: review and update. Arch Pathol Lab Med. 130(10):1448–53. PMID:17090186
**511.** Coit DG, Thompson JA, Algazi A, Andtbacka R, Bichakjian CK, Carson WE 3rd, et al. (2016). Melanoma, Version 2.2016, NCCN Clinical Practice Guidelines in Oncology. J Natl Compr Canc Netw. 14(4):450–73. PMID:27059193
**512.** Colburn DE, Welch MA, Giles FJ (2002). Skin infiltration with chronic lymphocytic leukemia is consistent with a good prognosis. Hematology. 7(3):187–8. PMID:12243983
**512A.** Colby TV, Burke JS, Hoppe RT (1981). Lymph node biopsy in mycosis fungoides.

Cancer. 47(2):351–9. PMID:7459823
**513.** Coleman WP 3rd, Loria PR, Reed RJ, Krementz ET (1980). Acral lentiginous melanoma. Arch Dermatol. 116(7):773–6. PMID:7396539
**514.** Collin M, Bigley V (2016). Monocyte, macrophage, and dendritic cell development: the human perspective. Microbiol Spectr. 4(5). PMID:27780016
**515.** Collin M, Bigley V, McClain KL, Allen CE (2015). Cell(s) of origin of Langerhans cell histiocytosis. Hematol Oncol Clin North Am. 29(5):825–38. PMID:26461145
**516.** Collin M, Milne P (2016). Langerhans cell origin and regulation. Curr Opin Hematol. 23(1):28–35. PMID:26554892
**517.** Collini P, Sampietro G, Bertulli R, Casali PG, Luksch R, Mezzelani A, et al. (2001). Cytokeratin immunoreactivity in 41 cases of ES/PNET confirmed by molecular diagnostic studies. Am J Surg Pathol. 25(2):273–4. PMID:11176079
**518.** Colomo L, Loong F, Rives S, Pittaluga S, Martínez A, López-Guillermo A, et al. (2004). Diffuse large B-cell lymphomas with plasmablastic differentiation represent a heterogeneous group of disease entities. Am J Surg Pathol. 28(6):736–47. PMID:15166665
**519.** Calonje E, Brenn T, Lazar A, McKee PH (2011). Tumors of the surface epithelium. In: McKee's pathology of the skin. 4th ed. Philadelphia: Saunders Elsevier; pp. 1086–7.
**520.** Conde-Sterling DA, Aguilera NS, Nandedkar MA, Abbondanzo SL (2000). Immunoperoxidase detection of CD10 in precursor T-lymphoblastic lymphoma/leukemia: a clinicopathologic study of 24 cases. Arch Pathol Lab Med. 124(5):704–8. PMID:10782151
**521.** Cook DL, Pugliano-Mauro MA, Schultz ZL (2013). Atypical pilar leiomyomatosis: an unusual presentation of multiple atypical cutaneous leiomyomas. J Cutan Pathol. 40(6):564–8. PMID:23550704
**522.** Cook MG, Massi D, Blokx WAM, Van den Oord J, Koljenović S, De Giorgi V, et al. (2017). New insights into naevoid melanomas: a clinicopathological reassessment. Histopathology. 71(6):943–950. PMID:28741688
**523.** Cooper JZ, Newman SR, Scott GA, Brown MD (2005). Metastasizing atypical fibroxanthoma (cutaneous malignant histiocytoma): report of five cases. Dermatol Surg. 31(2):221–5. PMID:15762219
**524.** Cooper PH (1992). Deep penetrating (plexiform spindle cell) nevus. A frequent participant in combined nevus. J Cutan Pathol. 19(3):172–80. PMID:1401342
**525.** Cooper PH, Adelson GL, Holthaus WH (1984). Primary cutaneous adenoid cystic carcinoma. Arch Dermatol. 120(6):774–7. PMID:6326693
**526.** Cooper PH, McAllister HA, Helwig EB (1979). Intravenous pyogenic granuloma. A study of 18 cases. Am J Surg Pathol. 3(3):221–8. PMID:575269
**527.** Cooper PH, Mills SE, Leonard DD, Santa Cruz DJ, Headington JT, Barr RJ, et al. (1985). Sclerosing sweat duct (syringomatous) carcinoma. Am J Surg Pathol. 9(6):422–33. PMID:4091180
**528.** Corbalán-Vélez R, Ruiz-Macia JA, Brufau C, López-Lozano JM, Martínez-Barba E, Carapeto FJ (2009). Clear cells in cutaneous squamous cell carcinoma. Actas Dermosifiliogr. 100(4):307–16. [Spanish] PMID:19463234
**529.** Cordiali-Fei P, Trento E, Giovanetti M, Lo Presti A, Latini A, Giuliani M, et al. (2015). Analysis of the ORFK1 hypervariable regions reveal distinct HHV-8 clustering in Kaposi's sarcoma and non-Kaposi's cases. J Exp Clin Cancer Res. 34(1):1. PMID:25592960
**530.** Correa R, Salpea P, Stratakis CA (2015). Carney complex: an update. Eur J Endocrinol. 173(4):M85–97. PMID:26130139
**531.** Corti M, Carolis LD, Solari R, Villafañe MF, Schtirbu R, Lewi D, et al. (2010). Non Hodgkin's lymphoma with cutaneous involvement in AIDS patients: report of five cases and review of the literature. Braz J Infect Dis. 14(1):81–5. PMID:20428660
**532.** Costa S, Byrne M, Pissaloux D, Haddad V, Paindavoine S, Thomas L, et al. (2016). Melanomas associated with blue nevi or mimicking cellular blue nevi: clinical, pathologic, and molecular study of 11 cases displaying a high frequency of GNA11 mutations, BAP1 expression loss, and a predilection for the scalp. Am J Surg Pathol. 40(3):368–77. PMID:26645730
**533.** Costache M, Desa LT, Mitrache LE, Pătraşcu OM, Dumitru A, Costache D, et al. (2014). Cutaneous verrucous carcinoma - report of three cases with review of literature. Rom J Morphol Embryol. 55(2):383–8. PMID:24969990
**534.** Costigan DC, Doyle LA (2016). Advances in the clinicopathological and molecular classification of cutaneous mesenchymal neoplasms. Histopathology. 68(6):776–95. PMID:26763770
**535.** Cota C, Vale E, Viana I, Requena L, Ferrara G, Anemona L, et al. (2010). Cutaneous manifestations of blastic plasmacytoid dendritic cell neoplasm-morphologic and phenotypic variability in a series of 33 patients. Am J Surg Pathol. 34(1):75–87. PMID:19956058
**537.** Coustan-Smith E, Mullighan CG, Onciu M, Behm FG, Raimondi SC, Pei D, et al. (2009). Early T-cell precursor leukaemia: a subtype of very high-risk acute lymphoblastic leukaemia. Lancet Oncol. 10(2):147–56. PMID:19147408
**538.** Couto JA, Vivero MP, Kozakewich HP, Taghinia AH, Mulliken JB, Warman ML, et al. (2015). A somatic MAP3K3 mutation is associated with verrucous venous malformation. Am J Hum Genet. 96(3):480–6. PMID:25728774
**539.** Cowen EW, Pichard DC, Garabedian E, Miettinen M (2016). Medallion-like dermal dendrocytic hamartoma, dermatofibrosarcoma protuberans, and adenosine deaminase-deficient severe combined immunodeficiency. Pediatr Dermatol. 33(3):359–60. PMID:27176810
**540.** Cox NH, Bloxham CA, Lawrence CM (1991). Halo eczema–resolution after excision of the central naevus alone. Clin Exp Dermatol. 16(1):66–7. PMID:2025942
**541.** Cox NH, Eedy DJ, Morton CA (2007). Guidelines for management of Bowen's disease: 2006 update. Br J Dermatol. 156(1):11–21. PMID:17199561
**542.** Cramer SF (1984). The histogenesis of acquired melanocytic nevi. Based on a new concept of melanocytic differentiation. Am J Dermatopathol. 6 Suppl:289–98. PMID:6528932
**543.** Cramer SF, Fesyuk A (2012). On the development of neurocutaneous units–implications for the histogenesis of congenital, acquired, and dysplastic nevi. Am J Dermatopathol. 34(1):60–81. PMID:22197860
**544.** Cramer SF, Heggeness LM (1989). Signet-ring squamous cell carcinoma. Am J Clin Pathol. 91(4):488–91. PMID:2467552
**545.** Crawford KM, Kobayashi T (2004). Nevoid basal cell carcinoma syndrome or multiple hereditary infundibulocystic basal cell carcinoma syndrome? J Am Acad Dermatol. 51(6):989–95. PMID:15583598
**546.** Criscione VD, Weinstock MA, Naylor MF, Luque C, Eide MJ, Bingham SF (2009). Actinic keratoses: natural history and risk of malignant transformation in the Veterans Affairs Topical Tretinoin Chemoprevention Trial. Cancer. 115(11):2523–30. PMID:19382202
**547.** Cronin DM, George TI, Reichard KK, Sundram UN (2012). Immunophenotypic analysis of myeloperoxidase-negative leukemia cutis and blastic plasmacytoid dendritic cell neoplasm. Am J Clin Pathol. 137(3):367–76. PMID:22338048
**548.** Croteau SE, Gupta D (2016). The clinical spectrum of kaposiform hemangioendothelioma and tufted angioma. Semin Cutan Med Surg. 35(3):147–52. PMID:27607323
**549.** Crotty KA, Scolyer RA, Li L, Palmer AA, Wang L, McCarthy SW (2002). Spitz naevus versus Spitzoid melanoma: when and how can they be distinguished? Pathology. 34(1):6–12. PMID:11902448
**550.** Crowson AN (2006). Basal cell carcinoma: biology, morphology and clinical implications. Mod Pathol. 19 Suppl 2:S127–47. PMID:16446711
**551.** Crum CP, Herrington CS, McCluggage WG, Regauer S, Wilkinson EJ (2014). Paget disease. In: Kurman RJ, Carcangiu ML, Herrington CS, Young RH, editors. WHO classification of tumours of female reproductive organs. 4th ed. Lyon: International Agency for Research on Cancer; pp. 236–7.
**552.** Cui L, Zhang J, Zhang X, Chang H, Qu C, Zhang J, et al. (2015). Angiosarcoma (Stewart-Treves syndrome) in postmastectomy patients: report of 10 cases and review of literature. Int J Clin Exp Pathol. 8(9):11108–15. PMID:26617830
**553.** Cullen D, Díaz Recuero JL, Cullen R, Rodríguez Peralto JL, Kutzner H, Requena L (2017). Superficial acral fibromyxoma: report of 13 cases with new immunohistochemical findings. Am J Dermatopathol. 39(1):14–22. PMID:28045748
**554.** Curtin JA, Busam K, Pinkel D, Bastian BC (2006). Somatic activation of KIT in distinct subtypes of melanoma. J Clin Oncol. 24(26):4340–6. PMID:16908931
**555.** Curtin JA, Fridlyand J, Kageshita T, Patel HN, Busam KJ, Kutzner H, et al. (2005). Distinct sets of genetic alterations in melanoma. N Engl J Med. 353(20):2135–47. PMID:16291983
**556.** Cust AE, Armstrong BK, Goumas C, Jenkins MA, Schmid H, Hopper JL, et al. (2011). Sunbed use during adolescence and early adulthood is associated with increased risk of early-onset melanoma. Int J Cancer. 128(10):2425–35. PMID:20669232
**557.** da Silva Almeida AC, Abate F, Khiabanian H, Martinez-Escala E, Guitart J, Tensen CP, et al. (2015). The mutational landscape of cutaneous T cell lymphoma and Sézary syndrome. Nat Genet. 47(12):1465–70. PMID:26551667
**558.** da Silva AD, Silva CA, de Camargo Moraes P, Thomaz LA, Furuse C, de Araújo VC (2011). Recurrent oral pyogenic granuloma in port-wine stain. J Craniofac Surg. 22(6):2356–8. PMID:22134277
**559.** Dabner M, McClure RJ, Harvey NT, Budgeon CA, Beer TW, Amanuel B, et al. (2014). Merkel cell polyomavirus and p63 status in Merkel cell carcinoma by immunohistochemistry: Merkel cell polyomavirus positivity is inversely correlated with sun damage, but neither is correlated with outcome. Pathology. 46(3):205–10. PMID:24614722
**560.** Dahlén A, Debiec-Rychter M, Pedeutour F, Domanski HA, Höglund M, Bauer HC, et al. (2003). Clustering of deletions on chromosome 13 in benign and low-malignant lipomatous tumors. Int J Cancer. 103(5):616–23. PMID:12494468
**561.** Dahlén A, Fletcher CD, Mertens F, Fletcher JA, Perez-Atayde AR, Hicks MJ, et al. (2004). Activation of the GLI oncogene through fusion with the beta-actin gene (ACTB) in a group of distinctive pericytic neoplasms: pericytoma with t(7;12). Am J Pathol. 164(5):1645–53. PMID:15111311
**562.** Dai B, Kong YY, Cai X, Shen XX, Kong JC (2014). Spiradenocarcinoma, cylindrocarcinoma and spiradenocylindrocarcinoma: a clinicopathological study of nine cases. Histopathology. 65(5):658–66. PMID:24796384
**563.** Dal Cin P, Sciot R, Polito P, Stas M, de Wever I, Cornelis A, et al. (1997). Lesions of 13q may occur independently of deletion of 16q in spindle cell/pleomorphic lipomas. Histopathology. 31(3):222–5. PMID:9354891
**564.** Daley T, Metcalfe DD, Akin C (2001). Association of the Q576R polymorphism in the interleukin-4 receptor alpha chain with indolent mastocytosis limited to the skin. Blood. 98(3):880–2. PMID:11468192
**565.** Dalia S, Sagatys E, Sokol L, Kubal T (2014). Rosai-Dorfman disease: tumor biology, clinical features, pathology, and treatment. Cancer Control. 21(4):322–7. PMID:25310213
**566.** Dalle S, Beylot-Barry M, Bagot M, Lipsker D, Machet L, Joly P, et al. (2010). Blastic plasmacytoid dendritic cell neoplasm: is transplantation the treatment of choice? Br J Dermatol. 162(1):74–9. PMID:19689477
**567.** Dalton SR, LeBoit PE (2008). Squamous cell carcinoma with clear cells: how often is there evidence of tricholemmal differentiation? Am J Dermatopathol. 30(4):333–9. PMID:18645304
**568.** Damato B, Coupland SE (2008). Conjunctival melanoma and melanosis: a reappraisal of terminology, classification and staging. Clin Exp Ophthalmol. 36(8):786–95. PMID:19128387
**569.** Damato B, Coupland SE (2009). Management of conjunctival melanoma. Expert Rev Anticancer Ther. 9(9):1227–39. PMID:19761427
**570.** Damato B, Eleuteri A, Taktak AF, Coupland SE (2011). Estimating prognosis for survival after treatment of choroidal melanoma. Prog Retin Eye Res. 30(5):285–95. PMID:21658465
**571.** Damato BE, Coupland SE (2012). Differences in uveal melanomas between men and women from the British Isles. Eye (Lond). 26(2):292–9. PMID:22079972
**572.** Danga ME, Yaar R, Bhawan J (2015). Melan-A positive dermal cells in malignant melanoma in situ. J Cutan Pathol. 42(6):388–93. PMID:25726939
**573.** Dangoor A, Seddon B, Gerrand C, Grimer R, Whelan J, Judson I (2016). UK guidelines for the management of soft tissue sarcomas. Clin Sarcoma Res. 6:20. PMID:27891213
**574.** Danialan R, Mutyambizi K, Aung P, Prieto VG, Ivan D (2015). Challenges in the diagnosis of cutaneous adnexal tumours. J Clin Pathol. 68(12):992–1002. PMID:26602416
**575.** Daniels BH, Ko JS, Rowe JJ, Downs-Kelly E, Billings SD (2017). Radiation-associated angiosarcoma in the setting of breast cancer mimicking radiation dermatitis: a diagnostic pitfall. J Cutan Pathol. 44(5):456–61. PMID:28169467
**576.** Daoud MA, Mete O, Al Habeeb A, Ghazarian D (2013). Neuroendocrine carcinoma of the skin–an updated review. Semin Diagn Pathol. 30(3):234–44. PMID:24144292
**577.** Dargent JL, Delannoy A, Pieron P, Husson B, Debecker C, Petrella T (2011). Cutaneous accumulation of plasmacytoid dendritic cells associated with acute myeloid leukemia: a rare condition distinct from blastic plasmacytoid dendritic cell neoplasm. J Cutan Pathol. 38(11):893–8. PMID:21883371
**578.** Dasgupta T, Wilson LD, Yu JB (2009). A retrospective review of 1349 cases of sebaceous carcinoma. Cancer. 115(1):158–65. PMID:18988294
**579.** Daud AI, Wolchok JD, Robert C, Hwu WJ, Weber JS, Ribas A, et al. (2016). Programmed death-ligand 1 expression and response to the anti-programmed death 1 antibody pembrolizumab in melanoma. J Clin Oncol.

34(34):4102–9. PMID:27863197
**580.** Davies H, Bignell GR, Cox C, Stephens P, Edkins S, Clegg S, et al. (2002). Mutations of the BRAF gene in human cancer. Nature. 417(6892):949–54. PMID:12068308
**581.** Davies JR, Chang YM, Bishop DT, Armstrong BK, Bataille V, Bergman W, et al. (2015). Development and validation of a melanoma risk score based on pooled data from 16 case-control studies. Cancer Epidemiol Biomarkers Prev. 24(5):817–24. PMID:25713022
**582.** Davis DA, Cohen PR (1995). Genitourinary tumors in men with the Muir-Torre syndrome. J Am Acad Dermatol. 33(5 Pt 2):909–12. PMID:7593809
**583.** Davis TH, Morton CC, Miller-Cassman R, Balk SP, Kadin ME (1992). Hodgkin's disease, lymphomatoid papulosis, and cutaneous T-cell lymphoma derived from a common T-cell clone. N Engl J Med. 326(17):1115–22. PMID:1532439
**584.** Dawe RS, Wainwright NJ, Evans AT, Lowe JG (1998). Multiple widespread eruptive Spitz naevi. Br J Dermatol. 138(5):872–4. PMID:9666837
**585.** de Bruin PC, Beljaards RC, van Heerde P, Van Der Valk P, Noorduyn LA, Van Krieken JH, et al. (1993). Differences in clinical behaviour and immunophenotype between primary cutaneous and primary nodal anaplastic large cell lymphoma of T-cell or null cell phenotype. Histopathology. 23(2):127–35. PMID:8406384
**586.** de Coninck EC, Kim YH, Varghese A, Hoppe RT (2001). Clinical characteristics and outcome of patients with extracutaneous mycosis fungoides. J Clin Oncol. 19(3):779–84. PMID:11157031
**587.** de la Garza Bravo MM, Patel KP, Loghavi S, Curry JL, Torres Cabala CA, Cason RC, et al. (2015). Shared clonality in distinctive lesions of lymphomatoid papulosis and mycosis fungoides occurring in the same patients suggests a common origin. Hum Pathol. 46(4):558–69. PMID:25666664
**588.** de la Fouchardière A, Cabaret O, Pètre J, Aydin S, Leroy A, de Potter P, et al. (2015). Primary leptomeningeal melanoma is part of the BAP1-related cancer syndrome. Acta Neuropathol. 129(6):921–3. PMID:25900292
**589.** de la Fouchardière A, Cabaret O, Savin L, Combemale P, Schvartz H, Penet C, et al. (2015). Germline BAP1 mutations predispose also to multiple basal cell carcinomas. Clin Genet. 88(3):273–7. PMID:25080371
**590.** de Planell-Mas E, Martínez-Garriga B, Zalacain AJ, Vinuesa T, Viñas M (2017). Human papillomaviruses genotyping in plantar warts. J Med Virol. 89(5):902–7. PMID:27736001
**591.** De Rose AF, Tosi M, Mantica G, Piol N, Toncini C, Terrone C (2016). Verruciform xanthoma of the penis: a rare benign lesion that simulates carcinoma. Arch Ital Urol Androl. 88(4):284–5. PMID:28073194
**592.** de Snoo FA, Bishop DT, Bergman W, van Leeuwen I, van der Drift C, van Nieuwpoort FA, et al. (2008). Increased risk of cancer other than melanoma in CDKN2A founder mutation (p16-Leiden)-positive melanoma families. Clin Cancer Res. 14(21):7151–7. PMID:18981015
**593.** de Feraudy S, Fletcher CD (2010). Intradermal nodular fasciitis: a rare lesion analyzed in a series of 24 cases. Am J Surg Pathol. 34(9):1377–81. PMID:20716998
**594.** de Feraudy S, Fletcher CD (2012). Fibroblastic connective tissue nevus: a rare cutaneous lesion analyzed in a series of 25 cases. Am J Surg Pathol. 36(10):1509–15. PMID:22892597
**595.** de Leval L, Harris NL, Longtine J, Ferry JA, Duncan LM (2001). Cutaneous B-cell lymphomas of follicular and marginal zone types: use of Bcl-6, CD10, Bcl-2, and CD21 in differential diagnosis and classification. Am J Surg Pathol. 25(6):732–41. PMID:11395550
**595A.** de Leval L, Parrens M, Le Bras F, Jais JP, Fataccioli V, Martin A, et al. (2015). Angioimmunoblastic T-cell lymphoma is the most common T-cell lymphoma in two distinct French information data sets. Haematologica. 100(9):e361–4. PMID:26045291
**596.** de Masson A, Velter C, Galicier L, Meignin V, Boutboul D, Guéry R, et al. (2016). Disseminated skin involvement in HIV-associated Burkitt lymphoma: a rare clinical feature with poor prognosis. Br J Dermatol. 174(1):184–6. PMID:26114450
**597.** de Souza A, el-Azhary RA, Camilleri MJ, Wada DA, Appert DL, Gibson LE (2012). In search of prognostic indicators for lymphomatoid papulosis: a retrospective study of 123 patients. J Am Acad Dermatol. 66(6):928–37. PMID:21982062
**598.** De Souza A, Ferry JA, Burghart DR, Tinguely M, Goyal A, Duncan LM, et al. (2017). IgG4 expression in primary cutaneous marginal zone lymphoma: a multicenter study. Appl Immunohistochem Mol Morphol. [EPUB ahead of print] PMID:28151793
**599.** De Wever I, Dal Cin P, Fletcher CD, Mandahl N, Mertens F, Mitelman F, et al. (2000). Cytogenetic, clinical, and morphologic correlations in 78 cases of fibromatosis: a report from the CHAMP Study Group. CHromosomes And Morphology. Mod Pathol. 13(10):1080–5. PMID:11048801
**600.** DeCoteau JF, Butmarc JR, Kinney MC, Kadin ME (1996). The t(2;5) chromosomal translocation is not a common feature of primary cutaneous CD30+ lymphoproliferative disorders: comparison with anaplastic large-cell lymphoma of nodal origin. Blood. 87(8):3437–41. PMID:8605362
**601.** Dehner LP (2003). Juvenile xanthogranulomas in the first two decades of life: a clinicopathologic study of 174 cases with cutaneous and extracutaneous manifestations. Am J Surg Pathol. 27(5):579–93. PMID:12717244
**602.** Dei Tos AP, Maestro R, Doglioni C, Gasparotto D, Boiocchi M, Laurino L, et al. (1994). Ultraviolet-induced p53 mutations in atypical fibroxanthoma. Am J Pathol. 145(1):11–7. PMID:8030743
**603.** Dei Tos AP, Mentzel T, Fletcher CD (1998). Primary liposarcoma of the skin: a rare neoplasm with unusual high grade features. Am J Dermatopathol. 20(4):332–8. PMID:9700369
**604.** Deisch J, Fuda FB, Chen W, Karandikar N, Arbini AA, Zhou XJ, et al. (2009). Segmental tandem triplication of the MLL gene in an intravascular large B-cell lymphoma with multisystem involvement: a comprehensive morphologic, immunophenotypic, cytogenetic, and molecular cytogenetic antemortem study. Arch Pathol Lab Med. 133(9):1477–82. PMID:19722759
**605.** del Pino M, Bleeker MC, Quint WG, Snijders PJ, Meijer CJ, Steenbergen RD (2012). Comprehensive analysis of human papillomavirus prevalence and the potential role of low-risk types in verrucous carcinoma. Mod Pathol. 25(10):1354–63. PMID:22684225
**606.** Delaplace M, Lhommet C, de Pinieux G, Vergier B, de Muret A, Machet L (2012). Primary cutaneous Ewing sarcoma: a systematic review focused on treatment and outcome. Br J Dermatol. 166(4):721–6. PMID:22098102
**607.** Delattre O, Zucman J, Melot T, Garau XS, Zucker JM, Lenoir GM, et al. (1994). The Ewing family of tumors–a subgroup of small-round-cell tumors defined by specific chimeric transcripts. N Engl J Med. 331(5):294–9. PMID:8022439
**608.** Demenais F, Mohamdi H, Chaudru V, Goldstein AM, Newton Bishop JA, Bishop DT, et al. (2010). Association of MC1R variants and host phenotypes with melanoma risk in CDKN2A mutation carriers: a GenoMEL study. J Natl Cancer Inst. 102(20):1568–83. PMID:20876876
**609.** Demirkesen C, Tüzüner N, Esen T, Lebe B, Ozkal S (2011). The expression of IgM is helpful in the differentiation of primary cutaneous diffuse large B cell lymphoma and follicle center lymphoma. Leuk Res. 35(9):1269–72. PMID:21700336
**610.** Deng A, Lee W, Pfau R, Harrington A, DiGiovani J, Prickett KA, et al. (2008). Primary cutaneous Langerhans cell sarcoma without Birbeck granules: indeterminate cell sarcoma? J Cutan Pathol. 35(9):849–54. PMID:18422973
**611.** Derheimer FA, Hicks JK, Paulsen MT, Canman CE, Ljungman M (2009). Psoralen-induced DNA interstrand cross-links block transcription and induce p53 in an ataxia-telangiectasia and rad3-related-dependent manner. Mol Pharmacol. 75(3):599–607. PMID:19064630
**612.** DeSimone RS, Zielinski CJ (2001). Calcifying aponeurotic fibroma of the hand. A case report. J Bone Joint Surg Am. 83-A(4):586–8. PMID:11315790
**613.** Dessars B, De Raeve LE, El Housni H, Debouck CJ, Sidon PJ, Morandini R, et al. (2007). Chromosomal translocations as a mechanism of BRAF activation in two cases of large congenital melanocytic nevi. J Invest Dermatol. 127(6):1468–70. PMID:17301836
**614.** Dey A, Allen J, Hankey-Giblin PA (2015). Ontogeny and polarization of macrophages in inflammation: blood monocytes versus tissue macrophages. Front Immunol. 5:683. PMID:25657646
**615.** Deyrup AT, Lee VK, Hill CE, Cheuk W, Toh HC, Kesavan S, et al. (2006). Epstein-Barr virus-associated smooth muscle tumors are distinctive mesenchymal tumors reflecting multiple infection events: a clinicopathologic and molecular analysis of 29 tumors from 19 patients. Am J Surg Pathol. 30(1):75–82. PMID:16330945
**616.** Deyrup AT, McKenney JK, Tighiouart M, Folpe AL, Weiss SW (2008). Sporadic cutaneous angiosarcomas: a proposal for risk stratification based on 69 cases. Am J Surg Pathol. 32(1):72–7. PMID:18162773
**617.** Deyrup AT, Tighiouart M, Montag AG, Weiss SW (2008). Epithelioid hemangioendothelioma of soft tissue: a proposal for risk stratification based on 49 cases. Am J Surg Pathol. 32(6):924–7. PMID:18551749
**618.** Dhomen N, Reis-Filho JS, da Rocha Dias S, Hayward R, Savage K, Delmas V, et al. (2009). Oncogenic Braf induces melanocyte senescence and melanoma in mice. Cancer Cell. 15(4):294–303. PMID:19345328
**619.** Di Giannatale A, Frezza AM, Le Deley MC, Marec-Bérard P, Benson C, Blay JY, et al. (2015). Primary cutaneous and subcutaneous Ewing sarcoma. Pediatr Blood Cancer. 62(9):1555–61. PMID:25894676
**620.** Di Napoli A, Giubettini M, Duranti E, Ferrari A, Guglielmi C, Uccini S, et al. (2011). Iatrogenic EBV-positive lymphoproliferative disorder with features of EBV+ mucocutaneous ulcer: evidence for concomitant TCRγ/IGH rearrangements in the Hodgkin-like neoplastic cells. Virchows Arch. 458(5):631–6. PMID:21399965
**621.** Di Tommaso L, Franchi G, Destro A, Broglia F, Minuti F, Rahal D, et al. (2008). Toker cells of the breast. Morphological and immunohistochemical characterization of 40 cases. Hum Pathol. 39(9):1295–300. PMID:18614197
**622.** Di Tommaso L, Rosai J (2005). The capillary lobule: a deceptively benign feature of post-radiation angiosarcoma of the skin: report of three cases. Am J Dermatopathol. 27(4):301–5. PMID:16121049
**623.** Diamandidou E, Colome M, Fayad L, Duvic M, Kurzrock R (1999). Prognostic factor analysis in mycosis fungoides/Sézary syndrome. J Am Acad Dermatol. 40(6 Pt 1):914–24. PMID:10365922
**624.** Diamond EL, Dagna L, Hyman DM, Cavalli G, Janku F, Estrada-Veras J, et al. (2014). Consensus guidelines for the diagnosis and clinical management of Erdheim-Chester disease. Blood. 124(4):483–92. PMID:24850756
**625.** Diamond EL, Durham BH, Haroche J, Yao Z, Ma J, Parikh SA, et al. (2016). Diverse and targetable kinase alterations drive histiocytic neoplasms. Cancer Discov. 6(2):154–65. PMID:26566875
**625A.** Diamond EL, Subbiah V, Lockhart AC, Blay JY, Puzanov I, Chau I, et al. (2018). Vemurafenib for BRAF V600-mutant Erdheim-Chester disease and Langerhans cell histiocytosis: analysis of data from the histology-independent, phase 2, open-label VE-BASKET study. JAMA Oncol. 4(3):384–8. PMID:29188284
**626.** Dickson BC, Pethe V, Chung CT, Howarth DJ, Bilbao JM, Fornasier VL, et al. (2008). Systemic Erdheim-Chester disease. Virchows Arch. 452(2):221–7. PMID:18188596
**627.** DiGiovanna JJ, Kraemer KH (2012). Shining a light on xeroderma pigmentosum. J Invest Dermatol. 132(3 Pt 2):785–96. PMID:22217736
**628.** DiGiovanna JJ, Patronas N, Katz D, Abangan D, Kraemer KH (1998). Xeroderma pigmentosum: spinal cord astrocytoma with 9-year survival after radiation and isotretinoin therapy. J Cutan Med Surg. 2(3):153–8. PMID:9479081
**629.** Dijkman R, Tensen CP, Jordanova ES, Knijnenburg J, Hoefnagel JJ, Mulder AA, et al. (2006). Array-based comparative genomic hybridization analysis reveals recurrent chromosomal alterations and prognostic parameters in primary cutaneous large B-cell lymphoma. J Clin Oncol. 24(2):296–305. PMID:16330669
**630.** Dijkman R, van Doorn R, Szuhai K, Willemze R, Vermeer MH, Tensen CP (2007). Gene-expression profiling and array-based CGH classify CD4+CD56+ hematodermic neoplasm and cutaneous myelomonocytic leukemia as distinct disease entities. Blood. 109(4):1720–7. PMID:17068154
**631.** Dim DC, Cooley LD, Miranda RN (2007). Clear cell sarcoma of tendons and aponeuroses: a review. Arch Pathol Lab Med. 131(1):152–6. PMID:17227118
**632.** Dinneen AM, Mehregan DR (1996). Sebaceous epithelioma: a review of twenty-one cases. J Am Acad Dermatol. 34(1):47–50. PMID:8543694
**633.** Diwan AH, Lazar AJ (2011). Nevoid melanoma. Clin Lab Med. 31(2):243–53. PMID:21549238
**634.** Do JE, Noh S, Jee HJ, Oh SH (2013). Familial multiple pilomatricomas showing clinical features of a giant mass without associated diseases. Int J Dermatol. 52(2):250–2. PMID:23347315
**635.** Dodds A, Chia A, Shumack S (2014). Actinic keratosis: rationale and management. Dermatol Ther (Heidelb). 4(1):11–31. PMID:24627245
**636.** Doeden K, Molina-Kirsch H, Perez E, Warnke R, Sundram U (2008). Hydroa-like lymphoma with CD56 expression. J Cutan Pathol. 35(5):488–94. PMID:17976208
**637.** Dogan S, Wang L, Ptashkin RN, Dawson RR, Shah JP, Sherman EJ, et al. (2016). Mammary analog secretory carcinoma of the thyroid gland: a primary thyroid adenocarcinoma harboring ETV6-NTRK3 fusion. Mod Pathol. 29(9):985–95. PMID:27282352
**638.** Dogru M, Matsuo H, Inoue M, Okubo K, Yamamoto M (1997). Management of eyelid sebaceous carcinomas. Ophthalmologica. 211(1):40–3. PMID:8958530
**639.** Döhner H, Stilgenbauer S, Benner

A, Leupolt E, Kröber A, Bullinger L, et al. (2000). Genomic aberrations and survival in chronic lymphocytic leukemia. N Engl J Med. 343(26):1910–6. PMID:11136261
**640.** Dojcinov SD, Venkataraman G, Pittaluga S, Wlodarska I, Schrager JA, Raffeld M, et al. (2011). Age-related EBV-associated lymphoproliferative disorders in the Western population: a spectrum of reactive lymphoid hyperplasia and lymphoma. Blood. 117(18):4726–35. PMID:21385849
**641.** Dojcinov SD, Venkataraman G, Raffeld M, Pittaluga S, Jaffe ES (2010). EBV positive mucocutaneous ulcer–a study of 26 cases associated with various sources of immunosuppression. Am J Surg Pathol. 34(3):405–17. PMID:20154586
**642.** Domoto H, Terahata S, Sato K, Tamai S (1998). Nodular hidradenoma of the breast: report of two cases with literature review. Pathol Int. 48(11):907–11. PMID:9832062
**643.** Dores GM, Huycke MM, Devesa SS, Garcia CA (2010). Primary cutaneous adenoid cystic carcinoma in the United States: incidence, survival, and associated cancers, 1976 to 2005. J Am Acad Dermatol. 63(1):71–8. PMID:20447723
**644.** Dorsey CS, Montgomery H (1954). Blue nevus and its distinction from Mongolian spot and the nevus of Ota. J Invest Dermatol. 22(3):225–36. PMID:13130904
**645.** Dossett LA, Harrington M, Cruse CW, Gonzalez RJ (2015). Cutaneous angiosarcoma. Curr Probl Cancer. 39(4):258–63. PMID:26276214
**646.** Doyle LA, Fletcher CD (2011). EMA positivity in epithelioid fibrous histiocytoma: a potential diagnostic pitfall. J Cutan Pathol. 38(9):697–703. PMID:21752057
**647.** Doyle LA, Fletcher CD (2013). Metastasizing "benign" cutaneous fibrous histiocytoma: a clinicopathologic analysis of 16 cases. Am J Surg Pathol. 37(4):484–95. PMID:23426120
**648.** Doyle LA, Fletcher CD, Hornick JL (2016). Nuclear expression of CAMTA1 distinguishes epithelioid hemangioendothelioma from histologic mimics. Am J Surg Pathol. 40(1):94–102. PMID:26414223
**649.** Doyle LA, Mariño-Enriquez A, Fletcher CD, Hornick JL (2015). ALK rearrangement and overexpression in epithelioid fibrous histiocytoma. Mod Pathol. 28(7):904–12. PMID:25857825
**650.** Doyle LA, Möller E, Dal Cin P, Fletcher CD, Mertens F, Hornick JL (2011). MUC4 is a highly sensitive and specific marker for low-grade fibromyxoid sarcoma. Am J Surg Pathol. 35(5):733–41. PMID:21415703
**651.** Dratviman-Storobinsky O, Cohen Y, Frenkel S, Pe'er J, Goldenberg-Cohen N (2010). Lack of oncogenic GNAQ mutations in melanocytic lesions of the conjunctiva as compared to uveal melanoma. Invest Ophthalmol Vis Sci. 51(12):6180–2. PMID:20631239
**652.** Dreizen S, McCredie KB, Keating MJ, Luna MA (1983). Malignant gingival and skin "infiltrates" in adult leukemia. Oral Surg Oral Med Oral Pathol. 55(6):572–9. PMID:6576290
**653.** Droupy S, Attias D, Eschwege P, Hammoudi Y, Benoit G, Jardin A (1999). Bilateral hydronephrosis in a patient with Erdheim-Chester disease. J Urol. 162(6):2084–5. PMID:10569576
**654.** Dubina M, Goldenberg G (2009). Viral-associated nonmelanoma skin cancers: a review. Am J Dermatopathol. 31(6):561–73. PMID:19590418
**655.** Duke WH, Sherrod TT, Lupton GP (2000). Aggressive digital papillary adenocarcinoma (aggressive digital papillary adenoma and adenocarcinoma revisited). Am J Surg Pathol. 24(6):775–84. PMID:10843279
**656.** Duong T, Grange F, Auffret N, Aractingi S, Bodemer C, Brousse N, et al. (2010). Cutaneous Richter's syndrome, prognosis, and clinical, histological and immunohistological patterns: report of four cases and review of the literature. Dermatology. 220(3):226–33. PMID:20145381
**657.** Dupré A, Carrère S, Bonafé JL, Christol B, Lassère J, Touron P (1981). Eruptive generalized syringomas, milium and atrophoderma vermiculata. Nicolau and Balus' syndrome (author's transl). Dermatologica. 162(4):281–6. [French] PMID:7262384
**658.** Duprez R, Lacoste V, Brière J, Couppié P, Frances C, Sainte-Marie D, et al. (2007). Evidence for a multiclonal origin of multicentric advanced lesions of Kaposi sarcoma. J Natl Cancer Inst. 99(14):1086–94. PMID:17623796
**659.** Dupuis L, Nezarati MM (2001). Neurofibromatosis type I as a model of autosomal dominant inheritance. Pediatr Dermatol. 18(5):445–7. PMID:11737695
**660.** Dupuy A, Sarasin A (2015). DNA damage and gene therapy of xeroderma pigmentosum, a human DNA repair-deficient disease. Mutat Res. 776:2–8. PMID:26255934
**661.** Dupuy A, Valton J, Leduc S, Armier J, Galetto R, Gouble A, et al. (2013). Targeted gene therapy of xeroderma pigmentosum cells using meganuclease and TALEN™. PLoS One. 8(11):e78678. PMID:24236034
**662.** Eberle FC, Song JY, Xi L, Raffeld M, Harris NL, Wilson WH, et al. (2012). Nodal involvement by cutaneous CD30-positive T-cell lymphoma mimicking classical Hodgkin lymphoma. Am J Surg Pathol. 36(5):716–25. PMID:22367293
**663.** Edelbroek JR, Vermeer MH, Jansen PM, Stoof TJ, van der Linden MM, Horváth B, et al. (2012). Langerhans cell histiocytosis first presenting in the skin in adults: frequent association with a second haematological malignancy. Br J Dermatol. 167(6):1287–94. PMID:22835048
**664.** Edinger JT, Kant JA, Swerdlow SH (2010). Cutaneous marginal zone lymphomas have distinctive features and include 2 subsets. Am J Surg Pathol. 34(12):1830–41. PMID:21107089
**665.** Egan CA, Stratakis CA, Turner ML (2001). Multiple lentigines associated with cutaneous myxomas. J Am Acad Dermatol. 44(2):282–4. PMID:11174387
**666.** Egawa N, Egawa K, Griffin H, Doorbar J (2015). Human papillomaviruses; epithelial tropisms, and the development of neoplasia. Viruses. 7(7):3863–90. PMID:26193301
**667.** Egeler RM, Neglia JP, Puccetti DM, Brennan CA, Nesbit ME (1993). Association of Langerhans cell histiocytosis with malignant neoplasms. Cancer. 71(3):865–73. PMID:8431870
**668.** Egemen A, Ikizoğlu T, Ergör S, Mete Asar G, Yilmaz O (2006). Frequency and characteristics of Mongolian spots among Turkish children in Aegean region. Turk J Pediatr. 48(3):232–6. PMID:17172067
**669.** Egozi-Reinman E, Avitan-Hersh E, Barzilai A, Indelman M, Bergman R (2016). Epidermolytic acanthoma of the genitalia does not show mutations in KRT1 or KRT10. Am J Dermatopathol. 38(2):164–5. PMID:26825163
**670.** El Shabrawi-Caelen L, Kerl H, Cerroni L (2004). Lymphomatoid papulosis: reappraisal of clinicopathologic presentation and classification into subtypes A, B, and C. Arch Dermatol. 140(4):441–7. PMID:15096372
**671.** El Demellawy D, Onuma K, Alowami S (2011). Signet ring squamous cell carcinoma–the forgotten variant: case report and review of the literature. J Cutan Pathol. 38(3):306–8. PMID:19751229
**672.** El-Naggar AK (2006). Clear cell hidradenoma of the skin–a third tumor type with a t(11;19)-associated TORC1-MAML2 gene fusion: Genes Chromosomes Cancer. 2005;43:202-205. Adv Anat Pathol. 13(2):80–2. PMID:16670462
**673.** El-Safadi S, Estel R, Mayser P, Muenstedt K (2014). Primary malignant melanoma of the urethra: a systematic analysis of the current literature. Arch Gynecol Obstet. 289(5):935–43. PMID:24370958
**674.** El-Shabrawi L, LeBoit PE (1997). Basal cell carcinoma with thickened basement membrane: a variant that resembles some benign adnexal neoplasms. Am J Dermatopathol. 19(6):568–74. PMID:9415612
**675.** Elco CP, Mariño-Enríquez A, Abraham JA, Dal Cin P, Hornick JL (2010). Hybrid myxoinflammatory fibroblastic sarcoma/hemosiderotic fibrolipomatous tumor: report of a case providing further evidence for a pathogenetic link. Am J Surg Pathol. 34(11):1723–7. PMID:20871391
**676.** Elder DE (1995). Skin cancer. Melanoma and other specific nonmelanoma skin cancers. Cancer. 75(1 Suppl):245–56. PMID:8000999
**677.** Elder DE (2006). Precursors to melanoma and their mimics: nevi of special sites. Mod Pathol. 19 Suppl 2:S4–20. PMID:16446715
**678.** Elder DE (2010). Dysplastic naevi: an update. Histopathology. 56(1):112–20. PMID:20055909
**679.** Elder DE (2014). Pathological staging of melanoma. Methods Mol Biol. 1102:325–51. PMID:24258986
**680.** Elder DE (2016). Melanoma progression. Pathology. 48(2):147–54. PMID:27020387
**681.** Elder DE, Goldman LI, Goldman SC, Greene MH, Clark WH Jr (1980). Dysplastic nevus syndrome: a phenotypic association of sporadic cutaneous melanoma. Cancer. 46(8):1787–94. PMID:7427881
**682.** Elder DE, Xu X (2004). The approach to the patient with a difficult melanocytic lesion. Pathology. 36(5):428–34. PMID:15370112
**683.** Ellis DL, Wheeland RG, Solomon H (1985). Estrogen and progesterone receptors in melanocytic lesions. Occurrence in patients with dysplastic nevus syndrome. Arch Dermatol. 121(10):1282–5. PMID:4037821
**684.** Elmore JG, Barnhill RL, Elder DE, Longton GM, Pepe MS, Reisch LM, et al. (2017). Pathologists' diagnosis of invasive melanoma and melanocytic proliferations: observer accuracy and reproducibility study. BMJ. 357:j2813. PMID:28659278
**685.** Emanuel PO, de Vinck D, Waldorf HA, Phelps RG (2007). Recurrent endocrine mucin-producing sweat gland carcinoma. Ann Diagn Pathol. 11(6):448–52. PMID:18022131
**686.** Emile JF, Abla O, Fraitag S, Horne A, Haroche J, Donadieu J, et al. (2016). Revised classification of histiocytoses and neoplasms of the macrophage-dendritic cell lineages. Blood. 127(22):2672–81. PMID:26966089
**687.** Emile JF, Diamond EL, Hélias-Rodzewicz Z, Cohen-Aubart F, Charlotte F, Hyman DM, et al. (2014). Recurrent RAS and PIK3CA mutations in Erdheim-Chester disease. Blood. 124(19):3016–9. PMID:25150293
**688.** Emory TS, Scheithauer BW, Hirose T, Wood M, Onofrio BM, Jenkins RB (1995). Intraneural perineurioma. A clonal neoplasm associated with abnormalities of chromosome 22. Am J Clin Pathol. 103(6):696–704. PMID:7785653
**689.** Endly DC, Weenig RH, Peters MS, Viswanatha DS, Comfere NI (2013). Indolent course of cutaneous gamma-delta T-cell lymphoma. J Cutan Pathol. 40(10):896–902. PMID:23379625
**690.** Engels EA, Frisch M, Goedert JJ, Biggar RJ, Miller RW (2002). Merkel cell carcinoma and HIV infection. Lancet. 359(9305):497–8. PMID:11853800
**691.** Enjolras O, Mulliken JB (1997). Vascular tumors and vascular malformations (new issues). Adv Dermatol. 13:375–423. PMID:9551150
**692.** Enjolras O, Mulliken JB, Boon LM, Wassef M, Kozakewich HP, Burrows PE (2001). Noninvoluting congenital hemangioma: a rare cutaneous vascular anomaly. Plast Reconstr Surg. 107(7):1647–54. PMID:11391180
**693.** Enjolras O, Mulliken JB, Wassef M, Frieden IJ, Rieu PN, Burrows PE, et al. (2000). Residual lesions after Kasabach-Merritt phenomenon in 41 patients. J Am Acad Dermatol. 42(2 Pt 1):225–35. PMID:10642677
**694.** Enzinger FM (1965). Clear-cell sarcoma of tendons and aponeuroses. An analysis of 21 cases. Cancer. 18(9):1163–74. PMID:14332545
**695.** Enzinger FM (1970). Epitheloid sarcoma. A sarcoma simulating a granuloma or a carcinoma. Cancer. 26(5):1029–41. PMID:5476785
**696.** Enzinger FM, Harvey DA (1975). Spindle cell lipoma. Cancer. 36(5):1852–9. PMID:1192370
**697.** Enzinger FM, Zhang RY (1988). Plexiform fibrohistiocytic tumor presenting in children and young adults. An analysis of 65 cases. Am J Surg Pathol. 12(11):818–26. PMID:2847569
**698.** Epelman S, Lavine KJ, Randolph GJ (2014). Origin and functions of tissue macrophages. Immunity. 41(1):21–35. PMID:25035951
**699.** Epinette WW, Norins AL, Drew AL, Zeman W, Patel V (1973). Angiokeratoma corporis diffusum with alpha-L-fucosidase deficiency. Arch Dermatol. 107(5):754–7. PMID:4634000
**700.** Erickson C, Miller SJ (2010). Treatment options in melanoma in situ: topical and radiation therapy, excision and Mohs surgery. Int J Dermatol. 49(5):482–91. PMID:20534080
**701.** Erickson-Johnson MR, Chou MM, Evers BR, Roth CW, Seys AR, Jin L, et al. (2011). Nodular fasciitis: a novel model of transient neoplasia induced by MYH9-USP6 gene fusion. Lab Invest. 91(10):1427–33. PMID:21826056
**702.** Erickson-Johnson MR, Seys AR, Roth CW, King AA, Hulshizer RL, Wang X, et al. (2009). Carboxypeptidase M: a biomarker for the discrimination of well-differentiated liposarcoma from lipoma. Mod Pathol. 22(12):1541–7. PMID:19820690
**703.** Errani C, Zhang L, Sung YS, Hajdu M, Singer S, Maki RG, et al. (2011). A novel WWTR1-CAMTA1 gene fusion is a consistent abnormality in epithelioid hemangioendothelioma of different anatomic sites. Genes Chromosomes Cancer. 50(8):644–53. PMID:21584898
**704.** Erverdi N, Terzier C, Bostanci B, Kulaçoğlu S (1995). Extra-ocular sebaceous gland carcinoma. Eur J Cancer. 31A(9):1546. PMID:7577087
**705.** Escalonilla P, Requena L (1996). Plaque variant of trichoblastic fibroma. Arch Dermatol. 132(11):1388–90. PMID:8915324
**706.** Escribano L, Orfao A, Díaz-Agustin B, Villarrubia J, Cerveró C, López A, et al. (1998). Indolent systemic mast cell disease in adults: immunophenotypic characterization of bone marrow mast cells and its diagnostic implications. Blood. 91(8):2731–6. PMID:9531582
**707.** Eskelin S, Kivelä T (2002). Mode of presentation and time to treatment of uveal melanoma in Finland. Br J Ophthalmol. 86(3):333–8. PMID:11864894
**708.** Esmaeli B, Roberts D, Ross M, Fellman M, Cruz H, Kim SK, et al. (2012). Histologic features of conjunctival melanoma predictive of metastasis and death (an American Ophthalmological thesis). Trans Am Ophthalmol Soc. 110: 64–73. PMID:23818735
**709.** Estela JR, Rico MT, Pérez A, Unamuno B, Garcías J, Cubells L, et al. (2014). Dermatofibroma of the face: a clinicopathologic study of

20 cases. Actas Dermosifiliogr. 105(2):172–7. PMID:24275565
**710.** Estrada-Veras JI, O'Brien KJ, Boyd LC, Dave RH, Durham B, Xi L, et al. (2017). The clinical spectrum of Erdheim-Chester disease: an observational cohort study. Blood Adv. 1(6):357–66. PMID:28553668
**711.** Estrozi B, Sanches JA Jr, Varela PC, Bacchi CE (2009). Primary cutaneous blastoid mantle cell lymphoma-case report. Am J Dermatopathol. 31(4):398–400. PMID:19461249
**712.** Etzkorn JR, Sobanko JF, Elenitsas R, Newman JG, Goldbach H, Shin TM, et al. (2015). Low recurrence rates for in situ and invasive melanomas using Mohs micrographic surgery with melanoma antigen recognized by T cells 1 (MART-1) immunostaining: tissue processing methodology to optimize pathologic staging and margin assessment. J Am Acad Dermatol. 72(5):840–50. PMID:25774012
**713.** Evangelista MT, North JP (2015). Comparative analysis of cytokeratin 15, TDAG51, cytokeratin 20 and androgen receptor in sclerosing adnexal neoplasms and variants of basal cell carcinoma. J Cutan Pathol. 42(11):824–31. PMID:26016446
**714.** Evangelista MT, North JP (2017). MYB, CD117 and SOX-10 expression in cutaneous adnexal tumors. J Cutan Pathol. 44(5):444–50. PMID:28098399
**715.** Evans DG, Howard E, Giblin C, Clancy T, Spencer H, Huson SM, et al. (2010). Birth incidence and prevalence of tumor-prone syndromes: estimates from a UK family genetic register service. Am J Med Genet A. 152A(2):327–32. PMID:20082463
**716.** Evans DG, Ladusans EJ, Rimmer S, Burnell LD, Thakker N, Farndon PA (1993). Complications of the naevoid basal cell carcinoma syndrome: results of a population based study. J Med Genet. 30(6):460–4. PMID:8326488
**717.** Evans HL (1979). Liposarcoma: a study of 55 cases with a reassessment of its classification. Am J Surg Pathol. 3(6):507–23. PMID:534388
**718.** Evans HL (1995). Desmoplastic fibroblastoma. A report of seven cases. Am J Surg Pathol. 19(9):1077–81. PMID:7661281
**719.** Evans HL (2002). Multinucleated giant cells in plantar fibromatosis. Am J Surg Pathol. 26(2):244–8. PMID:11812947
**720.** Evans HL (2007). Atypical lipomatous tumor, its variants, and its combined forms: a study of 61 cases, with a minimum follow-up of 10 years. Am J Surg Pathol. 31(1):1–14. PMID:17197914
**721.** Evans HL, Winkelmann RK, Banks PM (1979). Differential diagnosis of malignant and benign cutaneous lymphoid infiltrates: a study of 57 cases in which malignant lymphoma had been diagnosed or suspected in the skin. Cancer. 44(2):699–717. PMID:582573
**722.** Evans MJ, Gray ES, Blessing K (1998). Histopathological features of acral melanocytic nevi in children: study of 21 cases. Pediatr Dev Pathol. 1(5):388–92. PMID:9688763
**723.** Everett JN, Raymond VM, Dandapani M, Marvin M, Kohlmann W, Chittenden A, et al. (2014). Screening for germline mismatch repair mutations following diagnosis of sebaceous neoplasm. JAMA Dermatol. 150(12):1315–21. PMID:25006859
**724.** Exner JH, Dahod S, Pochi PE (1983). Pyogenic granuloma-like acne lesions during isotretinoin therapy. Arch Dermatol. 119(10):808–11. PMID:6225396
**725.** Fabrizi G, Pagliarello C, Parente P, Massi G (2007). Atypical nevi of the scalp in adolescents. J Cutan Pathol. 34(5):365–9. PMID:17448189
**726.** Fabrizi G, Pennacchia I, Pagliarello C, Massi G (2008). Sclerosing nevus with pseudomelanomatous features. J Cutan Pathol. 35(11):995–1002. PMID:18537860
**727.** Facchetti F, Pileri SA, Agostinelli C, Martelli MP, Paulli M, Venditti A, et al. (2009). Cytoplasmic nucleophosmin is not detected in blastic plasmacytoid dendritic cell neoplasm. Haematologica. 94(2):285–8. PMID:19066330
**728.** Facchetti F, Pileri SA, Lorenzi L, Tabanelli V, Rimsza L, Pittaluga S, et al. (2017). Histiocytic and dendritic cell neoplasms: what have we learnt by studying 67 cases. Virchows Arch. 471(4):467–89. PMID:28695297
**729.** Falchi M, Bataille V, Hayward NK, Duffy DL, Bishop JA, Pastinen T, et al. (2009). Genome-wide association study identifies variants at 9p21 and 22q13 associated with development of cutaneous nevi. Nat Genet. 41(8):915–9. PMID:19578365
**730.** Falini B, Lenze D, Hasserjian R, Coupland S, Jaehne D, Soupir C, et al. (2007). Cytoplasmic mutated nucleophosmin (NPM) defines the molecular status of a significant fraction of myeloid sarcomas. Leukemia. 21(7):1566–70. PMID:17443224
**731.** Fan Y, Lee S, Wu G, Easton J, Yergeau D, Dummer R, et al. (2016). Telomerase expression by aberrant methylation of the TERT promoter in melanoma arising in giant congenital nevi. J Invest Dermatol. 136(1):339–42. PMID:26763461
**732.** Fan YS, Carr RA, Sanders DS, Smith AP, Lazar AJ, Calonje E (2007). Characteristic Ber-EP4 and EMA expression in sebaceoma is immunohistochemically distinct from basal cell carcinoma. Histopathology. 51(1):80–6. PMID:17593083
**733.** Fanburg JC, Meis-Kindblom JM, Rosenberg AE (1995). Multiple enchondromas associated with spindle-cell hemangioendotheliomas. An overlooked variant of Maffucci's syndrome. Am J Surg Pathol. 19(9):1029–38. PMID:7661276
**734.** Fanburg-Smith JC, Devaney KO, Miettinen M, Weiss SW (1998). Multiple spindle cell lipomas: a report of 7 familial and 11 nonfamilial cases. Am J Surg Pathol. 22(1):40–8. PMID:9422314
**735.** Fanburg-Smith JC, Meis-Kindblom JM, Fante R, Kindblom LG (1998). Malignant granular cell tumor of soft tissue: diagnostic criteria and clinicopathologic correlation. Am J Surg Pathol. 22(7):779–94. PMID:9669341
**736.** Fanburg-Smith JC, Spiro IJ, Katapuram SV, Mankin HJ, Rosenberg AE (1999). Infiltrative subcutaneous malignant fibrous histiocytoma: a comparative study with deep malignant fibrous histiocytoma and an observation of biologic behavior. Ann Diagn Pathol. 3(1):1–10. PMID:9990107
**737.** Fang J, Dagenais SL, Erickson RP, Arlt MF, Glynn MW, Gorski JL, et al. (2000). Mutations in FOXC2 (MFH-1), a forkhead family transcription factor, are responsible for the hereditary lymphedema-distichiasis syndrome. Am J Hum Genet. 67(6):1382–8. PMID:11078474
**738.** Fargnoli MC, Suppa M, Micantonio T, Antonini A, Tambone S, Peris K (2014). Dermoscopic features and follow-up changes of acral melanocytic naevi in childhood and adolescence. Br J Dermatol. 170(2):374–81. PMID:24125566
**739.** Fariña MC, Piqué E, Olivares M, Escalonilla P, Martín L, Requena L, et al. (1995). Multiple hidrocystoma of the face: three cases. Clin Exp Dermatol. 20(4):323–7. PMID:8548991
**740.** Farrahi F, Egbert BM, Swetter SM (2005). Histologic similarities between lentigo maligna and dysplastic nevus: importance of clinicopathologic distinction. J Cutan Pathol. 32(6):405–12. PMID:15953373
**741.** Fava P, Stroppiana E, Savoia P, Bernengo MG (2010). Halo nevi related to treatment with imatinib in a dermatofibrosarcoma protuberans patient. J Eur Acad Dermatol Venereol. 24(2):244–5. PMID:19694892
**742.** Fedele M, Battista S, Manfioletti G, Croce CM, Giancotti V, Fusco A (2001). Role of the high mobility group A proteins in human lipomas. Carcinogenesis. 22(10):1583–91. PMID:11576996
**743.** Federico M, Rudiger T, Bellei M, Nathwani BN, Luminari S, Coiffier B, et al. (2013). Clinicopathologic characteristics of angioimmunoblastic T-cell lymphoma: analysis of the international peripheral T-cell lymphoma project. J Clin Oncol. 31(2):240–6. PMID:22869878
**744.** Feibleman CE, Stoll H, Maize JC (1980). Melanomas of the palm, sole, and nailbed: a clinicopathologic study. Cancer. 46(11):2492–504. PMID:7438021
**745.** Feldman AL (2013). Clonal relationships between malignant lymphomas and histiocytic/dendritic cell tumors. Surg Pathol Clin. 6(4):619–29. PMID:26839189
**746.** Feldman AL, Berthold F, Arceci RJ, Abramowsky C, Shehata BM, Mann KP, et al. (2005). Clonal relationship between precursor T-lymphoblastic leukaemia/lymphoma and Langerhans-cell histiocytosis. Lancet Oncol. 6(6):435–7. PMID:15925822
**747.** Feng CJ, Ma H, Liao WC (2015). Superficial or cutaneous malignant peripheral nerve sheath tumor–clinical experience at Taipei Veterans General Hospital. Ann Plast Surg. 74 Suppl 2:S85–8. PMID:25695445
**748.** Feng S, Jin P, Zeng X (2008). Hydroa vacciniforme-like primary cutaneous CD8-positive T-cell lymphoma. Eur J Dermatol. 18(3):364–5. PMID:18474490
**749.** Ferguson-Smith MA, Goudie DR (2014). Digenic/multilocus aetiology of multiple self-healing squamous epithelioma (Ferguson-Smith disease): TGFBR1 and a second linked locus. Int J Biochem Cell Biol. 53:520–5. PMID:24747516
**750.** Fernandez AP, Sun Y, Tubbs RR, Goldblum JR, Billings SD (2012). FISH for MYC amplification and anti-MYC immunohistochemistry: useful diagnostic tools in the assessment of secondary angiosarcoma and atypical vascular proliferations. J Cutan Pathol. 39(2):234–42. PMID:22121953
**751.** Fernandez-Figueras MT, Michal M, Kazakov DV (2010). Mammary-type tubulolobular carcinoma of anogenital mammary-like glands with prominent stromal elastosis. Am J Surg Pathol. 34(8):1224–6. PMID:20505503
**752.** Fernandez-Flores A (2009). Irritated seborrheic keratosis with coarse keratohyalin granules. Rom J Morphol Embryol. 50(4):583–7. PMID:19942951
**753.** Fernandez-Flores A (2012). Eponyms, morphology, and pathogenesis of some less mentioned types of melanocytic nevi. Am J Dermatopathol. 34(6):607–18. PMID:22699863
**754.** Fernandez-Flores A, Cassarino DS (2015). Endocrine mucin-producing sweat gland carcinoma: a study of three cases and CK8, CK18 and CD5/6 immunoexpression. J Cutan Pathol. 42(8):578–86. PMID:25925290
**755.** Fernandez-Flores A, Cassarino DS (2017). Histopathological diagnosis of acral lentiginous melanoma in early stages. Ann Diagn Pathol. 26:64–9. PMID:27601330
**756.** Fernandez-Flores A, Cassarino DS, Riveiro-Falkenbach E, Rodriguez-Peralto JL, Fernandez-Figueras MT, Monteagudo C (2017). Cutaneous dermal non-neural granular cell tumor is a granular cell dermal root sheath fibroma. J Cutan Pathol. 44(6):582–7. PMID:28266050
**757.** Fernandez-Flores A, Saeb-Lima M (2014). The inflammatory infiltrate of melanocytic nevus. Rom J Morphol Embryol. 55(4):1277–85. PMID:25611257
**758.** Fernández-Guarino M, Boixeda P, de Las Heras E, Aboin S, García-Millán C, Olasolo PJ (2008). Phakomatosis pigmentovascularis: clinical findings in 15 patients and review of the literature. J Am Acad Dermatol. 58(1):88–93. PMID:18045734
**759.** Ferneiny M, Pansé I, Schartz N, Battistella M, Verola O, Morel P, et al. (2012). Disseminated perinaevic Meyerson phenomenon revealing melanoma. Ann Dermatol Venereol. 139(2):137–41. [French] PMID:22325754
**760.** Ferrara G, Cusano F, Robson A, Stefanato CM (2011). Primary cutaneous marginal zone B-cell lymphoma with anetoderma: spontaneous involution plus de novo clonal expansion. J Cutan Pathol. 38(4):342–5. PMID:21219395
**761.** Ferreiro JA, Carney JA (1994). Myxomas of the external ear and their significance. Am J Surg Pathol. 18(3):274–80. PMID:8116795
**762.** Ferrell RE (2002). Research perspectives in inherited lymphatic disease. Ann N Y Acad Sci. 979(1):39–51, discussion 76–9. PMID:12543715
**763.** Ferrell RE, Levinson KL, Esman JH, Kimak MA, Lawrence EC, Barmada MM, et al. (1998). Hereditary lymphedema: evidence for linkage and genetic heterogeneity. Hum Mol Genet. 7(13):2073–8. PMID:9817924
**764.** Ferreri AJ, Dognini GP, Bairey O, Szomor A, Montalbán C, Horvath B, et al. (2008). The addition of rituximab to anthracycline-based chemotherapy significantly improves outcome in 'Western' patients with intravascular large B-cell lymphoma. Br J Haematol. 143(2):253–7. PMID:18699850
**765.** Ferreri AJ, Dognini GP, Campo E, Willemze R, Seymour JF, Bairey O, et al. (2007). Variations in clinical presentation, frequency of hemophagocytosis and clinical behavior of intravascular lymphoma diagnosed in different geographical regions. Haematologica. 92(4):486–92. PMID:17488659
**766.** Ferreri AJ, Dognini GP, Govi S, Crocchiolo R, Bouzani M, Bollinger CR, et al. (2008). Can rituximab change the usually dismal prognosis of patients with intravascular large B-cell lymphoma? J Clin Oncol. 26(31):5134–7. PMID:18838697
**767.** Ferry JA, Harris NL, Picker LJ, Weinberg DS, Rosales RK, Tapia J, et al. (1988). Intravascular lymphomatosis (malignant angioendotheliomatosis). A B-cell neoplasm expressing surface homing receptors. Mod Pathol. 1(6):444–52. PMID:3065781
**768.** Fetsch JF, Laskin WB, Hallman JR, Lupton GP, Miettinen M (2007). Neurothekeoma: an analysis of 178 tumors with detailed immunohistochemical data and long-term patient follow-up information. Am J Surg Pathol. 31(7):1103–14. PMID:17592278
**769.** Fetsch JF, Laskin WB, Miettinen M (2001). Superficial acral fibromyxoma: a clinicopathologic and immunohistochemical analysis of 37 cases of a distinctive soft tissue tumor with a predilection for the fingers and toes. Hum Pathol. 32(7):704–14. PMID:11486169
**770.** Fetsch JF, Laskin WB, Miettinen M (2005). Nerve sheath myxoma: a clinicopathologic and immunohistochemical analysis of 57 morphologically distinctive, S-100 protein- and GFAP-positive, myxoid peripheral nerve sheath tumors with a predilection for the extremities and a high local recurrence rate. Am J Surg Pathol. 29(12):1615–24. PMID:16327434
**771.** Fetsch JF, Laskin WB, Miettinen M (2005). Palmar-plantar fibromatosis in children and preadolescents: a clinicopathologic study of 56 cases with newly recognized demographics and extended follow-up information. Am J Surg Pathol. 29(8):1095–105. PMID:16006806
**772.** Fetsch JF, Laskin WB, Tavassoli FA

(1997). Superficial angiomyxoma (cutaneous myxoma): a clinicopathologic study of 17 cases arising in the genital region. Int J Gynecol Pathol. 16(4):325–34. PMID:9421071
**773.** Fetsch JF, Michal M, Miettinen M (2000). Pigmented (melanotic) neurofibroma: a clinicopathologic and immunohistochemical analysis of 19 lesions from 17 patients. Am J Surg Pathol. 24(3):331–43. PMID:10716146
**774.** Fetsch JF, Miettinen M (1997). Sclerosing perineurioma: a clinicopathologic study of 19 cases of a distinctive soft tissue lesion with a predilection for the fingers and palms of young adults. Am J Surg Pathol. 21(12):1433–42. PMID:9414186
**775.** Fetsch JF, Miettinen M (1998). Calcifying aponeurotic fibroma: a clinicopathologic study of 22 cases arising in uncommon sites. Hum Pathol. 29(12):1504–10. PMID:9865839
**776.** Fetsch JF, Weiss SW (1991). Observations concerning the pathogenesis of epithelioid hemangioma (angiolymphoid hyperplasia). Mod Pathol. 4(4):449–55. PMID:1924276
**777.** Feuillard J, Jacob MC, Valensi F, Maynadié M, Gressin R, Chaperot L, et al. (2002). Clinical and biologic features of CD4(+) CD56(+) malignancies. Blood. 99(5):1556–63. PMID:11861268
**778.** Fields RC, Busam KJ, Chou JF, Panageas KS, Pulitzer MP, Allen PJ, et al. (2011). Five hundred patients with Merkel cell carcinoma evaluated at a single institution. Ann Surg. 254(3):465–75. PMID:21865945
**779.** Fierro MT, Comessatti A, Quaglino P, Ortoncelli M, Osella Abate S, Ponti R, et al. (2006). Expression pattern of chemokine receptors and chemokine release in inflammatory erythroderma and Sézary syndrome. Dermatology. 213(4):284–92. PMID:17135733
**780.** Fink-Puches R, Chott A, Ardigó M, Simonitsch I, Ferrara G, Kerl H, et al. (2004). The spectrum of cutaneous lymphomas in patients less than 20 years of age. Pediatr Dermatol. 21(5):525–33. PMID:15461755
**781.** Finley AG, Musso LA (1972). Naevus lipomatosus cutaneus superficialis (Hoffman-Zurhelle). Br J Dermatol. 87(6):557–64. PMID:4648802
**782.** Fisher KR, Maize JC Jr, Maize JC Sr (2013). Histologic features of scalp melanocytic nevi. J Am Acad Dermatol. 68(3):466–72. PMID:23267721
**783.** Fitzgerald TL, Dennis S, Kachare SD, Vohra NA, Wong JH, Zervos EE (2015). Dramatic increase in the incidence and mortality from Merkel cell carcinoma in the United States. Am Surg. 81(8):802–6. PMID:26215243
**784.** Flanagan BP, Helwig EB (1977). Cutaneous lymphangioma. Arch Dermatol. 113(1):24–30. PMID:831620
**785.** Flann S, Orchard GE, Wain EM, Russell-Jones R (2006). Three cases of lymphomatoid papulosis with a CD56+ immunophenotype. J Am Acad Dermatol. 55(5):903–6. PMID:17052504
**786.** Fletcher CD (1989). Solitary circumscribed neuroma of the skin (so-called palisaded, encapsulated neuroma). A clinicopathologic and immunohistochemical study. Am J Surg Pathol. 13(7):574–80. PMID:2660609
**787.** Fletcher CD, Akerman M, Dal Cin P, de Wever I, Mandahl N, Mertens F, et al. (1996). Correlation between clinicopathological features and karyotype in lipomatous tumors. A report of 178 cases from the Chromosomes and Morphology (CHAMP) Collaborative Study Group. Am J Pathol. 148(2):623–30. PMID:8579124
**788.** Fletcher CD, Beham A, Bekir S, Clarke AM, Marley NJ (1991). Epithelioid angiosarcoma of deep soft tissue: a distinctive tumor readily mistaken for an epithelial neoplasm. Am J Surg Pathol. 15(10):915–24. PMID:1718176
**789.** Fletcher CD, Beham A, Schmid C (1991). Spindle cell haemangioendothelioma: a clinicopathological and immunohistochemical study indicative of a non-neoplastic lesion. Histopathology. 18(4):291–301. PMID:2071088
**790.** Fletcher CD, Davies SE, McKee PH (1987). Cellular schwannoma: a distinct pseudosarcomatous entity. Histopathology. 11(1):21–35. PMID:3557324
**791.** Fletcher CD, Martin-Bates E (1987). Spindle cell lipoma: a clinicopathological study with some original observations. Histopathology. 11(8):803–17. PMID:3623439
**792.** Fletcher CDM, Bridge JA, Hogendoorn PCW, Mertens F, editors (2013). WHO classification of tumours of soft tissue and bone. 4th ed. Lyon: International Agency for Research on Cancer.
**793.** Flieder A, Koerner FC, Pilch BZ, Maluf HM (1997). Endocrine mucin-producing sweat gland carcinoma: a cutaneous neoplasm analogous to solid papillary carcinoma of breast. Am J Surg Pathol. 21(12):1501–6. PMID:9414195
**794.** Florez-Vargas A, Vargas SO, Debelenko LV, Perez-Atayde AR, Archibald T, Kozakewich HP, et al. (2008). Comparative analysis of D2-40 and LYVE-1 immunostaining in lymphatic malformations. Lymphology. 41(3):103–10. PMID:19013877
**795.** Flucke U, Palmedo G, Blankenhorn N, Slootweg PJ, Kutzner H, Mentzel T (2011). EWSR1 gene rearrangement occurs in a subset of cutaneous myoepithelial tumors: a study of 18 cases. Mod Pathol. 24(11):1444–50. PMID:21725291
**796.** Flucke U, van Krieken JH, Mentzel T (2011). Cellular angiofibroma: analysis of 25 cases emphasizing its relationship to spindle cell lipoma and mammary-type myofibroblastoma. Mod Pathol. 24(1):82–9. PMID:20852591
**797.** Flucke U, Vogels RJ, de Saint Aubain Somerhausen N, Creytens DH, Riedl RG, van Gorp JM, et al. (2014). Epithelioid hemangioendothelioma: clinicopathologic, immunhistochemical, and molecular genetic analysis of 39 cases. Diagn Pathol. 9(1):131. PMID:24986479
**798.** Flux K (2017). Sebaceous neoplasms. Surg Pathol Clin. 10(2):367–82. PMID:28477886
**799.** Flux K, Brenn T (2017). Cutaneous sweat gland carcinomas with basaloid differentiation: an update with emphasis on differential diagnoses. Clin Lab Med. 37(3):587–601. PMID:28802502
**800.** Flux K, Kutzner H, Rütten A, Plaza JA, Gasparov S, Michal M, et al. (2016). Infundibulocystic structures and prominent squamous metaplasia in sebaceoma-a rare feature. A clinicopathologic study of 10 cases. Am J Dermatopathol. 38(9):678–82. PMID:26760686
**801.** Fogel AL, Sarin KY, Teng JMC (2017). Genetic diseases associated with an increased risk of skin cancer development in childhood. Curr Opin Pediatr. 29(4):426–33. PMID:28525403
**802.** Folberg R, Hendrix MJ, Maniotis AJ (2000). Vasculogenic mimicry and tumor angiogenesis. Am J Pathol. 156(2):361–81. PMID:10666364
**803.** Folberg R, Jakobiec FA, Bernardino VB, Iwamoto T (1989). Benign conjunctival melanocytic lesions. Clinicopathologic features. Ophthalmology. 96(4):436–61. PMID:2657539
**804.** Folberg R, McLean IW, Zimmerman LE (1985). Primary acquired melanosis of the conjunctiva. Hum Pathol. 16(2):129–35. PMID:3972395
**805.** Folpe AL, Billings SD, McKenney JK, Walsh SV, Nusrat A, Weiss SW (2002). Expression of claudin-1, a recently described tight junction-associated protein, distinguishes soft tissue perineurioma from potential mimics. Am J Surg Pathol. 26(12):1620–6. PMID:12459629
**806.** Folpe AL, Chand EM, Goldblum JR, Weiss SW (2001). Expression of Fli-1, a nuclear transcription factor, distinguishes vascular neoplasms from potential mimics. Am J Surg Pathol. 25(8):1061–6. PMID:11474291
**807.** Folpe AL, Fanburg-Smith JC, Miettinen M, Weiss SW (2001). Atypical and malignant glomus tumors: analysis of 52 cases, with a proposal for the reclassification of glomus tumors. Am J Surg Pathol. 25(1):1–12. PMID:11145243
**808.** Folpe AL, Goldblum JR, Rubin BP, Shehata BM, Liu W, Dei Tos AP, et al. (2005). Morphologic and immunophenotypic diversity in Ewing family tumors: a study of 66 genetically confirmed cases. Am J Surg Pathol. 29(8):1025–33. PMID:16006796
**809.** Folpe AL, Hill CE, Parham DM, O'Shea PA, Weiss SW (2000). Immunohistochemical detection of FLI-1 protein expression: a study of 132 round cell tumors with emphasis on CD99-positive mimics of Ewing's sarcoma/primitive neuroectodermal tumor. Am J Surg Pathol. 24(12):1657–62. PMID:11117787
**810.** Font RL, Stone MS, Schanzer MC, Lewis RA (1986). Apocrine hidrocystomas of the lids, hypodontia, palmar-plantar hyperkeratosis, and onychodystrophy. A new variant of ectodermal dysplasia. Arch Ophthalmol. 104(12):1811–3. PMID:2947556
**811.** Forlino A, Vetro A, Garavelli L, Ciccone R, London E, Stratakis CA, et al. (2014). PRKACB and Carney complex. N Engl J Med. 370(11):1065–7. PMID:24571725
**812.** Forman SB, Tyler WB, Ferringer TC, Elston DM (2007). Glomeruloid hemangiomas without POEMS syndrome: series of three cases. J Cutan Pathol. 34(12):956–7. PMID:18001423
**813.** Formicone F, Fargnoli MC, Pisani F, Rascente M, Famulari A, Peris K (2005). Cutaneous manifestations in Italian kidney transplant recipients. Transplant Proc. 37(6):2527–8. PMID:16182734
**814.** Foss HD, Herbst H, Araujo I, Hummel M, Berg E, Schmitt-Gräff A, et al. (1996). Monokine expression in Langerhans' cell histiocytosis and sinus histiocytosis with massive lymphadenopathy (Rosai-Dorfman disease). J Pathol. 179(1):60–5. PMID:8691347
**815.** Foster R, Byrnes E, Meldrum C, Griffith R, Ross G, Upjohn E, et al. (2008). Association of paediatric mastocytosis with a polymorphism resulting in an amino acid substitution (M541L) in the transmembrane domain of c-KIT. Br J Dermatol. 159(5):1160–9. PMID:18795925
**816.** Fouilloux B, Perrin C, Dutoit M, Cambazard F (2001). Clear cell syringofibroadenoma (of Mascaro) of the nail. Br J Dermatol. 144(3):625–7. PMID:11260030
**817.** Fox JC, Reed JA, Shea CR (2011). The recurrent nevus phenomenon: a history of challenge, controversy, and discovery. Arch Pathol Lab Med. 135(7):842–6. PMID:21732772
**818.** Fox MD, Gleason BC, Thomas AB, Victor TA, Cibull TL (2010). Extra-acral cutaneous/soft tissue sclerosing perineurioma: an under-recognized entity in the differential of CD34-positive cutaneous neoplasms. J Cutan Pathol. 37(10):1053–6. PMID:20412342
**819.** Fraga GR, Amin SM (2014). Large cell acanthoma: a variant of solar lentigo with cellular hypertrophy. J Cutan Pathol. 41(9):733–9. PMID:24917472
**820.** Franceschini D, Dinulos JG (2015). Dermal melanocytosis and associated disorders. Curr Opin Pediatr. 27(4):480–5. PMID:26087431
**821.** Franke FE, Steger K, Marks A, Kutzner H, Mentzel T (2004). Hobnail hemangiomas (targetoid hemosiderotic hemangiomas) are true lymphangiomas. J Cutan Pathol. 31(5):362–7. PMID:15059220
**822.** Frater JL, Maddox JS, Obadiah JM, Hurley MY (2006). Cutaneous Rosai-Dorfman disease: comprehensive review of cases reported in the medical literature since 1990 and presentation of an illustrative case. J Cutan Med Surg. 10(6):281–90. PMID:17241598
**823.** French CA, Mentzel T, Kutzner H, Fletcher CD (2000). Intradermal spindle cell/pleomorphic lipoma: a distinct subset. Am J Dermatopathol. 22(6):496–502. PMID:11190440
**824.** Freyer DR, Kennedy R, Bostrom BC, Kohut G, Dehner LP (1996). Juvenile xanthogranuloma: forms of systemic disease and their clinical implications. J Pediatr. 129(2):227–37. PMID:8765620
**825.** Friedman JM (1999). Epidemiology of neurofibromatosis type 1. Am J Med Genet. 89(1):1–6. PMID:10469430
**826.** Friedman PM, Friedman RH, Jiang SB, Nouri K, Amonette R, Robins P (1999). Microcystic adnexal carcinoma: collaborative series review and update. J Am Acad Dermatol. 41(2 Pt 1):225–31. PMID:10426893
**826A.** Fritz A, Percy C, Jack A, Shanmugaratnam K, Sobin L, Parkin DM, et al., editors (2013). International classification of diseases for oncology (ICD-O). 3rd ed. 1st revision. Geneva: World Health Organization.
**827.** Frost C, Williams G, Green A (2000). High incidence and regression rates of solar keratoses in a Queensland community. J Invest Dermatol. 115(2):273–7. PMID:10951246
**828.** Frost MW, Steiniche T, Damsgaard TE, Stolle LB (2014). Primary cutaneous myoepithelial carcinoma: a case report and review of the literature. APMIS. 122(5):369–79. PMID:23992447
**829.** Frouin E, Vignon-Pennamen MD, Balme B, Cavelier-Balloy B, Zimmermann U, Ortonne N, et al. (2015). Anatomoclinical study of 30 cases of sclerosing sweat duct carcinomas (microcystic adnexal carcinoma, syringomatous carcinoma and squamoid eccrine ductal carcinoma). J Eur Acad Dermatol Venereol. 29(10):1978–94. PMID:25873411
**830.** Fryssira H, Leventopoulos G, Psoni S, Kitsiou-Tzeli S, Stavrianeas N, Kanavakis E (2008). Tumor development in three patients with Noonan syndrome. Eur J Pediatr. 167(9):1025–31. PMID:18057963
**831.** Fu JM, McCalmont T, Yu SS (2009). Adenosquamous carcinoma of the skin: a case series. Arch Dermatol. 145(10):1152–8. PMID:19841403
**832.** Fu L, Lau S, Roy I, Ferenczy A (2011). Phyllodes tumor with malignant stromal morphology of the vulva: a case report and review of the literature. Int J Gynecol Pathol. 30(2):198–202. PMID:21293278
**833.** Fu W, Cockerell CJ (2003). The actinic (solar) keratosis: a 21st-century perspective. Arch Dermatol. 139(1):66–70. PMID:12533168
**834.** Fujiwara M, Morales AV, Seo K, Kim YH, Arber DA, Sundram UN (2013). Clonal identity and differences in primary cutaneous B-cell lymphoma occurring at different sites or time points in the same patient. Am J Dermatopathol. 35(1):11–8. PMID:22588547
**835.** Fujiwara M, Taube J, Sharma M, McCalmont TH, Kim J (2010). PAX8 discriminates ovarian metastases from adnexal tumors and other cutaneous metastases. J Cutan Pathol. 37(9):938–43. PMID:20492080
**836.** Fukunaga M, Suzuki K, Saegusa N, Folpe AL (2007). Composite hemangioendothelioma: report of 5 cases including one with associated Maffucci syndrome. Am J Surg Pathol. 31(10):1567–72. PMID:17895759
**837.** Fullen DR, Lowe L, Su LD (2003). Antibody to S100a6 protein is a sensitive immunohistochemical marker for neurothekeoma. J Cutan Pathol. 30(2):118–22. PMID:12641790
**838.** Furney SJ, Turajlic S, Stamp G, Nohadani

M, Carlisle A, Thomas JM, et al. (2013). Genome sequencing of mucosal melanomas reveals that they are driven by distinct mechanisms from cutaneous melanoma. J Pathol. 230(3):261–9. PMID:23620124

**839.** Furney SJ, Turajlic S, Stamp G, Thomas JM, Hayes A, Strauss D, et al. (2014). The mutational burden of acral melanoma revealed by whole-genome sequencing and comparative analysis. Pigment Cell Melanoma Res. 27(5):835–8. PMID:24913711

**840.** Fusco N, Bonometti A, Augello C, Fabris S, Boiocchi L, Fiori S, et al. (2017). Clonal reticulohistiocytosis of the skin and bone marrow associated with systemic mastocytosis and acute myeloid leukaemia. Histopathology. 70(6):1000–8. PMID:28074480

**841.** Gabillot-Carré M, Weill F, Mamelle G, Kolb F, Boitier F, Petrow P, et al. (2006). Microcystic adnexal carcinoma: report of seven cases including one with lung metastasis. Dermatology. 212(3):221–8. PMID:16549917

**842.** Gallager RL, Helwig EB (1980). Neurothekeoma–a benign cutaneous tumor of neural origin. Am J Clin Pathol. 74(6):759–64. PMID:7446487

**843.** Gallardo F, Bellosillo B, Espinet B, Pujol RM, Estrach T, Servitje O, et al. (2006). Aberrant nuclear BCL10 expression and lack of t(11;18)(q21;q21) in primary cutaneous marginal zone B-cell lymphoma. Hum Pathol. 37(7):867–73. PMID:16784987

**844.** Galyfos G, Karantzikos GA, Kavouras N, Sianou A, Palogos K, Filis K (2016). Extraosseous Ewing sarcoma: diagnosis, prognosis and optimal management. Indian J Surg. 78(1):49–53. PMID:27186040

**845.** Gandini S, Sera F, Cattaruzza MS, Pasquini P, Abeni D, Boyle P, et al. (2005). Meta-analysis of risk factors for cutaneous melanoma: I. Common and atypical naevi. Eur J Cancer. 41(1):28–44. PMID:15617989

**846.** Gandini S, Sera F, Cattaruzza MS, Pasquini P, Zanetti R, Masini C, et al. (2005). Meta-analysis of risk factors for cutaneous melanoma: III. Family history, actinic damage and phenotypic factors. Eur J Cancer. 41(14):2040–59. PMID:16125929

**847.** Garces S, Medeiros LJ, Patel KP, Li S, Pina-Oviedo S, Li J, et al. (2017). Mutually exclusive recurrent KRAS and MAP2K1 mutations in Rosai-Dorfman disease. Mod Pathol. 30(10):1367–77. PMID:28664935

**848.** Garcia C, Crowson AN (2011). Acantholytic squamous cell carcinoma: is it really a more-aggressive tumor? Dermatol Surg. 37(3):353–6. PMID:21410819

**849.** Garcia-Herrera A, Colomo L, Camós M, Carreras J, Balague O, Martinez A, et al. (2008). Primary cutaneous small/medium CD4+ T-cell lymphomas: a heterogeneous group of tumors with different clinicopathologic features and outcome. J Clin Oncol. 26(20):3364–71. PMID:18541895

**850.** Garcia-Herrera A, Song JY, Chuang SS, Villamor N, Colomo L, Pittaluga S, et al. (2011). Nonhepatosplenic γδ T-cell lymphomas represent a spectrum of aggressive cytotoxic T-cell lymphomas with a mainly extranodal presentation. Am J Surg Pathol. 35(8):1214–25. PMID:21753698

**851.** Gardie B, Remenieras A, Kattygnarath D, Bombled J, Lefèvre S, Perrier-Trudova V, et al. (2011). Novel FH mutations in families with hereditary leiomyomatosis and renal cell cancer (HLRCC) and patients with isolated type 2 papillary renal cell carcinoma. J Med Genet. 48(4):226–34. PMID:21398687

**852.** Gardner EW, Miller HM, Lowney ED (1979). Folded skin associated with underlying nevus lipomatosus. Arch Dermatol. 115(8):978–9. PMID:464627

**853.** Gardner JM, Dandekar M, Thomas D, Goldblum JR, Weiss SW, Billings SD, et al. (2012). Cutaneous and subcutaneous pleomorphic liposarcoma: a clinicopathologic study of 29 cases with evaluation of MDM2 gene amplification in 26. Am J Surg Pathol. 36(7):1047–51. PMID:22472959

**854.** Garib G, Siegal GP, Andea AA (2015). Autosomal-dominant familial angiolipomatosis. Cutis. 95(1):E26–9. PMID:25671454

**855.** Garnache-Ottou F, Feuillard J, Saas P (2007). Plasmacytoid dendritic cell leukaemia/lymphoma: towards a well defined entity? Br J Haematol. 136(4):539–48. PMID:17367408

**856.** Garrè ML, Cama A, Bagnasco F, Morana G, Giangaspero F, Brisigotti M, et al. (2009). Medulloblastoma variants: age-dependent occurrence and relation to Gorlin syndrome–a new clinical perspective. Clin Cancer Res. 15(7):2463–71. PMID:19276247

**857.** Garrett AB, Azmi FH, Ogburia KS (2004). Trichilemmal carcinoma: a rare cutaneous malignancy: a report of two cases. Dermatol Surg. 30(1):113–5. PMID:14692940

**858.** Garriga MM, Friedman MM, Metcalfe DD (1988). A survey of the number and distribution of mast cells in the skin of patients with mast cell disorders. J Allergy Clin Immunol. 82(3 Pt 1):425–32. PMID:3170991

**859.** Gaspar N, Hawkins DS, Dirksen U, Lewis IJ, Ferrari S, Le Deley MC, et al. (2015). Ewing sarcoma: current management and future approaches through collaboration. J Clin Oncol. 33(27):3036–46. PMID:26304893

**860.** Gasparini P, Facchinetti F, Boeri M, Lorenzetto E, Livio A, Gronchi A, et al. (2011). Prognostic determinants in epithelioid sarcoma. Eur J Cancer. 47(2):287–95. PMID:20932739

**861.** Gatta G, van der Zwan JM, Casali PG, Siesling S, Dei Tos AP, Kunkler I, et al. (2011). Rare cancers are not so rare: the rare cancer burden in Europe. Eur J Cancer. 47(17):2493–511. PMID:22033323

**862.** Gaulard P, Bourquelot P, Kanavaros P, Haioun C, Le Couedic JP, Divine M, et al. (1990). Expression of the alpha/beta and gamma/delta T-cell receptors in 57 cases of peripheral T-cell lymphomas. Identification of a subset of gamma/delta T-cell lymphomas. Am J Pathol. 137(3):617–28. PMID:1698028

**863.** Gauthier Y, Surléve-Bazeille JE, Texier L (1978). Halo nevi without dermal infiltrate. Arch Dermatol. 114(11):1718. PMID:718234

**864.** Gebhard S, Coindre JM, Michels JJ, Terrier P, Bertrand G, Trassard M, et al. (2002). Pleomorphic liposarcoma: clinicopathologic, immunohistochemical, and follow-up analysis of 63 cases: a study from the French Federation of Cancer Centers Sarcoma Group. Am J Surg Pathol. 26(5):601–16. PMID:11979090

**865.** Gellrich S, Rutz S, Golembowski S, Jacobs C, von Zimmermann M, Lorenz P, et al. (2001). Primary cutaneous follicle center cell lymphomas and large B cell lymphomas of the leg descend from germinal center cells. A single cell polymerase chain reaction analysis. J Invest Dermatol. 117(6):1512–20. PMID:11886516

**866.** Gemer O, Piura B, Segal S, Inbar IY (2003). Adenocarcinoma arising in a chondroid syringoma of vulva. Int J Gynecol Pathol. 22(4):398–400. PMID:14501823

**867.** Cancer Genome Atlas Network (2015). Genomic classification of cutaneous melanoma. Cell. 161(7):1681–96. PMID:26091043

**868.** Georgin-Lavialle S, Lhermitte L, Dubreuil P, Chandesris MO, Hermine O, Damaj G (2013). Mast cell leukemia. Blood. 121(8):1285–95. PMID:23243287

**869.** Gerami P, Busam K, Cochran A, Cook MG, Duncan LM, Elder DE, et al. (2014). Histomorphologic assessment and interobserver diagnostic reproducibility of atypical spitzoid melanocytic neoplasms with long-term follow-up. Am J Surg Pathol. 38(7):934–40. PMID:24618612

**870.** Gerami P, Cooper C, Bajaj S, Wagner A, Fullen D, Busam K, et al. (2013). Outcomes of atypical Spitz tumors with chromosomal copy number aberrations and conventional melanomas in children. Am J Surg Pathol. 37(9):1387–94. PMID:23797719

**871.** Gerami P, Pouryazdanparast P, Vemula S, Bastian BC (2010). Molecular analysis of a case of nevus of Ota showing progressive evolution to melanoma with intermediate stages resembling cellular blue nevus. Am J Dermatopathol. 32(3):301–5. PMID:20110797

**872.** Gerami P, Scolyer RA, Xu X, Elder DE, Abraham RM, Fullen D, et al. (2013). Risk assessment for atypical spitzoid melanocytic neoplasms using FISH to identify chromosomal copy number aberrations. Am J Surg Pathol. 37(5):676–84. PMID:23388126

**873.** Gerami P, Wickless SC, Querfeld C, Rosen ST, Kuzel TM, Guitart J (2010). Cutaneous involvement with marginal zone lymphoma. J Am Acad Dermatol. 63(1):142–5. PMID:20462658

**874.** Gerami P, Wickless SC, Rosen S, Kuzel TM, Ciurea A, Havey J, et al. (2008). Applying the new TNM classification system for primary cutaneous lymphomas other than mycosis fungoides and Sézary syndrome in primary cutaneous marginal zone lymphoma. J Am Acad Dermatol. 59(2):245–54. PMID:18486274

**875.** Gerami P, Yélamos O, Lee CY, Obregon R, Yazdan P, Sholl LM, et al. (2015). Multiple cutaneous melanomas and clinically atypical moles in a patient with a novel germline BAP1 mutation. JAMA Dermatol. 151(11):1235–9. PMID:26154183

**876.** Gerdsen R, Stockfleth E, Uerlich M, Fartasch M, Steen KH, Bieber T (2000). Papular palmoplantar hyperkeratosis following chronic medical exposure to arsenic: human papillomavirus as a co-factor in the pathogenesis of arsenical keratosis? Acta Derm Venereol. 80(4):292–3. PMID:11028865

**877.** Gerner N, Nørregaard JC, Jensen OA, Prause JU (1996). Conjunctival naevi in Denmark 1960-1980. A 21-year follow-up study. Acta Ophthalmol Scand. 74(4):334–7. PMID:8883545

**878.** Gescheidt-Shoshany H, Weltfriend S, Bergman R (2015). Nodular melanoma arising in a large segmental speckled lentiginous nevus. Am J Dermatopathol. 37(8):663–4. PMID:25072686

**879.** Ghadimi MP, Liu P, Peng T, Bolshakov S, Young ED, Torres KE, et al. (2011). Pleomorphic liposarcoma: clinical observations and molecular variables. Cancer. 117(23):5359–69. PMID:21598240

**880.** Giger OT, Lacoste E, Honegger C, Padberg B, Moch H, Varga Z (2007). Expression of the breast differentiation antigen NY-BR-1 in a phyllodes tumor of the vulva. Virchows Arch. 450(4):471–4. PMID:17318573

**881.** Gill PS (2007). The origin of Kaposi sarcoma. J Natl Cancer Inst. 99(14):1063. PMID:17623793

**882.** Gill S, Melosky B, Haley L, ChanYan C (2003). Use of random skin biopsy to diagnose intravascular lymphoma presenting as fever of unknown origin. Am J Med. 114(1):56–8. PMID:12543290

**883.** Gillet NA, Cook L, Laydon DJ, Hlela C, Verdonck K, Alvarez C, et al. (2013). Strongyloidiasis and infective dermatitis alter human T lymphotropic virus-1 clonality in vivo. PLoS Pathog. 9(4):e1003263. PMID:23592987

**884.** Gimotty PA, Elder DE, Fraker DL, Botbyl J, Sellers K, Elenitsas R, et al. (2007). Identification of high-risk patients among those diagnosed with thin cutaneous melanomas. J Clin Oncol. 25(9):1129–34. PMID:17369575

**885.** Ginter PS, Mosquera JM, MacDonald TY, D'Alfonso TM, Rubin MA, Shin SJ (2014). Diagnostic utility of MYC amplification and anti-MYC immunohistochemistry in atypical vascular lesions, primary or radiation-induced mammary angiosarcomas, and primary angiosarcomas of other sites. Hum Pathol. 45(4):709–16. PMID:24457083

**886.** Gleason BC, Calder KB, Cibull TL, Thomas AB, Billings SD, Morgan MB, et al. (2009). Utility of p63 in the differential diagnosis of atypical fibroxanthoma and spindle cell squamous cell carcinoma. J Cutan Pathol. 36(5):543–7. PMID:19476522

**887.** Gleason BC, Fletcher CD (2008). Deep "benign" fibrous histiocytoma: clinicopathologic analysis of 69 cases of a rare tumor indicating occasional metastatic potential. Am J Surg Pathol. 32(3):354–62. PMID:18300816

**888.** Gleason BC, Hirsch MS, Nucci MR, Schmidt BA, Zembowicz A, Mihm MC Jr, et al. (2008). Atypical genital nevi. A clinicopathologic analysis of 56 cases. Am J Surg Pathol. 32(1):51–7. PMID:18162770

**889.** Gleason BC, Nascimento AF (2007). HMB-45 and Melan-A are useful in the differential diagnosis between granular cell tumor and malignant melanoma. Am J Dermatopathol. 29(1):22–7. PMID:17284958

**890.** Glick JB, Alapati U, Khachemoune A (2016). Pilomatrix carcinoma mimicking a pigmented basal cell carcinoma. Skinmed. 14(6):475–7. PMID:28031142

**891.** Globerman H, Burstein S, Girardina PJ, Winchester P, Frankel S (1991). A xanthogranulomatous histiocytosis in a child presenting with short stature. Am J Pediatr Hematol Oncol. 13(1):42–6. PMID:1903027

**892.** Gloor P, Ansari I, Sinard J (1999). Sebaceous carcinoma presenting as a unilateral papillary conjunctivitis. Am J Ophthalmol. 127(4):458–9. PMID:10218701

**893.** Glusac EJ, Barr RJ, Everett MA, Pitha J, Santa Cruz DJ (1994). Epithelioid cell histiocytoma. A report of 10 cases including a new cellular variant. Am J Surg Pathol. 18(6):583–90. PMID:7909998

**894.** Glusac EJ, McNiff JM (1999). Epithelioid cell histiocytoma: a simulant of vascular and melanocytic neoplasms. Am J Dermatopathol. 21(1):1–7. PMID:10027517

**895.** Goecke T, Schulmann K, Engel C, Holinski-Feder E, Pagenstecher C, Schackert HK, et al. (2006). Genotype-phenotype comparison of German MLH1 and MSH2 mutation carriers clinically affected with Lynch syndrome: a report by the German HNPCC Consortium. J Clin Oncol. 24(26):4285–92. PMID:16908935

**896.** Goette DK (1980). Benign lichenoid keratosis. Arch Dermatol. 116(7):780–2. PMID:7396541

**897.** Goette DK (1986). Calcifying neurothekeoma. J Dermatol Surg Oncol. 12(9):958–60. PMID:3745622

**898.** Goette DK, Odom RB, Fitzwater JE Jr (1982). Diffuse cutaneous reticulohistiocytosis. Arch Dermatol. 118(3):173–6. PMID:6950687

**899.** Gogia A, Sharma MC, Bakhshi S (2013). Subcutaneous nodules as initial presentation of Burkitt lymphoma in HIV-negative child. J Pediatr Hematol Oncol. 35(8):e326–8. PMID:23426001

**900.** Goh G, Walradt T, Markarov V, Blom A, Riaz N, Doumani R, et al. (2016). Mutational landscape of MCPyV-positive and MCPyV-negative Merkel cell carcinomas with implications for immunotherapy. Oncotarget. 7(3):3403–15. PMID:26655088

**901.** Goh SG, Dayrit JF, Calonje E (2007).

Sarcomatoid eccrine porocarcinoma: report of two cases and a review of the literature. J Cutan Pathol. 34(1):55–60. PMID:17214856
**902.** Gokalp H, Gurer MA, Alan S (2013). Trichofolliculoma: a rare variant of hair follicle hamartoma. Dermatol Online J. 19(8):19264. PMID:24021443
**903.** Goldblum JR, Beals TF, Weiss SW (1994). Neuroblastoma-like neurilemoma. Am J Surg Pathol. 18(3):266–73. PMID:8116794
**904.** Goldblum JR, Weiss SW, Folpe AL (2013). Enzinger and Weiss's soft tissue tumors. 6th ed. Philadelphia: WB Saunders.
**905.** Goldenberg-Cohen N, Cohen Y, Rosenbaum E, Herscovici Z, Chowers I, Weinberger D, et al. (2005). T1799A BRAF mutations in conjunctival melanocytic lesions. Invest Ophthalmol Vis Sci. 46(9):3027–30. PMID:16123397
**906.** Goldgeier MH, Nordlund JJ, Lucky AW, Sibrack LA, McCarthy MJ, McGuire J (1982). Hydroa vacciniforme: diagnosis and therapy. Arch Dermatol. 118(8):588–91. PMID:7103528
**907.** Goldstein AM, Chan M, Harland M, Hayward NK, Demenais F, Bishop DT, et al. (2007). Features associated with germline CDKN2A mutations: a GenoMEL study of melanoma-prone families from three continents. J Med Genet. 44(2):99–106. PMID:16905682
**908.** Goldstein AM, Tucker MA (2013). Dysplastic nevi and melanoma. Cancer Epidemiol Biomarkers Prev. 22(4):528–32. PMID:23549396
**909.** Goldstein DJ, Barr RJ, Santa Cruz DJ (1982). Microcystic adnexal carcinoma: a distinct clinicopathologic entity. Cancer. 50(3):566–72. PMID:7093897
**910.** Golling P, Cozzio A, Dummer R, French L, Kempf W (2008). Primary cutaneous B-cell lymphomas - clinicopathological, prognostic and therapeutic characterisation of 54 cases according to the WHO-EORTC classification and the ISCL/EORTC TNM classification system for primary cutaneous lymphomas other than mycosis fungoides and Sezary syndrome. Leuk Lymphoma. 49(6):1094–103. PMID:18569636
**911.** Gonzalez CL, Medeiros LJ, Braziel RM, Jaffe ES (1991). T-cell lymphoma involving subcutaneous tissue. A clinicopathologic entity commonly associated with hemophagocytic syndrome. Am J Surg Pathol. 15(1):17–27. PMID:1985499
**912.** González-Guerra E, Haro MR, Fariña MC, Martín L, Manzarbeitia L, Requena L (2009). Glomeruloid haemangioma is not always associated with POEMS syndrome. Clin Exp Dermatol. 34(7):800–3. PMID:19077091
**913.** González-Vela MC, Val-Bernal JF, González-López MA, Drake M, Fernández-Llaca JH (2006). Pure sclerotic neurofibroma: a neurofibroma mimicking sclerotic fibroma. J Cutan Pathol. 33(1):47–50. PMID:16441412
**914.** Goodlad JR (2001). Spindle-cell B-cell lymphoma presenting in the skin. Br J Dermatol. 145(2):313–7. PMID:11531800
**915.** Goodlad JR, Davidson MM, Hollowood K, Ling C, MacKenzie C, Christie I, et al. (2000). Primary cutaneous B-cell lymphoma and Borrelia burgdorferi infection in patients from the Highlands of Scotland. Am J Surg Pathol. 24(9):1279–85. PMID:10976703
**916.** Goodlad JR, Krajewski AS, Batstone PJ, McKay P, White JM, Benton EC, et al. (2002). Primary cutaneous follicular lymphoma: a clinicopathologic and molecular study of 16 cases in support of a distinct entity. Am J Surg Pathol. 26(6):733–41. PMID:12023577
**917.** Goodlad JR, Krajewski AS, Batstone PJ, McKay P, White JM, Benton EC, et al. (2003). Primary cutaneous diffuse large B-cell lymphoma: prognostic significance of clinicopathological subtypes. Am J Surg Pathol. 27(12):1538–45. PMID:14657713
**918.** Gordon DK, Ponder EN, Berrey BH, Kubik MJ, Sindone J (2014). Verrucous carcinoma of the foot, not your typical plantar wart: a case study. Foot (Edinb). 24(2):94–8. PMID:24810296
**919.** Goto K (2015). Immunohistochemistry for CD117 (KIT) is effective in distinguishing cutaneous adnexal tumors with apocrine/eccrine or sebaceous differentiation from other epithelial tumors of the skin. J Cutan Pathol. 42(7):480–8. PMID:25864700
**920.** Gottfarstein-Maruani A, Michenet P, Kerdraon R, Estève E (2002). Benign vascular proliferations in previously irradiated skin. Am J Surg Pathol. 26(10):1372–3. PMID:12360056
**921.** Goyal A, Moore JB, Gimbel D, Carter JB, Kroshinsky D, Ferry JA, et al. (2015). PD-1, S-100 and CD1a expression in pseudolymphomatous folliculitis, primary cutaneous marginal zone B-cell lymphoma (MALT lymphoma) and cutaneous lymphoid hyperplasia. J Cutan Pathol. 42(1):6–15. PMID:25384543
**922.** Graadt van Roggen JF, Hogendoorn PC, Fletcher CD (1999). Myxoid tumours of soft tissue. Histopathology. 35(4):291–312. PMID:10564384
**923.** Grange F, Bekkenk MW, Wechsler J, Meijer CJ, Cerroni L, Bernengo M, et al. (2001). Prognostic factors in primary cutaneous large B-cell lymphomas: a European multicenter study. J Clin Oncol. 19(16):3602–10. PMID:11504742
**924.** Grange F, Beylot-Barry M, Courville P, Maubec E, Bagot M, Vergier B, et al. (2007). Primary cutaneous diffuse large B-cell lymphoma, leg type: clinicopathologic features and prognostic analysis in 60 cases. Arch Dermatol. 143(9):1144–50. PMID:17875875
**925.** Grange F, Joly P, Barbe C, Bagot M, Dalle S, Ingen-Housz-Oro S, et al. (2014). Improvement of survival in patients with primary cutaneous diffuse large B-cell lymphoma, leg type, in France. JAMA Dermatol. 150(5):535–41. PMID:24647650
**926.** Grange F, Petrella T, Beylot-Barry M, Joly P, D'Incan M, Delaunay M, et al. (2004). Bcl-2 protein expression is the strongest independent prognostic factor of survival in primary cutaneous large B-cell lymphomas. Blood. 103(10):3662–8. PMID:14726400
**927.** Granter SR, Badizadegan K, Fletcher CD (1998). Myofibromatosis in adults, glomangiopericytoma, and myopericytoma: a spectrum of tumors showing perivascular myoid differentiation. Am J Surg Pathol. 22(5):513–25. PMID:9591720
**928.** Granter SR, Seeger K, Calonje E, Busam K, McKee PH (2000). Malignant eccrine spiradenoma (spiradenocarcinoma): a clinicopathologic study of 12 cases. Am J Dermatopathol. 22(2):97–103. PMID:10770427
**929.** Grayson W (2011). Recognition of dual or multiple pathology in skin biopsies from patients with HIV/AIDS. Patholog Res Int. 2011:398546. PMID:21789262
**930.** Grayson W, Pantanowitz L (2008). Histological variants of cutaneous Kaposi sarcoma. Diagn Pathol. 3:31. PMID:18655700
**931.** Grayson W, Pantanowitz L (2010). Histological variants of Kaposi sarcoma. In: Pantanowitz L, Stebbing J, Dezube BJ, editors. Kaposi sarcoma: a model of oncogenesis. Kerala: Research Signpost; pp. 139–59.
**932.** Green A, McCredie M, MacKie R, Giles G, Young P, Morton C, et al. (1999). A case-control study of melanomas of the soles and palms (Australia and Scotland). Cancer Causes Control. 10(1):21–5. PMID:10334638
**933.** Greenblatt D, Ally M, Child F, Scarisbrick J, Whittaker S, Morris S, et al. (2013). Indolent CD8(+) lymphoid proliferation of acral sites: a clinicopathologic study of six patients with some atypical features. J Cutan Pathol. 40(2):248–58. PMID:23189944
**934.** Greenwald HS, Friedman EB, Osman I (2012). Superficial spreading and nodular melanoma are distinct biological entities: a challenge to the linear progression model. Melanoma Res. 22(1):1–8. PMID:22108608
**935.** Greisser J, Palmedo G, Sander C, Kutzner H, Kazakov DV, Roos M, et al. (2006). Detection of clonal rearrangement of T-cell receptor genes in the diagnosis of primary cutaneous CD30 lymphoproliferative disorders. J Cutan Pathol. 33(11):711–5. PMID:17083688
**936.** Griewank KG, Müller H, Jackett LA, Emberger M, Möller I, van de Nes JA, et al. (2017). SF3B1 and BAP1 mutations in blue nevus-like melanoma. Mod Pathol. 30(7):928–39. PMID:28409567
**937.** Griewank KG, Murali R, Schilling B, Scholz S, Sucker A, Song M, et al. (2013). TERT promoter mutations in ocular melanoma distinguish between conjunctival and uveal tumours. Br J Cancer. 109(2):497–501. PMID:23799844
**938.** Griewank KG, Schilling B, Murali R, Bielefeld N, Schwamborn M, Sucker A, et al. (2014). TERT promoter mutations are frequent in atypical fibroxanthomas and pleomorphic dermal sarcomas. Mod Pathol. 27(4):502–8. PMID:24030750
**939.** Griewank KG, Westekemper H, Murali R, Mach M, Schilling B, Wiesner T, et al. (2013). Conjunctival melanomas harbor BRAF and NRAS mutations and copy number changes similar to cutaneous and mucosal melanomas. Clin Cancer Res. 19(12):3143–52. PMID:23633454
**940.** Griffin JR, Wriston CC, Peters MS, Lehman JS (2013). Decreased expression of intercellular adhesion molecules in acantholytic squamous cell carcinoma compared with invasive well-differentiated squamous cell carcinoma of the skin. Am J Clin Pathol. 139(4):442–7. PMID:23525614
**941.** Groben PA, Harvell JD, White WL (2000). Epithelioid blue nevus: neoplasm sui generis or variation on a theme? Am J Dermatopathol. 22(6):473–88. PMID:11190438
**942.** Groesser L, Peterhof E, Evert M, Landthaler M, Berneburg M, Hafner C (2016). BRAF and RAS mutations in sporadic and secondary pyogenic granuloma. J Invest Dermatol. 136(2):481–6. PMID:26802240
**943.** Grogg KL, Jung S, Erickson LA, McClure RF, Dogan A (2008). Primary cutaneous CD4-positive small/medium-sized pleomorphic T-cell lymphoma: a clonal T-cell lymphoproliferative disorder with indolent behavior. Mod Pathol. 21(6):708–15. PMID:18311111
**944.** Gronchi A, Lo Vullo S, Colombo C, Collini P, Stacchiotti S, Mariani L, et al. (2010). Extremity soft tissue sarcoma in a series of patients treated at a single institution: local control directly impacts survival. Ann Surg. 251(3):506–11. PMID:20130465
**945.** Gronchi A, Miceli R, Shurell E, Eilber FC, Eilber FR, Anaya DA, et al. (2013). Outcome prediction in primary resected retroperitoneal soft tissue sarcoma: histology-specific overall survival and disease-free survival nomograms built on major sarcoma center data sets. J Clin Oncol. 31(13):1649–55. PMID:23530096
**946.** Gross RE, Wolbach SB (1943). Sclerosing hemangiomas: their relationship to dermatofibroma, histiocytoma, xanthoma and to certain pigmented lesions of the skin. Am J Pathol. 19(4):533–51. PMID:19970708
**947.** Grosshans E, Vetter JM, Capesius MC (1975). Malignant eccrine poromas (poro-epitheliomas, porocarcinomas). Ann Anat Pathol (Paris). 20(4):381–94. [French] PMID:1229958
**948.** Grossmann P, Vanecek T, Steiner P, Kacerovska D, Spagnolo DV, Cribier B, et al. (2013). Novel and recurrent germline and somatic mutations in a cohort of 67 patients from 48 families with Brooke-Spiegler syndrome including the phenotypic variant of multiple familial trichoepitheliomas and correlation with the histopathologic findings in 379 biopsy specimens. Am J Dermatopathol. 35(1):34–44. PMID:23249834
**948A.** Grossniklaus HE, Eberhart CG, Kivelä T, editors (2018). WHO classification of tumours of the eye. 4th ed. Lyon: International Agency for Research on Cancer.
**949.** Grouls V, Hey A (1988). Trichoblastic fibroma (fibromatoid trichoepithelioma). Pathol Res Pract. 183(4):462–8. PMID:3186547
**950.** Groussin L, Horvath A, Jullian E, Boikos S, Rene-Corail F, Lefebvre H, et al. (2006). A PRKAR1A mutation associated with primary pigmented nodular adrenocortical disease in 12 kindreds. J Clin Endocrinol Metab. 91(5):1943–9. PMID:16464939
**951.** Gru AA, Becker N, Dehner LP, Pfeifer JD (2014). Mucosal melanoma: correlation of clinicopathologic, prognostic, and molecular features. Melanoma Res. 24(4):360–70. PMID:24870295
**952.** Gru AA, Jaffe ES (2017). Cutaneous EBV-related lymphoproliferative disorders. Semin Diagn Pathol. 34(1):60–75. PMID:27988064
**953.** Gu M, Antonescu CR, Guiter G, Huvos AG, Ladanyi M, Zakowski MF (2000). Cytokeratin immunoreactivity in Ewing's sarcoma: prevalence in 50 cases confirmed by molecular diagnostic studies. Am J Surg Pathol. 24(3):410–6. PMID:10716155
**954.** Gualandri L, Betti R, Crosti C (2009). Clinical features of 36 cases of amelanotic melanomas and considerations about the relationship between histologic subtypes and diagnostic delay. J Eur Acad Dermatol Venereol. 23(3):283–7. PMID:19207640
**955.** Guenova E, Schanz S, Hoetzenecker W, DeSimone JA, Mehra T, Voykov B, et al. (2014). Systemic corticosteroids for subcutaneous panniculitis-like T-cell lymphoma. Br J Dermatol. 171(4):891–4. PMID:24725144
**956.** Guièze R, Wu CJ (2015). Genomic and epigenomic heterogeneity in chronic lymphocytic leukemia. Blood. 126(4):445–53. PMID:26065654
**957.** Aguilera-Barrantes I, Magro C, Nuovo GJ (2007). Verruca vulgaris of the vulva in children and adults: a nonvenereal type of vulvar wart. Am J Surg Pathol. 31(4):529–35. PMID:17414099
**958.** Guillou L, Calonje E, Speight P, Rosai J, Fletcher CD (1999). Hobnail hemangioma: a pseudomalignant vascular lesion with a reappraisal of targetoid hemosiderotic hemangioma. Am J Surg Pathol. 23(1):97–105. PMID:9888709
**959.** Guillou L, Wadden C, Coindre JM, Krausz T, Fletcher CD (1997). "Proximal-type" epithelioid sarcoma, a distinctive aggressive neoplasm showing rhabdoid features. Clinicopathologic, immunohistochemical, and ultrastructural study of a series. Am J Surg Pathol. 21(2):130–46. PMID:9042279
**960.** Guinee D Jr, Jaffe E, Kingma D, Fishback N, Wallberg K, Krishnan J, et al. (1994). Pulmonary lymphomatoid granulomatosis. Evidence for a proliferation of Epstein-Barr virus infected B-lymphocytes with a prominent T-cell component and vasculitis. Am J Surg Pathol. 18(8):753–64. PMID:8037289
**961.** Guinot-Moya R, Valmaseda-Castellon E, Berini-Aytes L, Gay-Escoda C (2011). Pilomatrixoma. Review of 205 cases. Med Oral Patol Oral Cir Bucal. 16(4):e552–5. PMID:20711110

**962.** Guitart J, Deonizio J, Bloom T, Martinez-Escala ME, Kuzel TM, Gerami P, et al. (2014). High incidence of gastrointestinal tract disorders and autoimmunity in primary cutaneous marginal zone B-cell lymphomas. JAMA Dermatol. 150(4):412–8. PMID:24500411
**962A.** Guitart J, Martinez-Escala ME, Subtil A, Duvic M, Pulitzer MP, Olsen EA, et al. (2017). Primary cutaneous aggressive epidermotropic cytotoxic T-cell lymphomas: reappraisal of a provisional entity in the 2016 WHO classification of cutaneous lymphomas. Mod Pathol. 30(5):761–72. PMID:28128277
**963.** Guitart J, Querfeld C (2009). Cutaneous CD30 lymphoproliferative disorders and similar conditions: a clinical and pathologic prospective on a complex issue. Semin Diagn Pathol. 26(3):131–40. PMID:20043512
**964.** Guitart J, Ramirez J, Laskin WB (2006). Cellular digital fibromas: what about superficial acral fibromyxoma? J Cutan Pathol. 33(11):762–4. PMID:17083699
**965.** Guitart J, Weisenburger DD, Subtil A, Kim E, Wood G, Duvic M, et al. (2012). Cutaneous γδ T-cell lymphomas: a spectrum of presentations with overlap with other cytotoxic lymphomas. Am J Surg Pathol. 36(11):1656–65. PMID:23073324
**966.** Gulia A, Saggini A, Wiesner T, Fink-Puches R, Argenyi Z, Ferrara G, et al. (2011). Clinicopathologic features of early lesions of primary cutaneous follicle center lymphoma, diffuse type: implications for early diagnosis and treatment. J Am Acad Dermatol. 65(5):991–1000. PMID:21704419
**967.** Guo R, Wang X, Chou MM, Asmann Y, Wenger DE, Al-Ibraheemi A, et al. (2016). PPP6R3-USP6 amplification: novel oncogenic mechanism in malignant nodular fasciitis. Genes Chromosomes Cancer. 55(8):640–9. PMID:27113271
**968.** Guo T, Zhang L, Chang NE, Singer S, Maki RG, Antonescu CR (2011). Consistent MYC and FLT4 gene amplification in radiation-induced angiosarcoma but not in other radiation-associated atypical vascular lesions. Genes Chromosomes Cancer. 50(1):25–33. PMID:20949568
**969.** Gupta D, Thappa DM (2013). Mongolian spots–a prospective study. Pediatr Dermatol. 30(6):683–8. PMID:23834326
**970.** Gupta D, Thappa DM (2013). Mongolian spots: how important are they? World J Clin Cases. 1(8):230–2. PMID:24340274
**971.** Gupta G, Man I, Kemmett D (2000). Hydroa vacciniforme: a clinical and follow-up study of 17 cases. J Am Acad Dermatol. 42(2 Pt 1):208–13. PMID:10642674
**972.** Gurbuz Y, Muezzinoglu B, Apaydin R, Yumbul AZ (2002). Acral arteriovenous tumor (cirsoid aneurysm): clinical and histopathological analysis of 6 cases. Adv Clin Path. 6(1):25–9. PMID:17582945
**973.** Gustafson P (1994). Soft tissue sarcoma. Epidemiology and prognosis in 508 patients. Acta Orthop Scand Suppl. 259:1–31. PMID:8042499
**974.** Gutiérrez-González E, Montero I, Sánchez-Aguilar D, Ginarte M, Toribio J (2014). Adult-onset verrucous nevus lipomatosus cutaneous superficialis. Int J Dermatol. 53(1):e69–71. PMID:23113758
**975.** Haas N, Audring H, Sterry W (2002). Carcinoma arising in a proliferating trichilemmal cyst expresses fetal and trichilemmal hair phenotype. Am J Dermatopathol. 24(4):340–4. PMID:12142616
**976.** Habougit C, Michiels-Marzais D, Wang Q, Pissaloux D, de la Fouchardiere A (2017). Linear variant of large plaque-type blue naevus with subcutaneous cellular nodules. Pathology. 49(5):542–4. PMID:28673427
**977.** Hachisuga T, Hashimoto H, Enjoji M (1984). Angioleiomyoma. A clinicopathologic reappraisal of 562 cases. Cancer. 54(1):126–30. PMID:6722737
**978.** Haddock ES, Cohen PR (2016). Fibroepithelioma of Pinkus revisited. Dermatol Ther (Heidelb). 6(3):347–62. PMID:27329375
**979.** HaDuong JH, Martin AA, Skapek SX, Mascarenhas L (2015). Sarcomas. Pediatr Clin North Am. 62(1):179–200. PMID:25435119
**980.** Haenssle HA, Mograby N, Ngassa A, Buhl T, Emmert S, Schön MP, et al. (2016). Association of patient risk factors and frequency of nevus-associated cutaneous melanomas. JAMA Dermatol. 152(3):291–8. PMID:26536613
**981.** Hafner C, Schmiemann V, Ruetten A, Coras B, Landthaler M, Reifenberger J, et al. (2007). PTCH mutations are not mainly involved in the pathogenesis of sporadic trichoblastomas. Hum Pathol. 38(10):1496–500. PMID:17597182
**982.** Hafner C, Stoehr R, van Oers JM, Zwarthoff EC, Hofstaedter F, Landthaler M, et al. (2009). FGFR3 and PIK3CA mutations are involved in the molecular pathogenesis of solar lentigo. Br J Dermatol. 160(3):546–51. PMID:19076977
**983.** Hafner C, Vogt T (2008). Seborrheic keratosis. J Dtsch Dermatol Ges. 6(8):664–77. PMID:18801147
**984.** Hagen JW, Magro CM (2014). Indolent CD8+ lymphoid proliferation of the face with eyelid involvement. Am J Dermatopathol. 36(2):137–41. PMID:24556898
**985.** Haghighi B, Smoller BR, LeBoit PE, Warnke RA, Sander CA, Kohler S (2000). Pagetoid reticulosis (Woringer-Kolopp disease): an immunophenotypic, molecular, and clinicopathologic study. Mod Pathol. 13(5):502–10. PMID:10824921
**986.** Hahn H, Wicking C, Zaphiropoulous PG, Gailani MR, Shanley S, Chidambaram A, et al. (1996). Mutations of the human homolog of Drosophila patched in the nevoid basal cell carcinoma syndrome. Cell. 85(6):841–51. PMID:8681379
**987.** Hahtola S, Tuomela S, Elo L, Häkkinen T, Karenko L, Nedoszytko B, et al. (2006). Th1 response and cytotoxicity genes are down-regulated in cutaneous T-cell lymphoma. Clin Cancer Res. 12(16):4812–21. PMID:16914566
**988.** Hall BD, Cadle RG, Morrill-Cornelius SM, Bay CA (2007). Phakomatosis pigmentovascularis: implications for severity with special reference to Mongolian spots associated with Sturge-Weber and Klippel-Trenaunay syndromes. Am J Med Genet A. 143A(24):3047–53. PMID:17937434
**989.** Hall BJ, LeBoit PE (2014). Suprabasal spread of melanocytes in dysplastic nevi and melanoma in situ: Ki-67-labeling rate of junctional melanocytes and suprabasal cells may be a helpful clue to the diagnosis. Am J Surg Pathol. 38(8):1111–7. PMID:24805862
**990.** Haller F, Knopf J, Ackermann A, Bieg M, Kleinheinz K, Schlesner M, et al. (2016). Paediatric and adult soft tissue sarcomas with NTRK1 gene fusions: a subset of spindle cell sarcomas unified by a prominent myopericytic/haemangiopericytic pattern. J Pathol. 238(5):700–10. PMID:26863915
**991.** Hallermann C, Kaune KM, Gesk S, Martin-Subero JI, Gunawan B, Griesinger F, et al. (2004). Molecular cytogenetic analysis of chromosomal breakpoints in the IGH, MYC, BCL6, and MALT1 gene loci in primary cutaneous B-cell lymphomas. J Invest Dermatol. 123(1):213–9. PMID:15191563
**992.** Hallermann C, Kaune KM, Siebert R, Vermeer MH, Tensen CP, Willemze R, et al. (2004). Chromosomal aberration patterns differ in subtypes of primary cutaneous B cell lymphomas. J Invest Dermatol. 122(6):1495–502. PMID:15175042
**993.** Halling AC, Wollan PC, Pritchard DJ, Vlasak R, Nascimento AG (1996). Epithelioid sarcoma: a clinicopathologic review of 55 cases. Mayo Clin Proc. 71(7):636–42. PMID:8656704
**994.** Hallor KH, Sciot R, Staaf J, Heidenblad M, Rydholm A, Bauer HC, et al. (2009). Two genetic pathways, t(1;10) and amplification of 3p11-12, in myxoinflammatory fibroblastic sarcoma, haemosiderotic fibrolipomatous tumour, and morphologically similar lesions. J Pathol. 217(5):716–27. PMID:19199331
**995.** Halpern AC, Guerry D 4th, Elder DE, Trock B, Synnestvedt M, Humphreys T (1993). Natural history of dysplastic nevi. J Am Acad Dermatol. 29(1):51–7. PMID:8315078
**996.** Hamad N, Armytage T, McIlroy K, Singh N, Ward C (2015). Primary cutaneous mantle-cell lymphoma: a case report and literature review. J Clin Oncol. 33(26):e104–8. PMID:24733805
**997.** Hamilton SN, Wai ES, Tan K, Alexander C, Gascoyne RD, Connors JM (2013). Treatment and outcomes in patients with primary cutaneous B-cell lymphoma: the BC Cancer Agency experience. Int J Radiat Oncol Biol Phys. 87(4):719–25. PMID:24001373
**998.** Han J, Kraft P, Colditz GA, Wong J, Hunter DJ (2006). Melanocortin 1 receptor variants and skin cancer risk. Int J Cancer. 119(8):1976–84. PMID:16721784
**999.** Hanaka T, Makihara K, Hachiya Y, Mukae H (2015). Primary lung sebaceous carcinoma. Intern Med. 54(3):351–2. PMID:25748747
**1000.** Hanau D, Grosshans E, Laplanche G (1984). A complex poroma-like adnexal adenoma. Am J Dermatopathol. 6(6):567–72. PMID:6098189
**1001.** Handley J, Carson D, Sloan J, Walsh M, Thornton C, Hadden D, et al. (1992). Multiple lentigines, myxoid tumours and endocrine overactivity; four cases of Carney's complex. Br J Dermatol. 126(4):367–71. PMID:1571257
**1002.** Hanft VN, Shea CR, McNutt NS, Pulitzer D, Horenstein MG, Prieto VG (2000). Expression of CD34 in sclerotic ("plywood") fibromas. Am J Dermatopathol. 22(1):17–21. PMID:10698210
**1003.** Haniffa M, Bigley V, Collin M (2015). Human mononuclear phagocyte system reunited. Semin Cell Dev Biol. 41:59–69. PMID:25986054
**1004.** Hanson M, Lupski JR, Hicks J, Metry D (2003). Association of dermal melanocytosis with lysosomal storage disease: clinical features and hypotheses regarding pathogenesis. Arch Dermatol. 139(7):916–20. PMID:12873889
**1005.** Hantschke M, Mentzel T, Rütten A, Palmedo G, Calonje E, Lazar AJ, et al. (2010). Cutaneous clear cell sarcoma: a clinicopathologic, immunohistochemical, and molecular analysis of 12 cases emphasizing its distinction from dermal melanoma. Am J Surg Pathol. 34(2):216–22. PMID:20087159
**1006.** Hapgood G, Mooney E, Dinh HV, Gin D, McLean C, Ting SB (2012). Leukaemia cutis in chronic lymphocytic leukaemia following varicella zoster virus reactivation. Intern Med J. 42(12):1355–8. PMID:23253001
**1007.** Happle R (2002). Speckled lentiginous nevus syndrome: delineation of a new distinct neurocutaneous phenotype. Eur J Dermatol. 12(2):133–5. PMID:11872407
**1008.** Haque AK, Myers JL, Hudnall SD, Gelman BB, Lloyd RV, Payne D, et al. (1998). Pulmonary lymphomatoid granulomatosis in acquired immunodeficiency syndrome: lesions with Epstein-Barr virus infection. Mod Pathol. 11(4):347–56. PMID:9578085
**1008A.** Harada H, Hashimoto K, Ko MS (1996). The gene for multiple familial trichoepithelioma maps to chromosome 9p21. J Invest Dermatol. 107(1):41–3. PMID:8752837
**1009.** Harbour JW, Onken MD, Roberson ED, Duan S, Cao L, Worley LA, et al. (2010). Frequent mutation of BAP1 in metastasizing uveal melanomas. Science. 330(6009):1410–3. PMID:21051595
**1010.** Harding-Jackson N, Sangueza M, Mackinnon A, Suster S, Plaza JA (2015). Spindle cell atypical fibroxanthoma: myofibroblastic differentiation represents a diagnostic pitfall in this variant of AFX. Am J Dermatopathol. 37(7):509–14. PMID:26098709
**1011.** Harland M, Petljak M, Robles-Espinoza CD, Ding Z, Gruis NA, van Doorn R, et al. (2016). Germline TERT promoter mutations are rare in familial melanoma. Fam Cancer. 15(1):139–44. PMID:26433962
**1012.** Harms KL, Healy MA, Nghiem P, Sober AJ, Johnson TM, Bichakjian CK, et al. (2016). Analysis of prognostic factors from 9387 Merkel cell carcinoma cases forms the basis for the new 8th edition AJCC Staging System. Ann Surg Oncol. 23(11):3564–71. PMID:27198511
**1013.** Harms PW, Fullen DR, Patel RM, Chang D, Shalin SC, Ma L, et al. (2015). Cutaneous basal cell carcinosarcomas: evidence of clonality and recurrent chromosomal losses. Hum Pathol. 46(5):690–7. PMID:25704628
**1014.** Harms PW, Hocker TL, Zhao L, Chan MP, Andea AA, Wang M, et al. (2016). Loss of p16 expression and copy number changes of CDKN2A in a spectrum of spitzoid melanocytic lesions. Hum Pathol. 58:152–60. PMID:27569296
**1015.** Harms PW, Hovelson DH, Cani AK, Omata K, Haller MJ, Wang ML, et al. (2016). Porocarcinomas harbor recurrent HRAS-activating mutations and tumor suppressor inactivating mutations. Hum Pathol. 51:25–31. PMID:27067779
**1016.** Haroche J, Abla O (2015). Uncommon histiocytic disorders: Rosai-Dorfman, juvenile xanthogranuloma, and Erdheim-Chester disease. Hematology Am Soc Hematol Educ Program. 2015(1):571–8. PMID:26637774
**1017.** Haroche J, Amoura Z, Dion E, Wechsler B, Costedoat-Chalumeau N, Cacoub P, et al. (2004). Cardiovascular involvement, an overlooked feature of Erdheim-Chester disease: report of 6 new cases and a literature review. Medicine (Baltimore). 83(6):371–92. PMID:15525849
**1018.** Haroche J, Arnaud L, Cohen-Aubart F, Hervier B, Charlotte F, Emile JF, et al. (2014). Erdheim-Chester disease. Curr Rheumatol Rep. 16(4):412. PMID:24532298
**1019.** Haroche J, Charlotte F, Arnaud L, von Deimling A, Hélias-Rodzewicz Z, Hervier B, et al. (2012). High prevalence of BRAF V600E mutations in Erdheim-Chester disease but not in other non-Langerhans cell histiocytoses. Blood. 120(13):2700–3. PMID:22879539
**1020.** Haroche J, Cluzel P, Toledano D, Montalescot G, Touitou D, Grenier PA, et al. (2009). Images in cardiovascular medicine. Cardiac involvement in Erdheim-Chester disease: magnetic resonance and computed tomographic scan imaging in a monocentric series of 37 patients. Circulation. 119(25):e597–8. PMID:19564564
**1021.** Haroche J, Cohen-Aubart F, Emile JF, Maksud P, Drier A, Tolédano D, et al. (2015). Reproducible and sustained efficacy of targeted therapy with vemurafenib in patients with BRAF(V600E)-mutated Erdheim-Chester disease. J Clin Oncol. 33(5):411–8. PMID:25422482
**1022.** Haroche J, Cohen-Aubart F, Rollins BJ, Donadieu J, Charlotte F, Idbaih A, et al. (2017). Histiocytoses: emerging neoplasia behind

inflammation. Lancet Oncol. 18(2):e113–25. PMID:28214412

1023. Harris DW, Ostlere LS, Rustin MH (1992). Cutaneous granulocytic sarcoma (chloroma) presenting as the first sign of relapse following autologous bone marrow transplantation for acute myeloid leukaemia. Br J Dermatol. 127(2):182–4. PMID:1390150

1024. Harris MN, Desai R, Chuang TY, Hood AF, Mirowski GW (2000). Lobular capillary hemangiomas: an epidemiologic report, with emphasis on cutaneous lesions. J Am Acad Dermatol. 42(6):1012–6. PMID:10827405

1025. Harrison B, Moore AM, Calfee R, Sammer DM (2013). The association between glomus tumors and neurofibromatosis. J Hand Surg Am. 38(8):1571–4. PMID:23849732

1026. Harrison B, Sammer D (2014). Glomus tumors and neurofibromatosis: a newly recognized association. Plast Reconstr Surg Glob Open. 2(9):e214. PMID:25426397

1027. Hart M, Thakral B, Yohe S, Balfour HH Jr, Singh C, Spears M, et al. (2014). EBV-positive mucocutaneous ulcer in organ transplant recipients: a localized indolent posttransplant lymphoproliferative disorder. Am J Surg Pathol. 38(11):1522–9. PMID:25007145

1028. Hartmann K, Escribano L, Grattan C, Brockow K, Carter MC, Alvarez-Twose I, et al. (2016). Cutaneous manifestations in patients with mastocytosis: consensus report of the European Competence Network on Mastocytosis; the American Academy of Allergy, Asthma & Immunology; and the European Academy of Allergology and Clinical Immunology. J Allergy Clin Immunol. 137(1):35–45. PMID:26476479

1029. Hartmann K, Wardelmann E, Ma Y, Merkelbach-Bruse S, Preussner LM, Woolery C, et al. (2005). Novel germline mutation of KIT associated with familial gastrointestinal stromal tumors and mastocytosis. Gastroenterology. 129(3):1042–6. PMID:16143141

1030. Hartschuh W, Schulz T (1995). Merkel cells are integral constituents of desmoplastic trichoepithelioma: an immunohistochemical and electron microscopic study. J Cutan Pathol. 22(5):413–21. PMID:8594073

1031. Hartschuh W, Schulz T (1997). Merkel cell hyperplasia in chronic radiation-damaged skin: its possible relationship to fibroepithelioma of Pinkus. J Cutan Pathol. 24(8):477–83. PMID:9331893

1032. Harvell JD (2003). Multiple spindle cell lipomas and dermatofibrosarcoma protuberans within a single patient: evidence for a common neoplastic process of interstitial dendritic cells? J Am Acad Dermatol. 48(1):82–5. PMID:12522375

1033. Harvell JD, Meehan SA, LeBoit PE (1997). Spitz's nevi with halo reaction: a histopathologic study of 17 cases. J Cutan Pathol. 24(10):611–9. PMID:9449488

1034. Harvey NT, Millward M, Macgregor K, Bucat RP, Wood BA (2016). Cutaneous metastatic melanoma resembling a halo nevus, in the setting of PD-1 inhibition. Am J Dermatopathol. 38(12):e159–62. PMID:27870733

1035. Harvey NT, Tabone T, Erber W, Wood BA (2016). Circumscribed sebaceous neoplasms: a morphological, immunohistochemical and molecular analysis. Pathology. 48(5):454–62. PMID:27311873

1036. Hasegawa SL, Davison JM, Rutten A, Fletcher JA, Fletcher CD (1998). Primary cutaneous Ewing's sarcoma: immunophenotypic and molecular cytogenetic evaluation of five cases. Am J Surg Pathol. 22(3):310–8. PMID:9500772

1037. Hasegawa T, Seki K, Yang P, Hirose T, Hizawa K (1994). Mechanism of pain and cytoskeletal properties in angioleiomyomas: an immunohistochemical study. Pathol Int. 44(1):66–72. PMID:8025650

1038. Hasegawa T, Shimoda T, Hirohashi S, Hizawa K, Sano T (1998). Collagenous fibroma (desmoplastic fibroblastoma): report of four cases and review of the literature. Arch Pathol Lab Med. 122(5):455–60. PMID:9593348

1039. Haskell HD, Haynes HA, McKee PH, Redston M, Granter SR, Lazar AJ (2005). Basal cell carcinoma with matrical differentiation: a case study with analysis of beta-catenin. J Cutan Pathol. 32(3):245–50. PMID:15701088

1040. Hassan SF, Stephens E, Fallon SC, Schady D, Hicks MJ, Lopez ME, et al. (2013). Characterizing pilomatricomas in children: a single institution experience. J Pediatr Surg. 48(7):1551–6. PMID:23895971

1041. Hassanein AM, Glanz SM (2004). Beta-catenin expression in benign and malignant pilomatrix neoplasms. Br J Dermatol. 150(3):511–6. PMID:15030335

1042. Hassim AM (1969). Bilateral fibroadenoma in supernumerary breasts of the vulva. J Obstet Gynaecol Br Commonw. 76(3):275–7. PMID:5775152

1043. Hattori R, Kubo T, Yano K, Tanemura A, Yamaguchi Y, Itami S, et al. (2003). Nevus lipomatosus cutaneous superficialis of the clitoris. Dermatol Surg. 29(10):1071–2. PMID:12974709

1044. Haupt HM, Stern JB, Berlin SJ (1992). Immunohistochemistry in the differential diagnosis of nodular hidradenoma and glomus tumor. Am J Dermatopathol. 14(4):310–4. PMID:1380207

1045. Haupt R, Minkov M, Astigarraga I, Schäfer E, Nanduri V, Jubran R, et al. (2013). Langerhans cell histiocytosis (LCH): guidelines for diagnosis, clinical work-up, and treatment for patients till the age of 18 years. Pediatr Blood Cancer. 60(2):175–84. PMID:23109216

1046. Hawley IC, Krausz T, Evans DJ, Fletcher CD (1994). Spindle cell lipoma–a pseudoangiomatous variant. Histopathology. 24(6):565–9. PMID:8063285

1047. Hayes MM, Konstantinova AM, Kacerovska D, Michal M, Kreuzberg B, Suvova B, et al. (2016). Bilateral gigantomastia, multiple synchronous nodular pseudoangiomatous stromal hyperplasia involving breast and bilateral axillary accessory breast tissue, and perianal mammary-type hamartoma of anogenital mammary-like glands: a case report. Am J Dermatopathol. 38(5):374–83. PMID:26863057

1048. Hayes MM, Matisic JP, Weir L (1996). Apocrine carcinoma of the lip: a case report including immunohistochemical and ultrastructural study, discussion of differential diagnosis, and review of the literature. Oral Surg Oral Med Oral Pathol Oral Radiol Endod. 82(2):193–9. PMID:8863310

1049. Hays JP, Malone CH, Goodwin BP, Wagner RF Jr (2018). Reactive eccrine syringofibroadenoma associated with basal cell carcinoma: a histologic mimicker of fibroepithelioma of Pinkus. Dermatol Surg. 44(5):738–40. PMID:28902033

1050. Hayward NK, Wilmott JS, Waddell N, Johansson PA, Field MA, Nones K, et al. (2017). Whole-genome landscapes of major melanoma subtypes. Nature. 545(7653):175–80. PMID:28467829

1051. Headington JT (1976). Tumors of the hair follicle. A review. Am J Pathol. 85(2):479–514. PMID:793411

1052. Headington JT, Teears R, Niederhuber JE, Slinger RP (1978). Primary adenoid cystic carcinoma of skin. Arch Dermatol. 114(3):421–4. PMID:204257

1053. Heath M, Jaimes N, Lemos B, Mostaghimi A, Wang LC, Peñas PF, et al. (2008). Clinical characteristics of Merkel cell carcinoma at diagnosis in 195 patients: the AEIOU features. J Am Acad Dermatol. 58(3):375–81. PMID:18280333

1054. Heenan PJ (2003). Nodular melanoma is not a distinct entity. Arch Dermatol. 139(3):387–8. PMID:12622643

1055. Heenan PJ, Bogle MS (1993). Eccrine differentiation in basal cell carcinoma. J Invest Dermatol. 100(3):295S–9S. PMID:8440908

1056. Heenan PJ, Quirk CJ, Papadimitriou JM (1986). Epithelioid sarcoma. A diagnostic problem. Am J Dermatopathol. 8(2):95–104. PMID:3717528

1057. Heidarpour M, Rajabi P, Sajadi F (2011). CD10 expression helps to differentiate basal cell carcinoma from trichoepithelioma. J Res Med Sci. 16(7):938–44. PMID:22279463

1058. Helbig D, Ihle MA, Pütz K, Tantcheva-Poor I, Mauch C, Büttner R, et al. (2016). Oncogene and therapeutic target analyses in atypical fibroxanthomas and pleomorphic dermal sarcomas. Oncotarget. 7(16):21763–74. PMID:26943575

1059. Helgadottir H, Höiom V, Jönsson G, Tuominen R, Ingvar C, Borg A, et al. (2014). High risk of tobacco-related cancers in CDKN2A mutation-positive melanoma families. J Med Genet. 51(8):545–52. PMID:24935963

1060. Helwig EB, May D (1986). Atypical fibroxanthoma of the skin with metastasis. Cancer. 57(2):368–76. PMID:3942970

1061. Henderson SA, Torres-Cabala CA, Curry JL, Bassett RL, Ivan D, Prieto VG, et al. (2014). p40 is more specific than p63 for the distinction of atypical fibroxanthoma from other cutaneous spindle cell malignancies. Am J Surg Pathol. 38(8):1102–10. PMID:25029117

1062. Henn A, Michel L, Fite C, Deschamps L, Ortonne N, Ingen-Housz-Oro S, et al. (2015). Sézary syndrome without erythroderma. J Am Acad Dermatol. 72(6):1003–9.e1. PMID:25981000

1063. Henner MS, Shapiro PE, Ritter JH, Leffell DJ, Wick MR (1995). Solitary syringoma. Report of five cases and clinicopathologic comparison with microcystic adnexal carcinoma of the skin. Am J Dermatopathol. 17(5):465–70. PMID:8599451

1064. Henning B, Stieger P, Kamarachev J, Dummer R, Goldinger SM (2016). Pyogenic granuloma in patients treated with selective BRAF inhibitors: another manifestation of paradoxical pathway activation. Melanoma Res. 26(3):304–7. PMID:27116335

1065. Henricks WH, Chu YC, Goldblum JR, Weiss SW (1997). Dedifferentiated liposarcoma: a clinicopathological analysis of 155 cases with a proposal for an expanded definition of dedifferentiation. Am J Surg Pathol. 21(3):271–81. PMID:9060596

1066. Herd RM, Hunter JA (1998). Familial halo naevi. Clin Exp Dermatol. 23(2):68–9. PMID:9692308

1067. Héritier S, Emile JF, Barkaoui MA, Thomas C, Fraitag S, Boudjemaa S, et al. (2016). BRAF mutation correlates with high-risk Langerhans cell histiocytosis and increased resistance to first-line therapy. J Clin Oncol. 34(25):3023–30. PMID:27382093

1068. Héritier S, Hélias-Rodzewicz Z, Lapillonne H, Terrones N, Garrigou S, Normand C, et al. (2017). Circulating cell-free $BRAF^{V600E}$ as a biomarker in children with Langerhans cell histiocytosis. Br J Haematol. 178(3):457–67. PMID:28444728

1069. Héritier S, Saffroy R, Radosevic-Robin N, Pothin Y, Pacquement H, Peuchmaur M, et al. (2015). Common cancer-associated PIK3CA activating mutations rarely occur in Langerhans cell histiocytosis. Blood. 125(15):2448–9. PMID:25858893

1070. Herling M, Jones D (2007). CD4+/CD56+ hematodermic tumor: the features of an evolving entity and its relationship to dendritic cells. Am J Clin Pathol. 127(5):687–700. PMID:17439829

1071. Herling M, Teitell MA, Shen RR, Medeiros LJ, Jones D (2003). TCL1 expression in plasmacytoid dendritic cells (DC2s) and the related CD4+ CD56+ blastic tumors of skin. Blood. 101(12):5007–9. PMID:12576313

1072. Hernández-Núñez A, Nájera Botello L, Romero Maté A, Martínez-Sánchez C, Utrera Busquets M, Calderón Komáromy A, et al. (2014). Retrospective study of pilomatricoma: 261 tumors in 239 patients. Actas Dermosifiliogr. 105(7):699–705. PMID:24838222

1073. Herrmann JL, Allan A, Trapp KM, Morgan MB (2014). Pilomatrix carcinoma: 13 new cases and review of the literature with emphasis on predictors of metastasis. J Am Acad Dermatol. 71(1):38–43.e2. PMID:24739254

1074. Herron MD, Coffin CM, Vanderhooft SL (2002). Tufted angiomas: variability of the clinical morphology. Pediatr Dermatol. 19(5):394–401. PMID:12383094

1075. Hervier B, Haroche J, Arnaud L, Charlotte F, Donadieu J, Néel A, et al. (2014). Association of both Langerhans cell histiocytosis and Erdheim-Chester disease linked to the BRAFV600E mutation. Blood. 124(7):1119–26. PMID:24894769

1076. Hes O, Perez-Montiel DM, Alvarado Cabrero I, Zamecnik M, Podhola M, Sulc M, et al. (2003). Thread-like bridging strands: a morphologic feature present in all adenomatoid tumors. Ann Diagn Pathol. 7(5):273–7. PMID:14571427

1077. Heslin MJ, Lewis JJ, Woodruff JM, Brennan MF (1997). Core needle biopsy for diagnosis of extremity soft tissue sarcoma. Ann Surg Oncol. 4(5):425–31. PMID:9259971

1078. Hidano A, Kajima H, Ikeda S, Mizutani H, Miyasato H, Niimura M (1967). Natural history of nevus of Ota. Arch Dermatol. 95(2):187–95. PMID:6018994

1079. Hilliard NJ, Wakefield DN, Krahl D, Sellheyer K (2009). p16 expression in conventional and desmoplastic trichilemmomas. Am J Dermatopathol. 31(4):342–9. PMID:19461237

1080. Hindocha S, McGrouther DA, Bayat A (2009). Epidemiological evaluation of Dupuytren's disease incidence and prevalence rates in relation to etiology. Hand (N Y). 4(3):256–69. PMID:19145463

1081. Hinds B, Agulló Pérez AD, LeBoit PE, McCalmont TH, North JP (2017). Loss of retinoblastoma in pleomorphic fibroma: an immunohistochemical and genomic analysis. J Cutan Pathol. 44(8):665–71. PMID:28543636

1082. Hinds GA, Heald P (2009). Cutaneous T-cell lymphoma in skin of color. J Am Acad Dermatol. 60(3):359–75. PMID:19231637

1083. Hingmire S, Narayanan P, Khadwal A, Maru D, Biswas G, Sastry PS, et al. (2007). Isolated cutaneous relapse of acute myeloid leukemia. J Assoc Physicians India. 55:131. PMID:17571743

1084. Hirai Y, Kodama Y, Moriwaki S, Noda A, Cullings HM, Macphee DG, et al. (2006). Heterozygous individuals bearing a founder mutation in the XPA DNA repair gene comprise nearly 1% of the Japanese population. Mutat Res. 601(1–2):171–8. PMID:16905156

1085. Hirai Y, Yamamoto T, Kimura H, Ito Y, Tsuji K, Miyake T, et al. (2012). Hydroa vacciniforme is associated with increased numbers of Epstein-Barr virus-infected γδT cells. J Invest Dermatol. 132(5):1401–8. PMID:22297643

1086. Hiramatsu K, Sasaki K, Matsuda M, Hashimoto M, Eguchi T, Tomikawa S, et al. (2015). A case of trichilemmal carcinoma with distant metastases in a kidney transplantation patient. Transplant Proc. 47(1):155–7. PMID:25645796

1087. Hirose T, Scheithauer BW, Sano T

(1998). Perineurial malignant peripheral nerve sheath tumor (MPNST): a clinicopathologic, immunohistochemical, and ultrastructural study of seven cases. Am J Surg Pathol. 22(11):1368–78. PMID:9808129

**1088.** Hisaoka M, Ishida T, Kuo TT, Matsuyama A, Imamura T, Nishida K, et al. (2008). Clear cell sarcoma of soft tissue: a clinicopathologic, immunohistochemical, and molecular analysis of 33 cases. Am J Surg Pathol. 32(3):452–60. PMID:18300804

**1089.** Histiocytosis syndromes in children. Writing Group of the Histiocyte Society. (1987). Lancet. 1(8526): 208–9. PMID:2880029

**1090.** Ho J, Bhawan J (2017). Folliculosebaceous neoplasms: a review of clinical and histological features. J Dermatol. 44(3):259–78. PMID:28256760

**1091.** Ho YK, Zhi H, Bowlin T, Dorjbal B, Philip S, Zahoor MA, et al. (2015). HTLV-1 Tax stimulates ubiquitin E3 ligase, ring finger protein 8, to assemble lysine 63-linked polyubiquitin chains for TAK1 and IKK activation. PLoS Pathog. 11(8):e1005102. PMID:26285145

**1092.** Hoang MP, Dresser KA, Kapur P, High WA, Mahalingam M (2008). Microcystic adnexal carcinoma: an immunohistochemical reappraisal. Mod Pathol. 21(2):178–85. PMID:18065959

**1093.** Hoang MP, Prieto VG, Burchette JL, Shea CR (2001). Recurrent melanocytic nevus: a histologic and immunohistochemical evaluation. J Cutan Pathol. 28(8):400–6. PMID:11493377

**1094.** Hocker T, Tsao H (2007). Ultraviolet radiation and melanoma: a systematic review and analysis of reported sequence variants. Hum Mutat. 28(6):578–88. PMID:17295241

**1095.** Brachtel E, Koerner F (2014). Paget disease of the nipple. In: Hoda SA, Brogi E, Koerner FC, Rosen PP, editors. Rosen's breast pathology. 4th ed. Philadelphia: Lippincott Williams & Wilkins; pp. 775–95.

**1096.** Hodak E, Feuerman H, Barzilai A, David M, Cerroni L, Feinmesser M (2010). Anetodermic primary cutaneous B-cell lymphoma: a unique clinicopathological presentation of lymphoma possibly associated with antiphospholipid antibodies. Arch Dermatol. 146(2):175–82. PMID:20157029

**1097.** Hodak E, Amitay-Laish I, Atzmony L, Prag-Naveh H, Yanichkin N, Barzilai A, et al. (2016). New insights into folliculotropic mycosis fungoides (FMF): a single-center experience. J Am Acad Dermatol. 75(2):347–55. PMID:27245278

**1098.** Hodis E, Watson IR, Kryukov GV, Arold ST, Imielinski M, Theurillat JP, et al. (2012). A landscape of driver mutations in melanoma. Cell. 150(2):251–63. PMID:22817889

**1099.** Hoefnagel JJ, Dijkman R, Basso K, Jansen PM, Hallermann C, Willemze R, et al. (2005). Distinct types of primary cutaneous large B-cell lymphoma identified by gene expression profiling. Blood. 105(9):3671–8. PMID:15308563

**1100.** Hoefnagel JJ, Vermeer MH, Jansen PM, Fleuren GJ, Meijer CJ, Willemze R (2003). Bcl-2, Bcl-6 and CD10 expression in cutaneous B-cell lymphoma: further support for a follicle centre cell origin and differential diagnostic significance. Br J Dermatol. 149(6):1183–91. PMID:14674895

**1101.** Hoefnagel JJ, Vermeer MH, Jansen PM, Heule F, van Voorst Vader PC, Sanders CJ, et al. (2005). Primary cutaneous marginal zone B-cell lymphoma: clinical and therapeutic features in 50 cases. Arch Dermatol. 141(9):1139–45. PMID:16172311

**1102.** Hoesly PM, Lowe GC, Lohse CM, Brewer JD, Lehman JS (2015). Prognostic impact of fibrosarcomatous transformation in dermatofibrosarcoma protuberans: a cohort study. J Am Acad Dermatol. 72(3):419–25. PMID:25582537

**1103.** Hofmann-Wellenhof R (2013). Special criteria for special locations 2: scalp, mucosal, and milk line. Dermatol Clin. 31(4):625–36, ix. PMID:24075550

**1104.** Hofvander J, Arbajian E, Stenkula KG, Lindkvist-Petersson K, Larsson M, Nilsson J, et al. (2017). Frequent low-level mutations of protein kinase D2 in angiolipoma. J Pathol. 241(5):578–82. PMID:28139834

**1105.** Holden CA, Wells RS, MacDonald DM (1982). Cutaneous lymphomatoid granulomatosis. Clin Exp Dermatol. 7(4):449–54. PMID:7127892

**1106.** Hollmann TJ, Bovée JV, Fletcher CD (2012). Digital fibromyxoma (superficial acral fibromyxoma): a detailed characterization of 124 cases. Am J Surg Pathol. 36(6):789–98. PMID:22367301

**1107.** Hollmann TJ, Brenn T, Hornick JL (2008). CD25 expression on cutaneous mast cells from adult patients presenting with urticaria pigmentosa is predictive of systemic mastocytosis. Am J Surg Pathol. 32(1):139–45. PMID:18162781

**1108.** Hollmann TJ, Hornick JL (2011). INI1-deficient tumors: diagnostic features and molecular genetics. Am J Surg Pathol. 35(10):e47–63. PMID:21934399

**1109.** Hollowood K, Holley MP, Fletcher CD (1991). Plexiform fibrohistiocytic tumour: clinicopathological, immunohistochemical and ultrastructural analysis in favour of a myofibroblastic lesion. Histopathology. 19(6):503–13. PMID:1723956

**1110.** Holmes RC, Fensom AH, McKee P, Cairns RJ, Black MM (1984). Angiokeratoma corporis diffusum in a patient with normal enzyme activities. J Am Acad Dermatol. 10(2 Pt 2):384–7. PMID:6423705

**1111.** Holst VA, Junkins-Hopkins JM, Elenitsas R (2002). Cutaneous smooth muscle neoplasms: clinical features, histologic findings, and treatment options. J Am Acad Dermatol. 46(4):477–90. PMID:11907496

**1112.** Honda A, Iwasaki T, Sata T, Kawashima M, Morishima T, Matsukura T (1994). Human papillomavirus type 60-associated plantar wart. Ridged wart. Arch Dermatol. 130(11):1413–7. PMID:7979443

**1113.** Hong YK, Shin JW, Detmar M (2004). Development of the lymphatic vascular system: a mystery unravels. Dev Dyn. 231(3):462–73. PMID:15376314

**1114.** Hönigsmann H, Schwarz T (2012). Ultraviolet therapy. In: Bolognia JL, Jorizzo JJ, Schaffer JV, Callen JP, Cerroni L, Heymann WR, et al., editors. Dermatology. 3rd ed. London: Elsevier; pp. 2219–36.

**1115.** Hönigsmann H, Wolff K, Gschnait F, Brenner W, Jaschke E (1980). Keratoses and nonmelanoma skin tumors in long-term photochemotherapy (PUVA). J Am Acad Dermatol. 3(4):406–14. PMID:7430462

**1116.** Hori Y, Kawashima M, Oohara K, Kukita A (1984). Acquired, bilateral nevus of Ota-like macules. J Am Acad Dermatol. 10(6):961–4. PMID:6736340

**1117.** Horn S, Figl A, Rachakonda PS, Fischer C, Sucker A, Gast A, et al. (2013). TERT promoter mutations in familial and sporadic melanoma. Science. 339(6122):959–61. PMID:23348503

**1118.** Horn TD, Vennos EM, Bernstein BD, Cooper PH (1995). Multiple tumors of follicular infundibulum with sweat duct differentiation. J Cutan Pathol. 22(3):281–7. PMID:7593824

**1119.** Horna P, Shao H, Idrees A, Glass LF, Torres-Cabala CA (2017). Indeterminate dendritic cell neoplasm of the skin: a 2-case report and review of the literature. J Cutan Pathol. 44(11):958–63. PMID:28880462

**1120.** Hornick JL, Bosenberg MW, Mentzel T, McMenamin ME, Oliveira AM, Fletcher CD (2004). Pleomorphic liposarcoma: clinicopathologic analysis of 57 cases. Am J Surg Pathol. 28(10):1257–67. PMID:15371941

**1121.** Hornick JL, Dal Cin P, Fletcher CD (2009). Loss of INI1 expression is characteristic of both conventional and proximal-type epithelioid sarcoma. Am J Surg Pathol. 33(4):542–50. PMID:19033866

**1122.** Hornick JL, Fletcher CD (2004). Cutaneous myoepithelioma: a clinicopathologic and immunohistochemical study of 14 cases. Hum Pathol. 35(1):14–24. PMID:14745720

**1123.** Hornick JL, Fletcher CD (2005). Intestinal perineuriomas: clinicopathologic definition of a new anatomic subset in a series of 10 cases. Am J Surg Pathol. 29(7):859–65. PMID:15958849

**1124.** Hornick JL, Fletcher CD (2005). Soft tissue perineurioma: clinicopathologic analysis of 81 cases including those with atypical histologic features. Am J Surg Pathol. 29(7):845–58. PMID:15958848

**1125.** Hornick JL, Fletcher CD (2006). Intraarticular nodular fasciitis–a rare lesion: clinicopathologic analysis of a series. Am J Surg Pathol. 30(2):237–41. PMID:16434899

**1126.** Hornick JL, Fletcher CD (2007). Cellular neurothekeoma: detailed characterization in a series of 133 cases. Am J Surg Pathol. 31(3):329–40. PMID:17325474

**1127.** Hornick JL, Fletcher CD (2011). Pseudomyogenic hemangioendothelioma: a distinctive, often multicentric tumor with indolent behavior. Am J Surg Pathol. 35(2):190–201. PMID:21263239

**1128.** Horny H-P, Akin C, Arber DA, Peterson LC, Tefferi A, Metcalfe DD, et al. (2017). Mastocytosis. In: Swerdlow SH, Campo E, Harris NL, Jaffe ES, Pileri SA, Stein H, et al., editors. WHO classification of tumours of haematopoietic and lymphoid tissues. Revised 4th ed. Lyon: International Agency for Research on Cancer; pp. 62–9.

**1129.** Horny HP, Sotlar K, Stellmacher F, Krokowski M, Agis H, Schwartz LB, et al. (2006). The tryptase positive compact round cell infiltrate of the bone marrow (TROCI-BM): a novel histopathological finding requiring the application of lineage specific markers. J Clin Pathol. 59(3):298–302. PMID:16505282

**1130.** Horvath A, Bertherat J, Groussin L, Guillaud-Bataille M, Tsang K, Cazabat L, et al. (2010). Mutations and polymorphisms in the gene encoding regulatory subunit type 1-alpha of protein kinase A (PRKAR1A): an update. Hum Mutat. 31(4):369–79. PMID:20358582

**1131.** Horvath A, Bossis I, Giatzakis C, Levine E, Weinberg F, Meoli E, et al. (2008). Large deletions of the PRKAR1A gene in Carney complex. Clin Cancer Res. 14(2):388–95. PMID:18223213

**1132.** Howrey RP, Lipham WJ, Schultz WH, Buckley EG, Dutton JJ, Klintworth GK, et al. (1998). Sebaceous gland carcinoma: a subtle second malignancy following radiation therapy in patients with bilateral retinoblastoma. Cancer. 83(4):767–71. PMID:9708943

**1133.** Hoy WE, Cestero RV, Freeman RB (1978). Lymphocyte subpopulations in maintenance hemodialysis patients. J Dial. 2(1):1–15. PMID:305928

**1134.** Hsi AC, Hurley MY, Lee SJ, Rosman IS, Pang X, Gru A, et al. (2016). Diagnostic utility of SOX11 immunohistochemistry in differentiating cutaneous spread of mantle cell lymphoma from primary cutaneous B-cell lymphomas. J Cutan Pathol. 43(4):354–61. PMID:26762898

**1135.** Hsi AC, Robirds DH, Luo J, Kreisel FH, Frater JL, Nguyen TT (2014). T-cell prolymphocytic leukemia frequently shows cutaneous involvement and is associated with gains of MYC, loss of ATM, and TCL1A rearrangement. Am J Surg Pathol. 38(11):1468–83. PMID:25310835

**1136.** Hsu YC, Li L, Fuchs E (2014). Emerging interactions between skin stem cells and their niches. Nat Med. 20(8):847–56. PMID:25100530

**1137.** Hu DN, Yu GP, McCormick SA, Schneider S, Finger PT (2005). Population-based incidence of uveal melanoma in various races and ethnic groups. Am J Ophthalmol. 140(4):612–7. PMID:16226513

**1138.** Hu Z, Medeiros LJ, Fang L, Sun Y, Tang Z, Tang G, et al. (2017). Prognostic significance of cytogenetic abnormalities in T-cell prolymphocytic leukemia. Am J Hematol. 92(5):441–7. PMID:28194886

**1139.** Hu-Lieskovan S, Zhang J, Wu L, Shimada H, Schofield DE, Triche TJ (2005). EWS-FLI1 fusion protein up-regulates critical genes in neural crest development and is responsible for the observed phenotype of Ewing's family of tumors. Cancer Res. 65(11):4633–44. PMID:15930281

**1140.** Huang D, Sumegi J, Dal Cin P, Reith JD, Yasuda T, Nelson M, et al. (2010). C11orf95-MKL2 is the resulting fusion oncogene of t(11;16)(q13;p13) in chondroid lipoma. Genes Chromosomes Cancer. 49(9):810–8. PMID:20607705

**1141.** Huang FW, Hodis E, Xu MJ, Kryukov GV, Chin L, Garraway LA (2013). Highly recurrent TERT promoter mutations in human melanoma. Science. 339(6122):957–9. PMID:23348506

**1142.** Huang KP, Weinstock MA, Clarke CA, McMillan A, Hoppe RT, Kim YH (2007). Second lymphomas and other malignant neoplasms in patients with mycosis fungoides and Sezary syndrome: evidence from population-based and clinical cohorts. Arch Dermatol. 143(1):45–50. PMID:17224541

**1143.** Huang L, Wang SA, Konoplev S, Bueso-Ramos CE, Thakral B, Miranda RN, et al. (2016). Well-differentiated systemic mastocytosis showed excellent clinical response to imatinib in the absence of known molecular genetic abnormalities: a case report. Medicine (Baltimore). 95(41):e4934. PMID:27741105

**1144.** Huang SC, Zhang L, Sung YS, Chen CL, Kao YC, Agaram NP, et al. (2016). Recurrent CIC gene abnormalities in angiosarcomas: a molecular study of 120 cases with concurrent investigation of PLCG1, KDR, MYC, and FLT4 gene alterations. Am J Surg Pathol. 40(5):645–55. PMID:26735859

**1145.** Huang SC, Zhang L, Sung YS, Chen CL, Krausz T, Dickson BC, et al. (2015). Frequent FOS gene rearrangements in epithelioid hemangioma: a molecular study of 58 cases with morphologic reappraisal. Am J Surg Pathol. 39(10):1313–21. PMID:26135557

**1146.** Hügel H (1993). Plaque-like dermal fibromatosis/dermatomyofibroma. J Cutan Pathol. 20(1):94. PMID:8468425

**1147.** Hügel H, Requena L (2003). Ductal carcinoma arising from a syringocystadenoma papilliferum in a nevus sebaceus of Jadassohn. Am J Dermatopathol. 25(6):490–3. PMID:14631190

**1148.** Hulsebos TJ, Plomp AS, Wolterman RA, Robanus-Maandag EC, Baas F, Wesseling P (2007). Germline mutation of INI1/SMARCB1 in familial schwannomatosis. Am J Hum Genet. 80(4):805–10. PMID:17357086

**1149.** Qiagen Bioinformatics (2017). The Human Gene Mutation Database (HGMD). Hilden: Qiagen Bioinformatics. Available from: https://portal.biobase-international.com/.

**1150.** Hung T, Argenyi Z, Erickson L, Guitart J, Horenstein MG, Lowe L, et al. (2016). Cellular blue nevomelanocytic lesions: analysis of clinical, histological, and outcome data in 37 cases. Am J Dermatopathol. 38(7):499–503.

PMID:26909585
**1151.** Hung T, Yang A, Mihm MC, Barnhill RL (2014). The plexiform spindle cell nevus nevi and atypical variants: report of 128 cases. Hum Pathol. 45(12):2369–78. PMID:25300464
**1152.** Hung YP, Fletcher CD, Hornick JL (2016). Evaluation of NKX2-2 expression in round cell sarcomas and other tumors with EWSR1 rearrangement: imperfect specificity for Ewing sarcoma. Mod Pathol. 29(4):370–80. PMID:26847175
**1153.** Hung YP, Fletcher CD, Hornick JL (2017). FOSB is a useful diagnostic marker for pseudomyogenic hemangioendothelioma. Am J Surg Pathol. 41(5):596–606. PMID:28009608
**1154.** Hung YP, Fletcher CDM (2017). Myopericytomatosis: clinicopathologic analysis of 11 cases with molecular identification of recurrent PDGFRB alterations in myopericytomatosis and myopericytoma. Am J Surg Pathol. 41(8):1034–44. PMID:28505006
**1155.** Hunt KM, Srivastava RK, Elmets CA, Athar M (2014). The mechanistic basis of arsenicosis: pathogenesis of skin cancer. Cancer Lett. 354(2):211–9. PMID:25173797
**1156.** Hunt SJ, Kilzer B, Santa Cruz DJ (1990). Desmoplastic trichilemmoma: histologic variant resembling invasive carcinoma. J Cutan Pathol. 17(1):45–52. PMID:2319039
**1157.** Hunt SJ, Santa Cruz DJ, Barr RJ (1991). Microvenular hemangioma. J Cutan Pathol. 18(4):235–40. PMID:1939781
**1158.** Hunt SJ, Santa Cruz DJ, Kerl H (1990). Giant eccrine acrospiroma. J Am Acad Dermatol. 23(4 Pt 1):663–8. PMID:2172332
**1159.** Huppmann AR, Xi L, Raffeld M, Pittaluga S, Jaffe ES (2013). Subcutaneous panniculitis-like T-cell lymphoma in the pediatric age group: a lymphoma of low malignant potential. Pediatr Blood Cancer. 60(7):1165–70. PMID:23382035
**1160.** Hurley MY, Ghahramani GK, Frisch S, Armbrecht ES, Lind AC, Nguyen TT, et al. (2013). Cutaneous myeloid sarcoma: natural history and biology of an uncommon manifestation of acute myeloid leukemia. Acta Derm Venereol. 93(3):319–24. PMID:23165700
**1161.** Husein-ElAhmed H, Fernandez-Pugnaire MA (2016). Dermatoscopy-guided therapy of pigmented basal cell carcinoma with imiquimod. An Bras Dermatol. 91(6):764–9. PMID:28099598
**1162.** Hussein MR (2005). Melanocytic dysplastic naevi occupy the middle ground between benign melanocytic naevi and cutaneous malignant melanomas: emerging clues. J Clin Pathol. 58(5):453–6. PMID:15858113
**1163.** Iarikov D, Duke W, Skiest D (2008). Extensive development of flat warts as a cutaneous manifestation of immune reconstitution syndrome. AIDS Read. 18(10):524–7. PMID:18975443
**1164.** Ichihashi N, Kitajima Y (2000). Loss of heterozygosity of adenomatous polyposis coli gene in cutaneous tumors as determined by using polymerase chain reaction and paraffin section preparations. J Dermatol Sci. 22(2):102–6. PMID:10674823
**1165.** Idriss MH, Elston DM (2014). Secondary neoplasms associated with nevus sebaceus of Jadassohn: a study of 707 cases. J Am Acad Dermatol. 70(2):332–7. PMID:24268309
**1166.** Igawa HH, Ohura T, Sugihara T, Ishikawa T, Kumakiri M (1994). Cleft lip Mongolian spot: Mongolian spot associated with cleft lip. J Am Acad Dermatol. 30(4):566–9. PMID:8157782
**1167.** Ikonomou IM, Aamot HV, Heim S, Fosså A, Delabie J (2007). Granulomatous slack skin with a translocation t(3;9)(q12;p24). Am J Surg Pathol. 31(5):803–6. PMID:17460466
**1168.** Iles MM, Law MH, Stacey SN, Han J, Fang S, Pfeiffer R, et al. (2013). A variant in FTO shows association with melanoma risk not due to BMI. Nat Genet. 45(4):428–32, e1. PMID:23455637
**1169.** Imko-Walczuk B, Cegielska A, Placek W, Kaszewski S, Fiedor P (2014). Human papillomavirus-related verrucous carcinoma in a renal transplant patient after long-term immunosuppression: a case report. Transplant Proc. 46(8):2916–9. PMID:25380950
**1170.** Imko-Walczuk B, Kryś A, Lizakowski S, Dębska-Ślizień A, Rutkowski B, Biernat W, et al. (2014). Sebaceous carcinoma in patients receiving long-term immunosuppresive treatment: case report and literature review. Transplant Proc. 46(8):2903–7. PMID:25380947
**1171.** Imperial R, Helwig EB (1967). Angiokeratoma of the scrotum (Fordyce type). J Urol. 98(3):379–87. PMID:6069899
**1172.** Imperial R, Helwig EB (1967). Angiokeratoma of the vulva. Obstet Gynecol. 29(3):307–12. PMID:6019084
**1173.** Imperial R, Helwig EB (1967). Angiokeratoma. A clinicopathological study. Arch Dermatol. 95(2):166–75. PMID:6018992
**1174.** Imperial R, Helwig EB (1967). Verrucous hemangioma. A clinicopathologic study of 21 cases. Arch Dermatol. 96(3):247–53. PMID:6038751
**1175.** Inaba H, Greaves M, Mullighan CG (2013). Acute lymphoblastic leukaemia. Lancet. 381(9881):1943–55. PMID:23523389
**1176.** Inalöz HS, Chowdhury MM, Knight AG (2001). Cutaneous lymphadenoma. J Eur Acad Dermatol Venereol. 15(5):481–3. PMID:11763398
**1177.** Inamadar AC, Palit A (2007). Persistent, aberrant Mongolian spots in Sjögren-Larsson syndrome. Pediatr Dermatol. 24(1):98–9. PMID:17300667
**1178.** Indinnimeo M, Impagnatiello A, D'Ettorre G, Bernardi G, Moschella CM, Gozzo P, et al. (2013). Buschke-Löwenstein tumor with squamous cell carcinoma treated with chemo-radiation therapy and local surgical excision: report of three cases. World J Surg Oncol. 11:231. PMID:24040860
**1179.** Inoue M, Ueda K, Hashimoto T (2002). Nevus lipomatosus cutaneus superficialis with follicular papules and hypertrophic pilo-sebaceous units. Int J Dermatol. 41(4):241–3. PMID:12031036
**1180.** Inoue T, Misago N, Asami A, Tokunaga O, Narisawa Y (2016). Myopericytoma proliferating in an unusual anastomosing multinodular fashion. J Dermatol. 43(5):557–9. PMID:26499100
**1181.** Ioannidou DJ, Stefanidou MP, Panayiotides JG, Tosca AD (2001). Nevus lipomatosus cutaneous superficialis (Hoffmann-Zurhelle) with localized scleroderma like appearance. Int J Dermatol. 40(1):54–7. PMID:11277956
**1182.** Iorizzo LJ 3rd, Brown MD (2011). Atypical fibroxanthoma: a review of the literature. Dermatol Surg. 37(2):146–57. PMID:21269345
**1183.** Iraji F, Kiani A, Shahidi S, Vahabi R (2002). Histopathology of skin lesions with warty appearance in renal allograft recipients. Am J Dermatopathol. 24(4):324–5. PMID:12142612
**1184.** Ireland AM, Harvey NT, Berry BD, Wood BA (2017). Paediatric cutaneous adnexal tumours: a study of 559 cases. Pathology. 49(1):50–4. PMID:27914683
**1185.** Irvine AD, Sweeney L, Corbett JR (1996). Lymphangioma circumscriptum associated with paravesical cystic retroperitoneal lymphangioma. Br J Dermatol. 134(6):1135–7. PMID:8763441
**1186.** Ishibashi M, Yamamoto K, Kudo S, Chen KR (2010). Mantle cell lymphoma with skin invasion characterized by the common variant in the subcutis and blastoid transformation in the overlying dermis. Am J Dermatopathol. 32(2):180–2. PMID:20010283
**1187.** Ishida M, Okabe H (2012). Intraepidermal sebaceous carcinoma occurring concurrently with actinic keratosis. J Cutan Pathol. 39(7):731–2. PMID:22416794
**1188.** Ishige T, Kikuchi K, Miyazaki Y, Hara H, Yoshino A, Terui T, et al. (2011). Differentiation and apoptosis in pilomatrixoma. Am J Dermatopathol. 33(1):60–4. PMID:21239898
**1189.** Ishikawa K (1971). Malignant hidroacanthoma simplex. Arch Dermatol. 104(5):529–32. PMID:5120180
**1190.** Ishimura E, Iwamoto H, Kobashi Y, Yamabe H, Ichijima K (1983). Malignant chondroid syringoma. Report of a case with widespread metastasis and review of pertinent literature. Cancer. 52(10):1966–73. PMID:6194872
**1191.** Islam MN, Bhattacharyya I, Proper SA, Glanz SM, Vega JM, Hassanein AM (2007). Melanocytic matricoma: a distinctive clinicopathologic entity. Dermatol Surg. 33(7):857–63. PMID:17598856
**1192.** Ivan D, Nash JW, Prieto VG, Calonje E, Lyle S, Diwan AH, et al. (2007). Use of p63 expression in distinguishing primary and metastatic cutaneous adnexal neoplasms from metastatic adenocarcinoma to skin. J Cutan Pathol. 34(6):474–80. PMID:17518775
**1193.** Iwata J, Fletcher CD (2000). Lipidized fibrous histiocytoma: clinicopathologic analysis of 22 cases. Am J Dermatopathol. 22(2):126–34. PMID:10770432
**1194.** Iwata S, Wada K, Tobita S, Gotoh K, Ito Y, Demachi-Okamura A, et al. (2010). Quantitative analysis of Epstein-Barr virus (EBV)-related gene expression in patients with chronic active EBV infection. J Gen Virol. 91(Pt 1):42–50. PMID:19793909
**1195.** Iwatsuki K, Ohtsuka M, Akiba H, Kaneko F (1999). Atypical hydroa vacciniforme in childhood: from a smoldering stage to Epstein-Barr virus-associated lymphoid malignancy. J Am Acad Dermatol. 40(2 Pt 1):283–4. PMID:10025766
**1196.** Iwatsuki K, Satoh M, Yamamoto T, Oono T, Morizane S, Ohtsuka M, et al. (2006). Pathogenic link between hydroa vacciniforme and Epstein-Barr virus-associated hematologic disorders. Arch Dermatol. 142(5):587–95. PMID:16702496
**1197.** Iwatsuki K, Xu Z, Takata M, Iguchi M, Ohtsuka M, Akiba H, et al. (1999). The association of latent Epstein-Barr virus infection with hydroa vacciniforme. Br J Dermatol. 140(4):715–21. PMID:10233328
**1198.** Iwaya M, Uehara T, Yoshizawa A, Kobayashi Y, Momose M, Honda T, et al. (2012). A case of primary signet-ring cell/histiocytoid carcinoma of the eyelid: immunohistochemical comparison with the normal sweat gland and review of the literature. Am J Dermatopathol. 34(8):e139–45. PMID:22935888
**1199.** Izumi M, Ohara K, Hoashi T, Nakayama H, Chiu CS, Nagai T, et al. (2008). Subungual melanoma: histological examination of 50 cases from early stage to bone invasion. J Dermatol. 35(11):695–703. PMID:19120763
**1200.** Izumi T, Oda Y, Hasegawa T, Nakanishi Y, Iwasaki H, Sonobe H, et al. (2006). Prognostic significance of dysadherin expression in epithelioid sarcoma and its diagnostic utility in distinguishing epithelioid sarcoma from malignant rhabdoid tumor. Mod Pathol. 19(6):820–31. PMID:16557275
**1201.** Jacob MC, Chaperot L, Mossuz P, Feuillard J, Valensi F, Leroux D, et al. (2003). CD4+ CD56+ lineage negative malignancies: a new entity developed from malignant early plasmacytoid dendritic cells. Haematologica. 88(8):941–55. PMID:12935983
**1201A.** Jacobsen E, Shanmugam V, Jagannathan J (2017). Rosai-Dorfman disease with activating KRAS mutation - response to cobimetinib. N Engl J Med. 377(24):2398–9. PMID:29236635
**1202.** Jacobson MA, Hutcheson AC, Hurray DH, Metcalf JS, Thiers BH (2006). Cutaneous involvement by Burkitt lymphoma. J Am Acad Dermatol. 54(6):1111–3. PMID:16713488
**1203.** Jacoby LB, MacCollin M, Barone R, Ramesh V, Gusella JF (1996). Frequency and distribution of NF2 mutations in schwannomas. Genes Chromosomes Cancer. 17(1):45–55. PMID:8889506
**1204.** Jaffe ES, Arber DA, Campo E, Harris NL, Quintanilla-Martinez L (2017). Primary cutaneous B-cell lymphomas. In: Hematopathology. 2nd ed. Oxford: Elsevier.
**1205.** Jaffe ES, Krenacs L, Raffeld M (2003). Classification of cytotoxic T-cell and natural killer cell lymphomas. Semin Hematol. 40(3):175–84. PMID:12876666
**1206.** Jaffe ES, Wilson WH (1997). Lymphomatoid granulomatosis: pathogenesis, pathology and clinical implications. Cancer Surv. 30:233–48. PMID:9547995
**1207.** Jaffer S, Ambrosini-Spaltro A, Mancini AM, Eusebi V, Rosai J (2009). Neurothekeoma and plexiform fibrohistiocytic tumor: mere histologic resemblance or histogenetic relationship? Am J Surg Pathol. 33(6):905–13. PMID:19342943
**1208.** Jain P, Aoki E, Keating M, Wierda WG, O'Brien S, Gonzalez GN, et al. (2017). Characteristics, outcomes, prognostic factors and treatment of patients with T-cell prolymphocytic leukemia (T-PLL). Ann Oncol. 28(7):1554–9. PMID:28379307
**1209.** Jakobiec FA, Folberg R, Iwamoto T (1989). Clinicopathologic characteristics of premalignant and malignant melanocytic lesions of the conjunctiva. Ophthalmology. 96(2):147–66. PMID:2649838
**1210.** James E, Sokhn JG, Gibson JF, Carlson K, Subtil A, Girardi M, et al. (2015). CD4 + primary cutaneous small/medium-sized pleomorphic T-cell lymphoma: a retrospective case series and review of literature. Leuk Lymphoma. 56(4):951–7. PMID:24996443
**1211.** James MP, Wells GC, Whimster IW (1978). Spreading pigmented actinic keratoses. Br J Dermatol. 98(4):373–9. PMID:638043
**1212.** James WD, Odom RB, Katzenstein AL (1981). Cutaneous manifestations of lymphomatoid granulomatosis. Report of 44 cases and a review of the literature. Arch Dermatol. 117(4):196–202. PMID:7212740
**1213.** Jamshidi F, Bashashati A, Shumansky K, Dickson B, Gokgoz N, Wunder JS, et al. (2016). The genomic landscape of epithelioid sarcoma cell lines and tumours. J Pathol. 238(1):63–73. PMID:26365879
**1214.** Jans SR, Schomerus E, Bygum A (2015). Neurofibromatosis type 1 diagnosed in a child based on multiple juvenile xanthogranulomas and juvenile myelomonocytic leukemia. Pediatr Dermatol. 32(1):e29–32. PMID:25516272
**1215.** Janssen D, Harms D (2005). Juvenile xanthogranuloma in childhood and adolescence: a clinicopathologic study of 129 patients from the Kiel Pediatric Tumor Registry. Am J Surg Pathol. 29(1):21–8. PMID:15613853
**1216.** Jardin F, Ruminy P, Parmentier F, Troussard X, Vaida I, Stamatoullas A, et al. (2011). TET2 and TP53 mutations are frequently observed in blastic plasmacytoid dendritic cell neoplasm. Br J Haematol. 153(3):413–6. PMID:21275969
**1217.** Jawhar M, Schwaab J, Schnittger S, Sotlar K, Horny HP, Metzgeroth G, et al. (2015). Molecular profiling of myeloid progenitor cells in multi-mutated advanced systemic mastocytosis identifies KIT D816V as a distinct and late event. Leukemia. 29(5):1115–22.

PMID:25567135
**1218.** Jaworski R (1987). Unusual proliferating trichilemmal cyst. Am J Dermatopathol. 9(5):459–61. PMID:3688371
**1219.** Jayaraman SS, Rayhan DJ, Hazany S, Kolodney MS (2014). Mutational landscape of basal cell carcinomas by whole-exome sequencing. J Invest Dermatol. 134(1):213–20. PMID:23774526
**1220.** Jaye DL, Geigerman CM, Herling M, Eastburn K, Waller EK, Jones D (2006). Expression of the plasmacytoid dendritic cell marker BDCA-2 supports a spectrum of maturation among CD4+ CD56+ hematodermic neoplasms. Mod Pathol. 19(12):1555–62. PMID:16998465
**1221.** Jedrych J, Nikiforova M, Kennedy TF, Ho J (2015). Epithelioid cell histiocytoma of the skin with clonal ALK gene rearrangement resulting in VCL-ALK and SQSTM1-ALK gene fusions. Br J Dermatol. 172(5):1427–9. PMID:25413595
**1222.** Jegalian AG, Buxbaum NP, Facchetti F, Raffeld M, Pittaluga S, Wayne AS, et al. (2010). Blastic plasmacytoid dendritic cell neoplasm in children: diagnostic features and clinical implications. Haematologica. 95(11):1873–9. PMID:20663945
**1223.** Jeltsch M, Kaipainen A, Joukov V, Meng X, Lakso M, Rauvala H, et al. (1997). Hyperplasia of lymphatic vessels in VEGF-C transgenic mice. Science. 276(5317):1423–5. PMID:9162011
**1224.** Jeon IS, Davis JN, Braun BS, Sublett JE, Roussel MF, Denny CT, et al. (1995). A variant Ewing's sarcoma translocation (7;22) fuses the EWS gene to the ETS gene ETV1. Oncogene. 10(6):1229–34. PMID:7700648
**1225.** Jessup CJ, Redston M, Tilton E, Reimann JD (2016). Importance of universal mismatch repair protein immunohistochemistry in patients with sebaceous neoplasia as an initial screening tool for Muir-Torre syndrome. Hum Pathol. 49:1–9. PMID:26826402
**1226.** Jha A, Khunger N, Malarvizhi K, Ramesh V, Singh A (2016). Familial disseminated cutaneous glomuvenous malformation: treatment with polidocanol sclerotherapy. J Cutan Aesthet Surg. 9(4):266–9. PMID:28163461
**1227.** Jha P, Moosavi C, Fanburg-Smith JC (2007). Giant cell fibroblastoma: an update and addition of 86 new cases from the Armed Forces Institute of Pathology, in honor of Dr. Franz M. Enzinger. Ann Diagn Pathol. 11(2):81–8. PMID:17349565
**1228.** Jiao Y, Pawlik TM, Anders RA, Selaru FM, Streppel MM, Lucas DJ, et al. (2013). Exome sequencing identifies frequent inactivating mutations in BAP1, ARID1A and PBRM1 in intrahepatic cholangiocarcinomas. Nat Genet. 45(12):1470–3. PMID:24185509
**1229.** Jin X, Li F, Li X, Zhu W, Mou Y, Huang Y, et al. (2017). Cutaneous presentation preceding acute monocytic leukemia: a CARE-compliant article. Medicine (Baltimore). 96(10):e6269. PMID:28272239
**1230.** Jo VY, Antonescu CR, Zhang L, Dal Cin P, Hornick JL, Fletcher CD (2013). Cutaneous syncytial myoepithelioma: clinicopathologic characterization in a series of 38 cases. Am J Surg Pathol. 37(5):710–8. PMID:23588365
**1231.** Jo VY, Fletcher CD (2015). Epithelioid malignant peripheral nerve sheath tumor: clinicopathologic analysis of 63 cases. Am J Surg Pathol. 39(5):673–82. PMID:25602794
**1232.** Johansson P, Aoude LG, Wadt K, Glasson WJ, Warrier SK, Hewitt AW, et al. (2016). Deep sequencing of uveal melanoma identifies a recurrent mutation in PLCB4. Oncotarget. 7(4):4624–31. PMID:26683228
**1233.** Johansson PA, Pritchard AL, Patch AM, Wilmott JS, Pearson JV, Waddell N, et al. (2017). Mutation load in melanoma is affected by MC1R genotype. Pigment Cell Melanoma Res. 30(2):255–8. PMID:28024115
**1234.** John AM, Schwartz RA (2016). Muir-Torre syndrome (MTS): an update and approach to diagnosis and management. J Am Acad Dermatol. 74(3):558–66. PMID:26892655
**1235.** John I, Folpe AL (2016). Anastomosing hemangiomas arising in unusual locations: a clinicopathologic study of 17 soft tissue cases showing a predilection for the paraspinal region. Am J Surg Pathol. 40(8):1084–9. PMID:26945338
**1236.** Johnson BL, Buerger GF Jr (1994). Syringocystadenoma papilliferum of the eyelid. Am J Ophthalmol. 118(6):822–3. PMID:7977619
**1237.** Johnson LW (1995). Communal showers and the risk of plantar warts. J Fam Pract. 40(2):136–8. PMID:7852935
**1238.** Johnson MD, Kamso-Pratt J, Federspiel CF, Whetsell WO Jr (1989). Mast cell and lymphoreticular infiltrates in neurofibromas. Comparison with nerve sheath tumors. Arch Pathol Lab Med. 113(11):1263–70. PMID:2479359
**1239.** Johnson WT, Patel P, Hernandez A, Grandinetti LM, Huen AC, Marks S, et al. (2016). Langerhans cell histiocytosis and Erdheim-Chester disease, both with cutaneous presentations, and papillary thyroid carcinoma all harboring the BRAF(V600E) mutation. J Cutan Pathol. 43(3):270–5. PMID:26454140
**1240.** Johnston EE, LeBlanc RE, Kim J, Chung J, Balagtas J, Kim YH, et al. (2015). Subcutaneous panniculitis-like T-cell lymphoma: pediatric case series demonstrating heterogeneous presentation and option for watchful waiting. Pediatr Blood Cancer. 62(11):2025–8. PMID:26146844
**1241.** Jokinen CH, Ragsdale BD, Argenyi ZB (2010). Expanding the clinicopathologic spectrum of palisaded encapsulated neuroma. J Cutan Pathol. 37(1):43–8. PMID:19614730
**1242.** Joly MO, Attignon V, Saurin JC, Desseigne F, Leroux D, Martin-Denavit T, et al. (2015). Somatic MMR gene mutations as a cause for MSI-H sebaceous neoplasms in Muir-Torre syndrome-like patients. Hum Mutat. 36(3):292–5. PMID:25504677
**1243.** Jones CL, Wain EM, Chu CC, Tosi I, Foster R, McKenzie RC, et al. (2010). Downregulation of Fas gene expression in Sézary syndrome is associated with promoter hypermethylation. J Invest Dermatol. 130(4):1116–25. PMID:19759548
**1244.** Jones EW, Cerio R, Smith NP (1989). Epithelioid cell histiocytoma: a new entity. Br J Dermatol. 120(2):185–95. PMID:2466472
**1245.** Jones EW, Marks R, Pongsehirun D (1975). Naevus superficialis lipomatosus. A clinicopathological report of twenty cases. Br J Dermatol. 93(2):121–33. PMID:1235780
**1246.** Jones EW, Orkin M (1989). Tufted angioma (angioblastoma). A benign progressive angioma, not to be confused with Kaposi's sarcoma or low-grade angiosarcoma. J Am Acad Dermatol. 20(2 Pt 1):214–25. PMID:2644316
**1247.** Jones MS, Helm KF, Maloney ME (1997). The immunohistochemical characteristics of the basosquamous cell carcinoma. Dermatol Surg. 23(3):181–4. PMID:9145960
**1248.** Joyce JC, Keith PJ, Szabo S, Holland KE (2014). Superficial hemosiderotic lymphovascular malformation (hobnail hemangioma): a report of six cases. Pediatr Dermatol. 31(3):281–5. PMID:24601986
**1249.** Julia F, Dalle S, Duru G, Balme B, Vergier B, Ortonne N, et al. (2014). Blastic plasmacytoid dendritic cell neoplasms: clinico-immunohistochemical correlations in a series of 91 patients. Am J Surg Pathol. 38(5):673–80. PMID:24441662
**1250.** Julia F, Petrella T, Beylot-Barry M, Bagot M, Lipsker D, Machet L, et al. (2013). Blastic plasmacytoid dendritic cell neoplasm: clinical features in 90 patients. Br J Dermatol. 169(3):579–86. PMID:23646868
**1251.** Jung HJ, Kweon SS, Lee JB, Lee SC, Yun SJ (2013). A clinicopathologic analysis of 177 acral melanomas in Koreans: relevance of spreading pattern and physical stress. JAMA Dermatol. 149(11):1281–8. PMID:24067997
**1252.** Jurecka W (1988). Pigmented neurofibroma. J Dermatol. 15(2):172–9. PMID:3049734
**1253.** Jurecka W (1988). Plexiforme neurofibroma of the skin. Am J Dermatopathol. 10(3):209–17. PMID:3068997
**1254.** Kaasinen E, Aavikko M, Vahteristo P, Patama T, Li Y, Saarinen S, et al. (2013). Nationwide registry-based analysis of cancer clustering detects strong familial occurrence of Kaposi sarcoma. PLoS One. 8(1):e55209. PMID:23365693
**1255.** Kacerovska D, Kazakov DV, Kutzner H, Michal M (2010). Spiradenoma with marked adenomyoepitheliomatous features. Am J Dermatopathol. 32(7):744–6. PMID:20859082
**1256.** Kacerovska D, Kazakov DV, Michal M (2010). Spindle-cell predominant trichodiscoma with a palisaded arrangement of stromal cells. Am J Dermatopathol. 32(7):743–4. PMID:20644461
**1257.** Kacerovska D, Nemcova J, Pomahacova R, Michal M, Kazakov DV (2008). Cutaneous and superficial soft tissue lesions associated with Albright hereditary osteodystrophy: clinicopathological and molecular genetic study of 4 cases, including a novel mutation of the GNAS gene. Am J Dermatopathol. 30(5):417–24. PMID:18806481
**1258.** Kacerovska D, Szepe P, Vanecek T, Nemcova J, Michal M, Mukensnabl P, et al. (2008). Spiradenocylindroma-like basaloid carcinoma of the anus and rectum: case report, including HPV studies and analysis of the CYLD gene mutations. Am J Dermatopathol. 30(5):472–6. PMID:18806492
**1259.** Kaddu S, Dong H, Mayer G, Kerl H, Cerroni L (2002). Warty dyskeratoma–"follicular dyskeratoma": analysis of clinicopathologic features of a distinctive follicular adnexal neoplasm. J Am Acad Dermatol. 47(3):423–8. PMID:12196754
**1260.** Kaddu S, Leinweber B (2009). Podoplanin expression in fibrous histiocytomas and cellular neurothekeomas. Am J Dermatopathol. 31(2):137–9. PMID:19318798
**1261.** Kaddu S, McMenamin ME, Fletcher CD (2002). Atypical fibrous histiocytoma of the skin: clinicopathologic analysis of 59 cases with evidence of infrequent metastasis. Am J Surg Pathol. 26(1):35–46. PMID:11756767
**1262.** Kaddu S, Smolle J, Cerroni L, Kerl H (1996). Prognostic evaluation of specific cutaneous infiltrates in B-chronic lymphocytic leukemia. J Cutan Pathol. 23(6):487–94. PMID:9001978
**1263.** Kaddu S, Zenahlik P, Beham-Schmid C, Kerl H, Cerroni L (1999). Specific cutaneous infiltrates in patients with myelogenous leukemia: a clinicopathologic study of 26 patients with assessment of diagnostic criteria. J Am Acad Dermatol. 40(6 Pt 1):966–78. PMID:10365929
**1264.** Kadin ME, Hughey LC, Wood GS (2014). Large-cell transformation of mycosis fungoides-differential diagnosis with implications for clinical management: a consensus statement of the US Cutaneous Lymphoma Consortium. J Am Acad Dermatol. 70(2):374–6. PMID:24438952
**1265.** Kadin ME, Pinkus JL, Pinkus GS, Duran IH, Fuller CE, Onciu M, et al. (2008). Primary cutaneous ALCL with phosphorylated/activated cytoplasmic ALK and novel phenotype: EMA/MUC1+, cutaneous lymphocyte antigen negative. Am J Surg Pathol. 32(9):1421–6. PMID:18670345
**1266.** Kadin ME, Vonderheid EC, Weiss LM (1993). Absence of Epstein-Barr viral RNA in lymphomatoid papulosis. J Pathol. 170(2):145–8. PMID:8393923
**1267.** Kakavand H, Wilmott JS, Long GV, Scolyer RA (2016). Targeted therapies and immune checkpoint inhibitors in the treatment of metastatic melanoma patients: a guide and update for pathologists. Pathology. 48(2):194–202. PMID:27020392
**1268.** Kalirai H, Dodson A, Faqir S, Damato BE, Coupland SE (2014). Lack of BAP1 protein expression in uveal melanoma is associated with increased metastatic risk and has utility in routine prognostic testing. Br J Cancer. 111(7):1373–80. PMID:25058347
**1269.** Kamalpour L, Brindise RT, Nodzenski M, Bach DQ, Veledar E, Alam M (2014). Primary cutaneous mucinous carcinoma: a systematic review and meta-analysis of outcomes after surgery. JAMA Dermatol. 150(4):380–4. PMID:24452370
**1270.** Kamarashev J, French LE, Dummer R, Kerl K (2009). Symplastic glomus tumor - a rare but distinct benign histological variant with analogy to other 'ancient' benign skin neoplasms. J Cutan Pathol. 36(10):1099–102. PMID:19602065
**1271.** Kamino H, Jacobson M (1990). Dermatofibroma extending into the subcutaneous tissue. Differential diagnosis from dermatofibrosarcoma protuberans. Am J Surg Pathol. 14(12):1156–64. PMID:2252106
**1272.** Kamino H, Lee JY, Berke A (1989). Pleomorphic fibroma of the skin: a benign neoplasm with cytologic atypia. A clinicopathologic study of eight cases. Am J Surg Pathol. 13(2):107–13. PMID:2916726
**1273.** Kamino H, Reddy VB, Gero M, Greco MA (1992). Dermatomyofibroma. A benign cutaneous, plaque-like proliferation of fibroblasts and myofibroblasts in young adults. J Cutan Pathol. 19(2):85–93. PMID:1597573
**1274.** Kamińska-Winciorek G, Szymszal J (2014). Dermoscopy of halo nevus in own observation. Postepy Dermatol Alergol. 31(3):152–8. PMID:25097486
**1275.** Kamyab-Hesari K, Seirafi H, Naraghi ZS, Shahshahani MM, Rahbar Z, Damavandi MR, et al. (2014). Diagnostic accuracy of punch biopsy in subtyping basal cell carcinoma. J Eur Acad Dermatol Venereol. 28(2):250–3. PMID:22989368
**1276.** Kanazawa T, Hiramatsu Y, Iwata S, Siddiquey M, Sato Y, Suzuki M, et al. (2014). Anti-CCR4 monoclonal antibody mogamulizumab for the treatment of EBV-associated T- and NK-cell lymphoproliferative diseases. Clin Cancer Res. 20(19):5075–84. PMID:25117294
**1277.** Kaneko Y, Yoshida K, Handa M, Toyoda Y, Nishihira H, Tanaka Y, et al. (1996). Fusion of an ETS-family gene, EIAF, to EWS by t(17;22)(q12;q12) chromosome translocation in an undifferentiated sarcoma of infancy. Genes Chromosomes Cancer. 15(2):115–21. PMID:8834175
**1278.** Kang HC, Quigley DA, Kim IJ, Wakabayashi Y, Ferguson-Smith MA, D'Alessandro M, et al. (2013). Multiple self-healing squamous epithelioma (MSSE): rare variants in an adjacent region of chromosome 9q22.3 to known TGFBR1 mutations suggest a digenic or multilocus etiology. J Invest Dermatol. 133(7):1907–10. PMID:23358096
**1279.** Kang Z, Xu F, Zhang QA, Wu Z, Zhang X, Xu J, et al. (2013). Oncogenic mutations in extramammary Paget's disease and their clinical relevance. Int J Cancer. 132(4):824–31. PMID:22821211

**1280.** Kanitakis J, Chouvet B (2007). Expression of p63 in cutaneous metastases. Am J Clin Pathol. 128(5):753–8. PMID:17951196
**1281.** Kanitakis J, Euvrard S, Sebbag L, Claudy A (2007). Trichilemmal carcinoma of the skin mimicking a keloid in a heart transplant recipient. J Heart Lung Transplant. 26(6):649–51. PMID:17543793
**1282.** Kao GF, Helwig EB, Graham JH (1987). Aggressive digital papillary adenoma and adenocarcinoma. A clinicopathological study of 57 patients, with histochemical, immunopathological, and ultrastructural observations. J Cutan Pathol. 14(3):129–46. PMID:3301927
**1283.** Kao GF, Laskin WB, Olsen TG (1989). Solitary cutaneous plexiform neurilemmoma (schwannoma): a clinicopathologic, immunohistochemical, and ultrastructural study of 11 cases. Mod Pathol. 2(1):20–6. PMID:2493641
**1284.** Karagas MR, Zens MS, Li Z, Stukel TA, Perry AE, Gilbert-Diamond D, et al. (2014). Early-onset basal cell carcinoma and indoor tanning: a population-based study. Pediatrics. 134(1):e4–12. PMID:24958589
**1285.** Karai LJ, Kadin ME, Hsi ED, Sluzevich JC, Ketterling RP, Knudson RA, et al. (2013). Chromosomal rearrangements of 6p25.3 define a new subtype of lymphomatoid papulosis. Am J Surg Pathol. 37(8):1173–81. PMID:23648461
**1286.** Kari L, Loboda A, Nebozhyn M, Rook AH, Vonderheid EC, Nichols C, et al. (2003). Classification and prediction of survival in patients with the leukemic phase of cutaneous T cell lymphoma. J Exp Med. 197(11):1477–88. PMID:12782714
**1287.** Kashima M, Takahama H, Baba T, Egawa K, Kitasato H, Murakami Y, et al. (2003). Detection of human papillomavirus type 57 in the tissue of a plantar epidermoid cyst. Dermatology. 207(2):185–7. PMID:12920371
**1288.** Kato H, Mizuno N, Nakagawa K, Furukawa M, Hamada T (1990). Microcystic adnexal carcinoma: a light microscopic, immunohistochemical and ultrastructural study. J Cutan Pathol. 17(2):87–95. PMID:2187025
**1289.** Kato I, Yoshida A, Ikegami M, Okuma T, Tonooka A, Horiguchi S, et al. (2016). FOSL1 immunohistochemistry clarifies the distinction between desmoplastic fibroblastoma and fibroma of tendon sheath. Histopathology. 69(6):1012–20. PMID:27442992
**1290.** Kato N, Ueno H (1993). Infundibulocystic basal cell carcinoma. Am J Dermatopathol. 15(3):265–7. PMID:8517497
**1291.** Katona TM, Perkins SM, Billings SD (2008). Does the panel of cytokeratin 20 and androgen receptor antibodies differentiate desmoplastic trichoepithelioma from morpheaform/infiltrative basal cell carcinoma? J Cutan Pathol. 35(2):174–9. PMID:18190441
**1292.** Katsuya H, Ishitsuka K, Utsunomiya A, Hanada S, Eto T, Moriuchi Y, et al. (2015). Treatment and survival among 1594 patients with ATL. Blood. 126(24):2570–7. PMID:26361794
**1293.** Katsuya H, Shimokawa M, Ishitsuka K, Kawai K, Amano M, Utsunomiya A, et al. (2017). Prognostic index for chronic- and smoldering-type adult T-cell leukemia-lymphoma. Blood. 130(1):39–47. PMID:28515095
**1294.** Katzenstein AL, Carrington CB, Liebow AA (1979). Lymphomatoid granulomatosis: a clinicopathologic study of 152 cases. Cancer. 43(1):360–73. PMID:761171
**1295.** Katzenstein AL, Doxtader E, Narendra S (2010). Lymphomatoid granulomatosis: insights gained over 4 decades. Am J Surg Pathol. 34(12):e35–48. PMID:21107080
**1296.** Kawabe S, Ito Y, Gotoh K, Kojima S, Matsumoto K, Kinoshita T, et al. (2012). Application of flow cytometric in situ hybridization assay to Epstein-Barr virus-associated T/natural killer cell lymphoproliferative diseases. Cancer Sci. 103(8):1481–8. PMID:22497716
**1297.** Kazakov DV (2012). Mammary Paget's disease. In: Kazakov DV, Michal M, Kacerovska D, McKee PH, editors. Cutaneous adnexal tumors. Philadelphia: Lippincott Williams & Wilkins; pp. 451–543.
**1298.** Kazakov DV (2016). Brooke-Spiegler syndrome and phenotypic variants: an update. Head Neck Pathol. 10(2):125–30. PMID:26971504
**1299.** Kazakov DV, Belousova IE, Bisceglia M, Calonje E, Emberger M, Grayson W, et al. (2007). Apocrine mixed tumor of the skin ("mixed tumor of the folliculosebaceous-apocrine complex"). Spectrum of differentiations and metaplastic changes in the epithelial, myoepithelial, and stromal components based on a histopathologic study of 244 cases. J Am Acad Dermatol. 57(3):467–83. PMID:17707152
**1300.** Kazakov DV, Belousova IE, Müller B, Palmedo G, Samtsov AV, Burg G, et al. (2002). Primary cutaneous plasmacytoma: a clinicopathological study of two cases with a long-term follow-up and review of the literature. J Cutan Pathol. 29(4):244–8. PMID:12028158
**1301.** Kazakov DV, Belousova IE, Sima R, Michal M (2006). Mammary type tubulolobular carcinoma of the anogenital area: report of a case of a unique tumor presumably originating in anogenital mammarylike glands. Am J Surg Pathol. 30(9):1193–6. PMID:16931966
**1302.** Kazakov DV, Bisceglia M, Calonje E, Hantschke M, Kutzner H, Mentzel T, et al. (2007). Tubular adenoma and syringocystadenoma papilliferum: a reappraisal of their relationship. An interobserver study of a series, by a panel of dermatopathologists. Am J Dermatopathol. 29(3):256–63. PMID:17519623
**1303.** Kazakov DV, Bisceglia M, Mukensnabl P, Michal M (2005). Pseudoangiomatous stromal hyperplasia in lesions involving anogenital mammary-like glands. Am J Surg Pathol. 29(9):1243–6. PMID:16096415
**1304.** Kazakov DV, Bisceglia M, Sima R, Michal M (2006). Adenosis tumor of anogenital mammary-like glands: a case report and demonstration of clonality by HUMARA assay. J Cutan Pathol. 33(1):43–6. PMID:16441411
**1305.** Kazakov DV, Bisceglia M, Spagnolo DV, Kutzner H, Belousova IE, Hes O, et al. (2007). Apocrine mixed tumors of the skin with architectural and/or cytologic atypia: a retrospective clinicopathologic study of 18 cases. Am J Surg Pathol. 31(7):1094–102. PMID:17592277
**1306.** Kazakov DV, Bouda J Jr, Kacerovska D, Michal M (2011). Vulvar syringomas with deep extension: a potential histopathologic mimic of microcystic adnexal carcinoma. Int J Gynecol Pathol. 30(1):92–4. PMID:21131826
**1307.** Kazakov DV, Calonje E, Rütten A, Glatz K, Michal M (2007). Cutaneous sebaceous neoplasms with a focal glandular pattern (seboapocrine lesions): a clinicopathological study of three cases. Am J Dermatopathol. 29(4):359–64. PMID:17667168
**1308.** Kazakov DV, Calonje E, Zelger B, Luzar B, Belousova IE, Mukensnabl P, et al. (2007). Sebaceous carcinoma arising in nevus sebaceus of Jadassohn: a clinicopathological study of five cases. Am J Dermatopathol. 29(3):242–8. PMID:17519621
**1309.** Kazakov DV, Grossmann P, Spagnolo DV, Vanecek T, Vazmitel M, Kacerovska D, et al. (2010). Expression of p53 and TP53 mutational analysis in malignant neoplasms arising in preexisting spiradenoma, cylindroma, and spiradenocylindroma, sporadic or associated with Brooke-Spiegler syndrome. Am J Dermatopathol. 32(3):215–21. PMID:20075707
**1310.** Kazakov DV, Hantschke M, Vanecek T, Kacerovska D, Michal M (2010). Mammary-type secretory carcinoma of the skin. Am J Surg Pathol. 34(8):1226–8. PMID:20631609
**1311.** Kazakov DV, Hügel H, Vanecek T, Michal M (2006). Unusual hyperplasia of anogenital mammary-like glands. Am J Dermatopathol. 28(2):134–7. PMID:16625075
**1312.** Kazakov DV, Ivan D, Kutzner H, Spagnolo DV, Grossmann P, Vanecek T, et al. (2009). Cutaneous hidradenocarcinoma: a clinicopathological, immunohistochemical, and molecular biologic study of 14 cases, including Her2/neu gene expression/amplification, TP53 gene mutation analysis, and t(11;19) translocation. Am J Dermatopathol. 31(3):236–47. PMID:19384064
**1313.** Kazakov DV, Kacerovska D, Hantschke M, Zelger B, Kutzner H, Requena L, et al. (2011). Cutaneous mixed tumor, eccrine variant: a clinicopathologic and immunohistochemical study of 50 cases, with emphasis on unusual histopathologic features. Am J Dermatopathol. 33(6):557–68. PMID:21697702
**1314.** Kazakov DV, Kacerovska D, Michal M (2011). Microcystic adnexal carcinoma with multiple areas of follicular differentiation toward germinative cells and specific follicular stroma (trichoblastomatous areas). Am J Dermatopathol. 33(4):e47–9. PMID:21252639
**1315.** Kazakov DV, Kacerovska D, Skalova A, Zelger B, Schaller J, Shelekhova K, et al. (2011). Cutaneous apocrine mixed tumor with intravascular tumor deposits: a diagnostic pitfall. Am J Dermatopathol. 33(8):775–9. PMID:21785330
**1316.** Kazakov DV, Kempf W, Michal M (2004). Low-grade trichoblastic carcinosarcoma of the skin. Am J Dermatopathol. 26(4):304–9. PMID:15249861
**1317.** Kazakov DV, Kutzner H, Rütten A, Mukensnabl P, Michal M (2005). Carcinoid-like pattern in sebaceous neoplasms: another distinctive, previously unrecognized pattern in extraocular sebaceous carcinoma and sebaceoma. Am J Dermatopathol. 27(3):195–203. PMID:15900121
**1318.** Kazakov DV, Kutzner H, Spagnolo DV, Kempf W, Zelger B, Mukensnabl P, et al. (2008). Sebaceous differentiation in poroid neoplasms: report of 11 cases, including a case of metaplastic carcinoma associated with apocrine poroma (sarcomatoid apocrine porocarcinoma). Am J Dermatopathol. 30(1):21–6. PMID:18212539
**1319.** Kazakov DV, Kutzner H, Spagnolo DV, Rütten A, Mukensnabl P, Michal M (2010). What is extraocular cutaneous sebaceous carcinoma in situ? Am J Dermatopathol. 32(8):857–8. PMID:20966738
**1320.** Kazakov DV, Magro G, Kutzner H, Spagnolo DV, Yang Y, Zaspa O, et al. (2008). Spiradenoma and spiradenocylindroma with an adenomatous or atypical adenomatous component: a clinicopathological study of 6 cases. Am J Dermatopathol. 30(5):436–41. PMID:18806484
**1321.** Kazakov DV, Mentzel T, Erlandson RA, Mukensnabl P, Michal M (2006). Clear cell trichoblastoma: a clinicopathological and ultrastructural study of two cases. Am J Dermatopathol. 28(3):197–201. PMID:16778484
**1322.** Kazakov DV, Michal M, Kacerovska D, McKee PH, editors (2012). Cutaneous adnexal tumors. Philadelphia: Lippincott Williams & Wilkins.
**1323.** Kazakov DV, Plaza JA, Suster S, Kacerovska D, Michal M (2011). Cutaneous cribriform carcinoma: a short comment. J Am Acad Dermatol. 64(3):599–601. PMID:21315957
**1324.** Kazakov DV, Requena L, Kutzner H, Fernandez-Figueras MT, Kacerovska D, Mentzel T, et al. (2010). Morphologic diversity of syringocystadenocarcinoma papilliferum based on a clinicopathologic study of 6 cases and review of the literature. Am J Dermatopathol. 32(4):340–7. PMID:20216201
**1325.** Kazakov DV, Sima R, Vanecek T, Kutzner H, Palmedo G, Kacerovska D, et al. (2009). Mutations in exon 3 of the CTNNB1 gene (beta-catenin gene) in cutaneous adnexal tumors. Am J Dermatopathol. 31(3):248–55. PMID:19384065
**1326.** Kazakov DV, Soukup R, Mukensnabl P, Boudova L, Michal M (2005). Brooke-Spiegler syndrome: report of a case with combined lesions containing cylindromatous, spiradenomatous, trichoblastomatous, and sebaceous differentiation. Am J Dermatopathol. 27(1):27–33. PMID:15677973
**1327.** Kazakov DV, Spagnolo DV, Kacerovska D, Michal M (2011). Lesions of anogenital mammary-like glands: an update. Adv Anat Pathol. 18(1):1–28. PMID:21169735
**1328.** Kazakov DV, Spagnolo DV, Stewart CJ, Thompson J, Agaimy A, Magro G, et al. (2010). Fibroadenoma and phyllodes tumors of anogenital mammary-like glands: a series of 13 neoplasms in 12 cases, including mammary-type juvenile fibroadenoma, fibroadenoma with lactation changes, and neurofibromatosis-associated pseudoangiomatous stromal hyperplasia with multinucleated giant cells. Am J Surg Pathol. 34(1):95–103. PMID:20035149
**1329.** Kazakov DV, Suster S, LeBoit PE, Calonje E, Bisceglia M, Kutzner H, et al. (2005). Mucinous carcinoma of the skin, primary, and secondary: a clinicopathologic study of 63 cases with emphasis on the morphologic spectrum of primary cutaneous forms: homologies with mucinous lesions in the breast. Am J Surg Pathol. 29(6):764–82. PMID:15897743
**1330.** Kazakov DV, Vanecek T, Nemcova J, Kacerovska D, Spagnolo DV, Mukensnabl P, et al. (2009). Spectrum of tumors with follicular differentiation in a patient with the clinical phenotype of multiple familial trichoepitheliomas: a clinicopathological and molecular biological study, including analysis of the CYLD and PTCH genes. Am J Dermatopathol. 31(8):819–27. PMID:19730223
**1331.** Kazakov DV, Vanecek T, Zelger B, Carlson JA, Spagnolo DV, Schaller J, et al. (2011). Multiple (familial) trichoepitheliomas: a clinicopathological and molecular biological study, including CYLD and PTCH gene analysis, of a series of 16 patients. Am J Dermatopathol. 33(3):251–65. PMID:21389835
**1332.** Kazakov DV, Vittay G, Michal M, Calonje E (2008). High-grade trichoblastic carcinosarcoma. Am J Dermatopathol. 30(1):62–4. PMID:18212548
**1333.** Kazakov DV, Zelger B, Rütten A, Vazmitel M, Spagnolo DV, Kacerovska D, et al. (2009). Morphologic diversity of malignant neoplasms arising in preexisting spiradenoma, cylindroma, and spiradenocylindroma based on the study of 24 cases, sporadic or occurring in the setting of Brooke-Spiegler syndrome. Am J Surg Pathol. 33(5):705–19. PMID:19194280
**1334.** Ke H, Kazi JU, Zhao H, Sun J (2016). Germline mutations of KIT in gastrointestinal stromal tumor (GIST) and mastocytosis. Cell Biosci. 6:55. PMID:27777718
**1335.** Keasbey LE (1953). Juvenile aponeurotic fibroma (calcifying fibroma); a distinctive tumor arising in the palms and soles of young children. Cancer. 6(2):338–46. PMID:13032926
**1336.** Keasbey LE, Hadley GG (1954). Clearcell hidradenoma; report of three cases with widespread metastases. Cancer. 7(5):934–52. PMID:13199772
**1337.** Kehrer-Sawatzki H, Farschtschi S, Mautner VF, Cooper DN (2017). The molecular pathogenesis of schwannomatosis, a paradigm for the co-involvement of multiple tumour suppressor genes in tumorigenesis. Hum Genet.

136(2):129–48. PMID:27921248
**1338.** Kempf W (2006). CD30+ lymphoproliferative disorders: histopathology, differential diagnosis, new variants, and simulators. J Cutan Pathol. 33 Suppl 1:58–70. PMID:16412214
**1339.** Kempf W (2014). Cutaneous CD30-positive lymphoproliferative disorders. Surg Pathol Clin. 7(2):203–28. PMID:26837199
**1340.** Kempf W (2017). A new era for cutaneous CD30-positive T-cell lymphoproliferative disorders. Semin Diagn Pathol. 34(1):22–35. PMID:27993440
**1341.** Kempf W, Kadin ME, Kutzner H, Lord CL, Burg G, Letvin NL, et al. (2001). Lymphomatoid papulosis and human herpesviruses–a PCR-based evaluation for the presence of human herpesvirus 6, 7 and 8 related herpesviruses. J Cutan Pathol. 28(1):29–33. PMID:11168749
**1342.** Kempf W, Kazakov DV, Baumgartner HP, Kutzner H (2013). Follicular lymphomatoid papulosis revisited: a study of 11 cases, with new histopathological findings. J Am Acad Dermatol. 68(5):809–16. PMID:23375516
**1343.** Kempf W, Kazakov DV, Buechner SA, Graf M, Zettl A, Zimmermann DR, et al. (2014). Primary cutaneous marginal zone lymphoma in children: a report of 3 cases and review of the literature. Am J Dermatopathol. 36(8):661–6. PMID:24698939
**1344.** Kempf W, Kazakov DV, Cozzio A, Kamarashev J, Kerl K, Plaza T, et al. (2013). Primary cutaneous CD8(+) small- to medium-sized lymphoproliferative disorder in extrafacial sites: clinicopathologic features and concept on their classification. Am J Dermatopathol. 35(2):159–66. PMID:22885550
**1345.** Kempf W, Kazakov DV, Hübscher E, Tinguely M (2015). Cutaneous borreliosis with a T-cell-rich infiltrate and simultaneous involvement by B-cell chronic lymphocytic leukemia with t(14;18)(q32;q21). Am J Dermatopathol. 37(9):715–8. PMID:25171429
**1346.** Kempf W, Kazakov DV, Schärer L, Rütten A, Mentzel T, Paredes BE, et al. (2013). Angioinvasive lymphomatoid papulosis: a new variant simulating aggressive lymphomas. Am J Surg Pathol. 37(1):1–13. PMID:23026936
**1347.** Kempf W, Ostheeren-Michaelis S, Paulli M, Lucioni M, Wechsler J, Audring H, et al. (2008). Granulomatous mycosis fungoides and granulomatous slack skin: a multicenter study of the Cutaneous Lymphoma Histopathology Task Force Group of the European Organization for Research and Treatment of Cancer (EORTC). Arch Dermatol. 144(12):1609–17. PMID:19075143
**1348.** Kempf W, Pfaltz K, Vermeer MH, Cozzio A, Ortiz-Romero PL, Bagot M, et al. (2011). EORTC, ISCL, and USCLC consensus recommendations for the treatment of primary cutaneous CD30-positive lymphoproliferative disorders: lymphomatoid papulosis and primary cutaneous anaplastic large-cell lymphoma. Blood. 118(15):4024–35. PMID:21841159
**1349.** Kenawy N, Lake SL, Coupland SE, Damato BE (2013). Conjunctival melanoma and melanocytic intra-epithelial neoplasia. Eye (Lond). 27(2):142–52. PMID:23222568
**1350.** Keough KM, Parsons CS, Tweeddale MG (1989). Interactions between plasma proteins and pulmonary surfactant: pulsating bubble studies. Can J Physiol Pharmacol. 67(6):663–8. PMID:2476209
**1351.** Kesserwan C, Sokolic R, Cowen EW, Garabedian E, Heselmeyer-Haddad K, Lee CC, et al. (2012). Multicentric dermatofibrosarcoma protuberans in patients with adenosine deaminase-deficient severe combined immune deficiency. J Allergy Clin Immunol. 129(3):762–9.e1. PMID:22153773
**1352.** Khalil FK, Keehn CA, Saeed S, Morgan MB (2005). Verrucous psoriasis: a distinctive clinicopathologic variant of psoriasis. Am J Dermatopathol. 27(3):204–7. PMID:15900122
**1353.** Khandelwal A, Seilstad KH, Magro CM (2006). Subclinical chronic lymphocytic leukaemia associated with a 13q deletion presenting initially in the skin: apropos of a case. J Cutan Pathol. 33(3):256–9. PMID:16466516
**1354.** Khoury JD, Medeiros LJ, Manning JT, Sulak LE, Bueso-Ramos C, Jones D (2002). CD56(+) TdT(+) blastic natural killer cell tumor of the skin: a primitive systemic malignancy related to myelomonocytic leukemia. Cancer. 94(9):2401–8. PMID:12015765
**1355.** Kiel MJ, Sahasrabuddhe AA, Rolland DC, Velusamy T, Chung F, Schaller M, et al. (2015). Genomic analyses reveal recurrent mutations in epigenetic modifiers and the JAK-STAT pathway in Sézary syndrome. Nat Commun. 6:8470. PMID:26415585
**1356.** Kikuchi I (1980). Mongolian spots remaining in schoolchildren a statistical survey in Central Okinawa. J Dermatol. 7(3):213–6. PMID:6997352
**1357.** Kikuchi I, Inoue S, Sakaguchi E, Ono T (1993). Regressing nevoid nail melanosis in childhood. Dermatology. 186(2):88–93. PMID:8428053
**1358.** Kilcline C, Frieden IJ (2008). Infantile hemangiomas: how common are they? A systematic review of the medical literature. Pediatr Dermatol. 25(2):168–73. PMID:18429772
**1359.** Kilkenny M, Merlin K, Young R, Marks R (1998). The prevalence of common skin conditions in Australian school students: 1. Common, plane and plantar viral warts. Br J Dermatol. 138(5):840–5. PMID:9666831
**1360.** Kim BK, Surti U, Pandya A, Cohen J, Rabkin MS, Swerdlow SH (2005). Clinicopathologic, immunophenotypic, and molecular cytogenetic fluorescence in situ hybridization analysis of primary and secondary cutaneous follicular lymphomas. Am J Surg Pathol. 29(1):69–82. PMID:15613857
**1361.** Kim DH, Kim MY, Park YM, Kim HO (2006). Agminated lobular capillary hemangiomas presumably associated with an acquired arteriovenous malformation. J Dermatol. 33(9):646–8. PMID:16958814
**1362.** Kim HJ, Lee M, Lee MG (2016). A twist on piloleiomyoma: segmental cutaneous leiomyomatosis. J Cutan Pathol. 43(11):1083–5. PMID:27584971
**1363.** Kim J, McCarthy SW, Thompson JF, Pupo GM, Vonthethoff L, Nash P, et al. (2012). Cellular blue naevus involving the urinary bladder. Pathology. 44(7):664–8. PMID:23172087
**1364.** Kim J, Taube JM, McCalmont TH, Glusac EJ (2011). Quantitative comparison of MiTF, Melan-A, HMB-45 and Mel-5 in solar lentigines and melanoma in situ. J Cutan Pathol. 38(10):775–9. PMID:21797920
**1365.** Kim NH, Choi YD, Seon HJ, Lee JB, Yun SJ (2017). Anatomic mapping and clinicopathologic analysis of benign acral melanocytic neoplasms: a comparison between adults and children. J Am Acad Dermatol. 77(4):735–45. PMID:28676327
**1366.** Kim SY, Yun SJ (2016). Cutaneous melanoma in Asians. Chonnam Med J. 52(3):185–93. PMID:27689028
**1367.** Kim YC, Lee MG, Choe SW, Lee MC, Chung HG, Cho SH (2003). Acral lentiginous melanoma: an immunohistochemical study of 20 cases. Int J Dermatol. 42(2):123–9. PMID:12709000
**1368.** Kim YD, Lee EJ, Song MH, Suhr KB, Lee JH, Park JK (2002). Multiple eccrine hidrocystomas associated with Graves' disease. Int J Dermatol. 41(5):295–7. PMID:12100710
**1368A.** Kim YH, Willemze R, Pimpinelli N, Whittaker S, Olsen EA, Ranki A, et al. (2007). TNM classification system for primary cutaneous lymphomas other than mycosis fungoides and Sezary syndrome: a proposal of the International Society for Cutaneous Lymphomas (ISCL) and the Cutaneous Lymphoma Task Force of the European Organization of Research and Treatment of Cancer (EORTC). Blood. 110(2):479–84. PMID:17339420
**1369.** Kim YM, Ramírez JA, Mick JE, Giebler HA, Yan JP, Nyborg JK (2007). Molecular characterization of the Tax-containing HTLV-1 enhancer complex reveals a prominent role for CREB phosphorylation in Tax transactivation. J Biol Chem. 282(26):18750–7. PMID:17449469
**1370.** Kimonis VE, Goldstein AM, Pastakia B, Yang ML, Kase R, DiGiovanna JJ, et al. (1997). Clinical manifestations in 105 persons with nevoid basal cell carcinoma syndrome. Am J Med Genet. 69(3):299–308. PMID:9096761
**1371.** Kimura H, Ito Y, Kawabe S, Gotoh K, Takahashi Y, Kojima S, et al. (2012). EBV-associated T/NK-cell lymphoproliferative diseases in nonimmunocompromised hosts: prospective analysis of 108 cases. Blood. 119(3):673–86. PMID:22096243
**1372.** Kindblom LG, Meis-Kindblom JM (1995). Chondroid lipoma: an ultrastructural and immunohistochemical analysis with further observations regarding its differentiation. Hum Pathol. 26(7):706–15. PMID:7628841
**1373.** Kindem S, Traves V, Requena C, Alcalá R, Llombart B, Serra-Guillén C, et al. (2014). Bilateral cauliflower ear as the presenting sign of B-cell chronic lymphocytic leukemia. J Cutan Pathol. 41(2):73–7. PMID:24460879
**1374.** King CM, Johnston JS, Ofili K, Tam M, Palefsky J, Da Costa M, et al. (2014). Human papillomavirus types 2, 27, and 57 identified in plantar verrucae from HIV-positive and HIV-negative individuals. J Am Podiatr Med Assoc. 104(2):141–6. PMID:24725033
**1375.** King R, Hayzen BA, Page RN, Googe PB, Zeagler D, Mihm MC Jr (2009). Recurrent nevus phenomenon: a clinicopathologic study of 357 cases and histologic comparison with melanoma with regression. Mod Pathol. 22(5):611–7. PMID:19270643
**1376.** Kinsler VA, Krengel S, Riviere JB, Waelchli R, Chapusot C, Al-Olabi L, et al. (2014). Next-generation sequencing of nevus spilus-type congenital melanocytic nevus: exquisite genotype-phenotype correlation in mosaic RASopathies. J Invest Dermatol. 134(10):2658–60. PMID:24751729
**1377.** Kinsler VA, O'Hare P, Bulstrode N, Calonje JE, Chong WK, Hargrave D, et al. (2017). Melanoma in congenital melanocytic naevi. Br J Dermatol. 176(5):1131–43. PMID:28078671
**1378.** Kinsler VA, Thomas AC, Ishida M, Bulstrode NW, Loughlin S, Hing S, et al. (2013). Multiple congenital melanocytic nevi and neurocutaneous melanosis are caused by postzygotic mutations in codon 61 of NRAS. J Invest Dermatol. 133(9):2229–36. PMID:23392294
**1379.** Kirby JS, Siebert Lucking SM, Billingsley EM (2012). Trichoblastic carcinoma associated with multiple familial trichoepithelioma. Dermatol Surg. 38(12):2018–21. PMID:22849566
**1380.** Kirschner LS, Carney JA, Pack SD, Taymans SE, Giatzakis C, Cho YS, et al. (2000). Mutations of the gene encoding the protein kinase A type I-alpha regulatory subunit in patients with the Carney complex. Nat Genet. 26(1):89–92. PMID:10973256
**1381.** Kirschner LS, Sandrini F, Monbo J, Lin JP, Carney JA, Stratakis CA (2000). Genetic heterogeneity and spectrum of mutations of the PRKAR1A gene in patients with the Carney complex. Hum Mol Genet. 9(20):3037–46. PMID:11115848
**1382.** Kiuru M, Hameed M, Busam KJ (2013). Compound clear cell sarcoma misdiagnosed as a Spitz nevus. J Cutan Pathol. 40(11):950–4. PMID:23980901
**1383.** Kiuru M, Jungbluth A, Kutzner H, Wiesner T, Busam KJ (2016). Spitz tumors: comparison of histological features in relationship to immunohistochemical staining for ALK and NTRK1. Int J Surg Pathol. 24(3):200–6. PMID:26873340
**1384.** Kiuru M, McDermott G, Berger M, Halpern AC, Busam KJ (2014). Desmoplastic melanoma with sarcomatoid dedifferentiation. Am J Surg Pathol. 38(6):864–70. PMID:24618614
**1385.** Kivelä T, Eskelin S (2006). Transformation of nevus to melanoma. Ophthalmology. 113(5):887–8.e1. PMID:16650691
**1386.** Kiyohara T, Kumakiri M, Kobayashi H, Shimizu T, Ohkawara A, Ohnuki M (2000). A case of intravascular large B-cell lymphoma mimicking erythema nodosum: the importance of multiple skin biopsies. J Cutan Pathol. 27(8):413–8. PMID:10955689
**1387.** Kleijer WJ, Laugel V, Berneburg M, Nardo T, Fawcett H, Gratchev A, et al. (2008). Incidence of DNA repair deficiency disorders in western Europe: xeroderma pigmentosum, Cockayne syndrome and trichothiodystrophy. DNA Repair (Amst). 7(5):744–50. PMID:18329345
**1388.** Klein JA, Barr RJ (1986). Diffuse lipomatosis and tuberous sclerosis. Arch Dermatol. 122(11):1298–302. PMID:3777976
**1389.** Kleinstiver BJ, Rodriguez HA (1968). Nodular fasciitis. A study of forty-five cases and review of the literature. J Bone Joint Surg Am. 50(6):1204–12. PMID:5675403
**1390.** Klemke CD, Booken N, Weiss C, Nicolay JP, Goerdt S, Felcht M, et al. (2015). Histopathological and immunophenotypical criteria for the diagnosis of Sézary syndrome in differentiation from other erythrodermic skin diseases: a European Organisation for Research and Treatment of Cancer (EORTC) Cutaneous Lymphoma Task Force Study of 97 cases. Br J Dermatol. 173(1):93–105. PMID:25864856
**1391.** Kluk J, Kai A, Koch D, Taibjee SM, O'Connor S, Persic M, et al. (2016). Indolent CD8-positive lymphoid proliferation of acral sites: three further cases of a rare entity and an update on a unique patient. J Cutan Pathol. 43(2):125–36. PMID:26423705
**1392.** Kluk J, Moonim M, Duran A, Costa Rosa J, Cabeçadas J, Alvarez R, et al. (2015). Cutaneous Richter syndrome: a better place to transform? Br J Dermatol. 172(2):513–21. PMID:24935194
**1393.** Knoeller SM, Haag M, Adler CP, Reichelt A (2004). Skeletal metastasis in tricholemmal carcinoma. Clin Orthop Relat Res. (423):213–6. PMID:15232451
**1394.** Ko CJ, Barr RJ, Subtil A, McNiff JM (2008). Acantholytic dyskeratotic acanthoma: a variant of a benign keratosis. J Cutan Pathol. 35(3):298–301. PMID:18251744
**1395.** Ko CJ, Bolognia JL, Glusac EJ (2011). "Clark/dysplastic" nevi with florid fibroplasia associated with pseudomelanomatous features. J Am Acad Dermatol. 64(2):346–51. PMID:21238828
**1396.** Ko CJ, Cochran AJ, Eng W, Binder SW (2006). Hidradenocarcinoma: a histological and immunohistochemical study. J Cutan Pathol. 33(11):726–30. PMID:17083691
**1397.** Ko CJ, Leffell DJ, McNiff JM (2009). Adenosquamous carcinoma: a report of nine cases with p63 and cytokeratin 5/6 staining. J Cutan Pathol. 36(4):448–52. PMID:19278431
**1398.** Ko JS, Daniels B, Emanuel PO, Elson P, Khachaturov V, McKenney JK, et al. (2017). Spindle cell lipomas in women: a report of 53 cases. Am J Surg Pathol. 41(9):1267–74. PMID:28719462
**1399.** Ko JY, Choi WJ, Kang HS, Yu HJ, Park MH (2011). Intravascular myopericytoma: an

interesting case of a long-standing large, painful subcutaneous tumor. Pathol Int. 61(3):161–4. PMID:21355959
**1400.** Kobayashi M, Tojo A (2014). The BRAF-V600E mutation in circulating cell-free DNA is a promising biomarker of high-risk adult Langerhans cell histiocytosis. Blood. 124(16):2610–1. PMID:25323687
**1401.** Koch BB, Trask DK, Hoffman HT, Karnell LH, Robinson RA, Zhen W, et al. (2001). National survey of head and neck verrucous carcinoma: patterns of presentation, care, and outcome. Cancer. 92(1):110–20. PMID:11443616
**1402.** Kodama K, Kobayashi H, Abe R, Ohkawara A, Yoshii N, Yotsumoto S, et al. (2001). A new case of alpha-N-acetylgalactosaminidase deficiency with angiokeratoma corporis diffusum, with Ménière's syndrome and without mental retardation. Br J Dermatol. 144(2):363–8. PMID:11251574
**1403.** Kodama K, Massone C, Chott A, Metze D, Kerl H, Cerroni L (2005). Primary cutaneous large B-cell lymphomas: clinicopathologic features, classification, and prognostic factors in a large series of patients. Blood. 106(7):2491–7. PMID:15947086
**1404.** Koens L, Senff NJ, Vermeer MH, Willemze R, Jansen PM (2014). Methotrexate-associated B-cell lymphoproliferative disorders presenting in the skin: a clinicopathologic and immunophenotypical study of 10 cases. Am J Surg Pathol. 38(7):999–1006. PMID:24805861
**1405.** Koens L, Vermeer MH, Willemze R, Jansen PM (2010). IgM expression on paraffin sections distinguishes primary cutaneous large B-cell lymphoma, leg type from primary cutaneous follicle center lymphoma. Am J Surg Pathol. 34(7):1043–8. PMID:20551823
**1406.** Koens L, Zoutman WH, Ngarmlertsirichai P, Przybylski GK, Grabarczyk P, Vermeer MH, et al. (2014). Nuclear factor-κB pathway-activating gene aberrancies in primary cutaneous large B-cell lymphoma, leg type. J Invest Dermatol. 134(1):290–2. PMID:23863863
**1407.** Koga H, Saida T, Uhara H (2011). Key point in dermoscopic differentiation between early nail apparatus melanoma and benign longitudinal melanonychia. J Dermatol. 38(1):45–52. PMID:21175755
**1408.** Koga H, Yoshikawa S, Shinohara T, Le Gal FA, Cortés B, Saida T, et al. (2016). Long-term follow-up of longitudinal melanonychia in children and adolescents using an objective discrimination index. Acta Derm Venereol. 96(5):716–7. PMID:26806608
**1409.** Kogushi-Nishi H, Kawasaki J, Kageshita T, Ishihara T, Ihn H (2009). The prevalence of melanocytic nevi on the soles in the Japanese population. J Am Acad Dermatol. 60(5):767–71. PMID:19389519
**1410.** Koh SH, Oh SJ, Chun H, Kim SG (2014). Pseudoangiosarcomatous squamous cell carcinoma developing on a burn scar: a case report and review of the literature. Burns. 40(7):e47–52. PMID:24768344
**1411.** Kohashi K, Yamamoto H, Kumagai R, Yamada Y, Hotokebuchi Y, Taguchi T, et al. (2014). Differential microRNA expression profiles between malignant rhabdoid tumor and epithelioid sarcoma: miR193a-5p is suggested to downregulate SMARCB1 mRNA expression. Mod Pathol. 27(6):832–9. PMID:24287458
**1412.** Koike T, Mikami T, Maegawa J, Iwai T, Wada H, Yamanaka S (2013). Recurrent endocrine mucin-producing sweat gland carcinoma in the eyelid. Australas J Dermatol. 54(2):e46–9. PMID:23582005
**1413.** Koizumi H, Kumakiri M, Yamanaka K, Tomizawa K, Endo M, Ohkawara A (1995). Dermal dendrocyte hamartoma with stubby white hair: a novel connective tissue hamartoma of infancy. J Am Acad Dermatol. 32(2 Pt 2):318–21. PMID:7530262
**1414.** Kolde G, Bröcker EB (1986). Multiple skin tumors of indeterminate cells in an adult. J Am Acad Dermatol. 15(4 Pt 1):591–7. PMID:3095403
**1415.** Kolenik SA 3rd, Bolognia JL, Castiglione FM Jr, Longley BJ (1996). Multiple tumors of the follicular infundibulum. Int J Dermatol. 35(4):282–4. PMID:8786188
**1416.** Kong YY, Kong JC, Shi DR, Lu HF, Zhu XZ, Wang J, et al. (2007). Cutaneous Rosai-Dorfman disease: a clinical and histopathologic study of 25 cases in China. Am J Surg Pathol. 31(3):341–50. PMID:17325475
**1417.** Konstantinova AM, Hayes MM, Stewart CJ, Plaza JA, Michal M, Kerl K, et al. (2016). Syringomatous structures in extramammary Paget disease: a potential diagnostic pitfall. Am J Dermatopathol. 38(9):653–7. PMID:26863060
**1418.** Konstantinova AM, Kacerovska D, Michal M, Kazakov DV (2013). A tumoriform lesion of the vulva with features of mammary-type fibrocystic disease. Am J Dermatopathol. 35(7):e124–7. PMID:23435363
**1419.** Konstantinova AM, Kacerovska D, Stewart CJ, Szepe P, Pitha J, Sulc M, et al. (2016). Syringocystadenocarcinoma papilliferum in situ-like changes in extramammary Paget disease: a report of 11 cases. Am J Dermatopathol. 38(12):882–6. PMID:26863065
**1420.** Konstantinova AM, Kyrpychova L, Belousova IE, Spagnolo DV, Kacerovska D, Michal M, et al. (2017). Anogenital mammary-like glands: a study of their normal histology with emphasis on glandular depth, presence of columnar epithelial cells, and distribution of elastic fibers. Am J Dermatopathol. 39(9):663–7. PMID:27759697
**1421.** Konstantinova AM, Michal M, Kacerovska D, Spagnolo DV, Stewart CJ, Kutzner H, et al. (2016). Hidradenoma papilliferum: a clinicopathologic study of 264 tumors from 261 patients, with emphasis on mammary-type alterations. Am J Dermatopathol. 38(8):598–607. PMID:26863059
**1422.** Konstantinova AM, Shelekhova KV, Imyanitov EN, Iyevleva A, Kacerovska D, Michal M, et al. (2017). Study of selected BRCA1, BRCA2, and PIK3CA mutations in benign and malignant lesions of anogenital mammary-like glands. Am J Dermatopathol. 39(5):358–62. PMID:28291131
**1423.** Konstantinova AM, Shelekhova KV, Stewart CJ, Spagnolo DV, Kutzner H, Kacerovska D, et al. (2016). Depth and patterns of adnexal involvement in primary extramammary (anogenital) Paget disease: a study of 178 lesions from 146 patients. Am J Dermatopathol. 38(11):802–8. PMID:26863064
**1424.** Konstantinova AM, Spagnolo DV, Stewart CJR, Kacerovska D, Shelekhova KV, Plaza JA, et al. (2017). Spectrum of changes in anogenital mammary-like glands in primary extramammary (anogenital) Paget disease and their possible role in the pathogenesis of the disease. Am J Surg Pathol. 41(8):1053–8. PMID:28614205
**1425.** Konstantinova AM, Stewart CJR, Kyrpychova L, Belousova IE, Michal M, Kazakov DV (2017). An immunohistochemical study of anogenital mammary-like glands. Am J Dermatopathol. 39(8):599–605. PMID:27655126
**1426.** Konstantinova AM, Vanecek T, Martinek P, Kyrpychova L, Spagnolo DV, Stewart CJR, et al. (2017). Molecular alterations in lesions of anogenital mammary-like glands and their mammary counterparts including hidradenoma papilliferum, intraductal papilloma, fibroadenoma and phyllodes tumor. Ann Diagn Pathol. 28:12–8. PMID:28648934
**1427.** Koopmans AE, Ober K, Dubbink HJ, Paridaens D, Naus NC, Belunek S, et al. (2014). Prevalence and implications of TERT promoter mutation in uveal and conjunctival melanoma and in benign and premalignant conjunctival melanocytic lesions. Invest Ophthalmol Vis Sci. 55(9):6024–30. PMID:25159205
**1428.** Kopf AW, Levine LJ, Rigel DS, Friedman RJ, Levenstein M (1985). Prevalence of congenital-nevus-like nevi, nevi spili, and café au lait spots. Arch Dermatol. 121(6):766–9. PMID:4004301
**1429.** Kopf AW, Weidman AI (1962). Nevus of Ota. Arch Dermatol. 85(2):195–208. PMID:14458325
**1430.** Koplin SA, Nielsen GP, Hornicek FJ, Rosenberg AE (2010). Epithelioid sarcoma with heterotopic bone: a morphologic review of 4 cases. Int J Surg Pathol. 18(3):207–12. PMID:20034988
**1431.** Korgavkar K, Xiong M, Weinstock M (2013). Changing incidence trends of cutaneous T-cell lymphoma. JAMA Dermatol. 149(11):1295–9. PMID:24005876
**1432.** Kornberg R, Ackerman AB (1975). Pseudomelanoma: recurrent melanocytic nevus following partial surgical removal. Arch Dermatol. 111(12):1588–90. PMID:1200664
**1433.** Koss MN, Hochholzer L, Langloss JM, Wehunt WD, Lazarus AA, Nichols PW (1986). Lymphomatoid granulomatosis: a clinicopathologic study of 42 patients. Pathology. 18(3):283–8. PMID:3785978
**1434.** Kossard S, Finley AG, Poyzer K, Kocsard E (1989). Eruptive infundibulomas. A distinctive presentation of the tumor of follicular infundibulum. J Am Acad Dermatol. 21(2 Pt 2):361–6. PMID:2474013
**1435.** Kossard S, Wilkinson B (1997). Small cell (naevoid) melanoma: a clinicopathologic study of 131 cases. Australas J Dermatol. 38 Suppl 1:S54–8. PMID:10994474
**1436.** Kossard S, Xenias SJ, Palestine RF, Scheen SR 3rd, Winkelmann RK (1980). Inflammatory changes in verruca vulgaris. J Cutan Pathol. 7(4):217–21. PMID:7430479
**1437.** Koutlas IG, Scheithauer BW (2010). Palisaded encapsulated ("solitary circumscribed") neuroma of the oral cavity: a review of 55 cases. Head Neck Pathol. 4(1):15–26. PMID:20237984
**1438.** Kovarik CL, Barrett T, Auerbach A, Cassarino DS (2008). Acral myxoinflammatory fibroblastic sarcoma: case series and immunohistochemical analysis. J Cutan Pathol. 35(2):192–6. PMID:18190444
**1439.** Kraemer KH, DiGiovanna JJ (1993). Xeroderma pigmentosum. In: Adam MP, Ardinger HH, Pagon RA, Wallace SE, Bean LJH, Stephens K, et al., editors. GeneReviews®. Seattle: University of Washington, Seattle. PMID:20301571
**1440.** Kraemer KH, Lee MM, Scotto J (1987). Xeroderma pigmentosum. Cutaneous, ocular, and neurologic abnormalities in 830 published cases. Arch Dermatol. 123(2):241–50. PMID:3545087
**1441.** Kraft S, Fletcher CD (2011). Atypical intradermal smooth muscle neoplasms: clinicopathologic analysis of 84 cases and a reappraisal of cutaneous "leiomyosarcoma". Am J Surg Pathol. 35(4):599–607. PMID:21358302
**1442.** Kraft S, Granter SR (2014). Molecular pathology of skin neoplasms of the head and neck. Arch Pathol Lab Med. 138(6):759–87. PMID:24878016
**1443.** Krahl D, Sellheyer K (2007). Monoclonal antibody Ber-EP4 reliably discriminates between microcystic adnexal carcinoma and basal cell carcinoma. J Cutan Pathol. 34(10):782–7. PMID:17880584
**1444.** Kratochvil FJ 3rd, Stewart JC, Moore SR (2012). Mammary analog secretory carcinoma of salivary glands: a report of 2 cases in the lips. Oral Surg Oral Med Oral Pathol Oral Radiol. 114(5):630–5. PMID:23021923
**1445.** Krauthammer M, Kong Y, Bacchiocchi A, Evans P, Pornputtapong N, Wu C, et al. (2015). Exome sequencing identifies recurrent mutations in NF1 and RASopathy genes in sun-exposed melanomas. Nat Genet. 47(9):996–1002. PMID:26214590
**1446.** Krenács L, Tiszalvicz L, Krenács T, Boumsell L (1993). Immunohistochemical detection of CD1A antigen in formalin-fixed and paraffin-embedded tissue sections with monoclonal antibody 010. J Pathol. 171(2):99–104. PMID:7506772
**1447.** Krishnan KG, Pinzer T, Schackert G (2005). Coverage of painful peripheral nerve neuromas with vascularized soft tissue: method and results. Neurosurgery. 56(2 Suppl):369–78. PMID:15794833
**1448.** Kruse R, Rütten A, Schweiger N, Jakob E, Mathiak M, Propping P, et al. (2003). Frequency of microsatellite instability in unselected sebaceous gland neoplasias and hyperplasias. J Invest Dermatol. 120(5):858–64. PMID:12713593
**1449.** Kryvenko ON, Chitale DA, VanEgmond EM, Gupta NS, Schultz D, Lee MW (2011). Angiolipoma of the female breast: clinicomorphological correlation of 52 cases. Int J Surg Pathol. 19(1):35–43. PMID:21087987
**1450.** Ku LS, Chong LY, Yau KC (2005). Giant annular dermatomyofibroma. Int J Dermatol. 44(12):1039–41. PMID:16409272
**1451.** Kuchelmeister C, Schaumburg-Lever G, Garbe C (2000). Acral cutaneous melanoma in Caucasians: clinical features, histopathology and prognosis in 112 patients. Br J Dermatol. 143(2):275–80. PMID:10951133
**1452.** Kuet K, Goodfield M (2014). Multiple halo naevi associated with tocilizumab. Clin Exp Dermatol. 39(6):717–9. PMID:24986573
**1453.** Kujala E, Mäkitie T, Kivelä T (2003). Very long-term prognosis of patients with malignant uveal melanoma. Invest Ophthalmol Vis Sci. 44(11):4651–9. PMID:14578381
**1454.** Kumar E, Patel NR, Demicco EG, Bovee JV, Olivera AM, Lopez-Terrada DH, et al. (2016). Cutaneous nodular fasciitis with genetic analysis: a case series. J Cutan Pathol. 43(12):1143–9. PMID:27686647
**1455.** Kumar R, Lefkowitz RA, Neto AD (2017). Myxoinflammatory fibroblastic sarcoma: clinical, imaging, management and outcome in 29 patients. J Comput Assist Tomogr. 41(1):104–15. PMID:27560024
**1456.** Kumar S, Fend F, Quintanilla-Martinez L, Kingma DW, Sorbara L, Raffeld M, et al. (2000). Epstein-Barr virus-positive primary gastrointestinal Hodgkin's disease: association with inflammatory bowel disease and immunosuppression. Am J Surg Pathol. 24(1):66–73. PMID:10632489
**1457.** Kumar S, Krenacs L, Medeiros J, Elenitoba-Johnson KS, Greiner TC, Sorbara L, et al. (1998). Subcutaneous panniculitic T-cell lymphoma is a tumor of cytotoxic T lymphocytes. Hum Pathol. 29(4):397–403. PMID:9563791
**1458.** Kummer JA, Vermeer MH, Dukers D, Meijer CJ, Willemze R (1997). Most primary cutaneous CD30-positive lymphoproliferative disorders have a CD4-positive cytotoxic T-cell phenotype. J Invest Dermatol. 109(5):636–40. PMID:9347791
**1459.** Kung IT, Gibson JB, Bannatyne PM (1984). Kimura's disease: a clinico-pathological study of 21 cases and its distinction from angiolymphoid hyperplasia with eosinophilia. Pathology. 16(1):39–44. PMID:6718071
**1460.** Kuno Y, Numata T, Kanzaki T (1999). Adenocarcinoma with signet ring cells of the axilla showing apocrine features: a case

report. Am J Dermatopathol. 21(1):37–41. PMID:10027525
**1461.** Kuo KY, Batra P, Cho HG, Li S, Chahal HS, Rieger KE, et al. (2017). Correlates of multiple basal cell carcinoma in a retrospective cohort study: sex, histologic subtypes, and anatomic distribution. J Am Acad Dermatol. 77(2):233–4.e2. PMID:28392289
**1462.** Kuo T (1980). Clear cell carcinoma of the skin. A variant of the squamous cell carcinoma that simulates sebaceous carcinoma. Am J Surg Pathol. 4(6):573–83. PMID:6163367
**1463.** Kuo TT, Hu S, Chan HL (1998). Keloidal dermatofibroma: report of 10 cases of a new variant. Am J Surg Pathol. 22(5):564–8. PMID:9591726
**1464.** Kurek KC, Pansuriya TC, van Ruler MA, van den Akker B, Luks VL, Verbeke SL, et al. (2013). R132C IDH1 mutations are found in spindle cell hemangiomas and not in other vascular tumors or malformations. Am J Pathol. 182(5):1494–500. PMID:23485734
**1465.** Kurli M, Finger PT (2005). Melanocytic conjunctival tumors. Ophthalmol Clin North Am. 18(1):15–24, vii. PMID:15763188
**1466.** Kurokawa I, Senba Y, Nishimura K, Habe K, Hakamada A, Isoda K, et al. (2006). Cytokeratin expression in trichilemmal carcinoma suggests differentiation towards follicular infundibulum. In Vivo. 20(5):583–5. PMID:17091763
**1467.** Kurzen H, Esposito L, Langbein L, Hartschuh W (2001). Cytokeratins as markers of follicular differentiation: an immunohistochemical study of trichoblastoma and basal cell carcinoma. Am J Dermatopathol. 23(6):501–9. PMID:11801790
**1468.** Küsters-Vandevelde HV, Creytens D, van Engen-van Grunsven AC, Jeunink M, Winnepenninckx V, Groenen PJ, et al. (2016). SF3B1 and EIF1AX mutations occur in primary leptomeningeal melanocytic neoplasms; yet another similarity to uveal melanomas. Acta Neuropathol Commun. 4:5. PMID:26769193
**1469.** Kutzner H, Kerl H, Pfaltz MC, Kempf W (2009). CD123-positive plasmacytoid dendritic cells in primary cutaneous marginal zone B-cell lymphoma: diagnostic and pathogenetic implications. Am J Surg Pathol. 33(9):1307–13. PMID:19718787
**1470.** Kutzner H, Mentzel T, Kaddu S, Soares LM, Sangueza OP, Requena L (2001). Cutaneous myoepithelioma: an under-recognized cutaneous neoplasm composed of myoepithelial cells. Am J Surg Pathol. 25(3):348–55. PMID:11224605
**1471.** Kutzner H, Mentzel T, Palmedo G, Hantschke M, Rütten A, Paredes BE, et al. (2010). Plaque-like CD34-positive dermal fibroma ("medallion-like dermal dendrocyte hamartoma"): clinicopathologic, immunohistochemical, and molecular analysis of 5 cases emphasizing its distinction from superficial, plaque-like dermatofibrosarcoma protuberans. Am J Surg Pathol. 34(2):190–201. PMID:20061935
**1472.** Kutzner H, Metzler G, Argenyi Z, Requena L, Palmedo G, Mentzel T, et al. (2012). Histological and genetic evidence for a variant of superficial spreading melanoma composed predominantly of large nests. Mod Pathol. 25(6):838–45. PMID:22388759
**1473.** Kutzner H, Requena L, Rütten A, Mentzel T (2006). Spindle cell predominant trichodiscoma: a fibrofolliculoma/trichodiscoma variant considered formerly to be a neurofollicular hamartoma: a clinicopathological and immunohistochemical analysis of 17 cases. Am J Dermatopathol. 28(1):1–8. PMID:16456317
**1474.** Kwiek B, Schwartz RA (2016). Keratoacanthoma (KA): an update and review. J Am Acad Dermatol. 74(6):1220–33. PMID:26853179
**1475.** Kyllo RL, Brady KL, Hurst EA (2015). Sebaceous carcinoma: review of the literature. Dermatol Surg. 41(1):1–15. PMID:25521100
**1476.** Kyrpychova L, Carr RA, Martinek P, Vanecek T, Perret R, Chottová-Dvořáková M, et al. (2017). Basal cell carcinoma with matrical differentiation: clinicopathologic, immunohistochemical, and molecular biological study of 22 cases. Am J Surg Pathol. 41(6):738–49. PMID:28368926
**1477.** Kyrpychova L, Kacerovska D, Vanecek T, Grossmann P, Michal M, Kerl K, et al. (2016). Cutaneous hidradenoma: a study of 21 neoplasms revealing neither correlation between the cellular composition and CRTC1-MAML2 fusions nor presence of CRTC3-MAML2 fusions. Ann Diagn Pathol. 23:8–13. PMID:27402217
**1478.** Lack EE, Worsham GF, Callihan MD, Crawford BE, Klappenbach S, Rowden G, et al. (1980). Granular cell tumor: a clinicopathologic study of 110 patients. J Surg Oncol. 13(4):301–16. PMID:6246310
**1479.** Lafferty KA, Nelson EL, Demuth RJ, Miller SH, Harrison MW (1986). Juvenile aponeurotic fibroma with disseminated fibrosarcoma. J Hand Surg Am. 11(5):737–40. PMID:3760506
**1480.** LaGrenade L, Hanchard B, Fletcher V, Cranston B, Blattner W (1990). Infective dermatitis of Jamaican children: a marker for HTLV-I infection. Lancet. 336(8727):1345–7. PMID:1978165
**1481.** Laharanne E, Oumouhou N, Bonnet F, Carlotti M, Gentil C, Chevret E, et al. (2010). Genome-wide analysis of cutaneous T-cell lymphomas identifies three clinically relevant classes. J Invest Dermatol. 130(6):1707–18. PMID:20130593
**1482.** Lai JP, Liu YC, Alimchandani M, Liu Q, Aung PP, Matsuda K, et al. (2013). The influence of DNA repair on neurological degeneration, cachexia, skin cancer and internal neoplasms: autopsy report of four xeroderma pigmentosum patients (XP-A, XP-C and XP-D). Acta Neuropathol Commun. 1:4. PMID:24252196
**1483.** Lake SL, Jmor F, Dopierala J, Taktak AF, Coupland SE, Damato BE (2011). Multiplex ligation-dependent probe amplification of conjunctival melanoma reveals common BRAF V600E gene mutation and gene copy number changes. Invest Ophthalmol Vis Sci. 52(8):5598–604. PMID:21693616
**1484.** Lam C, Ou JC, Billingsley EM (2013). "PTCH"-ing it together: a basal cell nevus syndrome review. Dermatol Surg. 39(11):1557–72. PMID:23725561
**1485.** Lambert I, Debiec-Rychter M, Guelinckx P, Hagemeijer A, Sciot R (2001). Acral myxoinflammatory fibroblastic sarcoma with unique clonal chromosomal changes. Virchows Arch. 438(5):509–12. PMID:11407481
**1486.** Lancerotto L, Salmaso R, Sartore L, Bassetto F (2012). Malignant glomus tumor of the leg developed in the context of a superficial typical glomus tumor. Int J Surg Pathol. 20(4):420–4. PMID:22228777
**1486A.** Landi MT, Bauer J, Pfeiffer RM, Elder DE, Hulley B, Minghetti P, et al. (2006). MC1R germline variants confer risk for BRAF-mutant melanoma. Science. 313(5786):521–2. PMID:16809487
**1487.** Landry M, Winkelmann RK (1972). An unusual tubular apocrine adenoma. Arch Dermatol. 105(6):869–79. PMID:4113017
**1488.** Lang PG Jr, McKelvey AC, Nicholson JH (1987). Three-dimensional reconstruction of the superficial multicentric basal cell carcinoma using serial sections and a computer. Am J Dermatopathol. 9(3):198–203. PMID:3631446
**1489.** Lange M, Gleń J, Zabłotna M, Nedoszytko B, Sokołowska-Wojdyło M, Rębała K, et al. (2017). Interleukin-31 polymorphisms and serum IL-31 level in patients with mastocytosis: correlation with clinical presentation and pruritus. Acta Derm Venereol. 97(1):47–53. PMID:27276346
**1490.** Lange M, Żawrocki A, Nedoszytko B, Wasąg B, Niedoszytko M, Jassem E, et al. (2014). Does the aberrant expression of CD2 and CD25 by skin mast cells truly correlate with systemic involvement in patients presenting with mastocytosis in the skin? Int Arch Allergy Immunol. 165(2):104–10. PMID:25402852
**1491.** Lanting R, Broekstra DC, Werker PM, van den Heuvel ER (2014). A systematic review and meta-analysis on the prevalence of Dupuytren disease in the general population of Western countries. Plast Reconstr Surg. 133(3):593–603. PMID:24263394
**1492.** Larre Borges A, Zalaudek I, Longo C, Dufrechou L, Argenziano G, Lallas A, et al. (2014). Melanocytic nevi with special features: clinical-dermoscopic and reflectance confocal microscopic-findings. J Eur Acad Dermatol Venereol. 28(7):833–45. PMID:24171788
**1493.** Larsen AC, Dahmcke CM, Dahl C, Siersma VD, Toft PB, Coupland SE, et al. (2015). A retrospective review of conjunctival melanoma presentation, treatment, and outcome and an investigation of features associated with BRAF mutations. JAMA Ophthalmol. 133(11):1295–303. PMID:26425792
**1494.** Laskin WB, Fetsch JF, Michal M, Miettinen M (2006). Sclerotic (fibroma-like) lipoma: a distinctive lipoma variant with a predilection for the distal extremities. Am J Dermatopathol. 28(4):308–16. PMID:16871033
**1495.** Laskin WB, Fetsch JF, Miettinen M (2000). The "neurothekeoma": immunohistochemical analysis distinguishes the true nerve sheath myxoma from its mimics. Hum Pathol. 31(10):1230–41. PMID:11070116
**1496.** Laskin WB, Fetsch JF, Miettinen M (2014). Myxoinflammatory fibroblastic sarcoma: a clinicopathologic analysis of 104 cases, with emphasis on predictors of outcome. Am J Surg Pathol. 38(1):1–12. PMID:24121178
**1497.** Laskin WB, Weiss SW, Bratthauer GL (1991). Epithelioid variant of malignant peripheral nerve sheath tumor (malignant epithelioid schwannoma). Am J Surg Pathol. 15(12):1136–45. PMID:1746681
**1498.** Lasota J, Fetsch JF, Wozniak A, Wasag B, Sciot R, Miettinen M (2001). The neurofibromatosis type 2 gene is mutated in perineurial cell tumors: a molecular genetic study of eight cases. Am J Pathol. 158(4):1223–9. PMID:11290539
**1499.** Lau PP, Wong OK, Lui PC, Cheung OY, Ho LC, Wong WC, et al. (2009). Myopericytoma in patients with AIDS: a new class of Epstein-Barr virus-associated tumor. Am J Surg Pathol. 33(11):1666–72. PMID:19675451
**1500.** Lauer DH, Enzinger FM (1980). Cranial fasciitis of childhood. Cancer. 45(2):401–6. PMID:7351023
**1500A.** Laurent C, Baron M, Amara N, Haioun C, Dandoit M, Maynadié M, et al. (2017). Impact of expert pathologic review of lymphoma diagnosis: study of patients from the French Lymphopath Network. J Clin Oncol. 35(18):2008–17. PMID:28459613
**1501.** Laurent R, Kienzler JL, Croissant O, Orth G (1982). Two anatomoclinical types of warts with plantar localization: specific cytopathogenic effects of papillomavirus. Type I (HPV-1) and type 2 (HPV-2). Arch Dermatol Res. 274(1–2):101–11. PMID:6299203
**1502.** Laury AR, Perets R, Piao H, Krane JF, Barletta JA, French C, et al. (2011). A comprehensive analysis of PAX8 expression in human epithelial tumors. Am J Surg Pathol. 35(6):816–26. PMID:21552115
**1503.** Law MH, Bishop DT, Lee JE, Brossard M, Martin NG, Moses EK, et al. (2015). Genome-wide meta-analysis identifies five new susceptibility loci for cutaneous malignant melanoma. Nat Genet. 47(9):987–95. PMID:26237428
**1504.** Lazar AJ, Fletcher CD (2005). Primitive nonneural granular cell tumors of skin: clinicopathologic analysis of 13 cases. Am J Surg Pathol. 29(7):927–34. PMID:15958858
**1505.** Lazova R, Lester B, Glusac EJ, Handerson T, McNiff J (2005). The characteristic histopathologic features of nevi on and around the ear. J Cutan Pathol. 32(1):40–4. PMID:15660654
**1506.** Lazova R, Pornputtapong N, Halaban R, Bosenberg M, Bai Y, Chai H, et al. (2017). Spitz nevi and Spitzoid melanomas: exome sequencing and comparison with conventional melanocytic nevi and melanomas. Mod Pathol. 30(5):640–9. PMID:28186096
**1507.** Lazova R, Yang Z, El Habr C, Lim Y, Choate KA, Seeley EH, et al. (2017). Mass spectrometry imaging can distinguish on a proteomic level between proliferative nodules within a benign congenital nevus and malignant melanoma. Am J Dermatopathol. 39(9):689–95. PMID:28248717
**1508.** Lazovich D, Isaksson Vogel R, Weinstock MA, Nelson HH, Ahmed RL, Berwick M (2016). Association between indoor tanning and melanoma in younger men and women. JAMA Dermatol. 152(3):268–75. PMID:26818409
**1509.** Le Huu AR, Jokinen CH, Rubin BP, Mihm MC, Weiss SW, North PE, et al. (2010). Expression of Prox1, lymphatic endothelial nuclear transcription factor, in Kaposiform hemangioendothelioma and tufted angioma. Am J Surg Pathol. 34(11):1563–73. PMID:20975337
**1510.** Le EN, Gerstenblith MR, Gelber AC, Manno RL, Ranasinghe PD, Sweren RJ, et al. (2008). The use of blind skin biopsy in the diagnosis of intravascular B-cell lymphoma. J Am Acad Dermatol. 59(1):148–51. PMID:18406005
**1511.** Le Loarer F, Zhang L, Fletcher CD, Ribeiro A, Singer S, Italiano A, et al. (2014). Consistent SMARCB1 homozygous deletions in epithelioid sarcoma and in a subset of myoepithelial carcinomas can be reliably detected by FISH in archival material. Genes Chromosomes Cancer. 53(6):475–86. PMID:24585572
**1512.** LeBlanc KG Jr, Wenner M, Davis LS (2011). Multiple nuchal fibromas in a 2-year-old without Gardner syndrome. Pediatr Dermatol. 28(6):695–6. PMID:21950671
**1513.** LeBoit PE (1994). Granulomatous slack skin. Dermatol Clin. 12(2):375–89. PMID:8045049
**1514.** LeBoit PE, Barr RJ, Burall S, Metcalf JS, Yen TS, Wick MR (1991). Primitive polypoid granular-cell tumor and other cutaneous granular-cell neoplasms of apparent nonneural origin. Am J Surg Pathol. 15(1):48–58. PMID:1985501
**1514A.** LeBoit PE, Burg G, Weedon D, Sarasin A, editors (2005). World Health Organization classification of tumours. Pathology and genetics of skin tumours. 3rd ed. Lyon: International Agency for Research on Cancer.
**1515.** LeBoit PE, Sexton M (1993). Microcystic adnexal carcinoma of the skin. A reappraisal of the differentiation and differential diagnosis of an underrecognized neoplasm. J Am Acad Dermatol. 29(4):609–18. PMID:7691906
**1516.** Leclaire Alirkilicarslan A, Dupuy A, Pujals A, Parrens M, Vergier B, Robson A, et al. (2017). Expression of TFH markers and detection of RHOA p.G17V and IDH2 p.R172K/S mutations in cutaneous localizations of angioimmunoblastic T-cell lymphomas. Am J Surg Pathol. 41(12):1581–92. PMID:28945625
**1517.** Leclerc S, Hamel-Teillac D, Oger P, Brousse N, Fraitag S (2005). Plexiform fibrohistiocytic tumor: three unusual cases occurring in infancy. J Cutan Pathol. 32(8):572–6.

PMID:16115057
1518. Leclerc-Mercier S, Pedeutour F, Fabas T, Glorion C, Brousse N, Fraitag S (2011). Plexiform fibrohistiocytic tumor with molecular and cytogenetic analysis. Pediatr Dermatol. 28(1):26–9. PMID:21261704
1519. Lee AY, Agaram NP, Qin LX, Kuk D, Curtin C, Brennan MF, et al. (2016). Optimal percent myxoid component to predict outcome in high-grade myxofibrosarcoma and undifferentiated pleomorphic sarcoma. Ann Surg Oncol. 23(3):818–25. PMID:26759307
1520. Lee AY, Kawashima M, Nakagawa H, Ishibashi Y (1991). Generalized eruptive syringoma. J Am Acad Dermatol. 25(3):570–1. PMID:1918498
1521. Lee CH, Chen JS, Sun YL, Liao WT, Zheng YW, Chai CZ, et al. (2006). Defective beta1-integrins expression in arsenical keratosis and arsenic-treated cultured human keratinocytes. J Cutan Pathol. 33(2):129–38. PMID:16420308
1522. Lee CH, Wu SB, Hong CH, Chen GS, Wei YH, Yu HS (2013). Involvement of mtDNA damage elicited by oxidative stress in the arsenical skin cancers. J Invest Dermatol. 133(7):1890–900. PMID:23370535
1523. Lee CS, Southey MC, Slater H, Auldist AW, Chow CW, Venter DJ (1995). Primary cutaneous Ewing's sarcoma/peripheral primitive neuroectodermal tumors in childhood. A molecular, cytogenetic, and immunohistochemical study. Diagn Mol Pathol. 4(3):174–81. PMID:7493136
1524. Lee EY, Williamson R, Watt P, Hughes MC, Green AC, Whiteman DC (2006). Sun exposure and host phenotype as predictors of cutaneous melanoma associated with neval remnants or dermal elastosis. Int J Cancer. 119(3):636–42. PMID:16572428
1525. Lee HW, Lee DK, Lee MW, Choi JH, Moon KC, Koh JK (2005). Two cases of angiomyxolipoma (vascular myxolipoma) of subcutaneous tissue. J Cutan Pathol. 32(5):379–82. PMID:15811126
1526. Lee JH, Lee JH, Lee SH, Do SI, Cho SD, Forslund O, et al. (2016). TPL2 is an oncogenic driver in keratocanthoma and squamous cell carcinoma. Cancer Res. 76(22):6712–22. PMID:27503930
1527. Lee JJ, Mochel MC, Piris A, Boussahmain C, Mahalingam M, Hoang MP (2014). p40 exhibits better specificity than p63 in distinguishing primary skin adnexal carcinomas from cutaneous metastases. Hum Pathol. 45(5):1078–83. PMID:24746214
1528. Lee JY, Jung KE, Kim HS, Lee JY, Kim HO, Park YM (2014). Langerhans cell sarcoma: a case report and review of the literature. Int J Dermatol. 53(2):e84–7. PMID:23557341
1529. Lee KH, Kim JE, Cho BK, Kim YC, Park CJ (2008). Malignant transformation of multiple familial trichoepithelioma: case report and literature review. Acta Derm Venereol. 88(1):43–6. PMID:18176750
1530. Lee MH, Moon IJ, Lee WJ, Won CH, Chang SE, Choi JH, et al. (2016). A case of cutaneous Epstein-Barr virus-associated diffuse large B-cell lymphoma in an angioimmunoblastic T-cell lymphoma. Ann Dermatol. 28(6):789–91. PMID:27904290
1531. Lee MW, Jee KJ, Gong GY, Choi JH, Moon KC, Koh JK (2005). Comparative genomic hybridization in extramammary Paget's disease. Br J Dermatol. 153(2):290–4. PMID:16086738
1532. Lee S, Barnhill RL, Dummer R, Dalton J, Wu J, Pappo A, et al. (2015). TERT promoter mutations are predictive of aggressive clinical behavior in patients with spitzoid melanocytic neoplasms. Sci Rep. 5:11200. PMID:26061100
1533. Lee SM, Zhang W, Fernandez MP (2014). Atypical fibroxanthoma arising in a young patient with Li-Fraumeni syndrome. J Cutan Pathol. 41(3):303–7. PMID:24299451
1534. Lee W, Teckie S, Wiesner T, Ran L, Prieto Granada CN, Lin M, et al. (2014). PRC2 is recurrently inactivated through EED or SUZ12 loss in malignant peripheral nerve sheath tumors. Nat Genet. 46(11):1227–32. PMID:25240281
1535. Lee WJ, Lee JH, Won CH, Chang SE, Choi JH, Moon KC, et al. (2015). Nail apparatus melanoma: a comparative, clinicoprognostic study of the initial clinical and morphological characteristics of 49 patients. J Am Acad Dermatol. 73(2):213–20. PMID:26028523
1536. Lee WJ, Lee MH, Won CH, Chang SE, Choi JH, Moon KC, et al. (2016). Comparative histopathologic analysis of cutaneous extranodal natural killer/T-cell lymphomas according to their clinical morphology. J Cutan Pathol. 43(4):324–33. PMID:26695102
1537. Lee WJ, Lee SH, Moon IJ, Won CH, Chang SE, Choi JH, et al. (2016). Relative frequency, clinical features, and survival outcomes of 395 patients with cutaneous lymphoma in Korea: a subgroup analysis per 10-year period. Acta Derm Venereol. 96(7):888–93. PMID:26975334
1538. Lee WJ, Moon HR, Won CH, Chang SE, Choi JH, Moon KC, et al. (2014). Precursor B- or T-lymphoblastic lymphoma presenting with cutaneous involvement: a series of 13 cases including 7 cases of cutaneous T-lymphoblastic lymphoma. J Am Acad Dermatol. 70(2):318–25. PMID:24314877
1539. Leeborg N, Thompson M, Rossmiller S, Gross N, White C, Gatter K (2010). Diagnostic pitfalls in syringocystadenocarcinoma papilliferum: case report and review of the literature. Arch Pathol Lab Med. 134(8):1205–9. PMID:20670144
1540. Leffell DJ, Braverman IM (1986). Familial multiple lipomatosis. Report of a case and a review of the literature. J Am Acad Dermatol. 15(2 Pt 1):275–9. PMID:3745530
1541. Leffell DJ, Headington JT, Wong DS, Swanson NA (1991). Aggressive-growth basal cell carcinoma in young adults. Arch Dermatol. 127(11):1663–7. PMID:1952969
1542. Legius E, Marchuk DA, Collins FS, Glover TW (1993). Somatic deletion of the neurofibromatosis type 1 gene in a neurofibrosarcoma supports a tumour suppressor gene hypothesis. Nat Genet. 3(2):122–6. PMID:8499945
1543. Lehtonen HJ (2011). Hereditary leiomyomatosis and renal cell cancer: update on clinical and molecular characteristics. Fam Cancer. 10(2):397–411. PMID:21404119
1544. Leibovitch I, Huilgol SC, Selva D, Richards S, Paver R (2005). Basal cell carcinoma treated with Mohs surgery in Australia III. Perineural invasion. J Am Acad Dermatol. 53(3):458–63. PMID:16112353
1545. Ngan V (2006) Lentigo simplex. DermNet New Zealand. Available from: https://www.dermnetnz.org/topics/lentigo-simplex.
1546. Leonard N, Chaggar R, Jones C, Takahashi M, Nikitopoulou A, Lakhani SR (2001). Loss of heterozygosity at cylindromatosis gene locus, CYLD, in sporadic skin adnexal tumours. J Clin Pathol. 54(9):689–92. PMID:11533075
1547. Leshin B, Whitaker DC, Foucar E (1986). Lymphangioma circumscriptum following mastectomy and radiation therapy. J Am Acad Dermatol. 15(5 Pt 2):1117–9. PMID:3771862
1548. Lesluyes T, Pérot G, Largeau MR, Brulard C, Lagarde P, Dapremont V, et al. (2016). RNA sequencing validation of the Complexity INdex in SARComas prognostic signature. Eur J Cancer. 57:104–11. PMID:26916546
1549. Lever L, Marks R (1989). The significance of the Darier-like solar keratosis and acantholytic change in preneoplastic lesions of the epidermis. Br J Dermatol. 120(3):383–9. PMID:2713258
1550. Levin C, Mirzamani N, Zwerner J, Kim Y, Schwartz EJ, Sundram U (2012). A comparative analysis of cutaneous marginal zone lymphoma and cutaneous chronic lymphocytic leukemia. Am J Dermatopathol. 34(1):18–23. PMID:22257836
1551. Levisohn D, Seidel D, Phelps A, Burgdorf W (1993). Solitary congenital indeterminate cell histiocytoma. Arch Dermatol. 129(1):81–5. PMID:8380541
1552. Lezcano C, Ho J, Seethala RR (2017). Sox10 and DOG1 expression in primary adnexal tumors of the skin. Am J Dermatopathol. 39(12):896–902. PMID:28394798
1553. Li JY, Guitart J, Pulitzer MP, Subtil A, Sundram U, Kim Y, et al. (2014). Multicenter case series of indolent small/medium-sized CD8+ lymphoid proliferations with predilection for the ear and face. Am J Dermatopathol. 36(5):402–8. PMID:24394306
1554. Li L, Zeng Y, Fang K, Xiao Y, Jin H, Ray H, et al. (2012). Anetodermic pilomatricoma: molecular characteristics and trauma in the development of its bullous appearance. Am J Dermatopathol. 34(4):e41–5. PMID:22307232
1555. Li Z, Lu L, Zhou Z, Xue W, Wang Y, Jin M, et al. (2018). Recurrent mutations in epigenetic modifiers and the PI3K/AKT/mTOR pathway in subcutaneous panniculitis-like T-cell lymphoma. Br J Haematol. 181(3):406–10. PMID:28294301
1556. Li Z, Yang JJ, Wu M (2015). Collision tumor of primary Merkel cell carcinoma and chronic lymphocytic leukemia/small lymphocytic lymphoma, diagnosed on ultrasound-guided fine-needle aspiration biopsy: a unique case report and review of literature. Diagn Cytopathol. 43(1):66–71. PMID:24610800
1557. Liang H, Wu H, Giorgadze TA, Sariya D, Bellucci KS, Veerappan R, et al. (2007). Podoplanin is a highly sensitive and specific marker to distinguish primary skin adnexal carcinomas from adenocarcinomas metastatic to skin. Am J Surg Pathol. 31(2):304–10. PMID:17255777
1558. Liau JY, Lan J, Hong JB, Tsai JH, Kuo KT, Chu CY, et al. (2016). Frequent PIK3CA-activating mutations in hidradenoma papilliferums. Hum Pathol. 55:57–62. PMID:27184479
1559. Lichter MD, Karagas MR, Mott LA, Spencer SK, Stukel TA, Greenberg ER (2000). Therapeutic ionizing radiation and the incidence of basal cell carcinoma and squamous cell carcinoma. Arch Dermatol. 136(8):1007–11. PMID:10926736
1560. Lieberman PH, Jones CR, Steinman RM, Erlandson RA, Smith J, Gee T, et al. (1996). Langerhans cell (eosinophilic) granulomatosis. A clinicopathologic study encompassing 50 years. Am J Surg Pathol. 20(5):519–52. PMID:8619419
1561. Lim KH, Tefferi A, Lasho TL, Finke C, Patnaik M, Butterfield JH, et al. (2009). Systemic mastocytosis in 342 consecutive adults: survival studies and prognostic factors. Blood. 113(23):5727–36. PMID:19363219
1562. Lin BT, Weiss LM, Medeiros LJ (1997). Neurofibroma and cellular neurofibroma with atypia: a report of 14 tumors. Am J Surg Pathol. 21(12):1443–9. PMID:9414187
1563. Lin L, Skacel M, Sigel JE, Bergfeld WF, Montgomery E, Fisher C, et al. (2003). Epithelioid sarcoma: an immunohistochemical analysis evaluating the utility of cytokeratin 5/6 in distinguishing superficial epithelioid sarcoma from spindled squamous cell carcinoma. J Cutan Pathol. 30(2):114–7. PMID:12641789
1564. Lin WM, Luo S, Muzikansky A, Lobo AZ, Tanabe KK, Sober AJ, et al. (2015). Outcome of patients with de novo versus nevus-associated melanoma. J Am Acad Dermatol. 72(1):54–8. PMID:25440436
1565. Lindegaard J, Isager P, Prause JU, Heegaard S (2006). Optic nerve invasion of uveal melanoma: clinical characteristics and metastatic pattern. Invest Ophthalmol Vis Sci. 47(8):3268–75. PMID:16877391
1566. Lindegaard J, Isager P, Prause JU, Heegaard S (2007). Optic nerve invasion of uveal melanoma. APMIS. 115(1):1–16. PMID:17223846
1567. Bosisio FM, Cerroni L (2015). Expression of T-follicular helper markers in sequential biopsies of progressive mycosis fungoides and other primary cutaneous T-cell lymphomas. Am J Dermatopathol. 37(2):115–21. PMID:25406852
1568. Linos K, Carter JM, Gardner JM, Folpe AL, Weiss SW, Edgar MA (2014). Myofibromas with atypical features: expanding the morphologic spectrum of a benign entity. Am J Surg Pathol. 38(12):1649–54. PMID:24921644
1569. Linos K, Csaposs J, Carlson JA (2013). Microvenular hemangioma presenting with numerous bilateral macules, patches, and plaques: a case report and review of the literature. Am J Dermatopathol. 35(1):98–101. PMID:22722465
1570. Linos K, Sedivcová M, Cerna K, Sima R, Kazakov DV, Nazeer T, et al. (2011). Extra nuchal-type fibroma associated with elastosis, traumatic neuroma, a rare APC gene missense mutation, and a very rare MUTYH gene polymorphism: a case report and review of the literature. J Cutan Pathol. 38(11):911–8. PMID:21752055
1571. Liu GY, Song H, Xu XL (2016). Multiple palisaded encapsulated neuromas in siblings: a case report and review of the published work. J Dermatol. 43(5):560–3. PMID:26460241
1572. Liu H, Chen S, Zhang F, Shi B, Shi Z, Zhang D, et al. (2010). Seborrheic keratosis or verruca plana? A pilot study with confocal laser scanning microscopy. Skin Res Technol. 16(4):408–12. PMID:21039905
1573. Liu HL, Hoppe RT, Kohler S, Harvell JD, Reddy S, Kim YH (2003). CD30+ cutaneous lymphoproliferative disorders: the Stanford experience in lymphomatoid papulosis and primary cutaneous anaplastic large cell lymphoma. J Am Acad Dermatol. 49(6):1049–58. PMID:14639383
1574. Liu W, Dowling JP, Murray WK, McArthur GA, Thompson JF, Wolfe R, et al. (2006). Rate of growth in melanomas: characteristics and associations of rapidly growing melanomas. Arch Dermatol. 142(12):1551–8. PMID:17178980
1575. Livi L, Shah N, Paiar F, Fisher C, Judson I, Moskovic E, et al. (2003). Treatment of epithelioid sarcoma at the Royal Marsden Hospital. Sarcoma. 7(3–4):149–52. PMID:18521379
1576. Patterson JW (2015). Tumors of the epidermis: actinic keratosis. In: Weedon's skin pathology. 4th ed. London: Elsevier; pp. 796–9.
1577. Patterson JW (2015). Tumors of the epidermis: arsenic keratosis. In: Weedon's skin pathology. 4th ed. London: Elsevier; p. 800.
1578. Llamas-Velasco M, Pérez-Gónzalez YC, Requena L, Kutzner H (2014). Histopathologic clues for the diagnosis of Wiesner nevus. J Am Acad Dermatol. 70(3):549–54. PMID:24373783
1579. Llamas-Velasco M, Requena L, Adam J, Frizzell N, Hartmann A, Mentzel T (2016). Loss of fumarate hydratase and aberrant protein succination detected with S-(2-succino)-cysteine staining to identify patients with multiple cutaneous and uterine leiomyomatosis and hereditary leiomyomatosis and renal cell cancer syndrome. Am J Dermatopathol. 38(12):887–91. PMID:27097334
1580. Llamas-Velasco M, Requena L, Kutzner

H, Schärer L, Rütten A, Hantschke M, et al. (2014). Fumarate hydratase immunohistochemical staining may help to identify patients with multiple cutaneous and uterine leiomyomatosis (MCUL) and hereditary leiomyomatosis and renal cell cancer (HLRCC) syndrome. J Cutan Pathol. 41(11):859–65. PMID:25292446
**1581.** Llamas-Velasco M, Requena L, Podda M, Weidenthaler-Barth B, Rütten A (2014). Apocrine intraductal carcinoma in situ in nevus sebaceus: two case reports. J Cutan Pathol. 41(12):944–9. PMID:25302933
**1582.** Llombart B, Serra-Guillén C, Monteagudo C, López Guerrero JA, Sanmartín O (2013). Dermatofibrosarcoma protuberans: a comprehensive review and update on diagnosis and management. Semin Diagn Pathol. 30(1):13–28. PMID:23327727
**1583.** Llombart-Bosch A, Machado I, Navarro S, Bertoni F, Bacchini P, Alberghini M, et al. (2009). Histological heterogeneity of Ewing's sarcoma/PNET: an immunohistochemical analysis of 415 genetically confirmed cases with clinical support. Virchows Arch. 455(5):397–411. PMID:19841938
**1584.** Lodish MB, Yuan B, Levy I, Braunstein GD, Lyssikatos C, Salpea P, et al. (2015). Germline PRKACA amplification causes variable phenotypes that may depend on the extent of the genomic defect: molecular mechanisms and clinical presentations. Eur J Endocrinol. 172(6):803–11. PMID:25924874
**1585.** Loeb KR, Asgari MM, Hawes SE, Feng Q, Stern JE, Jiang M, et al. (2012). Analysis of Tp53 codon 72 polymorphisms, Tp53 mutations, and HPV infection in cutaneous squamous cell carcinomas. PLoS One. 7(4):e34422. PMID:22545084
**1586.** Loh J, Kenny P (2010). Meyerson phenomenon. J Cutan Med Surg. 14(1):30–2. PMID:20128988
**1587.** Lohmann DR, Gillessen-Kaesbach G (2000). Multiple subcutaneous granular-cell tumours in a patient with Noonan syndrome. Clin Dysmorphol. 9(4):301–2. PMID:11045593
**1588.** Lomas A, Leonardi-Bee J, Bath-Hextall F (2012). A systematic review of worldwide incidence of nonmelanoma skin cancer. Br J Dermatol. 166(5):1069–80. PMID:22251204
**1589.** Lombardi R, Jovine E, Zanini N, Salone MC, Gambarotti M, Righi A, et al. (2013). A case of lung metastasis in myxoinflammatory fibroblastic sarcoma: analytical review of one hundred and thirty eight cases. Int Orthop. 37(12):2429–36. PMID:24158237
**1590.** López L, Vélez R (2016). Atypical fibroxanthoma. Arch Pathol Lab Med. 140(4):376–9. PMID:27028396
**1591.** López V, Martín JM, Monteagudo C, Jordá E (2010). Epidemiology of pediatric dermatologic surgery: a retrospective study of 996 children. Actas Dermosifiliogr. 101(9):771–7. [Spanish] PMID:21034707
**1592.** Lott JP, Elmore JG, Zhao GA, Knezevich SR, Frederick PD, Reisch LM, et al. (2016). Evaluation of the Melanocytic Pathology Assessment Tool and Hierarchy for Diagnosis (MPATH-Dx) classification scheme for diagnosis of cutaneous melanocytic neoplasms: results from the International Melanoma Pathology Study Group. J Am Acad Dermatol. 75(2):356–63. PMID:27189823
**1593.** Lott JP, Wititsuwannakul J, Lee JJ, Ariyan S, Narayan D, Kluger HH, et al. (2014). Clinical characteristics associated with Spitz nevi and Spitzoid malignant melanomas: the Yale University Spitzoid Neoplasm Repository experience, 1991 to 2008. J Am Acad Dermatol. 71(6):1077–82. PMID:25308882
**1594.** Lowe S, Ferrand RA, Morris-Jones R, Salisbury J, Mangeya N, Dimairo M, et al. (2010). Skin disease among human immunodeficiency virus-infected adolescents in Zimbabwe: a strong indicator of underlying HIV infection. Pediatr Infect Dis J. 29(4):346–51. PMID:19940800
**1595.** Lu C, Zhang J, Nagahawatte P, Easton J, Lee S, Liu Z, et al. (2015). The genomic landscape of childhood and adolescent melanoma. J Invest Dermatol. 135(3):816–23. PMID:25268584
**1596.** Lucas GL, Nordby EJ (1974). Sweat gland carcinoma of the hand. Hand. 6(1):98–102. PMID:4825405
**1597.** Lucioni M, Novara F, Fiandrino G, Riboni R, Fanoni D, Arra M, et al. (2011). Twenty-one cases of blastic plasmacytoid dendritic cell neoplasm: focus on biallelic locus 9p21.3 deletion. Blood. 118(17):4591–4. PMID:21900200
**1598.** Luskin MR, Huen AO, Brooks SA, Stewart C, Watt CD, Morrissette JJ, et al. (2015). NPM1 mutation is associated with leukemia cutis in acute myeloid leukemia with monocytic features. Haematologica. 100(10):e412–4. PMID:26113416
**1599.** Luz FB, Gaspar AP, Ramos-e-Silva M, Carvalho da Fonseca E, Villar EG, Cordovil Pires AR, et al. (2005). Immunohistochemical profile of multicentric reticulohistiocytosis. Skinmed. 4(2):71–7. PMID:15785133
**1600.** Luz FB, Gaspar NK, Gaspar AP, Carneiro S, Ramos-e-Silva M (2007). Multicentric reticulohistiocytosis: a proliferation of macrophages with tropism for skin and joints, part I. Skinmed. 6(4):172–8. PMID:17618169
**1601.** Luz FB, Kurizky PS, Ramos-e-Silva M (2007). Reticulohistiocytosis. Dermatol Clin. 25(4):625–32, x. PMID:17903621
**1602.** Luzar B, Calonje E (2009). Superficial acral fibromyxoma: clinicopathological study of 14 cases with emphasis on a cellular variant. Histopathology. 54(3):375–7. PMID:19236516
**1603.** Luzar B, Calonje E (2010). Morphological and immunohistochemical characteristics of atypical fibroxanthoma with a special emphasis on potential diagnostic pitfalls: a review. J Cutan Pathol. 37(3):301–9. PMID:19807823
**1604.** Luzar B, Falconieri G (2017). Cutaneous malignant peripheral nerve sheath tumor. Surg Pathol Clin. 10(2):337–43. PMID:28477884
**1605.** Luzar B, Shanesmith R, Calonje E (2015). Perineural growth of benign cutaneous sweat gland tumors: a hitherto unrecognized phenomenon unassociated with malignancy. J Cutan Pathol. 42(11):878–83. PMID:26260952
**1606.** Luzar B, Shanesmith R, Ramakrishnan R, Fisher C, Calonje E (2016). Cutaneous epithelioid malignant peripheral nerve sheath tumour: a clinicopathological analysis of 11 cases. Histopathology. 68(2):286–96. PMID:26096054
**1607.** Luzar B, Tanaka M, Schneider J, Calonje E (2016). Cutaneous microcystic/reticular schwannoma: a poorly recognized entity. J Cutan Pathol. 43(2):93–100. PMID:26350054
**1608.** Lv J, Dai B, Kong Y, Shen X, Kong J (2016). Acral melanoma in Chinese: a clinicopathological and prognostic study of 142 cases. Sci Rep. 6:31432. PMID:27545198
**1609.** Ly L, Christie M, Swain S, Winship I, Kelly JW (2011). Melanoma(s) arising in large segmental speckled lentiginous nevi: a case series. J Am Acad Dermatol. 64(6):1190–3. PMID:21571187
**1610.** Lynde CW, McLean DI, Wood WS (1984). Tumors of ceruminous glands. J Am Acad Dermatol. 11(5 Pt 1):841–7. PMID:6096419
**1611.** Lynnhtun K, Achan A, Shingde M, Chou S, Howle JR, Sharma R (2012). Plexiform fibrohistiocytic tumour: morphological changes and challenges in assessment of recurrent and metastatic lesions. Histopathology. 60(7):1156–8. PMID:22435737
**1612.** Lyons LL, North PE, Mac-Moune Lai F, Stoler MH, Folpe AL, Weiss SW (2004). Kaposiform hemangioendothelioma: a study of 33 cases emphasizing its pathologic, immunophenotypic, and biologic uniqueness from juvenile hemangioma. Am J Surg Pathol. 28(5):559–68. PMID:15105642
**1613.** Ma JE, Wieland CN, Tollefson MM (2017). Dermatomyofibromas arising in children: report of two new cases and review of the literature. Pediatr Dermatol. 34(3):347–51. PMID:28318057
**1614.** Macarenco AC, Macarenco RS (2008). Cutaneous lipomatous sclerosing perineurioma. Am J Dermatopathol. 30(3):291–4. PMID:18496437
**1615.** Macarenco RS, Erickson-Johnson M, Wang X, Jenkins RB, Nascimento AG, Oliveira AM (2007). Cytogenetic and molecular cytogenetic findings in dedifferentiated liposarcoma with neural-like whorling pattern and metaplastic bone formation. Cancer Genet Cytogenet. 172(2):147–50. PMID:17213023
**1616.** Macchia G, Trombetta D, Möller E, Mertens F, Storlazzi CT, Debiec-Rychter M, et al. (2012). FOSL1 as a candidate target gene for 11q12 rearrangements in desmoplastic fibroblastoma. Lab Invest. 92(5):735–43. PMID:22411068
**1617.** Macgregor S, Montgomery GW, Liu JZ, Zhao ZZ, Henders AK, Stark M, et al. (2011). Genome-wide association study identifies a new melanoma susceptibility locus at 1q21.3. Nat Genet. 43(11):1114–8. PMID:21983785
**1618.** Macgrogan G, Vergier B, Dubus P, Beylot-Barry M, Belleannee G, Delaunay MM, et al. (1996). CD30-positive cutaneous large cell lymphomas. A comparative study of clinicopathologic and molecular features of 16 cases. Am J Clin Pathol. 105(4):440–50. PMID:8604686
**1619.** Machado I, Llombart B, Calabuig-Fariñas S, Llombart-Bosch A (2011). Superficial Ewing's sarcoma family of tumors: a clinicopathological study with differential diagnoses. J Cutan Pathol. 38(8):636–43. PMID:21649689
**1620.** Machado I, Noguera R, Mateos EA, Calabuig-Fariñas S, López FI, Martínez A, et al. (2011). The many faces of atypical Ewing's sarcoma. A true entity mimicking sarcomas, carcinomas and lymphomas. Virchows Arch. 458(3):281–90. PMID:21181413
**1621.** Machan S, Molina-Ruiz AM, Fernández-Aceñero MJ, Encabo B, LeBoit P, Bastian BC, et al. (2015). Metastatic melanoma in association with a giant congenital melanocytic nevus in an adult: controversial CGH findings. Am J Dermatopathol. 37(6):487–94. PMID:25062263
**1622.** Madankumar R, Gumaste PV, Martires K, Schaffer PR, Choudhary S, Falto-Aizpurua L, et al. (2016). Acral melanocytic lesions in the United States: prevalence, awareness, and dermoscopic patterns in skin-of-color and non-Hispanic white patients. J Am Acad Dermatol. 74(4):724–30.e1. PMID:26803347
**1623.** Amador-Ortiz C, Hurley MY, Ghahramani GK, Frisch S, Klco JM, Lind AC, et al. (2011). Use of classic and novel immunohistochemical markers in the diagnosis of cutaneous myeloid sarcoma. J Cutan Pathol. 38(12):945–53. PMID:22050091
**1624.** Maeda M, Shimizu A, Ikuta K, Okamoto H, Kashihara M, Uchiyama T, et al. (1985). Origin of human T-lymphotrophic virus I-positive T cell lines in adult T cell leukemia. Analysis of T cell receptor gene rearrangement. J Exp Med. 162(6):2169–74. PMID:2866223
**1625.** Magaña M, Massone C, Magaña P, Cerroni L (2016). Clinicopathologic features of hydroa vacciniforme-like lymphoma: a series of 9 patients. Am J Dermatopathol. 38(1):20–5. PMID:26368647
**1626.** Maggiani F, Debiec-Rychter M, Vanbockrijck M, Sciot R (2007). Cellular angiofibroma: another mesenchymal tumour with 13q14 involvement, suggesting a link with spindle cell lipoma and (extra)-mammary myofibroblastoma. Histopathology. 51(3):410–2. PMID:17727484
**1627.** Maghari A, Ma N, Aisner S, Benevenia J, Hameed M (2009). Collagenous fibroma (desmoplastic fibroblastoma) with a new translocation involving 11q12: a case report. Cancer Genet Cytogenet. 192(2):73–5. PMID:19596257
**1628.** Magni M, Di Nicola M, Carlo-Stella C, Matteucci P, Lavazza C, Grisanti S, et al. (2002). Identical rearrangement of immunoglobulin heavy chain gene in neoplastic Langerhans cells and B-lymphocytes: evidence for a common precursor. Leuk Res. 26(12):1131–3. PMID:12443887
**1629.** Magro CM, Abraham RM, Guo R, Li S, Wang X, Proper S, et al. (2014). Deep penetrating nevus-like borderline tumors: a unique subset of ambiguous melanocytic tumors with malignant potential and normal cytogenetics. Eur J Dermatol. 24(5):594–602. PMID:25118781
**1630.** Magro CM, Crowson AN, Kovatich AJ, Burns F (2001). Lupus profundus, indeterminate lymphocytic lobular panniculitis and subcutaneous T-cell lymphoma: a spectrum of subcuticular T-cell lymphoid dyscrasia. J Cutan Pathol. 28(5):235–47. PMID:11401667
**1631.** Magro CM, Morrison CD, Heerema N, Porcu P, Sroa N, Deng AC (2006). T-cell prolymphocytic leukemia: an aggressive T cell malignancy with frequent cutaneous tropism. J Am Acad Dermatol. 55(3):467–77. PMID:16908353
**1632.** Magro CM, Yang A, Fraga G (2013). Blastic marginal zone lymphoma: a clinical and pathological study of 8 cases and review of the literature. Am J Dermatopathol. 35(3):319–26. PMID:23190506
**1633.** Magro G, Bisceglia M, Michal M, Eusebi V (2002). Spindle cell lipoma-like tumor, solitary fibrous tumor and myofibroblastoma of the breast: a clinico-pathological analysis of 13 cases in favor of a unifying histogenetic concept. Virchows Arch. 440(3):249–60. PMID:11889594
**1634.** Magro G, Caltabiano R, Di Cataldo A, Puzzo L (2007). CD10 is expressed by mammary myofibroblastoma and spindle cell lipoma of soft tissue: an additional evidence of their histogenetic linking. Virchows Arch. 450(6):727–8. PMID:17497167
**1635.** Mahalingam M (2017). MSH6, past and present and Muir-Torre syndrome-connecting the dots. Am J Dermatopathol. 39(4):239–49. PMID:28323777
**1636.** Mahalingam M, Alter JN, Bhawan J (2006). Multiple cellular neurothekeomas–a case report and review on the role of immunohistochemistry as a histologic adjunct. J Cutan Pathol. 33(1):51–6. PMID:16441413
**1637.** Mahalingam M, Goldberg LJ (2001). Atypical pilar leiomyoma: cutaneous counterpart of uterine symplastic leiomyoma? Am J Dermatopathol. 23(4):299–303. PMID:11481520
**1638.** Mahalingam M, Nguyen LP, Richards JE, Muzikansky A, Hoang MP (2010). The diagnostic utility of immunohistochemistry in distinguishing primary skin adnexal carcinomas from metastatic adenocarcinoma to skin: an immunohistochemical reappraisal using cytokeratin 15, nestin, p63, D2-40, and calretinin. Mod Pathol. 23(5):713–9. PMID:20190734
**1639.** Mahalingam M, Srivastava A, Hoang MP (2010). Expression of stem-cell markers (cytokeratin 15 and nestin) in primary adnexal neoplasms-clues to etiopathogenesis. Am J Dermatopathol. 32(8):774–9. PMID:20700038
**1640.** Mahima VG, Patil K, Srikanth HS (2011).

Recurrent oral angioleiomyoma. Contemp Clin Dent. 2(2):102–5. PMID:21957385

**1641.** Mahomed F, Blok J, Grayson W (2008). The squamous variant of eccrine porocarcinoma: a clinicopathological study of 21 cases. J Clin Pathol. 61(3):361–5. PMID:17704263

**1642.** Maize JC Jr, McCalmont TH, Carlson JA, Busam KJ, Kutzner H, Bastian BC (2005). Genomic analysis of blue nevi and related dermal melanocytic proliferations. Am J Surg Pathol. 29(9):1214–20. PMID:16096412

**1643.** Majewski S, Jablonska S (1997). Human papillomavirus-associated tumors of the skin and mucosa. J Am Acad Dermatol. 36(5 Pt 1):659–85. PMID:9146528

**1644.** Mäkitie T, Summanen P, Tarkkanen A, Kivelä T (2001). Tumor-infiltrating macrophages (CD68(+) cells) and prognosis in malignant uveal melanoma. Invest Ophthalmol Vis Sci. 42(7):1414–21. PMID:11381040

**1645.** Maldonado JL, Fridlyand J, Patel H, Jain AN, Busam K, Kageshita T, et al. (2003). Determinants of BRAF mutations in primary melanomas. J Natl Cancer Inst. 95(24):1878–90. PMID:14679157

**1646.** Malhotra B, Schuetze SM (2012). Dermatofibrosarcoma protruberans treatment with platelet-derived growth factor receptor inhibitor: a review of clinical trial results. Curr Opin Oncol. 24(4):419–24. PMID:22510939

**1647.** Malhotra P, Walia H, Singh A, Ramesh V (2010). Leiomyoma cutis: a clinicopathological series of 37 cases. Indian J Dermatol. 55(4):337–41. PMID:21430885

**1648.** Malik K, Patel P, Chen J, Khachemoune A (2015). Leiomyoma cutis: a focused review on presentation, management, and association with malignancy. Am J Clin Dermatol. 16(1):35–46. PMID:25605645

**1649.** Mallett RB, Matutes E, Catovsky D, Maclennan K, Mortimer PS, Holden CA (1995). Cutaneous infiltration in T-cell prolymphocytic leukaemia. Br J Dermatol. 132(2):263–6. PMID:7888364

**1650.** Mallone S, De Vries E, Guzzo M, Midena E, Verne J, Coebergh JW, et al. (2012). Descriptive epidemiology of malignant mucosal and uveal melanomas and adnexal skin carcinomas in Europe. Eur J Cancer. 48(8):1167–75. PMID:22119735

**1651.** Maly A, Epstein D, Meir K, Pe'er J (2008). Histological criteria for grading of atypia in melanocytic conjunctival lesions. Pathology. 40(7):676–81. PMID:18985522

**1652.** Mambo NC (1983). Eccrine spiradenoma: clinical and pathologic study of 49 tumors. J Cutan Pathol. 10(5):312–20. PMID:6313776

**1653.** Mandahl N, Heim S, Willén H, Rydholm A, Mitelman F (1990). Supernumerary ring chromosome as the sole cytogenetic abnormality in a dermatofibrosarcoma protuberans. Cancer Genet Cytogenet. 49(2):273–5. PMID:2208065

**1654.** Mandahl N, Höglund M, Mertens F, Rydholm A, Willén H, Brosjö O, et al. (1994). Cytogenetic aberrations in 188 benign and borderline adipose tissue tumors. Genes Chromosomes Cancer. 9(3):207–15. PMID:7515663

**1655.** Mandal RV, Murali R, Lundquist KF, Ragsdale BD, Heenan P, McCarthy SW, et al. (2009). Pigmented epithelioid melanocytoma: favorable outcome after 5-year follow-up. Am J Surg Pathol. 33(12):1778–82. PMID:19773637

**1656.** Mane DR, Kale AD, Hallikerimath S, Angadi P, Kotrashetti V (2010). Trichilemmal carcinoma associated with xeroderma pigmentosa: report of a rare case. J Oral Sci. 52(3):505–7. PMID:20881348

**1657.** Manner J, Radlwimmer B, Hohenberger P, Mössinger K, Küffer S, Sauer C, et al. (2010). MYC high level gene amplification is a distinctive feature of angiosarcomas after irradiation or chronic lymphedema. Am J Pathol. 176(1):34–9. PMID:20008140

**1658.** Mansoor A, Fidda N, Himoe E, Payne M, Lawce H, Magenis RE (2004). Myxoinflammatory fibroblastic sarcoma with complex supernumerary ring chromosomes composed of chromosome 3 segments. Cancer Genet Cytogenet. 152(1):61–5. PMID:15193443

**1659.** Mao X, Lillington DM, Czepulkowski B, Russell-Jones R, Young BD, Whittaker S (2003). Molecular cytogenetic characterization of Sézary syndrome. Genes Chromosomes Cancer. 36(3):250–60. PMID:12557225

**1660.** Marchese C, Montera M, Torrini M, Goldoni F, Mareni C, Forni M, et al. (2003). Granular cell tumor in a PHTS patient with a novel germline PTEN mutation. Am J Med Genet A. 120A(2):286–8. PMID:12833416

**1661.** Margolis RJ, Tong AK, Byers HR, Mihm MC Jr (1989). Comparison of acral nevomelanocytic proliferations in Japanese and whites. J Invest Dermatol. 92(5 Suppl):222S–6S. PMID:2715654

**1662.** Maric I, Pittaluga S, Dale JK, Niemela JE, Delsol G, Diment J, et al. (2005). Histologic features of sinus histiocytosis with massive lymphadenopathy in patients with autoimmune lymphoproliferative syndrome. Am J Surg Pathol. 29(7):903–11. PMID:15958855

**1663.** Markovic SN, Erickson LA, Rao RD, Weenig RH, Pockaj BA, Bardia A, et al. (2007). Malignant melanoma in the 21st century, part 1: epidemiology, risk factors, screening, prevention, and diagnosis. Mayo Clin Proc. 82(3):364–80. PMID:17352373

**1664.** Marks R (1997). Epidemiology of non-melanoma skin cancer and solar keratoses in Australia: a tale of self-immolation in Elysian Fields. Australas J Dermatol. 38 Suppl 1:S26–9. PMID:10994467

**1665.** Marque M, Bessis D, Pedeutour F, Viseux V, Guillot B, Fraitag-Spinner S (2009). Medallion-like dermal dendrocyte hamartoma: the main diagnostic pitfall is congenital atrophic dermatofibrosarcoma. Br J Dermatol. 160(1):190–3. PMID:19016705

**1666.** Marshall-Taylor C, Fanburg-Smith JC (2000). Hemosiderotic fibrohistiocytic lipomatous lesion: ten cases of a previously undescribed fatty lesion of the foot/ankle. Mod Pathol. 13(11):1192–9. PMID:11106076

**1667.** Martel P, Laroche L, Courville P, Larroche C, Wechsler J, Lenormand B, et al. (2000). Cutaneous involvement in patients with angioimmunoblastic lymphadenopathy with dysproteinemia: a clinical, immunohistological, and molecular analysis. Arch Dermatol. 136(7):881–6. PMID:10890990

**1668.** Martignetti JA, Tian L, Li D, Ramirez MC, Camacho-Vanegas O, Camacho SC, et al. (2013). Mutations in PDGFRB cause autosomal-dominant infantile myofibromatosis. Am J Hum Genet. 92(6):1001–7. PMID:23731542

**1669.** Martin Flores-Stadler E, Gonzalez-Crussi F, Greene M, Thangavelu M, Kletzel M, Chou PM (1999). Indeterminate-cell histiocytosis: immunophenotypic and cytogenetic findings in an infant. Med Pediatr Oncol. 32(4):250–4. PMID:10102017

**1670.** Martin M, Maßhöfer L, Temming P, Rahmann S, Metz C, Bornfeld N, et al. (2013). Exome sequencing identifies recurrent somatic mutations in EIF1AX and SF3B1 in uveal melanoma with disomy 3. Nat Genet. 45(8):933–6. PMID:23793026

**1671.** Martin RC, Murali R, Scolyer RA, Fitzgerald P, Colman MH, Thompson JF (2009). So-called "malignant blue nevus": a clinicopathologic study of 23 patients. Cancer. 115(13):2949–55. PMID:19472395

**1672.** Martín-Martín L, López A, Vidriales B, Caballero MD, Rodrigues AS, Ferreira SI, et al. (2015). Classification and clinical behavior of blastic plasmacytoid dendritic cell neoplasms according to their maturation-associated immunophenotypic profile. Oncotarget. 6(22):19204–16. PMID:26056082

**1673.** Martinez SR, Barr KL, Canter RJ (2011). Rare tumors through the looking glass: an examination of malignant cutaneous adnexal tumors. Arch Dermatol. 147(9):1058–62. PMID:21931043

**1674.** Martinez-Escala ME, Sidiropoulos M, Deonizio J, Gerami P, Kadin ME, Guitart J (2015). γδ T-cell-rich variants of pityriasis lichenoides and lymphomatoid papulosis: benign cutaneous disorders to be distinguished from aggressive cutaneous γδ T-cell lymphomas. Br J Dermatol. 172(2):372–9. PMID:25143223

**1675.** Marzano AV, Ghislanzoni M, Gianelli U, Caputo R, Alessi E, Berti E (2005). Fatal CD8+ epidermotropic cytotoxic primary cutaneous T-cell lymphoma with multiorgan involvement. Dermatology. 211(3):281–5. PMID:16205076

**1676.** Marzuka AG, Book SE (2015). Basal cell carcinoma: pathogenesis, epidemiology, clinical features, diagnosis, histopathology, and management. Yale J Biol Med. 88(2):167–79. PMID:26029015

**1677.** Paulson KG, Park SY, Vandeven NA, Lachance K, Thomas H, Chapuis AG, et al. (2018). Merkel cell carcinoma: current US incidence and projected increases based on changing demographics. J Am Acad Dermatol. 78(3):457–63.e2. PMID:29102486

**1678.** Mason A, Wititsuwannakul J, Klump VR, Lott J, Lazova R (2012). Expression of p16 alone does not differentiate between Spitz nevi and Spitzoid melanoma. J Cutan Pathol. 39(12):1062–74. PMID:23005921

**1679.** Massi D, Carli P, Franchi A, Santucci M (1999). Naevus-associated melanomas: cause or chance? Melanoma Res. 9(1):85–91. PMID:10338338

**1680.** Massi D, Franchi A, Alos L, Cook M, Di Palma S, Enguita AB, et al. (2010). Primary cutaneous leiomyosarcoma: clinicopathological analysis of 36 cases. Histopathology. 56(2):251–62. PMID:20102404

**1681.** Massi G, Leboit P, editors (2014). Histological diagnosis of nevi and melanoma. 2nd ed. Berlin: Springer.

**1682.** Massi G, Leboit PE (2014). Combined nevus. In: Histological diagnosis of nevi and melanoma. 2nd ed. Berlin: Springer; pp. 285–300.

**1683.** Massone C, Cerroni L (2014). Phenotypic variability in primary cutaneous anaplastic large T-cell lymphoma: a study on 35 patients. Am J Dermatopathol. 36(2):153–7. PMID:24394302

**1684.** Massone C, Chott A, Metze D, Kerl K, Citarella L, Vale E, et al. (2004). Subcutaneous, blastic natural killer (NK), NK/T-cell, and other cytotoxic lymphomas of the skin: a morphologic, immunophenotypic, and molecular study of 50 patients. Am J Surg Pathol. 28(6):719–35. PMID:15166664

**1685.** Massone C, Crisman G, Kerl H, Cerroni L (2008). The prognosis of early mycosis fungoides is not influenced by phenotype and T-cell clonality. Br J Dermatol. 159(4):881–6. PMID:18644018

**1686.** Massone C, El-Shabrawi-Caelen L, Kerl H, Cerroni L (2008). The morphologic spectrum of primary cutaneous anaplastic large T-cell lymphoma: a histopathologic study on 66 biopsy specimens from 47 patients with report of rare variants. J Cutan Pathol. 35(1):46–53. PMID:18095994

**1687.** Massone C, Kodama K, Kerl H, Cerroni L (2005). Histopathologic features of early (patch) lesions of mycosis fungoides: a morphologic study on 745 biopsy specimens from 427 patients. Am J Surg Pathol. 29(4):550–60. PMID:15767812

**1688.** Massone C, Kodama K, Salmhofer W, Abe R, Shimizu H, Parodi A, et al. (2005). Lupus erythematosus panniculitis (lupus profundus): clinical, histopathological, and molecular analysis of nine cases. J Cutan Pathol. 32(6):396–404. PMID:15953372

**1689.** Massone C, Lozzi GP, Egberts F, Fink-Puches R, Cota C, Kerl H, et al. (2006). The protean spectrum of non-Hodgkin lymphomas with prominent involvement of subcutaneous fat. J Cutan Pathol. 33(6):418–25. PMID:16776717

**1690.** Mastrangelo G, Coindre JM, Ducimetière F, Dei Tos AP, Fadda E, Blay JY, et al. (2012). Incidence of soft tissue sarcoma and beyond: a population-based prospective study in 3 European regions. Cancer. 118(21):5339–48. PMID:22517534

**1691.** Masuda T, Arata J (1987). An epithelioma with hair follicle and apocrine differentiation. J Dermatol. 14(1):81–4. PMID:3301956

**1692.** Mataix J, López N, Haro R, González E, Angulo J, Requena L (2007). Late-onset Ito's nevus: an uncommon acquired dermal melanocytosis. J Cutan Pathol. 34(8):640–3. PMID:17640235

**1693.** Mathew R, Morgan MB (2006). Dermal atypical lipomatous tumor/well-differentiated liposarcoma obfuscated by epidermal inclusion cyst: a wolf in sheep's clothing? Am J Dermatopathol. 28(4):338–40. PMID:16871039

**1694.** Mathew RA, Bennett JM, Liu JJ, Komrokji RS, Lancet JE, Naghashpour M, et al. (2012). Cutaneous manifestations in CMML: indication of disease acceleration or transformation to AML and review of the literature. Leuk Res. 36(1):72–80. PMID:21782240

**1695.** Mathiak M, Rütten A, Mangold E, Fischer HP, Ruzicka T, Friedl W, et al. (2002). Loss of DNA mismatch repair proteins in skin tumors from patients with Muir-Torre syndrome and MSH2 or MLH1 germline mutations: establishment of immunohistochemical analysis as a screening test. Am J Surg Pathol. 26(3):338–43. PMID:11859205

**1696.** Mathis ED, Honningford JB, Rodriguez HE, Wind KP, Connolly MM, Podbielski FJ (2001). Malignant proliferating trichilemmal tumor. Am J Clin Oncol. 24(4):351–3. PMID:11474259

**1697.** Matito A, Morgado JM, Álvarez-Twose I, Sánchez-Muñoz L, Pedreira CE, Jara-Acevedo M, et al. (2013). Serum tryptase monitoring in indolent systemic mastocytosis: association with disease features and patient outcome. PLoS One. 8(10):e76116. PMID:24155887

**1698.** Matsue K, Asada N, Odawara J, Aoki T, Kimura S, Iwama K, et al. (2011). Random skin biopsy and bone marrow biopsy for diagnosis of intravascular large B cell lymphoma. Ann Hematol. 90(4):417–21. PMID:20957365

**1699.** Matsuyama A, Hisaoka M, Hashimoto H (2007). Angioleiomyoma: a clinicopathologic and immunohistochemical reappraisal with special reference to the correlation with myopericytoma. Hum Pathol. 38(4):645–51. PMID:17270242

**1700.** Matt D, Xin H, Vortmeyer AO, Zhuang Z, Burg G, Böni R (2000). Sporadic trichoepithelioma demonstrates deletions at 9q22.3. Arch Dermatol. 136(5):657–60. PMID:10815860

**1701.** Matter MS, Bihl M, Juskevicius D, Tzankov A (2017). Is Rosai-Dorfman disease a reactve process? Detection of a MAP2K1 L115V mutation in a case of Rosai-Dorfman disease. Virchows Arch. 471(4):545–7. PMID:28597077

**1702.** Matutes E, Brito-Babapulle V, Swansbury J, Ellis J, Morilla R, Dearden C, et al. (1991). Clinical and laboratory features of 78 cases of T-prolymphocytic leukemia. Blood.

78(12):3269–74. PMID:1742486
**1703.** Maughan C, Kolker S, Markus B, Young J (2014). Leukemia cutis coexisting with dermatofibroma as the initial presentation of B-cell chronic lymphocytic leukemia/small lymphocytic lymphoma. Am J Dermatopathol. 36(1):e14–5. PMID:23974225
**1704.** Mayerl C, Del Frari B, Parson W, Boeck G, Piza-Katzer H, Wick G, et al. (2016). Characterisation of the inflammatory response in Dupuytren's disease. J Plast Surg Hand Surg. 50(3):171–9. PMID:26852784
**1705.** McArthur GA, Demetri GD, van Oosterom A, Heinrich MC, Debiec-Rychter M, Corless CL, et al. (2005). Molecular and clinical analysis of locally advanced dermatofibrosarcoma protuberans treated with imatinib: Imatinib Target Exploration Consortium Study B2225. J Clin Oncol. 23(4):866–73. PMID:15681532
**1706.** McBride SR, Leonard N, Reynolds NJ (2002). Loss of p21(WAF1) compartmentalisation in sebaceous carcinoma compared with sebaceous hyperplasia and sebaceous adenoma. J Clin Pathol. 55(10):763–6. PMID:12354803
**1707.** McCalmont TH (2010). Paranuclear dots of neurofilament reliably identify Merkel cell carcinoma. J Cutan Pathol. 37(8):821–3. PMID:20642632
**1708.** McCarthy SW, Scolyer RA, Palmer AA (2004). Desmoplastic melanoma: a diagnostic trap for the unwary. Pathology. 36(5):445–51. PMID:15370114
**1709.** McCluggage WG, Jamison J, Boyde A, Ganesan R (2009). Vulval intraepithelial neoplasia with mucinous differentiation: report of 2 cases of a hitherto undescribed phenomenon. Am J Surg Pathol. 33(6):945–9. PMID:19238078
**1709A.** McComb EN, Feely MG, Neff JR, Johansson SL, Nelson M, Bridge JA (2001). Cytogenetic instability, predominantly involving chromosome 1, is characteristic of elastofibroma. Cancer Genet Cytogenet. 126(1):68–72. PMID:11343783
**1710.** McCoppin HH, Christiansen D, Stasko T, Washington C, Martinez JC, Brown MD, et al. (2012). Clinical spectrum of atypical fibroxanthoma and undifferentiated pleomorphic sarcoma in solid organ transplant recipients: a collective experience. Dermatol Surg. 38(2):230–9. PMID:22129349
**1711.** McDonnell KJ, Gallanis GT, Heller KA, Melas M, Idos GE, Culver JO, et al. (2016). A novel BAP1 mutation is associated with melanocytic neoplasms and thyroid cancer. Cancer Genet. 209(3):75–81. PMID:26774355
**1712.** McGinness JL, Spicknall KE, Mutasim DF (2012). Azathioprine-induced EBV-positive mucocutaneous ulcer. J Cutan Pathol. 39(3):377–81. PMID:22236092
**1713.** McGirt LY, Jia P, Baerenwald DA, Duszynski RJ, Dahlman KB, Zic JA, et al. (2015). Whole-genome sequencing reveals oncogenic mutations in mycosis fungoides. Blood. 126(4):508–19. PMID:26082451
**1714.** McGovern VJ (1970). The classification of melanoma and its relationship with prognosis. Pathology. 2(2):85–98. PMID:5520514
**1715.** McKay KM, Doyle LA, Lazar AJ, Hornick JL (2012). Expression of ERG, an Ets family transcription factor, distinguishes cutaneous angiosarcoma from histological mimics. Histopathology. 61(5):989–91. PMID:22716285
**1716.** McKay KM, Sambrano BL, Fox PS, Bassett RL, Chon S, Prieto VG (2013). Thickness of superficial basal cell carcinoma (sBCC) predicts imiquimod efficacy: a proposal for a thickness-based definition of sBCC. Br J Dermatol. 169(3):549–54. PMID:23627639
**1717.** McKee PH, Fletcher CD, Rasbridge SA (1990). The enigmatic eccrine epithelioma (eccrine syringomatous carcinoma). Am J Dermatopathol. 12(6):552–61. PMID:2267993
**1718.** McKee PH, Wilkinson JD, Black MM, Whimster IW (1981). Carcinoma (epithelioma) cuniculatum: a clinico-pathological study of nineteen cases and review of the literature. Histopathology. 5(4):425–36. PMID:6168555
**1719.** McKenzie CA, Chen AC, Choy B, Fernández-Peñas P, Damian DL, Scolyer RA (2016). Classification of high risk basal cell carcinoma subtypes: experience of the ONTRAC study with proposed definitions and guidelines for pathological reporting. Pathology. 48(5):395–7. PMID:27311865
**1720.** McKinley E, Valles R, Bang R, Bocklage T (1998). Signet-ring squamous cell carcinoma: a case report. J Cutan Pathol. 25(3):176–81. PMID:9550318
**1721.** McMenamin ME, Fletcher CD (2001). Mammary-type myofibroblastoma of soft tissue: a tumor closely related to spindle cell lipoma. Am J Surg Pathol. 25(8):1022–9. PMID:11474286
**1722.** McMenamin ME, Fletcher CD (2002). Malignant myopericytoma: expanding the spectrum of tumours with myopericytic differentiation. Histopathology. 41(5):450–60. PMID:12405913
**1723.** McNiff JM, Cooper D, Howe G, Crotty PL, Tallini G, Crouch J, et al. (1996). Lymphomatoid granulomatosis of the skin and lung. An angiocentric T-cell-rich B-cell lymphoproliferative disorder. Arch Dermatol. 132(12):1464–70. PMID:8961876
**1724.** McNiff JM, Eisen RN, Glusac EJ (1999). Immunohistochemical comparison of cutaneous lymphadenoma, trichoblastoma, and basal cell carcinoma: support for classification of lymphadenoma as a variant of trichoblastoma. J Cutan Pathol. 26(3):119–24. PMID:10235376
**1725.** McNiff JM, Subtil A, Cowper SE, Lazova R, Glusac EJ (2005). Cellular digital fibromas: distinctive CD34-positive lesions that may mimic dermatofibrosarcoma protuberans. J Cutan Pathol. 32(6):413–8. PMID:15953374
**1726.** McWhorter HE, Woolner LB (1954). Pigmented nevi, juvenile melanomas and malignant melanomas in children. Cancer. 7(3):564–85. PMID:13160941
**1727.** Meara JG, Shah S, Li KK, Cunningham MJ (1998). The odontogenic keratocyst: a 20-year clinicopathologic review. Laryngoscope. 108(2):280–3. PMID:9473082
**1728.** Meberg R, Kenyon E, Bierman R, Loveland L, Barbosa P (1998). Characterization of plantar verrucae among individuals with human immunodeficiency virus. J Am Podiatr Med Assoc. 88(9):442–5. PMID:9770936
**1729.** Megahed M (1994). Histopathological variants of neurofibroma. A study of 114 lesions. Am J Dermatopathol. 16(5):486–95. PMID:7528474
**1730.** Mehregan AH (1984). Infundibular tumors of the skin. J Cutan Pathol. 11(5):387–95. PMID:6392372
**1731.** Mehregan AH, Brownstein MH (1978). Pilar sheath acanthoma. Arch Dermatol. 114(10):1495–7. PMID:718186
**1732.** Mehregan AH, Tavafoghi V, Ghandchi A (1975). Nevus lipomatosus cutaneus superficialis (Hoffmann-Zurhelle). J Cutan Pathol. 2(6):307–13. PMID:1219048
**1733.** Mehregan DA, Mehregan AH (1993). Deep penetrating nevus. Arch Dermatol. 129(3):328–31. PMID:8447669
**1734.** Mehregan DR, Hamzavi F, Brown K (2003). Large cell acanthoma. Int J Dermatol. 42(1):36–9. PMID:12581141
**1735.** Meis-Kindblom JM, Kindblom LG (1998). Acral myxoinflammatory fibroblastic sarcoma: a low-grade tumor of the hands and feet. Am J Surg Pathol. 22(8):911–24. PMID:9706971
**1736.** Melton JL, Rasmussen JE (1991). Clinical manifestations of human papillomavirus infection in nongenital sites. Dermatol Clin. 9(2):219–33. PMID:1647902
**1737.** Menezes J, Acquadro F, Wiseman M, Gómez-López G, Salgado RN, Talavera-Casañas JG, et al. (2014). Exome sequencing reveals novel and recurrent mutations with clinical impact in blastic plasmacytoid dendritic cell neoplasm. Leukemia. 28(4):823–9. PMID:24072100
**1738.** Menguy S, Gros A, Pham-Ledard A, Battistella M, Ortonne N, Comoz F, et al. (2016). MYD88 somatic mutation is a diagnostic criterion in primary cutaneous large B-cell lymphoma. J Invest Dermatol. 136(8):1741–4. PMID:27189828
**1739.** Menon K, Dusza SW, Marghoob AA, Halpern AC, Nehal KS (2006). Classification and prevalence of pigmented lesions in patients with total-body photographs at high risk of developing melanoma. J Cutan Med Surg. 10(2):85–91. PMID:17241580
**1740.** Mentzel T (2001). Cutaneous lipomatous neoplasms. Semin Diagn Pathol. 18(4):250–7. PMID:11757864
**1741.** Mentzel T, Beham A, Calonje E, Katenkamp D, Fletcher CD (1997). Epithelioid hemangioendothelioma of skin and soft tissues: clinicopathologic and immunohistochemical study of 30 cases. Am J Surg Pathol. 21(4):363–74. PMID:9130982
**1742.** Mentzel T, Beham A, Katenkamp D, Dei Tos AP, Fletcher CD (1998). Fibrosarcomatous ("high-grade") dermatofibrosarcoma protuberans: clinicopathologic and immunohistochemical study of a series of 41 cases with emphasis on prognostic significance. Am J Surg Pathol. 22(5):576–87. PMID:9591728
**1743.** Mentzel T, Calonje E, Nascimento AG, Fletcher CD (1994). Infantile hemangiopericytoma versus infantile myofibromatosis. Study of a series suggesting a continuous spectrum of infantile myofibroblastic lesions. Am J Surg Pathol. 18(9):922–30. PMID:8067513
**1744.** Mentzel T, Calonje E, Wadden C, Camplejohn RS, Beham A, Smith MA, et al. (1996). Myxofibrosarcoma. Clinicopathologic analysis of 75 cases with emphasis on the low-grade variant. Am J Surg Pathol. 20(4):391–405. PMID:8604805
**1745.** Mentzel T, Dei Tos AP, Sapi Z, Kutzner H (2006). Myopericytoma of skin and soft tissues: clinicopathologic and immunohistochemical study of 54 cases. Am J Surg Pathol. 30(1):104–13. PMID:16330949
**1746.** Mentzel T, Kutzner H (2005). Reticular and plexiform perineurioma: clinicopathological and immunohistochemical analysis of two cases and review of perineurial neoplasms of skin and soft tissues. Virchows Arch. 447(4):677–82. PMID:16133356
**1747.** Mentzel T, Kutzner H (2009). Dermatomyofibroma: clinicopathologic and immunohistochemical analysis of 56 cases and reappraisal of a rare and distinct cutaneous neoplasm. Am J Dermatopathol. 31(1):44–9. PMID:19155724
**1748.** Mentzel T, Kutzner H, Rütten A, Hügel H (2001). Benign fibrous histiocytoma (dermatofibroma) of the face: clinicopathologic and immunohistochemical study of 34 cases associated with an aggressive clinical course. Am J Dermatopathol. 23(5):419–26. PMID:11801774
**1749.** Mentzel T, Partanen TA, Kutzner H (1999). Hobnail hemangioma ("targetoid hemosiderotic hemangioma"): clinicopathologic and immunohistochemical analysis of 62 cases. J Cutan Pathol. 26(6):279–86. PMID:10472756
**1750.** Mentzel T, Requena L, Kaddu S, Soares de Aleida LM, Sangueza OP, Kutzner H (2003). Cutaneous myoepithelial neoplasms: clinicopathologic and immunohistochemical study of 20 cases suggesting a continuous spectrum ranging from benign mixed tumor of the skin to cutaneous myoepithelioma and myoepithelial carcinoma. J Cutan Pathol. 30(5):294–302. PMID:12753168
**1751.** Mentzel T, Schärer L, Kazakov DV, Michal M (2007). Myxoid dermatofibrosarcoma protuberans: clinicopathologic, immunohistochemical, and molecular analysis of eight cases. Am J Dermatopathol. 29(5):443–8. PMID:17890911
**1752.** Mentzel T, Schildhaus HU, Palmedo G, Büttner R, Kutzner H (2012). Postradiation cutaneous angiosarcoma after treatment of breast carcinoma is characterized by MYC amplification in contrast to atypical vascular lesions after radiotherapy and control cases: clinicopathological, immunohistochemical and molecular analysis of 66 cases. Mod Pathol. 25(1):75–85. PMID:21909081
**1753.** Mentzel T, Wiesner T, Cerroni L, Hantschke M, Kutzner H, Rütten A, et al. (2013). Malignant dermatofibroma: clinicopathological, immunohistochemical, and molecular analysis of seven cases. Mod Pathol. 26(2):256–67. PMID:22996372
**1754.** Merkel EA, Martini MC, Amin SM, Lee CY, Gerami P (2016). Evaluation of dermoscopic features for distinguishing melanoma from special site nevi of the breast. J Am Acad Dermatol. 75(2):364–70. PMID:27313053
**1755.** Mertens F, Dal Cin P, De Wever I, Fletcher CD, Mandahl N, Mitelman F, et al. (2000). Cytogenetic characterization of peripheral nerve sheath tumours: a report of the CHAMP study group. J Pathol. 190(1):31–8. PMID:10640989
**1756.** Mertens F, Fletcher CD, Dal Cin P, De Wever I, Mandahl N, Mitelman F, et al. (1998). Cytogenetic analysis of 46 pleomorphic soft tissue sarcomas and correlation with morphologic and clinical features: a report of the CHAMP Study Group. Chromosomes and MorPhology. Genes Chromosomes Cancer. 22(1):16–25. PMID:9591630
**1757.** Mesbah Ardakani N, O'Brien G, Wood B (2016). Symplastic pilar leiomyoma: description of a rare entity. Am J Dermatopathol. 38(10):787–9. PMID:26981742
**1758.** Metcalf JS, Maize JC (1999). Clark's nevus. Semin Cutan Med Surg. 18(1):43–6. PMID:10188841
**1759.** Metcalf JS, Maize JC, LeBoit PE (1991). Circumscribed storiform collagenoma (sclerosing fibroma). Am J Dermatopathol. 13(2):122–9. PMID:2029087
**1760.** Metzler G, Schaumburg-Lever G, Hornstein O, Rassner G (1996). Malignant chondroid syringoma: immunohistopathology. Am J Dermatopathol. 18(1):83–9. PMID:8721597
**1761.** Meyerson LB (1971). A peculiar papulosquamous eruption involving pigmented nevi. Arch Dermatol. 103(5):510–2. PMID:5580293
**1763.** Michal M (1998). Inflammatory myxoid tumor of the soft parts with bizarre giant cells. Pathol Res Pract. 194(8):529–33. PMID:9779486
**1764.** Michal M, Bisceglia M, Di Mattia A, Requena L, Fanburg-Smith JC, Mukensnabl P, et al. (2002). Gigantic cutaneous horns of the scalp: lesions with a gross similarity to the horns of animals: a report of four cases. Am J Surg Pathol. 26(6):789–94. PMID:12023585
**1765.** Michal M, Fetsch JF, Hes O, Miettinen M (1999). Nuchal-type fibroma: a clinicopathologic study of 52 cases. Cancer. 85(1):156–63. PMID:9921988
**1766.** Michal M, Kazakov DV, Hadravsky L, Michalova K, Grossmann P, Steiner P, et al. (2017). Lipoblasts in spindle cell and pleomorphic lipomas: a close scrutiny. Hum Pathol. 65:140–6. PMID:28546131

**1767.** Michal M, Michal M, Miesbauerova M, Hercogova J, Skopalikova B, Kazakov DV (2016). Penile analogue of stratified mucin-producing intraepithelial lesion of the cervix: the first described case. a diagnostic pitfall. Am J Dermatopathol. 38(5):e64–7. PMID:27097242
**1768.** Michal M, Miettinen M (1999). Myoepitheliomas of the skin and soft tissues. Report of 12 cases. Virchows Arch. 434(5):393–400. PMID:10389622
**1769.** Michaloglou C, Vredeveld LC, Mooi WJ, Peeper DS (2008). BRAF(E600) in benign and malignant human tumours. Oncogene. 27(7):877–95. PMID:17724477
**1770.** Middel P, Hemmerlein B, Fayyazi A, Kaboth U, Radzun HJ (1999). Sinus histiocytosis with massive lymphadenopathy: evidence for its relationship to macrophages and for a cytokine-related disorder. Histopathology. 35(6):525–33. PMID:10583576
**1771.** Miettinen M, Fanburg-Smith JC, Virolainen M, Shmookler BM, Fetsch JF (1999). Epithelioid sarcoma: an immunohistochemical analysis of 112 classical and variant cases and a discussion of the differential diagnosis. Hum Pathol. 30(8):934–42. PMID:10452506
**1772.** Miettinen M, Fetsch JF (1998). Collagenous fibroma (desmoplastic fibroblastoma): a clinicopathologic analysis of 63 cases of a distinctive soft tissue lesion with stellate-shaped fibroblasts. Hum Pathol. 29(7):676–82. PMID:9670823
**1773.** Miettinen M, Fetsch JF (2006). Reticulohistiocytoma (solitary epithelioid histiocytoma): a clinicopathologic and immunohistochemical study of 44 cases. Am J Surg Pathol. 30(4):521–8. PMID:16625100
**1774.** Miettinen M, Wang Z, Sarlomo-Rikala M, Abdullaev Z, Pack SD, Fetsch JF (2013). ERG expression in epithelioid sarcoma: a diagnostic pitfall. Am J Surg Pathol. 37(10):1580–5. PMID:23774169
**1775.** Miettinen M, Wang ZF (2012). Prox1 transcription factor as a marker for vascular tumors-evaluation of 314 vascular endothelial and 1086 nonvascular tumors. Am J Surg Pathol. 36(3):351–9. PMID:22067331
**1776.** Mihic-Probst D, Zhao J, Saremaslani P, Baer A, Oehlschlegel C, Paredes B, et al. (2004). CGH analysis shows genetic similarities and differences in atypical fibroxanthoma and undifferentiated high grade pleomorphic sarcoma. Anticancer Res. 24(1):19–26. PMID:15015571
**1777.** Mihm MC Jr, Lopansri S (1979). A review of the classification of malignant melanoma. J Dermatol. 6(3):131–42. PMID:393742
**1778.** Miller K, Goodlad JR, Brenn T (2012). Pleomorphic dermal sarcoma: adverse histologic features predict aggressive behavior and allow distinction from atypical fibroxanthoma. Am J Surg Pathol. 36(9):1317–26. PMID:22510760
**1779.** Miller SJ, Alam M, Andersen J, Berg D, Bichakjian CK, Bowen G, et al. (2010). Basal cell and squamous cell skin cancers. J Natl Compr Canc Netw. 8(8):836–64. PMID:20870631
**1780.** Millot F, Robert A, Bertrand Y, Mechinaud F, Laureys G, Ferster A, et al. (1997). Cutaneous involvement in children with acute lymphoblastic leukemia or lymphoblastic lymphoma. Pediatrics. 100(1):60–4. PMID:9200360
**1781.** Mills JA, Gonzalez RG, Jaffe R (2008). Case records of the Massachusetts General Hospital. Case 25-2008. A 43-year-old man with fatigue and lesions in the pituitary and cerebellum. N Engl J Med. 359(7):736–47. PMID:18703477
**1782.** Milne P, Bigley V, Bacon CM, Néel A, McGovern N, Bomken S, et al. (2017). Hematopoietic origin of Langerhans cell histiocytosis and Erdheim-Chester disease in adults. Blood. 130(2):167–75. PMID:28512190
**1783.** Minagawa A, Koga H, Uhara H, Yokokawa Y, Okuyama R (2013). Age-related prevalence of dermoscopic patterns in acquired melanocytic nevus on acral volar skin. JAMA Dermatol. 149(8):989–90. PMID:23804247
**1784.** Minagawa A, Omodaka T, Okuyama R (2016). Melanomas and mechanical stress points on the plantar surface of the foot. N Engl J Med. 374(24):2404–6. PMID:27305207
**1785.** Minkov M, Grois N, Heitger A, Pötschger U, Westermeier T, Gadner H (2002). Response to initial treatment of multisystem Langerhans cell histiocytosis: an important prognostic indicator. Med Pediatr Oncol. 39(6):581–5. PMID:12376981
**1786.** Mir R, Cortes E, Papantoniou PA, Heller K, Muehlhausen V, Kahn LB (1986). Metastatic trichomatricial carcinoma. Arch Pathol Lab Med. 110(7):660–3. PMID:3755030
**1787.** Miracco C, Raffaelli M, de Santi MM, Fimiani M, Tosi P (1988). Solitary cutaneous reticulum cell tumor. Enzyme-immunohistochemical and electron-microscopic analogies with IDRC sarcoma. Am J Dermatopathol. 10(1):47–53. PMID:2845833
**1788.** Mirza B, Weedon D (2005). Atypical fibroxanthoma: a clinicopathological study of 89 cases. Australas J Dermatol. 46(4):235–8. PMID:16197421
**1789.** Mirza I, Macpherson N, Paproski S, Gascoyne RD, Yang B, Finn WG, et al. (2002). Primary cutaneous follicular lymphoma: an assessment of clinical, histopathologic, immunophenotypic, and molecular features. J Clin Oncol. 20(3):647–55. PMID:11821444
**1790.** Misago N, Ansai SI, Fukumoto T, Anan T, Kimura T, Nakao T (2017). Chronological changes in trichofolliculoma: folliculosebaceous cystic hamartoma is not a very-late-stage trichofolliculoma. J Dermatol. 44(9):1050–4. PMID:28370423
**1791.** Misago N, Inoue T, Koba S, Narisawa Y (2013). Keratoacanthoma and other types of squamous cell carcinoma with crateriform architecture: classification and identification. J Dermatol. 40(6):443–52. PMID:23414327
**1792.** Misago N, Kimura T, Narisawa Y (2009). Fibrofolliculoma/trichodiscoma and fibrous papule (perifollicular fibroma/angiofibroma): a revaluation of the histopathological and immunohistochemical features. J Cutan Pathol. 36(9):943–51. PMID:19674199
**1793.** Misago N, Mihara I, Ansai S, Narisawa Y (2002). Sebaceoma and related neoplasms with sebaceous differentiation: a clinicopathologic study of 30 cases. Am J Dermatopathol. 24(4):294–304. PMID:12142607
**1794.** Misago N, Narisawa Y (2000). Sebaceous neoplasms in Muir-Torre syndrome. Am J Dermatopathol. 22(2):155–61. PMID:10770437
**1795.** Misago N, Satoh T, Narisawa Y (2004). Basal cell carcinoma with ductal and glandular differentiation: a clinicopathological and immunohistochemical study of 10 cases. Eur J Dermatol. 14(6):383–7. PMID:15564201
**1796.** Misago N, Suse T, Uemura T, Narisawa Y (2004). Basal cell carcinoma with sebaceous differentiation. Am J Dermatopathol. 26(4):298–303. PMID:15249860
**1797.** Misago N, Toda S (2016). Sebaceous carcinoma within rippled/carcinoid pattern sebaceoma. J Cutan Pathol. 43(1):64–70. PMID:26268140
**1798.** Mishima Y, Mevorah B (1961). Nevus Ota and nevus Ito in American Negroes. J Invest Dermatol. 36(2):133–54. PMID:13771275
**1799.** Mishima Y, Pinkus H (1960). Benign mixed tumor of melanocytes and malpighian cells. Melanoacanthoma: its relationship to Bloch's benign non-nevoid melanoepithelioma. Arch Dermatol. 81(4):539–50. PMID:14422903
**1800.** Missero C (2016). The genetic evolution of skin squamous cell carcinoma: tumor suppressor identity matters. Exp Dermatol. 25(11):863–4. PMID:27193637
**1801.** Amitay-Laish I, Feinmesser M, Ben-Amitai D, Fenig E, Sorin D, Hodak E (2016). Unilesional folliculotropic mycosis fungoides: a unique variant of cutaneous lymphoma. J Eur Acad Dermatol Venereol. 30(1):25–9. PMID:25405551
**1802.** Amitay-Laish I, Tavallaee M, Kim J, Hoppe RT, Million L, Feinmesser M, et al. (2017). Paediatric primary cutaneous marginal zone B-cell lymphoma: does it differ from its adult counterpart? Br J Dermatol. 176(4):1010–20. PMID:27501236
**1803.** Mitsui H, Kiecker F, Shemer A, Cannizzaro MV, Wang CQF, Gulati N, et al. (2016). Discrimination of dysplastic nevi from common melanocytic nevi by cellular and molecular criteria. J Invest Dermatol. 136(10):2030–40. PMID:27377700
**1804.** Miura T, Yamamoto T (2013). Perforating pilomatricoma with anetodermic epidermis in an adolescent with lymphoma. Pediatr Dermatol. 30(4):e68–9. PMID:22937738
**1805.** Miyake T, Yamamoto T, Hirai Y, Otsuka M, Hamada T, Tsuji K, et al. (2015). Survival rates and prognostic factors of Epstein-Barr virus-associated hydroa vacciniforme and hypersensitivity to mosquito bites. Br J Dermatol. 172(1):56–63. PMID:25234411
**1806.** Miyamoto T, Hagari Y, Inoue S, Watanabe T, Yoshino T (2005). Axillary apocrine carcinoma with benign apocrine tumours: a case report involving a pathological and immunohistochemical study and review of the literature. J Clin Pathol. 58(7):757–61. PMID:15976347
**1807.** Miyamoto Y, Ueda K, Sato M, Yasuno H (1979). Disseminated epidermolytic acanthoma. J Cutan Pathol. 6(4):272–9. PMID:500873
**1808.** Miyazaki A, Saida T, Koga H, Oguchi S, Suzuki T, Tsuchida T (2005). Anatomical and histopathological correlates of the dermoscopic patterns seen in melanocytic nevi on the sole: a retrospective study. J Am Acad Dermatol. 53(2):230–6. PMID:16021115
**1809.** Modena P, Lualdi E, Facchinetti F, Galli L, Teixeira MR, Pilotti S, et al. (2005). SMARCB1/INI1 tumor suppressor gene is frequently inactivated in epithelioid sarcomas. Cancer Res. 65(10):4012–9. PMID:15899790
**1810.** Mohamed A, Gonzalez RS, Lawson D, Wang J, Cohen C (2013). SOX10 expression in malignant melanoma, carcinoma, and normal tissues. Appl Immunohistochem Mol Morphol. 21(6):506–10. PMID:23197006
**1811.** Mojtahed A, Schrijver I, Ford JM, Longacre TA, Pai RK (2011). A two-antibody mismatch repair protein immunohistochemistry screening approach for colorectal carcinomas, skin sebaceous tumors, and gynecologic tract carcinomas. Mod Pathol. 24(7):1004–14. PMID:21499234
**1812.** Molho-Pessach V, Ramot Y, Camille F, Doviner V, Babay S, Luis SJ, et al. (2014). H syndrome: the first 79 patients. J Am Acad Dermatol. 70(1):80–8. PMID:24172204
**1813.** Molina-Ruiz AM, Busam KJ (2016). Primary cutaneous Ewing sarcoma with EWSR1-ERG fusion. J Cutan Pathol. 43(9):729–34. PMID:27526022
**1814.** Molina-Ruiz AM, Llamas-Velasco M, Rütten A, Cerroni L, Requena L (2016). "Apocrine hidrocystoma and cystadenoma"-like tumor of the digits or toes: a potential diagnostic pitfall of digital papillary adenocarcinoma. Am J Surg Pathol. 40(3):410–8. PMID:26523544
**1815.** Moloney FJ, Comber H, O'Lorcain P, O'Kelly P, Conlon PJ, Murphy GM (2006). A population-based study of skin cancer incidence and prevalence in renal transplant recipients. Br J Dermatol. 154(3):498–504. PMID:16445782
**1816.** Montero J, Stephansky J, Cai T, Griffin GK, Cabal-Hierro L, Togami K, et al. (2017). Blastic plasmacytoid dendritic cell neoplasm is dependent on BCL2 and sensitive to venetoclax. Cancer Discov. 7(2):156–64. PMID:27986708
**1817.** Montes-Moreno S, Ramos-Medina R, Martínez-López A, Barrionuevo Cornejo C, Parra Cubillos A, Quintana-Truyenque S, et al. (2013). SPIB, a novel immunohistochemical marker for human blastic plasmacytoid dendritic cell neoplasms: characterization of its expression in major hematolymphoid neoplasms. Blood. 121(4):643–7. PMID:23165482
**1818.** Montgomery E, Epstein JI (2009). Anastomosing hemangioma of the genitourinary tract: a lesion mimicking angiosarcoma. Am J Surg Pathol. 33(9):1364–9. PMID:19606014
**1819.** Montgomery E, Lee JH, Abraham SC, Wu TT (2001). Superficial fibromatoses are genetically distinct from deep fibromatoses. Mod Pathol. 14(7):695–701. PMID:11455002
**1820.** Montgomery EA, Devaney KO, Giordano TJ, Weiss SW (1998). Inflammatory myxohyaline tumor of distal extremities with virocyte or Reed-Sternberg-like cells: a distinctive lesion with features simulating inflammatory conditions, Hodgkin's disease, and various sarcomas. Mod Pathol. 11(4):384–91. PMID:9578090
**1821.** Moody BR, Bartlett NL, George DW, Price CR, Breer WA, Rothschild Y, et al. (2001). Cyclin D1 as an aid in the diagnosis of mantle cell lymphoma in skin biopsies: a case report. Am J Dermatopathol. 23(5):470–6. PMID:11801782
**1822.** Mooney MA, Barr RJ, Buxton MG (1995). Halo nevus or halo phenomenon? A study of 142 cases. J Cutan Pathol. 22(4):342–8. PMID:7499574
**1823.** Moore AR, Ceraudo E, Sher JJ, Guan Y, Shoushtari AN, Chang MT, et al. (2016). Recurrent activating mutations of G-protein-coupled receptor CYSLTR2 in uveal melanoma. Nat Genet. 48(6):675–80. PMID:27089179
**1824.** Moosavi C, Jha P, Fanburg-Smith JC (2007). An update on plexiform fibrohistiocytic tumor and addition of 66 new cases from the Armed Forces Institute of Pathology, in honor of Franz M. Enzinger, MD. Ann Diagn Pathol. 11(5):313–9. PMID:17870015
**1825.** Morales AV, Arber DA, Seo K, Kohler S, Kim YH, Sundram UN (2008). Evaluation of B-cell clonality using the BIOMED-2 PCR method effectively distinguishes cutaneous B-cell lymphoma from benign lymphoid infiltrates. Am J Dermatopathol. 30(5):425–30. PMID:18806482
**1826.** Morandi L, Pession A, Marucci GL, Foschini MP, Pruneri G, Viale G, et al. (2003). Intraepidermal cells of Paget's carcinoma of the breast can be genetically different from those of the underlying carcinoma. Hum Pathol. 34(12):1321–30. PMID:14691919
**1827.** Mordehai J, Kurzbart E, Shinhar D, Sagi A, Finaly R, Mares AJ (1998). Lymphangioma circumscriptum. Pediatr Surg Int. 13(2–3):208–10. PMID:9563054
**1828.** Moreno C, Jacyk WK, Judd MJ, Requena L (2001). Highly aggressive extraocular sebaceous carcinoma. Am J Dermatopathol. 23(5):450–5. PMID:11801779
**1829.** Moreno C, Requena L, Kutzner H, de la Cruz A, Jaqueti G, Yus ES (2000). Epithelioid blue nevus: a rare variant of blue nevus not always associated with the Carney complex. J Cutan Pathol. 27(5):218–23. PMID:10847545
**1830.** Morgado JM, Perbellini O, Johnson RC, Teodósio C, Matito A, Álvarez-Twose I, et al. (2013). CD30 expression by bone marrow mast

cells from different diagnostic variants of systemic mastocytosis. Histopathology. 63(6):780–7. PMID:24111625
**1831.** Morgan MB, Stevens GL, Switlyk S (2005). Benign lichenoid keratosis: a clinical and pathologic reappraisal of 1040 cases. Am J Dermatopathol. 27(5):387–92. PMID:16148406
**1832.** Morgan NV, Morris MR, Cangul H, Gleeson D, Straatman-Iwanowska A, Davies N, et al. (2010). Mutations in SLC29A3, encoding an equilibrative nucleoside transporter ENT3, cause a familial histiocytosis syndrome (Faisalabad histiocytosis) and familial Rosai-Dorfman disease. PLoS Genet. 6(2):e1000833. PMID:20140240
**1833.** Mortier L, Marchetti P, Delaporte E, Martin de Lassalle E, Thomas P, Piette F, et al. (2002). Progression of actinic keratosis to squamous cell carcinoma of the skin correlates with deletion of the 9p21 region encoding the p16(INK4a) tumor suppressor. Cancer Lett. 176(2):205–14. PMID:11804749
**1834.** Moshari A, McLean IW (2001). Uveal melanoma: mean of the longest nucleoli measured on silver-stained sections. Invest Ophthalmol Vis Sci. 42(6):1160–3. PMID:11328722
**1835.** Mosquera JM, Sboner A, Zhang L, Chen CL, Sung YS, Chen HW, et al. (2013). Novel MIR143-NOTCH fusions in benign and malignant glomus tumors. Genes Chromosomes Cancer. 52(11):1075–87. PMID:23999936
**1836.** Moulis G, Sailler L, Bonneville F, Wagner T (2014). Imaging in Erdheim-Chester disease: classic features and new insights. Clin Exp Rheumatol. 32(3):410–4. PMID:24428974
**1837.** Mowbray M, Schofield OM (2007). Juvenile xanthogranuloma en plaque. Pediatr Dermatol. 24(6):670–1. PMID:18036001
**1838.** Moxley KM, Fader AN, Rose PG, Case AS, Mutch DG, Berry E, et al. (2011). Malignant melanoma of the vulva: an extension of cutaneous melanoma? Gynecol Oncol. 122(3):612–7. PMID:21570710
**1839.** Mravic M, LaChaud G, Nguyen A, Scott MA, Dry SM, James AW (2015). Clinical and histopathological diagnosis of glomus tumor: an institutional experience of 138 cases. Int J Surg Pathol. 23(3):181–8. PMID:25614464
**1840.** Mraz-Gernhard S, Natkunam Y, Hoppe RT, LeBoit P, Kohler S, Kim YH (2001). Natural killer/natural killer-like T-cell lymphoma, CD56+, presenting in the skin: an increasingly recognized entity with an aggressive course. J Clin Oncol. 19(8):2179–88. PMID:11304770
**1841.** Mukherjee S, Bandyopadhyay G, Saha S, Choudhuri M (2010). Cytodiagnosis of glomus tumor. J Cytol. 27(3):104–5. PMID:21187877
**1842.** Mukhopadhyay AK (2004). Nevus of Ota associated with nevus of Ito. Indian J Dermatol Venereol Leprol. 70(2):112–3. PMID:17642580
**1843.** Mukhopadhyay AK (2013). Unilateral nevus of Ota with bilateral nevus of Ito and palatal lesion: a case report with a proposed clinical modification of Tanino's classification. Indian J Dermatol. 58(4):286–9. PMID:23918999
**1844.** Müller R, Theissig F (1995). Syringocystadenoma papilliferum of the outer ear canal. Laryngorhinootologie. 74(1):43–5. [German] PMID:7888022
**1845.** Mulliken JB, Enjolras O (2004). Congenital hemangiomas and infantile hemangioma: missing links. J Am Acad Dermatol. 50(6):875–82. PMID:15153887
**1846.** Munden A, Butschek R, Tom WL, Marshall JS, Poeltler DM, Krohne SE, et al. (2014). Prospective study of infantile haemangiomas: incidence, clinical characteristics and association with placental anomalies. Br J Dermatol. 170(4):907–13. PMID:24641194
**1847.** Murali R, McCarthy SW, Scolyer RA (2009). Blue nevi and related lesions: a review highlighting atypical and newly described variants, distinguishing features and diagnostic pitfalls. Adv Anat Pathol. 16(6):365–82. PMID:19851128
**1848.** Murali R, Shaw HM, Lai K, McCarthy SW, Quinn MJ, Stretch JR, et al. (2010). Prognostic factors in cutaneous desmoplastic melanoma: a study of 252 patients. Cancer. 116(17):4130–8. PMID:20564101
**1849.** Murali R, Wiesner T, Rosenblum MK, Bastian BC (2012). GNAQ and GNA11 mutations in melanocytomas of the central nervous system. Acta Neuropathol. 123(3):457–9. PMID:22307269
**1850.** Murali R, Wiesner T, Scolyer RA (2013). Tumours associated with BAP1 mutations. Pathology. 45(2):116–26. PMID:23277170
**1851.** Murali R, Zannino D, Synnott M, McCarthy SW, Thompson JF, Scolyer RA (2011). Clinical and pathological features of metastases of primary cutaneous desmoplastic melanoma. Histopathology. 58(6):886–95. PMID:21438911
**1852.** Murase T, Yamaguchi M, Suzuki R, Okamoto M, Sato Y, Tamaru J, et al. (2007). Intravascular large B-cell lymphoma (IVLBCL): a clinicopathologic study of 96 cases with special reference to the immunophenotypic heterogeneity of CD5. Blood. 109(2):478–85. PMID:16985183
**1853.** Murphy CM, Grau-Massanés M, Sánchez RL (1995). Multiple cutaneous myxomas. Report of a case without other elements of Carney's complex. J Cutan Pathol. 22(6):556–62. PMID:8835175
**1854.** Murphy M, Brierley T, Pennoyer J, Rozenski D, Grant-Kels JM (2007). Lymphotropic adamantinoid trichoblastoma. Pediatr Dermatol. 24(2):157–61. PMID:17461815
**1855.** Musette P, Bachelez H, Flageul B, Delarbre C, Kourilsky P, Dubertret L, et al. (1999). Immune-mediated destruction of melanocytes in halo nevi is associated with the local expansion of a limited number of T cell clones. J Immunol. 162(3):1789–94. PMID:9973443
**1856.** Mutasim DF (2007). Psoriasiform keratosis: a lesion mimicking psoriasis. Am J Dermatopathol. 29(5):482–4. PMID:17890921
**1857.** Mutgi KA, Chitgopeker P, Ciliberto H, Stone MS (2016). Hypocellular plaque-like CD34-positive dermal fibroma (medallion-like dermal dendrocyte hamartoma) presenting as a skin-colored dermal nodule. Pediatr Dermatol. 33(1):e16–9. PMID:26645569
**1858.** Mutter RW, Singer S, Zhang Z, Brennan MF, Alektiar KM (2012). The enigma of myxofibrosarcoma of the extremity. Cancer. 118(2):518–27. PMID:21717447
**1859.** Myhre-Jensen O (1981). A consecutive 7-year series of 1331 benign soft tissue tumours. Clinicopathologic data. Comparison with sarcomas. Acta Orthop Scand. 52(3):287–93. PMID:7282321
**1860.** Na JI, Park KC, Youn SW (2006). Familial eruptive lentiginosis. J Am Acad Dermatol. 55(2 Suppl):S38–40. PMID:16843122
**1861.** Nagai K, Nakano N, Iwai T, Iwai A, Tauchi H, Ohshima K, et al. (2014). Pediatric subcutaneous panniculitis-like T-cell lymphoma with favorable result by immunosuppressive therapy: a report of two cases. Pediatr Hematol Oncol. 31(6):528–33. PMID:24684413
**1862.** Nagamine N, Nohara Y, Ito E (1982). Elastofibroma in Okinawa. A clinicopathologic study of 170 cases. Cancer. 50(9):1794–805. PMID:7116305
**1863.** Nagarajan P, Curry JL, Ning J, Piao J, Torres-Cabala CA, Aung PP, et al. (2017). Tumor thickness and mitotic rate robustly predict melanoma-specific survival in patients with primary vulvar melanoma: a retrospective review of 100 cases. Clin Cancer Res. 23(8):2093–104. PMID:27864417
**1864.** Nagata H, Worobec AS, Oh CK, Chowdhury BA, Tannenbaum S, Suzuki Y, et al. (1995). Identification of a point mutation in the catalytic domain of the protooncogene c-kit in peripheral blood mononuclear cells of patients who have mastocytosis with an associated hematologic disorder. Proc Natl Acad Sci U S A. 92(23):10560–4. PMID:7479840
**1865.** Nagatsuka H, Rivera RS, Gunduz M, Siar CH, Tamamura R, Mizukawa N, et al. (2006). Microcystic adnexal carcinoma with mandibular bone marrow involvement: a case report with immunohistochemistry. Am J Dermatopathol. 28(6):518–22. PMID:17122497
**1866.** Nagore E, Sánchez-Motilla JM, Pérez-Vallés A, Martínez-Lahuerta C, Alegre V, Aliaga A (2000). Pseudovascular squamous cell carcinoma of the skin. Clin Exp Dermatol. 25(3):206–8. PMID:10844496
**1867.** Nakagawa M, Schmitz R, Xiao W, Goldman CK, Xu W, Yang Y, et al. (2014). Gain-of-function CCR4 mutations in adult T cell leukemia/lymphoma. J Exp Med. 211(13):2497–505. PMID:25488980
**1868.** Nakajima K, Kaneko T, Aizu T, Nakano H, Matsuzaki Y, Sawamura D (2013). Signet-ring cutaneous squamous cell carcinoma arising on the back of the finger. Case Rep Dermatol. 5(2):215–8. PMID:24019773
**1869.** Nakamura M, Fukunaga-Kalabis M, Yamaguchi Y, Furuhashi T, Nishida E, Kato H, et al. (2015). Site-specific migration of human fetal melanocytes in volar skin. J Dermatol Sci. 78(2):143–8. PMID:25818865
**1870.** Nakashima K, Yamada N, Yoshida Y, Yamamoto O (2008). Solitary sclerotic neurofibroma of the skin. Am J Dermatopathol. 30(3):278–80. PMID:18496433
**1871.** Namiki T, Miura K, Ueno M, Arima Y, Nishizawa A, Yokozeki H (2016). Four different tumors arising in a nevus sebaceous. Case Rep Dermatol. 8(1):75–9. PMID:27194974
**1872.** Namiki T, Takahashi M, Nojima K, Ueno M, Hanafusa T, Tokoro S, et al. (2017). Phakomatosis pigmentovascularis type IIb: a case with Klippel-Trenáunay syndrome and extensive dermal melanocytosis as nevus of Ota, nevus of Ito and ectopic Mongolian spots. J Dermatol. 44(3):e32–3. PMID:27374914
**1873.** Napekoski KM, Fernandez AP, Billings SD (2014). Microvenular hemangioma: a clinicopathologic review of 13 cases. J Cutan Pathol. 41(11):816–22. PMID:25263662
**1874.** Nappi O, Pettinato G, Wick MR (1989). Adenoid (acantholytic) squamous cell carcinoma of the skin. J Cutan Pathol. 16(3):114–21. PMID:2768593
**1875.** Nappi O, Wick MR (1986). Disseminated lobular capillary hemangioma (pyogenic granuloma). A clinicopathologic study of two cases. Am J Dermatopathol. 8(5):379–85. PMID:3777375
**1876.** Narducci MG, Scala E, Bresin A, Caprini E, Picchio MC, Remotti D, et al. (2006). Skin homing of Sézary cells involves SDF-1-CXCR4 signaling and down-regulation of CD26/dipeptidylpeptidase IV. Blood. 107(3):1108–15. PMID:16204308
**1877.** Nascimento AF, Bertoni F, Fletcher CD (2007). Epithelioid variant of myxofibrosarcoma: expanding the clinicomorphologic spectrum of myxofibrosarcoma in a series of 17 cases. Am J Surg Pathol. 31(1):99–105. PMID:17197925
**1878.** Nash JW, Barrett TL, Kies M, Ross MI, Sneige N, Diwan AH, et al. (2007). Metastatic hidradenocarcinoma with demonstration of Her-2/neu gene amplification by fluorescence in situ hybridization: potential treatment implications. J Cutan Pathol. 34(1):49–54. PMID:17214855
**1879.** Nashan D, Müller ML, Braun-Falco M, Reichenberger S, Szeimies RM, Bruckner-Tuderman L (2009). Cutaneous metastases of visceral tumours: a review. J Cancer Res Clin Oncol. 135(1):1–14. PMID:18560891
**1880.** Nasser H, Danforth RD Jr, Sunbuli M, Dimitrijevic O (2010). Malignant granular cell tumor: case report with a novel karyotype and review of the literature. Ann Diagn Pathol. 14(4):273–8. PMID:20637434
**1881.** Nasseri E, Piram M, McCuaig CC, Kokta V, Dubois J, Powell J (2014). Partially involuting congenital hemangiomas: a report of 8 cases and review of the literature. J Am Acad Dermatol. 70(1):75–9. PMID:24176519
**1882.** Bichakjian CK, Olencki T, Aasi SZ, Alam M, Andersen JS, Berg D, et al. (2016). Basal cell skin cancer, Version 1.2016, NCCN Clinical Practice Guidelines in Oncology. J Natl Compr Canc Netw. 14(5):574–97. PMID:27160235
**1883.** Natkunam Y, Goodlad JR, Chadburn A, de Jong D, Gratzinger D, Chan JK, et al. (2017). EBV-positive B-cell proliferations of varied malignant potential: 2015 SH/EAHP Workshop Report-Part 1. Am J Clin Pathol. 147(2):129–52. PMID:28395107
**1884.** Natkunam Y, Warnke RA, Haghighi B, Su LD, Le Boit PE, Kim YH, et al. (2000). Co-expression of CD56 and CD30 in lymphomas with primary presentation in the skin: clinicopathologic, immunohistochemical and molecular analyses of seven cases. J Cutan Pathol. 27(8):392–9. PMID:10955685
**1885.** Navarini AA, Kolm I, Calvo X, Kamarashev J, Kerl K, Conrad C, et al. (2010). Trauma as triggering factor for development of melanocytic nevi. Dermatology. 220(4):291–6. PMID:20424415
**1886.** Nayler SJ, Rubin BP, Calonje E, Chan JK, Fletcher CD (2000). Composite hemangioendothelioma: a complex, low-grade vascular lesion mimicking angiosarcoma. Am J Surg Pathol. 24(3):352–61. PMID:10716148
**1887.** Nazarian RM, Kapur P, Rakheja D, Piris A, Duncan LM, Mihm MC Jr, et al. (2009). Atypical and malignant hidradenomas: a histological and immunohistochemical study. Mod Pathol. 22(4):600–10. PMID:19252473
**1888.** Nedoszytko B, Niedoszytko M, Lange M, van Doormaal J, Gleń J, Zabłotna M, et al. (2009). Interleukin-13 promoter gene polymorphism -1112C/T is associated with the systemic form of mastocytosis. Allergy. 64(2):287–94. PMID:19178408
**1889.** Nelson AA, Harrington AM, Kroft S, Dahar MA, Hamadani M, Dhakal B (2016). Presentation and management of post-allogeneic transplantation EBV-positive mucocutaneous ulcer. Bone Marrow Transplant. 51(2):300–2. PMID:26457913
**1890.** Nelson DS, Quispel W, Badalian-Very G, van Halteren AG, van den Bos C, Bovée JV, et al. (2014). Somatic activating ARAF mutations in Langerhans cell histiocytosis. Blood. 123(20):3152–5. PMID:24652991
**1891.** Nelson DS, van Halteren A, Quispel WT, van den Bos C, Bovée JV, Patel B, et al. (2015). MAP2K1 and MAP3K1 mutations in Langerhans cell histiocytosis. Genes Chromosomes Cancer. 54(6):361–8. PMID:25899310
**1892.** Nelson MA, Einspahr JG, Alberts DS, Balfour CA, Wymer JA, Welch KL, et al. (1994). Analysis of the p53 gene in human precancerous actinic keratosis lesions and squamous cell cancers. Cancer Lett. 85(1):23–9. PMID:7923098
**1893.** Neuhold JC, Friesenhahn J, Gerdes N, Krengel S (2015). Case reports of fatal or metastasizing melanoma in children and adolescents: a systematic analysis of the literature. Pediatr Dermatol. 32(1):13–22. PMID:25487565
**1894.** Neumann MP, Frizzera G (1986). The

coexistence of Langerhans' cell granulomatosis and malignant lymphoma may take different forms: report of seven cases with a review of the literature. Hum Pathol. 17(10):1060–5. PMID:3759063

**1895.** Neuville A, Chibon F, Coindre JM (2014). Grading of soft tissue sarcomas: from histological to molecular assessment. Pathology. 46(2):113–20. PMID:24378389

**1896.** Newton-Bishop JA, Chang YM, Iles MM, Taylor JC, Bakker B, Chan M, et al. (2010). Melanocytic nevi, nevus genes, and melanoma risk in a large case-control study in the United Kingdom. Cancer Epidemiol Biomarkers Prev. 19(8):2043–54. PMID:20647408

**1897.** Nezelof C, Basset F (2004). An hypothesis Langerhans cell histiocytosis: the failure of the immune system to switch from an innate to an adaptive mode. Pediatr Blood Cancer. 42(5):398–400. PMID:15049008

**1898.** Ng WK, Cheung MF, Ma L (1996). Dermatomyofibroma: further support of its myofibroblastic nature by electronmicroscopy. Histopathology. 29(2):181–3. PMID:8872155

**1899.** Nguyen CM, Chong K, Cassarino D (2016). Clear cell atypical fibroxanthoma: a case report and review of the literature. J Cutan Pathol. 43(6):538–42. PMID:26956561

**1900.** Nguyen TL, Theos A, Kelly DR, Busam K, Andea AA (2013). Mitotically active proliferative nodule arising in a giant congenital melanocytic nevus: a diagnostic pitfall. Am J Dermatopathol. 35(1):e16–21. PMID:23348144

**1901.** Nickoloff BJ, Fleischmann HE, Carmel J, Wood CC, Roth RJ (1986). Microcystic adnexal carcinoma. Immunohistologic observations suggesting dual (pilar and eccrine) differentiation. Arch Dermatol. 122(3):290–4. PMID:3513708

**1902.** Nicol I, Boye T, Carsuzaa F, Feier L, Collet Villette AM, Xerri L, et al. (2003). Post-transplant plasmablastic lymphoma of the skin. Br J Dermatol. 149(4):889–91. PMID:14616390

**1903.** Nicolae-Cristea AR, Benner MF, Zoutman WH, van Eijk R, Jansen PM, Tensen CP, et al. (2015). Diagnostic and prognostic significance of CDKN2A/CDKN2B deletions in patients with transformed mycosis fungoides and primary cutaneous CD30-positive lymphoproliferative disease. Br J Dermatol. 172(3):784–8. PMID:25308604

**1904.** Niedermeyer HP, Peris K, Höfler H (1996). Pilomatrix carcinoma with multiple visceral metastases. Report of a case. Cancer. 77(7):1311–4. PMID:8608508

**1905.** Niedoszytko M, Bonadonna P, Oude Elberink JN, Golden DB (2014). Epidemiology, diagnosis, and treatment of Hymenoptera venom allergy in mastocytosis patients. Immunol Allergy Clin North Am. 34(2):365–81. PMID:24745680

**1906.** Nielsen GP, O'Connell JX, Dickersin GR, Rosenberg AE (1996). Collagenous fibroma (desmoplastic fibroblastoma): a report of seven cases. Mod Pathol. 9(7):781–5. PMID:8832562

**1907.** Nishikawa Y, Tokusashi Y, Saito Y, Ogawa K, Miyokawa N, Katagiri M (1994). A case of apocrine adenocarcinoma associated with hamartomatous apocrine gland hyperplasia of both axillae. Am J Surg Pathol. 18(8):832–6. PMID:8037297

**1908.** Nishio J, Iwasaki H, Nagatomo M, Naito M (2014). Fibroma of tendon sheath with 11q rearrangements. Anticancer Res. 34(9):5159–62. PMID:25202108

**1909.** Nishio J, Iwasaki H, Ohjimi Y, Ishiguro M, Kobayashi K, Nabeshima K, et al. (2004). Chromosomal imbalances in angioleiomyomas by comparative genomic hybridization. Int J Mol Med. 13(1):13–6. PMID:14654964

**1910.** Nishio JN, Iwasaki H, Ohjimi Y, Ishiguro M, Koga T, Isayama T, et al. (2002). Gain of Xq detected by comparative genomic hybridization in elastofibroma. Int J Mol Med. 10(3):277–80. PMID:12165800

**1911.** Nishioka M, Kunisada M, Fujiwara N, Oka M, Funasaka Y, Nishigori C (2015). Multiple apocrine poromas: a new case report. J Cutan Pathol. 42(11):894–6. PMID:26269431

**1912.** Niu HT, Zhou QM, Wang F, Shao Q, Guan YX, Wen XZ, et al. (2013). Identification of anaplastic lymphoma kinase break points and oncogenic mutation profiles in acral/mucosal melanomas. Pigment Cell Melanoma Res. 26(5):646–53. PMID:23751074

**1913.** Noel JC, Detremmerie O, Peny MO, Candaele M, Verhest A, Heenen M, et al. (1994). Transformation of common warts into squamous cell carcinoma on sun-exposed areas in an immunosuppressed patient. Dermatology. 189(3):308–11. PMID:7949492

**1914.** Noguchi T, Ota N, Mabuchi Y, Yagi S, Minami S, Okuhira H, et al. (2017). A case of malignant melanoma of the uterine cervix with disseminated metastases throughout the vaginal wall. Case Rep Obstet Gynecol. 2017:5656340. PMID:28197351

**1915.** Nomura H, Egami S, Kasai H, Mori M, Yokoyama T, Fujimoto A, et al. (2014). An elderly patient with chronic active Epstein-Barr virus infection with severe hydroa vacciniforme-like eruptions associated with αβT-cell proliferation. J Dermatol. 41(4):360–2. PMID:24628134

**1916.** Nomura H, Suzuki H, Egami S, Yokoyama T, Sugiura M, Tomita K, et al. (2015). A patient with elderly-onset atypical hydroa vacciniforme with an indolent clinical course. Br J Dermatol. 173(3):801–5. PMID:25965563

**1917.** Noonan V, Lerman MA, Woo SB, Kabani S (2014). Granular cell tumor. J Mass Dent Soc. 63(1):45. PMID:24941552

**1918.** North JP, McCalmont TH, Fehr A, van Zante A, Stenman G, LeBoit PE (2015). Detection of MYB alterations and other immunohistochemical markers in primary cutaneous adenoid cystic carcinoma. Am J Surg Pathol. 39(10):1347–56. PMID:26076064

**1919.** North PE, Kahn T, Cordisco MR, Dadras SS, Detmar M, Frieden IJ (2004). Multifocal lymphangioendotheliomatosis with thrombocytopenia: a newly recognized clinicopathological entity. Arch Dermatol. 140(5):599–606. PMID:15148106

**1920.** North PE, Waner M, James CA, Mizeracki A, Frieden IJ, Mihm MC Jr (2001). Congenital nonprogressive hemangioma: a distinct clinicopathologic entity unlike infantile hemangioma. Arch Dermatol. 137(12):1607–20. PMID:11735711

**1921.** North PE, Waner M, Mizeracki A, Mihm MC Jr (2000). GLUT1: a newly discovered immunohistochemical marker for juvenile hemangiomas. Hum Pathol. 31(1):11–22. PMID:10665907

**1922.** North PE, Waner M, Mizeracki A, Mrak RE, Nicholas R, Kincannon J, et al. (2001). A unique microvascular phenotype shared by juvenile hemangiomas and human placenta. Arch Dermatol. 137(5):559–70. PMID:11346333

**1923.** Noto G (1999). 'Benign' proliferating trichilemmal tumour: does it really exist? Histopathology. 35(4):386–7. PMID:10564395

**1924.** Nova MP, Zung M, Halperin A (1991). Neurofollicular hamartoma. A clinicopathological study. Am J Dermatopathol. 13(5):459–62. PMID:1659245

**1925.** Nowak M, Pathan A, Fatteh S, Fatteh S, Lopez J (1998). Syringocystadenoma papilliferum of the male breast. Am J Dermatopathol. 20(4):422–4. PMID:9700386

**1926.** Nugteren HM, Nijman JM, de Jong IJ, van Driel MF (2011). The association between Peyronie's and Dupuytren's disease. Int J Impot Res. 23(4):142–5. PMID:21633367

**1927.** Nuovo GJ, Ishag M (2000). The histologic spectrum of epidermodysplasia verruciformis. Am J Surg Pathol. 24(10):1400–6. PMID:11023102

**1928.** O'Brien KP, Seroussi E, Dal Cin P, Sciot R, Mandahl N, Fletcher JA, et al. (1998). Various regions within the alpha-helical domain of the COL1A1 gene are fused to the second exon of the PDGFB gene in dermatofibrosarcomas and giant-cell fibroblastomas. Genes Chromosomes Cancer. 23(2):187–93. PMID:9739023

**1929.** O'Connor N, Patel M, Umar T, Macpherson DW, Ethunandan M (2011). Head and neck pilomatricoma: an analysis of 201 cases. Br J Oral Maxillofac Surg. 49(5):354–8. PMID:20594627

**1930.** O'Donnell PJ, Pantanowitz L, Grayson W (2010). Unique histologic variants of cutaneous Kaposi sarcoma. Am J Dermatopathol. 32(3):244–50. PMID:20075709

**1931.** O'Grady TC, Barr RJ, Billman G, Cunningham BB (1999). Epithelioid blue nevus occurring in children with no evidence of Carney complex. Am J Dermatopathol. 21(5):483–6. PMID:10535581

**1932.** O'Malley DP, Agrawal R, Grimm KE, Hummel J, Glazyrin A, Dim DC, et al. (2015). Evidence of BRAF V600E in indeterminate cell tumor and interdigitating dendritic cell sarcoma. Ann Diagn Pathol. 19(3):113–6. PMID:25787243

**1933.** O'Shea C, Fitzpatrick JE, Koch PJ (2014). Desmosomal defects in acantholytic squamous cell carcinomas. J Cutan Pathol. 41(11):873–9. PMID:25264142

**1934.** Ogita A, Ansai SI, Misago N, Anan T, Fukumoto T, Saeki H (2016). Clinicopathological study of crateriform verruca: crateriform epithelial lesions histopathologically distinct from keratoacanthoma. J Dermatol. 43(10):1154–9. PMID:26970425

**1935.** Oguchi S, Saida T, Koganehira Y, Ohkubo S, Ishihara Y, Kawachi S (1998). Characteristic epiluminescent microscopic features of early malignant melanoma on glabrous skin. A videomicroscopic analysis. Arch Dermatol. 134(5):563–8. PMID:9606325

**1936.** Ogura K, Goto T, Nemoto T (2012). Painless giant angioleiomyoma in the subfascia of the lower leg. J Foot Ankle Surg. 51(1):99–102. PMID:21940181

**1937.** Oh CW, Ivan D, Curry JL, Ellis R, Gerber H, Duvic M, et al. (2016). A case of indeterminate dendritic cell tumor presenting with leonine facies. J Cutan Pathol. 43(2):158–63. PMID:26272726

**1938.** Ohn J, Choe YS, Mun JH (2016). Dermoscopic features of nail matrix nevus (NMN) in adults and children: a comparative analysis. J Am Acad Dermatol. 75(3):535–40. PMID:27177439

**1939.** Ohnishi T, Watanabe S (1999). Immunohistochemical analysis of cytokeratin expression in various trichogenic tumors. Am J Dermatopathol. 21(4):337–43. PMID:10446774

**1940.** Ohtsuka H, Nagamatsu S (2002). Microcystic adnexal carcinoma: review of 51 Japanese patients. Dermatology. 204(3):190–3. PMID:12037446

**1941.** Okamoto N, Aoto T, Uhara H, Yamazaki S, Akutsu H, Umezawa A, et al. (2014). A melanocyte–melanoma precursor niche in sweat glands of volar skin. Pigment Cell Melanoma Res. 27(6):1039–50. PMID:25065272

**1942.** Okawa Y, Yokota R, Yamauchi A (1979). On the extracellular sheath of dermal melanocytes in nevus fusco-ceruleus acromiodeltoideus (Ito) and Mongolian spot. An ultrastructural study. J Invest Dermatol. 73(3):224–30. PMID:572849

**1943.** Okonkwo L, Jaffe ES (2017). Intravascular large cell lymphoma of NK/T-cell type, EBV positive. Blood. 130(6):837. PMID:28798060

**1944.** Oliveira AM, Chou MM (2014). USP6-induced neoplasms: the biologic spectrum of aneurysmal bone cyst and nodular fasciitis. Hum Pathol. 45(1):1–11. PMID:23769422

**1945.** Oliveira AM, Hsi BL, Weremowicz S, Rosenberg AE, Dal Cin P, Joseph N, et al. (2004). USP6 (Tre2) fusion oncogenes in aneurysmal bone cyst. Cancer Res. 64(6):1920–3. PMID:15026324

**1946.** Olsen E, Vonderheid E, Pimpinelli N, Willemze R, Kim Y, Knobler R, et al. (2007). Revisions to the staging and classification of mycosis fungoides and Sezary syndrome: a proposal of the International Society for Cutaneous Lymphomas (ISCL) and the Cutaneous Lymphoma Task Force of the European Organization of Research and Treatment of Cancer (EORTC). Blood. 110(6):1713–22. PMID:17540844

**1947.** Olsen TG, Helwig EB (1985). Angiolymphoid hyperplasia with eosinophilia. A clinicopathologic study of 116 patients. J Am Acad Dermatol. 12(5 Pt 1):781–96. PMID:4008683

**1948.** Onaindia A, Montes-Moreno S, Rodríguez-Pinilla SM, Batlle A, González de Villambrosía S, Rodríguez AM, et al. (2015). Primary cutaneous anaplastic large cell lymphomas with 6p25.3 rearrangement exhibit particular histological features. Histopathology. 66(6):846–55. PMID:25131361

**1949.** Ong CS, Keogh AM, Kossard S, Macdonald PS, Spratt PM (1999). Skin cancer in Australian heart transplant recipients. J Am Acad Dermatol. 40(1):27–34. PMID:9922009

**1950.** Onken MD, Worley LA, Ehlers JP, Harbour JW (2004). Gene expression profiling in uveal melanoma reveals two molecular classes and predicts metastatic death. Cancer Res. 64(20):7205–9. PMID:15492234

**1951.** Opletalova K, Bourillon A, Yang W, Pouvelle C, Armier J, Despras E, et al. (2014). Correlation of phenotype/genotype in a cohort of 23 xeroderma pigmentosum-variant patients reveals 12 new disease-causing POLH mutations. Hum Mutat. 35(1):117–28. PMID:24130121

**1952.** Orlow I, Satagopan JM, Berwick M, Enriquez HL, White KA, Cheung K, et al. (2015). Genetic factors associated with naevus count and dermoscopic patterns: preliminary results from the Study of Nevi in Children (SONIC). Br J Dermatol. 172(4):1081–9. PMID:25307738

**1953.** Orrock JM, Abbott JJ, Gibson LE, Folpe AL (2009). INI1 and GLUT-1 expression in epithelioid sarcoma and its cutaneous neoplastic and nonneoplastic mimics. Am J Dermatopathol. 31(2):152–6. PMID:19318800

**1954.** Ortonne N, Huet D, Gaudez C, Marie-Cardine A, Schiavon V, Bagot M, et al. (2006). Significance of circulating T-cell clones in Sezary syndrome. Blood. 107(10):4030–8. PMID:16418328

**1955.** Ortonne N, Le Gouvello S, Mansour H, Poillet C, Martin N, Delfau-Larue MH, et al. (2008). CD158K/KIR3DL2 transcript detection in lesional skin of patients with erythroderma is a tool for the diagnosis of Sézary syndrome. J Invest Dermatol. 128(2):465–72. PMID:17703174

**1956.** Oschlies I, Lisfeld J, Lamant L, Nakazawa A, d'Amore ES, Hansson U, et al. (2013). ALK-positive anaplastic large cell lymphoma limited to the skin: clinical, histopathological and molecular analysis of 6 pediatric cases. A report from the ALCL99 study. Haematologica. 98(1):50–6. PMID:22773605

**1957.** Oschlies I, Simonitsch-Klupp I, Maldyk J, Konovalov D, Abramov D, Myakova N, et al. (2015). Subcutaneous panniculitis-like T-cell lymphoma in children: a detailed clinicopathological description of 11 multifocal cases with a high frequency of haemophagocytic syndrome. Br J Dermatol. 172(3):793–7. PMID:25456748

**1958.** Oshiro H, Iwai T, Hirota M, Mitsudo K, Tohnai I, Minamimoto R, et al. (2010). Primary sebaceous carcinoma of the tongue. Med Mol Morphol. 43(4):246–52. PMID:21267703

**1959.** Osio A, Fraitag S, Hadj-Rabia S, Bodemer C, de Prost Y, Hamel-Teillac D (2010). Clinical spectrum of tufted angiomas in childhood: a report of 13 cases and a review of the literature. Arch Dermatol. 146(7):758–63. PMID:20644037

**1960.** Osterlind A, Tucker MA, Hou-Jensen K, Stone BJ, Engholm G, Jensen OM (1988). The Danish case-control study of cutaneous malignant melanoma. I. Importance of host factors. Int J Cancer. 42(2):200–6. PMID:3403065

**1961.** Ostler DA, Prieto VG, Reed JA, Deavers MT, Lazar AJ, Ivan D (2010). Adipophilin expression in sebaceous tumors and other cutaneous lesions with clear cell histology: an immunohistochemical study of 117 cases. Mod Pathol. 23(4):567–73. PMID:20118912

**1962.** Otsuka A, Levesque MP, Dummer R, Kabashima K (2015). Hedgehog signaling in basal cell carcinoma. J Dermatol Sci. 78(2):95–100. PMID:25766766

**1963.** Ouban A, Dellis J, Salup R, Morgan M (2003). Immunohistochemical expression of Mdm2 and p53 in penile verrucous carcinoma. Ann Clin Lab Sci. 33(1):101–6. PMID:12661905

**1964.** Oudijk L, den Bakker MA, Hop WC, Cohen M, Charles AK, Alaggio R, et al. (2012). Solitary, multifocal and generalized myofibromas: clinicopathological and immunohistochemical features of 114 cases. Histopathology. 60(6B):E1–11. PMID:22486319

**1965.** Ozerdem U, McNiff JM, Tavassoli FA (2016). Cytokeratin 7-negative mammary Paget's disease: a diagnostic pitfall. Pathol Res Pract. 212(4):279–81. PMID:26944832

**1966.** Pagano L, Valentini CG, Pulsoni A, Fisogni S, Carluccio P, Mannelli F, et al. (2013). Blastic plasmacytoid dendritic cell neoplasm with leukemic presentation: an Italian multicenter study. Haematologica. 98(2):239–46. PMID:23065521

**1967.** Page RN, King R, Mihm MC Jr, Googe PB (2004). Microphthalmia transcription factor and NKI/C3 expression in cellular neurothekeoma. Mod Pathol. 17(2):230–4. PMID:14685254

**1968.** Palicka GA, Rhodes AR (2010). Acral melanocytic nevi: prevalence and distribution of gross morphologic features in white and black adults. Arch Dermatol. 146(10):1085–94. PMID:20956637

**1969.** Pallure V, Frouin E, Petrella T, Depaepe L, Dalle S, Dereure O (2014). Cutaneous indeterminate cell histiocytosis: two new observations including a case with paraneoplastic-like evolution. Eur J Dermatol. 24(4):505–6. PMID:25266746

**1970.** Palmedo G, Hantschke M, Rütten A, Mentzel T, Kempf W, Tomasini D, et al. (2007). Primary cutaneous marginal zone B-cell lymphoma may exhibit both the t(14;18)(q32;q21) IGH/BCL2 and the t(14;18)(q32;q21) IGH/MALT1 translocation: an indicator for clonal transformation towards higher-grade B-cell lymphoma? Am J Dermatopathol. 29(3):231–6. PMID:17519619

**1971.** Palmer LC, Strauch WG, Welton WA (1978). Lymphangioma circumscriptum. A case with deep lymphatic involvement. Arch Dermatol. 114(3):394–6. PMID:629576

**1972.** Pan H, Wang H, Fan Y (2011). Intracranial meningeal melanocytoma associated with nevus of Ota. J Clin Neurosci. 18(11):1548–50. PMID:21924617

**1973.** Pandey CR, Singh N, Tamang B (2017). Subungual glomus tumours: is magnetic resonance imaging or ultrasound necessary for diagnosis? Malays Orthop J. 11(1):47–51. PMID:28435574

**1974.** Paniago-Pereira C, Maize JC, Ackerman AB (1978). Nevus of large spindle and/or epithelioid cells (Spitz's nevus). Arch Dermatol. 114(12):1811–23. PMID:367281

**1975.** Pansuriya TC, van Eijk R, d'Adamo P, van Ruler MA, Kuijjer ML, Oosting J, et al. (2011). Somatic mosaic IDH1 and IDH2 mutations are associated with enchondroma and spindle cell hemangioma in Ollier disease and Maffucci syndrome. Nat Genet. 43(12):1256–61. PMID:22057234

**1976.** Pantanowitz L, Stebbing J, Dezube BJ, editors (2010). Overview of Kaposi sarcoma. In: Kaposi sarcoma: a model of oncogenesis. Kerala: Research Signpost; pp. 1–40.

**1977.** Papalas JA, Proia AD (2010). Primary mucinous carcinoma of the eyelid: a clinicopathologic and immunohistochemical study of 4 cases and an update on recurrence rates. Arch Ophthalmol. 128(9):1160–5. PMID:20837800

**1978.** Papeš D, Altarac S, Arslani N, Rajković Z, Antabak A, Ćaćić M (2014). Melanoma of the glans penis and urethra. Urology. 83(1):6–11. PMID:23978371

**1979.** Papo M, Diamond EL, Cohen-Aubart F, Emile JF, Roos-Weil D, Gupta N, et al. (2017). High prevalence of myeloid neoplasms in adults with non-Langerhans cell histiocytosis. Blood. 130(8):1007–13. PMID:28679734

**1980.** Papp G, Krausz T, Stricker TP, Szendrői M, Sápi Z (2014). SMARCB1 expression in epithelioid sarcoma is regulated by miR-206, miR-381, and miR-671-5p on both mRNA and protein levels. Genes Chromosomes Cancer. 53(2):168–76. PMID:24327545

**1981.** Paradela S, Castiñeiras I, Cuevas J, Almagro M, del Pozo J, Fonseca E (2008). Mucinous carcinoma of the skin: evaluation of lymphatic invasion with D2-40. Am J Dermatopathol. 30(5):504–8. PMID:18806501

**1982.** Paradela S, Fonseca E, Prieto VG (2011). Melanoma in children. Arch Pathol Lab Med. 135(3):307–16. PMID:21366453

**1983.** Paredes BE, Mentzel T (2011). Atypical lipomatous tumor/"well-differentiated liposarcoma" of the skin clinically presenting as a skin tag: clinicopathologic, immunohistochemical, and molecular analysis of 2 cases. Am J Dermatopathol. 33(6):603–7. PMID:21358383

**1984.** Parekh V, Guerrero CE, Knapp CF, Elmets CA, McKay KM (2016). A histological snapshot of hypothetical multistep progression from nevus sebaceus to invasive syringocystadenocarcinoma papilliferum. Am J Dermatopathol. 38(1):56–62. PMID:26317389

**1985.** Parham DM, Fisher C (1997). Angiosarcomas of the breast developing post radiotherapy. Histopathology. 31(2):189–95. PMID:9279573

**1986.** Paridaens AD, Minassian DC, McCartney AC, Hungerford JL (1994). Prognostic factors in primary malignant melanoma of the conjunctiva: a clinicopathological study of 256 cases. Br J Ophthalmol. 78(4):252–9. PMID:8199108

**1987.** Park BS, Yang SG, Cho KH (1997). Malignant proliferating trichilemmal tumor showing distant metastases. Am J Dermatopathol. 19(5):536–9. PMID:9335249

**1988.** Park EA, Hong SH, Choi JY, Lee MW, Kang HS (2005). Glomangiomatosis: magnetic resonance imaging findings in three cases. Skeletal Radiol. 34(2):108–11. PMID:15372213

**1989.** Park HJ, Kim YC, Cinn YW (2000). Nodular hidradenocarcinoma with prominent squamous differentiation: case report and immunohistochemical study. J Cutan Pathol. 27(8):423–7. PMID:10955691

**1990.** Park HJ, Park CJ, Yi JY, Kim TY, Kim CW (1997). Nevus lipomatosus superficialis on the face. Int J Dermatol. 36(6):435–7. PMID:9248887

**1991.** Park HK, Leonard DD, Arrington JH 3rd, Lund HZ (1987). Recurrent melanocytic nevi: clinical and histologic review of 175 cases. J Am Acad Dermatol. 17(2 Pt 1):285–92. PMID:3624565

**1992.** Park JM, Tsao H, Tsao S (2009). Acquired bilateral nevus of Ota-like macules (Hori nevus): etiologic and therapeutic considerations. J Am Acad Dermatol. 61(1):88–93. PMID:19539841

**1993.** Park SW, Jang KT, Lee JH, Park JH, Kwon GY, Mun GH, et al. (2016). Scattered atypical melanocytes with hyperchromatic nuclei in the nail matrix: diagnostic clue for early subungual melanoma in situ. J Cutan Pathol. 43(1):41–52. PMID:26423820

**1994.** Park SY, Jin SP, Yeom B, Kim SW, Cho SY, Lee JH (2011). Multiple fibromas of tendon sheath: unusual presentation. Ann Dermatol. 23 Suppl 1:S45–7. PMID:22028571

**1995.** Park SY, Lee JK, Jo S, Huh CH, Cho KH, Na JI (2014). Cutaneous epithelioid hemangioendothelioma presented as an ulcerated areolar mass. J Dermatol. 41(1):112–3. PMID:24354555

**1996.** Parkin DM, Whelan SL, Ferlay J, Teppo L, Thomas DB, editors (2002). Cancer incidence in five continents, Vol. VIII. Lyon: International Agency for Research on Cancer. IARC Scientific Publication No. 155.

**1997.** Parratt MT, Donaldson JR, Flanagan AM, Saifuddin A, Pollock RC, Skinner JA, et al. (2010). Elastofibroma dorsi: management, outcome and review of the literature. J Bone Joint Surg Br. 92(2):262–6. PMID:20130320

**1998.** Patchefsky AS, Enzinger FM (1981). Intravascular fasciitis: a report of 17 cases. Am J Surg Pathol. 5(1):29–36. PMID:7246849

**1999.** Patel KU, Szabo SS, Hernandez VS, Prieto VG, Abruzzo LV, Lazar AJ, et al. (2008). Dermatofibrosarcoma protuberans COL1A1-PDGFB fusion is identified in virtually all dermatofibrosarcoma protuberans cases when investigated by newly developed multiplex reverse transcription polymerase chain reaction and fluorescence in situ hybridization assays. Hum Pathol. 39(2):184–93. PMID:17950782

**2000.** Patel V, Squires SM, Liu DY, Fraga GR (2014). Cutaneous adenosquamous carcinoma: a rare neoplasm with biphasic differentiation. Cutis. 94(5):231–3. PMID:25474451

**2001.** Paties C, Taccagni GL, Papotti M, Valente G, Zangrandi A, Aloi F (1993). Apocrine carcinoma of the skin. A clinicopathologic, immunocytochemical, and ultrastructural study. Cancer. 71(2):375–81. PMID:7678545

**2002.** Paties C, Vassallo G, Taccagni GL (1997). Clear cell dermatofibroma. Am J Surg Pathol. 21(2):250–2. PMID:9042295

**2003.** Patrice SJ, Wiss K, Mulliken JB (1991). Pyogenic granuloma (lobular capillary hemangioma): a clinicopathologic study of 178 cases. Pediatr Dermatol. 8(4):267–76. PMID:1792196

**2004.** Patrick RJ, Fenske NA, Messina JL (2007). Primary mucosal melanoma. J Am Acad Dermatol. 56(5):828–34. PMID:17349716

**2005.** Patterson JW (2015). Tumors of the epidermis: actinic keratosis. In: Weedon's skin pathology. 4th ed. London: Elsevier; pp. 796–9.

**2006.** Patterson JW (2015). Weedon's skin pathology. 4th ed. London: Elsevier; p. 1149.

**2007.** Patterson JW (2015). Weedon's skin pathology. 4th ed. London: Elsevier; pp. 1166–70.

**2008.** Patterson JW, Jordan WP Jr (1987). Atypical fibroxanthoma in a patient with xeroderma pigmentosum. Arch Dermatol. 123(8):1066–70. PMID:3631985

**2009.** Patterson JW, Wick MR (2006). Nonmelanocytic tumors of the skin. In: AFIP atlas of tumor pathology. Series 4, Fascicle 4. Washington, DC: American Registry of Pathology Press; pp. 389–92.

**2010.** Patton KT, Deyrup AT, Weiss SW (2008). Atypical vascular lesions after surgery and radiation of the breast: a clinicopathologic study of 32 cases analyzing histologic heterogeneity and association with angiosarcoma. Am J Surg Pathol. 32(6):943–50. PMID:18551753

**2011.** Paul S, Majumdar S, Giri AK (2015). Genetic susceptibility to arsenic-induced skin lesions and health effects: a review. Genes Environ. 37:23. PMID:27350818

**2012.** Paulli M, Berti E, Rosso R, Boveri E, Kindl S, Klersy C, et al. (1995). CD30/Ki-1-positive lymphoproliferative disorders of the skin–clinicopathologic correlation and statistical analysis of 86 cases: a multicentric study from the European Organization for Research and Treatment of Cancer Cutaneous Lymphoma Project Group. J Clin Oncol. 13(6):1343–54. PMID:7751878

**2013.** Paulli M, Rosso R, Kindl S, Boveri E, Marocolo D, Chioda C, et al. (1992). Immunophenotypic characterization of the cell infiltrate in five cases of sinus histiocytosis with massive lymphadenopathy (Rosai-Dorfman disease). Hum Pathol. 23(6):647–54. PMID:1592387

**2014.** Paulson KG, Iyer JG, Simonson WT, Blom A, Thibodeau RM, Schmidt M, et al. (2014). CD8+ lymphocyte intratumoral infiltration as a stage-independent predictor of Merkel cell carcinoma survival: a population-based study. Am J Clin Pathol. 142(4):452–8. PMID:25239411

**2015.** Pavlidakey PG, Burroughs C, Karrs T, Somach SC (2011). Cutaneous epithelioid angiomatous nodule: a case with metachronous lesions. Am J Dermatopathol. 33(8):831–4. PMID:21931284

**2016.** Pavlova O, Fraitag S, Hohl D (2016). 5-Hydroxymethylcytosine expression in proliferative nodules arising within congenital nevi allows differentiation from malignant melanoma. J Invest Dermatol. 136(12):2453–61. PMID:27456754

**2017.** Pawlik TM, Paulino AF, McGinn CJ, Baker LH, Cohen DS, Morris JS, et al. (2003). Cutaneous angiosarcoma of the scalp: a multidisciplinary approach. Cancer. 98(8):1716–26. PMID:14534889

**2018.** Pawlikowski JS, McBryan T, van Tuyn J, Drotar ME, Hewitt RN, Maier AB, et al. (2013). Wnt signaling potentiates nevogenesis. Proc Natl Acad Sci U S A. 110(40):16009–14. PMID:24043806

**2019.** Pawson R, Dyer MJ, Barge R, Matutes E, Thornton PD, Emmett E, et al. (1997). Treatment of T-cell prolymphocytic leukemia with human CD52 antibody. J Clin Oncol. 15(7):2667–72. PMID:9215839

**2020.** Payal R, Gupta S, Aggarwal R, Handa S, Radotra BD, Arora SK (2006). Detection of high-risk human papillomavirus type 16/18 in cutaneous warts in immunocompetent patients, using polymerase chain reaction. Dermatol Online J. 12(6):1. PMID:17083881

**2021.** Payne DA, Sanchez R, Tyring SK (1997). Cutaneous verruca with genital human papillomavirus in a 2-year-old girl. Am J Dermatopathol. 19(3):258–60. PMID:9185912

**2022.** Peachey RD, Lim CC, Whimster IW (1970). Lymphangioma of skin. A review of 65 cases. Br J Dermatol. 83(5):519–27. PMID:5484713

**2023.** Pechère M, Roten S, Piletta P, Harms M, Krischer J (1998). Pigmented eccrine poroma. Ann Dermatol Venereol. 125(4):281. [French] PMID:9747272

**2024.** Pedeutour F, Coindre JM, Sozzi G, Nicolo G, Leroux A, Toma S, et al. (1994). Supernumerary ring chromosomes containing

chromosome 17 sequences. A specific feature of dermatofibrosarcoma protuberans? Cancer Genet Cytogenet. 76(1):1–9. PMID:8076341
**2025.** Pedeutour F, Forus A, Coindre JM, Berner JM, Nicolo G, Michiels JF, et al. (1999). Structure of the supernumerary ring and giant rod chromosomes in adipose tissue tumors. Genes Chromosomes Cancer. 24(1):30–41. PMID:9892106
**2026.** Pedeutour F, Simon MP, Minoletti F, Sozzi G, Pierotti MA, Hecht F, et al. (1995). Ring 22 chromosomes in dermatofibrosarcoma protuberans are low-level amplifiers of chromosome 17 and 22 sequences. Cancer Res. 55(11):2400–3. PMID:7757993
**2027.** Pedeutour F, Suijkerbuijk RF, Van Gaal J, Van de Klundert W, Coindre JM, Van Haelst A, et al. (1993). Chromosome 12 origin in rings and giant markers in well-differentiated liposarcoma. Cancer Genet Cytogenet. 66(2):133–4. PMID:8500103
**2028.** Pellacani G, Scope A, Ferrari B, Pupelli G, Bassoli S, Longo C, et al. (2009). New insights into nevogenesis: in vivo characterization and follow-up of melanocytic nevi by reflectance confocal microscopy. J Am Acad Dermatol. 61(6):1001–13. PMID:19833408
**2029.** Peloponese JM Jr, Kinjo T, Jeang KT (2007). Human T-cell leukemia virus type 1 Tax and cellular transformation. Int J Hematol. 86(2):101–6. PMID:17875521
**2030.** Pereira ES, Moraes ET, Siqueira DM, Santos MA (2015). Stewart Treves syndrome. An Bras Dermatol. 90(3 Suppl 1):229–31. PMID:26312725
**2031.** Pereira PR, Odashiro AN, Rodrigues-Reyes AA, Correa ZM, de Souza Filho JP, Burnier MN Jr (2005). Histopathological review of sebaceous carcinoma of the eyelid. J Cutan Pathol. 32(7):496–501. PMID:16008694
**2032.** Perkins P, Weiss SW (1996). Spindle cell hemangioendothelioma. An analysis of 78 cases with reassessment of its pathogenesis and biologic behavior. Am J Surg Pathol. 20(10):1196–204. PMID:8827025
**2033.** Perry AM, Warnke RA, Hu Q, Gaulard P, Copie-Bergman C, Alkan S, et al. (2013). Indolent T-cell lymphoproliferative disease of the gastrointestinal tract. Blood. 122(22):3599–606. PMID:24009234
**2034.** Pesce C, Scalora S (2000). Apoptosis in the areas of squamous differentiation of irritated seborrheic keratosis. J Cutan Pathol. 27(3):121–3. PMID:10728813
**2035.** Peter M, Couturier J, Pacquement H, Michon J, Thomas G, Magdelenat H, et al. (1997). A new member of the ETS family fused to EWS in Ewing tumors. Oncogene. 14(10):1159–64. PMID:9121764
**2036.** Peterdy GA, Huettner PC, Rajaram V, Lind AC (2002). Trichofolliculoma of the vulva associated with vulvar intraepithelial neoplasia: report of three cases and review of the literature. Int J Gynecol Pathol. 21(3):224–30. PMID:12068167
**2037.** Peterson CM, Ratz JL, Sangueza OP (2001). Microcystic adnexal carcinoma: first reported case in an African American man. J Am Acad Dermatol. 45(2):283–5. PMID:11464192
**2038.** Petersson F, Huang J (2011). Epstein-Barr virus–associated smooth muscle tumor mimicking cutaneous angioleiomyoma. Am J Dermatopathol. 33(4):407–9. PMID:21285860
**2039.** Petersson F, Ivan D, Kazakov DV, Michal M, Prieto VG (2009). Pigmented Paget disease–a diagnostic pitfall mimicking melanoma. Am J Dermatopathol. 31(3):223–6. PMID:19384061
**2040.** Petersson F, Kutzner H, Spagnolo DV, Bisceglia M, Kacerovska D, Vazmitel M, et al. (2009). Adenoid cystic carcinoma-like pattern in spiradenoma and spiradenocylindroma: a rare feature in sporadic neoplasms and those associated with Brooke-Spiegler syndrome. Am J Dermatopathol. 31(7):642–8. PMID:19633533
**2041.** Petersson F, Michal M, Kazakov DV, Grossmann P, Michal M (2016). A new hitherto unreported histopathologic manifestation of mammary analogue secretory carcinoma: "masked MASC" associated with low-grade mucinous adenocarcinoma and low-grade in situ carcinoma components. Appl Immunohistochem Mol Morphol. 24(9):e80–5. PMID:26808131
**2042.** Petersson F, Nga ME (2012). Spiradenocarcinoma with low-grade basal cell adenocarcinoma pattern: report of a case with varied morphology and wild type TP53. J Cutan Pathol. 39(3):372–6. PMID:22077486
**2043.** Petrella T, Bagot M, Willemze R, Beylot-Barry M, Vergier B, Delaunay M, et al. (2005). Blastic NK-cell lymphomas (agranular CD4+CD56+ hematodermic neoplasms): a review. Am J Clin Pathol. 123(5):662–75. PMID:15981806
**2044.** Petrella T, Comeau MR, Maynadié M, Couillault G, De Muret A, Maliszewski CR, et al. (2002). 'Agranular CD4+ CD56+ hematodermic neoplasm' (blastic NK-cell lymphoma) originates from a population of CD56+ precursor cells related to plasmacytoid monocytes. Am J Surg Pathol. 26(7):852–62. PMID:12131152
**2045.** Petrella T, Facchetti F (2010). Tumoral aspects of plasmacytoid dendritic cells: what do we know in 2009? Autoimmunity. 43(3):210–4. PMID:20166873
**2046.** Petrella T, Maubec E, Cornillet-Lefebvre P, Willemze R, Pluot M, Durlach A, et al. (2007). Indolent CD8-positive lymphoid proliferation of the ear: a distinct primary cutaneous T-cell lymphoma? Am J Surg Pathol. 31(12):1887–92. PMID:18043044
**2047.** Petronic-Rosic V, Shea CR, Krausz T (2004). Pagetoid melanocytosis: when is it significant? Pathology. 36(5):435–44. PMID:15370113
**2048.** Pflug N, Bahlo J, Shanafelt TD, Eichhorst BF, Bergmann MA, Elter T, et al. (2014). Development of a comprehensive prognostic index for patients with chronic lymphocytic leukemia. Blood. 124(1):49–62. PMID:24797299
**2049.** Pham-Ledard A, Beylot-Barry M, Barbe C, Leduc M, Petrella T, Vergier B, et al. (2014). High frequency and clinical prognostic value of MYD88 L265P mutation in primary cutaneous diffuse large B-cell lymphoma, leg-type. JAMA Dermatol. 150(11):1173–9. PMID:25055137
**2050.** Pham-Ledard A, Cappellen D, Martinez F, Vergier B, Beylot-Barry M, Merlio JP (2012). MYD88 somatic mutation is a genetic feature of primary cutaneous diffuse large B-cell lymphoma, leg type. J Invest Dermatol. 132(8):2118–20. PMID:22495176
**2051.** Pham-Ledard A, Cowppli-Bony A, Doussau A, Prochazkova-Carlotti M, Laharanne E, Jouary T, et al. (2015). Diagnostic and prognostic value of BCL2 rearrangement in 53 patients with follicular lymphoma presenting as primary skin lesions. Am J Clin Pathol. 143(3):362–73. PMID:25696794
**2052.** Pham-Ledard A, Prochazkova-Carlotti M, Andrique L, Cappellen D, Vergier B, Martinez F, et al. (2014). Multiple genetic alterations in primary cutaneous large B-cell lymphoma, leg type support a common lymphomagenesis with activated B-cell-like diffuse large B-cell lymphoma. Mod Pathol. 27(3):402–11. PMID:24030746
**2053.** Pham-Ledard A, Prochazkova-Carlotti M, Laharanne E, Vergier B, Jouary T, Beylot-Barry M, et al. (2010). IRF4 gene rearrangements define a subgroup of CD30-positive cutaneous T-cell lymphoma: a study of 54 cases. J Invest Dermatol. 130(3):816–25. PMID:19812605
**2054.** Phan A, Touzet S, Dalle S, Ronger-Savlé S, Balme B, Thomas L (2006). Acral lentiginous melanoma: a clinicoprognostic study of 126 cases. Br J Dermatol. 155(3):561–9. PMID:16911282
**2055.** Piamphongsant T (1999). Chronic environmental arsenic poisoning. Int J Dermatol. 38(6):401–10. PMID:10397578
**2056.** Piccaluga PP, Rossi M, Agostinelli C, Ricci F, Gazzola A, Righi S, et al. (2014). Platelet-derived growth factor alpha mediates the proliferation of peripheral T-cell lymphoma cells via an autocrine regulatory pathway. Leukemia. 28(8):1687–97. PMID:24480986
**2057.** Piepkorn MW, Barnhill RL, Elder DE, Knezevich SR, Carney PA, Reisch LM, et al. (2014). The MPATH-Dx reporting schema for melanocytic proliferations and melanoma. J Am Acad Dermatol. 70(1):131–41. PMID:24176521
**2058.** Pieri L, Bonadonna P, Elena C, Papayannidis C, Grifoni FI, Rondoni M, et al. (2016). Clinical presentation and management practice of systemic mastocytosis. A survey on 460 Italian patients. Am J Hematol. 91(7):692–9. PMID:27060898
**2059.** Pilarski R, Burt R, Kohlman W, Pho L, Shannon KM, Swisher E (2013). Cowden syndrome and the PTEN hamartoma tumor syndrome: systematic review and revised diagnostic criteria. J Natl Cancer Inst. 105(21):1607–16. PMID:24136893
**2060.** Pilarski R, Cebulla CM, Massengill JB, Rai K, Rich T, Strong L, et al. (2014). Expanding the clinical phenotype of hereditary BAP1 cancer predisposition syndrome, reporting three new cases. Genes Chromosomes Cancer. 53(2):177–82. PMID:24243779
**2061.** Pileri A, Facchetti F, Rütten A, Zumiani G, Boi S, Fink-Puches R, et al. (2011). Syringotropic mycosis fungoides: a rare variant of the disease with peculiar clinicopathologic features. Am J Surg Pathol. 35(1):100–9. PMID:21164293
**2062.** Pileri SA, Grogan TM, Harris NL, Banks P, Campo E, Chan JK, et al. (2002). Tumours of histiocytes and accessory dendritic cells: an immunohistochemical approach to classification from the International Lymphoma Study Group based on 61 cases. Histopathology. 41(1):1–29. PMID:12121233
**2063.** Pilichowska ME, Fleming MD, Pinkus JL, Pinkus GS (2007). CD4+/CD56+ hematodermic neoplasm ("blastic natural killer cell lymphoma"): neoplastic cells express the immature dendritic cell marker BDCA-2 and produce interferon. Am J Clin Pathol. 128(3):445–53. PMID:17709319
**2064.** Pilozzi E, Pulford K, Jones M, Müller-Hermelink HK, Falini B, Ralfkiaer E, et al. (1998). Co-expression of CD79a (JCB117) and CD3 by lymphoblastic lymphoma. J Pathol. 186(2):140–3. PMID:9924428
**2065.** Piotrowski A, Xie J, Liu YF, Poplawski AB, Gomes AR, Madanecki P, et al. (2014). Germline loss-of-function mutations in LZTR1 predispose to an inherited disorder of multiple schwannomas. Nat Genet. 46(2):182–7. PMID:24362817
**2066.** Piqué E, Aguilar A, Fariña MC, Gallego MA, Escalonilla P, Requena L (1995). Partial unilateral lentiginosis: report of seven cases and review of the literature. Clin Exp Dermatol. 20(4):319–22. PMID:8548990
**2067.** Piqué E, Olivares M, Espinel ML, Fariña M, Martín L, Barat A, et al. (1995). Malignant hidroacanthoma simplex. A case report and literature review. Dermatology. 190(1):72–6. PMID:7894103
**2068.** Piris A, Peng Y, Boussahmain C, Essary LR, Gudewicz TM, Hoang MP (2014). Cutaneous and mammary apocrine carcinomas have different immunoprofiles. Hum Pathol. 45(2):320–6. PMID:24342430
**2069.** Pitchford CW, Schwartz HS, Atkinson JB, Cates JM (2006). Soft tissue perineurioma in a patient with neurofibromatosis type 2: a tumor not previously associated with the NF2 syndrome. Am J Surg Pathol. 30(12):1624–9. PMID:17122521
**2070.** Plateroti AM, Scavella V, Abdolrahimzadeh B, Plateroti R, Rahimi S (2017). An update on oculodermal melanocytosis and rare associated conditions. Semin Ophthalmol. 32(4):524–8. PMID:27083007
**2071.** Plaza JA, Comfere NI, Gibson LE, Colgan M, Davis DM, Pittelkow MR, et al. (2009). Unusual cutaneous manifestations of B-cell chronic lymphocytic leukemia. J Am Acad Dermatol. 60(5):772–80. PMID:19389520
**2072.** Plaza JA, Sangueza M (2015). Hydroa vacciniforme-like lymphoma with primarily periorbital swelling: 7 cases of an atypical clinical manifestation of this rare cutaneous T-cell lymphoma. Am J Dermatopathol. 37(1):20–5. PMID:25162933
**2073.** Plaza JA, Torres-Cabala C, Evans H, Diwan HA, Suster S, Prieto VG (2010). Cutaneous metastases of malignant melanoma: a clinicopathologic study of 192 cases with emphasis on the morphologic spectrum. Am J Dermatopathol. 32(2):129–36. PMID:20010406
**2074.** Plumb SJ, Argenyi ZB, Stone MS, De Young BR (2004). Cytokeratin 5/6 immunostaining in cutaneous adnexal neoplasms and metastatic adenocarcinoma. Am J Dermatopathol. 26(6):447–51. PMID:15618924
**2075.** Poiares Baptista A, Tellechea O, Reis JP, Cunha MF, Figueiredo P (1993). Eccrine porocarcinoma. A review of 24 cases. Ann Dermatol Venereol. 120(1):107–15. [French] PMID:8338322
**2076.** Pollard WL, Beachkofsky TM, Kobayashi TT (2015). Novel R634W c-kit mutation identified in familial mastocytosis. Pediatr Dermatol. 32(2):267–70. PMID:25243845
**2077.** Pollock PM, Harper UL, Hansen KS, Yudt LM, Stark M, Robbins CM, et al. (2003). High frequency of BRAF mutations in nevi. Nat Genet. 33(1):19–20. PMID:12447372
**2078.** Pongpudpunth M, Rattanakaemakorn P, Fleischer AB Jr (2015). Usefulness of random skin biopsy as a diagnostic tool of intravascular lymphoma presenting with fever of unknown origin. Am J Dermatopathol. 37(9):686–90. PMID:26291417
**2079.** Poniecka AW, Alexis JB (1999). An immunohistochemical study of basal cell carcinoma and trichoepithelioma. Am J Dermatopathol. 21(4):332–6. PMID:10446773
**2080.** Ponti G, Losi L, Pedroni M, Lucci-Cordisco E, Di Gregorio C, Pellacani G, et al. (2006). Value of MLH1 and MSH2 mutations in the appearance of Muir-Torre syndrome phenotype in HNPCC patients presenting sebaceous gland tumors or keratoacanthomas. J Invest Dermatol. 126(10):2302–7. PMID:16826164
**2081.** Ponti G, Pellacani G, Seidenari S, Pollio A, Muscatello U, Tomasi A (2013). Cancer-associated genodermatoses: skin neoplasms as clues to hereditary tumor syndromes. Crit Rev Oncol Hematol. 85(3):239–56. PMID:22823951
**2082.** Ponti G, Ponz de Leon M (2005). Muir-Torre syndrome. Lancet Oncol. 6(12):980–7. PMID:16321766
**2083.** Ponti R, Quaglino P, Novelli M, Fierro MT, Comessatti A, Peroni A, et al. (2005). T-cell receptor gamma gene rearrangement by multiplex polymerase chain reaction/heteroduplex analysis in patients with cutaneous T-cell lymphoma (mycosis fungoides/Sézary syndrome) and benign inflammatory disease: correlation with clinical, histological and immunophenotypical findings. Br J Dermatol. 153(3):565–73. PMID:16120144

**2084.** Ponticelli C, Cucchiari D, Bencini P (2014). Skin cancer in kidney transplant recipients. J Nephrol. 27(4):385–94. PMID:24809813
**2085.** Ponzoni M, Arrigoni G, Gould VE, Del Curto B, Maggioni M, Scapinello A, et al. (2000). Lack of CD 29 (beta1 integrin) and CD 54 (ICAM-1) adhesion molecules in intravascular lymphomatosis. Hum Pathol. 31(2):220–6. PMID:10685637
**2086.** Ponzoni M, Ferreri AJ (2006). Intravascular lymphoma: a neoplasm of 'homeless' lymphocytes? Hematol Oncol. 24(3):105–12. PMID:16721900
**2087.** Ponzoni M, Ferreri AJ, Campo E, Facchetti F, Mazzucchelli L, Yoshino T, et al. (2007). Definition, diagnosis, and management of intravascular large B-cell lymphoma: proposals and perspectives from an international consensus meeting. J Clin Oncol. 25(21):3168–73. PMID:17577023
**2088.** Popova T, Hebert L, Jacquemin V, Gad S, Caux-Moncoutier V, Dubois-d'Enghien C, et al. (2013). Germline BAP1 mutations predispose to renal cell carcinomas. Am J Hum Genet. 92(6):974–80. PMID:23684012
**2089.** Portal C, Fang F, Kanner W, Wilson B (2013). Clear cell acanthoma. Cutis. 92(2):62, 77–9. PMID:24087787
**2090.** Potrony M, Badenas C, Aguilera P, Puig-Butille JA, Carrera C, Malvehy J, et al. (2015). Update in genetic susceptibility in melanoma. Ann Transl Med. 3(15):210. PMID:26488006
**2091.** Pradhan A, Grimer RJ, Spooner D, Peake D, Carter SR, Tillman RM, et al. (2011). Oncological outcomes of patients with Ewing's sarcoma: is there a difference between skeletal and extra-skeletal Ewing's sarcoma? J Bone Joint Surg Br. 93(4):531–6. PMID:21464495
**2092.** Pranteda G, Grimaldi M, Lombardi M, Pranteda G, Arcese A, Cortesi G, et al. (2014). Basal cell carcinoma: differences according to anatomic location and clinical-pathological subtypes. G Ital Dermatol Venereol. 149(4):423–6. PMID:25068230
**2093.** Prasad A, Rabionet R, Espinet B, Zapata L, Puiggros A, Melero C, et al. (2016). Identification of gene mutations and fusion genes in patients with Sézary syndrome. J Invest Dermatol. 136(7):1490–9. PMID:27039262
**2094.** Prescott RJ, Husain EA, Abdellaoui A, Al-Mahmoud RM, Khan M, Salman WD, et al. (2008). Superficial acral fibromyxoma: a clinicopathological study of new 41 cases from the U.K.: should myxoma (NOS) and fibroma (NOS) continue as part of 21st-century reporting? Br J Dermatol. 159(6):1315–21. PMID:18764846
**2095.** Price EB Jr, Silliphant WM, Shuman R (1961). Nodular fasciitis: a clinicopathologic analysis of 65 cases. Am J Clin Pathol. 35(2):122–36. PMID:13737962
**2096.** Price SK, Kahn LB, Saxe N (1993). Dermal and intravascular fasciitis. Unusual variants of nodular fasciitis. Am J Dermatopathol. 15(6):539–43. PMID:8311183
**2097.** Prieto VG, Reed JA, Shea CR (1995). Immunohistochemistry of dermatofibromas and benign fibrous histiocytomas. J Cutan Pathol. 22(4):336–41. PMID:7499573
**2098.** Prieto-Granada CN, Lezcano C, Scolyer RA, Mihm MC Jr, Piris A (2016). Lethal melanoma in children: a clinicopathological study of 12 cases. Pathology. 48(7):705–11. PMID:27956274
**2099.** Prieto-Granada CN, Wiesner T, Messina JL, Jungbluth AA, Chi P, Antonescu CR (2016). Loss of H3K27me3 expression is a highly sensitive marker for sporadic and radiation-induced MPNST. Am J Surg Pathol. 40(4):479–89. PMID:26645727
**2100.** Prieto-Granada CN, Zhang L, Antonescu CR, Henneberry JM, Messina JL (2017). Primary cutaneous adenoid cystic carcinoma with MYB aberrations: report of three cases and comprehensive review of the literature. J Cutan Pathol. 44(2):201–9. PMID:27859477
**2101.** Prince C, Mehregan AH, Hashimoto K, Plotnick H (1984). Large melanoacanthomas: a report of five cases. J Cutan Pathol. 11(4):309–17. PMID:6491009
**2102.** Proietti FA, Carneiro-Proietti AB, Catalan-Soares BC, Murphy EL (2005). Global epidemiology of HTLV-I infection and associated diseases. Oncogene. 24(39):6058–68. PMID:16155612
**2103.** Puig-Butillé JA, Carrera C, Kumar R, Garcia-Casado Z, Badenas C, Aguilera P, et al. (2013). Distribution of MC1R variants among melanoma subtypes: p.R163Q is associated with lentigo maligna melanoma in a Mediterranean population. Br J Dermatol. 169(4):804–11. PMID:23647022
**2104.** Pujol RM, LeBoit PE, Su WP (1997). Microcystic adnexal carcinoma with extensive sebaceous differentiation. Am J Dermatopathol. 19(4):358–62. PMID:9261470
**2105.** Pulitzer DR, Martin PC, Reed RJ (1995). Epithelioid glomus tumor. Hum Pathol. 26(9):1022–7. PMID:7672784
**2106.** Pulitzer MP, Amin BD, Busam KJ (2009). Merkel cell carcinoma: review. Adv Anat Pathol. 16(3):135–44. PMID:19395876
**2107.** Pulitzer MP, Brannon AR, Berger MF, Louis P, Scott SN, Jungbluth AA, et al. (2015). Cutaneous squamous and neuroendocrine carcinoma: genetically and immunohistochemically different from Merkel cell carcinoma. Mod Pathol. 28(8):1023–32. PMID:26022453
**2108.** Puls F, Hofvander J, Magnusson L, Nilsson J, Haywood E, Sumathi VP, et al. (2016). FN1-EGF gene fusions are recurrent in calcifying aponeurotic fibroma. J Pathol. 238(4):502–7. PMID:26691015
**2109.** Puntervoll HE, Yang XR, Vetti HH, Bachmann IM, Avril MF, Benfodda M, et al. (2013). Melanoma prone families with CDK4 germline mutation: phenotypic profile and associations with MC1R variants. J Med Genet. 50(4):264–70. PMID:23384855
**2110.** Pursley TV (1983). Nevus lipomatosus cutaneous superficialis. Int J Dermatol. 22(7):430–1. PMID:6629609
**2111.** Pyne JH, Myint E, Barr EM, Clark SP, David M, Na R (2017). Acantholytic invasive squamous cell carcinoma: tumor diameter, invasion depth, grade of differentiation, surgical margins, perineural invasion, recurrence and death rate. J Cutan Pathol. 44(4):320–7. PMID:27991679
**2112.** Quaglino P, Pimpinelli N, Berti E, Calzavara-Pinton P, Alfonso Lombardo G, Rupoli S, et al. (2012). Time course, clinical pathways, and long-term hazards risk trends of disease progression in patients with classic mycosis fungoides: a multicenter, retrospective follow-up study from the Italian Group of Cutaneous Lymphomas. Cancer. 118(23):5830–9. PMID:22674564
**2113.** Quante M, Patel NK, Hill S, Merchant W, Courtauld E, Newman P, et al. (1998). Epithelioid hemangioendothelioma presenting in the skin: a clinicopathologic study of eight cases. Am J Dermatopathol. 20(6):541–6. PMID:9855348
**2114.** Que SK, Weston G, Suchecki J, Ricketts J (2015). Pigmentary disorders of the eyes and skin. Clin Dermatol. 33(2):147–58. PMID:25704935
**2115.** Quint KD, Cleven AH, Vermeer MH (2017). Special variant of histiocytosis. BMJ Case Rep. 2017:bcr-2017-221538. PMID:29070620
**2116.** Quintanilla-Martinez L, Jansen PM, Kinney MC, Swerdlow SH, Willemze R (2013). Non-mycosis fungoides cutaneous T-cell lymphomas: report of the 2011 Society for Hematopathology/European Association for Haematopathology workshop. Am J Clin Pathol. 139(4):491–514. PMID:23525618
**2117.** Quintanilla-Martinez L, Ridaura C, Nagl F, Sáez-de-Ocariz M, Durán-McKinster C, Ruiz-Maldonado R, et al. (2013). Hydroa vacciniforme-like lymphoma: a chronic EBV+ lymphoproliferative disorder with risk to develop a systemic lymphoma. Blood. 122(18):3101–10. PMID:23982171
**2118.** Quist SR, Eckardt M, Kriesche A, Gollnick HP (2016). Expression of epidermal stem cell markers in skin and adnexal malignancies. Br J Dermatol. 175(3):520–30. PMID:26914519
**2119.** Qureshi HS, Ormsby AH, Lee MW, Zarbo RJ, Ma CK (2004). The diagnostic utility of p63, CK5/6, CK 7, and CK 20 in distinguishing primary cutaneous adnexal neoplasms from metastatic carcinomas. J Cutan Pathol. 31(2):145–52. PMID:14690459
**2120.** Qureshi HS, Salama ME, Chitale D, Bansal I, Ma CK, Raju U, et al. (2004). Primary cutaneous mucinous carcinoma: presence of myoepithelial cells as a clue to the cutaneous origin. Am J Dermatopathol. 26(5):353–8. PMID:15365364
**2121.** Rabenhorst A, Christopeit B, Leja S, Gerbaulet A, Kleiner S, Förster A, et al. (2013). Serum levels of bone cytokines are increased in indolent systemic mastocytosis associated with osteopenia or osteoporosis. J Allergy Clin Immunol. 132(5):1234–7.e7. PMID:23910691
**2122.** Rahbari H, Mehregan AH (1981). Sporadic atypical mole syndrome. A report of five nonfamilial B-K mole syndrome-like cases and histopathologic findings. Arch Dermatol. 117(6):329–31. PMID:7247423
**2123.** Rahimi AD, Shelton R, Dumas A, DiConstanzo D, Phelps R (2001). Mohs micrographic surgery of a plexiform fibrohistiocytic tumor. Dermatol Surg. 27(8):768–71. PMID:11493305
**2124.** Rahman MM, Chowdhury UK, Mukherjee SC, Mondal BK, Paul K, Lodh D, et al. (2001). Chronic arsenic toxicity in Bangladesh and West Bengal, India–a review and commentary. J Toxicol Clin Toxicol. 39(7):683–700. PMID:11778666
**2125.** Raj S, Calonje E, Kraus M, Kavanagh G, Newman PL, Fletcher CD (1997). Cutaneous pilar leiomyoma: clinicopathologic analysis of 53 lesions in 45 patients. Am J Dermatopathol. 19(1):2–9. PMID:9056647
**2126.** Rajyaguru DJ, Bhaskar C, Borgert AJ, Smith A, Parsons B (2017). Intravascular large B-cell lymphoma in the United States (US): a population-based study using Surveillance, Epidemiology, and End Results program and National Cancer Database. Leuk Lymphoma. 58(9):1–9. PMID:28278725
**2127.** Ramakrishna R, Sarathy K, Sarathy T (2013). Rituximab therapy in cutaneous infiltration of chronic lymphocytic leukaemia. Acta Haematol. 130(1):47–51. PMID:23406682
**2128.** Ramakrishnan R, Chaudhry IH, Ramdial P, Lazar AJ, McMenamin ME, Kazakov D, et al. (2013). Primary cutaneous adenoid cystic carcinoma: a clinicopathologic and immunohistochemical study of 27 cases. Am J Surg Pathol. 37(10):1603–11. PMID:24025525
**2129.** Ramani P, Shah A (1993). Lymphangiomatosis. Histologic and immunohistochemical analysis of four cases. Am J Surg Pathol. 17(4):329–35. PMID:8494102
**2130.** Ramesh P, Annapureddy SR, Khan F, Sutaria PD (2004). Angioleiomyoma: a clinical, pathological and radiological review. Int J Clin Pract. 58(6):587–91. PMID:15311559
**2131.** Ramolia P, Treadwell P, Haggstrom A (2009). Speckled lentiginous nevus syndrome associated with musculoskeletal abnormalities. Pediatr Dermatol. 26(3):298–301. PMID:19706091
**2132.** Ramos da Silva S, Ferraz da Silva AP, Bacchi MM, Bacchi CE, Elgui de Oliveira D (2011). KSHV genotypes A and C are more frequent in Kaposi sarcoma lesions from Brazilian patients with and without HIV infection, respectively. Cancer Lett. 301(1):85–94. PMID:21109347
**2133.** Ramos-Caro FA, Sexton FM, Browder JF, Flowers FP (1992). Acantholytic acanthomas in an immunosuppressed patient. J Am Acad Dermatol. 27(3):452–3. PMID:1401284
**2134.** Rangwala S, Tsai KY (2011). Roles of the immune system in skin cancer. Br J Dermatol. 165(5):953–65. PMID:21729024
**2135.** Rao NA, Hidayat AA, McLean IW, Zimmerman LE (1982). Sebaceous carcinomas of the ocular adnexa: a clinicopathologic study of 104 cases, with five-year follow-up data. Hum Pathol. 13(2):113–22. PMID:7076199
**2136.** Rapini RP, Golitz LE (1989). Sclerotic fibromas of the skin. J Am Acad Dermatol. 20(2 Pt 1):266–71. PMID:2464630
**2137.** Ratterman M, Kruczek K, Sulo S, Shanafelt TD, Kay NE, Nabhan C (2014). Extramedullary chronic lymphocytic leukemia: systematic analysis of cases reported between 1975 and 2012. Leuk Res. 38(3):299–303. PMID:24064196
**2138.** Ratzinger G, Burgdorf WH, Metze D, Zelger BG, Zelger B (2005). Indeterminate cell histiocytosis: fact or fiction? J Cutan Pathol. 32(8):552–60. PMID:16115054
**2139.** Raut CP, Miceli R, Strauss DC, Swallow CJ, Hohenberger P, van Coevorden F, et al. (2016). External validation of a multi-institutional retroperitoneal sarcoma nomogram. Cancer. 122(9):1417–24. PMID:26916507
**2140.** Read J, Wadt KA, Hayward NK (2016). Melanoma genetics. J Med Genet. 53(1):1–14. PMID:26337759
**2141.** Rebel HG, Bodmann CA, van de Glind GC, de Gruijl FR (2012). UV-induced ablation of the epidermal basal layer including p53-mutant clones resets UV carcinogenesis showing squamous cell carcinomas to originate from interfollicular epidermis. Carcinogenesis. 33(3):714–20. PMID:22227037
**2142.** Redono C, Rocamora A, Villoria F, Garcia M (1982). Malignant mixed tumor of the skin: malignant chondroid syringoma. Cancer. 49(8):1690–6. PMID:6279274
**2143.** Reed ML, Jacoby RA (1983). Cutaneous neuroanatomy and neuropathology. Normal nerves, neural-crest derivatives, and benign neural neoplasms in the skin. Am J Dermatopathol. 5(4):335–62. PMID:6638406
**2144.** Reed RJ (1976). Acral lentiginous melanoma. In: Hartman W, Kay S, Reed RJ, editors. New concepts in surgical pathology of the skin. New York: Wiley; pp. 89–90.
**2145.** Reed RJ, Fine RM, Meltzer HD (1972). Palisaded, encapsulated neuromas of the skin. Arch Dermatol. 106(6):865–70. PMID:4639250
**2146.** Reed RJ, Ichinose H, Clark WH Jr, Mihm MC Jr (1975). Common and uncommon melanocytic nevi and borderline melanomas. Semin Oncol. 2(2):119–47. PMID:1234372
**2147.** Regauer S, Beham-Schmid C, Okcu M, Hartner E, Mannweiler S (2000). Trichoblastic carcinoma ("malignant trichoblastoma") with lymphatic and hematogenous metastases. Mod Pathol. 13(6):673–8. PMID:10874673
**2148.** Rehman I, Takata M, Wu YY, Rees JL (1996). Genetic change in actinic keratoses. Oncogene. 12(12):2483–90. PMID:8700506
**2149.** Reifenberger J, Wolter M, Knobbe CB, Köhler B, Schönicke A, Scharwächter C, et al. (2005). Somatic mutations in the PTCH, SMOH, SUFUH and TP53 genes in sporadic basal cell carcinomas. Br J Dermatol. 152(1):43–51. PMID:15656799

2150. Reimann JD, Fletcher CD (2007). Myxoid dermatofibrosarcoma protuberans: a rare variant analyzed in a series of 23 cases. Am J Surg Pathol. 31(9):1371–7. PMID:17721193
2151. Reis JP, Tellechea O, Cunha MF, Baptista AP (1993). Trichilemmal carcinoma: review of 8 cases. J Cutan Pathol. 20(1):44–9. PMID:8468416
2152. Remstein ED, Arndt CA, Nascimento AG (1999). Plexiform fibrohistiocytic tumor: clinicopathologic analysis of 22 cases. Am J Surg Pathol. 23(6):662–70. PMID:10366148
2153. Requena C, Botella R, Nagore E, Sanmartín O, Llombart B, Serra-Guillén C, et al. (2012). Characteristics of spitzoid melanoma and clues for differential diagnosis with Spitz nevus. Am J Dermatopathol. 34(5):478–86. PMID:22257900
2154. Requena C, Requena L, Kutzner H, Sánchez Yus E (2009). Spitz nevus: a clinicopathological study of 349 cases. Am J Dermatopathol. 31(2):107–16. PMID:19318795
2155. Requena L, Gutiérrez J, Sánchez Yus E (1992). Multiple sclerotic fibromas of the skin. A cutaneous marker of Cowden's disease. J Cutan Pathol. 19(4):346–51. PMID:1430474
2156. Requena L, Hiromano K, Bernard A, Ackerman MD, Carter D, editors (1998). Neoplasm with apocrine differentiation. In: Ackerman's histologic diagnosis of neoplastic diseases. Philadelphia: Lippincott Williams & Wilkins.
2157. Requena L, Kutzner H, editors (2014). Cutaneous soft tissue tumors. Philadelphia: Lippincott Williams & Wilkins; pp. 33–42.
2158. Requena L, Kutzner H, Mentzel T, Durán R, Rodríguez-Peralto JL (2002). Benign vascular proliferations in irradiated skin. Am J Surg Pathol. 26(3):328–37. PMID:11859204
2159. Requena L, Luis Díaz J, Manzarbeitia F, Carrillo R, Fernández-Herrera J, Kutzner H (2008). Cutaneous composite hemangioendothelioma with satellitosis and lymph node metastases. J Cutan Pathol. 35(2):225–30. PMID:18190450
2160. Requena L, Marquina A, Alegre V, Aliaga A, Sanchez Yus E (1990). Sclerosing-sweat-duct (microcystic adnexal) carcinoma–a tumor from a single eccrine origin. Clin Exp Dermatol. 15(3):222–4. PMID:2163783
2161. Requena L, Prieto VG, Requena C, Sarasa JL, Manzano R, Seco M, et al. (2011). Primary signet-ring cell/histiocytoid carcinoma of the eyelid: a clinicopathologic study of 5 cases and review of the literature. Am J Surg Pathol. 35(3):378–91. PMID:21317710
2162. Requena L, Requena C (2010). Histopathology of the more common viral skin infections. Actas Dermosifiliogr. 101(3):201–16. [Spanish] PMID:20398595
2163. Requena L, Sánchez M, Aguilar A, Ambrojo P, Sánchez Yus E (1990). Periungual porocarcinoma. Dermatologica. 180(3):177–80. PMID:2160378
2164. Requena L, Sangüeza O (2017). Cutaneous adnexal neoplasms. Cham: Springer International Publishing; pp. 75–81.
2165. Requena L, Sangüeza O (2017). Cutaneous adnexal neoplasms. Cham: Springer International Publishing; pp. 12–38.
2166. Requena L, Sangüeza O (2017). Cutaneous adnexal neoplasms. Cham: Springer International Publishing; pp. 27–33.
2167. Requena L, Sangüeza O (2017). Cutaneous adnexal neoplasms. Cham: Springer International Publishing; pp. 179–95.
2168. Requena L, Sangüeza O (2017). Cutaneous adnexal neoplasms. Cham: Springer International Publishing; pp. 139–44.
2169. Requena L, Sangüeza O (2017). Cutaneous adnexal neoplasms. Cham: Springer International Publishing; pp. 107–26.
2170. Requena L, Sangüeza OP (1995). Benign neoplasms with neural differentiation: a review. Am J Dermatopathol. 17(1):75–96. PMID:7695017
2171. Requena L, Sarasa JL, Piqué E, Fariña MC, Olivares M, Martín L (1997). Clear-cell porocarcinoma: another cutaneous marker of diabetes mellitus. Am J Dermatopathol. 19(5):540–4. PMID:9335250
2172. Requena L, Sitthinamsuwan P, Fried I, Kaddu S, Schirren CG, Schärer L, et al. (2013). A benign cutaneous plexiform hybrid tumor of perineurioma and cellular neurothekeoma. Am J Surg Pathol. 37(6):845–52. PMID:23598966
2173. Requena L, Yus ES, Simón P, del Rio E (1996). Induction of cutaneous hyperplasias by altered stroma. Am J Dermatopathol. 18(3):248–68. PMID:8806959
2174. Resende C, Araújo C, Vieira AP, Brito C (2013). Late onset Ito's nevus. BMJ Case Rep. 2013:bcr2013009746. PMID:23729678
2175. Resnik KS, Kantor GR, DiLeonardo M (2005). Granular parakeratotic acanthoma. Am J Dermatopathol. 27(5):393–6. PMID:16148407
2176. Reymond JL, Stoebner P, Amblard P (1980). Nevus lipomatosus cutaneous superficialis. An electron microscopic study of four cases. J Cutan Pathol. 7(5):295–301. PMID:7430482
2177. Reza AM, Farahnaz GZ, Hamideh S, Alinaghi SA, Saeed Z, Mostafa H (2010). Incidence of Mongolian spots and its common sites at two university hospitals in Tehran, Iran. Pediatr Dermatol. 27(4):397–8. PMID:20653863
2178. Rezk SA, Spagnolo DV, Brynes RK, Weiss LM (2008). Indeterminate cell tumor: a rare dendritic neoplasm. Am J Surg Pathol. 32(12):1868–76. PMID:18813122
2179. Ribé A (2008). Melanocytic lesions of the genital area with attention given to atypical genital nevi. J Cutan Pathol. 35 Suppl 2:24–7. PMID:18976416
2180. Ribero S, Osella-Abate S, Reyes-Garcia D, Glass D, Bataille V (2017). Effects of sex on naevus body distribution and melanoma risk in two melanoma case-control studies at different latitudes. Br J Dermatol. 176(4):1093–4. PMID:27478920
2181. Riccardi VM (1981). Cutaneous manifestation of neurofibromatosis: cellular interaction, pigmentation, and mast cells. Birth Defects Orig Artic Ser. 17(2):129–45. PMID:6802200
2182. Riccardi VM (1981). Von Recklinghausen neurofibromatosis. N Engl J Med. 305(27):1617–27. PMID:6796886
2183. Riccardi VM, Margos VA (1981). Characteristics of skin and tumor fibroblasts from neurofibromatosis patients. Adv Neurol. 29:191–8. PMID:6798835
2184. Richert B, Theunis A, Norrenberg S, André J (2013). Tangential excision of pigmented nail matrix lesions responsible for longitudinal melanonychia: evaluation of the technique on a series of 30 patients. J Am Acad Dermatol. 69(1):96–104. PMID:23453241
2185. Richfield DF (1980). Tricholemmoma. True and false types. Am J Dermatopathol. 2(3):233–4. PMID:7258556
2186. Riethdorf S, Neffen EF, Cviko A, Löning T, Crum CP, Riethdorf L (2004). p16INK4A expression as biomarker for HPV 16-related vulvar neoplasias. Hum Pathol. 35(12):1477–83. PMID:15619206
2187. Rigaud C, Barkaoui MA, Thomas C, Bertrand Y, Lambilliotte A, Miron J, et al. (2016). Langerhans cell histiocytosis: therapeutic strategy and outcome in a 30-year nationwide cohort of 1478 patients under 18 years of age. Br J Haematol. 174(6):887–98. PMID:27273725
2188. Riggi N, Cironi L, Provero P, Suvà ML, Kaloulis K, Garcia-Echeverria C, et al. (2005). Development of Ewing's sarcoma from primary bone marrow-derived mesenchymal progenitor cells. Cancer Res. 65(24):11459–68. PMID:16357154
2189. Riggi N, Suvà ML, Suvà D, Cironi L, Provero P, Tercier S, et al. (2008). EWS-FLI-1 expression triggers a Ewing's sarcoma initiation program in primary human mesenchymal stem cells. Cancer Res. 68(7):2176–85. PMID:18381423
2190. Rijlaarsdam JU, van der Putte SC, Berti E, Kerl H, Rieger E, Toonstra J, et al. (1993). Cutaneous immunocytomas: a clinicopathologic study of 26 cases. Histopathology. 23(2):117–25. PMID:8406383
2191. Rijlaarsdam U, Bakels V, van Oostveen JW, Gordijn RJ, Geerts ML, Meijer CJ, et al. (1992). Demonstration of clonal immunoglobulin gene rearrangements in cutaneous B-cell lymphomas and pseudo-B-cell lymphomas: differential diagnostic and pathogenetic aspects. J Invest Dermatol. 99(6):749–54. PMID:1469288
2192. Ríos-Martín JJ, Delgado MD, Moreno-Ramírez D, García-Escudero A, González-Cámpora R (2007). Granular cell atypical fibroxanthoma: report of two cases. Am J Dermatopathol. 29(1):84–7. PMID:17284969
2193. Ritterhouse LL, Barletta JA (2015). BRAF V600E mutation-specific antibody: a review. Semin Diagn Pathol. 32(5):400–8. PMID:25744437
2194. Rizzi R, Curci P, Delia M, Rinaldi E, Chiefa A, Specchia G, et al. (2009). Spontaneous remission of "methotrexate-associated lymphoproliferative disorders" after discontinuation of immunosuppressive treatment for autoimmune disease. Review of the literature. Med Oncol. 26(1):1–9. PMID:18461290
2195. Robak E, Robak T (2007). Skin lesions in chronic lymphocytic leukemia. Leuk Lymphoma. 48(5):855–65. PMID:17487727
2196. Roberts ME, Riegert-Johnson DL, Thomas BC, Rumilla KM, Thomas CS, Heckman MG, et al. (2014). A clinical scoring system to identify patients with sebaceous neoplasms at risk for the Muir-Torre variant of Lynch syndrome. Genet Med. 16(9):711–6. PMID:24603434
2197. Roberts ME, Riegert-Johnson DL, Thomas BC, Thomas CS, Heckman MG, Krishna M, et al. (2013). Screening for Muir-Torre syndrome using mismatch repair protein immunohistochemistry of sebaceous neoplasms. J Genet Couns. 22(3):393–405. PMID:23212176
2198. Robertson AG, Shih J, Yau C, Gibb EA, Oba J, Mungall KL, et al. (2017). Integrative analysis identifies four molecular and clinical subsets in uveal melanoma. Cancer Cell. 32(2):204–20.e15. PMID:28810145
2199. Robinson MR, Honda KS, Bordeaux JS (2011). Angiosarcoma in an obese woman with worsening lymphedema after weight-loss and skin-reduction surgeries. J Am Acad Dermatol. 65(2):448–9. PMID:21763582
2200. Robles-Espinoza CD, Harland M, Ramsay AJ, Aoude LG, Quesada V, Ding Z, et al. (2014). POT1 loss-of-function variants predispose to familial melanoma. Nat Genet. 46(5):478–81. PMID:24686849
2201. Robles-Espinoza CD, Roberts ND, Chen S, Leacy FP, Alexandrov LB, Pornputtapong N, et al. (2016). Germline MC1R status influences somatic mutation burden in melanoma. Nat Commun. 7:12064. PMID:27403562
2202. Robson A, Assaf C, Bagot M, Burg G, Calonje E, Castillo C, et al. (2015). Aggressive epidermotropic cutaneous CD8+ lymphoma: a cutaneous lymphoma with distinct clinical and pathological features. Report of an EORTC Cutaneous Lymphoma Task Force Workshop. Histopathology. 67(4):425–41. PMID:24438036
2203. Robson A, Greene J, Ansari N, Kim B, Seed PT, McKee PH, et al. (2001). Eccrine porocarcinoma (malignant eccrine poroma): a clinicopathologic study of 69 cases. Am J Surg Pathol. 25(6):710–20. PMID:11395548
2204. Robson A, Lazar AJ, Ben Nagi J, Hanby A, Grayson W, Feinmesser M, et al. (2008). Primary cutaneous apocrine carcinoma: a clinico-pathologic analysis of 24 cases. Am J Surg Pathol. 32(5):682–90. PMID:18347508
2205. Robson A, Morley-Quante M, Hempel H, McKee PH, Calonje E (2003). Deep penetrating naevus: clinicopathological study of 31 cases with further delineation of histological features allowing distinction from other pigmented benign melanocytic lesions and melanoma. Histopathology. 43(6):529–37. PMID:14636253
2206. Robson AM, Calonje E (2000). Cutaneous perineurioma: a poorly recognized tumour often misdiagnosed as epithelioid histiocytoma. Histopathology. 37(4):332–9. PMID:11012740
2207. Roden AC, Hu X, Kip S, Parrilla Castellar ER, Rumilla KM, Vrana JA, et al. (2014). BRAF V600E expression in Langerhans cell histiocytosis: clinical and immunohistochemical study on 25 pulmonary and 54 extrapulmonary cases. Am J Surg Pathol. 38(4):548–51. PMID:24625419
2208. Rodig SJ, Payne EG, Degar BA, Rollins B, Feldman AL, Jaffe ES, et al. (2008). Aggressive Langerhans cell histiocytosis following T-ALL: clonally related neoplasms with persistent expression of constitutively active NOTCH1. Am J Hematol. 83(2):116–21. PMID:17874453
2209. Rodríguez Pinilla SM, Roncador G, Rodríguez-Peralto JL, Mollejo M, García JF, Montes-Moreno S, et al. (2009). Primary cutaneous CD4+ small/medium-sized pleomorphic T-cell lymphoma expresses follicular T-cell markers. Am J Surg Pathol. 33(1):81–90. PMID:18987541
2210. Rodríguez D, Cornejo KM, Sadow PM, Santiago-Lastra Y, Feldman AS (2015). Myopericytoma tumor of the glans penis. Can J Urol. 22(3):7830–3. PMID:26068635
2211. Rodríguez-Díaz E, Román C, Yuste M, Morán AG, Aramendi T (1998). Cutaneous lymphadenoma: an adnexal neoplasm with intralobular activated lymphoid cells. Am J Dermatopathol. 20(1):74–8. PMID:9504675
2212. Rodríguez-Jurado R, Palacios C, Durán-McKinster C, Mercadillo P, Orozco-Covarrubias L, Saez-de-Ocariz MdelM, et al. (2004). Medallion-like dermal dendrocyte hamartoma: a new clinically and histopathologically distinct lesion. J Am Acad Dermatol. 51(3):359–63. PMID:15337977
2213. Rodríguez-Pinilla SM, Barrionuevo C, Garcia J, Martínez MT, Pajares R, Montes-Moreno S, et al. (2010). EBV-associated cutaneous NK/T-cell lymphoma: review of a series of 14 cases from Peru in children and young adults. Am J Surg Pathol. 34(12):1773–82. PMID:21107082
2214. Rodríguez-Pinilla SM, Ortiz-Romero PL, Monsalvez V, Tomás IE, Almagro M, Sevilla A, et al. (2013). TCR-γ expression in primary cutaneous T-cell lymphomas. Am J Surg Pathol. 37(3):375–84. PMID:23348211
2215. Rogers A, Graves M, Toscano M, Davis L (2014). A unique cutaneous presentation of Burkitt lymphoma. Am J Dermatopathol. 36(12):997–1001. PMID:24562050
2216. Rogers HW, Weinstock MA, Harris AR, Hinckley MR, Feldman SR, Fleischer AB, et al. (2010). Incidence estimate of nonmelanoma skin cancer in the United States, 2006. Arch Dermatol. 146(3):283–7. PMID:20231499
2217. Rogozinski TT, Jablonska S, Jarzabek-Chorzelska M (1988). Role of cell-mediated immunity in spontaneous regression of plane warts. Int J Dermatol. 27(5):322–6. PMID:2839432

2218. Rokuhara S, Saida T, Oguchi M, Matsumoto K, Murase S, Oguchi S (2004). Number of acquired melanocytic nevi in patients with melanoma and control subjects in Japan: nevus count is a significant risk factor for nonacral melanoma but not for acral melanoma. J Am Acad Dermatol. 50(5):695–700. PMID:15097952
2219. Roland CL, Wang WL, Lazar AJ, Torres KE (2016). Myxofibrosarcoma. Surg Oncol Clin N Am. 25(4):775–88. PMID:27591498
2220. Rolland S, Kokta V, Marcoux D (2009). Meyerson phenomenon in children: observation in five cases of congenital melanocytic nevi. Pediatr Dermatol. 26(3):292–7. PMID:19706090
2221. Romero-Pérez D, García-Bustinduy M, Cribier B (2017). Clinicopathologic study of 90 cases of trichofolliculoma. J Eur Acad Dermatol Venereol. 31(3):e141–2. PMID:27608202
2222. Ronger S, Touzet S, Ligeron C, Balme B, Viallard AM, Barrut D, et al. (2002). Dermoscopic examination of nail pigmentation. Arch Dermatol. 138(10):1327–33. PMID:12374538
2223. Rongioletti F, Ball RA, Marcus R, Barnhill RL (2000). Histopathological features of flexural melanocytic nevi: a study of 40 cases. J Cutan Pathol. 27(5):215–7. PMID:10847544
2224. Rongioletti F, Gambini C, Lerza R (1994). Glomeruloid hemangioma. A cutaneous marker of POEMS syndrome. Am J Dermatopathol. 16(2):175–8. PMID:8030771
2225. Rongioletti F, Margaritescu I, Smoller BR, editors (2015). Rare malignant skin tumours. Berlin: Springer.
2226. Rongioletti F, Urso C, Batolo D, Chimenti S, Fanti PA, Filotico R, et al. (2004). Melanocytic nevi of the breast: a histologic case-control study. J Cutan Pathol. 31(2):137–40. PMID:14690457
2227. Rooney MT, Nascimento AG, Tung RL (1994). Ossifying plexiform tumor. Report of a cutaneous ossifying lesion with histologic features of neurothekeoma. Am J Dermatopathol. 16(2):189–92. PMID:8030774
2228. Roos-Weil D, Dietrich S, Boumendil A, Polge E, Bron D, Carreras E, et al. (2013). Stem cell transplantation can provide durable disease control in blastic plasmacytoid dendritic cell neoplasm: a retrospective study from the European Group for Blood and Marrow Transplantation. Blood. 121(3):440–6. PMID:23203822
2229. Rosai J (1982). Angiolymphoid hyperplasia with eosinophilia of the skin. Its nosological position in the spectrum of histiocytoid hemangioma. Am J Dermatopathol. 4(2):175–84. PMID:6980603
2230. Rosati LA, Fratamico FC, Eusebi V (1986). Cellular neurothekeoma. Appl Pathol. 4(3):186–91. PMID:3297114
2231. Roschewski M, Wilson WH (2012). Lymphomatoid granulomatosis. Cancer J. 18(5):469–74. PMID:23006954
2232. Rosen PP (1983). Syringomatous adenoma of the nipple. Am J Surg Pathol. 7(8):739–45. PMID:6660349
2233. Rosenberg AS, Morgan MB (2001). Cutaneous indeterminate cell histiocytosis: a new spindle cell variant resembling dendritic cell sarcoma. J Cutan Pathol. 28(10):531–7. PMID:11737523
2234. Rosner IA, Argenta AE, Washington KM (2017). Unusual volar pulp location of glomus tumor. Plast Reconstr Surg Glob Open. 5(1):e1215. PMID:28203512
2235. Ross AS, Whalen FM, Elenitsas R, Xu X, Troxel AB, Schmults CD (2009). Diameter of involved nerves predicts outcomes in cutaneous squamous cell carcinoma with perineural invasion: an investigator-blinded retrospective cohort study. Dermatol Surg. 35(12):1859–66. PMID:19889009
2236. Ross HM, Lewis JJ, Woodruff JM, Brennan MF (1997). Epithelioid sarcoma: clinical behavior and prognostic factors of survival. Ann Surg Oncol. 4(6):491–5. PMID:9309338
2237. Rossi R, Mori M, Lotti T (2007). Actinic keratosis. Int J Dermatol. 46(9):895–904. PMID:17822489
2238. Rossi S, Orvieto E, Furlanetto A, Laurino L, Ninfo V, Dei Tos AP (2004). Utility of the immunohistochemical detection of FLI-1 expression in round cell and vascular neoplasm using a monoclonal antibody. Mod Pathol. 17(5):547–52. PMID:15001993
2239. Rossini AA, Cahill GF Jr, Jeanioz DA, Jeanioz RW (1975). Anomeric specificty of 3-0-methyl-D-glycopyranose against alloxan diabetes. Science. 188(4183):70–1. PMID:1167978
2240. Rossini M, Zanotti R, Bonadonna P, Artuso A, Caruso B, Schena D, et al. (2011). Bone mineral density, bone turnover markers and fractures in patients with indolent systemic mastocytosis. Bone. 49(4):880–5. PMID:21782049
2241. Rossini M, Zanotti R, Orsolini G, Tripi G, Viapiana O, Idolazzi L, et al. (2016). Prevalence, pathogenesis, and treatment options for mastocytosis-related osteoporosis. Osteoporos Int. 27(8):2411–21. PMID:26892042
2242. Rosso S, Zanetti R, Martinez C, Tormo MJ, Schraub S, Sancho-Garnier H, et al. (1996). The multicentre south European study 'Helios'. II: Different sun exposure patterns in the aetiology of basal cell and squamous cell carcinomas of the skin. Br J Cancer. 73(11):1447–54. PMID:8645596
2243. Roten SV, Bhawan J (1995). Isolated dyskeratotic acanthoma. A variant of isolated epidermolytic acanthoma. Am J Dermatopathol. 17(1):63–6. PMID:7695013
2244. Roth MJ, Medeiros LJ, Elenitoba-Johnson K, Kuchnio M, Jaffe ES, Stetler-Stevenson M (1995). Extramedullary myeloid cell tumors. An immunohistochemical study of 29 cases using routinely fixed and processed paraffin-embedded tissue sections. Arch Pathol Lab Med. 119(9):790–8. PMID:7668936
2245. Roth MJ, Stern JB, Hijazi Y, Haupt HM, Kumar A (1996). Oncocytic nodular hidradenoma. Am J Dermatopathol. 18(3):314–6. PMID:8806968
2246. Rothman IL (2014). Michelin tire baby syndrome: a review of the literature and a proposal for diagnostic criteria with adoption of the name circumferential skin folds syndrome. Pediatr Dermatol. 31(6):659–63. PMID:25424205
2247. Rouhani P, Fletcher CD, Devesa SS, Toro JR (2008). Cutaneous soft tissue sarcoma incidence patterns in the U.S.: an analysis of 12,114 cases. Cancer. 113(3):616–27. PMID:18618615
2248. Rouzbahman M, Kamel-Reid S, Al Habeeb A, Butler M, Dodge J, Laframboise S, et al. (2015). Malignant melanoma of vulva and vagina: a histomorphological review and mutation analysis–a single-center study. J Low Genit Tract Dis. 19(4):350–3. PMID:26225944
2249. Royo C, Salaverria I, Hartmann EM, Rosenwald A, Campo E, Beà S (2011). The complex landscape of genetic alterations in mantle cell lymphoma. Semin Cancer Biol. 21(5):322–34. PMID:21945515
2250. Rozza-de-Menezes RE, Andrade RM, Israel MS, Gonçalves Cunha KS (2013). Intraoral nerve sheath myxoma: case report and systematic review of the literature. Head Neck. 35(12):E397–404. PMID:23616426
2251. Ruben BS (2010). Pigmented lesions of the nail unit: clinical and histopathologic features. Semin Cutan Med Surg. 29(3):148–58. PMID:21051008
2252. Rubin AI, Chen EH, Ratner D (2005). Basal-cell carcinoma. N Engl J Med. 353(21):2262–9. PMID:16306523
2253. Rubin AI, Yassaee M, Johnson W, Elenitsas R, Zaladonis J Jr, Seykora JT (2009). Multiple cutaneous sclerosing perineuriomas: an extensive presentation with involvement of the bilateral upper extremities. J Cutan Pathol. 36 Suppl 1:60–5. PMID:19187114
2254. Rüdiger T, Weisenburger DD, Anderson JR, Armitage JO, Diebold J, MacLennan KA, et al. (2002). Peripheral T-cell lymphoma (excluding anaplastic large-cell lymphoma): results from the Non-Hodgkin's Lymphoma Classification Project. Ann Oncol. 13(1):140–9. PMID:11863096
2255. Ruëff F, Przybilla B, Biló MB, Müller U, Scheipl F, Aberer W, et al. (2009). Predictors of severe systemic anaphylactic reactions in patients with Hymenoptera venom allergy: importance of baseline serum tryptase-a study of the European Academy of Allergology and Clinical Immunology Interest Group on Insect Venom Hypersensitivity. J Allergy Clin Immunol. 124(5):1047–54. PMID:19895993
2256. Ruhoy SM, Prieto VG, Eliason SL, Grichnik JM, Burchette JL Jr, Shea CR (2000). Malignant melanoma with paradoxical maturation. Am J Surg Pathol. 24(12):1600–14. PMID:11117780
2257. Ruiz-Villaverde R, Sanchez-Cano D, Martinez-Peinado CM, Galan-Gutierrez M (2016). Verrucous tumor mimicking squamous cell carcinoma in immunocompetent patient. Dermatol Online J. 22(2). PMID:27267196
2258. Rulon DB, Helwig EB (1973). Multiple sebaceous neoplasms of the skin: an association with multiple visceral carcinomas, especially of the colon. Am J Clin Pathol. 60(6):745–52. PMID:4758274
2259. Rulon DB, Helwig EB (1974). Cutaneous sebaceous neoplasms. Cancer. 33(1):82–102. PMID:4129561
2260. Arumi-Uria M, McNutt NS, Finnerty B (2003). Grading of atypia in nevi: correlation with melanoma risk. Mod Pathol. 16(8):764–71. PMID:12920220
2261. Russell B, Pridie RB (1967). Lymphoedema of scrotum–scrotectomy–lymphangiectasia of anogenital region–? Congenital lymphatic deficiency and past filariasis. Br J Dermatol. 79(5):298–9. PMID:6025577
2262. Rutkowski P, Van Glabbeke M, Rankin CJ, Ruka W, Rubin BP, Debiec-Rychter M, et al. (2010). Imatinib mesylate in advanced dermatofibrosarcoma protuberans: pooled analysis of two phase II clinical trials. J Clin Oncol. 28(10):1772–9. PMID:20194851
2263. Rütten A, Burgdorf W, Hügel H, Kutzner H, Hosseiny-Malayeri HR, Friedl W, et al. (1999). Cystic sebaceous tumors as marker lesions for the Muir-Torre syndrome: a histopathologic and molecular genetic study. Am J Dermatopathol. 21(5):405–13. PMID:10535567
2264. Rütten A, Kutzner H, Mentzel T, Hantschke M, Eckert F, Angulo J, et al. (2009). Primary cutaneous cribriform apocrine carcinoma: a clinicopathologic and immunohistochemical study of 26 cases of an under-recognized cutaneous adnexal neoplasm. J Am Acad Dermatol. 61(4):644–51. PMID:19751882
2265. Rütten A, Requena L (2008). Sweat gland carcinomas of the skin. Hautarzt. 59(2):151–60. [German] PMID:18214401
2266. Rutter JL, Bromley CM, Goldstein AM, Elder DE, Holly EA, Guerry D 4th, et al. (2004). Heterogeneity of risk for melanoma and pancreatic and digestive malignancies: a melanoma case-control study. Cancer. 101(12):2809–16. PMID:15529312
2267. Rydholm A, Gustafson P, Rööser B, Willén H, Berg NO (1991). Subcutaneous sarcoma. A population-based study of 129 patients. J Bone Joint Surg Br. 73(4):662–7. PMID:2071656
2268. Saad N, Skowron F, Dalle S, Forestier JY, Balme B, Thomas L (2006). Multiple adult xanthogranuloma: case report and literature review. Dermatology. 212(1):73–6. PMID:16319479
2269. Sachdeva MP, Goldblum JR, Rubin BP, Billings SD (2009). Low-fat and fat-free pleomorphic lipomas: a diagnostic challenge. Am J Dermatopathol. 31(5):423–6. PMID:19542913
2270. Sachdeva S (2011). Ulcerated cutaneous epithelioid hemangioendothelioma in an 8-month old infant. Dermatol Reports. 3(2):e17. PMID:25386269
2271. Sáchez Yus E, Requena L, Simón P, del Río E (1995). Sebomatricoma: a unifying term that encompasses all benign neoplasms with sebaceous differentiation. Am J Dermatopathol. 17(3):213–21. PMID:8599428
2272. Sadow PM, Priolo C, Nanni S, Karreth FA, Duquette M, Martinelli R, et al. (2014). Role of BRAFV600E in the first preclinical model of multifocal infiltrating myopericytoma development and microenvironment. J Natl Cancer Inst. 106(8):dju182. PMID:25063326
2273. Sáez Rodríguez M, Rodríguez-Martin M, Carnerero A, Sidro M, Rodríguez F, Cabrera R, et al. (2005). Naevus lipomatosus cutaneous superficialis on the nose. J Eur Acad Dermatol Venereol. 19(6):751–2. PMID:16268886
2274. Sagebiel RW (1993). Melanocytic nevi in histologic association with primary cutaneous melanoma of superficial spreading and nodular types: effect of tumor thickness. J Invest Dermatol. 100(3):322S–5S. PMID:8440914
2275. Sagebiel RW, Chinn EK, Egbert BM (1984). Pigmented spindle cell nevus. Clinical and histologic review of 90 cases. Am J Surg Pathol. 8(9):645–53. PMID:6476194
2276. Saggini A, Gulia A, Argenyi Z, Fink-Puches R, Lissia A, Magaña M, et al. (2010). A variant of lymphomatoid papulosis simulating primary cutaneous aggressive epidermotropic CD8+ cytotoxic T-cell lymphoma. Description of 9 cases. Am J Surg Pathol. 34(8):1168–75. PMID:20661014
2277. Saha KC (2003). Diagnosis of arsenicosis. J Environ Sci Health A Tox Hazard Subst Environ Eng. 38(1):255–72. PMID:12635831
2278. Sahm F, Capper D, Preusser M, Meyer J, Stenzinger A, Lasitschka F, et al. (2012). BRAFV600E mutant protein is expressed in cells of variable maturation in Langerhans cell histiocytosis. Blood. 120(12):e28–34. PMID:22859608
2279. Saida T, Koga H, Uhara H (2011). Key points in dermoscopic differentiation between early acral melanoma and acral nevus. J Dermatol. 38(1):25–34. PMID:21175752
2280. Saida T, Miyazaki A, Oguchi S, Ishihara Y, Yamazaki Y, Murase S, et al. (2004). Significance of dermoscopic patterns in detecting malignant melanoma on acral volar skin: results of a multicenter study in Japan. Arch Dermatol. 140(10):1233–8. PMID:15492186
2281. Saijo S, Hara M, Kuramoto Y, Tagami H (1991). Generalized eruptive histiocytoma: a report of a variant case showing the presence of dermal indeterminate cells. J Cutan Pathol. 18(2):134–6. PMID:1856341
2282. Sakamoto A, Oda Y, Itakura E, Oshiro Y, Nikaido O, Iwamoto Y, et al. (2001). Immunoexpression of ultraviolet photoproducts and p53 mutation analysis in atypical fibroxanthoma and superficial malignant fibrous histiocytoma. Mod Pathol. 14(6):581–8. PMID:11406660
2283. Sakamoto F, Ito M, Sato S, Sato Y (1985). Basal cell tumor with apocrine differentiation: apocrine epithelioma. J Am Acad Dermatol. 13(2 Pt 2):355–63. PMID:4031160
2284. Sakharpe A, Lahat G, Gulamhusein T, Liu P, Bolshakov S, Nguyen T, et al. (2011).

Epithelioid sarcoma and unclassified sarcoma with epithelioid features: clinicopathological variables, molecular markers, and a new experimental model. Oncologist. 16(4):512–22. PMID:21357725
**2285.** Saldanha G, Fletcher A, Slater DN (2003). Basal cell carcinoma: a dermatopathological and molecular biological update. Br J Dermatol. 148(2):195–202. PMID:12588368
**2286.** Salgado CM, Basu D, Nikiforova M, Hamilton RL, Gehris R, Jakacki R, et al. (2015). Amplification of mutated NRAS leading to congenital melanoma in neurocutaneous melanocytosis. Melanoma Res. 25(5):453–60. PMID:26266759
**2287.** Salgado R, Llombart B, M Pujol R, Fernández-Serra A, Sanmartín O, Toll A, et al. (2011). Molecular diagnosis of dermatofibrosarcoma protuberans: a comparison between reverse transcriptase-polymerase chain reaction and fluorescence in situ hybridization methodologies. Genes Chromosomes Cancer. 50(7):510–7. PMID:21484928
**2288.** Salhany KE, Macon WR, Choi JK, Elenitsas R, Lessin SR, Felgar RE, et al. (1998). Subcutaneous panniculitis-like T-cell lymphoma: clinicopathologic, immunophenotypic, and genotypic analysis of alpha/beta and gamma/delta subtypes. Am J Surg Pathol. 22(7):881–93. PMID:9669350
**2289.** Salman A, Yucelten AD, Seckin D, Ergun T, Demircay Z (2015). Cutaneous leishmaniasis mimicking verrucous carcinoma: a case with an unusual clinical course. Indian J Dermatol Venereol Leprol. 81(4):392–4. PMID:25994897
**2290.** Salomao DR, Nascimento AG (1997). Plexiform fibrohistiocytic tumor with systemic metastases: a case report. Am J Surg Pathol. 21(4):469–76. PMID:9130995
**2291.** Salpea P, Horvath A, London E, Faucz FR, Vetro A, Levy I, et al. (2014). Deletions of the PRKAR1A locus at 17q24.2-q24.3 in Carney complex: genotype-phenotype correlations and implications for genetic testing. J Clin Endocrinol Metab. 99(1):E183–8. PMID:24170103
**2292.** Samadian M, Nejad AM, Bakhtevari MH, Sabeti S, Sharifi G, Jabbari R, et al. (2015). Primary meningeal melanocytoma in the left temporal lobe associated with nevus Ota: a case report and review of the literature. World Neurosurg. 84(2):567–73. PMID:25862111
**2293.** Samaha H, Dumontet C, Ketterer N, Moullet I, Thieblemont C, Bouafia F, et al. (1998). Mantle cell lymphoma: a retrospective study of 121 cases. Leukemia. 12(8):1281–7. PMID:9697885
**2294.** Samara WA, Khoo CT, Say EA, Saktanasate J, Eagle RC Jr, Shields JA, et al. (2015). Juvenile xanthogranuloma involving the eye and ocular adnexa: tumor control, visual outcomes, and globe salvage in 30 patients. Ophthalmology. 122(10):2130–8. PMID:26189188
**2295.** Samols MA, Su A, Ra S, Cappel MA, Louissant A Jr, Knudson RA, et al. (2014). Intralymphatic cutaneous anaplastic large cell lymphoma/lymphomatoid papulosis: expanding the spectrum of CD30-positive lymphoproliferative disorders. Am J Surg Pathol. 38(9):1203–11. PMID:24805854
**2296.** Sanchez DF, Rodriguez IM, Piris A, Cañete S, Lezcano C, Velazquez EF, et al. (2016). Clear cell carcinoma of the penis: an HPV-related variant of squamous cell carcinoma: a report of 3 cases. Am J Surg Pathol. 40(7):917–22. PMID:26848799
**2297.** Sanchez DF, Soares F, Alvarado-Cabrero I, Cañete S, Fernández-Nestosa MJ, Rodríguez IM, et al. (2015). Pathological factors, behavior, and histological prognostic risk groups in subtypes of penile squamous cell carcinomas (SCC). Semin Diagn Pathol. 32(3):222–31. PMID:25677263
**2298.** Sánchez Yus E, Aguilar A, Urbina F, Cristóbal MC, Vázquez F, Requena L (1988). Malignant cutaneous mixed tumor. A new case with unusual clinical features. Am J Dermatopathol. 10(4):330–4. PMID:2843063
**2299.** Sandell RF, Carter JM, Folpe AL (2015). Solitary (juvenile) xanthogranuloma: a comprehensive immunohistochemical study emphasizing recently developed markers of histiocytic lineage. Hum Pathol. 46(9):1390–7. PMID:26220162
**2300.** Sander CA, Flaig MJ, Jaffe ES (2001). Cutaneous manifestations of lymphoma: a clinical guide based on the WHO classification. Clin Lymphoma. 2(2):86–102. PMID:11707848
**2301.** Sander CA, Medeiros LJ, Abruzzo LV, Horak ID, Jaffe ES (1991). Lymphoblastic lymphoma presenting in cutaneous sites. A clinicopathologic analysis of six cases. J Am Acad Dermatol. 25(6 Pt 1):1023–31. PMID:1810981
**2302.** Sandoval M, Carrasco-Zuber J, Gonzalez S (2015). Extradigital symplastic glomus tumor of the hand: report of 2 cases and literature review. Am J Dermatopathol. 37(7):560–2. PMID:25051107
**2303.** Sanfilippo R, Miceli R, Grosso F, Fiore M, Puma E, Pennacchioli E, et al. (2011). Myxofibrosarcoma: prognostic factors and survival in a series of patients treated at a single institution. Ann Surg Oncol. 18(3):720–5. PMID:20878245
**2304.** Sangle NA, Schmidt RL, Patel JL, Medeiros LJ, Agarwal AM, Perkins SL, et al. (2014). Optimized immunohistochemical panel to differentiate myeloid sarcoma from blastic plasmacytoid dendritic cell neoplasm. Mod Pathol. 27(8):1137–43. PMID:24390220
**2305.** Sangueza M, Plaza JA (2013). Hydroa vacciniforme-like cutaneous T-cell lymphoma: clinicopathologic and immunohistochemical study of 12 cases. J Am Acad Dermatol. 69(1):112–9. PMID:23541598
**2306.** Sangueza OP, Requena L (1994). Neurofollicular hamartoma. A new histogenetic interpretation. Am J Dermatopathol. 16(2):150–4. PMID:8030767
**2307.** Sangüeza OP, Requena L (1998). Neoplasms with neural differentiation: a review. Part II: Malignant neoplasms. Am J Dermatopathol. 20(1):89–102. PMID:9504678
**2308.** Sangüeza OP, Walsh SN, Sheehan DJ, Orland AF, Llombart B, Requena L (2008). Cutaneous epithelioid angiomatous nodule: a case series and proposed classification. Am J Dermatopathol. 30(1):16–20. PMID:18212538
**2309.** Santa Cruz DJ, Barr RJ, Headington JT (1991). Cutaneous lymphadenoma. Am J Surg Pathol. 15(2):101–10. PMID:1989457
**2310.** Santa Cruz DJ, Prioleau PG (1984). Adnexal carcinomas of the skin. J Cutan Pathol. 11(5):450–6. PMID:6096426
**2311.** Santos-Juanes J, Galache Osuna C, Sánchez Del Río J, Soto de Delás J, Requena L (2005). Apocrine hidrocystoma on the tip of a finger. Br J Dermatol. 152(2):379–80. PMID:15727664
**2312.** Santucci M, Pimpinelli N, Arganini L (1991). Primary cutaneous B-cell lymphoma: a unique type of low-grade lymphoma. Clinicopathologic and immunologic study of 83 cases. Cancer. 67(9):2311–26. PMID:2013039
**2313.** Santucci M, Pimpinelli N, Massi D, Kadin ME, Meijer CJ, Müller-Hermelink HK, et al. (2003). Cytotoxic/natural killer cell cutaneous lymphomas. Report of EORTC Cutaneous Lymphoma Task Force Workshop. Cancer. 97(3):610–27. PMID:12548603
**2314.** Sápi Z, Papp G, Szendrői M, Pápai Z, Plótár V, Krausz T, et al. (2016). Epigenetic regulation of SMARCB1 by miR-206, -381 and -671-5p is evident in a variety of SMARCB1 immunonegative soft tissue sarcomas, while miR-765 appears specific for epithelioid sarcoma. A miRNA study of 223 soft tissue sarcomas. Genes Chromosomes Cancer. 55(10):786–802. PMID:27223121
**2315.** Sapienza MR, Fuligni F, Agostinelli C, Tripodo C, Righi S, Laginestra MA, et al. (2014). Molecular profiling of blastic plasmacytoid dendritic cell neoplasm reveals a unique pattern and suggests selective sensitivity to NF-kB pathway inhibition. Leukemia. 28(8):1606–16. PMID:24504027
**2316.** Sarangarajan R, Dehner LP (1999). Cranial and extracranial fasciitis of childhood: a clinicopathologic and immunohistochemical study. Hum Pathol. 30(1):87–92. PMID:9923933
**2317.** Sargen MR, Kanetsky PA, Newton-Bishop J, Hayward NK, Mann GJ, Gruis NA, et al. (2015). Histologic features of melanoma associated with CDKN2A genotype. J Am Acad Dermatol. 72(3):496–507.e7. PMID:25592620
**2318.** Sarin KY, McNiff JM, Kwok S, Kim J, Khavari PA (2014). Activating HRAS mutation in nevus spilus. J Invest Dermatol. 134(6):1766–8. PMID:24390138
**2319.** Sariya D, Ruth K, Adams-McDonnell R, Cusack C, Xu X, Elenitsas R, et al. (2007). Clinicopathologic correlation of cutaneous metastases: experience from a cancer center. Arch Dermatol. 143(5):613–20. PMID:17515511
**2320.** Sarkozy A, Carta C, Moretti S, Zampino G, Digilio MC, Pantaleoni F, et al. (2009). Germline BRAF mutations in Noonan, LEOPARD, and cardiofaciocutaneous syndromes: molecular diversity and associated phenotypic spectrum. Hum Mutat. 30(4):695–702. PMID:19206169
**2321.** Sass U, Kolivras A, Richert B, Moulonguet I, Goettmann-Bonvallot S, Anseeuw M, et al. (2009). Acantholytic tumor of the nail: acantholytic dyskeratotic acanthoma. J Cutan Pathol. 36(12):1308–11. PMID:19602069
**2322.** Satake M, Iwanaga M, Sagara Y, Watanabe T, Okuma K, Hamaguchi I (2016). Incidence of human T-lymphotropic virus 1 infection in adolescent and adult blood donors in Japan: a nationwide retrospective cohort analysis. Lancet Infect Dis. 16(11):1246–54. PMID:27567105
**2323.** Sau P, Graham JH, Helwig EB (1993). Pigmented spindle cell nevus: a clinicopathologic analysis of ninety-five cases. J Am Acad Dermatol. 28(4):565–71. PMID:8463457
**2324.** Sau P, Graham JH, Helwig EB (1995). Proliferating epithelial cysts. Clinicopathological analysis of 96 cases. J Cutan Pathol. 22(5):394–406. PMID:8594071
**2325.** Sau P, Lupton GP, Graham JH (1993). Pilomatrix carcinoma. Cancer. 71(8):2491–8. PMID:8453573
**2325A.** Sausville EA, Worsham GF, Matthews MJ, Makuch RW, Fischmann AB, Schechter GP, et al. (1985). Histologic assessment of lymph nodes in mycosis fungoides/Sézary syndrome (cutaneous T-cell lymphoma): clinical correlations and prognostic import of a new classification system. Hum Pathol. 16(11):1098–109. PMID:3876976
**2326.** Savage KJ, Harris NL, Vose JM, Ullrich F, Jaffe ES, Connors JM, et al. (2008). ALK-anaplastic large-cell lymphoma is clinically and immunophenotypically different from both ALK+ ALCL and peripheral T-cell lymphoma, not otherwise specified: report from the International Peripheral T-Cell Lymphoma Project. Blood. 111(12):5496–504. PMID:18385450
**2327.** Savoia P, Fava P, Bernengo MG (2011). Cutaneous metastases from malignant melanoma: clinical features and new therapeutic perspectives. In: Morton R, editor. Treatment of metastatic melanoma. Rijeka: InTech; pp. 3–14.
**2328.** Savoia P, Fava P, Nardò T, Osella-Abate S, Quaglino P, Bernengo MG (2009). Skin metastases of malignant melanoma: a clinical and prognostic survey. Melanoma Res. 19(5):321–6. PMID:19641475
**2329.** Sawada Y (1986). Solitary nevus lipomatosus superficialis on the forehead. Ann Plast Surg. 16(4):356–8. PMID:3273051
**2330.** Sawada Y, Hino R, Hama K, Ohmori S, Fueki H, Yamada S, et al. (2011). Type of skin eruption is an independent prognostic indicator for adult T-cell leukemia/lymphoma. Blood. 117(15):3961–7. PMID:21325600
**2331.** Scarisbrick JJ, Prince HM, Vermeer MH, Quaglino P, Horwitz S, Porcu P, et al. (2015). Cutaneous Lymphoma International Consortium study of outcome in advanced stages of mycosis fungoides and Sézary syndrome: effect of specific prognostic markers on survival and development of a prognostic model. J Clin Oncol. 33(32):3766–73. PMID:26438120
**2332.** Scarisbrick JJ, Woolford AJ, Calonje E, Photiou A, Ferreira S, Orchard G, et al. (2002). Frequent abnormalities of the p15 and p16 genes in mycosis fungoides and Sezary syndrome. J Invest Dermatol. 118(3):493–9. PMID:11874489
**2333.** Scarisbrick JJ, Woolford AJ, Russell-Jones R, Whittaker SJ (2000). Loss of heterozygosity on 10q and microsatellite instability in advanced stages of primary cutaneous T-cell lymphoma and possible association with homozygous deletion of PTEN. Blood. 95(9):2937–42. PMID:10779442
**2334.** Schacht V, Ramirez MI, Hong YK, Hirakawa S, Feng D, Harvey N, et al. (2003). T1alpha/podoplanin deficiency disrupts normal lymphatic vasculature formation and causes lymphedema. EMBO J. 22(14):3546–56. PMID:12853470
**2335.** Schaefer IM, Fletcher CD, Hornick JL (2016). Loss of H3K27 trimethylation distinguishes malignant peripheral nerve sheath tumors from histologic mimics. Mod Pathol. 29(1):4–13. PMID:26585554
**2336.** Schäfer T, Merkl J, Klemm E, Wichmann HE, Ring J (2006). The epidemiology of nevi and signs of skin aging in the adult general population: results of the KORA-survey 2000. J Invest Dermatol. 126(7):1490–6. PMID:16645597
**2337.** Schaffer JV, Orlow SJ, Lazova R, Bolognia JL (2001). Speckled lentiginous nevus–classic congenital melanocytic nevus hybrid not the result of "collision". Arch Dermatol. 137(12):1655. PMID:11735724
**2338.** Schaffer JV, Orlow SJ, Lazova R, Bolognia JL (2001). Speckled lentiginous nevus: within the spectrum of congenital melanocytic nevi. Arch Dermatol. 137(2):172–8. PMID:11176689
**2339.** Schaller J, Rytina E, Rütten A, Hendricks C, Ha T, Requena L (2010). Sweat duct proliferation associated with aggregates of elastic tissue and atrophodermia vermiculata: a simulator of microcystic adnexal carcinoma. Report of two cases. J Cutan Pathol. 37(9):1002–9. PMID:20175822
**2339A.** Scheffer E, Meijer CJ, Van Vloten WA (1980). Dermatopathic lymphadenopathy and lymph node involvement in mycosis fungoides. Cancer. 45(1):137–48. PMID:7350998
**2340.** Scheffer E, Meijer CJ, van Vloten WA, Willemze R (1986). A histologic study of lymph nodes from patients with the Sézary syndrome. Cancer. 57(12):2375–80. PMID:2938724
**2341.** Scheithauer BW, Woodruff JM, Earlandson RA (1999). Tumors of the peripheral nervous system. In: AFIP atlas of tumor pathology. Series 3, Fascicle 24. Washington, DC: Armed Forces Institute of Pathology; pp. 7–27.
**2342.** Schepel JA, Wille J, Seldenrijk CA, van Ramshorst B (1998). Elastofibroma: a familial occurrence. Eur J Surg. 164(7):557–8. PMID:9696981

**2343.** Schepis C, Siragusa M, Palazzo R, Batolo D, Romano C (1994). Perforating milia-like idiopathic calcinosis cutis and periorbital syringomas in a girl with Down syndrome. Pediatr Dermatol. 11(3):258–60. PMID:7971561
**2344.** Schiller PI, Itin PH (1996). Angiokeratomas: an update. Dermatology. 193(4):275–82. PMID:8993949
**2345.** Schmid U, Eckert F, Griesser H, Steinke C, Cogliatti SB, Kaudewitz P, et al. (1995). Cutaneous follicular lymphoid hyperplasia with monotypic plasma cells. A clinicopathologic study of 18 patients. Am J Surg Pathol. 19(1):12–20. PMID:7802133
**2346.** Schmitt D, Ortonne JP, Haftek M, Thivolet J (1981). Halo nevus and halo melanoma: immunocytochemical study of the inflammatory cell infiltrate. In: Ackerman AB, editor. Pathology of malignant melanoma. New York: Masson; pp. 333–40.
**2347.** Schmoeckel C, Burg G (1988). Congenital spiradenoma. Am J Dermatopathol. 10(6):541–5. PMID:2851273
**2348.** Schmoeckel C, Castro CE, Braun-Falco O (1985). Nevoid malignant melanoma. Arch Dermatol Res. 277(5):362–9. PMID:4026378
**2349.** Schön MP, Heisterkamp T, Ahrens C, Megahed M, Ruzicka T (2000). Presternal verrucous carcinoma. Hautarzt. 51(10):766–9. [German] PMID:11153364
**2350.** Schoolmeester JK, Lastra RR (2015). Granular cell tumors overexpress TFE3 without corollary gene rearrangement. Hum Pathol. 46(8):1242–3. PMID:26009539
**2351.** Schrader AM, Chung YY, Jansen PM, Szuhai K, Bastidas Torres AN, Tensen CP, et al. (2016). No TP63 rearrangements in a selected group of primary cutaneous CD30+ lymphoproliferative disorders with aggressive clinical course. Blood. 128(1):141–3. PMID:27146432
**2531A.** Schrader AMR, Jansen PM, Willemze R, Vermeer MH, Cleton-Jansen AM, Somers SF, et al. (2018). High prevalence of MYD88 and CD79B mutations in intravascular large B-cell lymphoma. Blood. 131(18):2086–9. PMID:29514783
**2352.** Schrader KA, Nelson TN, De Luca A, Huntsman DG, McGillivray BC (2009). Multiple granular cell tumors are an associated feature of LEOPARD syndrome caused by mutation in PTPN11. Clin Genet. 75(2):185–9. PMID:19054014
**2353.** Schreuder MI, Hoefnagel JJ, Jansen PM, van Krieken JH, Willemze R, Hebeda KM (2005). FISH analysis of MALT lymphoma-specific translocations and aneuploidy in primary cutaneous marginal zone lymphoma. J Pathol. 205(3):302–10. PMID:15682432
**2354.** Schulman JM, Oh DH, Sanborn JZ, Pincus L, McCalmont TH, Cho RJ (2016). Multiple hereditary infundibulocystic basal cell carcinoma syndrome associated with a germline SUFU mutation. JAMA Dermatol. 152(3):323–7. PMID:26677003
**2355.** Schulz T, Hartschuh W (1997). Merkel cells are absent in basal cell carcinomas but frequently found in trichoblastomas. An immunohistochemical study. J Cutan Pathol. 24(1):14–24. PMID:9027628
**2356.** Schwartz LB, Metcalfe DD, Miller JS, Earl H, Sullivan T (1987). Tryptase levels as an indicator of mast-cell activation in systemic anaphylaxis and mastocytosis. N Engl J Med. 316(26):1622–6. PMID:3295549
**2357.** Schwartz RA (1995). Verrucous carcinoma of the skin and mucosa. J Am Acad Dermatol. 32(1):1–21. PMID:7822496
**2358.** Schwartz RA (1997). Arsenic and the skin. Int J Dermatol. 36(4):241–50. PMID:9169318
**2359.** Schwartz RA, Bridges TM, Butani AK, Ehrlich A (2008). Actinic keratosis: an occupational and environmental disorder. J Eur Acad Dermatol Venereol. 22(5):606–15. PMID:18410618
**2360.** Schwartz RA, Torre DP (1995). The Muir-Torre syndrome: a 25-year retrospect. J Am Acad Dermatol. 33(1):90–104. PMID:7601953
**2361.** Schwarz Y, Pitaro J, Waissbluth S, Daniel SJ (2016). Review of pediatric head and neck pilomatrixoma. Int J Pediatr Otorhinolaryngol. 85:148–53. PMID:27240514
**2362.** Schweitzer WJ, Goldin HM, Bronson DM, Brody PE (1989). Ulcerated tumor on the scalp. Clear-cell hidradenoma. Arch Dermatol. 125(7):985–6, 989. PMID:2545168
**2363.** Sciot R, Bekaert J (2001). Spindle cell lipoma with extramedullary haematopoiesis. Histopathology. 39(2):215–6. PMID:11493343
**2364.** Scolyer RA, Thompson JF (2005). Desmoplastic melanoma: a heterogeneous entity in which subclassification as "pure" or "mixed" may have important prognostic significance. Ann Surg Oncol. 12(3):197–9. PMID:15827808
**2365.** Scolyer RA, Thompson JF, Mahar A, Murali R (2015). Metastatic tumors involving the skin. In: Busam KJ, editor. Dermatopathology. 2nd ed. London: Elsevier.
**2366.** Scolyer RA, Zhuang L, Palmer AA, Thompson JF, McCarthy SW (2004). Combined naevus: a benign lesion frequently misdiagnosed both clinically and pathologically as melanoma. Pathology. 36(5):419–27. PMID:15370111
**2367.** Scott A, Metcalf JS (1988). Cutaneous malignant mixed tumor. Report of a case and review of the literature. Am J Dermatopathol. 10(4):335–42. PMID:2458054
**2368.** Seab JA, Graham JH (1987). Primary cutaneous adenoid cystic carcinoma. J Am Acad Dermatol. 17(1):113–8. PMID:3038974
**2369.** Seab JA Jr, Graham JH, Helwig EB (1989). Deep penetrating nevus. Am J Surg Pathol. 13(1):39–44. PMID:2909196
**2370.** Seçkin D, Barete S, Euvrard S, Francès C, Kanitakis J, Geusau A, et al. (2013). Primary cutaneous posttransplant lymphoproliferative disorders in solid organ transplant recipients: a multicenter European case series. Am J Transplant. 13(8):2146–53. PMID:23718915
**2371.** Seetharamu N, Ott PA, Pavlick AC (2010). Mucosal melanomas: a case-based review of the literature. Oncologist. 15(7):772–81. PMID:20571149
**2372.** Segal NH, Pavlidis P, Noble WS, Antonescu CR, Viale A, Wesley UV, et al. (2003). Classification of clear-cell sarcoma as a subtype of melanoma by genomic profiling. J Clin Oncol. 21(9):1775–81. PMID:12721254
**2373.** Seifert HW (1981). Ultrastructural investigation on cutaneous angioleiomyoma. Arch Dermatol Res. 271(1):91–9. PMID:7294885
**2374.** Seiji M, Takematsu H, Hosokawa M, Obata M, Tomita Y, Kato T, et al. (1983). Acral melanoma in Japan. J Invest Dermatol. 80 Suppl:56s–60s. PMID:6343519
**2375.** Sellam A, Desjardins L, Barnhill R, Plancher C, Asselain B, Savignoni A, et al. (2016). Fine needle aspiration biopsy in uveal melanoma: technique, complications, and outcomes. Am J Ophthalmol. 162:28–34.e1. PMID:26556006
**2376.** Sellheyer K, Nelson P, Kutzner H (2012). Fibroepithelioma of Pinkus is a true basal cell carcinoma developing in association with a newly identified tumour-specific type of epidermal hyperplasia. Br J Dermatol. 166(1):88–97. PMID:21910710
**2377.** Sellheyer K, Nelson P, Kutzner H, Patel RM (2013). The immunohistochemical differential diagnosis of microcystic adnexal carcinoma, desmoplastic trichoepithelioma and morpheaform basal cell carcinoma using BerEP4 and stem cell markers. J Cutan Pathol. 40(4):363–70. PMID:23398472
**2378.** Selmi C, Greenspan A, Huntley A, Gershwin ME (2015). Multicentric reticulohistiocytosis: a critical review. Curr Rheumatol Rep. 17(6):511. PMID:25900189
**2379.** Sen F, Medeiros LJ, Lu D, Jones D, Lai R, Katz R, et al. (2002). Mantle cell lymphoma involving skin: cutaneous lesions may be the first manifestation of disease and tumors often have blastoid cytologic features. Am J Surg Pathol. 26(10):1312–8. PMID:12360046
**2380.** Sener SF, Milos S, Feldman JL, Martz CH, Winchester DJ, Dieterich M, et al. (2001). The spectrum of vascular lesions in the mammary skin, including angiosarcoma, after breast conservation treatment for breast cancer. J Am Coll Surg. 193(1):22–8. PMID:11442250
**2381.** Senff NJ, Hoefnagel JJ, Jansen PM, Vermeer MH, van Baarlen J, Blokx WA, et al. (2007). Reclassification of 300 primary cutaneous B-cell lymphomas according to the new WHO-EORTC classification for cutaneous lymphomas: comparison with previous classifications and identification of prognostic markers. J Clin Oncol. 25(12):1581–7. PMID:17353548
**2382.** Senff NJ, Zoutman WH, Vermeer MH, Assaf C, Berti E, Cerroni L, et al. (2009). Fine-mapping chromosomal loss at 9p21: correlation with prognosis in primary cutaneous diffuse large B-cell lymphoma, leg type. J Invest Dermatol. 129(5):1149–55. PMID:19020554
**2383.** Serratrice J, Granel B, De Roux C, Pellissier JF, Swiader L, Bartoli JM, et al. (2000). "Coated aorta": a new sign of Erdheim-Chester disease. J Rheumatol. 27(6):1550–3. PMID:10852289
**2384.** Servitje O, Muniesa C, Benavente Y, Monsálvez V, Garcia-Muret MP, Gallardo F, et al. (2013). Primary cutaneous marginal zone B-cell lymphoma: response to treatment and disease-free survival in a series of 137 patients. J Am Acad Dermatol. 69(3):357–65. PMID:23796549
**2385.** Sexton M, Sexton CW (1991). Recurrent pigmented melanocytic nevus. A benign lesion, not to be mistaken for malignant melanoma. Arch Pathol Lab Med. 115(2):122–6. PMID:1992976
**2386.** Seyda B (1965). Influence of Italian medicine on the origin and development of medical teaching at Cracow. Atti Mem Accad Stor Arte Sanit. 31:26–30. [Italian] PMID:14307321
**2387.** Sgouros D, Piana S, Argenziano G, Longo C, Moscarella E, Karaarslan IK, et al. (2013). Clinical, dermoscopic and histopathological features of eccrine poroid neoplasms. Dermatology. 227(2):175–9. PMID:24080919
**2388.** Shah A, Safaya A (2012). Granulomatous slack skin disease: a review, in comparison with mycosis fungoides. J Eur Acad Dermatol Venereol. 26(12):1472–8. PMID:22435618
**2389.** Shahla A, Parvaneh V, Hossein HD (2004). Langerhans cells histiocytosis in one family. Pediatr Hematol Oncol. 21(4):313–20. PMID:15205093
**2390.** Shain AH, Bastian BC (2016). From melanocytes to melanomas. Nat Rev Cancer. 16(6):345–58. PMID:27125352
**2391.** Shain AH, Bastian BC (2016). The genetic evolution of melanoma. N Engl J Med. 374(10):995–6. PMID:26962740
**2392.** Shain AH, Garrido M, Botton T, Talevich E, Yeh I, Sanborn JZ, et al. (2015). Exome sequencing of desmoplastic melanoma identifies recurrent NFKBIE promoter mutations and diverse activating mutations in the MAPK pathway. Nat Genet. 47(10):1194–9. PMID:26343386
**2393.** Shain AH, Pollack JR (2013). The spectrum of SWI/SNF mutations, ubiquitous in human cancers. PLoS One. 8(1):e55119. PMID:23355908
**2394.** Shain AH, Yeh I, Kovalyshyn I, Sriharan A, Talevich E, Gagnon A, et al. (2015). The genetic evolution of melanoma from precursor lesions. N Engl J Med. 373(20):1926–36. PMID:26559571
**2395.** Shalin SC, Lyle S, Calonje E, Lazar AJ (2010). Sebaceous neoplasia and the Muir-Torre syndrome: important connections with clinical implications. Histopathology. 56(1):133–47. PMID:20055911
**2396.** Shan SJ, Chen S, Heller P, Guo Y (2014). Syringocystadenocarcinoma papilliferum with intraepidermal pagetoid spread on an unusual location. Am J Dermatopathol. 36(12):1007–10. PMID:24423933
**2397.** Shanley S, Ratcliffe J, Hockey A, Haan E, Oley C, Ravine D, et al. (1994). Nevoid basal cell carcinoma syndrome: review of 118 affected individuals. Am J Med Genet. 50(3):282–90. PMID:8042673
**2398.** Shanmugam V, Margolskee E, Kluk M, Giorgadze T, Orazi A (2016). Rosai-Dorfman disease harboring an activating KRAS K117N missense mutation. Head Neck Pathol. 10(3):394–9. PMID:26922062
**2399.** Shao L, Newell B, Quintanilla N (2007). Atypical fibroxanthoma and squamous cell carcinoma of the conjunctiva in xeroderma pigmentosum. Pediatr Dev Pathol. 10(2):149–52. PMID:17378688
**2400.** Shapiro L, Baraf CS (1970). Isolated epidermolytic acanthoma. A solitary tumor showing granular degeneration. Arch Dermatol. 101(2):220–3. PMID:5413257
**2400A.** Sharara NA, Alexander RA, Luthert PJ, Hungerford JL, Cree IA (2001). Differential immunoreactivity of melanocytic lesions of the conjunctiva. Histopathology. 39(4):426–31. PMID:11683945
**2401.** Sheidow TG, Nicolle DA, Heathcote JG (2000). Erdheim-Chester disease: two cases of orbital involvement. Eye (Lond). 14(Pt 4):606–12. PMID:11040908
**2402.** Shen AS, Peterhof E, Kind P, Rütten A, Zelger B, Landthaler M, et al. (2015). Activating mutations in the RAS/mitogen-activated protein kinase signaling pathway in sporadic trichoblastoma and syringocystadenoma papilliferum. Hum Pathol. 46(2):272–6. PMID:25532942
**2403.** Shen LI, Liu L, Yang Z, Jiang N (2016). Identification of genes and signaling pathways associated with squamous cell carcinoma by bioinformatics analysis. Oncol Lett. 11(2):1382–90. PMID:26893747
**2404.** Shen S, Wolfe R, McLean CA, Haskett M, Kelly JW (2014). Characteristics and associations of high-mitotic-rate melanoma. JAMA Dermatol. 150(10):1048–55. PMID:25142970
**2405.** Sheng W, Lu L, Wang J (2013). Cellular angiolipoma: a clinicopathological and immunohistochemical study of 12 cases. Am J Dermatopathol. 35(2):220–5. PMID:22935891
**2406.** Sheth S, Li X, Binder S, Dry SM (2011). Differential gene expression profiles of neurothekeomas and nerve sheath myxomas by microarray analysis. Mod Pathol. 24(3):343–54. PMID:21297585
**2407.** Shi J, Yang XR, Ballew B, Rotunno M, Calista D, Fargnoli MC, et al. (2014). Rare missense variants in POT1 predispose to familial cutaneous malignant melanoma. Nat Genet. 46(5):482–6. PMID:24686846
**2408.** Shields CL, Fasiuddin AF, Mashayekhi A, Shields JA (2004). Conjunctival nevi: clinical features and natural course in 410 consecutive patients. Arch Ophthalmol. 122(2):167–75. PMID:14769591
**2409.** Shields CL, Manchandia A, Subbiah R, Eagle RC Jr, Shields JA (2008). Pigmented squamous cell carcinoma in situ of the conjunctiva in 5 cases. Ophthalmology. 115(10):1673–8. PMID:18378314
**2410.** Shields CL, Shields JA, Gündüz K,

Cater J, Mercado GV, Gross N, et al. (2000). Conjunctival melanoma: risk factors for recurrence, exenteration, metastasis, and death in 150 consecutive patients. Arch Ophthalmol. 118(11):1497–507. PMID:11074806

**2411.** Shields JA, Shields CL, Mashayekhi A, Marr BP, Benavides R, Thangappan A, et al. (2008). Primary acquired melanosis of the conjunctiva: risks for progression to melanoma in 311 eyes. The 2006 Lorenz E. Zimmerman Lecture. Ophthalmology. 115(3):511–9.e2. PMID:17884168

**2412.** Shih B, Tassabehji M, Watson JS, Bayat A (2012). DNA copy number variations at chromosome 7p14.1 and chromosome 14q11.2 are associated with Dupuytren's disease: potential role for MMP and Wnt signaling pathway. Plast Reconstr Surg. 129(4):921–32. PMID:22183494

**2413.** Shim JH, Lee DW, Cho BK (1996). A case of Cobb syndrome associated with lymphangioma circumscriptum. Dermatology. 193(1):45–7. PMID:8864618

**2414.** Shimada K, Kinoshita T, Naoe T, Nakamura S (2009). Presentation and management of intravascular large B-cell lymphoma. Lancet Oncol. 10(9):895–902. PMID:19717091

**2415.** Shimada K, Matsue K, Yamamoto K, Murase T, Ichikawa N, Okamoto M, et al. (2008). Retrospective analysis of intravascular large B-cell lymphoma treated with rituximab-containing chemotherapy as reported by the IVL study group in Japan. J Clin Oncol. 26(19):3189–95. PMID:18506023

**2416.** Shimada K, Shimada S, Sugimoto K, Nakatochi M, Suguro M, Hirakawa A, et al. (2016). Development and analysis of patient-derived xenograft mouse models in intravascular large B-cell lymphoma. Leukemia. 30(7):1568–79. PMID:27001523

**2417.** Shimauchi T, Imai S, Hino R, Tokura Y (2005). Production of thymus and activation-regulated chemokine and macrophage-derived chemokine by CCR4+ adult T-cell leukemia cells. Clin Cancer Res. 11(6):2427–35. PMID:15788694

**2418.** Shimizu S, Hashimoto H, Enjoji M (1984). Nodular fasciitis: an analysis of 250 patients. Pathology. 16(2):161–6. PMID:6462780

**2419.** Shimokawa M, Haraguchi M, Kobayashi W, Higashi Y, Matsushita S, Kawai K, et al. (2013). The transcription factor Snail expressed in cutaneous squamous cell carcinoma induces epithelial-mesenchymal transition and down-regulates COX-2. Biochem Biophys Res Commun. 430(3):1078–82. PMID:23261444

**2420.** Shimoyama M (1991). Diagnostic criteria and classification of clinical subtypes of adult T-cell leukaemia-lymphoma. A report from the Lymphoma Study Group (1984-87). Br J Haematol. 79(3):428–37. PMID:1751370

**2421.** Shin D, Sinha M, Kondziolka DS, Kirkwood JM, Rao UN, Tarhini AA (2015). Intermediate-grade meningeal melanocytoma associated with nevus of Ota: a case report and review of the literature. Melanoma Res. 25(4):273–8. PMID:25933209

**2422.** Shin HT, Jang KT, Mun GH, Lee DY, Lee JB (2014). Histopathological analysis of the progression pattern of subungual melanoma: late tendency of dermal invasion in the nail matrix area. Mod Pathol. 27(11):1461–7. PMID:24743223

**2423.** Shinde GB, Viswanath V, Torsekar RG (2012). Multiple yellowish plaques in cerebriform pattern on the right elbow. Nevus lipomatosus cutaneous superficialis (NLCS)–classical type of Hoffmann and Zurhelle. Int J Dermatol. 51(6):662–4. PMID:22607282

**2424.** Shingde MV, Buckland M, Busam KJ, McCarthy SW, Wilmott J, Thompson JF, et al. (2009). Primary cutaneous Ewing sarcoma/primitive neuroectodermal tumour: a clinicopathological analysis of seven cases highlighting diagnostic pitfalls and the role of FISH testing in diagnosis. J Clin Pathol. 62(10):915–9. PMID:19783720

**2425.** Shinozaki A, Nagao T, Endo H, Kato N, Hirokawa M, Mizobuchi K, et al. (2008). Sebaceous epithelial-myoepithelial carcinoma of the salivary gland: clinicopathologic and immunohistochemical analysis of 6 cases of a new histologic variant. Am J Surg Pathol. 32(6):913–23. PMID:18425042

**2426.** Shiomi T, Noguchi T, Nakayama H, Yoshida Y, Yamamoto O, Hayashi N, et al. (2013). Clinicopathological study of invasive extramammary Paget's disease: subgroup comparison according to invasion depth. J Eur Acad Dermatol Venereol. 27(5):589–92. PMID:22364152

**2427.** Shitara D, Nascimento MM, Puig S, Yamada S, Enokihara MM, Michalany N, et al. (2014). Nevus-associated melanomas: clinicopathologic features. Am J Clin Pathol. 142(4):485–91. PMID:25239415

**2428.** Shmookler BM, Enzinger FM (1981). Pleomorphic lipoma: a benign tumor simulating liposarcoma. A clinicopathologic analysis of 48 cases. Cancer. 47(1):126–33. PMID:7459800

**2429.** Shon W, Ida CM, Boland-Froemming JM, Rose PS, Folpe A (2011). Cutaneous angiosarcoma arising in massive localized lymphedema of the morbidly obese: a report of five cases and review of the literature. J Cutan Pathol. 38(7):560–4. PMID:21518378

**2430.** Shon W, Salomão DR (2014). WT1 expression in endocrine mucin-producing sweat gland carcinoma: a study of 13 cases. Int J Dermatol. 53(10):1228–34. PMID:25219513

**2431.** Shon W, Sukov WR, Jenkins SM, Folpe AL (2014). MYC amplification and overexpression in primary cutaneous angiosarcoma: a fluorescence in-situ hybridization and immunohistochemical study. Mod Pathol. 27(4):509–15. PMID:24091875

**2432.** Shon W, Wada DA, Folpe AL, Pittelkow MR (2012). Angiosarcoma in a patient with congenital nonhereditary lymphedema. Cutis. 90(5):248–51. PMID:23270196

**2433.** Shoo BA, Shinkai K, McCalmont TH, Fox LP (2008). Xanthogranulomas associated with hematologic malignancy in adulthood. J Am Acad Dermatol. 59(3):488–93. PMID:18538449

**2434.** Shors AR, Kim S, White E, Argenyi Z, Barnhill RL, Duray P, et al. (2006). Dysplastic naevi with moderate to severe histological dysplasia: a risk factor for melanoma. Br J Dermatol. 155(5):988–93. PMID:17034530

**2435.** Shousha S, Eusebi V, Lester S (2012). Paget disease of the nipple. In: Lakhani SR, Ellis IO, Schnitt SJ, Tan PH, van der Vijver MJ, editors. WHO classification of tumours of the breast. 4th ed. Lyon: International Agency for Research on Cancer; pp. 152–3.

**2436.** Shu B, Shen XX, Chen P, Fang XZ, Guo YL, Kong YY (2016). Primary invasive extramammary Paget disease on penoscrotum: a clinicopathological analysis of 41 cases. Hum Pathol. 47(1):70–7. PMID:26508372

**2437.** Shugart RR, Soule EH, Johnson EW Jr (1963). Glomus tumor. Surg Gynecol Obstet. 117:334–40. PMID:14080348

**2438.** Shvili D, Rothem A (1986). Fulminant metastasizing chondroid syringoma of the skin. Am J Dermatopathol. 8(4):321–5. PMID:3021016

**2439.** Sibaud V, Beylot-Barry M, Thiébaut R, Parrens M, Vergier B, Delaunay M, et al. (2003). Bone marrow histopathologic and molecular staging in epidermotropic T-cell lymphomas. Am J Clin Pathol. 119(3):414–23. PMID:12645344

**2440.** Sidiropoulos M, Busam K, Guitart J, Laskin WB, Wagner AM, Gerami P (2013). Superficial paramucosal clear cell sarcoma of the soft parts resembling melanoma in a 13-year-old boy. J Cutan Pathol. 40(2):265–8. PMID:23228147

**2441.** Siegel JA, Korgavkar K, Weinstock MA (2017). Current perspective on actinic keratosis: a review. Br J Dermatol. 177(2):350–8. PMID:27500794

**2442.** Siegel RL, Miller KD, Jemal A (2017). Cancer statistics, 2017. CA Cancer J Clin. 67(1):7–30. PMID:28055103

**2443.** Sigg C, Pelloni F, Schnyder UW (1990). Frequency of congenital nevi, nevi spili and café-au-lait spots and their relation to nevus count and skin complexion in 939 children. Dermatologica. 180(3):118–23. PMID:2187718

**2444.** Signoretti S, Annessi G, Occhiuto S, Ruatti P, Faraggiana T (1996). Papular clear cell hyperplasia of the eccrine duct in a diabetic. Br J Dermatol. 135(1):139–43. PMID:8776379

**2445.** Sima R, Vanecek T, Kacerovska D, Trubac P, Cribier B, Rutten A, et al. (2010). Brooke-Spiegler syndrome: report of 10 patients from 8 families with novel germline mutations: evidence of diverse somatic mutations in the same patient regardless of tumor type. Diagn Mol Pathol. 19(2):83–91. PMID:20502185

**2446.** Simionescu O, Popescu BO, Costache M, Manole E, Spulber S, Gherghiceanu M, et al. (2012). Apoptosis in seborrheic keratoses: an open door to a new dermoscopic score. J Cell Mol Med. 16(6):1223–31. PMID:22404841

**2447.** Simon MP, Pedeutour F, Sirvent N, Grosgeorge J, Minoletti F, Coindre JM, et al. (1997). Deregulation of the platelet-derived growth factor B-chain gene via fusion with collagen gene COL1A1 in dermatofibrosarcoma protuberans and giant-cell fibroblastoma. Nat Genet. 15(1):95–8. PMID:8988177

**2448.** Singh AD, De Potter P, Fijal BA, Shields CL, Shields JA, Elston RC (1998). Lifetime prevalence of uveal melanoma in white patients with oculo(dermal) melanocytosis. Ophthalmology. 105(1):195–8. PMID:9442799

**2449.** Singh AD, Kalyani P, Topham A (2005). Estimating the risk of malignant transformation of a choroidal nevus. Ophthalmology. 112(10):1784–9. PMID:16154197

**2450.** Singh D, Garg RS, Vikas, Garg Y, Arora V (2016). Glomus tumor - a rarity; M.R.I- a big help in early diagnosis. J Orthop Case Rep. 6(3):38–9. PMID:28116265

**2451.** Singh Gomez C, Calonje E, Fletcher CD (1994). Epithelioid benign fibrous histiocytoma of skin: clinico-pathological analysis of 20 cases of a poorly known variant. Histopathology. 24(2):123–9. PMID:8181804

**2452.** Singh K, Sharma A, Chatterjee T (2016). Pigmented basal cell carcinoma: a rare case report. Indian J Cancer. 53(3):380–1. PMID:28244464

**2453.** Singh RS, Grayson W, Redston M, Diwan AH, Warneke CL, McKee PH, et al. (2008). Site and tumor type predicts DNA mismatch repair status in cutaneous sebaceous neoplasia. Am J Surg Pathol. 32(6):936–42. PMID:18551751

**2454.** Sington JD, Manek S, Hollowood K (2002). Fibroadenoma of the mammary-like glands of the vulva. Histopathology. 41(6):563–5. PMID:12460213

**2455.** Sini MC, Manca A, Cossu A, Budroni M, Botti G, Ascierto PA, et al. (2008). Molecular alterations at chromosome 9p21 in melanocytic naevi and melanoma. Br J Dermatol. 158(2):243–50. PMID:18028495

**2456.** Sirvent N, Perrin C, Lacour JP, Maire G, Attias R, Pedeutour F (2004). Monosomy 9q and trisomy 16q in a case of congenital solitary infantile myofibromatosis. Virchows Arch. 445(5):537–40. PMID:15365831

**2457.** N Sivrikoz O, Kandiloğlu G (2015). The effects of cyclin D1 and Bcl-2 expression on aggressive behavior in basal cell and basosquamous carcinoma. Iran J Pathol. 10(3):185–91. PMID:26351483

**2458.** Skala SL, Arps DP, Zhao L, Cha KB, Wang M, Harms PW, et al. (2018). Comprehensive histopathological comparison of epidermotropic/dermal metastatic melanoma and primary nodular melanoma. Histopathology. 72(3):472–80. PMID:28881040

**2459.** Skálová A, Vanecek T, Sima R, Laco J, Weinreb I, Perez-Ordonez B, et al. (2010). Mammary analogue secretory carcinoma of salivary glands, containing the ETV6-NTRK3 fusion gene: a hitherto undescribed salivary gland tumor entity. Am J Surg Pathol. 34(5):599–608. PMID:20410810

**2460.** Skender-Kalnenas TM, English DR, Heenan PJ (1995). Benign melanocytic lesions: risk markers or precursors of cutaneous melanoma? J Am Acad Dermatol. 33(6):1000–7. PMID:7490345

**2461.** Slager SL, Caporaso NE, de Sanjose S, Goldin LR (2013). Genetic susceptibility to chronic lymphocytic leukemia. Semin Hematol. 50(4):296–302. PMID:24246697

**2462.** Slater DN, Cotton DW, Azzopardi JG (1987). Oncocytic glomus tumour: a new variant. Histopathology. 11(5):523–31. PMID:3038728

**2463.** Smit DL, Mensenkamp AR, Badeloe S, Breuning MH, Simon ME, van Spaendonck KY, et al. (2011). Hereditary leiomyomatosis and renal cell cancer in families referred for fumarate hydratase germline mutation analysis. Clin Genet. 79(1):49–59. PMID:20618355

**2464.** Smith K, Mezebish D, Williams JP, Menon P, Rolfe A, Cobb M, et al. (1998). Cutaneous epithelioid schwannomas: a rare variant of a benign peripheral nerve sheath tumor. J Cutan Pathol. 25(1):50–5. PMID:9508344

**2465.** Smith KJ, Barrett TL, Skelton HG 3rd, Lupton GP, Graham JH (1989). Spindle cell and epithelioid cell nevi with atypia and metastasis (malignant Spitz nevus). Am J Surg Pathol. 13(11):931–9. PMID:2802011

**2466.** Smith KJ, Hamza S, Skelton H (2004). Histologic features in primary cutaneous squamous cell carcinomas in immunocompromised patients focusing on organ transplant patients. Dermatol Surg. 30(4 Pt 2):634–41. PMID:15061848

**2467.** Smith KJ, Williams J, Corbett D, Skelton H (2001). Microcystic adnexal carcinoma: an immunohistochemical study including markers of proliferation and apoptosis. Am J Surg Pathol. 25(4):464–71. PMID:11257620

**2468.** Smith ME, Fisher C, Weiss SW (1996). Pleomorphic hyalinizing angiectatic tumor of soft parts. A low-grade neoplasm resembling neurilemoma. Am J Surg Pathol. 20(1):21–9. PMID:8540605

**2469.** Smith MJ, Beetz C, Williams SG, Bhaskar SS, O'Sullivan J, Anderson B, et al. (2014). Germline mutations in SUFU cause Gorlin syndrome-associated childhood medulloblastoma and redefine the risk associated with PTCH1 mutations. J Clin Oncol. 32(36):4155–61. PMID:25403219

**2470.** Smith NP (1987). The pigmented spindle cell tumor of Reed: an underdiagnosed lesion. Semin Diagn Pathol. 4(1):75–87. PMID:3671907

**2471.** Smith SC, Poznanski AA, Fullen DR, Ma L, McHugh JB, Lucas DR, et al. (2013). CD34-positive superficial myxofibrosarcoma: a potential diagnostic pitfall. J Cutan Pathol. 40(7):639–45. PMID:23600956

**2472.** Smolle J, Kerl H (1983). Pilar sheath acanthoma - a benign follicular hamartoma. Dermatologica. 167(6):335–8. [German] PMID:6662259

2473. Snow S, Madjar DD, Hardy S, Bentz M, Lucarelli MJ, Bechard R, et al. (2001). Microcystic adnexal carcinoma: report of 13 cases and review of the literature. Dermatol Surg. 27(4):401–8. PMID:11298716

2474. Snow SN, Reizner GT (1992). Eccrine porocarcinoma of the face. J Am Acad Dermatol. 27(2 Pt 2):306–11. PMID:1325487

2475. Sofianos C, Chauke NY, Grubnik A (2016). Metastatic trichilemmal carcinoma in a patient with breast cancer. BMJ Case Rep. 2016:bcr2016217661. PMID:27872134

2476. Sokolowska-Wojdylo M, Wenzel J, Gaffal E, Steitz J, Roszkiewicz J, Bieber T, et al. (2005). Absence of CD26 expression on skin-homing CLA+ CD4+ T lymphocytes in peripheral blood is a highly sensitive marker for early diagnosis and therapeutic monitoring of patients with Sézary syndrome. Clin Exp Dermatol. 30(6):702–6. PMID:16197392

2477. Soler AP, Burchette JL, Bellet JS, Olson JA Jr (2007). Cell adhesion protein expression in melanocytic matricoma. J Cutan Pathol. 34(6):456–60. PMID:17518772

2478. Soler-Carrillo J, Estrach T, Mascaró JM (2001). Eruptive syringoma: 27 new cases and review of the literature. J Eur Acad Dermatol Venereol. 15(3):242–6. PMID:11683289

2479. Sommer LL, Barcia SM, Clarke LE, Helm KF (2011). Persistent melanocytic nevi: a review and analysis of 205 cases. J Cutan Pathol. 38(6):503–7. PMID:21362017

2480. Song JY, Pittaluga S, Dunleavy K, Grant N, White T, Jiang L, et al. (2015). Lymphomatoid granulomatosis–a single institute experience: pathologic findings and clinical correlations. Am J Surg Pathol. 39(2):141–56. PMID:25321327

2481. Sonnex TS, Hawk JL (1988). Hydroa vacciniforme: a review of ten cases. Br J Dermatol. 118(1):101–8. PMID:3342168

2482. Sordillo PP, Epremian B, Koziner B, Lacher M, Lieberman P (1982). Lymphomatoid granulomatosis: an analysis of clinical and immunologic characteristics. Cancer. 49(10):2070–6. PMID:6978760

2483. Sorensen PH, Lessnick SL, Lopez-Terrada D, Liu XF, Triche TJ, Denny CT (1994). A second Ewing's sarcoma translocation, t(21;22), fuses the EWS gene to another ETS-family transcription factor, ERG. Nat Genet. 6(2):146–51. PMID:8162068

2484. Sotlar K, Cerny-Reiterer S, Petat-Dutter K, Hessel H, Berezowska S, Müllauer L, et al. (2011). Aberrant expression of CD30 in neoplastic mast cells in high-grade mastocytosis. Mod Pathol. 24(4):585–95. PMID:21186345

2485. Soufir N, Ribojad M, Magnaldo T, Thibaudeau O, Delestaing G, Daya-Grosjean L, et al. (2002). Germline and somatic mutations of the INK4a-ARF gene in a xeroderma pigmentosum group C patient. J Invest Dermatol. 119(6):1355–60. PMID:12485439

2486. Soulard R, Nguyen AT, Souraud JB, Oddon PA, Fouet B, Cathelinaud O (2012). Osteochondrolipoma of the submandibular region: a case report and review of the literature. Head Neck Pathol. 6(4):486–91. PMID:22623084

2487. South CD, Hampel H, Comeras I, Westman JA, Frankel WL, de la Chapelle A (2008). The frequency of Muir-Torre syndrome among Lynch syndrome families. J Natl Cancer Inst. 100(4):277–81. PMID:18270343

2488. Southwick GJ, Schwartz RA (1979). The basal cell nevus syndrome: disasters occurring among a series of 36 patients. Cancer. 44(6):2294–305. PMID:509397

2489. Souvatzidis P, Sbano P, Mandato F, Fimiani M, Castelli A (2008). Malignant nodular hidradenoma of the skin: report of seven cases. J Eur Acad Dermatol Venereol. 22(5):549–54. PMID:18410617

2490. Soyer HP, Rigel DS, Wurm EMT (2012). Actinic keratosis, basal cell carcinoma and squamous cell carcinoma. In: Bolognia JL, Jorizzo JJ, Schaffer JV, Callen JP, Cerroni L, Heymann WR, et al., editors. Dermatology. 3rd ed. London: Elsevier; pp. 1773–93.

2491. Spatz A, Calonje E, Handfield-Jones S, Barnhill RL (1999). Spitz tumors in children: a grading system for risk stratification. Arch Dermatol. 135(3):282–5. PMID:10086449

2492. Spatz A, Ruiter D, Hardmeier T, Renard N, Wechsler J, Bailly C, et al. (1996). Melanoma in childhood: an EORTC-MCG multicenter study on the clinico-pathological aspects. Int J Cancer. 68(3):317–24. PMID:8903473

2493. Spencer JM, Kahn SM, Jiang W, DeLeo VA, Weinstein IB (1995). Activated ras genes occur in human actinic keratoses, premalignant precursors to squamous cell carcinomas. Arch Dermatol. 131(7):796–800. PMID:7611795

2494. Spencer KR, Mehnert JM (2016). Mucosal melanoma: epidemiology, biology and treatment. Cancer Treat Res. 167:295–320. PMID:26601869

2495. Sperr WR, Jordan JH, Fiegl M, Escribano L, Bellas C, Dirnhofer S, et al. (2002). Serum tryptase levels in patients with mastocytosis: correlation with mast cell burden and implication for defining the category of disease. Int Arch Allergy Immunol. 128(2):136–41. PMID:12065914

2496. Spillane AJ, Thomas JM, Fisher C (2000). Epithelioid sarcoma: the clinicopathological complexities of this rare soft tissue sarcoma. Ann Surg Oncol. 7(3):218–25. PMID:10791853

2497. Stålemark H, Laurencikas E, Karis J, Gavhed D, Fadeel B, Henter JI (2008). Incidence of Langerhans cell histiocytosis in children: a population-based study. Pediatr Blood Cancer. 51(1):76–81. PMID:18266220

2498. Stam H, Lohuis PJ, Zupan-Kajcovski B, Wouters MW, van der Hage JA, Visser O (2013). Increasing incidence and survival of a rare skin cancer in the Netherlands. A population-based study of 2,220 cases of skin adnexal carcinoma. J Surg Oncol. 107(8):822–7. PMID:23505050

2499. Staples MP, Elwood M, Burton RC, Williams JL, Marks R, Giles GG (2006). Non-melanoma skin cancer in Australia: the 2002 national survey and trends since 1985. Med J Aust. 184(1):6–10. PMID:16398622

2500. Starink TM (1984). Cowden's disease: analysis of fourteen new cases. J Am Acad Dermatol. 11(6):1127–41. PMID:6512057

2501. Starink TM (1997). Eccrine syringofibroadenoma: multiple lesions representing a new cutaneous marker of the Schöpf syndrome, and solitary nonhereditary tumors. J Am Acad Dermatol. 36(4):569–76. PMID:9092743

2502. Starink TM, Hausman R (1984). The cutaneous pathology of facial lesions in Cowden's disease. J Cutan Pathol. 11(5):331–7. PMID:6512062

2503. Staser K, Yang FC, Clapp DW (2010). Mast cells and the neurofibroma microenvironment. Blood. 116(2):157–64. PMID:20233971

2504. Stebbing J, Sanitt A, Nelson M, Powles T, Gazzard B, Bower M (2006). A prognostic index for AIDS-associated Kaposi's sarcoma in the era of highly active antiretroviral therapy. Lancet. 367(9521):1495–502. PMID:16679162

2505. Stefanato CM, Ferrara G, Chaudhry IH, Guevara Pineda C, Waschkowski G, Rose C, et al. (2012). Clear cell nodular hidradenoma involving the lymphatic system: a tumor of uncertain malignant potential or a novel example of "metastasizing" benign tumor? Am J Surg Pathol. 36(12):1835–40. PMID:23095508

2506. Stenzinger A, Endris V, Pfarr N, Andrulis M, Jöhrens K, Klauschen F, et al. (2014). Targeted ultra-deep sequencing reveals recurrent and mutually exclusive mutations of cancer genes in blastic plasmacytoid dendritic cell neoplasm. Oncotarget. 5(15):6404–13. PMID:25115387

2507. Stern JB, Haupt HM, Smith RR (1994). Fibroepithelioma of Pinkus. Eccrine duct spread of basal cell carcinoma. Am J Dermatopathol. 16(6):585–7. PMID:7864295

2508. Stern RS (2012). The risk of squamous cell and basal cell cancer associated with psoralen and ultraviolet A therapy: a 30-year prospective study. J Am Acad Dermatol. 66(4):553–62. PMID:22264671

2509. Stewart CJ (2008). Syringocystadenoma papilliferum-like lesion of the vulva. Pathology. 40(6):638–9. PMID:18752136

2510. Stewart DR, Pemov A, Van Loo P, Beert E, Brems H, Sciot R, et al. (2012). Mitotic recombination of chromosome arm 17q as a cause of loss of heterozygosity of NF1 in neurofibromatosis type 1-associated glomus tumors. Genes Chromosomes Cancer. 51(5):429–37. PMID:22250039

2511. Stewart DR, Sloan JL, Yao L, Mannes AJ, Moshyedi A, Lee CC, et al. (2010). Diagnosis, management, and complications of glomus tumours of the digits in neurofibromatosis type 1. J Med Genet. 47(8):525–32. PMID:20530151

2512. Stockfleth E (2017). The importance of treating the field in actinic keratosis. J Eur Acad Dermatol Venereol. 31 Suppl 2:8–11. PMID:28263021

2513. Stockfleth E, Sterry W (2002). New treatment modalities for basal cell carcinoma. Recent Results Cancer Res. 160:259–68. PMID:12079222

2514. Stockfleth E, Ulrich C, Meyer T, Christophers E (2002). Epithelial malignancies in organ transplant patients: clinical presentation and new methods of treatment. Recent Results Cancer Res. 160:251–8. PMID:12079221

2515. Stockman DL, Hornick JL, Deavers MT, Lev DC, Lazar AJ, Wang WL (2014). ERG and FLI1 protein expression in epithelioid sarcoma. Mod Pathol. 27(4):496–501. PMID:24072183

2516. Stockschlaeder M, Sucker C (2006). Adult Langerhans cell histiocytosis. Eur J Haematol. 76(5):363–8. PMID:16548916

2517. Stratakis CA, Kirschner LS, Carney JA (2001). Clinical and molecular features of the Carney complex: diagnostic criteria and recommendations for patient evaluation. J Clin Endocrinol Metab. 86(9):4041–6. PMID:11549623

2518. Stratton J, Billings SD (2014). Cellular neurothekeoma: analysis of 37 cases emphasizing atypical histologic features. Mod Pathol. 27(5):701–10. PMID:24186141

2519. Streubel B, Lamprecht A, Dierlamm J, Cerroni L, Stolte M, Ott G, et al. (2003). t(14;18)(q32;q21) involving IGH and MALT1 is a frequent chromosomal aberration in MALT lymphoma. Blood. 101(6):2335–9. PMID:12406890

2520. Streubel B, Simonitsch-Klupp I, Müllauer L, Lamprecht A, Huber D, Siebert R, et al. (2004). Variable frequencies of MALT lymphoma-associated genetic aberrations in MALT lymphomas of different sites. Leukemia. 18(10):1722–6. PMID:15356642

2521. Ströbel P, Zettl A, Ren Z, Starostik P, Riedmiller H, Störkel S, et al. (2002). Spiradenocylindroma of the kidney: clinical and genetic findings suggesting a role of somatic mutation of the CYLD1 gene in the oncogenesis of an unusual renal neoplasm. Am J Surg Pathol. 26(1):119–24. PMID:11756779

2522. Strungs I (2004). Common and uncommon variants of melanocytic naevi. Pathology. 36(5):396–403. PMID:15370108

2523. Stuart LN, Hiatt KM, Zaki Z, Gardner JM, Shalin SC (2014). Plaque-like CD34-positive dermal fibroma/medallion-like dermal dendrocyte hamartoma: an unusual spindle cell neoplasm. J Cutan Pathol. 41(8):625–9. PMID:25065391

2524. Su A, Low L, Li X, Zhou S, Mascarenhas L, Barnhill RL (2014). De novo congenital melanoma: analysis of 2 cases with array comparative genomic hybridization. Am J Dermatopathol. 36(11):915–9. PMID:25051103

2525. Su F, Viros A, Milagre C, Trunzer K, Bollag G, Spleiss O, et al. (2012). RAS mutations in cutaneous squamous-cell carcinomas in patients treated with BRAF inhibitors. N Engl J Med. 366(3):207–15. PMID:22256804

2526. Suarez-Vilela D, Izquierdo-Garcia FM (2003). Angioimmunoblastic lymphadenopathy-like T-cell lymphoma: cutaneous clinical onset with prominent granulomatous reaction. Am J Surg Pathol. 27(5):699–700. PMID:12717256

2527. Suchak R, Wang WL, Prieto VG, Ivan D, Lazar AJ, Brenn T, et al. (2012). Cutaneous digital papillary adenocarcinoma: a clinicopathologic study of 31 cases of a rare neoplasm with new observations. Am J Surg Pathol. 36(12):1883–91. PMID:23026931

2528. Sugianto JZ, Ralston JS, Metcalf JS, McFaddin CL, Smith MT (2016). Blue nevus and "malignant blue nevus:" A concise review. Semin Diagn Pathol. 33(4):219–24. PMID:27199078

2529. Sugita S, Hirano H, Kikuchi N, Kubo T, Asanuma H, Aoyama T, et al. (2016). Diagnostic utility of FOSB immunohistochemistry in pseudomyogenic hemangioendothelioma and its histological mimics. Diagn Pathol. 11(1):75. PMID:27515856

2530. Sugiura M, Colby KA, Mihm MC Jr, Zembowicz A (2007). Low-risk and high-risk histologic features in conjunctival primary acquired melanosis with atypia: clinicopathologic analysis of 29 cases. Am J Surg Pathol. 31(2):185–92. PMID:17255762

2531. Sullivan LM, Folpe AL, Pawel BR, Judkins AR, Biegel JA (2013). Epithelioid sarcoma is associated with a high percentage of SMARCB1 deletions. Mod Pathol. 26(3):385–92. PMID:23060122

2532. Sun P, Watanabe K, Fallahi M, Lee B, Afetian ME, Rheaume C, et al. (2014). Pygo2 regulates β-catenin-induced activation of hair follicle stem/progenitor cells and skin hyperplasia. Proc Natl Acad Sci U S A. 111(28):10215–20. PMID:24982158

2533. Suringa DW, Ackerman AB (1970). Cutaneous lymphangiomas with dyschondroplasia (Maffucci's syndrome). A unique variant of an unusual syndrome. Arch Dermatol. 101(4):472–4. PMID:5440820

2534. Suster S (1996). Clear cell tumors of the skin. Semin Diagn Pathol. 13(1):40–59. PMID:8834514

2535. Suster S, Fisher C (1997). Immunoreactivity for the human hematopoietic progenitor cell antigen (CD34) in lipomatous tumors. Am J Surg Pathol. 21(2):195–200. PMID:9042286

2536. Suster S, Fisher C, Moran CA (1998). Expression of bcl-2 oncoprotein in benign and malignant spindle cell tumors of soft tissue, skin, serosal surfaces, and gastrointestinal tract. Am J Surg Pathol. 22(7):863–72. PMID:9669348

2537. Suurmeijer AJ (2010). Papillary hemangiomas and glomeruloid hemangiomas are distinct clinicopathological entities. Int J Surg Pathol. 18(1):48–54. PMID:18805868

2538. Suurmeijer AJ, Fletcher CD (2007). Papillary haemangioma. A distinctive cutaneous haemangioma of the head and neck area containing eosinophilic hyaline globules. Histopathology. 51(5):638–48. PMID:17927585

2539. Suzaki R, Ishizaki S, Iyatomi H, Tanaka M (2014). Age-related prevalence of dermatoscopic patterns of acral melanocytic

nevi. Dermatol Pract Concept. 4(1):53–7. PMID:24520515
**2540.** Suzuki N, Konohana I, Fukushige T, Kanzaki T (2004). Beta-mannosidosis with angiokeratoma corporis diffusum. J Dermatol. 31(11):931–5. PMID:15729869
**2541.** Suzuki R, Nakamura S, Suzumiya J, Ichimura K, Ichikawa M, Ogata K, et al. (2005). Blastic natural killer cell lymphoma/leukemia (CD56-positive blastic tumor): prognostication and categorization according to anatomic sites of involvement. Cancer. 104(5):1022–31. PMID:15999368
**2542.** Švajdler M, Baník P, Poliaková K, Straka L, Hríbiková Z, Kinkor Z, et al. (2015). Sebaceous carcinoma of the breast: report of four cases and review of the literature. Pol J Pathol. 66(2):142–8. PMID:26247527
**2543.** Swanson PE, Cherwitz DL, Neumann MP, Wick MR (1987). Eccrine sweat gland carcinoma: an histologic and immunohistochemical study of 32 cases. J Cutan Pathol. 14(2):65–86. PMID:2439558
**2544.** Swerdlow SH (2017). Cutaneous marginal zone lymphomas. Semin Diagn Pathol. 34(1):76–84. PMID:27986434
**2545.** Swerdlow SH, Campo E, Harris NL, Jaffe ES, Pileri SA, Stein H, et al., editors (2017). WHO classification of tumours of haematopoietic and lymphoid tissues. Revised 4th ed. Lyon: International Agency for Research on Cancer.
**2546.** Swerdlow SH, Campo E, Harris NL, Jaffe ES, Pileri SA, Stein H, et al., editors (2008). WHO classification of tumours of haematopoietic and lymphoid tissues. 4th edition. Lyon: International Agency for Research on Cancer.
**2547.** Swerdlow SH, Campo E, Pileri SA, Harris NL, Stein H, Siebert R, et al. (2016). The 2016 revision of the World Health Organization classification of lymphoid neoplasms. Blood. 127(20):2375–90. PMID:26980727
**2548.** Swerdlow SH, Jaffe ES, Brousset P, Chan JK, de Leval L, Gaulard P, et al. (2014). Cytotoxic T-cell and NK-cell lymphomas: current questions and controversies. Am J Surg Pathol. 38(10):e60–71. PMID:25025449
**2549.** Swerdlow SH, Quintanilla-Martinez L, Willemze R, Kinney MC (2013). Cutaneous B-cell lymphoproliferative disorders: report of the 2011 Society for Hematopathology/European Association for Haematopathology workshop. Am J Clin Pathol. 139(4):515–35. PMID:23525619
**2550.** Swick BL, Baum CL, Venkat AP, Liu V (2011). Indolent CD8+ lymphoid proliferation of the ear: report of two cases and review of the literature. J Cutan Pathol. 38(2):209–15. PMID:21083681
**2551.** Szablewski V, Ingen-Housz-Oro S, Baia M, Delfau-Larue MH, Copie-Bergman C, Ortonne N (2016). Primary cutaneous follicle center lymphomas expressing BCL2 protein frequently harbor BCL2 gene break and may present 1p36 deletion: a study of 20 cases. Am J Surg Pathol. 40(1):127–36. PMID:26658664
**2552.** Szablewski V, Laurent-Roussel S, Rethers L, Rommel A, Van Eeckhout P, Camboni A, et al. (2014). Atypical fibrous histiocytoma of the skin with CD30 and p80/ALK1 positivity and ALK gene rearrangement. J Cutan Pathol. 41(9):715–9. PMID:24666231
**2553.** Szczepański T, Pongers-Willemse MJ, Langerak AW, van Dongen JJ (1999). Unusual immunoglobulin and T-cell receptor gene rearrangement patterns in acute lymphoblastic leukemias. Curr Top Microbiol Immunol. 246:205–15. PMID:10396058
**2554.** Tabanelli V, Valli R, Righi S, Nucera G, Zecchini Barrese T, Pileri S, et al. (2014). A unique case of an indolent myometrial T-cell lymphoproliferative disorder with phenotypic features resembling uterine CD8+ resident memory T cells. Pathobiology. 81(4):176–82. PMID:25138577
**2555.** Tacha D, Qi W, Ra S, Bremer R, Yu C, Chu J, et al. (2015). A newly developed mouse monoclonal SOX10 antibody is a highly sensitive and specific marker for malignant melanoma, including spindle cell and desmoplastic melanomas. Arch Pathol Lab Med. 139(4):530–6. PMID:25436903
**2556.** Tagami H, Takigawa M, Ogino A, Imamura S, Ofugi S (1977). Spontaneous regression of plane warts after inflammation: clinical and histologic studies in 25 cases. Arch Dermatol. 113(9):1209–13. PMID:900963
**2557.** Taher A, Pushpanathan C (2007). Plexiform fibrohistiocytic tumor: a brief review. Arch Pathol Lab Med. 131(7):1135–8. PMID:17617005
**2558.** Tajirian AL, Malik MK, Robinson-Bostom L, Lally EV (2006). Multicentric reticulohistiocytosis. Clin Dermatol. 24(6):486–92. PMID:17113966
**2559.** Takai T (2017). Advances in histopathological diagnosis of keratoacanthoma. J Dermatol. 44(3):304–14. PMID:28256761
**2560.** Takashima H, Toyoda M, Ikeda Y, Kagoura M, Morohashi M (2003). Nevus lipomatosus cutaneous superficialis with perifollicular fibrosis. Eur J Dermatol. 13(6):584–6. PMID:14721781
**2561.** Takata K, Hong ME, Sitthinamsuwan P, Loong F, Tan SY, Liau JY, et al. (2015). Primary cutaneous NK/T-cell lymphoma, nasal type and CD56-positive peripheral T-cell lymphoma: a cellular lineage and clinicopathologic study of 60 patients from Asia. Am J Surg Pathol. 39(1):1–12. PMID:25188863
**2562.** Takata M, Rehman I, Rees JL (1998). A trichilemmal carcinoma arising from a proliferating trichilemmal cyst: the loss of the wild-type p53 is a critical event in malignant transformation. Hum Pathol. 29(2):193–5. PMID:9490283
**2563.** Takino H, Li C, Hu S, Kuo TT, Geissinger E, Muller-Hermelink HK, et al. (2008). Primary cutaneous marginal zone B-cell lymphoma: a molecular and clinicopathological study of cases from Asia, Germany, and the United States. Mod Pathol. 21(12):1517–26. PMID:18820662
**2564.** Tallon B, Beer TW (2014). MITF positivity in atypical fibroxanthoma: a diagnostic pitfall. Am J Dermatopathol. 36(11):888–91. PMID:25238448
**2565.** Tamada S, Ackerman AB (1987). Dermatofibroma with monster cells. Am J Dermatopathol. 9(5):380–7. PMID:2825558
**2566.** Tamura D, DiGiovanna JJ, Khan SG, Kraemer KH (2014). Living with xeroderma pigmentosum: comprehensive photoprotection for highly photosensitive patients. Photodermatol Photoimmunol Photomed. 30(2–3):146–52. PMID:24417420
**2567.** Tan CY, Marks R (1982). Lichenoid solar keratosis–prevalence and immunologic findings. J Invest Dermatol. 79(6):365–7. PMID:7142736
**2568.** Tan CZ, Rieger KE, Sarin KY (2017). Basosquamous carcinoma: controversy, advances, and future directions. Dermatol Surg. 43(1):23–31. PMID:27340741
**2569.** Tan KB, Moncrieff M, Thompson JF, McCarthy SW, Shaw HM, Quinn MJ, et al. (2007). Subungual melanoma: a study of 124 cases highlighting features of early lesions, potential pitfalls in diagnosis, and guidelines for histologic reporting. Am J Surg Pathol. 31(12):1902–12. PMID:18043047
**2570.** Tan KW, Koh MJ, Tay YK (2010). Juvenile xanthogranuloma in monozygotic twins. Pediatr Dermatol. 27(6):666–7. PMID:21091658
**2571.** Tanas MR, Sboner A, Oliveira AM, Erickson-Johnson MR, Hespelt J, Hanwright PJ, et al. (2011). Identification of a disease-defining gene fusion in epithelioid hemangioendothelioma. Sci Transl Med. 3(98):98ra82. PMID:21885404
**2572.** Tanboon J, Manonukul J, Pattanaprichakul P (2014). Melanocytic matricoma: two cases of a rare entity in women. J Cutan Pathol. 41(10):775–82. PMID:24641267
**2573.** Tang JY, Ally MS, Chanana AM, Mackay-Wiggan JM, Aszterbaum M, Lindgren JA, et al. (2016). Inhibition of the hedgehog pathway in patients with basal-cell nevus syndrome: final results from the multicentre, randomised, double-blind, placebo-controlled, phase 2 trial. Lancet Oncol. 17(12):1720–31. PMID:27838224
**2574.** Tantcheva-Poór I, Vanecek T, Lurati MC, Rychly B, Kempf W, Michal M, et al. (2016). Report of three novel germline CYLD mutations in unrelated patients with Brooke-Spiegler syndrome, including classic phenotype, multiple familial trichoepitheliomas and malignant transformation. Dermatology. 232(1):30–7. PMID:26329847
**2575.** Tapia G, Mate JL, Fuente MJ, Navarro JT, Fernández-Figueras MT, Juncà J, et al. (2013). Cutaneous presentation of chronic lymphocytic leukemia as unique extramedullar involvement in a patient with normal peripheral blood lymphocyte count (monoclonal B-cell lymphocytosis). J Cutan Pathol. 40(8):740–4. PMID:23639136
**2576.** Tardío JC (2008). CD34-reactive tumors of the skin. An updated review of an ever-growing list of lesions. J Cutan Pathol. 35(12):1079–92. PMID:18976402
**2577.** Tardío JC (2009). CD34-reactive tumors of the skin. An updated review of an ever-growing list of lesions. J Cutan Pathol. 36(1):89–102. PMID:19125742
**2578.** Tardío JC, Azorín D, Hernández-Núñez A, Guzmán A, Torrelo A, Herráiz M, et al. (2011). Dermatomyofibromas presenting in pediatric patients: clinicopathologic characteristics and differential diagnosis. J Cutan Pathol. 38(12):967–72. PMID:21752049
**2579.** Tardío JC, Pinedo F, Aramburu JA, Martínez-González MA, Arias D, Khedaoui R, et al. (2016). Clear cell atypical fibroxanthoma: clinicopathological study of 6 cases and review of the literature with special emphasis on the differential diagnosis. Am J Dermatopathol. 38(8):586–92. PMID:26848640
**2580.** Tardío JC, Pinedo F, Aramburu JA, Suárez-Massa D, Pampín A, Requena L, et al. (2016). Pleomorphic dermal sarcoma: a more aggressive neoplasm than previously estimated. J Cutan Pathol. 43(2):101–12. PMID:26264237
**2581.** Tariq S, Hugenberg ST, Hirano-Ali SA, Tariq H (2016). Multicentric reticulohistiocytosis (MRH): case report with review of literature between 1991 and 2014 with in depth analysis of various treatment regimens and outcomes. Springerplus. 5:180. PMID:27026876
**2582.** Tas F, Keskin S, Karadeniz A, Dağoğlu N, Sen F, Kilic L, et al. (2011). Noncutaneous melanoma have distinct features from each other and cutaneous melanoma. Oncology. 81(5–6):353–8. PMID:22248874
**2583.** Tateishi U, Hasegawa T, Onaya H, Satake M, Arai Y, Moriyama N (2005). Myxoinflammatory fibroblastic sarcoma: MR appearance and pathologic correlation. AJR Am J Roentgenol. 184(6):1749–53. PMID:15908525
**2584.** Tateyama H, Eimoto T, Tada T, Inagaki H, Nakamura T, Yamauchi R (1995). p53 protein and proliferating cell nuclear antigen in eccrine poroma and porocarcinoma. An immunohistochemical study. Am J Dermatopathol. 17(5):457–64. PMID:8599450
**2585.** Tay YK, Tham SN, Teo R (1996). Localized vulvar syringomas–an unusual cause of pruritus vulvae. Dermatology. 192(1):62–3. PMID:8832956
**2586.** Taylor GB, Chan YF (2000). Subcutaneous primitive neuroectodermal tumour in the abdominal wall of a child: long-term survival after local excision. Pathology. 32(4):294–8. PMID:11186429
**2587.** Tbakhi A, Cowan DF, Kumar D, Kyle D (1993). Recurring phyllodes tumor in aberrant breast tissue of the vulva. Am J Surg Pathol. 17(9):946–50. PMID:8394655
**2588.** Tcheung WJ, Selim MA, Herndon JE 2nd, Abernethy AP, Nelson KC (2012). Clinicopathologic study of 85 cases of melanoma of the female genitalia. J Am Acad Dermatol. 67(4):598–605. PMID:22243767
**2589.** Tebcherani AJ, de Andrade HF Jr, Sotto MN (2012). Diagnostic utility of immunohistochemistry in distinguishing trichoepithelioma and basal cell carcinoma: evaluation using tissue microarray samples. Mod Pathol. 25(10):1345–53. PMID:22684216
**2590.** Tellechea O, Reis JP, Baptista AP (1992). Desmoplastic trichilemmoma. Am J Dermatopathol. 14(2):107–4. PMID:1373583
**2591.** Tellechea O, Reis JP, Marques C, Baptista AP (1995). Tubular apocrine adenoma with eccrine and apocrine immunophenotypes or papillary tubular adenoma? Am J Dermatopathol. 17(5):499–505. PMID:8599457
**2592.** Templeton SF, Solomon AR Jr (1996). Spindle cell lipoma is strongly CD34 positive. An immunohistochemical study. J Cutan Pathol. 23(6):546–50. PMID:9001985
**2593.** ten Berge RL, Oudejans JJ, Ossenkoppele GJ, Pulford K, Willemze R, Falini B, et al. (2000). ALK expression in extranodal anaplastic large cell lymphoma favours systemic disease with (primary) nodal involvement and a good prognosis and occurs before dissemination. J Clin Pathol. 53(6):445–50. PMID:10911802
**2594.** Ten Broek RW, Bekers EM, de Leng WWJ, Strengman E, Tops BBJ, Kutzner H, et al. (2017). Mutational analysis using Sanger and next generation sequencing in sporadic spindle cell hemangiomas: a study of 19 cases. Genes Chromosomes Cancer. 56(12):855–60. PMID:28845532
**2595.** Ten Dam EJ, van Beuge MM, Bank RA, Werker PM (2016). Further evidence of the involvement of the Wnt signaling pathway in Dupuytren's disease. J Cell Commun Signal. 10(1):33–40. PMID:26635199
**2596.** ten Kate GL, Kleibeuker JH, Nagengast FM, Craanen M, Cats A, Menko FH, et al. (2007). Is surveillance of the small bowel indicated for Lynch syndrome families? Gut. 56(9):1198–201. PMID:17409122
**2597.** Terrier-Lacombe MJ, Guillou L, Chibon F, Gallagher G, Benhattar J, Terrier P, et al. (2009). Superficial primitive Ewing's sarcoma: a clinicopathologic and molecular cytogenetic analysis of 14 cases. Mod Pathol. 22(1):87–94. PMID:18820660
**2598.** Terrier-Lacombe MJ, Guillou L, Maire G, Terrier P, Vince DR, de Saint Aubain Somerhausen N, et al. (2003). Dermatofibrosarcoma protuberans, giant cell fibroblastoma, and hybrid lesions in children: clinicopathologic comparative analysis of 28 cases with molecular data–a study from the French Federation of Cancer Centers Sarcoma Group. Am J Surg Pathol. 27(1):27–39. PMID:12502925
**2599.** Teruya-Feldstein J, Chiao E, Filippa DA, Lin O, Comenzo R, Coleman M, et al. (2004). CD20-negative large-cell lymphoma with plasmablastic features: a clinically heterogenous spectrum in both HIV-positive and -negative patients. Ann Oncol. 15(11):1673–9. PMID:15520070
**2600.** Tessier-Cloutier B, Asleh-Aburaya K,

Shah V, McCluggage WG, Tinker A, Gilks CB (2017). Molecular subtyping of mammary-like adenocarcinoma of the vulva shows molecular similarity to breast carcinomas. Histopathology. 71(3):446–52. PMID:28418164

**2601.** Testa JR, Cheung M, Pei J, Below JE, Tan Y, Sementino E, et al. (2011). Germline BAP1 mutations predispose to malignant mesothelioma. Nat Genet. 43(10):1022–5. PMID:21874000

**2602.** Tetzlaff MT, Singh RR, Seviour EG, Curry JL, Hudgens CW, Bell D, et al. (2016). Next-generation sequencing identifies high frequency of mutations in potentially clinically actionable genes in sebaceous carcinoma. J Pathol. 240(1):84–95. PMID:27287813

**2603.** Tetzlaff MT, Torres-Cabala CA, Pattanaprichakul P, Rapini RP, Prieto VG, Curry JL (2015). Emerging clinical applications of selected biomarkers in melanoma. Clin Cosmet Investig Dermatol. 8:35–46. PMID:25674009

**2604.** Thiagalingam S, Johnson MM, Colby KA, Zembowicz A (2008). Juvenile conjunctival nevus: clinicopathologic analysis of 33 cases. Am J Surg Pathol. 32(3):399–406. PMID:18300811

**2605.** Thiex R, Mulliken JB, Revencu N, Boon LM, Burrows PE, Cordisco M, et al. (2010). A novel association between RASA1 mutations and spinal arteriovenous anomalies. AJNR Am J Neuroradiol. 31(4):775–9. PMID:20007727

**2606.** Thomas AC, Zeng Z, Rivière JB, O'Shaughnessy R, Al-Olabi L, St-Onge J, et al. (2016). Mosaic activating mutations in GNA11 and GNAQ are associated with phakomatosis pigmentovascularis and extensive dermal melanocytosis. J Invest Dermatol. 136(4):770–8. PMID:26778290

**2607.** Thomas C, Somani N, Owen LG, Malone JC, Billings SD (2009). Cutaneous malignant peripheral nerve sheath tumors. J Cutan Pathol. 36(8):896–900. PMID:19586501

**2608.** Thompson SC, Jolley D, Marks R (1993). Reduction of solar keratoses by regular sunscreen use. N Engl J Med. 329(16):1147–51. PMID:8377777

**2609.** Thornton CM, Hunt SJ (1995). Sebaceous adenoma with a cutaneous horn. J Cutan Pathol. 22(2):185–7. PMID:7560356

**2610.** Thum C, Hollowood K, Birch J, Goodlad JR, Brenn T (2011). Aberrant Melan-A expression in atypical fibroxanthoma and undifferentiated pleomorphic sarcoma of the skin. J Cutan Pathol. 38(12):954–60. PMID:22050092

**2611.** Thum C, Husain EA, Mulholland K, Hornick JL, Brenn T (2013). Atypical fibroxanthoma with pseudoangiomatous features: a histological and immunohistochemical mimic of cutaneous angiosarcoma. Ann Diagn Pathol. 17(6):502–7. PMID:24080496

**2612.** Thway K, Flora RS, Fisher C (2012). Chondroid lipoma: an update and review. Ann Diagn Pathol. 16(3):230–4. PMID:22607659

**2613.** Thway K, Gibson S, Ramsay A, Sebire NJ (2009). Beta-catenin expression in pediatric fibroblastic and myofibroblastic lesions: a study of 100 cases. Pediatr Dev Pathol. 12(4):292–6. PMID:18939887

**2614.** Thway K, Jones RL, Noujaim J, Fisher C (2016). Epithelioid sarcoma: diagnostic features and genetics. Adv Anat Pathol. 23(1):41–9. PMID:26645461

**2615.** Thway K, Noujaim J, Jones RL, Fisher C (2016). Dermatofibrosarcoma protuberans: pathology, genetics, and potential therapeutic strategies. Ann Diagn Pathol. 25:64–71. PMID:27806849

**2616.** Tirode F, Laud-Duval K, Prieur A, Delorme B, Charbord P, Delattre O (2007). Mesenchymal stem cell features of Ewing tumors. Cancer Cell. 11(5):421–9. PMID:17482132

**2617.** Tirumalae R, Rout P, Jayaseelan E, Shet A, Devi S, Kumar KR (2011). Paraneoplastic multicentric reticulohistiocytosis: a clinicopathologic challenge. Indian J Dermatol Venereol Leprol. 77(3):318–20. PMID:21508571

**2618.** Titgemeyer C, Grois N, Minkov M, Flucher-Wolfram B, Gatterer-Menz I, Gadner H (2001). Pattern and course of single-system disease in Langerhans cell histiocytosis data from the DAL-HX 83- and 90-study. Med Pediatr Oncol. 37(2):108–14. PMID:11496348

**2619.** Tjalma WA, Siozopoulou V, Huizing MT (2017). A clitoral verrucous carcinoma in an area of lichen planus has aggressive features. World J Surg Oncol. 15(1):7. PMID:28061900

**2620.** Toker C (1972). Trabecular carcinoma of the skin. Arch Dermatol. 105(1):107–10. PMID:5009611

**2621.** Tokura Y, Ishihara S, Tagawa S, Seo N, Ohshima K, Takigawa M (2001). Hypersensitivity to mosquito bites as the primary clinical manifestation of a juvenile type of Epstein-Barr virus-associated natural killer cell leukemia/lymphoma. J Am Acad Dermatol. 45(4):569–78. PMID:11568749

**2622.** Tokura Y, Ito T, Kawakami C, Sugita K, Kasuya A, Tatsuno K, et al. (2015). Human T-lymphotropic virus 1 (HTLV-1)-associated lichenoid dermatitis induced by CD8+ T cells in HTLV-1 carrier, HTLV-1-associated myelopathy/tropical spastic paraparesis and adult T-cell leukemia/lymphoma. J Dermatol. 42(10):967–74. PMID:26077665

**2623.** Tokura Y, Yamanaka K, Wakita H, Kurokawa S, Horiguchi D, Usui A, et al. (1994). Halo congenital nevus undergoing spontaneous regression. Involvement of T-cell immunity in involution and presence of circulating anti-nevus cell IgM antibodies. Arch Dermatol. 130(8):1036–41. PMID:8053701

**2624.** Tomaszewski MM, Lupton GP (1998). Unusual expression of S-100 protein in histiocytic neoplasms. J Cutan Pathol. 25(3):129–35. PMID:9550310

**2625.** Tomlins SA, Palanisamy N, Brenner JC, Stall JN, Siddiqui J, Thomas DG, et al. (2013). Usefulness of a monoclonal ERG/FLI1 antibody for immunohistochemical discrimination of Ewing family tumors. Am J Clin Pathol. 139(6):771–9. PMID:23690120

**2626.** Torchia EC, Jaishankar S, Baker SJ (2003). Ewing tumor fusion proteins block the differentiation of pluripotent marrow stromal cells. Cancer Res. 63(13):3464–8. PMID:12839926

**2627.** Toribio J, Zulaica A, Peteiro C (1987). Tubular apocrine adenoma. J Cutan Pathol. 14(2):114–7. PMID:3036918

**2628.** Toro JR, Beaty M, Sorbara L, Turner ML, White J, Kingma DW, et al. (2000). Gamma delta T-cell lymphoma of the skin: a clinical, microscopic, and molecular study. Arch Dermatol. 136(8):1024–32. PMID:10926739

**2629.** Toro JR, Liewehr DJ, Pabby N, Sorbara L, Raffeld M, Steinberg SM, et al. (2003). Gamma-delta T-cell phenotype is associated with significantly decreased survival in cutaneous T-cell lymphoma. Blood. 101(9):3407–12. PMID:12522013

**2630.** Torrelo A, Juarez A, Hernández A, Colmenero I (2009). Multiple lichenoid juvenile xanthogranuloma. Pediatr Dermatol. 26(2):238–40. PMID:19419490

**2631.** Tosti A, Baran R, Morelli R, Fanti PA, Peserico A (1994). Progressive fading of longitudinal melanonychia due to a nail matrix melanocytic nevus in a child. Arch Dermatol. 130(8):1076–7. PMID:8053713

**2632.** Tosti A, Baran R, Piraccini BM, Cameli N, Fanti PA (1996). Nail matrix nevi: a clinical and histopathologic study of twenty-two patients. J Am Acad Dermatol. 34(5 Pt 1):765–71. PMID:8632071

**2633.** Totonchy MB, Tamura D, Pantell MS, Zalewski C, Bradford PT, Merchant SN, et al. (2013). Auditory analysis of xeroderma pigmentosum 1971-2012: hearing function, sun sensitivity and DNA repair predict neurological degeneration. Brain. 136(Pt 1):194–208. PMID:23365097

**2634.** Tourlaki A, Recalcati S, Boneschi V, Gaiani F, Colombo A, Mancuso R, et al. (2013). Anaplastic Kaposi's sarcoma: a study of eight patients. Eur J Dermatol. 23(3):382–6. PMID:23783037

**2635.** Toussaint S, Kamino H (1999). Dysplastic changes in different types of melanocytic nevi. A unifying concept. J Cutan Pathol. 26(2):84–90. PMID:10082398

**2636.** Toz B, Büyükbabani N, İnanç M (2016). Multicentric reticulohistiocytosis: rheumatology perspective. Best Pract Res Clin Rheumatol. 30(2):250–60. PMID:27886798

**2637.** Tozawa T, Ackerman AB (1987). Basal cell carcinoma with follicular differentiation. Am J Dermatopathol. 9(6):474–82. PMID:2981015

**2638.** Tozetto-Mendoza TR, Ibrahim KY, Tateno AF, Oliveira CM, Sumita LM, Sanchez MC, et al. (2016). Genotypic distribution of HHV-8 in AIDS individuals without and with Kaposi sarcoma: is genotype B associated with better prognosis of AIDS-KS? Medicine (Baltimore). 95(48):e5291. PMID:27902590

**2639.** Tracey L, Villuendas R, Dotor AM, Spiteri I, Ortiz P, Garcia JF, et al. (2003). Mycosis fungoides shows concurrent deregulation of multiple genes involved in the TNF signaling pathway: an expression profile study. Blood. 102(3):1042–50. PMID:12689942

**2640.** Traianou A, Ulrich M, Apalla Z, De Vries E, Bakirtzi K, Kalabalikis D, et al. (2012). Risk factors for actinic keratosis in eight European centres: a case-control study. Br J Dermatol. 167 Suppl 2:36–42. PMID:22881586

**2641.** Tran DC, Li S, Henry S, Wood DJ, Chang ALS (2017). An 18-year retrospective study on the outcomes of keratoacanthomas with different treatment modalities at a single academic centre. Br J Dermatol. 177(6):1749–51. PMID:27943239

**2642.** Tran LP, Velanovich V, Kaufmann CR (1994). Familial multiple glomus tumors: report of a pedigree and literature review. Ann Plast Surg. 32(1):89–91. PMID:8141540

**2643.** Tran TA, Deavers MT, Carlson JA, Malpica A (2015). Collision of ductal carcinoma in situ of anogenital mammary-like glands and vulvar sarcomatoid squamous cell carcinoma. Int J Gynecol Pathol. 34(5):487–94. PMID:26107561

**2644.** Tran TA, Hayner-Buchan A, Jones DM, McRorie D, Carlson JA (2007). Cutaneous balloon cell dermatofibroma (fibrous histiocytoma). Am J Dermatopathol. 29(2):197–200. PMID:17414448

**2645.** Tregnago AC, Furlan MV, Bezerra SM, Porto GC, Mendes GG, Henklain JV, et al. (2015). Orbital melanocytoma completely resected with conservative surgery in association with ipsilateral nevus of Ota: report of a case and review of the literature. Head Neck. 37(4):E49–55. PMID:24989678

**2646.** Triay E, Bergman L, Nilsson B, All-Ericsson C, Seregard S (2009). Time trends in the incidence of conjunctival melanoma in Sweden. Br J Ophthalmol. 93(11):1524–8. PMID:19628487

**2647.** Trindade F, Kutzner H, Requena L, Tellechea Ó, Colmenero I (2012). Microvenular hemangioma-an immunohistochemical study of 9 cases. Am J Dermatopathol. 34(8):810–2. PMID:23169416

**2648.** Trindade F, Kutzner H, Tellechea Ó, Requena L, Colmenero I (2012). Hobnail hemangioma reclassified as superficial lymphatic malformation: a study of 52 cases. J Am Acad Dermatol. 66(1):112–5. PMID:21821311

**2649.** Trindade F, Torrelo A, Kutzner H, Requena L, Tellechea Ó, Colmenero I (2014). An immunohistochemical study of angiokeratomas of children. Am J Dermatopathol. 36(10):796–9. PMID:25243395

**2650.** Tripoli M, Cordova A, Moschella F (2016). Update on the role of molecular factors and fibroblasts in the pathogenesis of Dupuytren's disease. J Cell Commun Signal. 10(4):315–30. PMID:27271552

**2651.** Trombetta D, Magnusson L, von Steyern FV, Hornick JL, Fletcher CD, Mertens F (2011). Translocation t(7;19)(q22;q13)–a recurrent chromosome aberration in pseudomyogenic hemangioendothelioma? Cancer Genet. 204(4):211–5. PMID:21536240

**2652.** Tronnier M, Vogelbruch M (2007). Atypical fibroxanthoma arising in an area of syringocystadenoma papilliferum associated with nevus sebaceus: positivity of the atypical fibroxanthoma component for CD31. J Cutan Pathol. 34 Suppl 1:58–63. PMID:17997741

**2653.** Trotter MJ, Whittaker SJ, Orchard GE, Smith NP (1997). Cutaneous histopathology of Sézary syndrome: a study of 41 cases with a proven circulating T-cell clone. J Cutan Pathol. 24(5):286–91. PMID:9194581

**2654.** Trovik CS, Bauer HC, Alvegård TA, Anderson H, Blomqvist C, Berlin O, et al. (2000). Surgical margins, local recurrence and metastasis in soft tissue sarcomas: 559 surgically-treated patients from the Scandinavian Sarcoma Group Register. Eur J Cancer. 36(6):710–6. PMID:10762742

**2655.** Trown K, Heenan PJ (1994). Malignant mixed tumor of the skin (malignant chondroid syringoma). Pathology. 26(3):237–43. PMID:7991276

**2656.** Troy JL, Ackerman AB (1984). Sebaceoma. A distinctive benign neoplasm of adnexal epithelium differentiating toward sebaceous cells. Am J Dermatopathol. 6(1):7–13. PMID:6703260

**2657.** Tsai JH, Hsiao TL, Chen YY, Hsiao CH, Liau JY (2014). Endocrine mucin-producing sweat gland carcinoma occurring on extra-facial site: a case report. J Cutan Pathol. 41(6):544–7. PMID:24673415

**2658.** Tsai JW, Huang HY, Lee JC, Yen YS, Tung CL, Huang CC, et al. (2011). Composite haemangioendothelioma: report of four cases with emphasis on atypical clinical presentation. Pathology. 43(2):176–80. PMID:21233686

**2659.** Tsang WY, Chan JK (1993). The family of epithelioid vascular tumors. Histol Histopathol. 8(1):187–212. PMID:8443431

**2660.** Tsao H, Bevona C, Goggins W, Quinn T (2003). The transformation rate of moles (melanocytic nevi) into cutaneous melanoma: a population-based estimate. Arch Dermatol. 139(3):282–8. PMID:12622618

**2661.** Tse JY, Nguyen AT, Le LP, Hoang MP (2013). Microcystic adnexal carcinoma versus desmoplastic trichoepithelioma: a comparative study. Am J Dermatopathol. 35(1):50–5. PMID:22722464

**2662.** Tse JY, Pawlak AC, Boussahmain C, Routhier CA, Dias-Santagata D, Kalomiris D, et al. (2013). Basal cell carcinoma with osteosarcomatous component. Am J Dermatopathol. 35(2):261–5. PMID:23221485

**2663.** Tse JY, Walls BE, Pomerantz H, Yoon CH, Buchbinder EI, Werchniak AE, et al. (2016). Melanoma arising in a nevus of Ito: novel genetic mutations and a review of the literature on cutaneous malignant transformation of dermal melanocytosis. J Cutan Pathol. 43(1):57–63. PMID:26260725

**2664.** Tseng D, Kim J, Warrick A, Nelson D,

Pukay M, Beadling C, et al. (2014). Oncogenic mutations in melanomas and benign melanocytic nevi of the female genital tract. J Am Acad Dermatol. 71(2):229–36. PMID:24842760
**2665.** Tsukamoto Y, Katsunobu Y, Omura Y, Maeda I, Hirai M, Teshima H, et al. (2006). Subcutaneous panniculitis-like T-cell lymphoma: successful initial treatment with prednisolone and cyclosporin A. Intern Med. 45(1):21–4. PMID:16467600
**2666.** Tsukasaki K, Tsushima H, Yamamura M, Hata T, Murata K, Maeda T, et al. (1997). Integration patterns of HTLV-I provirus in relation to the clinical course of ATL: frequent clonal change at crisis from indolent disease. Blood. 89(3):948–56. PMID:9028326
**2667.** Tucker MA, Halpern A, Holly EA, Hartge P, Elder DE, Sagebiel RW, et al. (1997). Clinically recognized dysplastic nevi. A central risk factor for cutaneous melanoma. JAMA. 277(18):1439–44. PMID:9145715
**2668.** Tuomaala S, Eskelin S, Tarkkanen A, Kivelä T (2002). Population-based assessment of clinical characteristics predicting outcome of conjunctival melanoma in whites. Invest Ophthalmol Vis Sci. 43(11):3399–408. PMID:12407149
**2669.** Turnbull JR, Assaf Ch, Zouboulis C, Tebbe B (2004). Bilateral naevus of Ota: a rare manifestation in a Caucasian. J Eur Acad Dermatol Venereol. 18(3):353–5. PMID:15096155
**2670.** Turnbull JR, Husak R, Treudler R, Zouboulis CC, Orfanos CE (2002). Regression of multiple viral warts in a human immunodeficiency virus-infected patient treated by triple antiretroviral therapy. Br J Dermatol. 146(2):330. PMID:11903251
**2671.** Turner J, Couts K, Sheren J, Saichaemchan S, Ariyawutyakorn W, Avolio I, et al. (2017). Kinase gene fusions in defined subsets of melanoma. Pigment Cell Melanoma Res. 30(1):53–62. PMID:27864876
**2672.** Tuttle R, Kane JM 3rd (2015). Biopsy techniques for soft tissue and bowel sarcomas. J Surg Oncol. 111(5):504–12. PMID:25663366
**2673.** Ud Din N, Zhang P, Sukov WR, Sattler CA, Jenkins SM, Doyle LA, et al. (2016). Spindle cell lipomas arising at atypical locations. Am J Clin Pathol. 146(4):487–95. PMID:27686175
**2674.** Udager AM, Ishikawa MK, Lucas DR, McHugh JB, Patel RM (2016). MYC immunohistochemistry in angiosarcoma and atypical vascular lesions: practical considerations based on a single institutional experience. Pathology. 48(7):697–704. PMID:27780597
**2675.** Uddin S, Katzav S, White MF, Platanias LC (1995). Insulin-dependent tyrosine phosphorylation of the vav protooncogene product in cells of hematopoietic origin. J Biol Chem. 270(13):7712–6. PMID:7535775
**2676.** Uguen A, Talagas M, Costa S, Duigou S, Bouvier S, De Braekeleer M, et al. (2015). A p16-Ki-67-HMB45 immunohistochemistry scoring system as an ancillary diagnostic tool in the diagnosis of melanoma. Diagn Pathol. 10:195. PMID:26503349
**2677.** Ungewickell A, Bhaduri A, Rios E, Reuter J, Lee CS, Mah A, et al. (2015). Genomic analysis of mycosis fungoides and Sézary syndrome identifies recurrent alterations in TNFR2. Nat Genet. 47(9):1056–60. PMID:26258847
**2678.** Urosevic M, Conrad C, Kamarashev J, Asagoe K, Cozzio A, Burg G, et al. (2005). CD4+CD56+ hematodermic neoplasms bear a plasmacytoid dendritic cell phenotype. Hum Pathol. 36(9):1020–4. PMID:16153467
**2679.** Ushijima M, Tsuneyoshi M, Enjoji M (1984). Dupuytren type fibromatoses. A clinicopathologic study of 62 cases. Acta Pathol Jpn. 34(5):991–1001. PMID:6507097
**2680.** Vaillo-Vinagre A, Ballestin-Carcavilla C, Madero-Garcia S, Pastor Garcia S, Checa Garcia A, Martinez-Tello FJ (2000). Primary angioleiomyoma of the iliac bone: clinical pathological study of one case with flow cytometric DNA content and S-phase fraction analysis. Skeletal Radiol. 29(3):181–5. PMID:10794558
**2681.** Vakilzadeh F (1987). Pilar sheath acanthoma. Hautarzt. 38(1):40–2. [German] PMID:3557980
**2682.** Val-Bernal JF, de sa Dehesa J, Garijo MF, Val D (2002). Cutaneous lipomatous neurofibroma. Am J Dermatopathol. 24(3):246–50. PMID:12140442
**2683.** Val-Bernal JF, Figols J, Vázquez-Barquero A (1995). Cutaneous plexiform schwannoma associated with neurofibromatosis type 2. Cancer. 76(7):1181–6. PMID:8630895
**2684.** Val-Bernal JF, González-Vela MC (2005). Cutaneous lipomatous neurofibroma: characterization and frequency. J Cutan Pathol. 32(4):274–9. PMID:15769276
**2685.** Val-Bernal JF, Mira C (1996). Dermatofibroma with granular cells. J Cutan Pathol. 23(6):562–5. PMID:9001988
**2686.** Valent P, Akin C, Hartmann K, Nilsson G, Reiter A, Hermine O, et al. (2017). Advances in the classification and treatment of mastocytosis: current status and outlook toward the future. Cancer Res. 77(6):1261–70. PMID:28254862
**2687.** Valent P, Akin C, Metcalfe DD (2017). Mastocytosis: 2016 updated WHO classification and novel emerging treatment concepts. Blood. 129(11):1420–7. PMID:28031180
**2688.** Valent P, Escribano L, Broesby-Olsen S, Hartmann K, Grattan C, Brockow K, et al. (2014). Proposed diagnostic algorithm for patients with suspected mastocytosis: a proposal of the European Competence Network on Mastocytosis. Allergy. 69(10):1267–74. PMID:24836395
**2689.** van der Horst MP, Garcia-Herrera A, Markiewicz D, Martin B, Calonje E, Brenn T (2016). Squamoid eccrine ductal carcinoma: a clinicopathologic study of 30 cases. Am J Surg Pathol. 40(6):755–60. PMID:26796504
**2690.** van der Horst MP, Marusic Z, Hornick JL, Luzar B, Brenn T (2015). Morphologically low-grade spiradenocarcinoma: a clinicopathologic study of 19 cases with emphasis on outcome and MYB expression. Mod Pathol. 28(7):944–53. PMID:25857824
**2691.** van der Putte SC (1994). Mammary-like glands of the vulva and their disorders. Int J Gynecol Pathol. 13(2):150–60. PMID:8005737
**2692.** van der Zwan JM, Trama A, Otter R, Larrañaga N, Tavilla A, Marcos-Gragera R, et al. (2013). Rare neuroendocrine tumours: results of the Surveillance of Rare Cancers in Europe project. Eur J Cancer. 49(11):2565–78. PMID:23541566
**2693.** van Dijk MC, Bernsen MR, Ruiter DJ (2005). Analysis of mutations in B-RAF, N-RAS, and H-RAS genes in the differential diagnosis of Spitz nevus and spitzoid melanoma. Am J Surg Pathol. 29(9):1145–51. PMID:16096402
**2694.** van Haalen FM, Bruggink SC, Gussekloo J, Assendelft WJ, Eekhof JA (2009). Warts in primary schoolchildren: prevalence and relation with environmental factors. Br J Dermatol. 161(1):148–52. PMID:19438464
**2695.** van Kester MS, Borg MK, Zoutman WH, Out-Luiting JJ, Jansen PM, Dreef EJ, et al. (2012). A meta-analysis of gene expression data identifies a molecular signature characteristic for tumor-stage mycosis fungoides. J Invest Dermatol. 132(8):2050–9. PMID:22513784
**2696.** van Kester MS, Tensen CP, Vermeer MH, Dijkman R, Mulder AA, Szuhai K, et al. (2010). Cutaneous anaplastic large cell lymphoma and peripheral T-cell lymphoma NOS show distinct chromosomal alterations and differential expression of chemokine receptors and apoptosis regulators. J Invest Dermatol. 130(2):563–75. PMID:19710685
**2697.** Van Neer FJ, Toonstra J, Van Voorst Vader PC, Willemze R, Van Vloten WA (2001). Lymphomatoid papulosis in children: a study of 10 children registered by the Dutch Cutaneous Lymphoma Working Group. Br J Dermatol. 144(2):351–4. PMID:11251571
**2698.** van Praag MC, Bavinck JN, Bergman W, Rosendaal FR, Mommaas AM, Bruynzeel I, et al. (1993). PUVA keratosis. A clinical and histopathologic entity associated with an increased risk of nonmelanoma skin cancer. J Am Acad Dermatol. 28(3):412–7. PMID:8445056
**2699.** Van Raamsdonk CD, Bezrookove V, Green G, Bauer J, Gaugler L, O'Brien JM, et al. (2009). Frequent somatic mutations of GNAQ in uveal melanoma and blue naevi. Nature. 457(7229):599–602. PMID:19078957
**2700.** Van Raamsdonk CD, Griewank KG, Crosby MB, Garrido MC, Vemula S, Wiesner T, et al. (2010). Mutations in GNA11 in uveal melanoma. N Engl J Med. 363(23):2191–9. PMID:21083380
**2701.** van Vugt LJ, van der Vleuten CJM, Flucke U, Blokx WAM (2017). The utility of GLUT1 as a diagnostic marker in cutaneous vascular anomalies: a review of literature and recommendations for daily practice. Pathol Res Pract. 213(6):591–7. PMID:28552538
**2702.** van Zuuren EJ, Posma AN (2003). Diffuse neurofibroma on the lower back. J Am Acad Dermatol. 48(6):938–40. PMID:12789188
**2703.** van Doorn R, Dijkman R, Vermeer MH, Out-Luiting JJ, van der Raaij-Helmer EM, Willemze R, et al. (2004). Aberrant expression of the tyrosine kinase receptor EphA4 and the transcription factor twist in Sézary syndrome identified by gene expression analysis. Cancer Res. 64(16):5578–86. PMID:15313894
**2704.** van Doorn R, Scheffer E, Willemze R (2002). Follicular mycosis fungoides, a distinct disease entity with or without associated follicular mucinosis: a clinicopathologic and follow-up study of 51 patients. Arch Dermatol. 138(2):191–8. PMID:11843638
**2705.** van Doorn R, Van Haselen CW, van Voorst Vader PC, Geerts ML, Heule F, de Rie M, et al. (2000). Mycosis fungoides: disease evolution and prognosis of 309 Dutch patients. Arch Dermatol. 136(4):504–10. PMID:10768649
**2706.** van Gorp J, van der Putte SC (1993). Periungual eccrine porocarcinoma. Dermatology. 187(1):67–70. PMID:8391881
**2707.** Van Hoyweghen I, Horstman K, Schepers R (2007). Genetic 'risk carriers' and lifestyle 'risk takers'. Which risks deserve our legal protection in insurance? Health Care Anal. 15(3):179–93. PMID:17922196
**2708.** van Maldegem F, van Dijk R, Wormhoudt TA, Kluin PM, Willemze R, Cerroni L, et al. (2008). The majority of cutaneous marginal zone B-cell lymphomas expresses class-switched immunoglobulins and develops in a T-helper type 2 inflammatory environment. Blood. 112(8):3355–61. PMID:18687986
**2709.** van Santen S, Roach RE, van Doorn R, Horváth B, Bruijn MS, Sanders CJ, et al. (2016). Clinical staging and prognostic factors in folliculotropic mycosis fungoides. JAMA Dermatol. 152(9):992–1000. PMID:27276223
**2710.** van Santen S, van Doorn R, Neelis KJ, Daniëls LA, Horváth B, Bruijn MS, et al. (2017). Recommendations for treatment in folliculotropic mycosis fungoides: report of the Dutch Cutaneous Lymphoma Group. Br J Dermatol. 177(1):223–8. PMID:28132406
**2711.** Vang R, Cohen PR (1999). Ectopic hidradenoma papilliferum: a case report and review of the literature. J Am Acad Dermatol. 41(1):115–8. PMID:10411423
**2712.** Vanni R, Fletcher CD, Sciot R, Dal Cin P, De Wever I, Mandahl N, et al. (2000). Cytogenetic evidence of clonality in cutaneous benign fibrous histiocytomas: a report of the CHAMP study group. Histopathology. 37(3):212–7. PMID:10971696
**2713.** Vano-Galvan S, Moreno C, Vano-Galvan E, Arrazola JM, Muñoz-Zato E, Jaen P (2008). Solitary naevus lipomatosus cutaneous superficialis on the sole. Eur J Dermatol. 18(3):353–4. PMID:18474480
**2714.** Vaqué JP, Gómez-López G, Monsálvez V, Varela I, Martínez N, Pérez C, et al. (2014). PLCG1 mutations in cutaneous T-cell lymphomas. Blood. 123(13):2034–43. PMID:24497536
**2715.** Varey AHR, Goumas C, Hong AM, Mann GJ, Fogarty GB, Stretch JR, et al. (2017). Neurotropic melanoma: an analysis of the clinicopathological features, management strategies and survival outcomes for 671 patients treated at a tertiary referral center. Mod Pathol. 30(11):1538–50. PMID:28731051
**2716.** Alvarez-Cuesta CC, Raya-Aguado C, Vázquez-López F, García PB, Pérez-Oliva N (2002). Nevus of Ota associated with ipsilateral deafness. J Am Acad Dermatol. 47(5 Suppl):S257–9. PMID:12399743
**2717.** Alvarez-Twose I, González P, Morgado JM, Jara-Acevedo M, Sánchez-Muñoz L, Matito A, et al. (2012). Complete response after imatinib mesylate therapy in a patient with well-differentiated systemic mastocytosis. J Clin Oncol. 30(12):e126–9. PMID:22370312
**2718.** Álvarez-Twose I, Jara-Acevedo M, Morgado JM, García-Montero A, Sánchez-Muñoz L, Teodósio C, et al. (2016). Clinical, immunophenotypic, and molecular characteristics of well-differentiated systemic mastocytosis. J Allergy Clin Immunol. 137(1):168–78.e1. PMID:26100086
**2719.** Varikatt W, Soper J, Simmons G, Dave C, Munk J, Bonar F (2008). Superficial acral fibromyxoma: a report of two cases with radiological findings. Skeletal Radiol. 37(6):499–503. PMID:18327578
**2720.** Varshney A, Goyal T, Zawar V, Tinguely M, Kempf W (2016). Disseminated anetoderma in a patient with nodal Epstein-Barr virus-associated classical Hodgkin lymphoma: anetodermic form of a concurrent discordant cutaneous marginal zone lymphoma. Int J Dermatol. 55(7):739–44. PMID:26945704
**2721.** Vasmatzis G, Johnson SH, Knudson RA, Ketterling RP, Braggio E, Fonseca R, et al. (2012). Genome-wide analysis reveals recurrent structural abnormalities of TP63 and other p53-related genes in peripheral T-cell lymphomas. Blood. 120(11):2280–9. PMID:22855598
**2722.** Vassallo R, Ryu JH, Colby TV, Hartman T, Limper AH (2000). Pulmonary Langerhans'-cell histiocytosis. N Engl J Med. 342(26):1969–78. PMID:10877650
**2723.** Vazmitel M, Pavlovsky M, Kacerovska D, Michal M, Kazakov DV (2009). Pseudoangiomatous stromal hyperplasia in a complex neoplastic lesion involving anogenital mammary-like glands. J Cutan Pathol. 36(10):1117–20. PMID:19508499
**2724.** Vázquez-Bayo MC, Rodríguez-Bujaldón A, Jiménez-Puya R, Galán M, Vélez A, Moreno JC, et al. (2006). Diffuse cutaneous reticulohistiocytosis. Actas Dermosifiliogr. 97(2):118–21. [Spanish] PMID:16595113
**2725.** Vázquez-Doval J, Sola MA, Contreras-Mejuto F, Redondo P, Soto J, Quintanilla E (1995). Malignant melanoma developing in a speckled lentiginous nevus. Int J Dermatol. 34(9):637–8. PMID:7591464
**2726.** Velez MJ, Billings SD, Weaver JA (2016). Fibroblastic connective tissue nevus. J Cutan Pathol. 43(1):75–9. PMID:26268513
**2727.** Vella JE, Taibjee SM, Sanders DS, Stellakis M, Carr RA (2008). Fibroadenoma of the

anogenital region. J Clin Pathol. 61(7):871–2. PMID:18587019
**2728.** Velusamy T, Kiel MJ, Sahasrabuddhe AA, Rolland D, Dixon CA, Bailey NG, et al. (2014). A novel recurrent NPM1-TYK2 gene fusion in cutaneous CD30-positive lymphoproliferative disorders. Blood. 124(25):3768–71. PMID:25349176
**2729.** Vencio EF, Jenkins RB, Schiller JL, Huynh TV, Wenger DD, Inwards CY, et al. (2007). Clonal cytogenetic abnormalities in Erdheim-Chester disease. Am J Surg Pathol. 31(2):319–21. PMID:17255779
**2730.** Vener C, Soligo D, Berti E, Gianelli U, Servida F, Ceretti E, et al. (2007). Indeterminate cell histiocytosis in association with later occurrence of acute myeloblastic leukaemia. Br J Dermatol. 156(6):1357–61. PMID:17459045
**2731.** Vente C, Neumann C, Bertsch H, Rupprecht R, Happle R (2004). Speckled lentiginous nevus syndrome: report of a further case. Dermatology. 209(3):228–9. PMID:15459538
**2732.** Vergier B, Belaud-Rotureau MA, Benassy MN, Beylot-Barry M, Dubus P, Delaunay M, et al. (2004). Neoplastic cells do not carry bcl2-JH rearrangements detected in a subset of primary cutaneous follicle center B-cell lymphomas. Am J Surg Pathol. 28(6):748–55. PMID:15166666
**2733.** Vergier B, de Muret A, Beylot-Barry M, Vaillant L, Ekouevi D, Chene G, et al. (2000). Transformation of mycosis fungoides: clinicopathological and prognostic features of 45 cases. Blood. 95(7):2212–8. PMID:10733487
**2734.** Vergier B, Laharanne E, Prochazkova-Carlotti M, de la Fouchardière A, Merlio JP, Kadlub N, et al. (2016). Proliferative nodules vs melanoma arising in giant congenital melanocytic nevi during childhood. JAMA Dermatol. 152(10):1147–51. PMID:27486690
**2735.** Verkouteren JAC, Ramdas KHR, Wakkee M, Nijsten T (2017). Epidemiology of basal cell carcinoma: scholarly review. Br J Dermatol. 177(2):359–72. PMID:28220485
**2736.** Vermeer MH, Geelen FA, Kummer JA, Meijer CJ, Willemze R (1999). Expression of cytotoxic proteins by neoplastic T cells in mycosis fungoides increases with progression from plaque stage to tumor stage disease. Am J Pathol. 154(4):1203–10. PMID:10233858
**2737.** Vermeer MH, Geelen FA, van Haselen CW, van Voorst Vader PC, Geerts ML, van Vloten WA, et al. (1996). Primary cutaneous large B-cell lymphomas of the legs. A distinct type of cutaneous B-cell lymphoma with an intermediate prognosis. Arch Dermatol. 132(11):1304–8. PMID:8915307
**2738.** Vermeer MH, van Doorn R, Dijkman R, Mao X, Whittaker S, van Voorst Vader PC, et al. (2008). Novel and highly recurrent chromosomal alterations in Sézary syndrome. Cancer Res. 68(8):2689–98. PMID:18413736
**2739.** Vermi W, Facchetti F, Rosati S, Vergoni F, Rossi E, Festa S, et al. (2004). Nodal and extranodal tumor-forming accumulation of plasmacytoid monocytes/interferon-producing cells associated with myeloid disorders. Am J Surg Pathol. 28(5):585–95. PMID:15105645
**2740.** Veugelers M, Wilkes D, Burton K, McDermott DA, Song Y, Goldstein MM, et al. (2004). Comparative PRKAR1A genotype-phenotype analyses in humans with Carney complex and prkar1a haploinsufficient mice. Proc Natl Acad Sci U S A. 101(39):14222–7. PMID:15371594
**2741.** Veyssier-Belot C, Cacoub P, Caparros-Lefebvre D, Wechsler J, Brun B, Remy M, et al. (1996). Erdheim-Chester disease. Clinical and radiologic characteristics of 59 cases. Medicine (Baltimore). 75(3):157–69. PMID:8965684
**2742.** Vezzoli P, Fiorani R, Girgenti V, Fanoni D, Tavecchio S, Balice Y, et al. (2011). Cutaneous T-cell/histiocyte-rich B-cell lymphoma: a case report and review of the literature. Dermatology. 222(3):225–30. PMID:21540569
**2743.** Vilain RE, McCarthy SW, Thompson JF, Scolyer RA (2015). BAP1-inactivated spitzoid naevi. Am J Surg Pathol. 39(5):722. PMID:25871468
**2744.** Virgili A, Marzola A, Corazza M (2000). Vulvar hidradenoma papilliferum. A review of 10.5 years' experience. J Reprod Med. 45(8):616–8. PMID:10986678
**2745.** Virgili G, Gatta G, Ciccolallo L, Capocaccia R, Biggeri A, Crocetti E, et al. (2007). Incidence of uveal melanoma in Europe. Ophthalmology. 114(12):2309–15. PMID:17498805
**2746.** Viros A, Fridlyand J, Bauer J, Lasithiotakis K, Garbe C, Pinkel D, et al. (2008). Improving melanoma classification by integrating genetic and morphologic features. PLoS Med. 5(6):e120. PMID:18532874
**2747.** Vitte F, Fabiani B, Bénet C, Dalac S, Balme B, Delattre C, et al. (2012). Specific skin lesions in chronic myelomonocytic leukemia: a spectrum of myelomonocytic and dendritic cell proliferations: a study of 42 cases. Am J Surg Pathol. 36(9):1302–16. PMID:22895265
**2748.** Vivancos A, Caratú G, Matito J, Muñoz E, Ferrer B, Hernández-Losa J, et al. (2016). Genetic evolution of nevus of Ota reveals clonal heterogeneity acquiring BAP1 and TP53 mutations. Pigment Cell Melanoma Res. 29(2):247–53. PMID:26701415
**2749.** Vocke CD, Ricketts CJ, Merino MJ, Srinivasan R, Metwalli AR, Middelton LA, et al. (2017). Comprehensive genomic and phenotypic characterization of germline FH deletion in hereditary leiomyomatosis and renal cell carcinoma. Genes Chromosomes Cancer. 56(6):484–92. PMID:28196407
**2750.** von Hochstetter AR, Meyer VE, Grant JW, Honegger HP, Schreiber A (1991). Epithelioid sarcoma mimicking angiosarcoma: the value of immunohistochemistry in the differential diagnosis. Virchows Arch A Pathol Anat Histopathol. 418(3):271–8. PMID:1900974
**2751.** von Levetzow C, Jiang X, Gwye Y, von Levetzow G, Hung L, Cooper A, et al. (2011). Modeling initiation of Ewing sarcoma in human neural crest cells. PLoS One. 6(4):e19305. PMID:21559395
**2752.** Vonderheid EC, Pavlov I, Delgado JC, Martins TB, Telang GH, Hess AD, et al. (2014). Prognostic factors and risk stratification in early mycosis fungoides. Leuk Lymphoma. 55(1):44–50. PMID:23547839
**2753.** Vonderheid EC, Pena J, Nowell P (2006). Sézary cell counts in erythrodermic cutaneous T-cell lymphoma: implications for prognosis and staging. Leuk Lymphoma. 47(9):1841–56. PMID:17064997
**2754.** Vourc'h-Jourdain M, Martin L, Barbarot S (2013). Large congenital melanocytic nevi: therapeutic management and melanoma risk: a systematic review. J Am Acad Dermatol. 68(3):493–8.e1–14. PMID:23182059
**2755.** Wada DA, Law ME, Hsi ED, Dicaudo DJ, Ma L, Lim MS, et al. (2011). Specificity of IRF4 translocations for primary cutaneous anaplastic large cell lymphoma: a multicenter study of 204 skin biopsies. Mod Pathol. 24(4):596–605. PMID:21169992
**2756.** Wada M, Ito T, Tsuji G, Nakahara T, Hagihara A, Furue M, et al. (2017). Acral lentiginous melanoma versus other melanoma: a single-center analysis in Japan. J Dermatol. 44(8):932–8. PMID:28342269
**2757.** Wada T, Toga A, Sakakibara Y, Toma T, Hasegawa M, Takehara K, et al. (2012). Clonal expansion of Epstein-Barr virus (EBV)-infected γδ T cells in patients with chronic active EBV disease and hydroa vacciniforme-like eruptions. Int J Hematol. 96(4):443–9. PMID:22886572
**2758.** Wadhera A, Fazio M, Bricca G, Stanton O (2006). Metastatic basal cell carcinoma: a case report and literature review. How accurate is our incidence data? Dermatol Online J. 12(5):7. PMID:16962022
**2759.** Wadt K, Choi J, Chung JY, Kiilgaard J, Heegaard S, Drzewiecki KT, et al. (2012). A cryptic BAP1 splice mutation in a family with uveal and cutaneous melanoma, and paraganglioma. Pigment Cell Melanoma Res. 25(6):815–8. PMID:22889334
**2760.** Wadt KA, Aoude LG, Johansson P, Solinas A, Pritchard A, Crainic O, et al. (2015). A recurrent germline BAP1 mutation and extension of the BAP1 tumor predisposition spectrum to include basal cell carcinoma. Clin Genet. 88(3):267–72. PMID:25225168
**2761.** Wahl CE, Todd DH, Binder SW, Cassarino DS (2009). Apocrine hidradenocarcinoma showing Paget's disease and mucinous metaplasia. J Cutan Pathol. 36(5):582–5. PMID:19476529
**2762.** Walling HW (2009). Primary hyperhidrosis increases the risk of cutaneous infection: a case-control study of 387 patients. J Am Acad Dermatol. 61(2):242–6. PMID:19395123
**2763.** Walsh N, Ackerman AB (1990). Infundibulocystic basal cell carcinoma: a newly described variant. Mod Pathol. 3(5):599–608. PMID:2235986
**2764.** Walsh N, Crotty K, Palmer A, McCarthy S (1998). Spitz nevus versus spitzoid malignant melanoma: an evaluation of the current distinguishing histopathologic criteria. Hum Pathol. 29(10):1105–12. PMID:9781649
**2765.** Walsh NM (2001). Primary neuroendocrine (Merkel cell) carcinoma of the skin: morphologic diversity and implications thereof. Hum Pathol. 32(7):680–9. PMID:11486166
**2766.** Walsh NM (2016). Complete spontaneous regression of Merkel cell carcinoma (1986-2016): a 30 year perspective. J Cutan Pathol. 43(12):1150–4. PMID:27596690
**2767.** Walsh SN, Hurt MA, Santa Cruz DJ (2007). Psoriasiform keratosis. Am J Dermatopathol. 29(2):137–40. PMID:17414434
**2768.** Walther BS, Gibbons G, Chan EF, Ziselman E, Rothfleisch JE, Willard RJ, et al. (2009). Leukemia cutis (involving chronic lymphocytic leukemia) within excisional specimens: a series of 6 cases. Am J Dermatopathol. 31(2):162–5. PMID:19318802
**2769.** Walther C, Hofvander J, Nilsson J, Magnusson L, Domanski HA, Gisselsson D, et al. (2015). Gene fusion detection in formalin-fixed paraffin-embedded benign fibrous histiocytomas using fluorescence in situ hybridization and RNA sequencing. Lab Invest. 95(9):1071–6. PMID:26121314
**2770.** Walther C, Tayebwa J, Lilljebjörn H, Magnusson L, Nilsson J, von Steyern FV, et al. (2014). A novel SERPINE1-FOSB fusion gene results in transcriptional up-regulation of FOSB in pseudomyogenic haemangioendothelioma. J Pathol. 232(5):534–40. PMID:24374978
**2771.** Wambacher-Gasser B, Zelger B, Zelger BG, Steiner H (1997). Clear cell dermatofibroma. Histopathology. 30(1):64–9. PMID:9023559
**2772.** Wang AR, May D, Bourne P, Scott G (1999). PGP9.5: a marker for cellular neurothekeoma. Am J Surg Pathol. 23(11):1401–7. PMID:10555009
**2773.** Wang E, Lee JS, Kazakov DV (2013). A rare combination of sebaceoma with carcinomatous change (sebaceous carcinoma), trichoblastoma, and poroma arising from a nevus sebaceus. J Cutan Pathol. 40(7):676–82. PMID:23550845
**2774.** Wang HH, Myers T, Lach LJ, Hsieh CC, Kadin ME (1999). Increased risk of lymphoid and nonlymphoid malignancies in patients with lymphomatoid papulosis. Cancer. 86(7):1240–5. PMID:10506709
**2775.** Wang L, Gao T, Wang G (2014). Verrucous hemangioma: a clinicopathological and immunohistochemical analysis of 74 cases. J Cutan Pathol. 41(11):823–30. PMID:25263605
**2776.** Wang L, Li C, Gao T (2011). Cutaneous intravascular anaplastic large cell lymphoma. J Cutan Pathol. 38(2):221–6. PMID:20337769
**2777.** Wang L, Ni X, Covington KR, Yang BY, Shiu J, Zhang X, et al. (2015). Genomic profiling of Sézary syndrome identifies alterations of key T cell signaling and differentiation genes. Nat Genet. 47(12):1426–34. PMID:26551670
**2778.** Wang L, Yuan W, Geng S, Xiong Y, Zhang D, Zhao X, et al. (2014). Expression of lymphatic markers in angiokeratomas. J Cutan Pathol. 41(7):576–81. PMID:24666194
**2779.** Wang WL, Bones-Valentin RA, Prieto VG, Pollock RE, Lev DC, Lazar AJ (2012). Sarcoma metastases to the skin: a clinicopathologic study of 65 patients. Cancer. 118(11):2900–4. PMID:21989966
**2780.** Wang WL, Mayordomo E, Zhang W, Hernandez VS, Tuvin D, Garcia L, et al. (2009). Detection and characterization of EWSR1/ATF1 and EWSR1/CREB1 chimeric transcripts in clear cell sarcoma (melanoma of soft parts). Mod Pathol. 22(9):1201–9. PMID:19561568
**2781.** Wang WL, Torres-Cabala C, Curry JL, Ivan D, McLemore M, Tetzlaff M, et al. (2015). Metastatic atypical fibroxanthoma: a series of 11 cases including with minimal and no subcutaneous involvement. Am J Dermatopathol. 37(6):455–61. PMID:25590287
**2782.** Wang Y, Zhao Y, Ma S (2016). Racial differences in six major subtypes of melanoma: descriptive epidemiology. BMC Cancer. 16:691. PMID:27576582
**2783.** Warkel RL, Helwig EB (1978). Apocrine gland adenoma and adenocarcinoma of the axilla. Arch Dermatol. 114(2):198–203. PMID:629545
**2784.** Warner J, Jones EW (1968). Pyogenic granuloma recurring with multiple satellites. A report of 11 cases. Br J Dermatol. 80(4):218–27. PMID:5647967
**2785.** Warrick E, Garcia M, Chagnoleau C, Chevallier O, Bergoglio V, Sartori D, et al. (2012). Preclinical corrective gene transfer in xeroderma pigmentosum human skin stem cells. Mol Ther. 20(4):798–807. PMID:22068429
**2786.** Wartchow EP, Goin L, Schreiber J, Mierau GW, Terella A, Allen GC (2009). Plexiform fibrohistiocytic tumor: ultrastructural studies may aid in discrimination from cellular neurothekeoma. Ultrastruct Pathol. 33(6):286–92. PMID:19929176
**2787.** Wasco MJ, Fullen D, Su L, Ma L (2008). The expression of MUM1 in cutaneous T-cell lymphoproliferative disorders. Hum Pathol. 39(4):557–63. PMID:18234282
**2788.** Watanabe S, Sawada M, Dekio I, Ishizaki S, Fujibayashi M, Tanaka M (2016). Chronology of lichen planus-like keratosis features by dermoscopy: a summary of 17 cases. Dermatol Pract Concept. 6(2):29–35. PMID:27222769
**2789.** Watson P, Vasen HFA, Mecklin JP, Bernstein I, Aarnio M, Järvinen HJ, et al. (2008). The risk of extra-colonic, extra-endometrial cancer in the Lynch syndrome. Int J Cancer. 123(2):444–9. PMID:18398828
**2790.** Watts CG, Madronio C, Morton RL, Goumas C, Armstrong BK, Curtin A, et al. (2017). Clinical features associated with individuals at higher risk of melanoma: a population-based study. JAMA Dermatol. 153(1):23–9. PMID:27829101
**2791.** Wayte DM, Helwig EB (1968). Halo nevi. Cancer. 22(1):69–90. PMID:5659416
**2792.** Weedon D, Little JH (1977). Spindle and epithelioid cell nevi in children and adults. A review of 211 cases of the Spitz nevus. Cancer.

40(1):217–25. PMID:880553
**2793.** Wehkamp U, Pott C, Unterhalt M, Koch K, Weichenthal M, Klapper W, et al. (2015). Skin involvement of mantle cell lymphoma may mimic primary cutaneous diffuse large B-cell lymphoma, leg type. Am J Surg Pathol. 39(8):1093–101. PMID:26034867
**2794.** Wehner MR, Shive ML, Chren MM, Han J, Qureshi AA, Linos E (2012). Indoor tanning and non-melanoma skin cancer: systematic review and meta-analysis. BMJ. 345:e5909. PMID:23033409
**2795.** Wehrli BM, Weiss SW, Yandow S, Coffin CM (2001). Gardner-associated fibromas (GAF) in young patients: a distinct fibrous lesion that identifies unsuspected Gardner syndrome and risk for fibromatosis. Am J Surg Pathol. 25(5):645–51. PMID:11342777
**2796.** Wei L, Liu S, Conroy J, Wang J, Papanicolau-Sengos A, Glenn ST, et al. (2015). Whole-genome sequencing of a malignant granular cell tumor with metabolic response to pazopanib. Cold Spring Harb Mol Case Stud. 1(1):a000380. PMID:27148567
**2797.** Weigand DA, Burgdorf WH (1980). Perianal apocrine gland adenoma. Arch Dermatol. 116(9):1051–3. PMID:7416759
**2798.** Weinreb I, Bergfeld WF, Patel RM, Ghazarian DM (2009). Apocrine carcinoma in situ of sweat duct origin. Am J Surg Pathol. 33(1):155–7. PMID:18971780
**2799.** Weinreb I, Shaw AJ, Perez-Ordoñez B, Goldblum JR, Rubin BP (2009). Nodular fasciitis of the head and neck region: a clinicopathologic description in a series of 30 cases. J Cutan Pathol. 36(11):1168–73. PMID:19469872
**2800.** Weiss J, Heine M, Grimmel M, Jung EG (1995). Malignant proliferating trichilemmal cyst. J Am Acad Dermatol. 32(5 Pt 2):870–3. PMID:7722047
**2801.** Weiss SW, Enzinger FM (1977). Myxoid variant of malignant fibrous histiocytoma. Cancer. 39(4):1672–85. PMID:192434
**2802.** Weiss SW, Enzinger FM (1982). Epithelioid hemangioendothelioma: a vascular tumor often mistaken for a carcinoma. Cancer. 50(5):970–81. PMID:7093931
**2803.** Weiss SW, Enzinger FM (1986). Spindle cell hemangioendothelioma. A low-grade angiosarcoma resembling a cavernous hemangioma and Kaposi's sarcoma. Am J Surg Pathol. 10(8):521–30. PMID:3740350
**2804.** Weitzman S, Jaffe R (2005). Uncommon histiocytic disorders: the non-Langerhans cell histiocytoses. Pediatr Blood Cancer. 45(3):256–64. PMID:15547923
**2805.** Weitzner S (1968). Solitary nevus lipomatosus cutaneus superficialis of scalp. Arch Dermatol. 97(5):540–2. PMID:5647029
**2806.** Welborn J, Fenner S, Parks R (2010). Angioleiomyoma: a benign tumor with karyotypic aberrations. Cancer Genet Cytogenet. 199(2):147–8. PMID:20471520
**2807.** Welch HG, Black WC (2010). Overdiagnosis in cancer. J Natl Cancer Inst. 102(9):605–13. PMID:20413742
**2808.** Wermker K, Roknic N, Goessling K, Klein M, Schulze HJ, Hallermann C (2015). Basosquamous carcinoma of the head and neck: clinical and histologic characteristics and their impact on disease progression. Neoplasia. 17(3):301–5. PMID:25810014
**2809.** West DS, Dogan A, Quint PS, Tricker-Klar ML, Porcher JC, Ketterling RP, et al. (2013). Clonally related follicular lymphomas and Langerhans cell neoplasms: expanding the spectrum of transdifferentiation. Am J Surg Pathol. 37(7):978–86. PMID:23759932
**2810.** Whimster IW (1976). The pathology of lymphangioma circumscriptum. Br J Dermatol. 94(5):473–86. PMID:1268059
**2811.** White WL, Hitchcock MG (1998). Dying dogma: the pathological diagnosis of epidermotropic metastatic malignant melanoma. Semin Diagn Pathol. 15(3):176–88. PMID:9711667
**2812.** Whitehead KJ, Smith MC, Li DY (2013). Arteriovenous malformations and other vascular malformation syndromes. Cold Spring Harb Perspect Med. 3(2):a006635. PMID:23125071
**2813.** Whiteman DC, Watt P, Purdie DM, Hughes MC, Hayward NK, Green AC (2003). Melanocytic nevi, solar keratoses, and divergent pathways to cutaneous melanoma. J Natl Cancer Inst. 95(11):806–12. PMID:12783935
**2814.** Whittaker SJ, Smith NP (1992). Diagnostic value of T-cell receptor beta gene rearrangement analysis on peripheral blood lymphocytes of patients with erythroderma. J Invest Dermatol. 99(3):361–2. PMID:1324964
**2815.** Whittaker SJ, Smith NP, Jones RR, Luzzatto L (1991). Analysis of beta, gamma, and delta T-cell receptor genes in mycosis fungoides and Sezary syndrome. Cancer. 68(7):1572–82. PMID:1654197
**2816.** Wick MR (1990). Malignant peripheral nerve sheath tumors of the skin. Mayo Clin Proc. 65(2):279–82. PMID:2304365
**2817.** Wick MR, Cooper PH, Swanson PE, Kaye VN, Sun TT (1990). Microcystic adnexal carcinoma. An immunohistochemical comparison with other cutaneous appendage tumors. Arch Dermatol. 126(2):189–94. PMID:1689137
**2818.** Wick MR, Mills SE, Ritter JH, Lind AC (1999). Postoperative/posttraumatic spindle cell nodule of the skin: the dermal analogue of nodular fasciitis. Am J Dermatopathol. 21(3):220–4. PMID:10380041
**2819.** Wick MR, Swanson PE (1986). Primary adenoid cystic carcinoma of the skin. A clinical, histological, and immunocytochemical comparison with adenoid cystic carcinoma of salivary glands and adenoid basal cell carcinoma. Am J Dermatopathol. 8(1):2–13. PMID:3010759
**2820.** Wiechers T, Rabenhorst A, Schick T, Preussner LM, Förster A, Valent P, et al. (2015). Large maculopapular cutaneous lesions are associated with favorable outcome in childhood-onset mastocytosis. J Allergy Clin Immunol. 136(6):1581–90.e3. PMID:26152315
**2821.** Wieselthier JS, White WL (1996). Cutaneous metastasis of ocular malignant melanoma. An unusual presentation simulating blue nevi. Am J Dermatopathol. 18(3):289–95. PMID:8806964
**2822.** Wieser I, Oh CW, Talpur R, Duvic M (2016). Lymphomatoid papulosis: treatment response and associated lymphomas in a study of 180 patients. J Am Acad Dermatol. 74(1):59–67. PMID:26518172
**2823.** Wiesner T, Fried I, Ulz P, Stacher E, Popper H, Murali R, et al. (2012). Toward an improved definition of the tumor spectrum associated with BAP1 germline mutations. J Clin Oncol. 30(32):e337–40. PMID:23032617
**2824.** Wiesner T, He J, Yelensky R, Esteve-Puig R, Botton T, Yeh I, et al. (2014). Kinase fusions are frequent in Spitz tumours and spitzoid melanomas. Nat Commun. 5:3116. PMID:24445538
**2825.** Wiesner T, Kiuru M, Scott SN, Arcila M, Halpern AC, Hollmann T, et al. (2015). NF1 mutations are common in desmoplastic melanoma. Am J Surg Pathol. 39(10):1357–62. PMID:26076063
**2826.** Wiesner T, Kutzner H, Cerroni L, Mihm MC Jr, Busam KJ, Murali R (2016). Genomic aberrations in spitzoid melanocytic tumours and their implications for diagnosis, prognosis and therapy. Pathology. 48(2):113–31. PMID:27020384
**2827.** Wiesner T, Murali R, Fried I, Cerroni L, Busam K, Kutzner H, et al. (2012). A distinct subset of atypical Spitz tumors is characterized by BRAF mutation and loss of BAP1 expression. Am J Surg Pathol. 36(6):818–30. PMID:22367297
**2828.** Wiesner T, Obenauf AC, Murali R, Fried I, Griewank KG, Ulz P, et al. (2011). Germline mutations in BAP1 predispose to melanocytic tumors. Nat Genet. 43(10):1018–21. PMID:21874003
**2829.** Wigle JT, Oliver G (1999). Prox1 function is required for the development of the murine lymphatic system. Cell. 98(6):769–78. PMID:10499794
**2830.** Wilk M, Schmoeckel C, Kaiser HW, Hepple R, Kreysel HW (1995). Cutaneous angiomyxoma: a benign neoplasm distinct from cutaneous focal mucinosis. J Am Acad Dermatol. 33(2 Pt 2):352–5. PMID:7615884
**2831.** Wilk M, Zelger BG, Zelger B (2015). Fibrosarcomatous dermatofibrosarcoma protuberans with myoid nodules. J Cutan Pathol. 42(10):782–5. PMID:26076821
**2832.** Willemze R, Jaffe ES, Burg G, Cerroni L, Berti E, Swerdlow SH, et al. (2005). WHO-EORTC classification for cutaneous lymphomas. Blood. 105(10):3768–85. PMID:15692063
**2833.** Willemze R, Jansen PM, Cerroni L, Berti E, Santucci M, Assaf C, et al. (2008). Subcutaneous panniculitis-like T-cell lymphoma: definition, classification, and prognostic factors: an EORTC Cutaneous Lymphoma Group Study of 83 cases. Blood. 111(2):838–45. PMID:17934071
**2834.** Willemze R, Kerl H, Sterry W, Berti E, Cerroni L, Chimenti S, et al. (1997). EORTC classification for primary cutaneous lymphomas: a proposal from the Cutaneous Lymphoma Study Group of the European Organization for Research and Treatment of Cancer. Blood. 90(1):354–71. PMID:9207472
**2835.** Willemze R, Meijer CJ (2003). Primary cutaneous CD30-positive lymphoproliferative disorders. Hematol Oncol Clin North Am. 17(6):1319–32, vii–viii. PMID:14710887
**2836.** Williams RF, Fernandez-Pineda I, Gosain A (2016). Pediatric sarcomas. Surg Clin North Am. 96(5):1107–25. PMID:27542645
**2837.** Wilson WH, Kingma DW, Raffeld M, Wittes RE, Jaffe ES (1996). Association of lymphomatoid granulomatosis with Epstein-Barr viral infection of B lymphocytes and response to interferon-alpha 2b. Blood. 87(11):4531–7. PMID:8639820
**2838.** Winchester DS, Gardner KH, Lehman JS, Otley CC (2016). Superficial liposarcoma: a retrospective review of 13 cases. J Am Acad Dermatol. 74(2):391–3. PMID:26775787
**2839.** Winkelmann RK, McLeod WA (1966). The dermal duct tumor. Arch Dermatol. 94(1):50–5. PMID:5938222
**2840.** Winkelmann RR, Rigel DS (2015). Management of dysplastic nevi: a 14-year follow-up survey assessing practice trends among US dermatologists. J Am Acad Dermatol. 73(6):1056–9. PMID:26568339
**2841.** Winnes M, Mölne L, Suurküla M, Andrén Y, Persson F, Enlund F, et al. (2007). Frequent fusion of the CRTC1 and MAML2 genes in clear cell variants of cutaneous hidradenomas. Genes Chromosomes Cancer. 46(6):559–63. PMID:17334997
**2842.** Wise SR, Capra G, Martin P, Wallace D, Miller C (2010). Malignant melanoma transformation within a nevus of Ito. J Am Acad Dermatol. 62(5):869–74. PMID:20074832
**2843.** Wobser M, Petrella T, Kneitz H, Kerstan A, Goebeler M, Rosenwald A, et al. (2013). Extrafacial indolent CD8-positive cutaneous lymphoid proliferation with unusual symmetrical presentation involving both feet. J Cutan Pathol. 40(11):955–61. PMID:24102688
**2844.** Wobser M, Roth S, Reinartz T, Rosenwald A, Goebeler M, Geissinger E (2015). CD68 expression is a discriminative feature of indolent cutaneous CD8-positive lymphoid proliferation and distinguishes this lymphoma subtype from other CD8-positive cutaneous lymphomas. Br J Dermatol. 172(6):1573–80. PMID:25524664
**2845.** Woestenborghs H, Van Eyken P, Dans A (2006). Syringocystadenocarcinoma papilliferum in situ with pagetoid spread: a case report. Histopathology. 48(7):869–70. PMID:16722938
**2846.** Wolfe JT 3rd, Yeatts RP, Wick MR, Campbell RJ, Waller RR (1984). Sebaceous carcinoma of the eyelid. Errors in clinical and pathologic diagnosis. Am J Surg Pathol. 8(8):597–606. PMID:6465419
**2847.** Wolff K, Komar M, Petzelbauer P (2001). Clinical and histopathological aspects of cutaneous mastocytosis. Leuk Res. 25(7):519–28. PMID:11377676
**2848.** Wolter NE, Adil E, Irace AL, Werger A, Perez-Atayde AR, Weldon C, et al. (2017). Malignant glomus tumors of the head and neck in children and adults: evaluation and management. Laryngoscope. 127(12):2873–82. PMID:28294349
**2849.** Wong CY, Helm MA, Kalb RE, Helm TN, Zeitouni NC (2013). The presentation, pathology, and current management strategies of cutaneous metastasis. N Am J Med Sci. 5(9):499–504. PMID:24251266
**2850.** Wong TY, Suster S (1994). Tricholemmal carcinoma. A clinicopathologic study of 13 cases. Am J Dermatopathol. 16(5):463–73. PMID:7528473
**2851.** Wong TY, Suster S, Mihm MC (1997). Squamoid eccrine ductal carcinoma. Histopathology. 30(3):288–93. PMID:9088963
**2852.** Wong TY, Suster S, Nogita T, Duncan LM, Dickersin RG, Mihm MC Jr (1994). Clear cell eccrine carcinomas of the skin. A clinicopathologic study of nine patients. Cancer. 73(6):1631–43. PMID:7512435
**2853.** Wong WK, Lim DH, Ong CW (2015). Epithelioid angiomatous nodule of the nasal cavity: report of 2 cases. Auris Nasus Larynx. 42(4):341–4. PMID:25728975
**2854.** Wong YP, Chia WK, Low SF, Mohamed-Haflah NH, Sharifah NA (2014). Dendritic fibromyxolipoma: a variant of spindle cell lipoma with extensive myxoid change, with cytogenetic evidence. Pathol Int. 64(7):346–51. PMID:25047505
**2855.** Wongchaowart NT, Kim B, Hsi ED, Swerdlow SH, Tubbs RR, Cook JR (2006). t(14;18)(q32;q21) involving IGH and MALT1 is uncommon in cutaneous MALT lymphomas and primary cutaneous diffuse large B-cell lymphomas. J Cutan Pathol. 33(4):286–92. PMID:16630178
**2856.** Woo DK, Jones CR, Vanoli-Storz MN, Kohler S, Reddy S, Advani R, et al. (2009). Prognostic factors in primary cutaneous anaplastic large cell lymphoma: characterization of clinical subset with worse outcome. Arch Dermatol. 145(6):667–74. PMID:19528422
**2857.** Wood A, Mentzel T, van Gorp J, Flucke U, Huschka U, Schneider J, et al. (2015). The spectrum of rare morphological variants of cutaneous epithelioid angiosarcoma. Histopathology. 66(6):856–63. PMID:25330326
**2858.** Wood GS, Hu CH, Beckstead JH, Turner RR, Winkelmann RK (1985). The indeterminate cell proliferative disorder: report of a case manifesting as an unusual cutaneous histiocytosis. J Dermatol Surg Oncol. 11(11):1111–9. PMID:3902927
**2859.** Wood GS, Kamath NV, Guitart J, Heald P, Kohler S, Smoller BR, et al. (2001). Absence of Borrelia burgdorferi DNA in cutaneous B-cell lymphomas from the United States. J Cutan Pathol. 28(10):502–7. PMID:11737518
**2860.** Woodman SE (2012). Metastatic uveal melanoma: biology and emerging treatments. Cancer J. 18(2):148–52. PMID:22453016

**2861.** Woodman SE, Davies MA (2010). Targeting KIT in melanoma: a paradigm of molecular medicine and targeted therapeutics. Biochem Pharmacol. 80(5):568–74. PMID:20457136
**2862.** Woollard WJ, Pullabhatla V, Lorenc A, Patel VM, Butler RM, Bayega A, et al. (2016). Candidate driver genes involved in genome maintenance and DNA repair in Sézary syndrome. Blood. 127(26):3387–97. PMID:27121473
**2863.** Wu G, Barnhill RL, Lee S, Li Y, Shao Y, Easton J, et al. (2016). The landscape of fusion transcripts in spitzoid melanoma and biologically indeterminate spitzoid tumors by RNA sequencing. Mod Pathol. 29(4):359–69. PMID:26892443
**2864.** Wu YH, Su HY, Hsieh YJ (2000). Survey of infectious skin diseases and skin infestations among primary school students of Taitung County, eastern Taiwan. J Formos Med Assoc. 99(2):128–34. PMID:10770027
**2865.** Xi Y, Shen W, Ma L, Zhao M, Zheng J, Bu S, et al. (2016). HMGA2 promotes adipogenesis by activating C/EBPβ-mediated expression of PPARγ. Biochem Biophys Res Commun. 472(4):617–23. PMID:26966068
**2866.** Xie J, Murone M, Luoh SM, Ryan A, Gu Q, Zhang C, et al. (1998). Activating Smoothened mutations in sporadic basal-cell carcinoma. Nature. 391(6662):90–2. PMID:9422511
**2867.** Xing X, Feldman AL (2015). Anaplastic large cell lymphomas: ALK positive, ALK negative, and primary cutaneous. Adv Anat Pathol. 22(1):29–49. PMID:25461779
**2868.** Xiong MY, Rabkin MS, Piepkorn MW, Barnhill RL, Argenyi Z, Erickson L, et al. (2014). Diameter of dysplastic nevi is a more robust biomarker of increased melanoma risk than degree of histologic dysplasia: a case-control study. J Am Acad Dermatol. 71(6):1257–8.e4. PMID:25454033
**2869.** Xu S, Zhao Q, Wei S, Wu Y, Liu J, Shi T, et al. (2015). Next generation sequencing uncovers potential genetic driver mutations of malignant pulmonary granular cell tumor. J Thorac Oncol. 10(10):e106–9. PMID:26398830
**2870.** Xu XL, Xu CR, Chen H, Cao YH, Zeng XS, Sun JF, et al. (2010). Eruptive microvenular hemangiomas in 4 Chinese patients: clinicopathologic correlation and review of the literature. Am J Dermatopathol. 32(8):837–40. PMID:20881833
**2871.** Xu Z, Lian S (2010). Epstein-Barr virus-associated hydroa vacciniforme-like cutaneous lymphoma in seven Chinese children. Pediatr Dermatol. 27(5):463–9. PMID:20497358
**2872.** Yamaguchi U, Hasegawa T, Hirose T, Fugo K, Mitsuhashi T, Shimizu M, et al. (2003). Sclerosing perineurioma: a clinicopathological study of five cases and diagnostic utility of immunohistochemical staining for GLUT1. Virchows Arch. 443(2):159–63. PMID:12836021
**2873.** Yamakawa N, Fujimoto M, Kawabata D, Terao C, Nishikori M, Nakashima R, et al. (2014). A clinical, pathological, and genetic characterization of methotrexate-associated lymphoproliferative disorders. J Rheumatol. 41(2):293–9. PMID:24334644
**2874.** Yamamoto O, Nakayama K, Asahi M (1992). Sweat gland carcinoma with mucinous and infiltrating duct-like patterns. J Cutan Pathol. 19(4):334–9. PMID:1331212
**2875.** Yamamoto O, Yasuda H (1999). An immunohistochemical study of the apocrine type of cutaneous mixed tumors with special reference to their follicular and sebaceous differentiation. J Cutan Pathol. 26(5):232–41. PMID:10408348
**2876.** Yamamoto T, Hirai Y, Miyake T, Hamada T, Yamasaki O, Morizane S, et al. (2016). Epstein-Barr virus reactivation is induced, but abortive, in cutaneous lesions of systemic hydroa vacciniforme and hypersensitivity to mosquito bites. J Dermatol Sci. 82(3):153–9. PMID:27039668
**2877.** Yanagihara M, Oiso N, Tanaka H, Narita T, Enoki E, Kimura M, et al. (2015). Aleukemic solitary cutaneous myeloid sarcoma. J Dermatol. 42(8):844–5. PMID:25958929
**2878.** Yang QX, Pei XJ, Tian XY, Li Y, Li Z (2012). Secondary cutaneous Epstein-Barr virus-associated diffuse large B-cell lymphoma in a patient with angioimmunoblastic T-cell lymphoma: a case report and review of literature. Diagn Pathol. 7:7. PMID:22260632
**2879.** Yang Y, Lin J, Fang S, Han S, Song Z (2017). What's new in dermoscopy of Bowen's disease: two new dermoscopic signs and its differential diagnosis. Int J Dermatol. 56(10):1022–5. PMID:28832993
**2880.** Yazdan P, Haghighat Z, Guitart J, Gerami P (2013). Epithelioid and fusiform blue nevus of chronically sun-damaged skin, an entity distinct from the epithelioid blue nevus of the Carney complex. Am J Surg Pathol. 37(1):81–8. PMID:22892599
**2881.** Yeatman JM, Kilkenny M, Marks R (1997). The prevalence of seborrhoeic keratoses in an Australian population: does exposure to sunlight play a part in their frequency? Br J Dermatol. 137(3):411–4. PMID:9349339
**2882.** Yeh I, Botton T, Talevich E, Shain AH, Sparatta AJ, de la Fouchardiere A, et al. (2015). Activating MET kinase rearrangements in melanoma and Spitz tumours. Nat Commun. 6:7174. PMID:26013381
**2883.** Yeh I, Fang Y, Busam KJ (2012). Melanoma arising in a large plaque-type blue nevus with subcutaneous cellular nodules. Am J Surg Pathol. 36(8):1258–63. PMID:22790865
**2884.** Yeh I, Lang UE, Durieux E, Tee MK, Jorapur A, Shain AH, et al. (2017). Combined activation of MAP kinase pathway and β-catenin signaling cause deep penetrating nevi. Nat Commun. 8(1):644. PMID:28935960
**2885.** Yeh I, McCalmont TH (2010). Fingerprint CD34 immunopositivity. J Cutan Pathol. 37(11):1127–9. PMID:20849453
**2886.** Yeh I, Tee MK, Botton T, Shain AH, Sparatta AJ, Gagnon A, et al. (2016). NTRK3 kinase fusions in Spitz tumours. J Pathol. 240(3):282–90. PMID:27477320
**2887.** Yeh S (1973). Skin cancer in chronic arsenicism. Hum Pathol. 4(4):469–85. PMID:4750817
**2888.** Yélamos O, Arva NC, Obregon R, Yazdan P, Wagner A, Guitart J, et al. (2015). A comparative study of proliferative nodules and lethal melanomas in congenital nevi from children. Am J Surg Pathol. 39(3):405–15. PMID:25517953
**2889.** Yélamos O, Busam KJ, Lee C, Meldi Sholl L, Amin SM, Merkel EA, et al. (2015). Morphologic clues and utility of fluorescence in situ hybridization for the diagnosis of nevoid melanoma. J Cutan Pathol. 42(11):796–806. PMID:26356543
**2890.** Yi S, Zou D, Li C, Zhong S, Chen W, Li Z, et al. (2015). High incidence of MYC and BCL2 abnormalities in mantle cell lymphoma, although only MYC abnormality predicts poor survival. Oncotarget. 6(39):42362–71. PMID:26517511
**2891.** Yilmaz I, Gamsizkan M, Sari SO, Yaman B, Demirkesen C, Heper A, et al. (2015). Molecular alterations in malignant blue nevi and related blue lesions. Virchows Arch. 467(6):723–32. PMID:26403583
**2892.** Yim IH, Will MB, Carnochan FM, Walker WS (2016). A glomus tumor with recurrence and malignant transformation in the chest wall: a cautionary tale of seeding? Ann Thorac Surg. 102(5):e397–9. PMID:27772590
**2893.** Yonekawa Y, Kim IK (2012). Epidemiology and management of uveal melanoma. Hematol Oncol Clin North Am. 26(6):1169–84. PMID:23116575
**2894.** Yoon JH, Park HJ, Park SY, Park BK (2013). Langerhans cell histiocytosis in non-twin siblings. Pediatr Int. 55(3):e73–6. PMID:23782385
**2895.** Yoshida A, Sekine S, Tsuta K, Fukayama M, Furuta K, Tsuda H (2012). NKX2.2 is a useful immunohistochemical marker for Ewing sarcoma. Am J Surg Pathol. 36(7):993–9. PMID:22446943
**2896.** Yoshikawa H, Ueda T, Mori S, Araki N, Myoui A, Uchida A, et al. (1996). Dedifferentiated liposarcoma of the subcutis. Am J Surg Pathol. 20(12):1525–30. PMID:8944047
**2897.** Youlden DR, Soyer HP, Youl PH, Fritschi L, Baade PD (2014). Incidence and survival for Merkel cell carcinoma in Queensland, Australia, 1993-2010. JAMA Dermatol. 150(8):864–72. PMID:24943712
**2898.** Yu GP, Hu DN, McCormick S, Finger PT (2003). Conjunctival melanoma: is it increasing in the United States? Am J Ophthalmol. 135(6):800–6. PMID:12788119
**2899.** Yu JB, Zuo Z, Tang Y, Zhao S, Zhang YC, Bi CF, et al. (2009). Extranodal nasal-type natural killer/T-cell lymphoma of the skin: a clinicopathologic study of 16 cases in China. Hum Pathol. 40(6):807–16. PMID:19200574
**2899A.** Yu LL, Heenan PJ (1999). The morphological features of locally recurrent melanoma and cutaneous metastases of melanoma. Hum Pathol. 30(5):551–5. PMID:10333226
**2900.** Yun SJ, Kim EJ, Kim SJ, Lee SC, Won YH, Lee JB (2005). The association of naevus lipomatosus with pilosebaceous abnormalities including fibrofolliculoma. Br J Dermatol. 153(1):209–10. PMID:16029355
**2901.** Yun SJ, Kim SJ (2011). Images in clinical medicine. Hutchinson's nail sign. N Engl J Med. 364(18):e38. PMID:21542738
**2902.** Zaenglein AL, Heintz P, Kamino H, Zisblatt M, Orlow SJ (2002). Congenital Spitz nevus clinically mimicking melanoma. J Am Acad Dermatol. 47(3):441–4. PMID:12196758
**2903.** Zagars GK, Ballo MT, Pisters PW, Pollock RE, Patel SR, Benjamin RS, et al. (2003). Prognostic factors for patients with localized soft-tissue sarcoma treated with conservation surgery and radiation therapy: an analysis of 1225 patients. Cancer. 97(10):2530–43. PMID:12733153
**2904.** Zaiac MN, Mlacker S, Shah VV, Simmons BJ (2016). Clinical pearl: the squeeze maneuver. Cutis. 97(3):202, 204. PMID:27023088
**2905.** Zaim MT (1988). Sebocrine adenoma. An adnexal adenoma with sebaceous and apocrine poroma-like differentiation. Am J Dermatopathol. 10(4):311–8. PMID:2843062
**2906.** Zala L, Ettlin C, Krebs A (1975). Focal dermal hypoplasia with keratoconus, papillomatosis of esophagus and hidrocystomas (author's transl). Dermatologica. 150(3):176–85. [German] PMID:1158014
**2907.** Zalaudek I, Kreusch J, Giacomel J, Ferrara G, Catricalà C, Argenziano G (2010). How to diagnose nonpigmented skin tumors: a review of vascular structures seen with dermoscopy: part II. Nonmelanocytic skin tumors. J Am Acad Dermatol. 63(3):377–86. PMID:20708470
**2908.** Zalaudek I, Piana S, Moscarella E, Longo C, Zendri E, Castagnetti F, et al. (2014). Morphologic grading and treatment of facial actinic keratosis. Clin Dermatol. 32(1):80–7. PMID:24314380
**2909.** Zamecnik M, Michal M (2007). Angiomatous spindle cell lipoma: report of three cases with immunohistochemical and ultrastructural study and reappraisal of former 'pseudoangiomatous' variant. Pathol Int. 57(1):26–31. PMID:17199739
**2910.** Zamir E, Mechoulam H, Micera A, Levi-Schaffer F, Pe'er J (2002). Inflamed juvenile conjunctival naevus: clinicopathological characterisation. Br J Ophthalmol. 86(1):28–30. PMID:11801498
**2911.** Zayour M, Bolognia JL, Lazova R (2012). Multiple Spitz nevi: a clinicopathologic study of 9 patients. J Am Acad Dermatol. 67(3):451–8, 458.e1–2. PMID:22300833
**2912.** Zbacnik AP, Rawal A, Lee B, Werling R, Knapp D, Mesa H (2015). Cutaneous basal cell carcinosarcoma: case report and literature review. J Cutan Pathol. 42(11):903–10. PMID:26268472
**2913.** Zeff RA, Freitag A, Grin CM, Grant-Kels JM (1997). The immune response in halo nevi. J Am Acad Dermatol. 37(4):620–4. PMID:9344203
**2914.** Zelger B, Kazakov DV, Zelger BG (2014). Clinical presentation of cutaneous adnexal tumors. Pathologe. 35(5):487–96. [German] PMID:25154603
**2915.** Zelger B, Sidoroff A, Stanzl U, Fritsch PO, Ofner D, Zelger B, et al. (1994). Deep penetrating dermatofibroma versus dermatofibrosarcoma protuberans. A clinicopathologic comparison. Am J Surg Pathol. 18(7):677–86. PMID:8017562
**2916.** Zelger B, Weinlich G, Zelger B (2000). Perineuroma. A frequently unrecognized entity with emphasis on a plexiform variant. Adv Clin Path. 4(1):25–33. PMID:10936896
**2917.** Zelger B, Zelger BG, Burgdorf WH (2004). Dermatofibroma-a critical evaluation. Int J Surg Pathol. 12(4):333–44. PMID:15494859
**2918.** Zelger BG, Sidoroff A, Zelger B (2000). Combined dermatofibroma: co-existence of two or more variant patterns in a single lesion. Histopathology. 36(6):529–39. PMID:10849095
**2919.** Zelger BG, Stelzmueller I, Dunst KM, Zelger B (2008). Solid apocrine carcinoma of the skin: report of a rare adnexal neoplasm mimicking lobular breast carcinoma. J Cutan Pathol. 35(3):332–6. PMID:18251751
**2920.** Zelger BG, Zelger B, Steiner H, Mikuz G (1995). Solitary giant xanthogranuloma and benign cephalic histiocytosis–variants of juvenile xanthogranuloma. Br J Dermatol. 133(4):598–604. PMID:7577591
**2921.** Zelger BW, Sidoroff A, Orchard G, Cerio R (1996). Non-Langerhans cell histiocytoses. A new unifying concept. Am J Dermatopathol. 18(5):490–504. PMID:8902096
**2922.** Zelger BW, Zelger BG, Plörer A, Steiner H, Fritsch PO (1995). Dermal spindle cell lipoma: plexiform and nodular variants. Histopathology. 27(6):533–40. PMID:8838333
**2923.** Zelger BW, Zelger BG, Rappersberger K (1997). Prominent myofibroblastic differentiation. A pitfall in the diagnosis of dermatofibroma. Am J Dermatopathol. 19(2):138–46. PMID:9129698
**2924.** Zelger BW, Zelger BG, Steiner H, Ofner D (1996). Aneurysmal and haemangiopericytoma-like fibrous histiocytoma. J Clin Pathol. 49(4):313–8. PMID:8655708
**2925.** Zembowicz A (2017). Blue nevi and related tumors. Clin Lab Med. 37(3):401–15. PMID:28802492
**2926.** Zembowicz A, Carney JA, Mihm MC (2004). Pigmented epithelioid melanocytoma: a low-grade melanocytic tumor with metastatic potential indistinguishable from animal-type melanoma and epithelioid blue nevus. Am J Surg Pathol. 28(1):31–40. PMID:14707861
**2927.** Zembowicz A, Garcia CF, Tannous ZS, Mihm MC, Koerner F, Pilch BZ (2005). Endocrine mucin-producing sweat gland carcinoma: twelve new cases suggest that it is a precursor of some invasive mucinous carcinomas. Am J Surg Pathol. 29(10):1330–9. PMID:16160476

**2928.** Zembowicz A, Knoepp SM, Bei T, Stergiopoulos S, Eng C, Mihm MC, et al. (2007). Loss of expression of protein kinase a regulatory subunit 1alpha in pigmented epithelioid melanocytoma but not in melanoma or other melanocytic lesions. Am J Surg Pathol. 31(11):1764–75. PMID:18059235
**2929.** Zembowicz A, Mandal RV, Choopong P (2010). Melanocytic lesions of the conjunctiva. Arch Pathol Lab Med. 134(12):1785–92. PMID:21128776
**2930.** Zembowicz A, McCusker M, Chiarelli C, Dei Tos AP, Granter SR, Calonje E, et al. (2001). Morphological analysis of nevoid melanoma: a study of 20 cases with a review of the literature. Am J Dermatopathol. 23(3):167–75. PMID:11391094
**2931.** Zeren-Bilgin I, Gür S, Aydin O, Ermete M (2006). Melanoma arising in a hairy nevus spilus. Int J Dermatol. 45(11):1362–4. PMID:17076727
**2932.** Zhang YH, Wang WL, Rapini RP, Torres-Cabala C, Prieto VG, Curry JL (2012). Syringocystadenocarcinoma papilliferum with transition to areas of squamous differentiation: a case report and review of the literature. Am J Dermatopathol. 34(4):428–33. PMID:22343110
**2933.** Zhao T, Matsuoka M (2012). HBZ and its roles in HTLV-1 oncogenesis. Front Microbiol. 3:247. PMID:22787458
**2934.** Zhou P, Zhang H, Bu H, Yin X, Zhang R, Fu J, et al. (2009). Paravertebral glomangiomatosis. Case report. J Neurosurg. 111(2):272–7. PMID:19267531
**2935.** Zhou S, Zhou J, Liu S, Wang R, Wang Z (2015). Arsenical keratosis caused by medication: a case report and literature. Int J Clin Exp Med. 8(1):1487–90. PMID:25785160
**2936.** Zhu GA, Danial C, Liu A, Li S, Su Chang AL (2014). Overall and progression-free survival in metastatic basosquamous cancer: a case series. J Am Acad Dermatol. 70(6):1145–6. PMID:24831322
**2937.** Zhuang SM, Zhang GH, Chen WK, Chen SW, Wang LP, Li H, et al. (2013). Survival study and clinicopathological evaluation of trichilemmal carcinoma. Mol Clin Oncol. 1(3):499–502. PMID:24649199
**2938.** Ziemer M (2012). Atypical fibroxanthoma. J Dtsch Dermatol Ges. 10(8):537–50. PMID:22709412
**2939.** Ziemer M, Bornkessel A, Hahnfeld S, Weyers W (2005). 'Specific' cutaneous infiltrate of B-cell chronic lymphocytic leukemia at the site of a florid herpes simplex infection. J Cutan Pathol. 32(8):581–4. PMID:16115059
**2940.** Zinzani PL, Quaglino P, Pimpinelli N, Berti E, Baliva G, Rupoli S, et al. (2006). Prognostic factors in primary cutaneous B-cell lymphoma: the Italian Study Group for Cutaneous Lymphomas. J Clin Oncol. 24(9):1376–82. PMID:16492713
**2941.** Zreik RT, Carter JM, Sukov WR, Ahrens WA, Fritchie KJ, Montgomery EA, et al. (2016). TGFBR3 and MGEA5 rearrangements are much more common in "hybrid" hemosiderotic fibrolipomatous tumor-myxoinflammatory fibroblastic sarcomas than in classical myxoinflammatory fibroblastic sarcomas: a morphological and fluorescence in situ hybridization study. Hum Pathol. 53:14–24. PMID:26980036
**2942.** Zukerberg LR, Nickoloff BJ, Weiss SW (1993). Kaposiform hemangioendothelioma of infancy and childhood. An aggressive neoplasm associated with Kasabach-Merritt syndrome and lymphangiomatosis. Am J Surg Pathol. 17(4):321–8. PMID:8494101
**2943.** Zvulunov A, Barak Y, Metzker A (1995). Juvenile xanthogranuloma, neurofibromatosis, and juvenile chronic myelogenous leukemia. World statistical analysis. Arch Dermatol. 131(8):904–8. PMID:7632061

# Subject index

## F



## G



## H

## Q



## R



## S

## T



## U



## V



## W



## X



## Y

# List of abbreviations

| | |
|---|---|
| 3D | three-dimensional |
| AJCC | American Joint Committee on Cancer |
| BCL2 | B-cell lymphoma 2 protein |
| BCL6 | B-cell lymphoma 6 protein |
| cAMP | cyclic adenosine monophosphate |
| CDK4 | cyclin-dependent kinase 4 |
| CNS | central nervous system |
| CT | computed tomography |
| DNA | deoxyribonucleic acid |
| EBER | Epstein–Barr virus–encoded small ribonucleic acid |
| EBV | Epstein–Barr virus |
| EGFR | epidermal growth factor receptor |
| EMA | epithelial membrane antigen |
| FISH | fluorescence in situ hybridization |
| GFAP | glial fibrillary acidic protein |
| H&E | haematoxylin and eosin |
| HHV8 | human herpesvirus 8 |
| HIV | human immunodeficiency virus |
| HPV | human papillomavirus |
| ICD-O | International Classification of Diseases for Oncology |
| Ig | immunoglobulin |
| MAPK | mitogen-activated protein kinase |
| MART1 | melanoma antigen recognized by T cells 1 |
| MDM2 | mouse double minute 2 homologue |
| MRI | magnetic resonance imaging |
| mRNA | messenger ribonucleic acid |
| N:C ratio | nuclear-to-cytoplasmic ratio |
| NK cell | natural killer cell |
| PAS | periodic acid–Schiff |
| PCR | polymerase chain reaction |
| PET | positron emission tomography |
| RB1 | retinoblastoma protein |
| RNA | ribonucleic acid |
| RT-PCR | reverse transcriptase polymerase chain reaction |
| SEER Program | Surveillance, Epidemiology, and End Results Program |
| SMA | smooth muscle actin |
| SMARCB1 | SWI/SNF-related matrix-associated actin-dependent regulator of chromatin subfamily B member 1 |
| STAT6 | signal transducer and activator of transcription 6 |
| TdT | terminal deoxynucleotidyl transferase |
| TNM | tumour, node, metastasis |